MODERN
COLPOSCOPY
Textbook & Atlas

THIRD EDITION

MODERN
COLPOSCOPY
Textbook & Atlas

THIRD EDITION

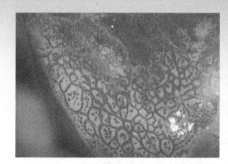
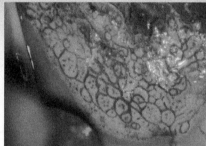

EDITED BY

E.J. Mayeaux Jr, MD

Professor and Chair of the Department of Family and Preventive Medicine
Professor of Obstetrics and Gynecology
University of South Carolina School of Medicine
Columbia, South Carolina

J. Thomas Cox, MD

Director, Women's Clinic (Retired)
Student Health Services
University of California Santa Barbara
Santa Barbara, California
Past-President, American Society for Colposcopy and Cervical Pathology (ASCCP)
Frederick, Maryland

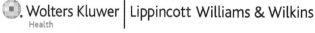
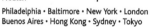
Wolters Kluwer | Lippincott Williams & Wilkins
Health

Philadelphia • Baltimore • New York • London
Buenos Aires • Hong Kong • Sydney • Tokyo

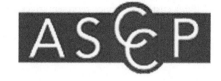
ASCCP

Acquisitions Editor: Sonya Seigafuse
Product Manager: Nicole Walz
Vendor Manager: Alicia Jackson
Senior Manufacturing Manager: Benjamin Rivera
Marketing Manager: Kimberly Schonberger
Design Coordinator: Doug Smock
Production Service: SPi Global

Printed in the United States of America

Library of Congress Cataloging-in-Publication Data
Modern colposcopy : textbook & atlas / [edited by] E.J. Mayeaux, Jr.,
J. Thomas Cox. — 3rd ed.
    p. ; cm.
  Includes bibliographical references and index.
  ISBN 978-1-60831-547-5 (hardback)
  I. Mayeaux, E. J. II. Cox, J. Thomas.
  [DNLM: 1. Colposcopy—methods. 2. Uterine Cervical Diseases—diagnosis. 3. Uterine Cervical Diseases—prevention & control. WP 250]
  LC classifcation not assigned
  618.1'407545—dc23

                                                                    2011031887

This textbook and atlas has been designed as an educational resource and as such does not define a standard of care, nor is it intended to dictate an exclusive course of treatment or procedure to be followed. It presents methods and techniques of clinical practice that are acceptable and used by recognized authorities, for consideration by licensed healthcare professionals to incorporate into their practice. Variations of practice, taking in account the needs of the individual patient, resources, and limitations unique to the institution or type of practice, may be appropriate. The statements and opinions expressed within this textbook are those of the authors and editors and not necessarily those of the American Society for Colposcopy and Cervical Pathology (ASCCP). ASCCP disclaims any responsibility and/or liability for such information.

Care has been taken to confirm the accuracy of the information presented and to describe generally accepted practices. However, the authors, editors, and publisher are not responsible for errors or omissions or for any consequences from application of the information in this book and make no warranty, expressed or implied, with respect to the currency, completeness, or accuracy of the contents of the publication. Application of the information in a particular situation remains the professional responsibility of the practitioner.

The authors, editors, and publisher have exerted every effort to ensure that drug selection and dosage set forth in this text are in accordance with current recommendations and practice at the time of publication. However, in view of ongoing research, changes in government regulations, and the constant flow of information relating to drug therapy and drug reactions, the reader is urged to check the package insert for each drug for any change in indications and dosage and for added warnings and precautions. This is particularly important when the recommended agent is a new or infrequently employed drug.

Some drugs and medical devices presented in the publication have Food and Drug Administration (FDA) clearance for limited use in restricted research settings. It is the responsibility of the health care provider to ascertain the FDA status of each drug or device planned for use in their clinical practice.

To purchase additional copies of this book, call our customer service department at (800) 638-3030 or fax orders to (301) 223-2320. International customers should call (301) 223-2300.

Visit Lippincott Williams & Wilkins on the Internet: at LWW.com. Lippincott Williams & Wilkins customer service representatives are available from 8:30 am to 6 pm, EST.

10 9 8

DE

The editors of this book would ...
the health care providers who throu...
and dedication continually provide and ...
around the world. Kudos and ...

J. Michael Berry, MD
Associate Clinical Professor
Department of Medicine
University of California San Francisco
Associate Director HPV-Related Clinical Studies
UCSF Anal Neoplasia Clinic
UCSF Helen Diller Family Comprehensive Cancer Center
San Francisco, California

J. Thomas Cox, MD
Director, Women's Clinic (Retired)
Student Health Services
University of California Santa Barbara
Santa Barbara, California
Past-President, American Society for Colposcopy and
    Cervical Pathology (ASCCP)
Frederick, MD

David P. Chelmow, MD
Leo J. Dunn Distinguished Professor of Obstetrics and
    Gynecology,
Virginia Commonwealth University School of Medicine
Richmond, VA

Miriam Cremer, MD, MPH
Assistant Professor
Director, Global Health Fellowship
Department of Obstetrics, Gynecology and Reproductive
    Sciences
Magee-Womens Hospital
Pittsburgh, Pennsylvania

Teresa M. Darragh, MD
Professor of Clinical Pathology
Departments of Pathology and Obstetrics, Gynecology and
    Reproductive Sciences
University of California, San Francisco
UCSF Medical Center at Mount Zion
San Francisco, California

Daron G. Ferris, MD
Professor
Departments of Family Medicine and Obstetrics and
    Gynecology
Georgia Health Sciences University
Augusta, Georgia

Francisco Garcia, MD, MPH
Distinguished Outreach Professor of Public Health,
    Obstetrics & Gynecology, Mexican American Studies and
    Clinical Pharmacy
University of Arizona
Tucson, Arizona

Michael A. Gold, MD
Associate Professor
Department of Obstetrics and Gynecology
Vanderbilt University Medical Center
Director
Division of Gynecologic Oncology
Vanderbilt University Medical Center
Nashville, Tennessee

Richard Guido, MD
Associate Professor, Chair IRB University of Pittsburgh
Obstetrics, Gynecology, and Reproductive Sciences
University of Pittsburgh
Associate Professor
Obstetrics, Gynecology, and Reproductive Sciences
Magee-Womens Hospital of the UPMC Health System
Pittsburgh, Pennsylvania

Hope K. Haefner, MD
Professor
Department of Obstetrics and Gynecology
The University of Michigan Hospitals
L 4000 Women's Hospital
Ann Arbor, Michigan

Naomi Jay, RN, NP, PhD
Medicine/HPV Research Studies
University of California San Francisco
Mount Zion Hospital
San Francisco, California

Edward J. Mayeaux, Jr., MD
Professor and Chair of the Department of Family and
    Preventive Medicine
Professor of Obstetrics and Gynecology
University of South Carolina School of Medicine
Columbia, South Carolina

Anna-Barbara Moscicki, MD
Professor
Department of Pediatrics
University of California, San Francisco
San Francisco, California

Dennis M. O'Connor, MD
Associate Clinical Professor
Departments of Obstetrics and Gynecology,
    and Pathology
University of Louisville School of Medicine
Staff Pathologist
Department of Pathology
Clinical Associates dbi CPA Lab
Louisville, Kentucky

Joel M. Palefsky, MD, CM
Professor of Medicine
Department of Medicine
University of California, San Francisco
San Francisco, California

V. Cecil Wright, MD
Professor Emeritus
Department of Obstetrics and Gynaecology
Schulich School of Medicine and Dentistry
The University of Western Ontario
London, Ontario, Canada

Thomas C. Wright, Jr., MD
Professor
Department of Pathology
Columbia University Medical Center
College of Physicians and Surgeons
Director
Obstetrical and Gynecological Pathology
Department of Obstetrics and Gynecology
New York Presbyterian Hospital
New York, New York

The American Society for Colposcopy and Cervical Pathology (ASCCP) is committed to providing excellence in education with respect to management of women with lower genital tract disease and men and women with anal and perianal disease. The first and second editions of *Modern Colposcopy* were extremely popular because of their unique and complete approach to colposcopy education. You will find that *Modern Colposcopy*, third edition, continues the tradition of encompassing complete coverage of human papillomavirus (HPV)-related diseases, colposcopy, and related topics. In addition, chapters have been added on adolescents and on the expanding field of anal screening, diagnosis of anal HPV-related precancer and cancer through high-resolution anoscopy, and treatment of anal and perianal neoplastic disease. New information on the rapidly expanding area of vulvar and vaginal HPV-related diseases is provided in this edition. *Modern Colposcopy*, third edition, has also been updated to include the 2012 American Cancer Society/ASCCP/American Society for Clinical Pathology (ACS/ASCCP/ASCP) primary cervical screening guidelines and the new 2012/2013 ASCCP updated guidelines for the management of abnormal cervical cytology and cervical precancer. We have strived to include the most up-to-date information, guidelines, and thinking in the production of this book.

Modern Colposcopy, third edition, is a collaboration of many teachers, researchers, and writers respected in the field of diagnosis, treatment, and prevention of lower genital tract benign and neoplastic disease. With 21 chapters, hundreds of color images, world-class medical illustrations, and helpful graphics, this educational resource is clearly the most comprehensive available. All the colposcopic images are printed in beautiful full color. In many cases, we have included images at various levels of magnification; some filtered by red-free light or stained with Lugol iodine, so that the book demonstrates concepts just as one would observe during a typical colposcopic examination. *Modern Colposcopy*, third edition, is poised to become the cornerstone of the extensive collection of educational resources available from the ASCCP. We hope you enjoy *Modern Colposcopy*, third edition. It has been our pleasure to make it available for you.

J. Thomas Cox, MD
E.J. Mayeaux Jr, MD

Disclaimer
The clinical history given with images in Modern Colposcopy, 3rd Ed. may represent an actual case, but not always. To improve educational quality, some gross, cytological, or histological images may come from photographic libraries that are not from the same patient. This provides protection of patient identity while optimizing the education of clinicians in the care of their patients. Some images are derived from Cervigrams rather than colpophotographs.

Many wonderful individuals and groups contributed to the production of this textbook, in addition to the authors and editors. We would like to thank Drs. Vesna Kesic, Gordon Davis, Ken Hatch, Ken Noller, and Duane Townsend for contributing many colpophotograph and Cervigrams for use in this book. We are particularly grateful to our reviewers, L. Stewart Massad, MD, Herschel W. Lawson, MD, Patricia Cason, RN, MS, FNP, and Elizabeth A. Stier, MD, for their critical and helpful review. We would also like to recognize David G. Weismiller, MD, for his review of some chapters. This book is enormously better for their incisive critiques of the work that helped us be as accurate and up-to-date as possible. We also thank our colleagues at Lippincott for their patience with us and their careful editorial review of the textbook. Finally, we would be remiss to not recognize Mrs. Kathy Poole, executive director of the ASCCP, for keeping us all on task. Neither this book nor the previous edition (*Modern Colposcopy*, 2nd ed.) could have happened without her patience, support, and central coordination of this effort.

The editors would also like to individually thank:

My partner in life, Deborah, and our children, Jonathan and Jamie, for all the love, support, and the many missed walks on the beach.

J. Thomas Cox, MD

My wonderful wife, Michelle, son, Jason, and supportive parents, Ed and Pat, and all of the extended family. Your presence, thoughtfulness, and patience with long days and evenings with the computer in my lap made this work possible. You are truly appreciated.

E.J. Mayeaux Jr, MD

CONTENTS

Contributing Authors *vii*

Preface *ix*

Acknowledgments *xi*

1 The Road to Cervical Cancer Prevention: Historical Perspective 1
J. Thomas Cox

2 Anatomy and Histology of the Normal Female Lower Genital Tract 14
Dennis M. O'Connor

3 The Cytology and Histology of Cervicovaginal Abnormalities 37
Dennis M. O'Connor

4 Cervical Cancer: Epidemiology and Etiology 61
Thomas C. Wright and J. Thomas Cox

5 The Biology and Importance of Human Papillomavirus Infection 74
J. Thomas Cox and Edward J. Mayeaux, Jr.

6 Colposcopic Equipment, Supplies, and Data Management 102
Daron G. Ferris and Edward J. Mayeaux, Jr.

7 The Colposcopic Examination 120
Daron G. Ferris, Edward J. Mayeaux, Jr., and J. Thomas Cox

8 Normal and Abnormal Colposcopic Features 150
Daron G. Ferris, Edward J. Mayeaux, Jr., and J. Thomas Cox

9 Colposcopy of Cervical Intraepithelial Neoplasia 234
Daron G. Ferris, J. Thomas Cox, and Edward J. Mayeaux, Jr.

10 Colposcopic, Clinical, and Etiologic Predictors of Invasive Squamous Cell Carcinoma of the Uterine Cervix 306
V. Cecil Wright

11 Colposcopy of Adenocarcinoma *In Situ* and Adenocarcinoma of the Uterine Cervix 322
V. Cecil Wright

12 Colposcopy and Pregnancy 343
Daron G. Ferris, J. Thomas Cox, and Edward J. Mayeaux, Jr.

13 Colposcopy in Special Situations 376
J. Thomas Cox and Edward J. Mayeaux, Jr.

14 Colposcopy of the Vagina 399
J. Thomas Cox and Michael A. Gold

15 Vulvar Abnormalities 432
Hope K. Haefner and Edward J. Mayeaux, Jr.

16 HPV Infections in Adolescents 472
Anna-Barbara Moscicki

17 The Anal Canal and Perianus: HPV-Related Disease 484
Teresa M. Darragh, J. Michael Berry, Naomi Jay, and Joel M. Palefsky

18 Primary and Secondary Prevention: HPV Vaccination and Cervical Cancer Screening 539
J. Thomas Cox

19 Management of Abnormal Cervical Cancer Screening Results 571
J. Thomas Cox, David P. Chelmow, and Anna-Barbara Moscicki

20 Management of Lower Genital Tract Neoplasia 599
J. Thomas Cox, Francisco Garcia, David P. Chelmow, Daron G. Ferris, V. Cecil Wright, Edward J. Mayeaux, Jr., Richard Guido, and Miriam Cremer

21 Preventing Errors during Colposcopy and Management of Lower Genital Tract Neoplasia 667
Daron G. Ferris, J. Thomas Cox, and Edward J. Mayeaux, Jr.

Index *685*

The Road to Cervical Cancer Prevention: Historical Perspective

1.1 INTRODUCTION
1.2 THE BIRTH OF COLPOSCOPY
1.3 DEVELOPING METHODS FOR CERVICAL CANCER SCREENING
    1.3.1 The Birth of Screening with Cervical Cytology
    1.3.2 The Short Life of Screening with Schiller's Test
1.4 GROWTH AND ACCEPTANCE OF COLPOSCOPY
1.5 INTEGRATION OF COLPOSCOPY INTO MANAGEMENT ALGORITHMS FOR ABNORMAL PAP RESULTS
    1.5.1 Management of Abnormal Cervical Cytology before the Introduction of Colposcopy

1.5.2 Management after the Introduction of Colposcopy
1.5.3 HPV and the Screening and Diagnosis of Cervical Disease
1.6 NEW CHALLENGES IN COLPOSCOPY
    1.6.1 Expansion of the Practice of Colposcopy to a Broader Clinical Base
    1.6.2 Challenges to the Accuracy of Colposcopy
1.7 ROLE OF COLPOSCOPY IN THE 21ST CENTURY

1.1 INTRODUCTION

Chronic diseases of the uterine corpus and cervix have been known throughout the ages, but the concept of cancer as disordered cell growth has only developed over the past 150 years. Hippocrates' writings provided the first description of cervical cancer in the years following 400 BC, but not until 1842 did Rigoni-Stern observe in Verona, Italy, that nuns had an increased incidence of breast cancer but seldom developed cervical cancer. However, the latter was a frequent disease among prostitutes, raising the possibility that this cancer might have something to do with coitus.[1] Consistent with medical theories of the time, he attributed this association to "nervous irritability" rather than to "licentiousness." It was not until 1950 that a clinician providing gynecologic services to nuns in Quebec confirmed Rigoni-Stern's observation when he noted that he had never seen a case of cervical cancer in a nun.[2] The pursuit was on to find the sexually transmitted disease that might be associated with cervical carcinogenesis. Starting in the late 1960s, significant advances were made in understanding the cellular changes leading to invasive cervical cancer, but for almost two decades herpes simplex virus type 2 was the leading contender for causation.[3] This belief held sway well beyond the 1976 publication by Meisels and Fortin establishing human papillomavirus (HPV) as the etiologic agent in an abnormal cervical cytologic finding (koilocytotic atypia).[4] Despite early skepticism, the mid-1970s prediction by zur Hausen that HPV was a likely cause of cervical cancer,[5,6] and his team's subsequent documentation of the presence of HPV within cervical neoplastic lesions[7,8] eventually led to the establishment of HPV as the etiologic agent in most, if not all, cervical cancers. For his contributions to this major breakthrough, Harold zur Hausen received the 2008 Nobel Prize in Medicine.

1.2 THE BIRTH OF COLPOSCOPY

Cervical cancer, once the 2nd most common cancer in women in both incidence and mortality, is now no greater than 11th in incidence and 13th in mortality in the United States, with similar reductions seen in countries with well-established cervical cancer screening and management programs.[9] This unparalleled success in cancer prevention has come in large part from the ability to detect and treat the precursor lesion to cervical cancer (cervical intraepithelial neoplasia grade 3 [CIN 3]) before it acquires the capacity to invade surrounding structures. Most important has been the partnership between cervical cytology screening and treatment of colposcopically detected high-grade neoplasia.[9]

Although the earliest speculum documented was found in the ruins of Pompeii (1st century BC), the study of the cervix in vivo began only after Recamier's invention of the modern speculum in the early 1800s. Beginning in the first half of the 19th century, the concept of cancer as uncontrolled cell growth began to develop through examination of pathology specimens under the microscope, initially by Virchow and subsequently by many others.[3] However, it was nearly a century before reports of white lesions on the cervix, termed *leukoplakia* (Figure 1.1), began to appear in the literature. Several of these had been observed to progress to invasive cancer.[10,11] Von Franque, a Viennese investigator, assigned his assistant, Hans Hinselmann, to study leukoplakia (Table 1.1). Hinselmann's conclusion was that leukoplakia was always a sign of either a precancerous or a cancerous condition but that he needed better illumination and magnification for adequate study.[12] Hence, he set out to devise an instrument that would illuminate and magnify the cervix.[13] He mounted a Leitz binocular dissecting microscope with an attached light source to a stand. Using 3.5× to 30× magnification, Hinselmann was able not only to detect the smallest possible invasive cancer but also to begin describing the characteristics of the normal cervix and of intraepithelial lesions (carcinoma *in situ* [CIS] and lesser grades of CIN) (Figure 1.2). While evaluating the effect of dilute acetic acid in removing cervical mucous, he discovered the colposcopic sign of acetowhitening.

During the same period, advances were made in understanding the histologic appearance of cervical precancer.

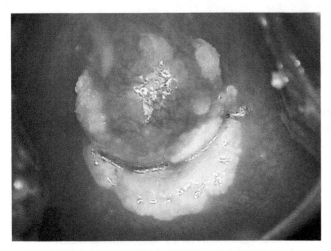

FIGURE 1.1. The earliest changes on the cervix noted with the naked eye were white lesions, termed leukoplakia. Although it is currently known that most areas of leukoplakia are not associated with cervical neoplasia, the initial reports of this finding concluded that it was always secondary to a precancerous or a cancerous process. This photomicrograph demonstrates an area of leukoplakia associated with a low-grade HPV lesion. (Colpophotograph courtesy of J.T. Cox, MD.)

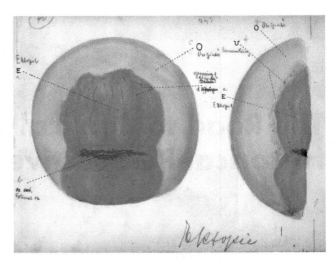

FIGURE 1.2. Hinselmann watercolor of cervical ectopy.

CIS, both in the absence of invasive carcinoma and at the periphery of such lesions, had been studied histologically by von Franque,[14] Schauenstein,[15] Schottlander and Kermauner,[16] and Cullen. Hinselmann's colposcope now made it possible to describe the fine detail of the morphologic changes and to compare the visual findings with the histologic detail.[17] With this capability, punctation and mosaic were described and related to histologic disturbances noted in the epithelial architecture. The colposcopic finding of punctation was called the *ground leukoplakia or Leukoplakiegrund* and mosaic was termed the *Mosaic leukoplakia or Felderung* (Figure 1.3).[18,19] Early investigators tried to explain all such *atypical* colposcopic patterns as part of the same process leading to cervical cancer. But over time it became apparent that some atypical patterns represented only benign disorders. This misperception resulted in the grouping of benign disorders of maturation, characterized only by wide bands of typical-appearing prickle cells, with CIN, characterized by similar bulky epithelial pegs of mostly atypical undifferentiated cells. These abnormal areas, recognized as involving primarily the transformation zone,[13,20] were labeled the *matrix area of carcinoma*.[21]

Areas of typical, immature or reactive metaplasia were originally characterized as *simple atypical* and what is

now termed CIN was called *marked atypical*, but it was not recognized that these were two distinct entities until the 1950s. Glatthar subdivided marked atypical epithelium into categories that have more recently been termed histologically as CIN grades 1, 2, and 3 or cytologically as low-grade and high-grade squamous intraepithelial lesions (LSIL and HSIL, respectively).[22] Subsequently, Dietel[23] reported on the long-term follow-up of 390 women originally diagnosed as having simple atypical cells within the matrix area of the cervix, with no malignancies occurring in any over a period of up to 23 years. These observations began to explain why many matrix areas, which we now call the *atypical transformation zone*, failed to consistently indicate a premalignant state. For those not destined to progress, histological sections often exhibited only florid metaplasia, often with underlying stromal inflammation, or reactive epithelial change, such as that found in both immature metaplasia and in the congenital transformation zone (see Chapter 2).

The colposcopic differentiation of CIN from metaplasia and benign disorders of maturation continues to be a perplexing problem. When the colposcope is used for primary screening, as done in a few countries in South America and Europe, or the threshold for referral to colposcopy is set at the level of minor cytologic changes, as has occurred in the United States and in the majority of countries with cytologic cervical screening, it becomes readily apparent that colposcopic differentiation of immature metaplasia and CIN is less accurate than originally anticipated. During the first few

TABLE 1.1	THE BIRTH OF COLPOSCOPY
1901	von Franque and others describe the earliest histologic changes of cervical cancer as *surface carcinoma* or *intraepithelial carcinoma*.[10]
1924	Hinselmann collaborates with Leitz to produce a binocular microscope with an attached light source on a movable stand.[11]
1931	Emmert (USA) introduces colposcopy to the United States in an article in the *Journal of the American Medical Association*.[37]
1932–1939	Colposcopy clinics are established in Switzerland (Mestwerdt and Wespi), England (Shaw), Spain (Usandizaga), Brazil (de Morales), Germany (Hinselmann), and Argentina (Jakob).[45]
1939	Kraatz (Germany) describes the use of colored filters.[45]
1943	Hinselmann collaborates with Eduard Wirths, the chief camp physician (SS-Standortarzt), and his brother, Helmut Wirths, gynecologist of Hamburg-Altona in medical experiments on Jewish women in Auschwitz.[24]

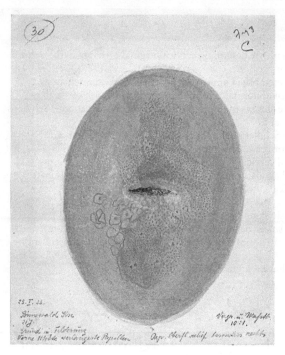

FIGURE 1.3.   Hinselmann watercolor of mosaic (*Mosaic leukoplakia or Felderung*) and punctation (*ground leukoplakia or Leukoplakiegrund*).

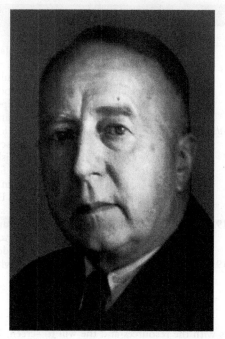

FIGURE 1.4.   Hans Hinselmann (1884–1959). *Father of Colposcopy*. His accomplishments are forever tarnished by his complicity in medical experiments on Jewish women in Auschwitz Block 10. This media file is in the public domain in the United States.

decades in the history of colposcopy, the prevailing impression that colposcopy could accurately predict histology was essentially correct because colposcopy was reserved primarily for evaluation of high-grade cytology and the underlying high-grade lesions were often the more advanced, large prevalent lesions commonly found in populations just beginning screening.

Hans Hinselmann's invention of the colposcope and his endeavors to understand the histologic basis of colposcopic findings establishes his place as the *Father of Colposcopy*. (Figure 1.4) However, his place in history will be forever sullied by his complicity in unethical medical experiments that resulted in unbearable suffering inflicted on Jewish women during World War II in Auschwitz's Block 10.[24] After the war, Hinselmann was sentenced to 3 years of imprisonment in recognition of his egregious role in medical experimentation, following which he immigrated to Argentina. He continued to lecture and promote colposcopy until his death in 1959. His legacy encompasses both *irony* and *pathos* in that he accomplished so much for the protection of women from cervical cancer, yet destroyed the lives of so many women through unethical and immoral experimentation.

1.3 DEVELOPING METHODS FOR CERVICAL CANCER SCREENING

1.3.1 The Birth of Screening with Cervical Cytology

As is common in scientific discoveries, two individuals without knowledge of a similar endeavor by another were concurrently evaluating cervical cell changes found in the vaginal pool. In 1926 at the Colthea Hospital in Romania, Aurel Babes introduced cytologic sampling as a means for detecting cervical cancer (Table 1.2). During this same period, Cornell University's George Papanicolaou (Figure 1.5) discovered during evaluation of the hormonal effects on vaginal cells that abnormal cells were present in the vaginal pool of women with early cervical cancer. In 1928, Babes published his methods of cytologic sampling[25] in the same year that Papanicolaou first presented his data on vaginal smears.[26] By quirk of fate, the work of Papanicolaou was to receive the bulk of recognition; otherwise, the Pap "smear" might have been the Babes "smear"! Unfortunately, it was many years before cervical cancer screening with the Pap smear became established, for its introduction to the United States did not occur until after the 1943 publication of Papanicolaou and Traut's *Diagnosis of Uterine Cancer by the Vaginal Smear*[27] (Figure 1.6).

1.3.1.1 Collection Devices for Obtaining Cervical Cytology Samples

Papanicolaou's method of sampling the vaginal pool was further refined by Ayre in 1947 with the introduction of a wooden spatula to physically scrape cells directly from the cervical surface.[28] Subsequently, routine practice came to include sampling of the endocervical canal by using a cotton-tipped applicator, an implement later replaced by the cytobrush, whose greater abrasiveness produces a significantly greater yield of endocervical cells.[29] These improvements significantly reduced the false-negative rate of cervical cytology.[30]

Although screening with cervical cytology was never the subject of a prospective, randomized study, the reduction in cervical cancer incidence after the introduction of large-scale mass screening programs established the Pap smear as the most successful cancer preventative test to date. For example, an organized cervical screening program was instituted during the 1950s in British Columbia, and by 1984 cervical cancer incidence was reduced by threefold and mortality by fourfold.[31] The Pap test was quick, simple, associated with low morbidity and low cost and was therefore embraced in most

TABLE 1.2	DEVELOPMENT OF METHODS FOR CERVICAL CANCER SCREENING
1926	Babes (Rumania) precedes Papanicolaou by several months in describing cervical/vaginal cytology in the detection of cervical carcinoma.[25]
1927	Fischer-Wasels reports on the particular importance of metaplasia in the process of cervical carcinogenesis.[45]
1928	Papanicolaou presents his observations on association of abnormal cells in the vaginal pool with cervical carcinoma.[26] Schiller (Germany) reports that an iodine stain is useful in screening for cervical cancer.[33] Schiller's test is subsequently used as an additional colposcopic aid.
1930s–1940s	Low-cost primary screening for cervical neoplasia with Schiller's solution is established in North America. Colposcopy becomes the primary screening method for cervical neoplasia in Europe.[45]
1941	Papanicolaou and Traut (USA) publish early findings on cervical cytology.[45]
1943	Papanicolaou and Traut publish the first book on the diagnosis of cervical neoplasia by vaginal pool smears.[27] Colposcopists in Switzerland and in Austria use cervical cytology to identify women who need colposcopy.[45]
1944	Cytologic screening is introduced to Europe.
1947	Ayre (Canada) introduces a wooden spatula for cytologic sampling of the cervix.[28]
1949–1954	Cervical cancer screening with the Papanicolaou (Pap) smear begins to gain acceptance in the United States.
1950	Glatthar subdivides *markedly atypical* epithelium into categories that more closely resembled the subsequent histologic designations of CIN grades 1, 2, and 3.[22]
1954–1955	Dietel documents that not all acetowhite *matrix areas* have a premalignant potential.[23]
1955	Koss describes the *koilocyte*.[65]

countries with the resources and the will to screen. It should also be noted that other changes in medical practice occurring during the same period may have also contributed to some of the reduction in cervical cancer incidence and mortality, particularly the switch in the late 1930s and 1940s from subtotal to total hysterectomy, thereby removing a large pool of at-risk women.[32]

Papanicolaou's pioneering work in cervical cytology occurred virtually simultaneously with the development of the colposcope, and both were initially intended to detect cervical cancer at an earlier stage than when women presented with symptoms.[12,26] However, correlation of colposcopic appearances with histology soon documented that the most important role of colposcopy was its capacity to detect preinvasive cervical disease. Similar conclusions about the role of cervical cytology were developed concurrently.

1.3.2 The Short Life of Screening with Schiller's Test

During the same period, Walter Schiller at the II Universitäts Frauenklinik in Vienna proposed the application of an iodine solution to the cervix as an inexpensive alternative cervical screen.[33] Schiller used Lugol's iodine, also known as Lugol's solution, first made in 1829 by the French physician J.G.A. Lugol. Lugol made his iodine solution with 5 g iodine (I_2) and 10 g potassium iodide (KI) mixed with 85-mL distilled water. Schiller based his iodine test on the observation that normal squamous epithelium stains mahogany brown with Lugol's solution due to the interaction of iodine with the glycogen present in normal mature squamous epithelium. In contrast, neoplastic tissue remains "unstained" (Figure 1.7).[34] Schiller

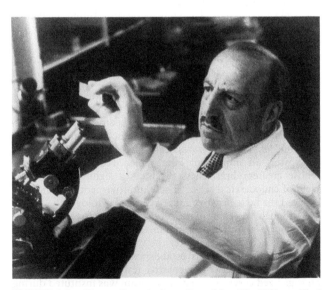

FIGURE 1.5. George Papanicolaou: Born May 13, 1883, at Kimi on the island of Evia, in Greece, died on February 19, 1962. (Photo courtesy of Corbis.)

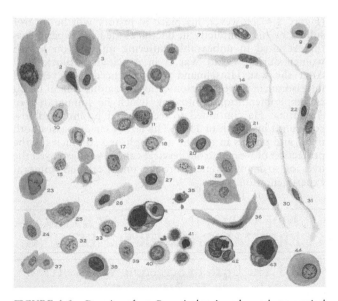

FIGURE 1.6. Drawings from Papanicolaou's early work on cervical cytology in the vaginal pool illustrate cells ranging from normal to cancer. (From Papanicolaou GN, Traut HF. *Diagnosis of Uterine Cancer by the Vaginal Smear.* New York, NY: Commonwealth Fund, 1943;vii:46, with permission.)

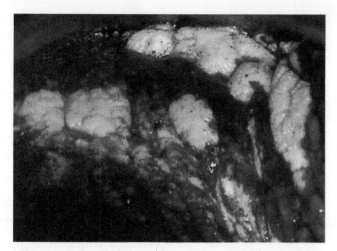

FIGURE 1.7. Schiller's iodine stained normal glycogen containing cells, but did not fully stain columnar, metaplastic, or neoplastic cells. Both metaplastic and neoplastic cells took on a yellow mustard stain, whereas columnar cells completely rejected the iodine uptake. Both maturing metaplasia and low-grade HPV-associated changes often were stained in a variegated or "tortoise shell" effect. This complex transformation zone demonstrates all of these degrees of iodine rejection, and partial and complete uptake. (Colpophotograph courtesy of J.T. Cox, MD.)

also noted that columnar epithelium did not take up any stain, nor did poorly estrogenized squamous epithelium. Colposcopists subsequently began to evaluate the use of Schiller's stain during the colposcopic examination. This technique was brought to the United States in 1932 by Schiller when he immigrated to Boston.[35] Graves,[36] during 9-month experience with Schiller's test, discovered three early cases of cancer of the cervix. This work led to his 1933 prediction that cervical cancer passes through a period in its life history during which it is theoretically 100% curable and his conclusion that "patients must repeatedly be on our examining tables who without impairment of health, and often without symptoms,

harbor a disease which at the same time is invisible to the keenest eye and intangible to the most sensitive touch."[36] However, despite its role in promulgating insights into the natural history of cervical carcinogenesis, Schiller's iodine test was soon found to be too nonspecific for primary screening of the cervix since many nonneoplastic conditions, including immature metaplasia and normal repair, also resulted in nonstaining areas. With the advent of Papanicolaou testing during the 1940s, Schiller's testing in primary cervical cancer screening fell out of use, but the stain was often used during the years following the introduction of cervical cytology screening to decide where to biopsy when the Pap result was appreciably abnormal. Once colposcopy was introduced for evaluation of the cervix in managing abnormal cervical cytology, Schiller's test was relegated to the role of an adjunct to the colposcopic evaluation.

1.4 GROWTH AND ACCEPTANCE OF COLPOSCOPY

Colposcopy was first introduced to the United States with the publication of an article by Emmert in the *Journal of the American Medical Association* in 1931.[37] However, it was not until the 1960s that colposcopy gained a small foothold in the United States, flourishing much earlier in Europe under the guidance of further pioneering work of Coupez,[38] Ganse,[39] Kolstad,[40] Limburg,[41] Mestwerdt,[42] Navratil,[43] and Wespi[44] (Table 1.3). However, until the 1950s colposcopy was rarely performed outside Germany and the German-speaking areas of Austria, Switzerland, and areas settled by Germans in South America. Improved equipment with better optics and illumination and the advent of colpophotography led to more precise descriptions of the capillary vascular bed of both normal and neoplastic cervical epithelium. These improvements eventually led to wider acceptance of colposcopy and establishment of colposcopy departments in Japan by Ando and Masubuchi (1950), in France by Palmer (1952), and in England by Stallworthy (1955).[45] In contrast, as late as 1952, Novak's obstetrical and gynecologic textbook continued resistance to

TABLE 1.3	GROWTH AND ACCEPTANCE OF COLPOSCOPY
1933–1950	The conflict in Europe ends the development of colposcopy in the United States as war interrupts the dialogue between European colposcopy pioneers and North American clinicians. Despite the war, advances in colposcopy continue to be made in Europe and South America.
1942	Triete (Germany) produces the first colpophotographs.[45]
1944	De la Riva (Spain) describes the value of colposcopy in the detection and treatment of cervical precancerous changes in the prevention of cervical carcinoma. Europeans begin screening with cervical cytology.[45]
1949	Hinselmann visits South America giving stimulus to the burgeoning practice of colposcopy in Argentina, Brazil, and other countries.[45]
1950	Ando and Masubichi introduce colposcopy to Japan. Primary mass screening with the colposcope becomes standard in Hungary 10 years before cervical cytology is used for the same purpose. Navratil establishes colposcopy as a routine technique in Austria.[45]
1953–1954	Mestwerdt produces the first atlas on colposcopy.[42] Bolten moves from Germany to the United States and establishes the first U.S. colposcopy clinics in Philadelphia and New Orleans.[45] A small nucleus of U.S. enthusiasts is trained (Lang, Weese, Torres, Ward, Schneider, Dampier, Bise, and Hull).[45]
1954	Stallworthy (England) sets up the first colposcopy department at Oxford in the United Kingdom. Colposcopy begins to flourish under advocates such as Anderson (1962), Jordan (1969), and Singer (1973).[45]
1961	Matew-Aragones and Usandizagas (Spain) describe colposcopic findings in pregnancy.[45]
1962	Vence comes from Columbia to Miami where he trains Scott and establishes the third center for colposcopy in the United States.[45]
1963	Koller advocates a saline wash with colposcopic evaluation prior to the application of acetic acid and iodine stain, noting that the angioarchitecture is more easily identified prior to the application of these stains. Kolstad (Norway) develops photographic techniques to document fine angioarchitecture and describes the relationship between intercapillary distance and the degree of histologic abnormality.[45]
1964	Disciples of Bolten and Vence establish the American Society for Colposcopy and Colpomicroscopy.[45]

this procedure in the United States with his statement that any discussion of colposcopic technique and terminology would "scarcely be profitable."[46] In 1953, the German colposcopist Bolten immigrated to Philadelphia, paving the way for eventual acceptance of colposcopy in the United States.[47] Bolten established colposcopy clinics at Jefferson Medical College, where he trained Lang,[48] and then at Louisiana State University Medical School in 1954, where he trained a nucleus of disciples—Bise, Dampier, Schneider, Torres, Ward, and Weese. These individuals would eventually be very important in establishing the role of colposcopy in the United States.[45]

Vence came to Miami in 1962 from Columbia, South America, and trained Scott in colposcopy. Scott joined with the small nucleus of colposcopists trained by Bolten to set up the American Society for Colposcopy and Colpomicroscopy in 1964.[45] However, barriers to acceptance of colposcopy in the United States continued well into the 1960s, at least partly secondary to the immense change in traditional management of abnormal cervical cytology that came with colposcopic triage (discussed in 1.4 below). It was not until the early work of Coppleson,[49-51] Stafl,[52,53] Burke,[54] Richart,[55,56] and Townsend[57] in improved understanding of the natural history of carcinogenesis, along with new colposcopic terminology, that the interest in colposcopy began to significantly increase. Coppleson et al.[49] and Stafl[53] were particularly instrumental in changing the ponderous German terminology to one based on English and Latin, thereby making the terminology more descriptive and communicative for modern colposcopists. Tireless teaching by these contemporary colposcopists helped to rapidly expand the cadre of colposcopic enthusiasts. By the late 1970s, colposcopy had become widely recognized in the United States as a complementary and necessary response to abnormal cervical cytology. In North America, and in much of Europe, colposcopy was used almost exclusively in the triage of women with abnormal cervical cytology. In contrast, in Germany, and in much of Latin America, colposcopy was incorporated into the routine gynecologic examination as a primary screen for cervical disease.

1.5 INTEGRATION OF COLPOSCOPY INTO MANAGEMENT ALGORITHMS FOR ABNORMAL PAP RESULTS

1.5.1 Management of Abnormal Cervical Cytology before the Introduction of Colposcopy

The wide acceptance of colposcopy in the 1970s as a method for localizing lesions on the cervix brought a more rational approach to the management of women with abnormal Papanicolaou tests. Prior to this time, the response to an abnormal Pap result depended entirely on the grade of the cytologic abnormality (Table 1.4). The response to *minor* cytologic abnormalities was to simply repeat the Pap test in 6 to 12 months. This was because minor cytologic abnormalities were thought to be rarely associated with high-grade cervical intraepithelial neoplasia (CIN 2,3), adenocarcinoma *in situ* (AIS), or invasive cancer. It was not until the 1980s that published studies demonstrated a high rate (10% to 30%) of CIN 2,3 and occasional invasive cervical cancer in women with minor cytologic abnormalities.[58] Cancer was occasionally missed by the failure of some women to return for recommended follow-up Pap tests or by failure of the test to detect the disease (false negative Pap) for some who did return.[59]

In contrast, high-grade (HSIL) Pap test results, including those suspicious for cancer, were managed aggressively by cervical conization because blind four-quadrant biopsy was known

TABLE 1.4	MANAGEMENT OF VARIOUS PAPANICOLAOU (PAP) CLASSIFICATIONS BEFORE THE INTRODUCTION OF COLPOSCOPY
■ PAP CLASS	**■ MANAGEMENT**
Class I	Repeat Pap at 12 mo
Class IIA	Vaginal Sulfa cream daily for 7 d followed by repeat Pap in 6–12 mo
IIB	Repeat Pap in 3–6 mo
Class III	Conization (some just repeated the Pap)
Class IV	Conization
Class V	Conization

to occasionally miss significant lesions. Although diagnosis of lesser grades of cervical dysplasia on conization was usually considered a "cure," the diagnosis of *CIS* most commonly prompted hysterectomy, even for very young patients who desired to maintain their fertility. Conization was expensive, as it required anesthesia and operating room time. Additionally, conization had the potential for significant complications, including bleeding, infection, cervical stenosis, and the risk of cervical incompetence. Because cytology is subjective, many women without significant precancer were exposed to these risks.

Therefore, prior to the widespread use of colposcopy, women with cytologic abnormalities were often either underevaluated or overtreated. Only those lesions correctly interpreted as high grade on cytology were actually triaged correctly to confirmatory diagnostic and therapeutic procedures, while many significant lesions remained undetected because of inadequate evaluation of lower-grade cytology. Moreover, harm was likely caused by the widespread use of conization and hysterectomy to manage high-grade Pap test interpretations and CIS lesions.

1.5.2 Management after the Introduction of Colposcopy

1.5.2.1 Management before The Bethesda System

The introduction of colposcopy and colposcopically directed biopsy noticeably changed the management of high-grade cytologic abnormalities and the treatment of diagnosed cervical neoplasia. Colposcopy facilitated the detection of all grades of preinvasive disease and invasive cancer. More importantly, colposcopists were able to delineate the location of neoplasia on the cervix and in the vagina. As a result, less radical treatment methods, such as cryotherapy and laser ablation, largely supplanted cold-knife conization for the treatment of CIN.[60-63] Additionally, beginning in the late 1960s, noteworthy advances were made in understanding the pathogenesis of invasive cervical cancer. In 1967, Richart and Barron published their work on the natural history of cervical carcinogenesis as a continuum of disease from mild dysplasia to cervical cancer[64] (Table 1.5). This work began to change the concept that dysplasia and CIS require different treatments. Although Koss identified the cytologic finding of koilocytotic atypia in 1955, it was not until 1976 that Meisels and Fortin established the role of HPV in the etiology of this cytologic abnormality.[4,65] At about the same time, Harold zur Hausen proposed HPV as the causative agent in the development of cervical cancer,[5,6] and subsequent development of HPV DNA probes during the early 1980s provided the tools to confirm his prediction.[7,8] The management of cervical preinvasive disease changed as these breakthroughs increased understanding of the disease process and as colposcopy and conservative outpatient treatment methods became acceptable and widely available.[66]

TABLE 1.5	THE ROLE OF COLPOSCOPY IN CONSERVATIVE MANAGEMENT OF CERVICAL NEOPLASIA BEFORE THE INTRODUCTION OF THE BETHESDA SYSTEM
1960s	Richart and Barron publish their work on the natural history of cervical carcinogenesis as a continuum of disease from mild dysplasia to cervical cancer, breaking down the concept that dysplasia and CIS must be treated differently.[56] Publications begin to promote more conservative approaches to treating cervical intraepithelial neoplasia (CIN 1,2, and 3 or mild, moderate, and severe dysplasia).[60] Coppleson and Reid popularize colposcopy in Australia.[49,50]
1970s	Colposcopy with directed cervical biopsy is reported to reduce the need for cone biopsy in the majority of women with abnormal Papanicolaou (Pap) smear results. Cryotherapy becomes the dominant outpatient treatment modality for CIN.[61] Canadian gynecologists establish colposcopy clinics.[45]
1971	Coppleson, Pixley, and Reid publish the first edition of their colposcopy text and further the understanding of the transformation zone in the development of CIN.[49]
1972	Argentina hosts the First World Congress of Colposcopy and Uterine Cervical Pathology following which the International Federation of Cervical Pathology and Colposcopy (IFCPC) is founded to provide a worldwide organization of colposcopy societies.[45]
1974	The CO_2 laser is introduced for the ablation of CIN. The IFCPC standardizes colposcopic terminology and publishes its International Nomenclature of Colposcopic Findings.[45]
1975	Zur Hausen (Germany) suggests that cervical neoplasia may be associated with HPV.[5,6]
1980s	CO_2 laser begins to dominate outpatient treatment of CIN.[62]
1983	Cartier describes electrodiathermy loop excision of cervical lesions, and later Prendiville promotes this as large loop excision of the transformation zone.[63]
1985	Ueki (Japan) publishes the first book on cervical adenocarcinoma.[45]

Until the late 1980s, only women with *dysplastic* cervical cytology were referred for colposcopy. Minor cervical cytologic abnormalities were still managed with repeat cervical cytology. This included cellular changes secondary to HPV (koilocytotic atypia) that did not have dysplastic features and cellular changes that were not completely normal, but not clearly abnormal either. This restrictive approach had the benefit of keeping the volume of women referred for colposcopy within a manageable range. However, cytologic terminology was about to change, and this change would lead to an expanding role for colposcopy.

1.5.2.2 Management after the Bethesda System

A public outcry followed the 1987 article in the *Wall Street Journal* titled "Lax Laboratories: The Pap Test Misses Much Cervical Cancer Through Lab Errors," in which problems inherent in cervical cytologic screening at the time were identified. These included shoddy laboratory oversight, overworked laboratory personnel, and false-negative Pap test results resulting in missed cervical cancers.[67] The U.S. government responded by changing regulations for cytology laboratories in the form of the 1988 Clinical Laboratories Improvement Act (CLIA 88).[68] Additionally, recognition that the Class System of Pap test terminology did not adequately address risks inherent in the subjectivity of cervical cytologic interpretation prompted the National Cancer Institute to convene a conference in Bethesda, Maryland for the purpose of revising cervical cytologic terminology (Table 1.6). The Bethesda System (TBS), as the new terminology was named, dramatically changed cervical cytologic classification and reporting, with similar impact

TABLE 1.6	CERVICAL CANCER PREVENTION FROM THE ERA OF THE BETHESDA SYSTEM INTO THE 21ST CENTURY
1988	The first Bethesda system for reporting cervical cytology is published in the *Journal of the American Medical Association*.[65] The colposcopic pool is greatly expanded to women with lesser degrees of cytologic atypia.
1990s	LEEP using smaller-size loops is adopted in the United States and widely criticized for overuse. A balance between use of LEEP for major and cryotherapy for minor lesions is accepted. Laser treatment of CIN falls out of favor due to higher cost and greater need for expertise.
1991	The Second Bethesda Conference refines TBS for reporting cervical cytology.
1995	The IARC confirms that HPV is necessary in the etiology of most cervical cancers.
1996	Several new cervical cancer screening technologies are introduced, including liquid-based cervical cytology and automated computer-based rescreening of Papanicolaou (Pap) tests.
Late 1990s	Intense efforts to evaluate low-cost cervical cancer screening modalities for resource-poor countries begin. Computer-based digital imaging systems, improved molecular probes for HPV, and computer analysis of differences in electromagnetic wavelengths of light and electrical stimulation emitted by normal and neoplastic tissues undergo intense study.
2001	The 2001 Bethesda Workshop further refines TBS cervical cytology terminology of 1988 and 1991.[129] The American Society for Colposcopy and Cervical Pathology hosts the ASCCP Consensus Conference for the Management of Abnormal Cervical Cytology and Cervical Cancer Precursors in Bethesda, MD.[98,99] Comprehensive evidence-based management guidelines for abnormal cytology and histology are developed for the first time by a consensus process involving 29 major national and international organizations with interest in cervical cancer screening.
2002	First report documenting efficacy of a prophylactic HPV vaccine is published in the *New England Journal of Medicine*.[130]
2006	The American Society for Colposcopy and Cervical Pathology hosts the second Consensus Conference for the Management of Abnormal Cervical Cytology and Cervical Cancer Precursors in Bethesda, MD.[100,101] Comprehensive evidence-based management guidelines for abnormal cytology and histology are refined and extended by a consensus process involving 29 major national and international organizations.
2006	The quadrivalent HPV vaccine is the first HPV vaccine to be licensed by the U.S. Food and Drug Administration and to be approved by the U.S. Advisory Committee on Immunization Practices for routine use in girls and women aged 9–26.

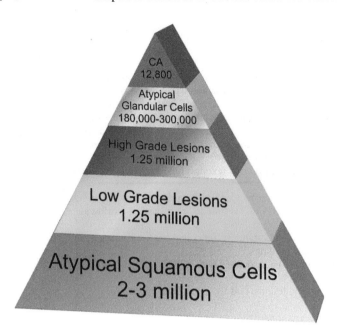

FIGURE 1.8. Many have argued that TBS more than doubled the number of women considered to have abnormal Pap results by including atypical cells in the epithelial abnormality category. This expanded the potential colposcopic pool by at least 2,000,000 Pap findings of ASCUS, which was previously part of the Papanicolaou Class IIA category. Additionally, another 500,000 Pap findings of koilocytotic atypia, originally part of Papanicolaou Class IIB, were included with CIN 1 in the category LSIL, increasing the concern for this Pap interpretation as well. Since most protocols considered the Pap result of ASCUS to be only atypical and not abnormal, the general recommendation was to repeat these Paps and to colposcopically examine only those women with abnormalities on repeat Pap testing. HSIL, high-grade squamous intraepithelial lesions; LSIL, low-grade squamous intraepithelial lesions.

on modern colposcopic practice.[69] Not only was koilocytotic atypia now included with low-grade dysplasia in a single abnormal category called LSIL, but even atypia that could not be reliably designated as *within normal limits* but also not reliably designated as *abnormal* was placed in its own category termed atypical squamous cells of undetermined significance (ASCUS). The inclusion of these minor cellular changes in an equivocal Pap classification, along with increased insecurity regarding the potential for false-negative repeat Pap test results, changed the traditional colposcopic triage guidelines.[58,70–75] The result was the referral of up to three times more women to colposcopy than would have been referred when the threshold for colposcopic referral began with mild dysplasia/CIN 1[75] (Figure 1.8). Although some women with CIN 2,3, AIS, and invasive cervical cancer that might have previously been missed were now evaluated and treated, so were many normal women and women with transient low-grade lesions that had little clinical significance. Biopsy of trivial colposcopic changes may result in histologic overcall, since differentiation between variants of the normal metaplastic process and cervical neoplasia is often quite difficult.[76–78] Improved sensitivity came at the price of subsequent overdiagnosis that led to unnecessary treatment with high financial and psychological costs. Additionally, initial enthusiasm for easy excision in the office of the abnormal transformation zone often led to loop electrosurgical excision procedure (LEEP) of women, including adolescents, with CIN 1 or CIN 2 that might have resolved spontaneously without treatment over time.

As a consequence of this lowered threshold for referral, modern colposcopists have a much more difficult task than did their predecessors, who had to respond only to markedly abnormal cervical cytology that carried a high probability of finding high-grade disease at colposcopy. Only a well-trained colposcopist can capably minimize both the risks of failed detection of cervical neoplasia and the risk of overcall inherent in the colposcopic examination of normal women. Fortunately, improved understanding of the potential for spontaneous remission of minor cervical lesions led to guidelines recommending follow-up rather than treatment for such lesions.[79]

1.5.3 HPV and the Screening and Diagnosis of Cervical Disease

1.5.3.1 Discovery of the Role of HPV in Cervical Carcinogenesis

These dilemmas were at least partially ameliorated by the introduction of HPV testing as an intermediate triage for women with ASCUS Pap results, as testing equivocal cytology for the virus that causes cervical cancer reduced colposcopic referral of many HPV-negative women not at risk for cervical neoplasia. Although Leopold Koss[65] described the koilocyte in 1955, and Meisels and Fortin[4] established HPV as the etiologic agent in Koss's koilocytotic atypia in 1976, it was not until Harold zur Hausen's 1983 isolation of HPV 16 in cervical cancers that this virus began to be accepted as the prime suspect in the etiology of this cancer.[7,8] However, at that time herpes simplex virus type 2 (HSV2) was the prime suspect in the etiology of cervical cancer and koilocytotic atypia was considered a benign cellular change.[80] Following zur Hausen's discoveries, the ability to document the presence of HPV within cervical neoplastic lesions led to the establishment of HPV as the etiologic agent in virtually all cervical cancers and to[81,82] the International Agency for Research on Cancer (IARC) statement that cervical cancer may be the first human cancer to have a single necessary cause. Having a single necessary viral cause raised the hopeful prospect that cervical cancer might someday be eliminated.[81] The race was on to find pathways to make this a reality. By 1989, research in both HPV primary prevention and secondary detection began to show the road ahead.[80] In that year, Ian Frazier and colleagues, working in Australia, demonstrated that the L1 gene in the HPV genome, when inserted into a yeast plasmid, could generate the HPV protein capsid of the virus without the DNA. This discovery paved the way to the eventual development of the HPV vaccine[82] (Figure 1.9). The other pathway led to the evaluation of the clinical use of HPV DNA probes in the detection of CIN.

1.5.3.2 The Early Years: Exploring the Potential for Clinical Utility in HPV Testing

As early as 1984, a number of studies evaluated the use of filter hybridization techniques for detection of HPV DNA in cervical scrape specimens collected in parallel with samples for routine cytology.[83–90] In 1988, the first comprehensive study of cytology, colposcopy, and cervicography, in addition to the collection of exfoliated cells for HPV testing, compared PCR testing for HPVs 6, 11, 16, 18, and 33 with dot blot hybridization techniques to determine the suitability of the PCR test for implementation in routine clinical settings.[89] The results were favorable enough for the authors to predict that it was possible that such tests might gain widespread use in cervical cancer screening. Other studies of HPV testing in clinical management were initiated in the late 1980s. The first to be published was an evaluation of the use of a non–FDA-approved HPV test using Southern Blot, in combination with cervicography (expert evaluation of cervical photography) and/or repeat cytology.[91] The second of these early

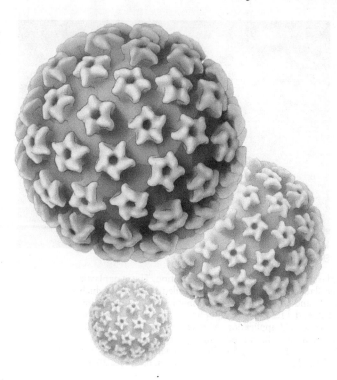

FIGURE 1.9.   Drawing of a HPV capsid.

clinical studies evaluated the first FDA-approved HPV test for clinical use (ViraPap, Life Technologies, Silver Spring, MD) in a colposcopy clinic overburdened with referrals.[92] Both studies demonstrated lower test sensitivity of cytology than with HPV testing and the second study indicated that women with ASCUS Pap results might benefit by triage to colposcopy based on HPV test results; HPV-negative ASCUS clearly did not require colposcopy, reducing the colposcopic burden for this clinic by 32%.

ASCUS was the first logical clinical application for HPV testing, as only about 50% of ASCUS HPV results were positive and the risk for cervical neoplasia existed largely in this group.[93] Hence, testing ASCUS for HPV offered the prospect of immediately decreasing colposcopic referral by half of the approximately 3 million ASCUS Pap results annually. During the 1990s, several studies demonstrating favorable results in HPV triage of ASCUS were published.[94–97] However, it was not until data from the ASCUS LSIL Triage Study (ALTS) began to be available in 2001[97] that management guidelines for abnormal cervical cytology began to include the option of testing for HPV in a variety of precolposcopy, postcolposcopy, and posttreatment settings.[98–101]

1.5.3.3 Integrating HPV Testing into Colposcopic Triage

The early studies on the use of HPV testing in colposcopic triage were encouraging but small numbers did not ensure generalizability of the findings sufficient for a paradigm shift in clinical management.[92–96] ALTS results provided the basis for such a paradigm change. The purpose of this large multicenter randomized trial was to evaluate whether ASCUS and LSIL cytology results would be most efficiently and safely managed by immediate referral to colposcopy, by triage to colposcopy based on testing positive for HPV, or by repeating the Pap test.[97] The results on 3488 women with ASCUS and 1572 women with LSIL were conclusive. ALTS established HPV testing as the preferred management option

for ASCUS, particularly when the test could be "reflexed" from the remaining sample of a liquid-based Pap specimen.[102] HPV triage was found to be at least as sensitive as immediate colposcopy for detecting CIN 3, but accomplished this with referring only about half as many women to colposcopy. Repeat cytology required two additional office visits and two repeat Pap tests to achieve sensitivity similar to that of a single HPV test for detection of CIN 3 and required more colposcopies than HPV triage.[97,102] In contrast, too many young women with LSIL tested positive for high-risk HPV for HPV testing to be a cost-effective triage.[103,104] Additionally, a single HPV test at 12 months was found to be as sensitive as two repeat Pap tests (at 6 and 12 months) in the referral back to colposcopy of women not found to have CIN 2,3 at initial colposcopy.[102] HPV testing was now firmly placed in both initial colposcopic triage of this common equivocal cytologic abnormality and as an option in postcolposcopy and, subsequently, posttreatment management.[98–101,105]

1.6 NEW CHALLENGES IN COLPOSCOPY

1.6.1 Expansion of the Practice of Colposcopy to a Broader Clinical Base

Colposcopy was once the exclusive domain of gynecologists and gynecologic oncologists. However, in the early 1990s in the interest of making medical care more available and less costly, the ASCCP began to teach colposcopy in some family practice and internal medicine residencies and to advanced practice clinicians (nurse practitioners, midwives, and physician assistants). While expanding colposcopic expertise to all clinicians who care for women provides an opportunity for a more cost-effective and accessible response to abnormal cervical cytology, providing equal training has been a challenge. Additionally, the pool of colposcopists has expanded during the same period in which the number of cervical cancers has dramatically declined, providing fewer and fewer opportunities for all but gynecologic oncologists to see invasive disease. These trends have diminished the number of cervical cancers seen in one's career to very few, if any. Therefore, colposcopists have had to obtain adequate exposure to the colposcopic findings of early invasive cervical and other lower genital tract cancers by other means. To ensure this level of exposure, several organizations have developed multimedia continuing education programs in the field of colposcopy, assisted by self-study of colposcopic atlases and other teaching aids.

Hence, expertise has been difficult for many to obtain, even when colposcopic training is made available during residency. When available, residency programs and postgraduate colposcopy courses have provided at least a baseline familiarity with colposcopic principles and, for some, a substantial basis of excellence. However, provision of an adequate understanding of the histologic and cytologic basis of disease recognition and management, an imperative for the practice of expert colposcopy, is often missing from colposcopy training.

1.6.2 Challenges to the Accuracy of Colposcopy

1.6.2.1 Increasing Incidence of Glandular Neoplasia

Contemporary colposcopists also confront the dilemma of an apparently increasing incidence of AIS and adenocarcinoma of the cervix.[106–110] Both cytology and colposcopy have long been understood to be less sensitive and, as a result, less reliable in

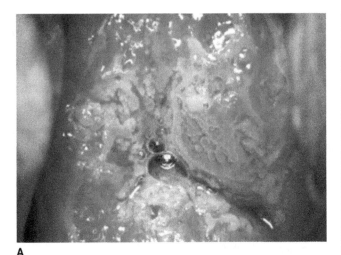
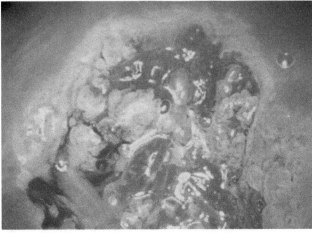

A   **B**

FIGURE 1.10.   **A:** A colpophotograph of immature metaplasia taken after acetic acid application. The metaplastic process has produced glazed, acetowhite fusing villi, some flat, others in mounds (also called bouquets), which overlie columnar epithelium. Coupled with the variegated red and white appearance, it mimics a glandular lesion (AIS/adenocarcinoma). Compare with Figures 11.4A,B, 11.9, and 11.22. **B:** A colpophotograph of an AIS lesion (histologically proven on an excised specimen) taken after acetic acid application. Mounds (bouquets) of acetowhite AIS tissue, some with papillary projections, overlie columnar epithelium producing a variegated red and white appearance. It mimics immature metaplasia. Compare with Figures 11.17 and 11.35A. (Reprinted with permission from Wright VC. *Color Atlas of Colposcopy – Cervix, Vagina and Vulva.* Houston, TX: Biomedical Communications, 2000.)

detecting cervical glandular neoplasia than in detecting CIN 2,3. Part of this is due to the fact that, when present, AIS often found in the canal and, if not, typically has a more subtle colposcopic appearance.[109] Attention of the colposcopist is often drawn away from glandular abnormalities by the more dramatic colposcopic findings of squamous lesions that are often adjacent. AIS is often so subtle that even experienced colposcopists may be challenged to find it (see Chapter 11). For the novice colposcopist, this difficulty is compounded by inexperience in recognizing colposcopic patterns associated with the abnormal transformation zone, and for any colposcopist, by failure to biopsy the most abnormal area, and by failure to take a sufficient number of biopsies.[111] Understanding these issues is particularly crucial in reducing the potential of missing glandular neoplasia because AIS can look like a normal ectopy (Figure 1.10A,B).

1.6.2.2 The Hunt for Ever Smaller CIN 2,3

Despite this success in the partnership of cytology and colposcopy in reducing cervical cancer morbidity and mortality, there have recently been questions regarding the accuracy of colposcopy.[111,112] The majority of studies questioning the accuracy of colposcopy have come from assessment of static colpophotographs or cervigrams, rather than real-time colposcopy.[113–116] However, the performance of online assessment of static cervigrams from ALTS was shown to not be significantly lower than that of same-day enrollment colposcopy.[116] Even studies of real-time colposcopy have documented sensitivity of the procedure for detection of CIN 3 varying from 54% in ALTS[102] to 85% documented in a meta-analysis of studies from 1960 to 1996.[117] Earlier studies likely demonstrated higher accuracy because they predated the continuing trend toward detection of increasingly small high-grade lesions, which are much more difficult to detect.[111] In contrast, recent studies, such as ALTS, followed the introduction of increasingly sensitive cervical cancer screening tests with a lowered threshold for triage to colposcopy. Additionally, the 54% estimated sensitivity of the initial colposcopy for CIN 3 in ALTS did not account for the likelihood that some of the CIN 3 subsequently detected during 2-year follow-up was probably

either newly incident or so small as to not be discernable at initial colposcopy.[111,118] These changes have placed colposcopists in the difficult position of finding lesions that may be below, or precisely at, the limits of detection.

Where does this leave us in relation to the practice of colposcopy? Fortunately, the median time between peak detection of CIN 3 (29 years) and microinvasive cervical cancer (42 years) gives reassurance that the oncogenic process typically spans many years.[111,118] Lesions in young women are generally small. The median length of CIN 3 in ALTS was only 6.5 mm and lesions in 1/3 of them were so small that colposcopic biopsy did not leave any residual CIN 3 to be detected in the LEEP specimen.[118] Hence, the finding of extensive CIN 3 at colposcopy when the referral Pap result was ASCUS or LSIL is unusual.[118] CIN 3 associated with invasion has been reported to be, on average, seven times the size of CIN 3 not associated with invasion.[119] Given the rarity of cervical cancer detected in follow-up to colposcopy not initially showing CIN 3 or cancer, the increased sensitivity of colposcopy for larger high-grade lesions, and the association of lesion size with risk of invasion, pushing the limits of detection of small lesions by colposcopy may have little impact on the overall cervical cancer rate.[111]

However, as the sensitivity of screening modalities increases, colposcopists will be challenged to detect all CIN 3, regardless of size, because risk of invasion is cumulative over time and unpredictable in a given patient.[118] Fortunately, a number of studies now document that the sensitivity of colposcopy for CIN 3 can be improved significantly by taking two or more biopsies.[120,121] Therefore, in this era where the challenge is to find increasingly earlier, smaller high-grade lesions, the solution lies in taking more biopsies (Figure 1.11). Eventually, new procedures or tests that are better equipped to triage at-risk women identified by increasingly sensitive tests may augment or even replace the colposcope.

1.6.2.3 The Impact of HPV Vaccines

As the cohorts of women receiving prophylactic HPV 16/18 or HPV 6/11/16/18 vaccine series reach the age to begin screening, the reduction in abnormal cervical cytology will likely decrease

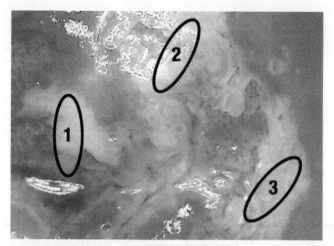

FIGURE 1.11. Many studies have documented that taking more biopsies increases detection of CIN 2,3. In this colpophotograph, three obvious sites for biopsy are circled. In addition, biopsy of areas of normal appearing transformation zone may also increase detection. (Colpophotograph courtesy of J.T. Cox, MD.)

colposcopic referrals by 40% to 60%, decreasing the positive predictive value (PPV) of cytology, colposcopy, and HPV testing.[9] However, this impact will be greatest on cytology and colposcopy because of their subjective nature.[122] The need for screening women and evaluation of those with abnormal results will continue, as some women will not have received the vaccine, some may have received the vaccine after already being exposed to HPV types in the vaccine, some may not have received the requisite series of three vaccinations, and not all carcinogenic HPV types are covered by the available vaccines. Future HPV vaccines will likely contain additional oncogenic HPV types, further reducing the PPV of cytology and colposcopy. Teaching both cytopathologists and colposcopists may become increasingly challenging as important cervical lesions become increasingly uncommon. While we welcome the potential demise of cervical neoplasia, a prolonged transition period during which women will continue to need to be screened may increasingly challenge the modern colposcopist. Additionally, vigilance will need to be maintained against the possibility that in the era of HPV vaccination women may assume that they do not need cervical screening.

1.7 ROLE OF COLPOSCOPY IN THE 21ST CENTURY

In this age of molecular medicine, it is essential that the modern colposcopist keeps abreast of the many advances regularly occurring in the understanding of cervical carcinogenesis that are being rapidly translated into clinical practice. In addition to advances in the fields of molecular biology and molecular pathology, technical advances in optics, electromagnetic imaging, and image analysis will likely provide new tools for the colposcopist.[123–125] Although colposcopes used by clinicians today are much better than the original instruments, they are probably more similar to the first colposcope than they will be to the devices that will be used to evaluate the cervix as this century progresses. It appears unlikely that colposcopic evaluation of the cervix in the 21st century will be limited to use of visible light, acetic acid, and magnification. Digital imaging computer systems and computer analysis of different wavelengths of light and electrical stimulation reflected by normal, cancerous, and precancerous tissues are but a few of the new

technologies likely to play a significant role in cervical cancer screening in the near future. Additionally, molecular biology will aid colposcopy in identifying women at greatest risk for cervical neoplasia that may already exist, or may develop over time. Burgeoning research in markers such as p16, a tumor suppressor gene product, and DNA methylation silencing certain genes necessary in protecting against carcinogenesis are providing a look at the direction cervical cancer prevention is moving.[126–128]

The future is exciting and full of hope for increasingly effective cervical cancer prevention. It is our aim in *Modern Colposcopy*, 3rd edition, to provide a scientific and clinical foundation that will enable novice as well as experienced colposcopists to move confidently through the early decades of the 21st century and become ever-evolving "modern colposcopists."

References

1. Scotto J, Bailar JC. Rigoni-Stern and medical statistics. A nineteenth-century approach to cancer research. *J Hist Med Allied Sci* 1969;24:65–75.
2. Gagnon F. Contribution to the study of the etiology and prevention of cancer of the cervix of the uterus. *Am J Obstet Gynecol* 1950;50:516–22.
3. Frazier IH. Chapter 21: Human papillomaviruses. In: Artensen AW, ed. *Vaccines: A Biography*. New York, NY: Springer, 2010:361–73.
4. Meisels A, Fortin R. Condylomatous lesions of the cervix and vagina. I. Cytologic patterns. *Acta Cytol* 1976;20;505–9.
5. zur Hausen H, Gissmann L, Steiner W, et al. Human papilloma viruses and cancer. *Bibl Haematol* 1975;(43):569–71.
6. zur Hausen H. Condylomata acuminata and human genital cancer. *Cancer Res* 1976;36(2 pt 2):794.
7. Dürst M, Gissmann L, Ikenberg H, et al. A papillomavirus DNA from a cervical carcinoma and its prevalence in cancer biopsy samples from different geographic regions. *Proc Natl Acad Sci U S A* 1983;80(12):3812–5.
8. Boshart M, Gissmann L, Ikenberg H, et al. A new type of papillomavirus DNA, its presence in genital cancer biopsies and in cell lines derived from cervical cancer. *EMBO J* 1984;3(5):1151–7.
9. Kitchener HC, Castle PE, Cox JT. Chapter 7: Achievements and limitations of cervical cytology screening. *Vaccine* 2006;24(suppl 3):S63–70.
10. von Franque O. Leukoplakia und carcinoma vaginae et uteri. *Z Geburtshilfe* 1907;60:237–9.
11. Hinselmann H. Zur kenntnis der pracancerosen veranderungen der portio. *Zentralbl Gynakol* 1927;51:901–2.
12. Hinselmann H. Die atiologie, symptomatologie und diagnostik des uteruscarcinoms. In: Veit J, Stockel W, eds. *Handbuch der Gynekologie*. Munich, Germany: Bergmann, 1930:854–856: Vol 6:1.
13. Hinselmann H. Verbessrung der inspektionsmoglichkeiten von vulva, vagina und portio. *Munchner Med Wochenschr* 1925;72:1733–6.
14. von Franque O. Das beginnende portiokankroid und die ausbreitungswege des gebarmutterhalskrebses. *Z Geburtshilfe* 1901;44:173–7.
15. Schauenstein W. Histologie untersuchungen uber atypisches plattenepithel an der portio und an der innenflache der cervix uteri. *Arch Gynakol* 1908;85:576–9.
16. Schottlander J, Kermauner F. *Zur Kenntnis des Uteruskarzinoms*. Berlin, Germany: Karger, 1912.
17. Hinselmann H. Ausgewahlte gesichtspunlte zur beurteilung des zusammenhanges der "matrixbezirke" und des karzinomsder sichtbaren abschnitte des weiblichen genitaltrakes. *Z Geburtshilfe* 1933;104:228–30.
18. Hinselmann H. Die Kolposkopie. In: *Klinische Fortbildung. Neue Deutsche Klinik* 1936;(suppl 4):717.
19. Hinselmann H. *Einfurung in die Kolposkopie*. Hamburg, Germany: Hartung, 1933.
20. Hinselmann H. Der begriff der umwandlungszone der portio. *Arch Gynakol* 1927;131:422–4.
21. Hinselmann H. Die linische und mikroskopische fruhdiagnose des portiokarzinoms. *Arch Gynakol* 1934:156:239–40.
22. Glatthaar E. Studien Uber die Morphogenese des Plattenepithelkarzinoms der Portio Vaginalis Uteri. Basel, Switzerland: Karger, 1950.
23. Dietel H, Focken A. Das schicksal des atypischen epithels an der portio. *Geburtshilfe Frauenheilkd* 1955;15:593–5.
24. Halioua B. The participation of Hans Hinselmann in medical experiments at Auschwitz. *J Low Gen Tract Dis* 2010;1:1–4.
25. Babes A. Diagnostic du cancer du col uterine par les frottis. *La Presse Medicale* 1928;36:451. [Reprinted in English *Acta Cytol* 1967;11:217.]
26. Papanicolaou GN. New cancer diagnosis. Proceedings Third Race Betterment Conference, Battle Creek, Michigan. Race Betterment Foundation, 1928.
27. Papanicolaou GN, Traut HF. *Diagnosis of Uterine Cancer by the Vaginal Smear*. New York, NY: Commonwealth Fund, 1943.
28. Ayre JE. Selective cytologic smear for the diagnosis of cancer. *Am J Obstet Gynecol* 1947;53:609–19.

29. Lai-Goldman M, Nieberg RK, Mulcahy D, et al. The cytobrush for evaluating routine cervicovaginal-endocervical smears. *J Reprod Med* 1990;35:959–63.

30. Martin-Hirsch P, Jarvis G, Kitchener H, et al. Collection devices for obtaining cervical cytology samples. *Cochrane Database Syst Rev* 2000;(2):CD001036.

31. Vasilev S. Commentary: Kaiser permanente medicine 50 years ago: the gynecological cancer detection clinic. *Permanente J* 2000;4(3).

32. Baskett TF. Hysterectomy: evolution and trends. *Best Pract Res Clin Obstet Gynaecol* 2005;19:295–305.

33. Schiller J. Jodpinselung und abschabung des portioepithels. *Zentralbl Gynakol* 1929;53:1056.

34. Karl Bolten's Introduction to Colposcopy. A Diagnostic Aid in Benign and Preclinical Cancerous Lesions of the Cervix Uteri, chapter 3. New York, NY: Grune & Stratton, Inc., 381 Fourth Avenue, 1960.

35. Schiller W. Early diagnosis of carcinoma of the cervix. *Surg Gyn and Obs.* 1933;56:210–22.

36. Graves WD. Detection of the clinically latent cancer of the cervix. *Surg Gyn Obs.* 1933;56:317–22.

37. Emmert F. The recognition of cancer of the uterus in its earliest stages. *JAMA* 1931;97:1684.

38. Coupez F. Dysplasia of the cervix uteri. *Rev Franc Gynec Obstet* 1965;60:579.

39. Ganse R. The influence of indirect metaplasia on the formation of carcinoma in situ of the portio. *Acta Un Int Cancer* 1963;19:1375–8.

40. Kolstad P. Carcinoma of the cervix. Stage 0. Diagnosis and treatment. *Am J Obstet Gynecol* 1966;96:1098–103.

41. Limburg H. *Die Fruhdiagnose des iteruscarcinoms.* Stuttgart, Germany: Theime, 1956.

42. Mestwerdt G. *Atlas der Kolposkopie.* Jena, Germany: Fischer, 1953.

43. Navratil E. Colposcopy. In: Gray LA, ed. *Dysplasia, carcinoma in situ and microinvasive carcinoma of the cervix uteri.* Springfield, IL: Thomas, 1964:228–83.

44. Wespi H. *Early Carcinoma of the Uterine Cervix: Pathogenesis and Detection.* New York, NY: Grune and Stratton, 1949.

45. Torres JE, Riopelle MA. History of colposcopy in the United States. In: Wright VC, ed. *Contemporary Colposcopy.* Philadelphia, PA. *Obstet Gynecol Clin N Am* 1993;20:1–12.

46. Novak E. *Gynecologic and Obstetric Pathology.* Philadelphia, PA: W.B. Saunders, 1952.

47. Scheffery LC, Bolten KA, Lang WR. Colposcopy. *Obstet Gynecol* 1955;5:294.

48. Bise JR. In memorium Karl August Bolten. *Colposcopist* 1972;1:1.

49. Coppleson M, Pixley E, Reid B. Colposcopy. *A Scientific and Practical Approach to the Cervix in Health and Disease.* Springfield, IL: Charles C.Thomas, 1971.

50. Coppleson M, Reid B. The colposcopic study of the cervix during pregnancy and the puerperium. *J Obstet Gynaecol Br Commonw* 1966;73:375.

51. Coppleson M, Reid BL. *Pre-clinical Carcinoma of the Cervix Uteri; Its Origin, Nature and Management.* Oxford: Pergamon, 1967.

52. Stafl A. Colposcopy in diagnosis of cervical neoplasia. *Am J Obstet Gynecol* 1973;115(2):286–7.

53. Stafl A. The clinical diagnosis of early cervical cancer. *Obstet Gynec Surv* 1969;24:976–82.

54. Burke L, Mathews B. *Colposcopy in Clinical Practice.* Philadelphia, PA: FA Davis, 1977.

55. Richart RM. A clinical staining test for the in vivo delineation of dysplasia and carcinoma in situ. *Am J Obstet Gynecol* 1963;86:703–4.

56. Richart RM. Observations on the biology of cervical dysplasia. *Bull Sloane Hosp Women* 1964;10:170–4.

57. Townsend DE, Ostergard D, Mishell D. Abnormal Papanicolaou smears: evaluation by colposcopy, biopsies, and endocervical curettage. *Am J Obstet Gynecol* 1970;108:429–36.

58. Jones DED, Creaseman WT, Dombroski RA, et al. Evaluation of the atypical Pap smear. *Am J Obstet Gynecol* 1987;157:544–9.

59. Mayeaux EJ, Harper MB, Abreo F, et al. A comparison of the reliability of repeat cervical smears and colposcopy in patients with abnormal cervical cytology. *J Fam Pract* 1995;40:57–62.

60. Richart RM, Sciarra JJ. Treatment of cervical dysplasia by outpatient electrocauterization. *Am J Obstet Gynecol* 1968;101:200–3.

61. Creaseman WT, Weed JC, Curry SL, et al. Efficacy of cryosurgical treatment of severe cervical intraepithelial neoplasia. *Obstet Gynecol* 1972;41:501–5.

62. Wright VC, Davies E, Riopelle MA. Laser surgery for cervical intraepithelial neoplasia: principles and results. *Am J Obstet Gynecol* 1983;145–81.

63. Prendiville W, Cullimore J, Norman S. Large loop excision of the transformation zone (LLETZ): a new method of management for women with intraepithelial neoplasia. *Br J Obstet Gynecol* 1989;96:1054–60.

64. Richart RM, Barron BA. A follow-up study of patients with cervical dysplasia. *Am J Obstet Gynecol* 1969;105:386–93.

65. Koss LG, Durfee GR. Cytological changes preceding the appearance of in situ carcinoma of the uterine cervix. *Cancer* 1955;8(2):295–301.

66. Shafti MI, Luesley DM. Management of low grade lesions: follow-up or treat? Cervical intraepithelial neoplasia. In: Jones HW, ed. *Balliere's Clinical Obstetrics and Gynecology.* London, UK: Bailliere Tindall, 1995;9:121–33.

67. Bogdanich W. Lax Laboratories: The Pap Test Misses Much Cervical Cancer Through Labs Errors. *Wall Street J* 1967.

68. Centers for Medicare & Medicaid Services (CMS) Clinical Laboratory Improvement Amendments (CLIA) Page. http://www.cms.gov/CLIA/ (Accessed August 22, 2011).

69. National Cancer Institute Workshop. The 1988 Bethesda System for reporting cervical/vaginal cytologic diagnosis. *JAMA* 1989;262:931–4.

70. Yobs AR, Swanson RA, Lamotte LC. Laboratory reliability of the Papanicolaou smear. *Obstet Gynecol* 1985;65:235–43.

71. Davey DD, Naryshkin S, Nielsen ML, et al. Atypical squamous cells of undetermined significance: interlaboratory comparisons and quality assurance monitors. *Diagn Cytopathol* 1994;11:390–6.

72. Van der Graaf Y, Vooijs GP, Gailland HLJ, et al. Screening errors in cervical cytologic screening. *Acta Cytol* 1987;31:434–8.

73. Lindheim SR, Smith-Nguyen G. Aggressive evaluation for atypical squamous cells in Papanicolaou smears. *J Reprod Med* 1990;35:971–3.

74. Slawson DC, Bennett JH, Herman JM. Follow-up Papanicolaou smear for cervical atypia. Are we missing significant disease? *J Fam Pract* 1993;36:289–293.

75. Gordon P, Hatch K. Survey of colposcopy practices by obstetricians gynecologists. *J Reprod Med* 1992;37:861–3.

76. Robertson AJ, Anderson JM, Swanson Beck J, et al. Observer variability in histopathological reporting of cervical biopsy specimens. *J Clin Pathol* 1989;42:231–8.

77. Ishmail SM, Colcough AB, Dinnen JS, et al. Observer variation in histopathological diagnosis and grading of cervical intraepithelial neoplasia. *BMJ* 1989;298:707–10.

78. Ishmail SM, Colclough AB, Dennen JS, et al. Reporting cervical intraepithelial neoplasia (CIN): intra- and interpathologist variation and factors associated with disagreement. *Histol Pathol* 1990;16:371–6.

79. Wright TC Jr, Massad LS, Dunton CJ, et al. 2006 consensus guidelines for the management of women with abnormal cervical cancer screening tests. *Am J Obstet Gynecol* 2007;197:346–55.

80. Cox JT. History of the Use of HPV testing in cervical screening and in the management of abnormal cervical screening results. *J Clin Virol* 2009;45(Suppl 1):S3–12.

81. Walboomers JM, Jacobs MV, Manos MM, et al. Human papillomavirus is a necessary cause of invasive cervical cancer worldwide. *J Pathol* 1999;189:12–9.

82. Zhou J, Sun XY, Davies H, et al. Definition of linear antigenic regions of the HPV16 L1 capsid protein using synthetic virion-like particles. *Virology* 1992;189:592–9.

83. Wagner D, Ikenberg H, Boehm N, et al. Identification of human papillomavirus in cervical swabs by deoxyribonucleic acid in situ hybridization. *Obstet Gynecol* 1984;64:767–72.

84. Wickenden C, Steele A, Malcolm ADB, et al. Screening for wart virus infection in normal and abnormal cervices by DNA hybridization of cervical scrapes. *Lancet* 1984;i:65–7.

85. Schneider A, Kraus H, Schumann R, et al. Papillomavirus infection of the lower genital tract: detection of viral DNA in gynecological swabs. *Int J Cancer* 1985;35:443–8.

86. Burk RD, Kadish AS, Calderin S, et al. Human papillomavirus infection of the cervix detected by cervicovaginal lavage and molecular hybridization. Correlation with biopsy results in Papanicolaou smear. *Am J Obstet Gyencol* 1986;154:982–9.

87. Webb DH, Rogers RE, Fife KH. A one-step method for detecting and typing human papillomavirus DNA in cervical specimens from women with cervical dysplasia. *J Infect Dis* 1987;156:912–9.

88. Henderson BR, Thompson CH, Rose BR, et al. Detection of specific types of human papillomavirus in cervical scrapes, anal scrapes, and anogenital biopsies by DNA hybridization. *J Med Virol* 1987;12:381–98.

89. Morris BJ, Flanagan JL, McKinnon KJ. Nightengale BN letter. *Lancet* 1988:1368.

90. Dallas PB, Flanagan JL, Nightingale, et al. Polymerase chain reaction for fast, nonradioactive detection of high- and low-risk papillomavirus types in routine cervical specimens and in biopsies. *J Med Virol* 1989;27:105–11.

91. Reid R, Greenberg MD, Lorincz A, et al. Should cervical cytologic testing be augmented by cervicography or human papillomavirus deoxyribonucleic acid detection. *Am J Obstet Gynecol* 1991;164:1461–9.

92. Cox JT, Schiffman MH, Winzelberg AJ, et al. An evaluation of human papillomavirus testing as part of referral to colposcopy clinics. *Obstet Gynecol* 1992;80:389–95.

93. Wright TC, Sun XW, Koulos J. Comparison of management algorithms for the evaluation of women with low-grade cytologic abnormalities. *Obstet Gynecol* 1995;85:202–10.

94. Cox JT, Lorincz AT, Schiffman MH, et al. Human papillomavirus testing by hybrid capture appears to be useful in triaging women with a cytologic diagnosis of atypical squamous cells of undetermined significance. *Am J Obstet Gynecol* 1995;172:946–54.

95. Wright TC, Lorincz AT, Ferris DG, et al. Reflex human papillomavirus deoxyribonucleic acid testing in women with abnormal Pap smears. *Am J Obstet Gynecol* 1998;178:962–66.

96. Manos MM, Kinney WK, Hurley LB, et al. Identifying women with cervical neoplasia: using human papillomavirus testing for equivocal Papanicolaou results. *J Amer Med Assoc* 1999;281:1605–10.

97. Solomon D, Schiffman MH, Tarone B for the ALTS Group. Comparison of HPV testing, repeat cytology, and immediate colposcopy in ASCUS triage: baseline results from a randomized trial. *J Natl Cancer Inst* 2001;93:293–99.

98. Wright TC Jr, Cox JT, Massad LS, et al. 2001 ASCCP-Sponsored Consensus Conference. 2001 Consensus guidelines for the management of women with cervical cytological abnormalities. *J Am Med Assoc* 2002;287:2120–9.

99. Wright TC Jr, Cox JT, Massad LS, et al.; American Society for Colposcopy and Cervical Pathology. 2001 consensus guidelines for the management of women with cervical intraepithelial neoplasia. *Am J Obstet Gynecol* 2003;189:295–304.

100. Wright TC Jr, Massad LS, Dunton CJ, et al.; 2006 ASCCP-Sponsored Consensus Conference. 2006 consensus guidelines for the management of women with abnormal cervical screening tests. *J Low Genit Tract Dis* 2007;11:201–22.

101. Wright TC Jr, Massad LS, Dunton CJ, et al.; 2006 American Society for Colposcopy and Cervical Pathology-sponsored Consensus Conference. 2006 consensus guidelines for the management of women with cervical intraepithelial neoplasia or adenocarcinoma in situ. *J Low Genit Tract Dis* 2007;11:223–39.

102. The ASCUS-LSIL Triage Study (ALTS)* Group. Results of a randomized trial on the management of cytology interpretations of atypical squamous cells of undetermined significance. *Am J Obstet Gynecol* 2003;188:1383–92.

103. The ASCUS-LSIL Triage Study (ALTS)* Group. Human papillomavirus testing for triage of women with cytologic evidence of low-grade squamous intraepithelial lesions: baseline data from a randomized trial. The Atypical Squamous Cells of Undetermined Significance/Low-Grade Squamous Intraepithelial Lesions Triage Study (ALTS) Group. *J Natl Cancer Inst* 2000;92(1):397–402.

104. ASCUS-LSIL Triage Study (ALTS) Group. A randomized trial on the management of LSIL cytology interpretations. *Am J Obstet Gynecol* 2003;188:1393–400.

105. Guido R, Schiffman M, Solomon D, et al., ASCUS LSIL Triage Study Group. Postcolposcopy management strategies for patients referred with low-grade squamous intraepithelial lesions or human papillomavirus DNA–positive atypical squamous cells of undetermined significance: a two-year prospective study. *Am J Obstet Gynecol* 2003;188:1401–5.

106. Peters RK, Mack TM, Thomas D, et al. Increased frequency of adenocarcinoma of the uterine cervix in young women in Los Angeles County. *J Natl Cancer Inst* 1986;76:423–8.

107. Wang SS, Sherman ME, Hildesheim A, et al. Cervical adenocarcinoma and squamous cell carcinoma incidence trends among white women and black women in the United States for 1976–2000. *Cancer.* 2004;100(5):1035–44.

108. Sherman ME, Wang SS, Carreon J, et al. Cancer. Mortality trends for cervical squamous and adenocarcinoma in the United States. Relation to incidence and survival. 2005;103:1258–64.

109. Gari A, Lotocki R, Krepart G, et al. Cervical cancer in the province of Manitoba: a 30-year experience. *J Obstet Gynaecol Can* 2008;30(9):788–95.

110. Luesley DM, Jordan JA, Woodman CBJ, et al. A retrospective review of adenocarcinoma in situ and glandular atypia of the uterine cervix. *Br J Obstet Gynecol* 1987;94:699–703.

111. Cox JT. More questions about the accuracy of colposcopy: what does this mean for cervical cancer prevention? *Obstet Gynecol* 2008;111:1266–7.

112. Chase DM, Kalouyan M, DiSaia PJ. Colposcopy to evaluate abnormal cervical cytology in 2008. *Am J Obstet Gynecol* 2009;200:472–80.

113. Jeronimo J, Massad LS, Castle PE, et al.; National Institutes of Health (NIH)-American Society for Colposcopy and Cervical Pathology (ASCCP) Research Group. Interobserver agreement in the evaluation of digitized cervical images. *Obstet Gynecol* 2007;110:833–40.

114. Ferris DG, Litaker MS; ALTS Group. Prediction of cervical histologic results using an abbreviated Reid Colposcopic Index during ALTS. *Am J Obstet Gynecol* 2006;194:704–10.

115. Massad LS, Jeronimo J, Katki HA, et al.; National Institutes of Health/American Society for Colposcopy and Cervical Pathology (The NIH/ASCCP) Research Group. The accuracy of colposcopic grading for detection of high-grade cervical intraepithelial neoplasia. *J Low Genit Tract Dis* 2009;13:137–44.

116. Massad LS, Jeronimo J, Katki HA, et al.; National Institutes of Health/American Society for Colposcopy and Cervical Pathology Research Group. The accuracy of colposcopic grading for detection of high-grade cervical intraepithelial neoplasia. *J Low Genit Tract Dis* 2009;13(3):137–44.

117. Mitchell MF, Schottenfeld D, Tortolero-Luna G, et al. Colposcopy for the diagnosis of squamous intraepithelial lesions: a meta-analysis. *Obstet Gynecol* 1998;91:626–31.

118. Sherman ME, Wang SS, Tarone R, et al. Histopathologic extent of CIN 3 lesions in ALTS: implications for subject safety and lead-time bias. *Cancer Epidemiol Biomarkers Prev* 2003;12:372–9.

119. Tidbury P, Singer A, Jenkins D. CIN 3: the role of lesion size in invasion. *Br J Obstet Gynaecol.* 1992;99:583–6.

120. Gage JC, Hanson VW, Abbey K, et al.; ASCUS LSIL Triage Study (ALTS) Group. Number of cervical biopsies and sensitivity of colposcopy. *Obstet Gynecol* 2006;108:264–72.

121. Pretorius RG, Zhang WH, Belinson JL, et al. Colposcopically directed biopsy, random cervical biopsy, and endocervical curettage in the diagnosis of cervical intraepithelial neoplasia II or worse. *Am J Obstet Gynecol* 2004;191:430–4.

122. Cuzick J, Arbyn M, Sankaranarayanan R, et al. Overview of human papillomavirus-based and other novel options for cervical cancer screening in developed and developing countries. *Vaccine.* 2008;26(Suppl 10):K29–41.

123. Mitchell MF, Cantor SB, Ramanujam N, et al. Fluorescence spectroscopy for diagnosis of squamous intraepithelial lesions of the cervix. *Obstet Gynecol* 1999;93:462.

124. Siddiqi AM, Li H, Faruque F, et al. Use of hyperspectral imaging to distinguish normal, precancerous, and cancerous cells. *Cancer* 2008;114:13–21.

125. Cardenas-Turanzas M, Freeberg JA, Benedet JL, et al. The clinical effectiveness of optical spectroscopy for the in vivo diagnosis of cervical intraepithelial neoplasia: where are we? *Gynecol Oncol* 2007;107:S138–46.

126. Wentzensen N, Bergeron C, Cas F, et al. Triage of women with ASCUS and LSIL cytology: use of qualitative assessment of p16INK4a positive cells to identify patients with high-grade cervical intraepithelial neoplasia. *Cancer* 2007;111:58–66.

127. Horn LC, Reichert A, Oster A, et al. Immunostaining for p16INK4a used as a conjunctive tool improves interobserver agreement of the histologic diagnosis of cervical intraepithelial neoplasia. *Am J Surg Pathol* 2008;32:502–12.

128. Kahn SL, Ronnett BM, Gravitt PE, et al. Cancer. Quantitative methylation-specific PCR for the detection of aberrant DNA methylation in liquid-based Pap tests. *Cancer* 2008;114:57–64.

129. Solomon D, Davey D, Kurman R, et al. for the Forum Group Members and the Bethesda 2001 Workshop. The 2001 Bethesda System: terminology for reporting results of cervical cytology. *JAMA* 2002;287:2114–9.

130. Koutsky LA, Ault KA, Wheeler CM, et al.; Proof of Principle Study Investigators. A controlled trial of a human papillomavirus type 16 vaccine. *N Engl J Med* 2002;347:1645–51.

Anatomy and Histology of the Normal Female Lower Genital Tract

2.1 INTRODUCTION
2.2 THE CERVIX
    2.2.1 Embryology
    2.2.2 Anatomy
    2.2.3 Histology
    2.2.4 The Transformation Zone
    2.2.5 Cytology
2.3 THE VAGINA
    2.3.1 Embryology
    2.3.2 Anatomy

2.3.3 Histology
2.3.4 Cytology
2.4 THE VULVA
    2.4.1 Embryology
    2.4.2 Anatomy
    2.4.3 Histology
2.5 BIOPSY SPECIMEN COLLECTION, PROCESSING, AND INTERPRETATION
2.6 CYTOLOGY SPECIMEN COLLECTION, PROCESSING, AND INTERPRETATION

2.1 INTRODUCTION

The female lower genital tract includes the cervix, vagina, and vulva and is unique in that these areas are readily accessible for evaluation. A medical subspecialty (cytopathology) and a procedure (colposcopy) are devoted to the screening, diagnosis, and management of intraepithelial lesions and cancers of these sites. To better understand the significance of female lower genital tract abnormalities and the basis for colposcopy, it is necessary to have an understanding of the normal anatomy, histology, and cytology of this region.

2.2 THE CERVIX

2.2.1 Embryology

The female genital tract begins developing approximately 4 weeks after conception. In the female, a lack of testicular development results in an absence of müllerian-inhibiting substance. Müllerian ducts form as invaginations from the urogenital folds. These ducts extend caudally through the mesenchyme lateral to the mesonephros. By the seventh week, the müllerian ducts turn medial and anterior to the mesonephros, meeting at the midline. Continued caudal growth results in the fused ducts eventually joining the urogenital sinus. The solid tip enlarges at the urogenital sinus and becomes the müllerian tubercle. The midline septum within the ducts is lost, forming a single uterovaginal canal lined by columnar epithelium. By the 11th week of gestation, stratified squamous cells partially replace the columnar cells, and by the 16th week, a rudimentary cervix is recognizable (Figure 2.1).[1,2]

The point at which the columnar and squamous cells meet is the *original* or *native squamocolumnar junction (SCJ)*.[1,3] The location of the original SCJ varies throughout fetal life. By 24 to 32 weeks' gestation, the junction is located within the endocervical canal. After 32 weeks' gestation, it extends toward the vagina but by term (40 weeks' gestation) regresses back into the canal.[4] In some individuals, however, it remains on the outer cervix and can be located on the vaginal surface at the time of delivery.[1,4]

It is unclear why squamous cells partially replace the müllerian columnar cells in the fetal cervix. The squamous cells may originate from a cranial extension of the urogenital sinus or from reserve cells beneath the original columnar cells coordinated by the p63 protein.[5] The degree of squamous replacement probably is also influenced by the adjacent vaginal stroma and further modulated by the presence or absence of sex steroid hormones, particularly estrogen. Increased estrogen is known to cause delayed caudal extension of the müllerian duct and disruption of squamous cell development.[6]

2.2.2 Anatomy

The term cervix is derived from the Latin for *neck*. It is the inferior extension of the uterus and is divided into two portions. The lower portion (*portio*, or vaginal cervix) extends into the vagina and is the structure that can be visualized after speculum placement. The upper or supravaginal cervix extends from the vaginal attachment to the lower uterine segment. The cervix is oriented obliquely in the vagina. Consequently, the posterior cervix represents the majority of the portio and comprises one-half of the total cervix volume.[3,7,8] When examined through the opened speculum, the cervix appears as a raised oval to circular structure. Accordingly, topographic areas on the cervical surface are conventionally identified using the numbers on a clock face (Figure 2.2). In the nulliparous patient, the cylindrical cervix comprises approximately 50% of the total uterine size.[8,9] It is approximately 3 cm in length and approximately 2 cm in diameter. The centrally located external cervical os, or beginning of the endocervical canal, is round and measures 3 to 5 mm in diameter. During pregnancy, the cervix enlarges because of vascular congestion and proliferation of elastic fibers and smooth muscle cells. After vaginal delivery, the external os broadens into a horizontal slit with stellate lines attributable to scarring from cervical lacerations.[7-9] The cervical canal is approximately 3 cm in length and extends from the external os to the lower uterine segment or

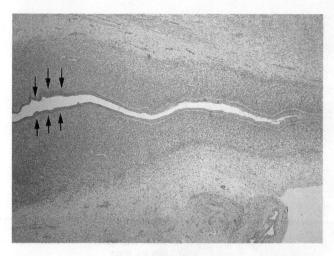

FIGURE 2.1. Junction of the embryonic lower uterine segment and cervix in a fetus at 4 to 5 months' gestation. The *arrows* point to the area of transition from columnar to squamous epithelium. The fused vagina is toward the right. A cross section of an embryonic fallopian tube is present in the lower portion of the photograph (hematoxylin and eosin, low power magnification).

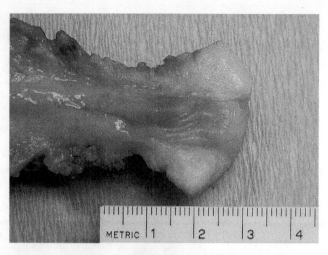

FIGURE 2.3. Gross photograph of a lower uterine segment and endocervix. The parallel plicae palmatae ridges are best seen near the external os. The remaining canal is covered by glistening, clear mucus.

isthmus. The canal has a fusiform shape and the diameter varies, being approximately 8 mm at its widest point. At the cervicouterine junction, the canal narrows and becomes rounded. This portion is known as the *internal cervical os*. The cervical canal contains ridges known as *plicae palmatae* or *arbor vitae uteri*. These small ridges are no longer apparent after vaginal delivery (Figure 2.3).[3,7]

The cervix is supported by the parametrial soft tissue, the uterosacral ligaments, and the cardinal ligaments of Mackenrodt. The latter provide the major source of cervical support and extend from the lateral cervix through the broad ligament base to the levator ani muscle.[7,8]

The cervix is perfused by the descending cervicovaginal branches of the uterine artery, which enter the cervix laterally through the parametrial soft tissues (Figure 2.4A). Venous drainage parallels the arterial supply and likewise courses laterally through the parametria into the uterine and hypogastric veins.[9] The lymphatic drainage of the cervix originates from the superficial stromal lymphatic spaces and extends into the parametrial tissues (Figure 2.4B). These efferent channels continue to the paracervical, obturator, hypogastric, iliac, and eventually to the paraaortic lymph nodes.[10] Sensory nerves from the cervix and lower vagina arise from the deep stroma and endocervical canal. They then proceed through the paracervical and uterosacral plexus (Frankenhäuser's ganglion) and the pelvic nerves to the second, third, and fourth sacral nerve roots.[7-9] The lack of ectocervical surface innervation relative to the endocervix may account for the minimal discomfort noted with an ectocervical biopsy or cryotherapy, compared with the significant cramping that can result from an endocervical curettage or loop excision (Figure 2.4C).

2.2.3 Histology

2.2.3.1 Squamous Epithelium

The majority of the cervix portio is covered by stratified squamous epithelium. This area is also known as the *ectocervix* or *exocervix*. As the squamous cells mature, they enlarge and increase in overall volume, while the amount of nuclear material decreases. The overall effect is a characteristic basketweave pattern.[3]

Cervical squamous cells are arbitrarily divided into four distinct layers (Figure 2.5).[3,11] The *basal* or germinal cell layer is composed of one to two layers of small cuboidal cells that contain large darkly staining round- to oval-shaped nuclei. Mitotic figures are occasionally seen here. The *parabasal* or prickle cell layer is composed of irregular polyhedral cells with large, dark, oval nuclei. Nucleoli can be seen in the majority of these cells. On electron microscopy, tonofilaments are present, indicating a squamous differentiation. Numerous desmosomes (cell adhesion sites) are also seen. The *intermediate* or navicular cell layer consists of flattened cells with glycogen-rich clear cytoplasm, and comprises the majority of the squamous cells. The nuclei are small, dark, and round, and nucleoli are no longer seen. The *superficial* or stratum corneum layer is composed of flat, elongated cells with small pyknotic nuclei. Collagen is present in the more superficial cells. Scanning electron microscopy of these squamous cells indicates numerous small ridges on the cell surface, which may suggest the presence of

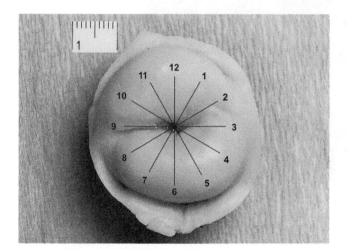

FIGURE 2.2. Gross photograph of an adult parous cervix. Lateral scars are indicative of prior vaginal deliveries. By convention, identification of a lesion site is by the nearest clock-face number.

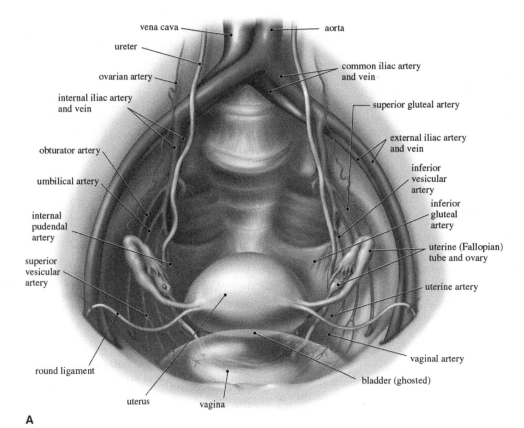

A

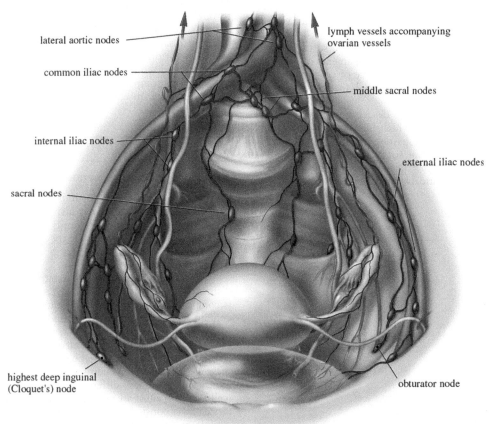

B

FIGURE 2.4. Vascular supply, support, and lymphatic drainage of the cervix. **A:** Vascular supply: blood flow is primarily through the descending branches of the uterine arteries, which arise from the hypogastric arteries. **B:** The lymphatic drainage flows through the adjacent parametrial nodes into the hypogastric and iliac nodes, which eventually drain into the paraaortic nodes.

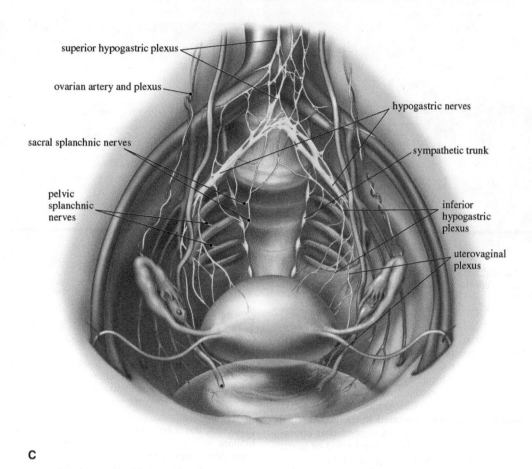

superior hypogastric plexus

ovarian artery and plexus

sacral splanchnic nerves

pelvic splanchnic nerves

hypogastric nerves

sympathetic trunk

inferior hypogastric plexus

uterovaginal plexus

C

FIGURE 2.4.   *(Continued)* **C:** Innervation of the pelvis and female genital tract.

keratin filaments.[3] Since maturation of squamous cells varies considerably, only basal and the superficial cells can be consistently identified.[3,7,11] Langerhans cells and rare melanocytes are interspersed among the squamous cells.[3,7]

Maturation of squamous cells, which is estrogen dependent, can take as little as 4 days. In the premenopausal and postmenopausal state, the less mature squamous cells (basal and parabasal) predominate (Figure 2.6).[3,12] These cells contain numerous receptors for epidermal growth factor and estrogen. Epidermal growth factor stimulates mitotic activity, induces keratinization, and promotes squamous cell differentiation. Estrogen stimulates DNA synthesis and shortens the cell cycle.[13]

The cytoskeleton of a cell consists of three types of filaments: microtubules, intermediate filaments, and microfilaments. The intermediate filaments, which are insoluble proteins with unique biochemical properties, make up the majority of

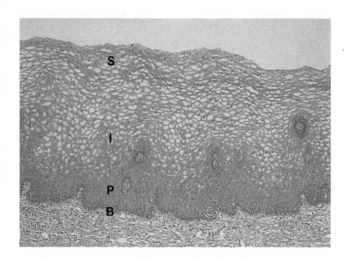

FIGURE 2.5.   Normal ectocervix. The stratified squamous cells are divided into four more or less distinct layers. *B*, basal cell layer; *P*, parabasal cell layer; *I*, intermediate cell layer; *S*, superficial cell layer. The latter two (outer) layers have clear cytoplasm, consistent with glycogenation (hematoxylin and eosin, medium-power magnification).

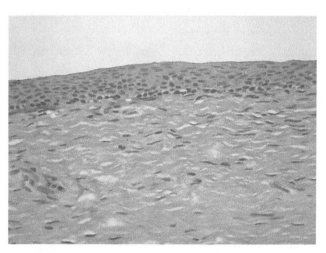

FIGURE 2.6.   Atrophic ectocervix. The number of squamous cell layers is decreased and parabasal cells predominate (hematoxylin and eosin, high-power magnification).

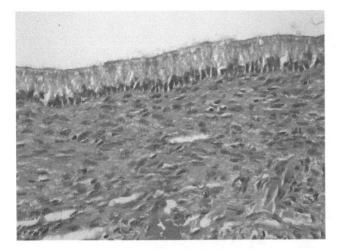

FIGURE 2.7. Normal endocervix. A single layer of columnar cells with basal nuclei covers the surface (hematoxylin and eosin, high-power magnification).

the cytoskeleton matrix. The cytokeratins are intermediate filament proteins unique to epithelial cells. Excluding hair keratins, there are at least 20 different polypeptides. These cytokeratins maintain their integrity during cell transformation, including malignant change. Nevertheless, they may vary depending on epithelial cell type. Cytokeratins 1, 4, 5, 6, 10, 13, 14, 15, 16, 19, and 20 are expressed in the ectocervical squamous cells.[11,14–16] Some investigators suggest that alterations of cytokeratins contribute to the contrast effect of acetic acid, which is used during colposcopic examination.[15]

The basement membrane lies beneath the basal cells. On electron microscopy, it usually measures 3 μm in thickness and consists of a *lamina densa* that borders the underlying cervical stroma and a *lamina lucida* that borders the basal cell. The basal cells contain foot processes that anchor the cell into the basement membrane.[12]

2.2.3.2 Columnar Epithelium

A single layer of tall columnar cells lines the endocervical canal. Some pathologists may refer to these cells as glandular cells. The nuclei in these cells are round to oval in shape and basal in position (Figure 2.7). The majority of these columnar cells secrete mucus (called mucin) using apocrine and merocrine

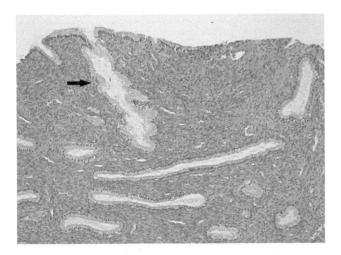

FIGURE 2.8. Endocervical glands. Although they are called glands because of their appearance in cross section, the structures should be considered crypts (*arrow*) (hematoxylin and eosin, medium-power magnification).

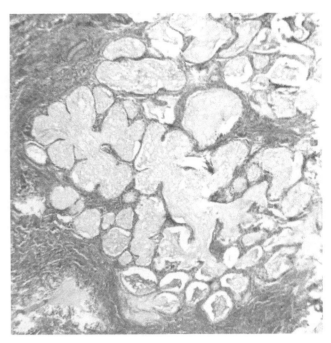

FIGURE 2.9. Tunnel clusters. Closely packed endocervical glands with compressed surface epithelium are present (hematoxylin and eosin, medium-power magnification).

processes, but a few columnar cells are ciliated and may participate in sperm transport.[3,7] Transmission electron microscopy demonstrates the presence of cilia, mucin droplets, and secretory granules of varying sizes.[12] Endocervical columnar cells consistently express cytokeratins 7, 8, 16, 18, and 19.[11,16]

Endocervical cells invaginate into the cervical stroma to a depth of approximately 5 to 8 mm (Figure 2.8). Since there are no ductal and acinar structures, this process technically represents crypt formation, but, by convention, they are called endocervical glands because of their rounded shape seen on cross section.[3] Compression of a group of arborizing glands can result in the formation of *tunnel clusters*, which can be mistaken for atypical glandular hyperplasia because of a superficial architectural complexity (Figure 2.9). However, these

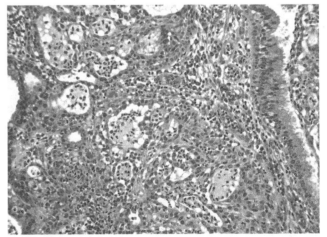

FIGURE 2.10. Microglandular hyperplasia. Numerous small glands are present. The nuclei are uniform, with frequent subnuclear vacuolization, and no mitoses are seen. There is squamous metaplasia and acute inflammation present (hematoxylin and eosin, medium power). (Courtesy of Debra Heller, MD.)

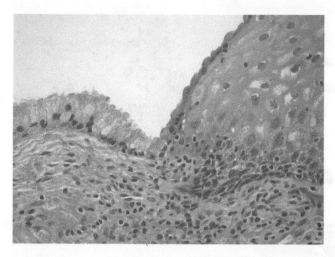

FIGURE 2.11.   The squamocolumnar junction. A single layer of columnar cells (**left**) abruptly meets multiple layers of stratified squamous cells. A few degenerated columnar cells are present on the immediately adjacent squamous cells (hematoxylin and eosin, high-power magnification).

columnar cell clusters are benign. *Microglandular hyperplasia* is another form of benign gland proliferation that results in sheets of endocervical cells that coalesce to form individual cell spaces and small gland-like structures. The benign nature of this condition is reflected by the lack of mitoses and benign nuclear features (Figure 2.10). Microglandular hyperplasia is often seen in pregnant women or young women using hormonal contraception.[3,7]

The intersection of the stratified squamous and columnar cells is known as the SCJ (Figure 2.11). This junction is abrupt in about one-third of examined specimens. The remainder have evidence of a gradual transformation from one cell type to the other (see Section 2.2.4).[3,8]

The cervical stroma is composed of fibrous connective tissue, with lesser amounts of smooth muscle and elastic fibers. In approximately 1% of cervices, small rounded structures lined by flattened cuboidal cells can be seen deep within the stroma at the 3 o'clock and at the 9 o'clock regions. These represent embryologic mesonephric or wolffian remnants (Figure 2.12).[3] Capillary arcades are located in the superficial stroma. Straight

vessel loops branch from these arcades and extend into the basal and parabasal layers of the squamous epithelium. In the endocervix, the small capillary loops are located directly beneath the columnar cells.

2.2.4 The Transformation Zone

2.2.4.1 Formation of Squamous Metaplasia

Metaplasia is defined as a transformation from one mature cell type to a different mature cell type. The process usually involves conversion from a columnar cell to a stratified squamous cell, although conversion from one glandular cell type to another also occurs. Metaplasia occurs in several human organ sites, such as the bronchus, stomach, bladder, and salivary gland. However, metaplasia in the uterine cervix has consistently generated great interest because it is the site for the development of cervical intraepithelial neoplasia or carcinoma.[14]

Historically, areas of cervical squamous metaplasia were originally misidentified either as early-differentiated carcinomas or as folds in the upper squamous epithelium.[17] In the late 19th century, German pathologists described the process of metaplasia using terms such as epidermidalization or epidermoidalization to identify these areas. Later, it was variously reclassified as reserve cell hyperplasia, squamocolumnar prosoplasia, or metaplasia.[18]

Factors that induce squamous metaplasia in the cervix are still poorly understood but may include environmental conditions, mechanical irritation, chronic inflammation, pH changes, or changes in sex steroid hormone balance.[3] Metaplasia probably begins when the original SCJ moves onto the portio and exposes the delicate columnar cells to an acidic bacteria-laden vaginal environment (Figure 2.13). Gradually, immature and then mature metaplastic squamous cells replace the columnar cells. These metaplastic cells eventually replicate and evolve into stratified squamous cells, which normally exist here.[3,7,8,19] During a woman's lifetime, the SCJ returns to the endocervical canal, which has the more neutral pH of cervical mucus. As stated earlier, the position of the SCJ at birth is known as the original or native SCJ. Following metaplasia-induced migration, it is known as the new SCJ or, simply, the SCJ. The transformation zone, then, is technically defined as the area between the original or native SCJ and the new SCJ.[20]

For decades, it was unclear how this transformation took place. The mechanism of squamous replacement has been described as proliferation of subcolumnar nests of squamous basal cells or development from undifferentiated embryonic nests within the superficial cervical stroma.[21,22] The evolution of the transformation zone may require several mechanisms. The two most commonly accepted involve the continued epithelialization with new squamous cells derived from previously formed squamous epithelium and development of metaplasia from the subcolumnar reserve cells. The origin of reserve cells remains obscure. Suggested parent cells include embryonal urogenital crest cells, fetal squamous cells, and stromal fibroblasts.[21] Presently, investigators believe that these reserve cells probably arise from the dedifferentiation of overlying columnar cells.[14,20] The presence of cytokeratins 5, 6, 8, 13, 14, 15, 16, 17, 18, and 19 in variable amounts indicates an epithelial origin of these cells.[11,23]

Initially, reserve cells appear as a single cell layer directly beneath the columnar cells to be replaced. Over time, these flattened cuboidal cells proliferate into multiple layers of immature squamoid metaplastic cells and push the columnar cells away from their underlying capillary vascular supply. These cells eventually degenerate and slough off the

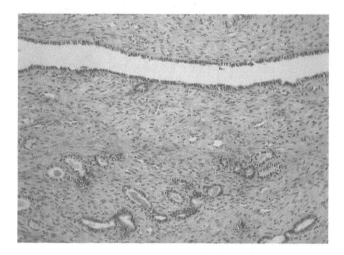

FIGURE 2.12.   Müllerian remnants. A large duct is surrounded by smaller cyst-like spaces, many of which contain eosinophilic material. All structures are lined by cuboidal cells (hematoxylin and eosin, medium-power magnification).

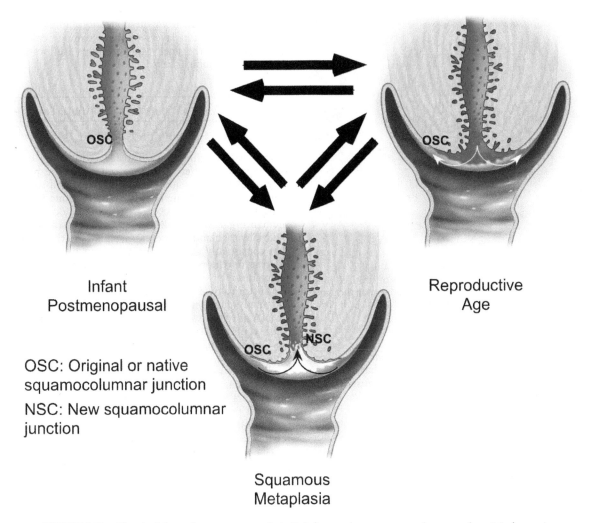

Infant
Postmenopausal

Reproductive
Age

OSC: Original or native
squamocolumnar junction

NSC: New squamocolumnar
junction

Squamous
Metaplasia

FIGURE 2.13.   The physiology of squamous metaplasia. In infants and postmenopausal women, the original or native SCJ is located in the endocervical canal. In reproductive-age women, this junction moves out on the portio, exposing the delicate columnar surface to the acidic vagina. Over time, the columnar cells are replaced by squamous cells (metaplasia), which create a new SCJ that moves back into the canal. The area between the original SCJ and the newly formed SCJ after metaplasia is complete is known as the transformation zone. (Modified with permission from Ferenzy and Wright.[7])

underlying immature metaplasia. As the reserve cells proliferate and differentiate into immature squamous cells, cytokeratins 8 and 18 (unique to reserve and columnar cells) are lost, and cytokeratin 19 predominates throughout the entire epithelial thickness.[14,23] As the immature metaplastic cells mature into squamous cells, cytokeratins 15 and 19 become limited to the basal and parabasal cells, while the surface cells begin to express other cytokeratins (4, 10, 13, and 14) commonly seen in intermediate and superficial squamous cells. In contrast, cytokeratins 6 and 16 predominate in metaplastic cells that have the potential to become dysplastic.[14,21,23] Other predictors of dysplastic potential in squamous metaplasia include the degree of metaplastic proliferation and rate of metaplastic change.[8,24,25]

2.2.4.2 The Histology of Squamous Metaplasia

Sixty percent of cervices will have a gradual transformation from columnar to mature squamous epithelium. Metaplasia is most commonly seen in the lower third of the endocervical canal.[8] The first evidence of squamous metaplasia is the identification of a single layer of subcolumnar reserve cells, known histologically as reserve cell hyperplasia (Figure 2.14).

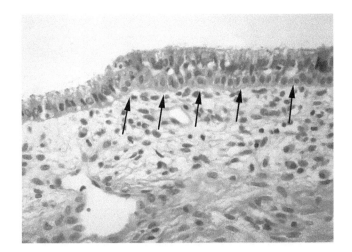

FIGURE 2.14.   Reserve cells. A second layer of round cells has formed under the columnar endocervical cells (*arrows*). Alternately, this is known as *reserve cell hyperplasia* (hematoxylin and eosin, high-power magnification).

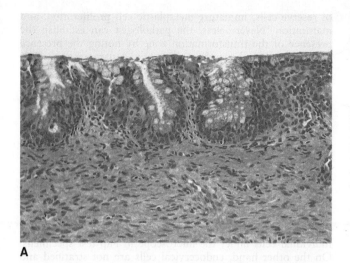

A

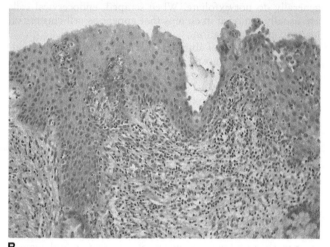

B

FIGURE 2.15 Development of squamous metaplasia. **A:** Proliferation of reserve cells leads to the presence of immature squamous cells directly underneath the remaining columnar cells (hematoxylin and eosin, high power). **B:** As metaplasia progresses, the immature cells acquire more cytoplasm and develop squamous cell characteristics. The remaining columnar cells degenerate and are lost. Chronic inflammatory cells are present in the superficial stroma (hematoxylin and eosin, medium-power magnification).

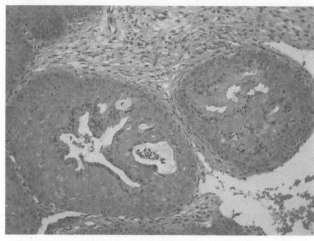

FIGURE 2.16. Partial replacement of glandular epithelium by immature squamous cells. The small spaces give the glands an adenomatous appearance (hematoxylin and eosin, medium-power magnification).

by nonmetaplastic columnar epithelium (Figure 2.17). Other areas can show well-developed mature squamous epithelium overlying endocervical glands with little or no metaplastic proliferation.[3,7]

Since metaplasia is brought about by irritation or inflammation, it is common to see plasma cells and lymphocytes. Occasionally, acute inflammatory cells are present in the underlying stroma and the surface metaplastic cells. Extensive chronic inflammation can result in the formation of small lymphoid follicles within the superficial stroma (Figure 2.18). This is known as *chronic follicular cervicitis*; investigators have noted this change in women with *Chlamydia trachomatis* infections of the cervix.[28]

Pathologists usually observe a continual blending of all the metaplastic processes when examining large cervical specimens from conization procedures and hysterectomies, although occasionally, there is an abrupt transition from columnar to squamous epithelium, which may represent squamous epithelialization. Smaller biopsy specimens usually lack evidence of all the features common to metaplasia, such as the presence

The reserve cells are cuboidal with scant cytoplasm and large round to oval nuclei. They can be seen beneath the surface columnar cells and the endocervical glands (Figure 2.15A). As the reserve cells proliferate, the amount of cytoplasm increases. The nuclei decrease somewhat in size, develop sharp nuclear membranes, and acquire prominent nucleoli. As the process continues, the cells flatten toward the surface and acquire cytoplasmic glycogen; the nuclei become small and round with uniform chromatin and lose their nucleoli.[3,7,26,27] The remaining surface columnar cells degenerate and slough (Figure 2.15B). As metaplasia evolves within the endocervical glands, there is squamous bridging across the lumens, resulting in smaller gland structures. In the past, this has been called adenomatous hyperplasia or mucoid degeneration (Figure 2.16).[3] Lastly, the endocervical glands undergoing metaplasia become solid round structures that converge into the surface squamous cells.

The process of metaplasia is highly variable and it is common to see islands of well-developed metaplasia interspersed

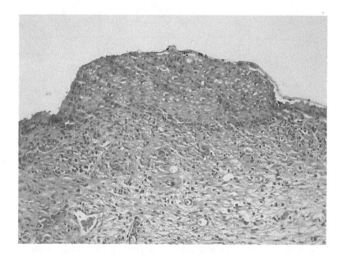

FIGURE 2.17. Focal squamous metaplasia. The area of squamous metaplasia is bordered on each side by a single layer of columnar cells (hematoxylin and eosin, high-power magnification).

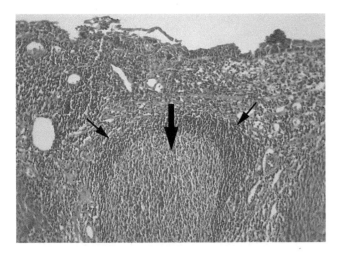

FIGURE 2.18. Follicular cervicitis. A central germinal follicle (*large arrow*) is surrounded by numerous chronic inflammatory cells (*small arrows*). Reactive squamous metaplastic cells cover the surface (hematoxylin and eosin, medium-power magnification).

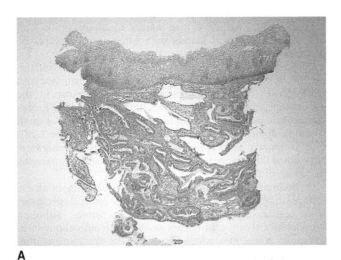

A

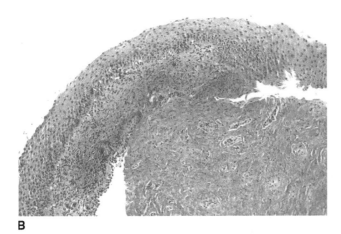

B

FIGURE 2.19. Cervical biopsies. **A:** The presence of endocervical glands beneath squamous epithelial cells signifies the transformation zone (hematoxylin and eosin, low power). **B:** A lack of endocervical cells signifies the microscopic absence of the transformation zone (hematoxylin and eosin, low-power magnification) (Courtesy of Debra Heller, MD.)

of reserve cells, immature metaplastic cell proliferation, and maturation. Nevertheless, the pathologist can establish the presence of the transformation zone by noting the presence of columnar cells beneath or adjacent to squamous epithelium (Figure 2.19A,B).

2.2.5 Cytology

Papanicolaou (Pap) test sampling of the cervix involves scraping of the ectocervical surface and a portion of the nonvisualized endocervical canal using various sampling devices. Stratified squamous cells are markedly cohesive. As maturation continues, however, functional desmosomes diminish, and individual squamous cells separate from each other. Therefore, the ectocervical cells removed for cytologic examination are those that have exfoliated from the surface and appear as individual cells under the microscope in Pap test specimens. On the other hand, endocervical cells are not stratified and generally do not exfoliate. When scraped, endocervical cells are usually removed in clumps that appear as cell clusters on microscopic examination.

In a background of abundant estrogen, the cytologic specimen will contain mostly superficial and intermediate cells (Figure 2.20). These cells are navicular in shape with a diameter of approximately 40 μm. The cytoplasm is abundant and usually eosinophilic (pink after staining using the Pap method). When glycogenated, the cells show a perinuclear yellow color. The nucleus of the superficial cell is centrally located, small (5 μm), round, and dark. An intermediate cell nucleus is slightly larger (8 to 10 μm) and contains fine, evenly distributed chromatin. The amount of cell exfoliation varies with the menstrual cycle.[11] During the proliferative phase, there is an increased exfoliation of well-glycogenated superficial cells. However, intermediate cells predominate in the progesterone enhanced secretory phase, and there is less glycogen.[29]

Parabasal cells and rare intermediate cells are more common in the cytologic specimens of postmenopausal women (Figure 2.21). Parabasal cells do not exfoliate as readily as do more mature squamous cells, and, like columnar cells, are often removed in groups. These cells are smaller and more rounded than mature squamous cells with large centrally located nuclei. The nuclear membranes in these cells are smooth, and

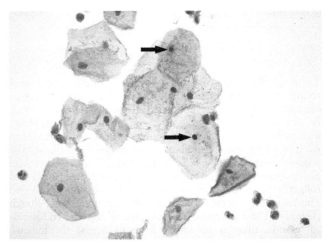

FIGURE 2.20. Superficial and intermediate cells. Although the squamous cells all have the same polygonal shape, there is a difference in nuclear sizes. The cells with the smaller pyknotic nuclei (*arrows*) are the superficial cells. Also present are scattered neutrophils (liquid preparation, Papanicolaou stain, high-power magnification).

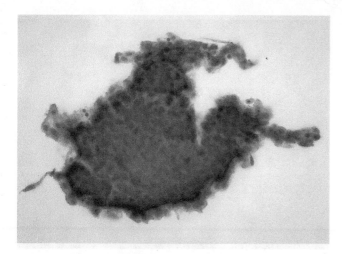

FIGURE 2.21.   Atrophic smear. A sheet of uniformly round parabasal cells (best seen in the periphery) in an otherwise clean background (liquid preparation, Papanicolaou stain, high-power magnification).

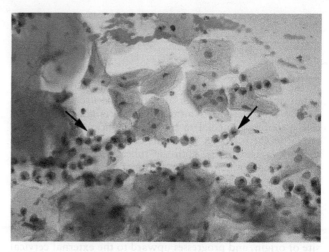

FIGURE 2.23.   Reserve cells. The small round to oval cells (*arrows*) are linear in arrangement. Note the small basophilic nuclei and the finely vacuolated cytoplasm (conventional preparation, Papanicolaou stain, high-power magnification).

the nuclear chromatin is usually granular or finely stippled. Air-drying is more commonly seen in conventional specimens from postmenopausal women, as there is little background mucus present. Consequently, the nuclei tend to enlarge and show smudging of the chromatin, which can be confused with intraepithelial lesions.[7,11] When present, the columnar cells are either arranged in a linear fashion or grouped in a honeycomb pattern when seen on end (Figure 2.22). The nuclei are basal, relatively large and round, and contain one to two micronucleoli. The chromatin is uniform and finely granular. Occasionally multinucleation occurs, and cilia are infrequently seen.[11]

Although basal cells are almost never present on a cytologic specimen, reserve cells can be seen. They are usually found within a mucoid background in linear sheets. They are commonly seen adjacent to columnar cells, which attest to their subcolumnar origin. Reserve cells are round to oval with irregular cell borders and finely vacuolated cytoplasm. The small nuclei are round to bean shaped and have prominent chromatin. Because of their arrangement and size, these cells can be difficult to discriminate from a high-grade squamous intraepithelial lesion

(Figure 2.23). However, squamous dysplastic cells will have irregularly shaped nuclei and lack smooth nuclear membranes.

The presence of metaplastic cells is considered minimal cytologic evidence that a specimen contains the transformation zone elements. The cells are typically seen in small individual cell groups or sheets (Figure 2.24). They have cyanophilic (blue-green) cytoplasm and are smaller in size than the mature squamous epithelial cells. The nuclei are slightly larger than intermediate cell nuclei. The nuclear membranes are smooth and round, and the chromatin is granular to finely stippled. Micronucleoli may be present.[7,23]

The appearance of metaplastic cells can be cytologically similar to that of parabasal cells. Because of this, it is difficult to differentiate metaplastic cells from parabasal cells in a postmenopausal woman; however, parabasal cells tend to be more cohesive and eosinophilic, and they are rarely seen in a woman of reproductive age. Therefore, the presence of small oval to polyhedral cells with cyanophilic cytoplasm and slightly enlarged nuclei in a background of mature squamous cells represents evidence of squamous metaplasia.

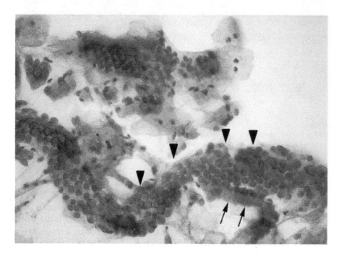

FIGURE 2.22.   Endocervical cells. Although some cells demonstrate the typical "picket fence" tall, columnar architecture (*small arrows*), the majority are seen on-end in a "honeycomb" arrangement (*arrowheads*). The nuclei are slightly larger than the normal intermediate cell nucleus (liquid preparation, Papanicolaou stain, high-power magnification).

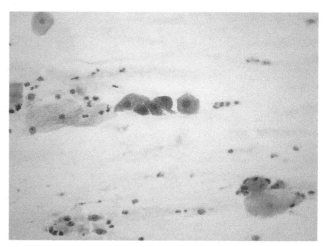

FIGURE 2.24.   Metaplastic cells. The cyanophilic cells (**center**) are smaller than the mature squamous cell (**lower right corner**) and have a more rounded shape. The nuclei are slightly larger than an intermediate cell nucleus (conventional preparation, Papanicolaou stain, high-power magnification).

2.3 THE VAGINA

2.3.1 Embryology

By the seventh week postconception, the solid tip of the müllerian duct reaches the dorsal wall of the urogenital sinus. As the tip enlarges to form the müllerian tubercle, sinus cells proliferate medial to the mesonephric ducts and just lateral to the tubercle. This sinus-cell proliferation becomes the sinovaginal bulbs. Both the tubercle and the sinovaginal bulbs continue to enlarge and cavitate, forming the rudimentary vagina by the 10th week of gestation. Although originally lined by columnar epithelium, replacement by squamous cells begins at around 11 weeks, coincidental to the appearance of estrogen receptors along the vaginal wall. The replacement begins at the urogenital sinus, probably the site of origin, and progresses upward to the external cervical os. Proliferation and stratification of the squamous cells leads to secondary occlusion of the vaginal lumen (Figure 2.25). By the 16th week of gestation, under continued estrogen modulation, the vaginal squamous cells mature, glycogenate, and begin to exfoliate. This exfoliative process results in secondary cavitation of the essentially solid vaginal plate. Vaginal development is practically complete by the fifth month of pregnancy.[6,30]

The process by which squamous cells replace the original columnar cells lining the rudimentary uterovaginal canal and the extent to which this occurs is not completely understood but may be similar to the formation of the urethral lining (see also Section 2.4.3).[6,31] Nevertheless, evolution of the terminal müllerian ducts and urogenital sinus into the cervix and vagina becomes hormonally dependent after completion of gonadal differentiation. Specifically, the reaction of these ducts to estrogen depends on the intensity and timing of the exposure. Exposure to large pharmacologic levels of estrogen during vaginal development in mice has resulted in delayed vaginal growth and retarded squamous replacement of the original columnar cells.[32] In the human, exposure to exogenous estrogen early in the second trimester can result in persistent glandular epithelium, known as adenosis, and other anomalies, such as transverse vaginal ridges and cobblestone mucosal surfaces.[20]

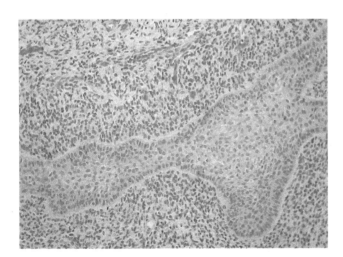

FIGURE 2.25.   Vaginal plate, fetus of 18 to 20 weeks' gestation. Cavitation has not occurred yet, although the original columnar cells have been replaced by immature squamous cells. Immature mesenchyme borders the squamous cells laterally (hematoxylin and eosin, medium-power magnification).

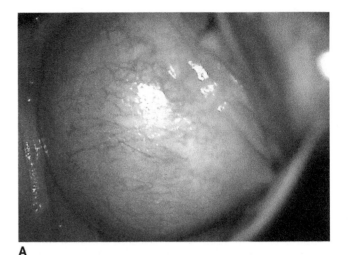

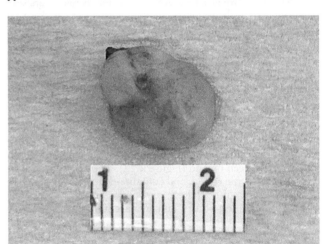

FIGURE 2.26.   Gartner's duct cyst. **A:** A large vaginal cyst in the left vaginal wall obscures the cervix. **B:** This excised cyst is unilocular and smooth walled. A small amount of elliptical vaginal mucosa is attached to the outer surface. **C:** Microscopically, the cyst is lined by a single layer of cuboidal cells (hematoxylin and eosin, medium-power magnification).

Persistence of the adjacent mesonephric ducts may lead to formation of cysts in the vaginal stroma, known as Gartner's duct cysts. Although usually asymptomatic, these cysts can grow to considerable size, compressing the vaginal lumen and extending into the broad ligament (Figure 2.26A–C).

2.3.2 Anatomy

The vagina, which is Latin for *sheath*, is a mucosa-lined tube that extends from the vulva to the cervix. It separates the bladder neck and urethra from the rectum and anus. Normally, the anterior and posterior walls of the vagina lie in close approximation centrally while being more lax peripherally. This results in the nondistended vagina having an "H" shape on cross section. The vagina is extremely pliable and can stretch considerably during intercourse and childbirth.[6,9]

The vagina is positioned perpendicular to the uterus and is offset approximately 60 degrees from the vestibule. The uterus is attached to the upper vagina at the recessed vaginal fornices. Because of the angle of attachment, the posterior fornix is usually longer than the anterior fornix. Accordingly, the anterior vaginal wall is shorter than the posterior wall, the former measuring 6 to 8 cm and the latter measuring 7 to 10 cm in length (Figure 2.27). In nulliparous women, small transverse ridges known as *rugae* cover the surface. These mucosal folds are usually not apparent after a vaginal birth and during the postmenopausal period. In the nonpregnant state, the mucosal surface is kept moist by cervical secretions. The amount of vaginal secretions increases considerably during sexual arousal and excitement, probably through direct passage of fluids through the mucosa. A mixture of cervical mucus and exfoliated surface epithelial cells can result in a thin-layered milky discharge known as a leukorrhea. During pregnancy, under the influence of increased estrogen levels, the amount of physiologic discharge can increase considerably. In an adult woman, the vagina is normally acidic at a pH between 3.5 and 4.5. This acidic environment is derived through the breakdown of surface epithelial cell glycogen into lactic acid by lactobacilli. Estrogen also has some minor direct influence on the pH of the vagina, which is lowest during midcycle and highest just before menses.[6,9]

The vagina is surrounded by an ill-defined muscular coat, which is divided into an outer layer composed of longitudinal fibers and an inner coat that contains circular fibers. Most of the mid and lower vaginal support comes from the pubovaginalis and iliococcygeus portion of the levator ani muscle and the transverse perineal muscles. The cardinal and uterosacral ligaments provide support to the upper vagina and the cervix.[6]

The vascular supply of the vagina is complex and has contributions from the arteries that supply the cervix (descending cervicovaginal arteries), bladder (inferior vesical arteries), and vulva (middle hemorrhoidal and internal pudendal arteries). The venous drainage starts in plexus found in the vaginal stroma and progresses parallel to the arterial system to enter the hypogastric veins. Lymphatic drainage of the vagina is also site dependent: the upper vagina drains into the paracervical and hypogastric nodes, while the lower vagina drains into the superficial iliac and deep pelvic nodes, in a route similar

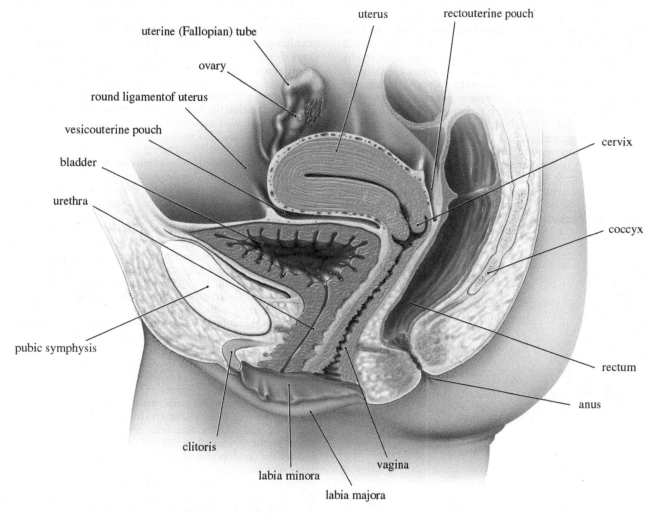

FIGURE 2.27. Sagittal section of the female pelvis, showing the relationship of the vagina to the cervix and adjacent pelvic organs (bladder and rectum).

to that of the vulva. The anterior midvagina drains into the paravesical nodes and the posterior midvagina drains into the pararectal nodes.[10]

Innervation of the vagina is through the sacral plexus, particularly S 2–5. The vagina is devoid of specialized receptors seen in the vulva; however, free nerve endings, which register pain, are occasionally found, primarily in the lower third of the vagina. The vagina is unable to sense temperature.[9]

2.3.3 Histology

The histology of the vagina recapitulates the cervix, in that stratified squamous epithelial cells cover the surface (Figure 2.28). As in the cervix, the cells are divided into different layers that reflect the various degrees of squamous cell maturity. The basal cells are small oval cells with large nuclei arranged in a palisade against the basement membrane. The parabasal cells are slightly larger and make up an additional two to three layers above the basal cells. The intermediate cells correspond to the similar layer in the cervix. As they mature, the cytoplasm acquires abundant glycogen, and their orientation is more parallel to the basement membrane and surface. The superficial squamous cells are glycogenated flattened cells with small pyknotic nuclei. Other cell types found in the vagina include rare melanocytes at the base and Langerhans cells throughout the epithelial surface. Epithelial cells are arranged in layers that average 26 to 28 rows. The majority of epithelial cells are in the superficial and intermediate layers, each averaging about 10 rows.[6] The thickness of the vaginal epithelium is hormonally dependent; during the nonovulatory portion of the menstrual cycle, it averages 24 cell layers, and during ovulation, 29.[33] A lack of estrogen results in epithelial cell atrophy. The surface cell layers are thinned; basal and parabasal cells predominate. As such, the amount of glycogen present in the epithelium is greatly diminished. Langerhans cell numbers, which reflect the immune status of the vagina, do not change with cyclic alterations in levels of estrogen or progesterone.

Cytokeratin expression in the vagina is similar to that in the cervix and reflects squamous cell maturity. Cells in the basal and adjacent suprabasal layers show early differentiation and express cytokeratin 13. The intermediate cells express a combination of cytokeratin 13 and 10, while the superficial cells express cytokeratin 10, exclusively.[34]

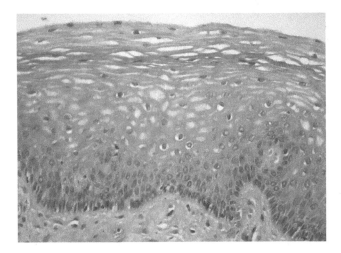

FIGURE 2.28. Vaginal squamous mucosa. The surface epithelial cells are similar in appearance to the cervix (hematoxylin and eosin, medium-power magnification).

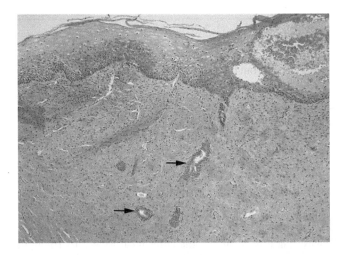

FIGURE 2.29. Vaginal adenosis. Small gland-like structures (*arrows*) directly lined by endocervical-type cells are present beneath the squamous mucosa (hematoxylin and eosin, medium-power magnification).

The vaginal stroma is composed of a mixture of elastic tissue and abundant lymph-vascular spaces. Occasionally, a thin layer of slightly enlarged fibroblastic cells is found directly beneath the epithelial surface. The nuclei of these stromal cells can also be mildly atypical, and it is important that the pathologist not confuse this layer with a vaginal sarcoma.[10]

Theoretically, the vagina is devoid of glandular elements or columnar cells. Nevertheless, mesonephric or wolffian remnants can occasionally be found in the lateral vaginal walls. As with mesonephric remnants in the cervix, these vestiges are usually composed of a central duct surrounded by small gland-like structures. The lining is composed of flattened bland cells with round nuclei; the lumens are commonly filled with inspissated proteinaceous material. Occasionally, endocervical-type glandular cells are also seen in the vagina, a finding known as *adenosis* (Figure 2.29).[3] During embryogenesis, the müllerian lining of the original tubo-uterovaginal canal is composed of columnar type cells that have the potential to differentiate into the various cells that line the adult tube, endometrium, and endocervix. Accordingly, the columnar cells found in adenosis can recapitulate these same glandular structures. However about 70% of adenosis is an endocervical cell type.[3] Adenosis acquired considerable notoriety from its association with *in utero* diethylstilbestrol exposure and its potential to develop into clear cell adenocarcinoma (for more information, see Chapters 13 and 14).[30] Nevertheless, it can also be seen in normal vaginas, particularly during the healing process after ablative or erosive therapy (5-fluorouracil cream). As in the cervix, the glandular cells of adenosis eventually are replaced with squamous epithelium by squamous metaplasia.

2.3.4 Cytology

Exfoliated squamous cells in the vagina are morphologically identical to those seen in the ectocervix. In well-estrogenized women, superficial and intermediate cells predominate; in postmenopausal women, primarily parabasal cells are seen. Historically, prior to the development of direct estrogen assays, a maturation index was calculated to infer estrogen levels by quantifying the degree of hormonal influence on the vagina. One hundred vaginal squamous cells would be counted and characterized as ratios of superficial, intermediate, and parabasal cells. This indirect assessment of estrogen levels can be inaccurate because of contamination by cervical metaplastic cells and is rarely used today.

The presence of glandular cells on a vaginal cytologic specimen is consistent with adenosis. It is therefore important that colposcopists identify the correct source of a cytologic specimen and provide appropriate history, particularly regarding surgical removal of the uterus or cervix. Since vaginal metaplasia can occur only in the presence of adenosis, pathologists must be careful not to misinterpret small parabasal-type cells, more commonly seen in postmenopausal women, as metaplastic cells.

2.4 THE VULVA

2.4.1 Embryology

The mesoderm along the anterior cloaca proliferates and creates a mound beneath the overlying ectoderm around the fourth week after conception. At the same time, small folds develop lateral to the central cloacal membrane of the urogenital sinus. By the sixth week of gestation, the rudimentary external genitalia are recognizable and consist of a urogenital membrane, a genital tubercle, two urogenital folds, and two labial scrotal swellings. The urogenital and labioscrotal folds fuse anteriorly to form the mons pubis by the seventh week. Posterior fusion separates the urogenital membrane from the anal membrane and results in formation of the posterior fourchette and perineum. By the end of the seventh week of gestation, the urogenital membrane disappears, exteriorizing the urogenital sinus. At 8 to 9 weeks, if testes are present, Leydig cells begin producing testosterone. If the target cells in the external genitalia contain the enzyme 5-alpha reductase, testosterone is converted into dihydrotestosterone and, by 10 weeks' gestation, male structures develop. If no testosterone is produced or the reductase enzyme is not found in the epithelial cells, a vulva develops. Specifically, the genital tubercle folds posteriorly and becomes the clitoris, the urogenital sinus becomes a portion of the vestibule that includes the introitus and hymenal membrane, the urogenital folds become the remaining vestibule and labia minora, and the labial scrotal swellings become the labia majora. The entire conversion to female structures is completed by 20 weeks' gestational age (Figure 2.30).[2,35]

The vulva represents the fusion of ectodermal elements (the surface epithelia of the labia majora and minora) and endodermal elements (the epithelia of the vestibule and vagina). Ectodermal squamous epithelium is keratinized while endodermal epithelium is not. The point where these two types of epithelia meet is known as *Hart's line*. Although this line represents a transition from one surface type to another, it does not have the same degree of significance as the transformation zone in the cervix, because both surfaces on the vulva consist only of squamous cells. Also, overall cell proliferation here is minimal and has no neoplastic potential. In addition, ectodermal glandular structures are more representative of skin adnexa, while the vestibular glands are derived from endoderm. Table 2.1 describes the male homologues of the different female vestibular glands.

As described previously, the period between 10 and 20 weeks' gestation is critical to the development of the vulva. Epithelial contact with androgens at this time results in a variable

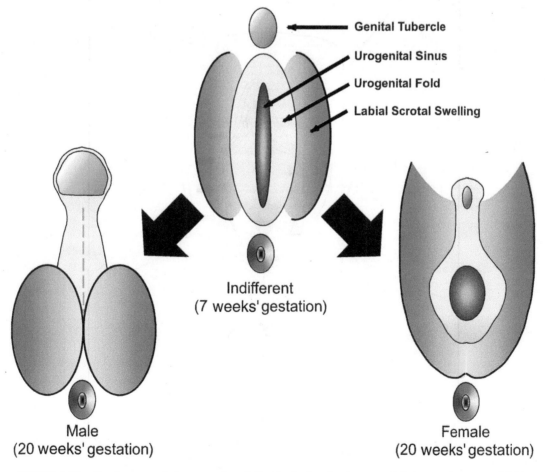

Genital Tubercle

Urogenital Sinus

Urogenital Fold

Labial Scrotal Swelling

Indifferent
(7 weeks' gestation)

Male
(20 weeks' gestation)

Female
(20 weeks' gestation)

FIGURE 2.30. Development of the external genitalia. In the female, the urogenital sinus and urogenital folds remain open, forming the labia minora, vestibule, and introitus.

TABLE 2.1	MALE AND FEMALE EXTERNAL GENITALIA HOMOLOGOUS GLANDULAR STRUCTURES	
■ **FEMALE**	■ **MALE**
Skene's glands	Prostate
Minor vestibular glands	Penile glands of Littre
Bartholin's glands	Cowper's glands

androgenic influence on the external genitalia. Reasons for androgen exposure may include drug or exogenous hormone intake, placental aromatase deficiency, maternal androgenic tumors, and congenital adrenal hyperplasia. The end result is a female pseudohermaphrodite with ambiguous genital development characterized by clitoral hypertrophy, hypospadias, and scrotalization of nonfused labia (Figure 2.31).[35]

2.4.2 Anatomy

Vulva, the Latin word for *covering*, is the area of the female external genital tract that extends from the symphysis pubis anteriorly to the anus posteriorly and lateral to the inguinal-gluteal folds. The area includes the mons pubis, the labia minora, and labia majora, the clitoris, the vestibule and associated structures, the posterior fourchette, and the perineum. The *vestibule* represents that portion of the vulva medial to the

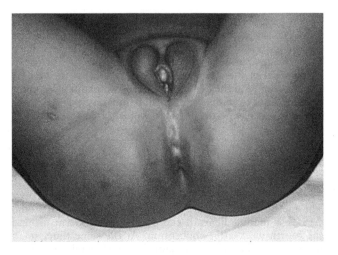

FIGURE 2.31. Ambiguous genitalia. There is enlargement of the labia majora and clitoromegaly, with enlargement of the clitoral hood.

labia minora that extends from the clitoral region anteriorly to the area of labia fusion beneath the introitus (the *posterior fourchette*). The urethral meatus and the introitus lie within the vestibule. The *pilosebaceous line* is the border separating the lateral skin covered by pubic hair from the medial non–hair-bearing skin (Figure 2.32).[36]

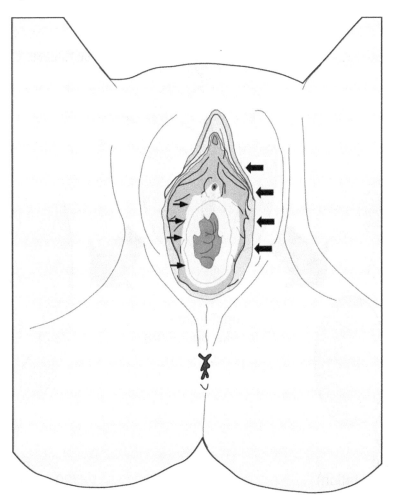

FIGURE 2.32.   Normal vulva. The *large arrows* delineate the pilosebaceous line. The *smaller arrows* delineate Hart's line.

The labia majora are lateral skin folds that vary in size depending on the amount of underlying adipose tissue. After childbearing, they decrease in size and become almost completely absent in postmenopausal women. They diverge anteriorly and blend into the mons. The labia minora are small folds located medially to the labia majora. The labia minora have numerous sebaceous glands visible clinically as small, white, slightly elevated, smooth areas known as *Fordyce spots*. The labia minora fuse anteriorly to form the frenulum of the clitoris. The portion of the clitoris that is visible is a small cylindrical nodule about 0.5 cm in diameter. It contains erectile tissue and enlarges during sexual arousal, but rarely exceeds 1 cm in diameter. Beneath the clitoris is the urethral opening or urinary meatus, a slit-like opening 0.5 cm in diameter.[36,37]

The hymenal ring represents the remnant of the urogenital membrane. Prior to intercourse, the hymen is commonly a plate-like structure with small areas of perforation (Figure 2.33A–C). After intercourse or vaginal delivery, small peripheral mucosal tags known as *myrtiform caruncles* represent the remnants of the hymenal plate. Rare cases of imperforate hymen, in which the hymenal plate remains intact, lead to accumulation of both menstrual efflux and vaginal material known as hematocolpos.[37]

The vestibule contains numerous gland openings. The two Skene's ducts are located just inferior and lateral to the urethra. The two Bartholin's ducts are located lateral to the posterior fourchette. The Skene's and Bartholin's ducts are small (less than 0.5 mm in diameter), and are not recognizable clinically unless obstructed and secondarily infected. The minor vestibular glands are located in a semicircular area that approximates Hart's line. The number of minor vestibular glands varies from 1 to 100, but usually averages between 2 and 10 in examined vestibulectomy specimens. These glands are also not recognizable clinically unless inflamed, when they appear as reddened spots. Near the

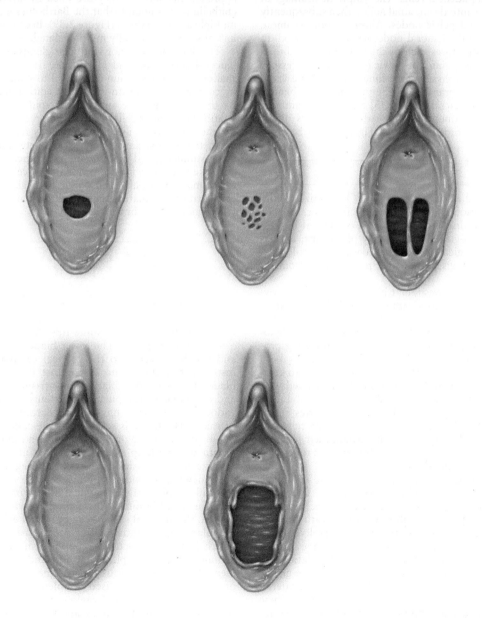

FIGURE 2.33.   Types of hymenal perforations. The size and shape are indicative of the amount of degeneration in the urogenital membrane. A lack of degeneration will result in a solid hymenal plate, which can lead to a hematocolpos (collection of menstrual efflux in the vagina). Large perforations are usually the result of tampon insertion, intercourse, or vaginal deliveries, but can occur spontaneously.

introitus are variable numbers of raised micropapillae, known as micropapillomatosis labialis. Although similar in appearance to a small vulvar condyloma, normal micropapillae do not contain human papillomavirus DNA (see Chapters 13 and 15).

Hair growth begins at puberty and reaches adult amounts by late adolescence. Hair distribution over the vulva, or the escutcheon, is shaped like an inverted triangle, with the base located at the upper mons pubis. The hair shafts arise from the mons and the lateral labia majora. The medial labia majora and the labia minora do not contain pilosebaceous units. The amount of pubic hair decreases after menopause.

The arterial supply of the vulva is mainly through branches of the pudendal and hemorrhoidal arteries. In general, the venous drainage parallels the arterial vessels. The exception is the convoluted venous plexus of the vestibular bulb. The apex of this teardrop-shaped bulb is the clitoral vein; the base is in the vicinity of Bartholin's gland. These plexus drain laterally into the labial and pudendal veins. The lymphatic drainage of the vulva is initially into the inguinal nodes, then subsequently into the femoral and pelvic nodes. Although not common, direct drainage into the femoral nodes has been reported. In addition, central structures such as the introitus and clitoris can rarely drain directly into the pelvic nodes using accessory channels over the symphysis pubis. Innervation of the vulva is through superficial branches of the pudendal and hemorrhoidal nerves from sacral roots 2, 3, and 4. The anterior portion of the vulva (mons) is supplied by branches of the ilioinguinal and genitofemoral nerves (Figure 2.34A,B).[9,36]

2.4.3 Histology

The majority of the vulva consists of keratinized skin. Because of its location and the fact that it is subject to various dermatological diseases, it is an area of clinical interest not only to gynecologists, but to family physicians, dermatologists, general surgical pathologists, dermatopathologists, gynecological pathologists, and other providers of women's health care.

The surface of the nonvestibular hair-bearing vulva is covered by keratinized stratified squamous epithelial cells or keratinocytes. Small projections of epidermal cells known as rete pegs extend into the superficial stroma or dermis.[36] Melanocytes are neuroepithelial cells responsible for producing protective pigmentation. They are distributed along the basal cell layer in a ratio ranging from 1:10 to 1:50 melanocytes to keratinocytes (Figure 2.35A,B). Langerhans cells, associated with skin immunity, are located suprabasally in a distribution ratio of approximately 1 Langerhans cell to 5 keratinocytes (Figure 2.36). Merkel cells, which are neuroendocrine-type cells, can also be identified within the vulvar epithelium; their function is unknown although they may be involved in light touch and establishing spatial relationships.[37]

The dermis consists of collagen, capillaries, and myofibroblastic type cells and is divided into two regions. The papillary dermis is the portion found between the rete pegs; the reticular dermis is the solid confluent area beneath the rete pegs. Within the reticular dermis are hair-bearing follicles with associated sebaceous glands, apocrine, and eccrine glands. The apocrine glands are sensitive to hormonal stimulation and release material by cytoplasmic secretion. The eccrine glands produce a watery sweat. They secrete by release of material through myoepithelial cell contraction into sweat ducts. These glands are not modulated by hormonal activity. Once the transition to non–hair-bearing skin occurs, the dermis of the labia minora contains only sebaceous glands and rare eccrine glands (Figure 2.37).[37,38]

The epithelium overlying the vestibule and the portion of the labia minora within Hart's line also consists of stratified squamous cells. This epithelium, however, has no surface keratin, and the mature squamous epithelial cells become glycogen rich (Figure 2.38). This is particularly true of the hymenal squamous epithelium; mild nuclear enlargement and the impression of cytoplasmic clearing can lead to a false diagnosis of human papillomavirus cytopathic effect. The dermis is highly vascular and rich in elastic fibers and erectile tissue. Here, adnexal structures are essentially absent.

The periurethral or Skene's glands are typically no more than 1.5 cm in length. Like the urethra, the ducts are lined with transitional-type epithelium that merges with the stratified squamous epithelium of the vestibular surface. The glands themselves are lined by mucin-producing columnar epithelium.

The major vestibular or Bartholin's gland area consists of acini lined by columnar epithelium and of ducts lined by columnar and transitional cell–type epithelium. As these ducts approach the surface, they are lined by stratified squamous epithelium. It is notable that the Bartholin's gland usually has multiple acini and ducts (Figure 2.39). Because of this, Bartholin's abscesses are usually multiloculated.[37,38]

The ducts of the minor vestibular glands exit directly to the mucosal surface around Hart's line. The tubular glands are shallow with a maximum depth of 3 to 4 mm. They are lined by columnar-type mucin-producing epithelium (Figure 2.40). As they approach the surface, the epithelia merge into the stratified squamous cells of the vulvar epidermis. It is common for these glands to undergo squamous metaplasia. In some cases, the metaplasia may cause complete transformation of the vestibular gland into squamous epithelium, producing a cleft-like structure. The transitional-type cells commonly seen in the major vestibular and periurethral glands are not present. Further information on the anatomy and histology of the vulva can be found in Chapter 15.

2.5 BIOPSY SPECIMEN COLLECTION, PROCESSING, AND INTERPRETATION

Various instruments have been designed to obtain cervical biopsies. All have scissors-like tips that can excise a 3- to 5-mm tissue fragment. The lower blade is slightly extended and can be placed into the cervical canal to stabilize the instrument. Little or no discomfort is felt if the forceps blades are sharp; dull blades cause tissue pulling, crushing, and subsequent cramping. Instruments designed to obtain endocervical material have the appearance of small baskets or rakes. The tissue is scraped off the canal surface, resulting in tiny tissue fragments of blood and mucus. Specimens obtained using loop excisional devices are similar in shape to large-shave biopsies. Biopsies of the vagina and vulva can be somewhat difficult to obtain because of their relatively flat and pliable surface. Cervical biopsy instruments can be used for raised lesions at these sites. For vaginal lesions that are flat, the mucosal surface can be tented using small hooks. Macular vulvar lesions can be removed using a Keyes punch, which is a trephine-cutter–type instrument that removes a cylinder of surface epithelium and underlying dermis. Pigmented lesions suspicious for malignancy, as on other parts of the body, are best excised completely using a sharp knife. Tissue from the proximal vagina adjacent to the cervix can usually be removed without anesthesia. Biopsies from the distal vagina and vulva usually require local anesthetic injection.

After removal, the tissue pieces are placed in formalin-filled containers labeled with the patient's name and the type of specimen submitted ("cervix biopsy," "labial biopsy,"

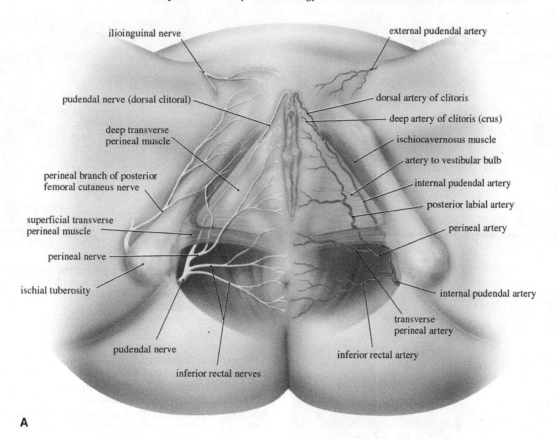

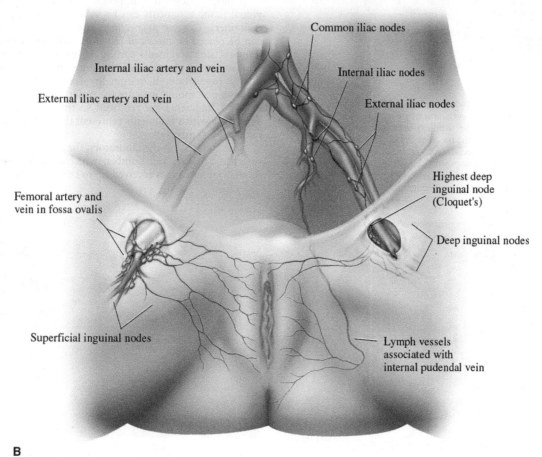

FIGURE 2.34. **A:** Arterial supply and innervation of the vulva and superficial perineum. **B:** Lymphatic drainage of the vulva and superficial perineum.

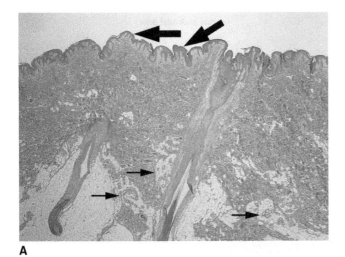

A

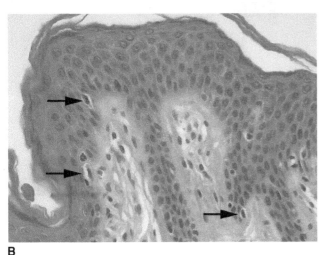

B

FIGURE 2.35. Vulvar surface covering the labia majora. **A:** Low power. Note the epidermal evaginations or rete pegs (*large arrows*) that interdigitate between the papillary dermis. Two hair shafts are found in the more eosinophilic reticular dermis. Eccrine glands (*small arrows*) are also present. Subcutaneous fat is present below the dermis (hematoxylin and eosin, low-power magnification). **B:** High power. Note the scattered melanocytes (*arrows*) in the epidermal basal layer (hematoxylin and eosin, high-power magnification).

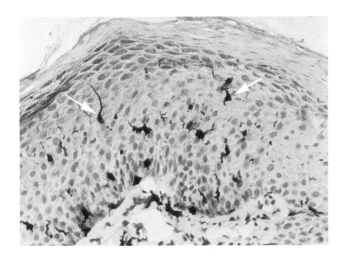

FIGURE 2.36. Langerhans cells. Individual dendritic type cells (*arrows*) are scattered among the surface epithelial cells (immunoperoxidase stain for S100 protein marker, hematoxylin counter stain, high-power magnification).

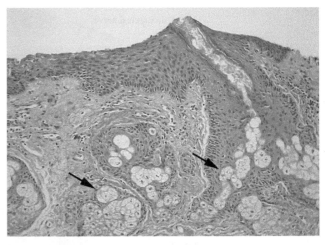

FIGURE 2.37. Vulvar surface covering the vestibule. Numerous sebaceous glands (*arrows*) are present beneath the epidermis. There are, however, no accompanying hair shafts (hematoxylin and eosin, medium-power magnification).

"endocervical curettage (ECC)"). At the same time, a requisition form should be completed. This should include the patient's name, date of birth, age, and pertinent history. Helpful additional information includes pregnancy status, hormone usage, the colposcopic impression, cytology result, and any prior lower genital tract abnormalities and treatment.

If biopsy location is important to the colposcopist, individual tissue fragments can be submitted in separate labeled containers. To assist in specimen orientation, the biopsy pieces can be placed on pieces of paper or Gelfoam. Larger cervical loop excision fragments can be oriented by dotting the edge with ink or by placing a small suture and noting the location on the requisition. If margin involvement is important, the colposcopist should indicate the order in which multiple loop excision fragments are removed so that the pathologist can determine which fragments represent the true ectocervical and endocervical margins.

Once received in the laboratory, the specimen is logged and assigned an accession number, which usually represents the number of specimens received up to that point for a particular

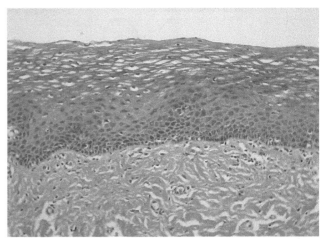

FIGURE 2.38. Vulva surface near the introitus. The epithelial surface is similar in appearance to the squamous mucosa of the vulva and vagina. Note the absence of rete pegs (hematoxylin and eosin, medium-power magnification).

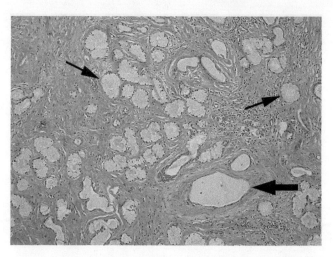

FIGURE 2.39. Major vestibular (Bartholin's) glands. Numerous acini (*small arrows*) lined by mucinous type epithelial cells are present. Scattered larger ductal structures (*large arrow*) are lined by urothelial-type cells (hematoxylin and eosin, medium-power magnification).

year. The specimen is then examined and described by a pathologist or an assistant, who notes the size, number, color, and consistency of the tissue pieces from a particular container. Larger tissue pieces, such as those removed during loop excisional procedures, are cut into smaller serial cross sections, a process known as "bread-loafing" (Figure 2.41). The fragments are then placed in small rectangular plastic cassettes. The process of describing and transferring the tissue into cassettes is known as prosection, "grossing," or "cutting in" the material.

After grossing is completed, a histotechnologist places the individual cassettes in a tissue processor that dehydrates the tissue and replaces any water with a medium that allows for optimal tissue cutting. This procedure is time dependent and takes approximately 4 to 9 hours. The tissue is then embedded into a modified paraffin material and sectioned by a microtome into small 5-μm ribbons. Before embedding, the histotechnologist must orient the biopsy specimen by hand; the larger the fragment, the easier it is to obtain sections that include surface epithelium and underlying stroma. The wax strips with the tissue are then transferred to glass slides. The surrounding wax is removed, and the remaining tissue is stained using hematoxylin and eosin dyes, and coverslipped (Figure 2.42).

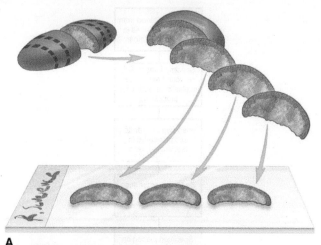

A

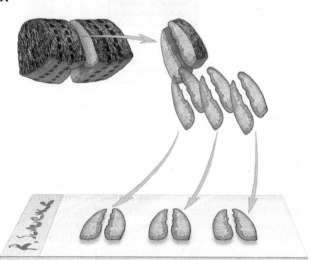

B

FIGURE 2.41. Specimen preparation. **A:** Sectioning small biopsy specimens for microscopic examination. **B:** Sectioning larger specimens obtained by means of cone and loop excision for microscopic examination.

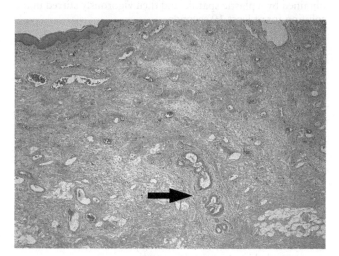

FIGURE 2.40. Minor vestibular glands. The small gland cluster (*arrow*) is found approximately 2 to 3 mm beneath the surface (hematoxylin and eosin, low-power magnification).

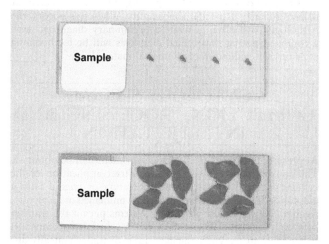

FIGURE 2.42. Glass slides stained with hematoxylin and eosin. The slide with the smaller pieces represents a cervical biopsy. The slide with the larger sections represents a loop excision.

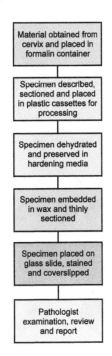

FIGURE 2.43. Processing of histology material by a pathology laboratory.

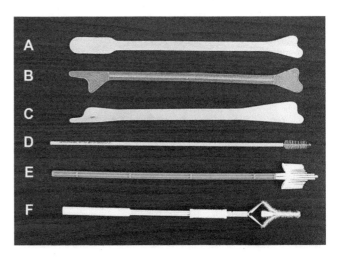

FIGURE 2.44. Different cervical cytologic sampling devices. *A–C*, Spatulas; *D*, Cytobrush®; *E*, Cervex-Brush® or Papette®; *F*, Accellon Combi® device.

Preparing biopsy material for microscopic examination takes about 6 to 10 hours. The pathologist then examines the glass slide after consulting the matching pathology requisition form for any pertinent clinical information and reports the result as a microscopic or final diagnosis. This process is known as "signing out" the specimens. The total process from specimen receipt and accession by the laboratory to provision of a diagnostic report to the colposcopist takes on average 18 to 24 hours (Figure 2.43).[39]

Since a single random 5-μm thin section may miss an intraepithelial lesion that partially covers a 3- to 4-mm biopsy fragment, most surgical pathology laboratories will cut two to three strips through different layers of the fragment, called "levels" or "step sections." Occasionally, a pathologist will request additional levels if diagnostic questions are raised during the initial microscopic interpretation or the specimen is not well oriented. In addition, special stains may be ordered if the presence of bacterial or fungal organisms is suspected, or to better clarify a specific abnormality. When this occurs, the pathologist will often generate a preliminary diagnosis, with a comment noting that a final diagnosis will be forthcoming after further evaluation of additional material.

2.6 CYTOLOGY SPECIMEN COLLECTION, PROCESSING, AND INTERPRETATION

At present, two types of cytologic specimens can be obtained. The conventional Pap test involves direct application of the cellular material collected from the cervix or vagina onto a glass slide. The slide is then sprayed or immersed in an alcohol fixative. Newer liquid processing systems permit the transfer of a collected cellular specimen into a solution for transport to the laboratory, where the material is then mechanically dispersed and a representative thin layer of cells is transferred to a glass slide (see Sections 3.2.1 and 19.2.4.5). The majority of providers use three types of sampling devices for specimen collection: the Ayre spatula (Surgipath Medical Industries Inc., P.O. Box 528, Richmond, IL 60071), the Cytobrush® (Cooper Surgical, Inc., 95 Corporate Drive, Trumbull, CT 06611), and the Cervex-brush® (Unimar, Inc. 475 Danbury Rd, Wilton, CT 06897) or Papette® (Wallach Surgical Devices, Inc. 235 Edison Rd. Orange, CT 06477) (Figure 2.44).

The wooden spatula is widely available, inexpensive, causes minimal discomfort, and only rarely causes cervical trauma. It cannot, however, sample an SCJ located in the endocervical canal and is not recommended for collection of liquid-based cytology specimens. Therefore, the original Ayre tip has been lengthened in some devices, and plastic spatulas have been introduced to improve cell capture and transfer. Use of the spatula is straightforward. It is placed against the cervix, rotated 360 degrees at least once, and the collected material spread across a glass slide. In some cases, however, the long end of the spatula is not always placed into the os. For women with a large ectropion, the spatula should not only sample the center as described above, but also be swiped around the peripheral margins of the ectopy to sample the red-to-pink interface representing the SCJ. Transfer of the material to the slide must be quick and deliberate to minimize air-drying–induced cell distortion. If a liquid processing system is used, the material is obtained by a plastic spatula and then vigorously stirred in the solution for at least 10 seconds.

The Cytobrush® has replaced the cotton swab or cotton-tipped applicator as an endocervical sampling device, as the cotton fibers of the latter cause cell trapping and may result in insufficient cell transfer (Figure 2.45).[40] The Cytobrush® has perpendicular pliable plastic bristles at the end of a thin wire applicator. For maximal sampling of the entire cervix, it should be used in conjunction with the spatula. The narrow tip of the brush can be inserted into a narrowed cervical os to sample the endocervical canal. To minimize bleeding, the brush should be rotated only one-fourth (90 degrees) to one-half (180 degrees) of a complete turn. Optimal cell transfer is accomplished by rolling the brush across a slide. If a liquid preparation system is used, the brush is stirred in the preservative for 10 seconds and then rolled around the wall of the collection jar at least 10 times. Some providers will also scrape the bristles with a spatula to improve cell transfer. A recent study has shown that the Cytobrush® is safe for use during pregnancy, but this is not recommended by the manufacturer.[41]

The Cervex-brush® or Papette® has bristles that are softer, thicker, and longer centrally than those of the Cytobrush®.

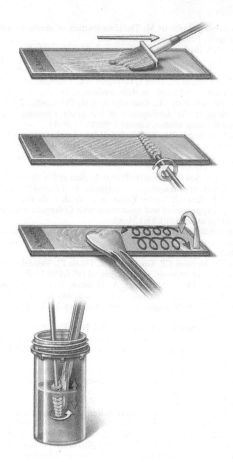

FIGURE 2.45. (Top) Transfer of cervical material to glass slides for preparation of conventional smears and (bottom) transfer of cervical material to liquid medium for preparation of monolayer smears.

The device resembles a paintbrush, except that the central bristles are longer than the short lateral bristles. Because of its shape, many clinicians refer to this device simply as "the broom." The longer bristles are inserted into the canal, while the shorter strands spread over the portio and lateral ectocervix. The technique for using this device is the most meticulous of the three instruments in use today. The cervix must first be wiped with a large cotton swab to remove any mucus adherent to the external cervical os. The Cervex-brush® is applied to the cervix with the central bristles inserted into the canal and rotated clockwise five times. It is then spread longitudinally across the glass slide in a single motion, turned to the opposite side, and again swept across the slide. If a liquid preparation system is used, the broom is stirred in the solution for at least 10 seconds, pressed against the bottom, and then stirred again for 10 seconds. Some systems require that the broom tip be removed and sent in the liquid container.

Many comparative studies have evaluated the efficacy of different collection devices. Most have concluded that the combination of a Cytobrush® and spatula is the best technique for sampling the cervix, followed by the broom.[42,43] An evidenced-based review evaluated different sampling devices to determine the best technique to detect the presence of cervical intraepithelial lesions.[44] Although not universally accepted, this review concluded that intraepithelial lesions were much more likely to be detected when individual preparations contained endocervical cells, as the number of Pap tests with endocervical cells increased, so also did the number of tests that contained high-grade intraepithelial lesions. While the extended tip spatula, Cervex-brush®, and the Cytobrush® were

better than the classic Ayre spatula for sampling the canal, the best technique for identification of cervical intraepithelial lesions was a combination of the spatula and Cytobrush®.[44]

In general, women should not douche, use vaginal creams, or have intercourse within 24 hours of specimen collection. The cytologic specimen should be obtained before the bimanual examination. Water or a thin film of water-soluble gel can be used as a speculum lubricant, but not at the tip. Once the specimen is obtained, the slide should be quickly fixed using an alcohol-based solution, labeled with the patient's name, and submitted to a laboratory with a requisition sheet that also includes the patient's name and any pertinent history. Important information for optimal Pap test interpretation includes the specimen source, the patient's age, last menstrual period, any hormonal usage or, if pregnant, gestational age, any history of prior abnormal cytologic specimens, or treatment of cervical or vaginal abnormalities.

Once received by the laboratory, conventional and liquid processed slides are stained by the Pap method, which uses variable combinations of hematoxylin, eosin, and orange G dyes, and coverslipped.[45] Slides are then screened by a cytotechnologist, an individual specifically trained to examine cytologic specimens. The cytotechnologist either reports the Pap test as normal, after which a report is generated, or identifies possible abnormalities that require final interpretation by the pathologist. In addition, laboratories are required by the U.S. Federal Clinical Laboratory Improvements Amendments of 1988 to randomly review 10% of all slides initially reported as normal. This is commonly done by a second senior cytotechnologist. As screening Pap tests is tedious and labor-intensive, laboratories are limited by law to the number of slides that can be screened by individual cytotechnologists over a 24-hour period. Most laboratories set a limit of 50 to 80 slides per day for each technologist. Therefore, the time from receipt of the cytologic specimen by the laboratory to the delivery of

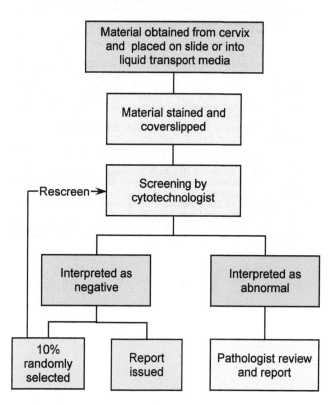

FIGURE 2.46. Standard processing of cytology specimens by a pathology laboratory.

a final diagnostic report to the colposcopist can span several days, depending on the slide review volume of the laboratory and the number of cytotechnologists employed (Figure 2.46).

References

1. Robboy SJ, Bernhardt PF, Parmley T. Embryology of the female genital tract and disorders of abnormal sexual development. In: Kurman RJ, ed. *Blaustein's Pathology of the Female Genital Tract* (4th ed.). New York, NY: Springer-Verlag, 1994:8–10.
2. Larsen WJ. *Human Embryology*. New York, NY: Churchill Livingstone, 1993:253–8.
3. Hendrickson MR, Atkins KA, Kempson RL. Uterus and fallopian tubes. In: Mills SM, ed. *Histology for Pathologists* (3rd ed.). Philadelphia-New York: Lippincott-Raven Publishers, 2007:1011–3.
4. Linhartova A. Extent of columnar epithelium on the ectocervix between the ages of 1 and 13 years. *Obstet Gynecol* 1978;52:451–6.
5. Ince TA, Cviko AP, Quade BJ, et al. p63 coordinates anogenital modeling and epithelial cell differentiation in the developing female urogenital tract. *Am J Pathol* 2002;161:1111–7.
6. Robboy SJ, Bentley RC. Vagina. In: Mills SM, ed. *Histology for Pathologists* (3rd ed.). Philadelphia-New York: Lippincott-Raven Publishers, 2007:999–1010.
7. Wright TC, Ronnett BM, Ferenczy A. Benign diseases of the cervix. In: Kurman RJ, Ellenson LH, Ronnett BM, eds. *Blaustein's Pathology of the Female Genital Tract* (6th ed.). New York, NY: Springer-Verlag, 2011:156–61.
8. Singer A. Anatomy of the cervix and physiological changes in cervical epithelium. In: Fox H, Well M. eds. *Haines and Taylor Obstetrical and Gynaecological Pathology*. New York, NY: Churchill Livingstone, 1995:225–48.
9. Hellman LM, Pritchard JA. *Williams Obstetrics* (14th ed.). New York, NY: Appleton-Century-Crofts, 1970:19–30.
10. Kurman RJ, Norris HJ, Wilkinson E. *Tumors of the Cervix, Vagina and Vulva. Atlas of Tumor Pathology* (Series 3, Volume 4). Bethesda, MD: Armed Forces Institute of Pathology (monograph), 1992:1–12.
11. Vooijs GP. Benign proliferative reactions, intraepithelial neoplasia and invasive cancer of the uterine cervix. In: Bibbo M, ed. *Diagnostic Cytopathology* (2nd ed.). Philadelphia, PA: WB Saunders Co., 1997:161–8.
12. Feldman D, Romney SL, Edgcomb J, Valentine T. Ultrastructure of normal, metaplastic, and abnormal human uterine cervix: use of montages to study the topographical relationship of epithelial cells. *Am J Obstet Gynecol* 1984;150:573–688.
13. Kupryjanczyk J. Epidermal growth factor receptor expression in the normal and inflamed cervix uteri: a comparison with estrogen receptor expression. *Int J Gynecol Pathol* 1990;9:263–71.
14. Gigi-Leiter O, Geiger B, Levy R, Czernobilsky B. Cytokeratin expression in squamous metaplasia of the human uterine cervix. *Differentiation* 1986;31:191–205.
15. Maddox P, Szarewski A, Dyson J, Cuzick J. Cytokeratin expression and acetowhite change in cervical epithelium. *J Clin Pathol* 1994;47:15–7.
16. Smedts F, Ramaekers F, Leube RE, Keijser K, Link M, Vooijs P. Expression of keratins 1, 6, 15, 16 and 20 in normal cervical epithelium, squamous metaplasia, cervical intraepithelial neoplasia and cervical carcinoma. *Am J Pathol* 1993;142:403–12.
17. Cullen TS. *Cancer of the Uterus*. New York, NY: D. Appleton and Co., 1900:180–7.
18. Fluhmann CF. *The Cervix Uteri and Its Diseases*. Philadelphia, PA: WB Saunders, 1961:56–78.
19. Lawrence WD, Shingleton HM. Early physiologic squamous metaplasia of the cervix: light and electron microscopic observation. *Am J Obstet Gynecol* 1980;137:661–71.
20. Burke L, Antonioli DA, Ducatman BS. *Colposcopy, Text and Atlas*. Norwalk, CT: Appleton and Lange, 1991:29–59.
21. Smedts F, Ramaekers F, Troyanovsky S, et al. Basal-cell keratins in cervical reserve cells and a comparison to their expression in cervical intraepithelial neoplasia. *Am J Pathol* 1992;140:601–12.
22. Szamborski J, Liebhart M. The ultrastructure of squamous metaplasia in endocervix. *Pathol Eur* 1973;1:13–20.
23. Vooijs GP. Benign proliferative reactions, intraepithelial neoplasia and invasive cancer of the uterine cervix. In: Bibbo M, ed. *Diagnostic Cytopathology* (2nd ed.). Philadelphia, PA: WB Saunders Co., 1997:169–74.
24. Autier P, Coibion M, Huet F, Grivegnee AR. Transformation zone location and intraepithelial neoplasia of the cervix uteri. *Br J Cancer* 1996;74:488–90.
25. Moscicki A-B, Burt VG, Kanowitz S, et al. The significance of squamous metaplasia in the development of low grade squamous intraepithelial lesions in young women. *Cancer* 1999;85:1139–44.
26. Gould PR, Barter RA, Papadimitriou JM. An ultrastructural, cytochemical and autoradiographic study of the mucous membrane of the human cervical canal with reference to subcolumnar basal cells. *Am J Pathol* 1979;95:1–16.
27. Tsutsumi K, Sun Q, Yasumoto S, et al. In vitro and in vivo analysis of cellular origin of cervical squamous metaplasia. *Am J Pathol* 1993;143:1150–8.
28. Hare MJ, Toone E, Taylor-Robinson D, et al. Follicular cervicitis—colposcopic appearances and association with *Chlamydia trachomatis. Br J Obstet Gynaecol* 1981;88:174–80.
29. Papanicolaou GN, Traut HF, Marchetti AA. *The Epithelia of Woman's Reproductive Organs*. New York, NY: The Commonwealth Fund, 1948:30–6.
30. Prins RP, Morrow CP, Townsend DE, Disaia PJ. Vaginal embryogenesis, estrogens, and adenosis. *Obstet Gynecol* 1976;48:246–50.
31. Patton DL, Thwin SS, Meier A, Houston TM, et al. Epithelial cell layer thickness and immune cell populations in the normal human vagina at different stages of the menstrual cycle. *Am J Obstet Gynecol* 1976;183:967–73.
32. Tsai P-S, Uchima F-D, Hamamoto ST, Bern HA. Proliferation of differentiation of prepubertal mouse vaginal epithelial cells in vitro and the specificity of estrogen-induced growth retardation. *In Vitro Cell Dev Biol* 1991;27A:461–8.
33. Boyd TK, Quade BJ, Crum CP. Female genital tract development and disorders of childhood. In: Crum CP, Nucci MR, Lee KR, eds. *Diagnostic Gynecologic and Obstetric Pathology* (2nd ed.). Philadelphia, PA: Elsevier Saunders, 2011:5–9.
34. Schaller G, Lengyel E, Pantel K, et al. Keratin expression reveals mosaic differentiation in vaginal epithelium. *Am J Obstet Gynecol* 1993;169:1603–7.
35. Speroff L, Glass RH, Kase NG. *Clinical Gynecologic Embryology and Infertility* (5th ed.). Baltimore, MD: Williams and Wilkins, 1994:326–9.
36. Wilkinson EJ, Massoll NA. Benign diseases of the vulva. In: Kurman RJ, Ellenson LH, Ronnett BM, eds. *Blaustein's Pathology of the Female Genital Tract* (6th ed.). New York, NY: Springer-Verlag, 2011:3–4.
37. Wilkinson EJ, Hart NS. Vulva. In: Mills SM, ed. *Histology for Pathologists* (3rd ed.). Philadelphia-New York: Lippincott-Raven Publishers, 2007:984–95.
38. Lever WF, Lever-Schaumburg G. *Histopathology of the Skin* (6th ed.). Philadelphia, PA: JB Lippincott, 1983:90–3.
39. Prophet EB, Mills B, Arrington JB, Sobin LH, eds. *Laboratory Methods in Histotechnology*. Washington, DC: Armed Forces Institute of Pathology, American Registry of Pathology, 1992:25–45.
40. Rubio CA. The false negative smear II. The trapping effect of collecting instruments. *Obstet Gynecol* 1976;49:576–9.
41. Lieberman RW, Henry MR, Laskin WB, et al. Colposcopy in pregnancy: directed brush cytology compared with cervical biopsy. *Obstet Gynecol* 1999;94:198–203.
42. Boon ME, de Graff Guilloud JC, Rietveld WJ. Analysis of five sampling methods for the preparation of cervical smears. *Acta Cytol* 1988;33:843–8.
43. Germain M, Heaton R, Erickson D, et al. A comparison of the three most common Papanicolaou smear collection techniques. *Obstet Gynecol* 1994;84:168–73.
44. Martin-Hirsch P, Jarvis G, Ketchener H, Lilford R. Collection devices for obtaining cervical cytology samples. *Cochrane Libr* 1999;2:1–25.
45. Mikel UV, ed. *Advanced Laboratory Methods in Histology and Pathology* (monograph). Washington, DC: Armed Forces Institute of Pathology, American Registry of Pathology, 1994:221–4.

The Cytology and Histology of Cervicovaginal Abnormalities

3.1 INTRODUCTION
3.2 CYTOLOGY OF CERVICOVAGINAL ABNORMALITIES
   3.2.1 The Bethesda System
   3.2.2 New Technologies in Cervicovaginal Cytology
3.3 HISTOLOGY OF SQUAMOUS ABNORMALITIES
   3.3.1 Reactive and Reparative Changes
   3.3.2 Intraepithelial Lesions
   3.3.3 Invasive Carcinoma
3.4 HISTOLOGY OF GLANDULAR ABNORMALITIES
   3.4.1 Reactive Changes
   3.4.2 Intraepithelial Lesions

3.4.3 Invasive Adenocarcinoma
3.4.4 Biomarkers for Cervical Squamous and Glandular
     Neoplasias
3.5 INTERPRETING PATHOLOGY REPORTS
3.6 NEW TERMINOLOGY FOR SQUAMOUS INTRAEPITHE-
   LIAL LESIONS THROUGHOUT THE LOWER GENITAL
   TRACT

3.1 INTRODUCTION

Cervicovaginal neoplasia has generated considerable attention throughout the past century. Much of this interest has been possible due to easy access to clinical inspection, the discovery of a premalignant condition, and, in most instances, the slow progression from a normal healthy mucosa to invasive carcinoma. The identification of small surface vascular changes in early cervicovaginal carcinomas led to the development of the technique of colposcopy by Hinselmann.[1] The matching of abnormal exfoliated cervical squamous and glandular cells to dysplastic and malignant abnormalities led to the eventual development of the specialty of cytopathology. Continued investigation into these abnormalities has resulted in the identification of human papillomavirus (HPV) as the major causative agent for these lesions. This chapter details the specific benign, intraepithelial, and malignant alterations that can occur in the cervix and vagina.

3.2 CYTOLOGY OF CERVICOVAGINAL ABNORMALITIES

The ability to identify atypical cells that represent squamous cell carcinoma in patients with abnormal vaginal bleeding was first reported by Papanicolaou in 1928.[2] The concept was revisited in a monograph published by Papanicolaou and Traut in 1942.[3] The introduction of a sampling device by Ayre improved the collection of cervical cells, increasing detection of preinvasive lesions and small cancers in asymptomatic women. Regional population-based trials such as those conducted in central Kentucky confirmed the value of examining cervicovaginal cells as a screening test.[4] Eventually the Papanicolaou (Pap) smear, or Pap test, became widely accepted in this country as the prototypical technique for the early detection of cervical dysplasia and cancer.

The Pap test is based on a relatively simple mechanism. Cells from squamous epithelium exfoliate over time. Thus, the cells removed for cytologic examination represent epithelial cells, normal or abnormal, found at the surface. Large numbers of cells with abundant cytoplasm and small nuclei would be compatible with superficial cells found in an area of glycogenated mature squamous epithelium. Smaller cells with slightly enlarged nuclei would suggest sampling over an area of squamous metaplasia, or removal of exfoliated cells from an estrogen-deprived cervix where the epithelial surface consists of parabasal cells. In the case of mild dysplasia, the exfoliated cells consist of koilocytic cells. As the dysplasia worsens, however, smaller atypical basaloid cells begin to reach the surface and exfoliate. Finally, abnormal cell forms from rapid growth exfoliate in squamous cell carcinoma (Figure 3.1). Endocervical cells tend to be more cohesive and are usually removed in clumps from the endocervical canal.

3.2.1 The Bethesda System

The discovery that HPV was associated with lower genital lesions directed investigators to reevaluate many lesions originally considered early dysplasias and reclassify them as pure viral infections, or koilocytotic or condylomatous atypias.[5] Table 3.1 compares the different classification systems used from 1950 until 1988. The association of HPV with high-grade cervical intraepithelial neoplasia (CIN) and cervix cancers created confusion about how HPV related to various cervicovaginal abnormalities and how they should be classified.[6,7] As a result, individual laboratories used their own unique classification systems, which were not reproducible. As the problem of multiple diagnostic terms in cervicovaginal cytology became pervasive, a workshop was convened in 1988 on the campus of the National Institutes of Health in Bethesda, Maryland, to standardize the reporting system for Pap tests. The result of this meeting and subsequent ones in 1991 and 2001 became known as the Bethesda System for reporting cervicovaginal cytologic abnormalities.[8-10] The 2001 Bethesda terminology classifies a Pap test report as either negative for intraepithelial lesions or malignancy, or demonstrating an epithelial cell abnormality.[11] This latter category is subdivided into atypical squamous and glandular cells of undetermined significance,

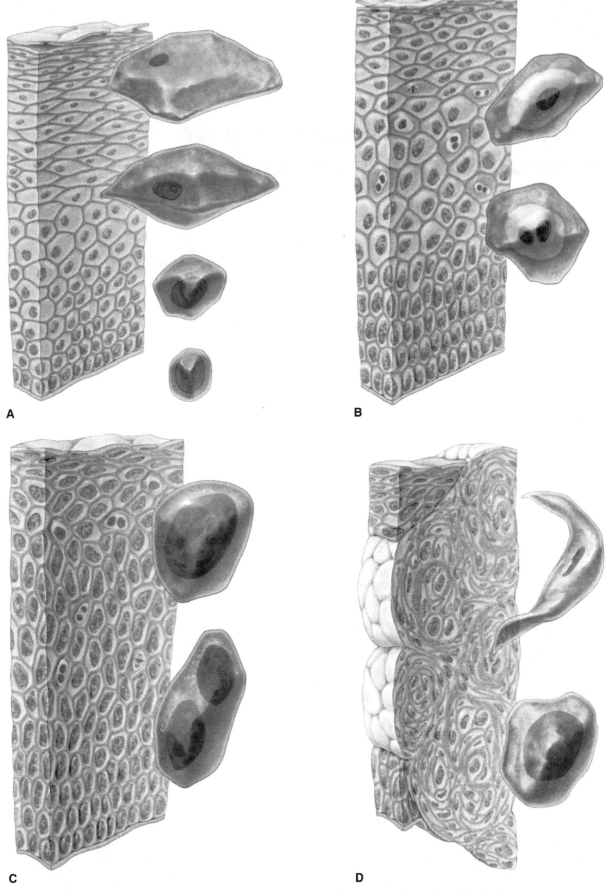

FIGURE 3.1. The cytology of individual normal and abnormal squamous cells and their histologic counterparts. **A:** Normal squamous epithelium and corresponding superficial, intermediate, parabasal, and basal cells. **B:** Low-grade squamous dysplasia and corresponding low-grade squamous intraepithelial cells. **C:** High-grade squamous dysplasia and corresponding high-grade squamous intraepithelial cells. **D:** Squamous cell carcinoma and corresponding malignant squamous cells.

TABLE 3.1	COMPARISON OF THE DIFFERENT CYTOLOGIC CLASSIFICATION SYSTEMS FOR CERVICOVAGINAL ABNORMALITIES		
■ PAPANICOLAOU	■ DYSPLASIA	■ CERVICAL INTRAEPITHELIAL NEOPLASIA	■ PAPILLOMAVIRUS
Class 1		Normal	
Class 2		Atypical	
Class 3	Mild dysplasia	CIN 1	Koilocytotic atypia CIN 1
	Moderate dysplasia	CIN 2	
	Severe dysplasia	CIN 3	
Class 4	Carcinoma *in situ*		
Class 5		Malignancy	

low- and high-grade squamous intraepithelial lesions (SIL), endocervical adenocarcinoma *in situ* (AIS), and squamous and glandular malignancies. Additionally, the Bethesda System requires comments on the specimen quality, using terms such as *satisfactory*, and *unsatisfactory* to indicate the interpretability of a submitted slide. Table 3.2 summarizes the Bethesda System currently in use.[11]

3.2.1.1 Quality of the Specimen

Specimen quality can affect the sensitivity of a cytologic specimen to identify cervicovaginal abnormalities.[12] The Bethesda System originally introduced three descriptors for the quality of the Pap test: *Satisfactory for Examination*, *Less than Optimal*, and *Unsatisfactory for Examination*.[8] Over time, *Satisfactory for Examination but Limited By (SBLB)* replaced the term *Less than Optimal*.[9] Although the latter term was considered more clinically useful than *Less than Optimal*, confusion persisted among providers that a satisfactory Pap test would still be limited in some way and, therefore, not be completely acceptable. This confusion led to the most recent revision of the Bethesda System terminology: elimination of this intermediate category altogether except for a descriptive comment. Hence, even if the specimen is satisfactory for examination, the reviewer should note whether a cellular component representing the transformation zone (TZ) (at least 10 metaplastic or 10 endocervical cells) is present. In addition, partially obscuring blood or inflammation, poor preservation of the cellular material, or lack of relevant clinical information can be noted as *Quality Indicators*.[11]

Reasons to label a specimen *Unsatisfactory for Examination* include the receipt of a broken slide, a slide with no patient identification (designated as *Rejected for Examination*), complete obscuration by blood or inflammation, or less than the minimally acceptable amount of cellular material on the slide. In the past, the amount of evaluable material on a slide was measured in percentages, with 10% being the minimum acceptable cellular amount, provided 50% to 75% of cells were well preserved.[9] Following the introduction and widespread adoption of specimens prepared using a liquid-based system, it has been recommended that an absolute number of cells be used as a minimally acceptable amount. For conventional specimens, the acceptable number is considered to be 10,000 to 12,000 cells; for liquid-based monolayer specimens, the minimal number is 5000.[11]

If abnormalities are identified on a specimen that would otherwise be considered unsatisfactory, the Bethesda System stipulates that they be reported rather than ignored even though the specimen is otherwise compromised.[9]

3.2.1.2 Negative for Squamous Intraepithelial Lesions or Malignancy

In the past, the descriptor *Benign Cellular Change* was used for epithelial cell alterations that reflect changes in the cervicovaginal environment from hormonal variations, shifts in pH, inflammation, overgrowth of vaginal flora, and exposure to external factors such as radiation and foreign material.[9] Although cells influenced by these issues do not appear to be normal, they reflect the effect of these benign influences rather than neoplasia. Nondysplastic epithelial cells that did not show these minimal variations were considered *Within Normal Limits*. *Benign Cellular Change* represented a compromise for pathologists who desired a category that encompassed cellular changes outside the realm of normal, yet did not represent premalignant potential. However, clinicians found the category confusing because the cells in question were qualified as not being normal. As a result, the most recent Bethesda System Workshop (2001) recommended combining the general categories *Within Normal Limits* and *Benign Cell Change* into one general category: *Negative for Intraepithelial Lesion or Malignancy*. This category can then be qualified by descriptors indicating the presence of various organisms or nonspecific reactive or reparative changes. The latter qualification is used to identify slides that require review and interpretation by a pathologist.[11,13]

3.2.1.3 Organisms

The cervicovaginal surface is polymicrobial and contains a large number of obligate and facultative organisms. Normally, the *Lactobacillus acidophilus* (Döderlein's bacillus) is present in large numbers and helps maintain an acidic pH (3.5 to 4.5). Organisms seen in fewer numbers include *Streptococcus viridans*, *Staphylococcus epidermidis*, *Bacteroides fecalis*, *Gardnerella (Hemophilus) vaginalis* and *Candida albicans*. These organisms vary depending on the hormonal milieu and pH of the vagina. Foreign material, such as tampons and intrauterine contraceptive device (IUD) strings, also can affect the number and type of organisms present. If there is an overgrowth of certain organisms normally found in the vagina, or if other pathogenic organisms are introduced by sexual activity, symptoms of a vaginal infection (discharge, odor, pruritus) may develop. In many cases, the causative organism or cellular changes indicative of a specific infection can be identified cytologically.[10,14]

Monilia, or yeast infections, are characterized by vaginal pruritus and a clumpy "cottage cheese" discharge. The etiologic agents are *Candida albicans* and, to a lesser extent, *Candida glabrata* and *Candida tropicalis*. The presence of these organisms is usually confirmed by examination of potassium hydroxide–treated wet mounts of the discharge or by culture. In a Papanicolaou-stained specimen, *Candida albicans* appears as pseudohyphae with buds. Epithelial cells cluster around the yeast forms in a rouleau formation. *Candida glabrata* are usually present in budding forms only, and *Candida tropicalis* in short stubby pseudohyphae with buds. The presence of yeast forms on Pap tests correlates highly with wet mount preparations in patients with symptomatic monilial infections (Figure 3.2).[14]

Specimen Type
 I. Conventional
 II. Liquid-based thin-layer preparation
 III. Other

Specimen Adequacy
 I. Satisfactory for evaluation (describe presence or absence of endocervical/TZ component and any other quality-limiting factors)
 II. Unsatisfactory for evaluation (specify reason)
 III. Specimen rejected (specify reason)
 IV. Specimen processed and examined, but unsatisfactory for evaluation of epithelial abnormality (specify reason)

General Categorization (Optional)
 I. Negative for intraepithelial lesion or malignancy
 II. Other: see interpretation/diagnosis (e.g., endometrial cells in a woman 40 y of age or older)
 III. Epithelial cell abnormality: see interpretation/diagnosis (specify "squamous" or ' "glandular," as appropriate)

Automated Review
If case is examined by automated device, specify device and result.

Ancillary Testing
Provide a brief description of the test methods and report the result so that the clinician easily understands it.

Descriptive Interpretations/Results
 I. Negative for intraepithelial lesion or malignancy (when there is no cellular evidence of neoplasia, state this in the General
    Categorization above and/or in the Interpretation/Diagnosis section of the report, whether or not there are organisms or other
    nonneoplastic findings)
 II. Organisms:
    A. *Trichomonas vaginalis*
    B. Fungal organisms morphologically consistent with *Candida spp.*
    C. Shift in vaginal flora suggestive of bacterial vaginosis
    D. Bacteria morphologically consistent with *Actinomyces spp.*
    E. Cellular changes associated with herpes simplex virus
 III. Other nonneoplastic findings (optional to report; list not inclusive)
    A. Reactive cellular changes associated with
       1. Inflammation (including typical repair)
       2. Radiation
       3. Intrauterine contraceptive device
    B. Benign-appearing glandular cells status post hysterectomy
    C. Atrophy
 IV. Other
    Endometrial cells (in a woman 40 y of age or older, specify if "negative for squamous intraepithelial lesion")
 V. Epithelial cell abnormalities
    A. Squamous cell
       1. Atypical squamous cells
          a. of undetermined significance (ASCUS)
          b. Cannot exclude a high-grade SIL (ASCH)
       2. Low-grade squamous intraepithelial lesion
          Encompassing HPV cytopathic effect/mild dysplasia/cervical intraepithelial neoplasia 1
       3. High-grade squamous intraepithelial lesion
          a. Encompassing: moderate and severe dysplasia, CIN 2, CIN 3 and CIS
          b. With features suspicious for invasion (if invasion is suspected)
       4. Squamous cell carcinoma
    B. Glandular cell
       1. Atypical
          a. Endocervical cells (not otherwise specified)
          b. Endometrial cells (not otherwise specified)
          c. Glandular cells (not otherwise specified)
       2. Atypical
          a. Endocervical cells, favor neoplastic
          b. Glandular cells, favor neoplastic
       3. Endocervical adenocarcinoma *in situ*
       4. Adenocarcinoma
          a. Endocervical
          b. Endometrial
          c. Extrauterine
          d. Not otherwise specified
    C. Other malignant neoplasms (specify)

Educational Notes and Recommendations (optional)
Suggestions should be concise and consistent with clinical follow-up guidelines published by professional organizations (references
to relevant publications may be included).

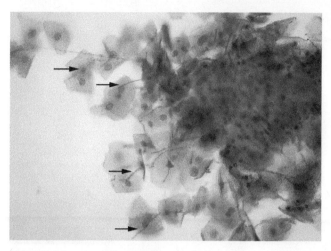

FIGURE 3.2. *Candida.* Branching hyphae are seen in a cluster of superficial and intermediate cells (*arrows*) (liquid preparation, Papanicolaou stain, high-power magnification).

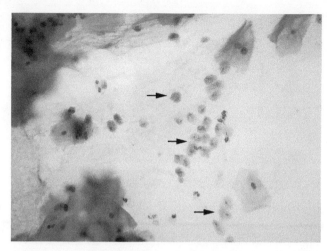

FIGURE 3.4. *Trichomonas.* The small protozoa are characterized by a cyanophilic cytoplasm and eccentric round to oval nuclei (*arrows*) (conventional preparation, Papanicolaou stain, high-power magnification).

Bacterial vaginosis is characterized by a malodorous gray adherent discharge; vaginal itching is variable. An increase in the vaginal pH leads to an overgrowth of the initiating organism, which is usually *G. vaginalis* (a gram-negative coccobacillus), and associated anaerobic vaginal flora. On wet mounts and cytologic specimens, the characteristic feature is bacteria-covered squamous epithelial cells called *clue cells.* For positive diagnosis, the bacteria must completely cover the cell and extend beyond the cell border, which gives the cell a moth-eaten appearance. In addition, the background is filmy or granular. If strict criteria are used to identify clue cells, bacterial vaginosis can be confirmed in 90% of patients with symptoms (Figure 3.3).[14,15]

Trichomonas vaginitis is characterized by vaginal itching and a greenish frothy discharge. Of the four *Trichomonas* species (*T. tenax, T hominis, T. fecalis, Trichomonas vaginalis*), *T. vaginalis* is most commonly associated with vaginal infections. The organism is sexually transmitted with an incubation time of 4 to 28 days. Factors that encourage proliferation of the trichomonads include endocervical mucus and associated vaginal flora. Clinical diagnosis consists of identifying the characteristic alkaline discharge, and motile organisms on wet-mount examination. Often, severe inflammation produces ecchymoses on the surface of the cervix and vagina ("strawberry cervix" or "strawberry spots"). On Pap tests, the organisms appear as pale amphophilic oval unicellular structures 100 μm in size. The nucleus is elongated and acentric and the cytoplasm contains red granules in well-preserved specimens. The trichomonads tend to cluster around the epithelial cell edge. Additionally, a cluster of leukocytes ("BB shot clusters") and a granular background are present. There is a high correlation among wet-mount preparations and vaginal cultures with trichomonads if strict criteria are used to identify *T. vaginalis* on cytologic specimens (Figure 3.4).[10,14,16]

Although often considered a fungus, the different actinomyces organisms (*Actinomyces israelii, Actinomyces bovis, and Actinomyces naeslundii*) actually represent a higher-order bacteria that also include the *Mycobacteriaceae* and *Streptomycetaceae. Actinomyces* infections are usually associated with foreign objects. Ten percent of women with IUDs become colonized with actinomyces, and the organism may persist 12 months after its removal. Histologically, actinomycosis is characterized by small yellow granules (sulfur granules). In cytologic specimens, small basophilic cotton ball clusters are identified on low-power examination; high-power inspection demonstrates acute angle branching of thin filamentous organisms (Figure 3.5A,B).[14]

Genital herpes virus infects the cervix in the immature squamous, metaplastic, or columnar cells. Once infected, the epithelial cells enlarge and fuse as a result of alterations in the cell membranes. The nuclei also enlarge and the nuclear membranes are accentuated because of margination of the nuclear chromatin. The nuclei cluster and the nuclear membranes compress each other. The chromatin-parachromatin interphase is lost and the chromatin material disperses. Pap tests from patients with herpetic infections will demonstrate multinucleated giant cells with nuclear molding (Figure 3.6), prominent nuclear membranes, and a homogenous "groundglass" nucleoplasm.[9,14]

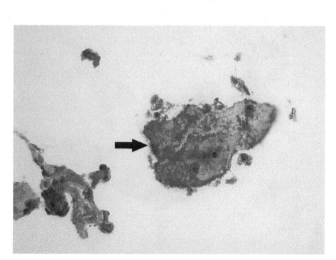

FIGURE 3.3. Bacterial vaginosis. A cluster of squamous cells is covered by bacterial organisms (clue cells), giving the cytoplasm a "moth-eaten" appearance (*arrow*) (liquid preparation, Papanicolaou stain, high-power magnification).

3.2.1.4 Reactive or Reparative Changes

Nonspecific cellular alterations have previously been classified as *cytologic atypias.* Atypia is a descriptive pathologic term that means "not in the range of normal." Cellular atypia could

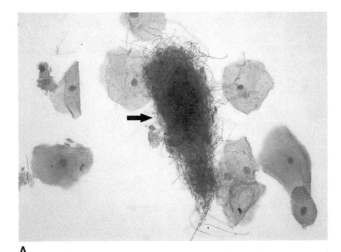

A

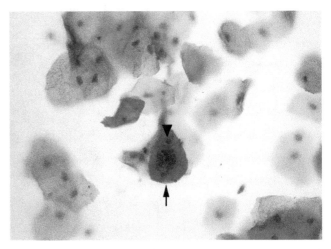

FIGURE 3.6.   Herpes simplex virus. A single teardrop-shaped squamous cell contains multiple nuclei with prominent central (Cowdry A) bodies (*arrow*). Nuclear molding (when adjacent cell nuclei conform to one another) is also present (liquid preparation, Papanicolaou stain, high-power magnification).

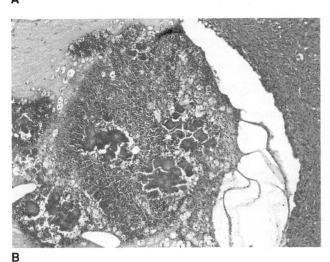

B

FIGURE 3.5.   Actinomyces. **A:** A central mass of thin filamentous strands is present (*arrow*) (liquid preparation, Papanicolaou stain, high-power magnification). **B:** On histology, small granules with radial filaments are present in a background of acute inflammatory cells (hematoxylin and eosin, medium-power magnification).

histologically to early metaplasia. The cells are arranged in sheets with recognizable cell borders. The nuclei are enlarged and hyperchromatic with slightly coarse chromatin. Nucleoli are recognizable (Figure 3.8A,B).[14]

Postmenopausal women not using hormone replacement therapy (HRT) can demonstrate reactive changes related to atrophy, which is characterized by sheets of parabasal cells with mild nuclear enlargement in an inflammatory background. Because of drying artifact in a high proportion of these specimens, the nuclei can be moderately enlarged and have smudged chromatin. Naked nuclei, which consist of basophilic amorphous material ("blue blobs"), represent degenerated parabasal cells. These changes can resolve with the application of a short course of topical estrogen.[17] Pap test results for patients who have undergone radiation treatment to the cervix and vagina will show increased cell size, multinucleation, and bizarre cell shapes. The cytoplasm is vacuolated and polychromatic. The nuclei demonstrate chromatin smudging and prominent single or multiple nucleoli (Figure 3.9).[10]

represent a number of conditions, including benign factors (inflammatory atypia, reactive atypia). However, historically clinicians equated atypia with premalignant changes. The confusion over different implications of the word "atypia" led to the introduction of the descriptive diagnosis *reactive or reparative change* as a substitute for atypical changes from benign processes.

Cytologically, reactive change caused by inflammation can occur in squamous or glandular cells and is usually represented by nuclear enlargement. In squamous cells, the enlargement is minimal—usually about 1.5 to 2 times the size of a normal intermediate cell nucleus. Glandular nuclei can show significant enlargement, along with multinucleation. The nuclei are hyperchromatic but lack coarseness. Mild cytoplasmic vacuolization is present, but there is no peripheral cytoplasmic accentuation (Figure 3.7). Hyperkeratosis and parakeratosis represent abnormal keratin production by mature and immature squamous epithelial cells. Cytologically, hyperkeratosis is characterized by the presence of mature orangeophilic or polychromatic squamous cells that lack nuclei ("ghost cells"). Parakeratotic cells are small orangeophilic cells with dark pyknotic nuclei. Reparative changes represent a healing process seen after severe or erosive inflammation and correspond

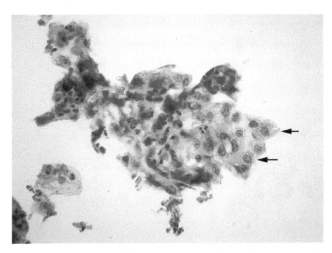

FIGURE 3.7.   Reactive squamous cells. A cohesive sheet of metaplastic-type cells demonstrates nuclei that are mildly enlarged with peripheral chromatin clumping and prominent nucleoli (*arrow*) (liquid preparation, Papanicolaou stain, high-power magnification).

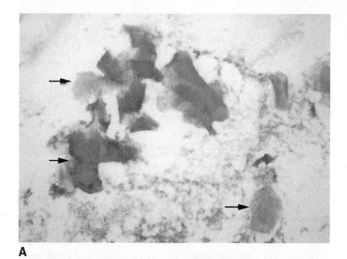

A

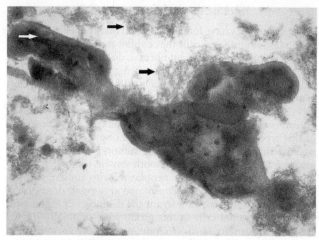

FIGURE 3.9.   Radiation change. A central cluster of large cells with enlarged round nuclei containing prominent nucleoli is seen. Cytoplasmic vacuoles are present (*white arrow*). The background contains numerous red blood cells (*black arrows*) (liquid preparation, Papanicolaou stain, high-power magnification).

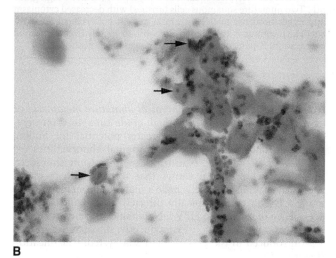

B

FIGURE 3.8.   **A:** Hyperkeratosis. A cluster of orangeophilic squamous cells that lack nuclear material is present (*arrow*) (conventional preparation, Papanicolaou stain, high-power magnification). **B:** Parakeratosis. Individual small orangeophilic cells with pyknotic ("dot-like") nuclei are present (*arrow*) (conventional preparation, Papanicolaou stain, high-power magnification).

of endometrial cells on a cytologic specimen was considered abnormal if these cells were present in the luteal phase of a reproductive-aged woman, or in a postmenopausal woman. It was thought that the presence of these cells indicated abnormal proliferation of the endometrium and could represent endometrial atypias or malignancies. However, the ability of the cytobrush, with its narrow tip, to easily remove endometrial cells from the lower uterine segment cavity, along with the presence of endometrial cells in postmenopausal women using HRT, made the presence of these cells not reliably predictive of uterine abnormalities. While most women with normal endometrial cells found on a Pap test will have no underlying abnormalities,[19] a number of published studies have indicated that a small number of women aged 40 or older with these cells may have underlying endometrial hyperplasia or/and carcinoma.[20-22] The present Bethesda System revision, therefore, recommended the reporting of normal endometrial cells in a woman aged 40 years or older, regardless of whether she is cycling normally or using hormonal therapy.[11]

In addition to actinomycosis, specimens from women with IUDs may show metaplastic cell clusters with high nuclear-to-cytoplasmic ratios and prominent nucleoli. These cells will have large cytoplasmic vacuoles that displace the nucleus. Psammomatous-type calcifications are occasionally seen. IUDs can also generate small endometrial-like cells known as IUD cells.[14]

3.2.1.5 Cytologic Evidence of Vaginal Glandular Cells or Normal Endometrial Cells

Prior to the most recent 2001 TBS changes, endocervical-type cells seen on vaginal specimen were considered a cytologic form of adenosis and were classified as a glandular cell abnormality. Since it is now known that women with normal endocervical cells on a vaginal specimen do not necessarily have underlying vaginal dysplasias or malignancies, this finding is no longer considered atypical. It is important for the provider, however, to report the precise source of the specimen so that glandular cells from the endocervix are not interpreted as vaginal cells.[3,18]

Normal endometrial cells are characterized cytologically as small cell clusters with diminutive round nuclei and minimally apparent nucleoli (Figure 3.10).[10] Traditionally, the presence

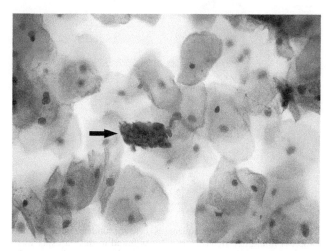

FIGURE 3.10.   Endometrial cells. A small cluster of benign round cells with sparse cytoplasm and round to oval basophilic nuclei is present (*arrow*) (liquid preparation, Papanicolaou stain, high-power magnification).

3.2.1.6 Atypical Squamous Cells

Cytopathologists have long understood that there is a category of squamous epithelial cells that exhibit nuclear and cytoplasmic variations that, while not normal, do not clearly represent morphology consistent with either benign cell changes or dysplasia. In other words, the behavior of these groups of cells cannot be determined by the usual assessment of cytologic features. Because of this, the category *Atypical Squamous Cells of Undetermined Significance (ASC-US)* was created.[8] Categories of this type have existed in other areas of gynecologic pathology. Epithelial ovarian borderline tumors, vulvar aggressive angiomyxomas, and uterine smooth muscle tumors of uncertain malignant potential are neoplasms with similar atypical features. Although they are considered abnormal, their histologies are not sufficient to warrant the diagnosis of malignant. The cervicovaginal cells in this group were originally named *Atypical Squamous Cells of Undetermined Significance,* and until 2001, qualifiers such as "favor reactive" and "favor neoplastic" were used to suggest potential behavior.[9,10,23] Presently, there are two categories of ASC: *Atypical Squamous Cells of Undetermined Significance (ASC-US)* and *Atypical Cells, Cannot Exclude a High-Grade Squamous Intraepithelial Lesions (ASC-H).*[11]

As defined by the Bethesda System, cells categorized as ASC-US have nuclear enlargement that is 2.5 to 3 times the normal intermediate cell nucleus. There is mild variation in nuclear size and shape and mild to moderate hyperchromasia of the nucleoplasm, but the chromatin is evenly distributed. The cytoplasm can show evidence of mild clearing, but the peripheral halo borders are poorly defined (Figure 3.11). In atrophy, the nuclei can show significant enlargement, irregular shapes, and hyperchromasia; however, these features usually resolve with topical estrogen treatment. ASC-US also encompasses atypical or pleomorphic parakeratosis, which consists of irregularly shaped orangeophilic cells with enlarged darkly stained nuclei.[10] Unfortunately, in spite of established morphologic changes, the diagnosis of ASC-US is poorly reproducible, as different pathologists use uniquely personal criteria to signify this diagnosis.[24]

Recently, cytopathologists have recognized that ASC characterized by small immature metaplastic cells with dark

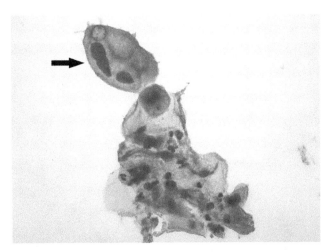

FIGURE 3.11. Atypical squamous cells of undetermined significance. A multinucleate cell (*arrow*) was found in this Pap specimen. The nuclei are mildly enlarged and irregularly shaped. However, the nuclear membranes are smooth, and the chromatin is uniform (liquid preparation, Papanicolaou stain, high-power magnification).

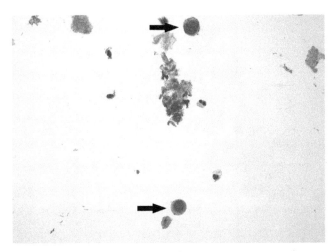

FIGURE 3.12. Atypical squamous cells, cannot exclude a high-grade SIL. Two immature squamous cells (*arrows*) with decreased cytoplasm and hyperchromatic nuclei with mild nuclear enlargement are present. The membranes are otherwise smooth to slightly irregular (liquid preparation, Papanicolaou stain, high-power magnification).

irregular nuclei, often called *atypical immature metaplasia* or *atypical cells-suspicious for a high-grade squamous intraepithelial lesion,* may indicate a greater potential for finding significant underlying cervical and vaginal abnormalities.[25,26] Analysis of a completed National Cancer Institute-sponsored prospective clinical trial shows that women with cytologic specimens having these cells have a higher percentage of high-grade CIN on colposcopically directed biopsy and a higher prevalence of oncogenic HPV DNA than do women with cells consistent with ASC-US.[27] Consequently, the qualifier ASC-H was introduced in the present Bethesda System Classification (Figure 3.12).[11]

3.2.1.7 Low-grade Squamous Intraepithelial Lesions

The finding of dysplastic cells on a Pap test indicates the presence of these cells on the surface of the cervix or vagina. For any degree of dysplasia, the hallmark cytologic feature is abnormal nuclear transformation. The nucleus enlarges, there is wrinkling of the nuclear membrane, and the chromatin becomes more distinct (coarse). If mild air-drying is present, the nuclear chromatin will appear hyperchromatic and smudged. As with histologic evidence of dysplasia, the degree or grade of dysplasia is dependent cytologically on the size of the dysplastic cell and, to a lesser extent, the number of dysplastic cells. The latter will be related to cell sampling, which reflects the skill of the examiner, the size of the abnormality, and the type of processing. Although it was previously thought that the interval between Pap tests might affect the cell yield on the slide, recent data from the ASCUS LSIL Triage Study (ALTS) have proven this to not be true.[28] Low-grade dysplasia is characterized by the transformation of mature (superficial or intermediate) epithelial cells, whereas high-grade dysplasia is characterized by transformation of immature (metaplastic or parabasal/basal) cells.

The term *low-grade squamous intraepithelial lesion* (LSIL) encompasses the categories of mild dysplasia, CIN 1, and various descriptors indicating the presence of HPV, such as condylomatous dysplasia or koilocytotic atypia. The category LSIL reflects evidence that these diverse descriptors demonstrate the same progression rates when compared to notable abnormalities (high-grade dysplasia or carcinoma) and the inability of

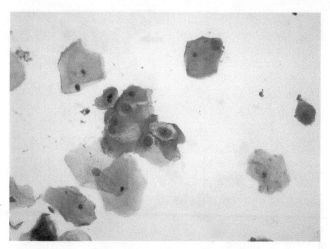

FIGURE 3.13. Low-grade SIL. The nuclei in these dysplastic cells are moderately enlarged compared to the nuclei of the adjacent normal squamous cells. In addition, there is perinuclear clearing and accentuation of the peripheral cytoplasm (koilocytosis). The cell size is equivalent to that of a mature squamous cell (liquid preparation, Papanicolaou stain, high-power magnification).

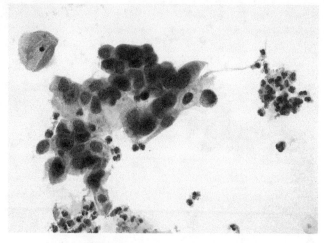

FIGURE 3.14. High-grade SIL (moderate dysplasia). Clusters of immature dysplastic cells are present that have enlarged, abnormally shaped hyperchromatic nuclei with irregular nuclear borders. The cell size is equivalent to a metaplastic cell (liquid preparation, Papanicolaou stain, high-power magnification).

pathologists to differentiate mild dysplasias from supposedly pure HPV infections.

The nuclear size of a cell interpreted as LSIL is at least three times the size of a normal intermediate cell or polymorphonucleocyte nucleus. The nuclear appearance is "raisinoid," with irregular nuclear shapes and membrane wrinkling. The nucleoplasm demonstrates hyperchromasia and smudging. Multinucleation along with variation of nuclear size is also present. Nucleoli are absent. LSIL is confined to intermediate or superficial-type cells. Although enlarged, the nucleus occupies only one-third the total cell area. Many of these cells will have perinuclear clearing and aggregation of the cytoplasm into the cell periphery, consistent with koilocytosis. As with koilocytes seen in biopsy specimens, the border between the clear space and the cytoplasm is distinct (Figure 3.13).[10,18]

3.2.1.8 High-grade Squamous Intraepithelial Lesions

The term *high-grade squamous intraepithelial lesion (HSIL)* encompasses cytologically the categories of moderate and severe dysplasia, CIN 2 and 3, and carcinoma *in situ* (CIS). The primary reason given to combine these categories into one (HSIL) is the impression that while the degree of dysplasia appears different histologically, the subjective nature of cytology makes subdivision of the HSIL category less exact. Because this concept is not universally accepted, the histologic grading of high-grade dysplasia remains separated into three major tiers,[29] and cytologists are encouraged to qualify, when possible, a diagnosis of HSIL into a moderate dysplasia (CIN 2), severe dysplasia (CIN 3), or CIS.[8,10]

Cytologic specimens from patients with CIN 2 consist of cells with nuclear features similar to those in LSIL. The cell size, however, is the equivalent of an immature metaplastic cell. The nucleus can occupy up to half the total cell area. Because of this decrease in cytoplasmic amount, the nuclear-to-cytoplasmic ratio (N/C ratio) is decreased. The cells are arranged singly, in sheets, or in syncytial-like aggregates (Figure 3.14). Specimens from patients having CIN 3 contain cells that are similar to parabasal or reserve cell in size. Although the nuclei have dysplastic features similar to those of LSIL, the nuclear size is smaller. Because of the smaller cell size

and the relatively large nuclear area in relation to the amount of cell cytoplasm, the N/C ratio is markedly increased. The cells are either isolated or have a characteristic linear arrangement. Cells with negligible cytoplasm ("stripped nuclei") or large syncytial aggregates containing mostly nuclei ("microtissue fragments") are cytologically consistent with CIS (Figure 3.15).[10,18]

3.2.1.9 Invasive Squamous Cell Carcinoma

Invasive squamous cell carcinoma indicates disruption of the basement membrane and invasion into the underlying stroma. For this to occur, the squamous cells proliferate rapidly and may outgrow their blood supply. This may lead to necrosis or a tumor diathesis. The background of a specimen with invasive carcinoma is often described as "dirty." There is marked inflammation, hemorrhage, and fragments of degenerated cytoplasmic

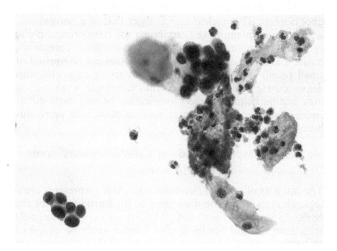

FIGURE 3.15. High-grade SIL (severe dysplasia or CIS). Two clusters of dysplastic cells from different areas are present. The small basaloid cells have minimal cytoplasm, and the irregularly shaped hyperchromatic nuclei are enlarged relative to the overall cell size. The nuclear to cytoplasmic ratio, therefore, is markedly increased (liquid preparation, Papanicolaou stain, high-power magnification).

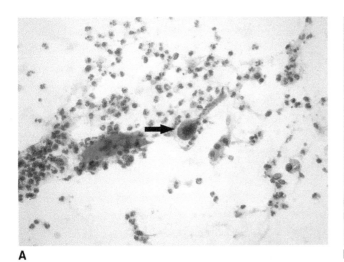
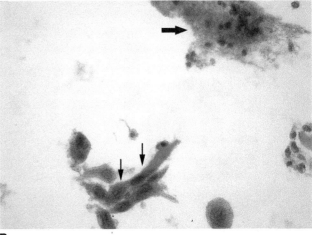

A   B

FIGURE 3.16.   Squamous cell carcinoma. **A:** A tadpole-shaped (caudate) cell (*arrow*) is present in the center of the field (conventional preparation, Papanicolaou stain, high-power magnification). **B:** A cluster of elongated cells that have enlarged nuclei with distinct nucleoli are present (*thin arrows*). Focal orangeophilic staining indicates abnormal keratin production. There is also patchy ("cotton-candy") necrosis (*thick arrow*) in the upper right of the photomicrograph as indicated by the *thick arrow* (liquid preparation, Papanicolaou stain, high-power magnification).

and nuclear material. The diathesis in a liquid-based specimen is subtler; and the degenerated elements are more condensed. The appearance of the degenerated elements is described as having a "cotton candy" consistency (Figure 3.16A,B). Squamous cell carcinomas that invade between 3 mm and 5 mm can also demonstrate cytologic evidence of a tumor diathesis.[29]

The individual malignant cells reflect the capability to invade adjacent stromal tissues or to "metastasize." This is particularly true in microinvasive squamous cell carcinoma, which is often localized in a background of CIN. Specifically, the cells are arranged in syncytial aggregates similar to that in CIS. In contrast to CIS, however, nucleoli are present; macronucleoli can also be seen but are infrequent.[18]

In invasive squamous cell carcinoma, the cells have abnormal forms. The shape is dependent on the surface tension, viscosity of the cytoplasm, and rigidity of the cell membrane, and is more common in the keratinizing squamous cell carcinomas. The cells can be arranged in syncytial masses with indistinct borders. The nuclear area is twice that of a normal cell. Keratinizing squamous cell carcinoma will have orangeophilic cytoplasm. The nuclei are dark and contain dense chromatin; nucleoli are not seen. Small-cell carcinomas are comprised of small round cells that consist almost entirely of nuclei with dense coarse granular chromatin. Cytologic examination may not be helpful in the identification of very well differentiated squamous carcinomas, such as those with verrucous histology.[18]

3.2.1.10 Atypical Glandular Cells/Adenocarcinoma *In Situ*

The category of atypical glandular cells (AGC) represents cytologic changes not recognized prior to the introduction of the Bethesda System. As with ASC, AGC represents glandular cells with morphologic variations that cannot easily be classified as benign, premalignant, or malignant.[9,10] Under the present Bethesda system revision, any atypical glandular cells should be categorized as either endocervical or endometrial in origin if possible.[14] Also, it should be noted if a glandular dysplastic process is favored. As with ASC, the reproducibility of this diagnosis is also poor.[30] Sensitive and specific biomarkers may have future discriminatory use similar to that of squamous atypias and intraepithelial neoplasias.[31]

In conventional specimens, atypical endocervical cells tend to shed in sheets or clusters. However, the cell borders and consistent spacing normally seen between benign glandular cells are lost. The nuclei are enlarged and demonstrate mild variation in size and shape. The chromatin is increased in density, nucleoli are usually not seen, and mitoses may be noted. The overall nuclear-to-cytoplasmic ratio is increased because of nuclear enlargement; however, a reactive endocervical cell can also show a marked increase in nuclear size.[27] Other differential interpretations include degenerative changes in immature metaplastic cells caused by infections such as trichomoniasis, lower uterine segment endometrial cells that are commonly obtained post conization, cervical endometriosis, and reactive change due to vigorous rotation of the cytobrush. In the past, the cytologic diagnosis of AIS had been included in the broad category of AGUS. Recently, however, specific cytologic features (nuclear rosettes that "feather" or palisade peripherally) that are unique to AIS have been described. This interpretation can now be reported separately from AGC (Figure 3.17A,B).[10]

Atypical endometrial cells are seen in small clusters usually containing five to ten cells. The nuclei are slightly enlarged and the nuclear-to-cytoplasmic ratios are increased. Nucleoli are usually present (Figure 3.18).[10]

3.2.1.11 Invasive Adenocarcinoma

The cytologic features of invasive adenocarcinoma can be similar to AIS, but in the former, nucleoli are readily evident and the nuclear chromatin is irregular in consistency. There also may be considerable variation in nuclear size, and a tumor diathesis may be present. Specialized endocervical adenocarcinomas, such as clear cell and serous change, may appear as poorly differentiated carcinomas. Minimum deviation adenocarcinoma, or adenoma malignum, is a well-differentiated adenocarcinoma with malignant cells that have bland features. Because of this, cytologic changes useful in diagnosing this entity have not been consistently described (Figure 3.19).[10,32]

In endometrial adenocarcinomas, the malignant cells are in small clusters. Although comparatively small, there is variation in nuclear size and nucleoli are evident. Poorly differentiated carcinoma cells in a clean background characterize adenocarcinomas that are metastatic to the cervix (Figure 3.20).[32]

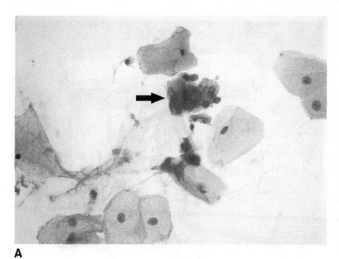

A

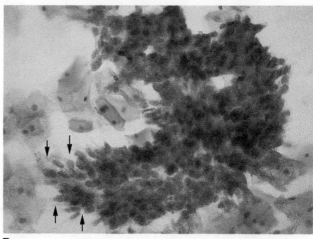

B

FIGURE 3.17.   Atypical endocervical cells. **A:** A small central cluster of atypical glandular cells is present (*arrow*). The nuclei are slightly enlarged, and the chromatin is coarse (liquid preparation, Papanicolaou stain, high-power magnification). **B:** A large group of atypical glandular cells. Note the peripheral palisading known as "feathering." (*arrow*) These features are indicative of an endocervical AIS (conventional preparation, Papanicolaou stain, high-power magnification).

3.2.2 New Technologies in Cervicovaginal Cytology

In the past decade, various ancillary technologies have been developed to augment the way cervical cytologic specimens are prepared and screened. Technologies used today fall into two general categories: specimen preparation (liquid-based, thin-layer systems) and computerized systems. The latter have been divided into methods that target certain slide areas for manual interpretation (digital imaging systems) and those that identify slides requiring manual rescreening for potential abnormalities (computer-assisted screening).

3.2.2.1 Processing Systems

Presently, there are two systems FDA approved for Pap test preparation: ThinPrep® Pap test (Hologic, Inc., Bedford, MA, Figure 3.21) and the SurePath™ Pap test (BD Diagnostics

Corporation, Franklin Lakes, NJ, Figure 3.22). Collection devices approved for ThinPrep® include the Cervex-Brush or Papette, or a combination of a Cytobrush and plastic spatula. These devices are also acceptable for the SurePath™ system, although with this system the heads are designed to be detachable and must be transported to the lab in the liquid medium. Both systems use a cell-preservative solution (Figure 3.23A,B). For ThinPrep®, stirring the devices in the solution transfers the material. For SurePath™, the device tip is also sent in the solution to the laboratory. The transference of cells from the solution to the slide differs for the two systems. With ThinPrep®, the material is dispersed by spinning, suctioned onto a Nuclepore filter to remove debris, and transferred onto a glass slide. For SurePath™, the cells are dispersed by withdrawing the material into a syringe containing a cell enrichment solution. The material is then centrifuged and vortexed to remove debris. Finally, the cells are transferred to a glass slide through gravitation. Regardless of the preparation method, the slides are screened in the conventional fashion (Figure 3.24).

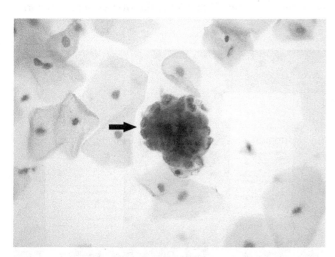

FIGURE 3.18.   Atypical endometrial cells. In contrast to benign endometrial cells, the nuclei are enlarged and irregularly shaped (*arrow*). In addition, the chromatin is coarse and small, but distinct nucleoli can be detected (liquid preparation, Papanicolaou stain, high-power magnification).

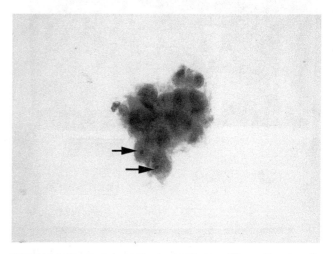

FIGURE 3.19.   Endocervical adenocarcinoma. The malignant cells maintain a rounded glandular shape. Note the prominent nucleoli in this rounded cluster of malignant cells (*arrow*) (liquid preparation, Papanicolaou stain, high-power magnification).

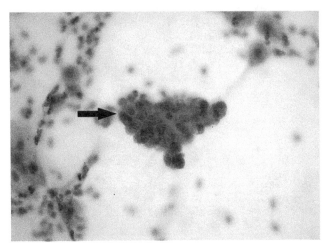

FIGURE 3.20. Endometrial adenocarcinoma (*arrow*). The cells are smaller than malignant endocervical cells, but they maintain their glandular shape. The nuclei are enlarged, irregularly shaped, have coarse chromatin, and have distinct but small nucleoli (liquid preparation, Papanicolaou stain, high-power magnification).

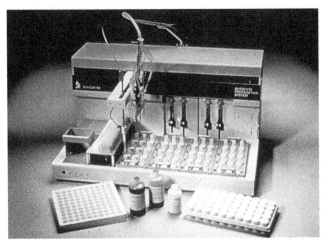

FIGURE 3.22. SurePath™ processing machine. The device can process and stain up to 48 specimens at one time, but the slides and liquid tubes have to be individually loaded by hand. (BD Corporation, Franklin Lakes, NJ; used with permission).

There are obvious advantages to liquid-based, thin-layered specimens. Air-dried and obscured slides should be eliminated. The material is well preserved and abnormal cells are easily recognizable. Numerous split-sample (preparing a conventional smear and a liquid-based monolayer slide from material obtained from the same cervix) and direct-to-vial (all material placed in the liquid medium) studies have shown a decrease in the number of specimens limited by obscuring blood,

inflammation, or drying artifact.[33–35] Some investigators have also reported a decrease in the number of specimens interpreted as ASC and a corresponding increase in SIL in several split-sample studies, corresponding to an increase in CIN on colposcopically directed biopsy.[36,37] However, the largest meta-analysis of liquid-based cytology studies has not demonstrated benefit over conventional cytology.[38] Nevertheless, an additional advantage of LBC is that the suspension can be used to create multiple slides if outside consultation is necessary or if additional studies, such as HPV DNA typing or screening for chlamydia and gonococcal organisms, are requested.

There are, however, disadvantages to both systems. Cytotechnologists and pathologists need additional training to screen and interpret these slides. Screening must be deliberate, as fewer normal and abnormal cells are available for review. These systems are expensive for laboratories to institute, and the continuous use of disposables (filters, vials with preservatives, collection devices, slides) leads to additional costs. These expenses may be at least partially offset by the decrease in the number of patient visits necessary for reevaluation of Pap tests with unclear results.[39] Presently, the overwhelming majority

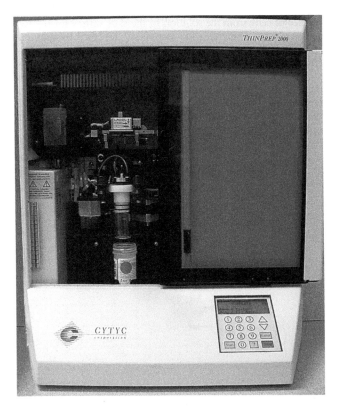

FIGURE 3.21. ThinPrep® processing machine (T-2000). The device can only process one specimen at a time; staining is completed in the usual fashion. It takes about 1 to 2 minutes to transfer the material from the liquid container to a glass slide. (Hologic, Inc., Bedford, MA; used with permission).

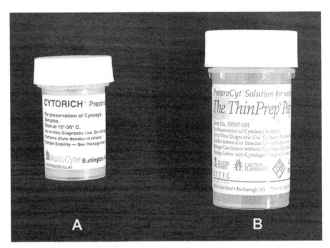

FIGURE 3.23. Liquid preservatives. **A:** Cytorich solution (TRIPATH Corporation, Burlington, NC, used with permission). **B:** PreservCyt solution. (Hologic, Inc., Bedford, MA; used with permission).

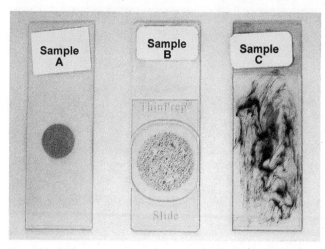

FIGURE 3.24. Comparison slides. **A:** SurePath™ slide. The button is approximately 13 mm in diameter. (BD Corporation, Franklin Lakes, NJ; used with permission). **B:** ThinPrep® slide. The button is approximately 22 mm in diameter (Hologic, Inc., Bedford, MA; used with permission). **C:** Conventional slide. Note the uneven thickness and staining.

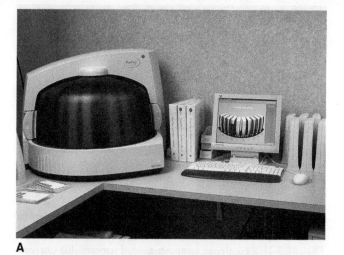

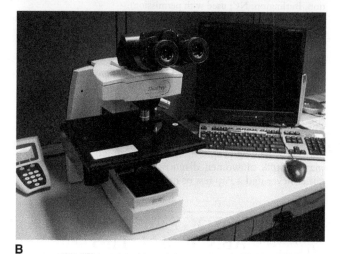

FIGURE 3.25. Hologic ThinPrep® imaging system. **A:** The computer-assisted imager. **B:** A microscope with a motorized stage networked to the imager. (Hologic, Inc., Bedford, MA; used with permission.)

of specimens screened in cytopathology laboratories in the United States are liquid based.

3.2.2.2 Digital Imaging Systems

These systems use an optical scanner to examine a specimen and identify areas of the slide with cells that require further evaluation. These areas are then captured as a digital image and presented on a computer monitor for examination. If needed, the original glass slide sample can also be examined and correlated with the computer images. Numerous studies using an early model system consistently demonstrated the accuracy and effectiveness of digital image analysis.[40–42] Presently, two systems are approved for use in the United States. One is the BD FocalPoint GS ("Guided Screening") Imaging System (BD Diagnostics Corporation, Franklin Lakes, NJ), which presents 10 fields of view that contain cells identified by the BD Focal-Point Slide Profiler (see below) as the most likely to contain abnormal features. If confirmed as atypical, the entire slide is then reviewed and interpreted by the cytotechnologist. The second is the ThinPrep® Imaging System (Hologic, Inc., Bedford, MA, Figure 3.25A,B), which identifies 22 fields with potentially abnormal cells. These fields are presented to the cytotechnologist on a microscope with a motorized stage. Using computer-generated coordinates, the cells in question are quickly assessed and evaluated. If any field is considered abnormal by the technologist, the entire slide is then screened and interpreted. The advantage of these systems is the ability of cytotechnologists to direct their attention to those areas identified by the computer as potentially abnormal. Screening time can therefore be reduced and the cytotechnologist's efforts more focused. However, the equipment has been expensive to install and maintain, and cytotechnologists and pathologists need additional training to operate the equipment and interpret the slides.[43] In addition, while identification of important abnormalities such as ASC-H, LSIL and HSIL is improved, the diagnosis of minimal abnormalities is not necessarily decreased.[44]

3.2.2.3 Computer Analysis and Reporting Systems

The only system FDA approved for commercial use is Focal-Point Slide Profiler (BD Diagnostics Corporation, Franklin Lakes, NJ, Figure 3.26). The FocalPoint Profiler uses a high-resolution digital scanner to image individual cells on a Pap

test. The computer uses a Bayesian Belief Network Technology to classify cells as normal or abnormal. It then quantifies ("scores") the degree of abnormality to a threshold percentage programmed by the company or the laboratory (10%, 20%, 30%). This represents a percentage of slides that the scanner will identify for manual screening.[45] In a typical laboratory setting, the Profiler can substitute as a primary screening system in low-risk patients at a setting of 20% manual screen threshold, and for a random rescreening system of 10% normal tests. In the latter, the Profiler can rescreen all normal Pap tests and, using a threshold percentage point of 10%, would identify slides requiring manual rescreening. Initial studies evaluating the FocalPoint system demonstrated a three- to fourfold improvement over manual rescreening of specimens originally interpreted as normal.[46,47] The FocalPoint Profiler, using a threshold percentage of 20%, has also been approved for primary screening of low-risk patients and can now screen liquid-based slides prepared using the SurePath™ system. Major disadvantages include the considerable purchase and maintenance expense for this device, which is unaffordable to all but the largest laboratories.

Much concern has been expressed recently over the cost of these various new technologies and whether they should be considered standard of care.[47–50] Various cost-efficiency models have been developed to compare liquid-based screening, digital imaging, and computer-assisted screening methods to each

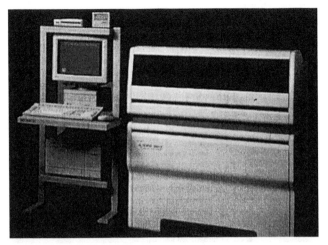

FIGURE 3.26. Focalpoint computer-assisted screener. (BD Corporation, Burlington, NC; used with permission).

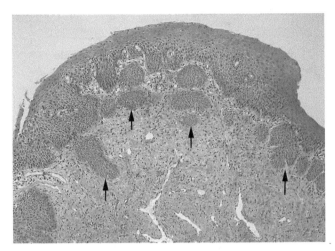

FIGURE 3.27. Cervical biopsy with squamous metaplasia. Although no endocervical cells are seen, the presence of immature squamous cell nests in the superficial stroma (*arrows*) is consistent with squamous metaplasia (hematoxylin and eosin, medium-power magnification).

other and to various other screening and preventative systems. Most have demonstrated that the new technologies can be of value in reducing the ill-defined costs of patient visits for evaluation and management of poor-quality Pap tests and unclear diagnoses.[39,51–53] Whether these cost savings will translate into reduction in the overall incidence of cervical cancer is unclear. It must be remembered that the most reliable way to reduce deaths from this malignancy is to encourage women to participate in a periodic screening program, since in the United States, approximately 50% of women diagnosed with cervical cancer have either never had a Pap test or not had one in the past 5 years.

3.3 HISTOLOGY OF SQUAMOUS ABNORMALITIES

The diagnostic specimens usually submitted by colposcopists for histologic examination are directed biopsies, loop excision or conization specimens, and endocervix curettings. Although small, these samples can supply a great deal of valuable information.

Colposcopically directed biopsies of the cervix are examined for the presence of the TZ. By convention, this is defined as the presence of endocervical gland elements adjacent to, or beneath, squamous epithelium. In some cases, nonglycogenated immature squamous cells replacing superficial glands can also represent squamous metaplasia (Figure 3.27). Orientation of the fragment is important; ideally, an intact basement membrane and surface should be identifiable. This is necessary for grading any surface intraepithelial neoplasia, as the severity is determined by assessing the proportion of basaloid dysplastic cells extending from the basement membrane toward the surface. Because endocervical curettage specimens contain small and unoriented fragments, the pathologist usually can indicate only that dysplasia is either present or absent (Figure 3.28A,B).

Unless stated to be an excisional biopsy, a pathologist will consider small biopsy specimens to be diagnostic only and will not comment on the presence or absence of abnormalities at the resection margins. On the other hand, by convention, all loop electrosurgical excision procedures (LEEP) and conization

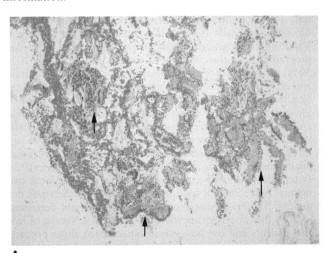

A

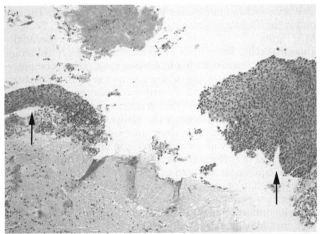

B

FIGURE 3.28. Endocervical curettings. **A:** Scattered fragments of endocervical gland epithelia (*arrow*) are seen in a background of mucus and red blood cells (hematoxylin and eosin, medium-power magnification). **B:** Fragments of detached dysplasia are present (*arrow*). As there is no surface or basement membrane, an accurate grade cannot be given. Nevertheless, the proliferation of squamous cells with enlarged atypical nuclei and scant cell cytoplasm suggests a high-grade dysplasia (hematoxylin and eosin, medium-power magnification).

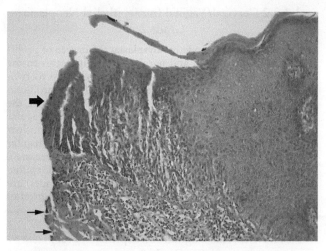

FIGURE 3.29.   Loop excisional specimen. There is high-grade dysplasia that extends to the specimen edge (*thick arrow*). The presence of black ink on the surface (*thin arrows*) and thermal damage (cell distortion) marks this edge as a resection margin (hematoxylin and eosin, medium-power magnification).

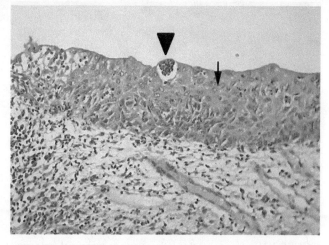

FIGURE 3.30.   Reactive cervicitis. The immature metaplastic cells have enlarged nuclei and prominent nucleoli. Considerable cytoplasm is present (*thin arrow*), and cell borders are recognizable. Acute inflammatory cells are present in the epithelium, and there is a small microabscess (*thick arrow*) (hematoxylin and eosin, medium-power magnification).

specimens are considered excisional unless stated otherwise. Because multipass LEEP specimens often cut through intraepithelial neoplasia, it can be difficult to determine the true resection margins unless specifically marked on the specimen by the clinician or illustrated on the requisition form. The presence of thermal artifact (char) along the edge of a loop excision specimen is useful to identify the line of excision (Figure 3.29). Traditional conization specimens are marked with colored ink along the nonmucosal cut edge before the specimen is sectioned for processing. When seen under the microscope, the presence of ink along a tissue edge differentiates a true resection margin from one created by tissue processing.

A pathologist should provide the following information on a diagnostic biopsy: degree of intraepithelial neoplasia if the specimen is oriented; histologic type and grade; and presence of lymphatic and vascular space invasion by tumor cells, if invasive carcinoma is identified. For excisional biopsies, such as LEEP or conization specimen oriented by the colposcopist, the pathologist should report the degree of intraepithelial neoplasia, its extent (usually reported as numbers on a clock face), and completeness of excision. If invasive squamous cell carcinoma is identified, the histologic type, grade, depth of invasion, horizontal extent, completeness of excision, and presence of lymphatic and vascular space invasion should be reported.

3.3.1 Reactive and Reparative Changes

It is common for areas of squamous metaplasia to demonstrate evidence of acute or, more frequently, chronic inflammation. The changes are generally nonspecific but can be related to various infectious organisms. In some instances, lymphoid follicles (collections of lymphocytes in the tissue) can be identified in the superficial stroma, a condition known as chronic follicular cervicitis.[54] Depending on the degree of inflammation, the surface epithelium can slough (erosive cervicitis). Immature metaplastic squamous cells quickly replace the lost squamous or glandular epithelia through a process known as repair. Typically, these cells have larger nuclei than the usual metaplastic cell. Nuclear chromatin is more granular, and nucleoli are prominent (Figure 3.30). These reactive squamous changes can be distinguished from squamous dysplasia by the presence of smooth nuclear borders, general uniformity of nuclear size, presence of distinct cell borders, and lack of

nuclear overlap. Mitoses are uncommon and, if present, are usually found along the basal cell layer. No abnormal mitotic forms are identified.[18,54]

3.3.2 Intraepithelial Lesions

Squamous intraepithelial neoplastic abnormalities, also referred to as squamous dysplasia, are associated with the presence of HPV. The degree of surface abnormality reflects the type of viral interaction with the immature squamous cell. In mild degrees of dysplasia, HPV produces proteins that direct the host cell to undergo maturation and cell death. The end result is a cell that exfoliates, disintegrates, and releases large numbers of intact viral particles. Higher degrees of dysplasia reflect actual disruption of the HPV DNA and integration into the host cell genome. Unregulated production of oncogenic viral proteins results in transformation and proliferation of the immature basal or parabasal cells that contain the viral DNA. Squamous dysplastic cells commonly contain cytokeratins 10, 11, 13, and 16, which reflect the squamous origin of these cells. As dysplasia worsens, however, the cytokeratin distribution becomes more consistent with those found in immature metaplastic cells.[18]

The hallmark of surface dysplasia is the presence of variable abnormal cytologic features in the squamous epithelial cells. These dysplastic cells may extend into and fill superficial endocervical glands (Figure 3.31). The basement membrane, nevertheless, remains intact along the affected surface and around the involved glands. The World Health Organization recognizes two general classification systems: cervical or vaginal dysplasia graded as mild, moderate, and severe, and CIS, or cervical or vaginal intraepithelial neoplasia (CIN/VaIN) graded as 1, 2, and 3.[18,55–59]

3.3.2.1 Cervical/Vaginal Intraepithelial Neoplasia Grade 1

The hallmark cell of CIN 1/VaIN 1, or mild dysplasia, is the *koilocyte*. This cell reflects marked degeneration of a mature squamous cell with a nucleus filled with particles of HPV. Koilocytes are located in the upper two-thirds of the squamous surface and are characterized by superficial or intermediate-type cells with nuclei that are enlarged three times the size of

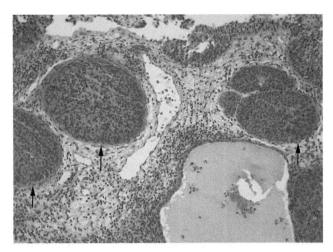

FIGURE 3.31.   Squamous dysplasia present in superficial endocervical glands (*arrows*). Although highly cellular, the basement membrane is intact. Dysplasia is also present on the surface (hematoxylin and eosin, medium-power magnification).

a normal intermediate cell nucleus. The nuclei are dark with coarse chromatin that fills the nucleus or aggregates in the periphery (vesicular change). Nucleoli usually are not seen. The nuclear membrane is markedly wrinkled, giving the enlarged nucleus a raisin-like appearance. Often, a single cell will contain multiple nuclei. The area adjacent to the nucleus appears transparent because the cytoplasm aggregates in the periphery of the cell, giving the appearance of a perinuclear halo.[5,29] The remaining peripheral cytoplasm is condensed into a border at the edge of the halo. Electron microscopic imaging of koilocytes indicates that the nuclei are filled with numerous encapsulated Papillomavirus virions. The cytoplasmic alterations represent aggregation of cytoskeleton filaments and organelles into the periphery. Koilocytosis, then, signifies an intermediate step towards cell death. Therefore, the diagnosis of koilocytosis can be made only when the nuclei demonstrate unmistakable abnormal cytologic features.[29]

At the base, there is proliferation of the immature basal and parabasal cells; however, the degree of proliferation is limited to the lower third of the epithelial surface. Mitoses can be seen, but the mitotic figures are limited to the layer where proliferation is seen. Abnormal forms are absent (Figure 3.32).[29]

3.3.2.2 Cervical/Vaginal Intraepithelial Neoplasia Grade 2

In CIN 2/VaIN 2, or moderate dysplasia, the degree of proliferation among the basal and parabasal cells increases to the point where the layer of abnormal cells reaches up to two-thirds of the epithelial surface. Very commonly, the proliferation occupies half of the surface epithelium. Cytologically, the nuclei within these immature cells are enlarged and irregular in shape. The nuclear size varies among the cells and nuclear overlapping is common. The nuclear membrane is irregular and nuclear chromatin is dark and granular. Nucleoli are small or absent. Mitotic figures now extend to one half of the epithelial surface, and abnormal forms (tripolar or ring shapes) are now present. Koilocytes can be found in the upper portion of the epithelial surface (Figure 3.33).[57,58,60]

3.3.2.3 Cervical/Vaginal Intraepithelial Neoplasia Grade 3

In CIN 3/VaIN 3 or severe dysplasia/CIS, the proliferation of immature cells involves almost the full thickness of the epithelium. The cytologic appearance of these cells is similar to those seen in CIN 2. Mitoses, including abnormal forms, are now found at or near the top of the epithelial surface. The differentiation between severe dysplasia and CIS is related to the presence of one or two residual layers of mature cells at the upper surface. The ability to differentiate a persistent layer of mature cells from degenerated superficial dysplastic cells is not consistent among pathologists, and the prognostic significance of a few residual "mature" cells is unclear. Consequently, most pathologists prefer the designation CIN 3 or VaIN 3 to include all proliferations of abnormal immature cells that occupy more than two-thirds of the epithelial surface (Figure 3.34).[29,57,58]

3.3.3 Invasive Carcinoma

Invasion is characterized by disruption of the basement membrane between the epithelial surface cells and the underlying stroma. Invasion occurs as finger-like extensions of malignant cells from adjacent epithelium extend into the stroma or irregularly shaped nests of malignant cells disperse throughout

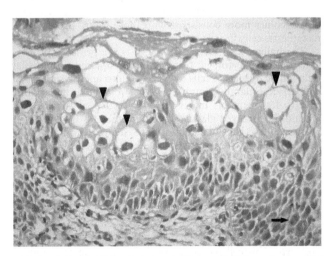

FIGURE 3.32.   Mild dysplasia (cervical intraepithelial neoplasia or CIN 1). Basal cell proliferation extends through one-third of the squamous surface. Note the mitosis (*arrows*). The remaining two-thirds contain koilocytic cells (hematoxylin and eosin, high-power magnification).

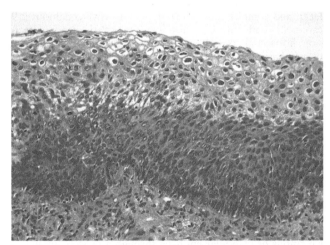

FIGURE 3.33.   Moderate dysplasia (cervical intraepithelial neoplasia or CIN 2). The basal proliferation of dysplastic cells extends through approximately one half of the surface epithelium. Mitoses are also present at the epithelial surface midpoint. Koilocytic cells are still present near the surface (hematoxylin and eosin, medium-power magnification).

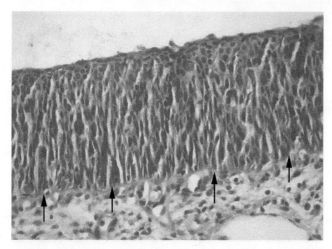

FIGURE 3.34. Severe dysplasia/CIS (cervical intraepithelial neoplasia or CIN 3). There is proliferation of dysplastic cells throughout the squamous epithelium from the basement membrane toward the surface. The basement membrane (*arrows*), however, remains intact (hematoxylin and eosin, high-power magnification).

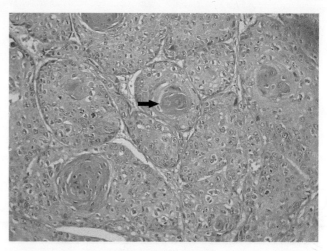

FIGURE 3.36. Keratinizing squamous cell carcinoma. Keratinizing pearls (*arrow*) are present in the malignant nests (hematoxylin and eosin, medium-power magnification).

the stroma. A rim of fibrosis and inflammation known as desmoplasia is commonly seen around these malignant nests. The malignant cells are often larger than the adjacent dysplastic cells. The nuclei are also large with dense peripheral chromatin and prominent nucleoli. The cytoplasm is eosinophilic and contains keratins 5, 8, 10, 13, 18, and 19, signifying squamous differentiation. The overall appearance suggests a process of "cellular maturation in the wrong direction," as the larger malignant cells are directed away from the surface (Figure 3.35).[18]

Squamous cell carcinomas are separated into keratinizing and nonkeratinizing types. Keratinizing tumors are characterized by the presence of squamous pearls in tumor nests (Figure 3.36). Carcinoma grading is based on the ability of the malignant cells to recapitulate normal squamous epithelium, and on cell size, morphology, and the interface between the

invasive neoplasm and the adjacent stroma. Well-differentiated carcinomas are usually keratinizing types that have large cohesive cells with a pushing interface. Poorly differentiated squamous carcinomas are usually nonkeratinizing and characterized by small cells that lack cohesion and infiltrate throughout the surrounding stroma (Figure 3.37).[61]

Because depth of invasion and horizontal spread have treatment and prognostic implications, small nests of invasive squamous cell carcinomas found in excisional biopsies should be measured with an ocular micrometer. The depth of invasion is measured from the nearest basement membrane of origin, which, in some cases, may be an endocervical gland that contains CIN. The measured tumor size, however, can be considered accurate only if any existing cancer and dysplasia are completely excised. The pathologist should report the presence of any lymphatic and vascular space invasion by tumor cells (Figure 3.38).[58,61,62]

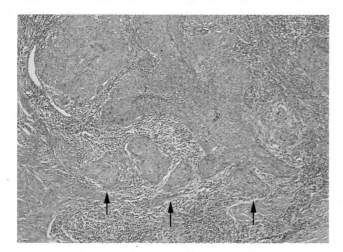

FIGURE 3.35. Early invasive squamous cell carcinoma. In contrast to the small cells in the surface squamous dysplasia, the invasive squamous cells have larger nuclei and abundant eosinophilic cytoplasm. The borders are irregular as small malignant nests extend into the surrounding stroma (*arrow*). If the depth of invasion and horizontal spread was <5 mm and <7 mm, respectively, and the lesion was completely excised, the focus would qualify as a microinvasive squamous cell carcinoma (hematoxylin and eosin, medium-power magnification).

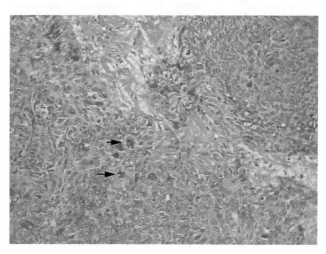

FIGURE 3.37. Poorly differentiated nonkeratinizing squamous cell carcinoma. Note the absence of keratin pearls in the nests of malignant cells. Numerous mitotic figures (*arrows*), including abnormal forms, are easily seen. The surrounding stroma demonstrates a fibrotic (desmoplastic) response (hematoxylin and eosin, medium-power magnification).

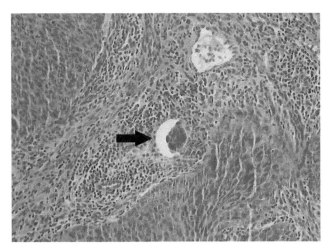

FIGURE 3.38. Lymphatic and vascular space invasion by tumor cells (*arrow*). The centrally located capillary-like space contains a cluster of malignant cells (hematoxylin and eosin, medium-power magnification).

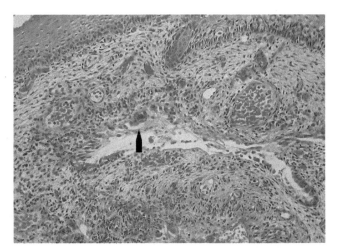

FIGURE 3.39. Reactive endocervical cells (*arrow*). The reactive cells (*arrow*) have slightly enlarged, irregularly shaped hyperchromatic nuclei. Features of AIS (mitoses, stratification), however, are absent (hematoxylin and eosin, medium-power magnification)

3.4 HISTOLOGY OF GLANDULAR ABNORMALITIES

Although glandular lesions can arise anywhere along the endocervical canal, the majority are found in the area of the TZ. Nonetheless, glandular lesions can occur outside the TZ and can be multifocal. If AIS is noted in an excisional specimen, the two-dimensional extent of the abnormality should be measured, its location in relation to the TZ should be reported, and the presence of abnormal glands at a resection margin should be noted. If invasive adenocarcinoma is found, the pathologist should report the cell type, tumor grade, lesion size, margin status, and presence of lymphatic and vascular space invasion.

3.4.1 Reactive Changes

These changes are similar to those identified in squamous metaplastic cells (see Chapter 2, The Histology of Squamous Metaplasia). The nuclei of the affected glandular cells are enlarged, and multinucleation can occur. The nuclear membranes, however, are smooth, and the nuclear shapes are generally round to oval. Micronuclei are present. Mitotic activity is generally not found (Figure 3.39).[18,54]

Microglandular hyperplasia is a benign condition commonly seen in women who are pregnant or who use oral contraceptives. Commonly seen in endocervical polyps and areas of immature metaplasia, the glandular cells proliferate and coalesce to form small lumens. Individual cells also demonstrate small intracellular gland-like spaces. Although the pattern appears architecturally neoplastic, the nuclei are small and uniform, and mitoses are rare.[63] In some cases, microglandular hyperplasia will form polypoid masses. These endocervical polyps contain central fibrovascular cores with surface glandular proliferation and immature metaplasia (Figure 3.40).[64]

3.4.2 Intraepithelial Lesions

Endocervical AIS is characterized by endocervical glands that, in general, are architecturally normal in size and location but contain cells that are cytologically abnormal. The cells contain less cytoplasm than does a normal glandular cell. The nuclei are

enlarged, nonuniform in size and shape, and dark, with dense granular chromatin. Nucleoli are difficult to identify. The cells stratify, and mitoses are common. In some cases, the proliferating cells form bridges, resulting in a cribriform pattern (multiple small round glands within a larger single gland). The basement membrane, however, is always intact (Figure 3.41).[61,65]

Although the majority of AIS is confined to the TZ, approximately 20% of these lesions can be multifocal. For excisional specimens, the pathologist should report the extent of the AIS and whether the margins are free of glandular abnormalities, but the colposcopist must remember that this information does not necessarily imply completeness of excision.[61,65]

3.4.3 Invasive Adenocarcinoma

Invasive adenocarcinoma, like invasive squamous cell carcinoma, implies disruption of the basement membrane and infiltration of abnormal glandular cells into the surrounding stroma. As with AIS, invasive endocervical adenocarcinoma can be multifocal and can originate anywhere along the endocervical canal.

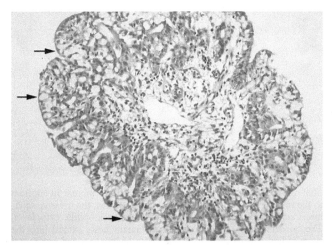

FIGURE 3.40. Endocervical polyp. The rounded polyp contains endocervical cells forming multiple small glands (microglandular hyperplasia) (*arrows*) (hematoxylin and eosin, medium-power magnification).

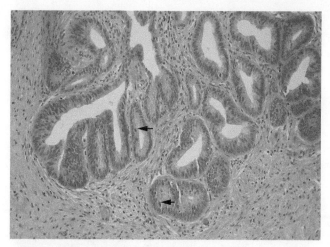

FIGURE 3.41. Endocervical adenocarcinoma *in situ*. There is stratification of the dysplastic glandular cells and numerous mitotic figures (*arrows*). The gland architecture, however, is normal and the basement membrane is intact (hematoxylin and eosin, medium-power magnification).

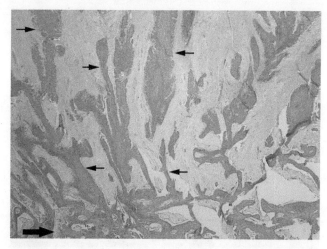

FIGURE 3.43. Villoglandular adenocarcinoma. Eosinophilic mucin separates thin villous-like extensions (*arrows*) that arise from the superficial endocervix (hematoxylin and eosin, low-power magnification).

In invasive adenocarcinoma, the malignant cells contain enlarged, irregular-shaped nonuniform nuclei with dense chromatin, commonly aggregated along the nuclear periphery (vesicular change). Prominent nucleoli are present, and mitoses, including abnormal forms, are common. A desmoplastic stromal response is present and helps to identify these glands as malignant. Because the malignant cells have the potential to recapitulate the lining cells of various crypts and tubules of the genitourinary and gastrointestinal tracts, the different malignant cell types can include mucinous (colonic), endometrioid (endometrium), clear cell (renal tubule), and serous (fallopian tube) (Figure 3.42).[61,65]

Endocervical adenocarcinomas are graded according to architectural appearance and the ability of the malignant cells to form recognizable glands. Well-differentiated adenocarcinomas contain numerous regular glands with minimal stratification and infrequent mitotic figures. Poorly differentiated adenocarcinomas, on the other hand, have solid sheets of malignant cells with few recognizable glands. Bizarre nuclei are common, and mitoses are frequent. Special types of well-differentiated endocervical adenocarcinoma include the minimum-deviation adenocarcinoma (or adenoma malignum) and the villoglandular types. Minimum-deviation adenocarcinomas consist of deeply

infiltrating glands with bland, almost normal-appearing cells. They can be diagnosed only in cervices removed by conization or hysterectomy and are often associated with polyposis syndromes and sex cord–stromal ovarian neoplasms. Villoglandular adenocarcinomas are superficial neoplasms characterized by thin villous outgrowths (Figure 3.43).[61]

It is unclear whether superficially invasive endocervical adenocarcinomas have the same prognostic significance as microinvasive squamous cell carcinomas. Regardless, the pathologist can provide useful information in excisional specimens by estimating the size of the invasive carcinoma, its location in relation to the TZ, and whether AIS or invasive adenocarcinoma involves a resection margin. This information should always be qualified by the fact that these lesions can be multifocal. Lymphatic and vascular space involvement by adenocarcinoma should also be reported.

3.4.4 Biomarkers for Cervical Squamous and Glandular Neoplasias

While it is generally assumed that pathologists can accurately differentiate benign from dysplastic and malignant abnormalities, it must be remembered that the result rendered on a histologic report represents only a best impression based on the history provided, the quality of submitted material, and the experience and expertise of the pathologist. While reproducibility of diagnoses among pathologists is best for high-grade intraepithelial neoplasias and invasive carcinomas, it can be only fair to poor for low-grade intraepithelial neoplasias.[24,66] Because of this, various biomarkers have been developed to differentiate reactive squamous and glandular lesions from true neoplastic processes. Among those commonly used by many surgical pathology laboratories are immunohistochemical assays for p16, Pro-EX C assay, Ki-67, and carcinoembryonic antigen (CEA).

p16 protein is produced in the normal cell to inhibit the production of cyclin D, a kinase enzyme necessary for phosphorylation of the retinoblastoma gene product. This product regulates the production of cyclin E, which results in activation of DNA synthesis in the growth cycle. Exposure of the HPV E7 gene product results in a bond between that protein and the retinoblastoma gene product, which inhibits the latter from undergoing phosphorylation. The lack of a phosphorylated retinoblastoma protein activates an overproduction of cyclin D. To counteract this, p16 is generated to inhibit the cyclin D protein.

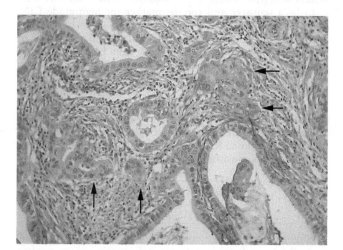

FIGURE 3.42. Invasive endocervical adenocarcinoma. Nests of malignant glandular cells (*arrows*) are present in the reactive endocervical stroma (hematoxylin and eosin, medium-power magnification).

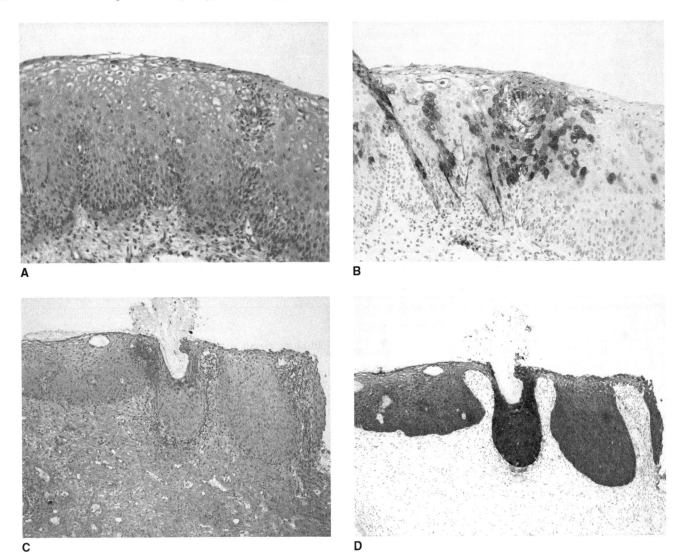

FIGURE 3.44. **A:** A low-grade squamous intraepithelial lesion (LSIL). **B:** The lesion is block negative by p16 staining (focal or "noncontinuous" staining). **C:** A questionable high-grade squamous intraepithelial lesion (HSIL) by H&E staining. **D:** The same lesion stains block positive by p16 (diffuse intense staining greater than one-third of the epithelial surface) confirming that this is a high-grade lesion.

Thus, an overexpression of p16 would indirectly indicate the presence of E7 protein seen with the integration of oncogenic HPV into the host cell genome. p16 protein is detected by immunohistochemical staining, which utilizes color changes that are detected when known antibodies to various protein products are detected. The most common color change seen is the presence of brown within the nucleus and/or cytoplasm of the cell that has the protein in question. A positive test is represented by a diffuse brown stain within the cells that have p16 (Figure 3.44D). Focal positivity (a brown stain in scattered cells) is not considered enough evidence to indicate the presence of this protein. A number of studies have shown that utilization of p16 immunostaining can help differentiate reactive immature metaplasia or atrophic squamous epithelium from high grade dysplasia with very good sensitivity and specificity.[67–69] In addition, p16 might have some value in predicting the outcome of LSILs.[70,71]

ProEx C is an assay for two proteins overexpressed in neoplastic lesions of the cervix: topoisomerase 2 alpha and minichromosome maintenance protein (MCM) 2. Identification of these proteins also uses immunohistochemical staining, with results similar to that seen with p16. However, the staining with ProEx C is limited to the nucleus, which yields a cleaner, more precise stain that some find easier to interpret than the results with p16. A number of investigators have shown ProEx C to be a sensitive and specific marker for high grade CIN, comparable to p16.[72,73]

As with high grade SILs, endocervical glandular neoplasia or AIS can also be difficult to distinguish from benign or reactive glandular changes. In such cases, immunostaining for CEA and Ki-67 may have some utility. CEA is generally absent in benign cervical lesions, but is positive in AIS. Nevertheless, this marker is not entirely sensitive or specific. To improve the reliability of diagnosis, Ki-67, a marker for cell proliferation, can be added. A high proliferation index (>40% of glandular cells show positive immunostaining for Ki67) along with a positive immunostain for CEA is consistent with a glandular neoplasia.[74]

3.5 INTERPRETING PATHOLOGY REPORTS

A clinician receiving a cytology or histopathology report will typically scan it for the microscopic diagnosis and, more often than not, accept that portion of the report as the final and complete result. Nevertheless, other portions of the report contain information that will expand the microscopic diagnosis and, in some cases, indicate that more information may be necessary to clarify what the diagnosis represents.

Since the inception of the Bethesda System, the cytology report has become structured to the point that the results as detailed vary little from different laboratories. Although the order may vary, all reports must contain the specimen source (conventional or liquid processed), the method of analysis (traditional or computer assisted), a statement regarding the specimen adequacy, the final interpretation, and any comments or suggestions. Thus, all necessary information is available. In addition, the diagnostic terminology is standardized. Any deviation from the accepted terminology must be explained in a comment or supplementary note.

In contrast, the surgical pathology report, while containing a somewhat standard format, will vary in organization and content from laboratory to laboratory. Attempts have been made to standardize elements of a report using a synoptic list. However, at present these synoptic reports are required only for malignancies. In general, the report will contain a microscopic diagnosis, a comment or explanatory notes, and a gross description. While the microscopic diagnosis is important, the clinician should read the gross description to ensure that the specimens listed and their description are consistent with the diagnoses rendered. The clinician should also note whether the specimen was processed appropriately based on the clinical history given to the pathologist. For example, if a woman with a history of cervical dysplasia has a hysterectomy for benign disease, the clinician should check to see that the vaginal cuff margins were marked for identification, and that the entire cervix was submitted.

In the end, if any question arises regarding a particular cytologic or histologic (surgical) report, the clinician should not hesitate to call the pathologist for clarification.

3.6 NEW TERMINOLOGY FOR SQUAMOUS INTRAEPITHELIAL LESIONS THROUGHOUT THE LOWER GENITAL TRACT

A consensus workshop was convened in 2012 to recommend terminology unified across all male and female lower anogenital tract (LAT) sites. The goal was to create a histopathologic nomenclature system that more accurately reflects current knowledge of HPV biology, optimally uses available biomarkers, and facilitates clear communication across different medical specialties.[75] The Lower Anogenital Squamous Terminology (LAST) Project was cosponsored by the College of American Pathologists (CAP) and the American Society for Colposcopy and Cervical Pathology (ASCCP). The final, approved recommendations standardize biologically relevant histopathologic terminology for HPV-associated squamous intraepithelial lesions (SIL) across all LAT sites. Specifically, a two-tiered histopathologic terminology similar to that used in cytology, which also consists of low-grade and high-grade SIL (LSIL and HSIL), was adopted for all HPV-associated abnormalities. LSIL and HSIL may be further qualified by use of more traditional terminology or by location, that is, various grades of cervical, vaginal, vulvar, anal, and penile intraepithelial neoplasia (CIN, VaIN, VIN, AIN, and PeIN) (Table 3.3).

The LAST workshop also recommended the application of a molecular marker whose overexpression is associated with cell dysregulation in neoplastic processes (cell growth cycle protein p16). This marker is most useful when the pathologist is having difficulty differentiating between LSIL and HSIL (CIN, VaIN, VIN, AIN, PeIN 2 under the old terminology) or to differentiate whether a lesion is an HSIL or a mimic not related to a neoplastic process such as reactive squamous metaplasia or atrophy. Other uses include cases where there is a professional disagreement in interpretation of the histology, or when there is a higher risk of a missed significant lesion (i.e., when the cytologic interpretation implies the presence of a high-grade squamous or glandular abnormality but the corresponding histology is not confirmatory) (Table 3.4)[75]. A diffuse intense ("block-positive") p16 result by immunoperoxidase staining supports a categorization of HSIL, whereas absence or focal ("block-negative") staining strongly favors an interpretation of LSIL or a non–HPV-associated pathology (Figure 3.44A–D).[75]

New terminology was also developed for minimally invasive squamous cell carcinoma (SCC) of the LAT, which is now to be called superficially invasive squamous cell carcinoma (SISCCA) (Table 3.5).[75] Definitions for what constitutes this diagnosis will vary depending on the LAT site. A full discussion of all of the new recommendations can be found in reference 75.

TABLE 3.3	SUMMARY OF RECOMMENDATIONS FOR SIL

■ RECOMMENDATION	■ COMMENT
1. A unified histopathologic nomenclature with a single set of diagnostic terms is recommended for all HPV-associated preinvasive squamous lesions of the LAT.	-IN refers to the generic intraepithelial neoplasia terminology, without specifying the location. For a specific location, the appropriate complete term should be used. Thus, for an -IN 3 lesion, cervix = CIN 3; vagina = VaIN 3; vulva = VIN 3; anus = AIN 3; perianus = PAIN 3; and penis = PeIN 3
2. A two-tiered nomenclature is recommended for noninvasive HPV-associated squamous proliferations of the LAT, which may be further qualified with the appropriate -IN terminology	
3. The recommended terminology for HPV-associated squamous lesions of the LAT is LSIL and HSIL, which may be further classified by the applicable -IN subcategorization.	

From Darragh TM, Colgan TJ, Cox JT, et al.; Members of LAST Project Work Groups. The Lower Anogenital Squamous Terminology Standardization Project for HPV-Associated Lesions: background and consensus recommendations from the College of American Pathologists and the American Society for Colposcopy and Cervical Pathology. *J Low Genit Tract Dis* 2012;16(3):205–42. Review. Erratum in: *J Low Genit Tract Dis* 2013;17(3):368, with permission.

TABLE 3.4	SUMMARY OF RECOMMENDATIONS FOR THE USE OF BIOMARKERS IN HPV-ASSOCIATED LAT LESIONS

■ RECOMMENDATION	■ COMMENT
1. p16 IHC is recommended when the H&E morphologic differential diagnosis is between precancer (YIN 2 or YIN 3) and a mimic of precancer (e.g., processes known to be not related to neoplastic risk such as immature squamous metaplasia, atrophy, reparative epithelial changes, tangential cutting).	Strong and diffuse block-positive p16 results support a categorization of precancerous disease.
2. If the pathologist is entertaining an H&E morphologic interpretation of -IN 2 (under the old terminology, which is a biologically equivocal lesion falling between the morphologic changes of HPV infection [low-grade lesion] and precancer), p16 IHC is recommended to help clarify the situation. Strong and diffuse block-positive p16 results support a categorization of precancer. Negative or non–block-positive staining strongly favors an interpretation of low-grade disease or a non–HPV-associated pathology.	
3. p16 is recommended for use as an adjudication tool for cases in which there is a professional disagreement in histologic specimen interpretation, with the caveat that the differential diagnosis includes a precancerous lesion (-IN 2 or -IN 3).	
4. Recommend against the use of p16 IHC as a routine adjunct to histologic assessment of biopsy specimens with morphologic interpretations of negative, -IN 1, and -IN 3.	
a. SPECIAL CIRCUMSTANCE: p16 IHC is recommended as an adjunct to morphologic assessment for biopsy specimens interpreted as ≤ -IN 1 that are at high risk for missed high-grade disease, which is defined as a prior cytologic interpretation of HSIL, ASC-H, ASC-US/HPV-16+, or AGC (NOS).	Any identified p16-positive area must meet H&E morphologic criteria for a high-grade lesion to be reinterpreted as such.

From Darragh TM, Colgan TJ, Cox JT, et al.; Members of LAST Project Work Groups. The Lower Anogenital Squamous Terminology Standardization Project for HPV-Associated Lesions: background and consensus recommendations from the College of American Pathologists and the American Society for Colposcopy and Cervical Pathology. *J Low Genit Tract Dis*. 2012;16(3):205–42. Review. Erratum in: *J Low Genit Tract Dis* 2013;17(3):368, with permission.

TABLE 3.5	SUMMARY OF RECOMMENDATIONS FOR SISCCA

■ RECOMMENDATION	■ COMMENT
1. The term SISCCA is recommended for minimally invasive SCC of the LAT that has been completely excised and is potentially amenable to conservative surgical therapy.	Note: Lymph–vascular invasion (LVI) and pattern of invasion is not part of the definition of SISCCA, with the exception of penile carcinoma.
2. For cases of invasive squamous carcinoma with positive biopsy/resection margins, the pathology report should state whether: The examined invasive tumor exceeds the dimensions for a SISCCA (defined below). OR The examined invasive tumor component is less than or equal to the dimensions for a SISCCA and conclude that the tumor is "At least a superficially invasive squamous carcinoma."	
3. In cases of SISCCA, the following parameters should be included in the pathology report: The presence or absence of lymphatic or vascular involvement (LVI) The presence, number, and size of independent multifocal carcinomas (after excluding the possibility of a single carcinoma)	
4. CERVIX: SISCCA of the cervix is defined as an invasive squamous carcinoma that: Is not a grossly visible lesion Has an invasive depth of ≤3 mm from the basement membrane of the point of origin Has a horizontal spread of ≤7 mm in maximal extent Has been completely excised	
5. VAGINA: No recommendation is offered for early invasive squamous carcinoma of the vagina.	Owing to the rarity of primary SCC of the vagina, there are insufficient data to define early invasive squamous carcinoma in the vagina.

TABLE 3.5 SUMMARY OF RECOMMENDATIONS FOR SISCCA *(CONTINUED)*

■ RECOMMENDATION	■ COMMENT
6. ANAL CANAL: The suggested definition of SISCCA of the anal canal is an invasive squamous carcinoma that: Has an invasive depth of ≤3 mm from the basement membrane of the point of origin Has a horizontal spread of ≤7 mm in maximal extent Has been completely excised	
7. VULVA: Vulvar SISCCA is defined as an AJCC T1a (FIGO *1A*) vulvar cancer. No change in the current definition of T1a vulvar cancer is recommended. Note: The depth of invasion is defined as the measurement of the tumor from the epithelial–stromal junction of the adjacent most superficial dermal papilla to the deepest point of invasion.	Current AJCC definition of T1a vulvar carcinoma: Tumor ≤2 cm in size, confined to the vulva or perineum AND Stromal invasion ≤1 mm
8. PENIS: Penile SISCCA is defined as an AJCC T1a. No change in the current definition of T1a penile cancer is recommended.	Current AJCC definition of T1a penile carcinoma: Tumor that invades only the subepithelial connective tissue, AND No LVI AND Is not poorly differentiated (i.e., grade 3–4)
9. SCROTUM: No recommendation is offered for early invasive squamous carcinoma of the scrotum.	Owing to the rarity of primary SCC of the scrotum, there is insufficient literature to make a recommendation regarding the current AJCC staging of early scrotal cancers.

From Darragh TM, Colgan TJ, Cox JT, et al.; Members of LAST Project Work Groups. The Lower Anogenital Squamous Terminology Standardization Project for HPV-Associated Lesions: background and consensus recommendations from the College of American Pathologists and the American Society for Colposcopy and Cervical Pathology. *J Low Genit Tract Dis* 2012;16(3):205–42. Review. Erratum in: *J Low Genit Tract Dis* 2013;17(3):368, with permission.

References

1. Kolstad P, Stafl A. *Atlas of Colposcopy*. Baltimore, MD: University Park Press, 1972:13–5.
2. Vilos GA. The history of the papanicolaou smear and the odyssey of George and Andormache Papanicolaou. *Obstet Gynecol* 1998;91:479–83.
3. Papanicolaou GN, Traut HF. *Diagnosis of Uterine Cancer by the Vaginal Smear*. New York: The Commonwealth Fund, 1943:19–45.
4. Christopherson WM. Parker JE, Drye JC. Control of cervical cancer: preliminary report on community program. *JAMA* 1962;182:179–82.
5. Meisels A, Fortin R. Condylomatous lesions of the cervix and vagina I: cytologic patterns. *Acta Cytol* 1976;20:505–9.
6. Fujii T, Crum C, Winkler B, Fu YS, Richart RM. Human papillomavirus infection and cervical intraepithelial neoplasia: histopathology and DNA content. *Obstet Gynecol* 1984;63:99–104.
7. Loning T, Ikenberg H, Becker J, Gissmann L, Hoepfer I, zur Hausen H. Analysis of oral papillomas, leukoplakias, and invasive carcinomas for human papillomavirus type related DNA. *J Invest Dermatol* 1985;84:417–20.
8. The 1988 Bethesda System for reporting cervical/vaginal cytologic diagnoses. Developed and approved at the National Cancer Institute Workshop, Bethesda, Maryland, U.S.A., December 12–13, 1988. *Acta Cytol* 1989;33:567–74.
9. The revised Bethesda System for reporting cervical/vaginal cytologic diagnoses: report of the 1991 Bethesda workshop. *Acta Cytol* 1992; 36:273–6.
10. Kurman RJ, Solomon D. *The Bethesda System for Reporting Cervical/ Vaginal Cytologic Diagnoses*. New York: Springer-Verlag, 1994;99:1–81.
11. Solomon D, Davey D, Kurman R, et al. The Bethesda System 2001: terminology for reporting the results of cervical cytology. *JAMA* 2002;287:2114–9.
12. Mintzer M, Curtis P, Resnick JC, Morrell D. The effect of quality of Papanicolaou smears on the detection of cytologic abnormalities. *Cancer Cytopathol* 1999;87:113–7.
13. Allen KA, Zaleski S, Cohen MB. Laboratory use of the diagnosis "reactive/reparative" in gynecologic smears: impact of CLIA 88. *Mod Pathol* 1995;8:266–9.
14. Gupta PK. Microbiology, inflammation and viral infections. In: Bibbo M, ed. *Comprehensive Cytopathology* (2nd ed.). Philadelphia, PA: WB Saunders Co, 1997:125–41.
15. Davis JD, Connor EE, Clark P, Wilkinson EJ, Duff P. Correlation between cervical cytologic results and Gram stain as diagnostic tests for bacterial vaginosis. *Am J Obstet Gynecol* 1997;177:532–5.
16. Weinberger MW, Harger JH. Accuracy of the Papanicolaou smear in the diagnosis of asymptomatic infection with *Trichomonas vaginalis*. *Obstet Gynecol* 1993;82:425–9.
17. Keebler CM, Wied GL. The estrogen test: an aid in differential cytodiagnosis. *Acta Cytol* 1974;18:482–93.
18. Voorjis PG. Benign proliferative reactions, intraepithelial neoplasia and invasive cancer of the cervix. In: Bibbo M, ed. *Comprehensive Cytopathology* (2nd ed.). Philadelphia, PA: WB Saunders Company, 1997:161–230.
19. Montz FJ. Significance of "normal" endometrial cells in cervical cytology from asymptomatic postmenopausal women receiving hormone replacement therapy. *Gynecol Oncol* 2001;81:33–9.
20. Gomez-Fernandez CR, Ganjei-Azar P, Behshid K, Averette HE, Nadji M. Normal endometrial cells in Papanicolaou smears: prevalence in women with and without endometrial disease. *Obstet Gynecol* 2000;96:874–8.
21. Cherkis RC, Patten SF, Andrews TJ, et al. Significance of normal endometrial cells detected by cervical cytology. *Obstet Gynecol* 1998;71:242–44.
22. Gondos B, King EB. Significance of endometrial cells in cervicovaginal smears. *Ann Clin Lab Sci* 1977;7:486–90.
23. Sheils LA, Wilbur DC. Atypical squamous cells of undetermined significance. Stratification of the risk of association with, or progression to, squamous intraepithelial lesions based on morphologic subcategorization. *Acta Cytol* 1997;41:1065–72.
24. Stoler MH, Schiffman M. Interobserver reproducibility of cervical cytologic and histologic interpretations: realistic estimates from the ASCUS-LSIL Triage Study. *JAMA* 2001;285:1500–5.
25. Geng L, Connolly DC, Isacson C, Ronnett BC, Cho KR. Atypical immature metaplasia (AIM) of the cervix: is it related to high-grade squamous intraepithelial lesion (HSIL)? *Human Pathol* 1999;30:345–51.
26. Sherman ME, Tabbara SO, Scott DR, et al. "ASCUS, rule out HSIL": cytologic features, histologic correlates, and human papillomavirus detection. *Mod Pathol* 1999;12:335–42.
27. Sherman ME, Solomon D, Schiffman M for the ALTS Group. Qualification of ASCUS: a comparison of equivocal LSIL and equivocal HSIL cervical cytology in the ASCUS LSIL Triage Study. *Am J Clin Pathol* 2001;116:386–94.
28. Jeronimo J, Khan MJ, Schiffman M, Solomon D, ALTS Group. Does the interval between Papanicolaou tests influence the quality of cytology? *Cancer* 2005;105(3):133–8.
29. Wright TC, Kurman RJ, Ferenczy A. Precancerous lesions of the cervix. In: Kurman RJ, ed. New York: Springer-Verlag, 1994:245–9.
30. Raab SS, Snider TE, Potts SA, et al. Atypical glandular cells of undetermined significance: diagnostic accuracy and interobserver variability using select cytologic criteria. *Am J Clin Pathol* 1997;107:299–307.
31. Liao SY, Stanbridge EJ. Expression of MN/CA 9 protein in Papanicolaou smears containing atypical glandular cells of undetermined significance

is a diagnostic biomarker of cervical dysplasia and neoplasia. *Cancer* 2000;88:1108–21.

32. Pacey NF, Ng ABP. Glandular neoplasms of the uterine cervix. In: Bibbo M. *Comprehensive Cytopathology* (2nd ed.). Philadelphia, PA: WB Saunders Co., 1997:231–50.

33. Lee KR, Ashfaq R, Birdsong GG, et al. Comparison of conventional Papanicolaou smears and a fluid-based, thin-layer system for cervical cancer screening. *Obstet Gynecol* 1997;90:278–84.

34. Corkill M, Knapp D, Martin J, Hutchinson ML. Specimen adequacy of ThinPrep sample preparations in a direct-to-vial study. *Acta Cytol*. 1997; 41:39–44.

35. Vassilakos P, Saurel J, Rondez R. Direct-to-vial use of the AutoCyte PREP liquid based preparation for cervical-vaginal specimens in three European laboratories. *Acta Cytol* 1999;43:650–8.

36. Papillo PL, Zarka MA, St. John TL. Evaluation of the ThinPrep pap test in clinical practice: a seven month, 16,314-case experience in northern Vermont. *Acta Cytol* 1998;42:203–8.

37. Vassilakos P, Schwartz D, de Marval F, et al. Biopsy-based comparison of liquid based, thin-layer preparations to conventional Pap smear. *J Reprod Med* 2000;45:11–6.

38. Arbyn M, Bergeron C, Klinkhamer P, Martin-Hirsch P, Siebers A, Bulten J. Liquid compared with conventional cervical cytology: a systematic review and meta-analysis. *Obstet Gynecol* 2008;111:167–77.

39. Evaluation of cervical cytology. Evidence Report/Technology Assessment #5. Washington, DC: Agency for Health Care Policy and Research. AHCPR Publication 99-E010, 1999.

40. Sherman ME, Mango LJ, Kelly D, et al. PAPNET analysis of reportedly negative smears preceding the diagnosis of a high-grade squamous intraepithelial lesion or carcinoma. *Mod Pathol* 1994;7:578–81.

41. Ashfaq R, Salinger F, Solares B. Evaluation of the PAPNET system for prescreening triage of cervicovaginal smears. *Acta Cytol* 1997;41:1058–64.

42. Michelow PM, Hlongwane NF, Lieman G. Simulation of primary cervical cancer screening by the PAPNET system in an unscreened, high-risk community. *Acta Cytol* 1997;41:88–92.

43. O'Leary TJ, Tellado M, Buckner S, Ali IS, Stevens A, Ollayos CW. PAPNET assisted rescreening of cervical smears: cost and accuracy with a 100% manual rescreening strategy. *JAMA* 1998;279:235–7.

44. Duby JM, DiFurio MJ. Implementation of the ThinPrep Imaging System in a tertiary military medical center. *Cancer Cytopathol* 2009;117:264–70.

45. Sedlacek TV. Automated cervical cytology. *Colposcopist* 1996;27:1–4.

46. Colgan TJ, Patten SF, Lee JSJ. A clinical trial of the AutoPap 300 QC system for quality control of cervicovaginal cytology in the clinical laboratory. *Acta Cytol* 1995;39:1191–98.

47. Wilbur DC, Bonfiglio TA, Rutkowski MA, et al. Sensitivity of the AutoPap 300 QC system for cervical cytologic screening. *Acta Cytol* 1996;40:127–32.

48. Brown AD, Garber AM. Cost effectiveness of three adjunctive methods to enhance the sensitivity of Papanicolaou testing. *JAMA* 1999;281:347–53.

49. Statement on technical devices for innovation in cervical cytology screening (editorial). *Am J Clin Pathol* 1996;169:441.

50. Bartels PH, Bibbo M, Hutchinson ML, et al. Computerized screening devices and performance assessment: development of a policy towards automation (IAC Task Force summary). *Acta Cytol* 1998;42:59–68.

51. Hutchinson ML. Assessing the costs and benefits of alternative rescreening strategies. *Acta Cytol* 1996;40:4–7.

52. Radensky PW, Mango LJ. Interactive neural network-assisted screening: an economic assessment. *Acta Cytol* 1998;42:246–52.

53. Schechter CB. Cost-effectiveness of rescreening conventionally prepared cervical smears by PAPNET testing. *Acta Cytol* 1996;40:1272–82.

54. Wright TC, Ferenczy A. Benign diseases of the cervix. In: Kurman RJ, ed. *Blaustein's Pathology of the Female Genital Tract*. New York: Springer-Verlag, 1994: 205–6.

55. Wright TC, Kurman RJ, Ferenczy A. Precancerous lesions of the cervix. In: Kurman RJ, ed. *Blaustein's Pathology of the Female Genital Tract*. New York: Springer-Verlag, 1994:229–32.

56. Reagan JW, Seidemand IL, Saracusa Y. The cellular morphology of carcinoma in situ and dysplasia or atypical hyperplasia of the uterine cervix. *Cancer* 1953;6:224–35.

57. Richart RM. Cervical intraepithelial neoplasia: a review. In: Sommers SC, ed. *Pathology Annual*. New York: Appleton-Century-Crofts, 1973:301–28.

58. Scully RE, Bonfiglio TA, Silverberg SG. *Histologic Typing of Female Genital Tract Tumours. World Health Organization International Histological Classification of Tumours* (2nd ed.). New York: Springer-Verlag, 1994:39–46.

59. Zaino RJ, Robboy SJ, Bentley R, Kurman RJ. Diseases of the vagina. In: Kurman RJ, ed. *Blaustein's Pathology of the Female Genital Tract*. New York: Springer-Verlag, 1994:156–70.

60. Wright TC, Kurman RJ, Ferenczy A. Precancerous lesions of the cervix. In: Kurman RJ, ed. New York: Springer-Verlag, 1994:249–53.

61. Kurman RJ, Norris HJ, Wilkinson E. Tumors of the cervix, vagina and vulva. In: *Atlas of Tumor Pathology* (Third Series: Fascicle 4). Washington, DC: American Registry of Pathology, Armed Forces Institute of Pathology, 1992:37–157.

62. Wright TC, Ferenczy A, Kurman RJ. Carcinoma and other tumors of the cervix. In: Kurman RJ, ed. *Blaustein's Pathology of the Female Genital Tract*. New York: Springer-Verlag, 1994:280–97.

63. Wright TC, Ferenczy A. Benign diseases of the cervix. In: Kurman RJ, ed. *Blaustein's Pathology of the Female Genital Tract*. New York: Springer-Verlag, 1994:212–4.

64. Wright TC, Ferenczy A. Benign diseases of the cervix. In: Kurman RJ, ed. *Blaustein's Pathology of the Female Genital Tract*. New York: Springer-Verlag, 1994:218–9.

65. Wright TC, Ferenczy A, Kurman RJ. Carcinoma and other tumors of the cervix. In: Kurman RJ, ed. *Blaustein's Pathology of the Female Genital Tract*. New York: Springer-Verlag, 1994:300–9.

66. Kato I, Santamaria M, De Ruiz PA, et al. Inter-observer variation in cytological and histological diagnoses of cervical neoplasia and its epidemiologic implication. *J Clin Epidemiol* 1995;48:1167–74.

67. O'Neill CJ, McCluggage WG. p16 in the female genital tract and its value in diagnosis. *Adv Anat Pathol* 2006;13:8–15.

68. Finegan MM, Han HC, Edelson MI, Rosenblum NG. p16 expression in squamous lesions of the female genital tract. *J Mol Histol* 2004;35:111–4.

69. Volgareva G, Zavalishina L, Andreeva Y, et al. Protein p16 as a marker of dysplastic and neoplastic alterations in cervical epithelial cells. *BMC Cancer* 2004;31:58.

70. Hariri J, Ostor A. The negative predictive value of p16ink4a to assess the outcome of cervical intraepithelial 1 in the uterine cervix. *Int J Gynecol Pathol* 2007;26:223–8.

71. del Pino M, Garcia S, Fuste V, et al. Value of p16ink4a as a marker of progression/regression in cervical intraepithelial neoplasia grade 1. *Am J Obstet Gynecol* 2009;201:488.e1–7.

72. Badr RE, Walts AE, Chung F, Bose S. BD ProEx C: a sensitive and specific marker for HPV-associated squamous lesions of the cervix. *Am J Surg Pathol* 2008;32:899–906.

73. Conesa-Zamora P, Domenech-Peris A, Orantes-Casado FJ, et al. Effect of human papillomavirus on cell cycle related proteins p16, Ki-67, Cyclin D1, p53 and ProEx C on precursor lesions of cervical carcinoma: a tissue microarray study. *Am J Clin Pathol* 2009;132:378–90.

74. Deavers MT, Malpica A, Silva EG. Immunohistochemistry in gynecological pathology. *Int J Gynecol Cancer* 2003;13:567–79.

75. Darragh TM, Colgan TJ, Cox JT, et al.; Members of LAST Project Work Groups. The Lower Anogenital Squamous Terminology Standardization Project for HPV-Associated Lesions: background and consensus recommendations from the College of American Pathologists and the American Society for Colposcopy and Cervical Pathology. *J Low Genit Tract Dis* 2012;16(3):205–42. Review. Erratum in: *J Low Genit Tract Dis* 2013;17(3):368.

CHAPTER 4

THOMAS C. WRIGHT, JR.,
J. THOMAS COX

Cervical Cancer: Epidemiology and Etiology

4.1 INTRODUCTION
4.2 DESCRIPTIVE EPIDEMIOLOGY
    4.2.1 Prevalence of Invasive Cervical Cancer Worldwide
    4.2.2 Time Trends and Impact of Cytologic Screening
    4.2.3 Other Factors Affecting Geographic Variations

4.3 RISK FACTORS FOR INVASIVE CERVICAL CANCER
    4.3.1 Human Papillomavirus
    4.3.2 Cofactors to HPV-Induced Oncogenesis
4.4 SUMMARY: EPIDEMIOLOGIC EVIDENCE FOR THE ETIOLOGY OF CERVICAL CANCER

4.1 INTRODUCTION

During the last three decades, our understanding of the epidemiology and pathogenesis of invasive cervical cancer has changed dramatically. For many years, it has been recognized that women who have had multiple sexual partners, who began sexual activity at an early age, and who were of lower socioeconomic status were at greatest risk for cervical cancer. At the other end of the spectrum, virgins and women with limited sexual exposure were recognized to be at low risk. These observations strongly suggested that a sexually transmitted agent was responsible for invasive cervical cancer, and over the years a number of potential agents were proposed including herpes simplex virus (HSV), *Chlamydia trachomatis*, and even sperm. However, each of these potential risks was subsequently ruled out as the causative agent of cervical cancer. In the 1970s, Harald zur Hausen used modern molecular biologic methods to study the pathogenesis of cervical cancer and found that specific types of human papillomavirus (HPV) could be identified in the majority of invasive cervical cancers. Based on this, he hypothesized that cervical cancer was caused by sexually transmitted HPV infections.[1] Since then, numerous molecular and epidemiologic studies have shown that specific "oncogenic" types of HPV act as carcinogens in humans and are responsible for the development of almost all invasive cervical cancers.[2] Because of his pioneering work in demonstrating the role of HPV in cervical cancer, Dr. zur Hausen was awarded the Nobel Prize in Physiology or Medicine 2008.[3]

4.2 DESCRIPTIVE EPIDEMIOLOGY

4.2.1 Prevalence of Invasive Cervical Cancer Worldwide

Worldwide, cervical cancer is the second most common cancer among women. It is estimated that each year there are approximately 529,828 cases globally (Table 4.1).[4] It occurs in relatively young women, accounting for an average of 17 potential years of life lost for every death from invasive cervical cancer occurring before the age of 70.[5] Globally, the mortality:incidence ratio is 52%, and there are approximately 275,128 deaths from cervical cancer annually.[4] Approximately 3.4 million women-years of life before age 70 are lost

yearly from cervical cancer throughout the world.[5] Other HPV-associated squamous cell malignancies of the lower genital tract account for another 150,000 cases.[5]

There are marked global disparities in both the incidence of, and mortality from, cervical cancer.[6] More than 85% of the cases of cervical cancer occur in developing countries where it accounts for 13% of all cancers in women (Table 4.1).[7,8] Highest risk regions include Eastern and Western Africa where the age-standardized incidence rates (ASIRs) are over 30 per 100,000.[7,8] Other high-risk regions with ASIRs of over 20 per 100,000 include South Africa, South-Central Asia, South America, Melanesia, Middle Africa, Central America, and the Caribbean. Rates are lowest in Western Asia, North America, and Australia/New Zealand, all with ASIRs <6 per 100,000.[7] India and China combined account for 39% of all cases of cervical cancer globally. In large part, these global disparities reflect differences in cervical cancer screening rates as well as rates of infection with high-risk HPV types.[4]

Invasive cervical cancer is predominately a disease of women older than age 30 years. In the United States, the Surveillance, Epidemiology, and End Results (SEER) Program of the National Cancer Institute has monitored the incidence, mortality, and age distribution of invasive cervical cancer since 1973.[9] From 2004 to 2008 the median age at diagnosis in the United States was 48 years (Figure 4.1). Approximately 0.2% were diagnosed under age 20, 14.5% between 20 and 34, 26.1% between 35 and 44, 23.7% between 45 and 54, 16.3% between 55 and 64, and 9.3% in women 65 years and older. In the United States, it is estimated that in 2010 there were approximately 12,200 new cases of cervical cancer, and approximately 4210 women died of cervical cancer.[10] ASIRs for all regions in the world show an increasing trend with age and ASIRs plateau after age 45 to 50 in most countries.

4.2.2 Time Trends and Impact of Cytologic Screening

During the last four decades, there have been dramatic reductions in the incidence of invasive cervical cancer in North America and Western Europe. Much of the reduction in incidence and mortality rates for cervical cancer reflects the widespread availability of cytologic screening. In the United States, the incidence of cervical cancer has decreased

TABLE 4.1	ESTIMATED NUMBERS OF CASES AND DEATHS FROM CERVICAL CANCER IN 2008	
■ REGION	■ CASES	■ DEATHS
World	529,828	275,125
More developed regions	76,000	32,000
Less developed regions	453,000	242,000
WHO Africa region	75,000	50,000
WHO Americas region	80,000	36,000
European Union	31,000	13,000
United States	11,000	3000
China	75,000	33,000
India	134,000	72,000

Adapted from Ferlay J, Shin HR, Bray F, Forman D, Mathers C, Parkin DM. Estimates of worldwide burden of cancer in 2008: GLOBOCAN 2008. *Int J Cancer* 2010;127:2893–917. Reference 8.

75% and mortality has decreased 74% since the implementation of Papanicolaou (Pap) cervical cytology screening in 1949.[11] Between 1975 and 2008, the age-adjusted incidence rates for invasive cervical cancer in the United States declined from 14.79 to 6.43 per 100,000 women, representing a 57% decrease (Figure 4.2). Decreases were even more marked for black women who showed a 75% reduction during this time period (from 33.06 to 8.41 per 100,000 women) (Figure 4.2). Incidence rates have continued to drop since 2000 for both white and black women, although rates for black women remain higher than for white women.

Women who do not get regular screening with Pap tests are particularly vulnerable to cervical cancer. A woman in the United States who has never been screened has an estimated lifetime risk of developing cervical cancer of 3.7% (3748 cases per 100,000 women).[12] With annual cytologic screening, the lifetime risk drops to 0.3%, or 305 cases per 100,000 women.[12] Reviews of cervical cancer screening histories of

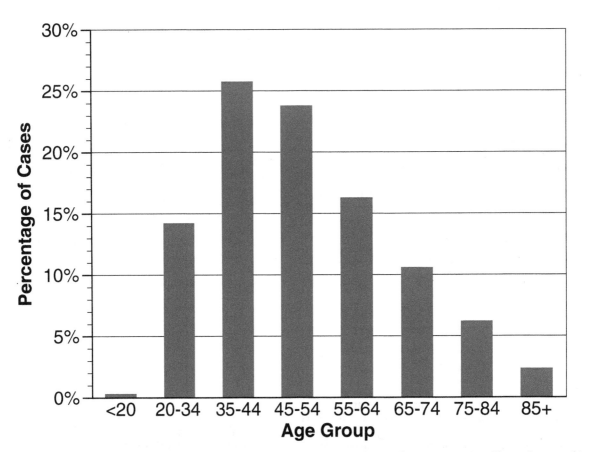

FIGURE 4.1. Age distribution of incident cases of invasive cervical cancer in the United States from 2004 to 2008. The median age of incident cases of invasive cervical cancer is 48 years. Only 0.2% of cases are diagnosed in women 20 years and younger. Based on SEER summary data tables.[9]

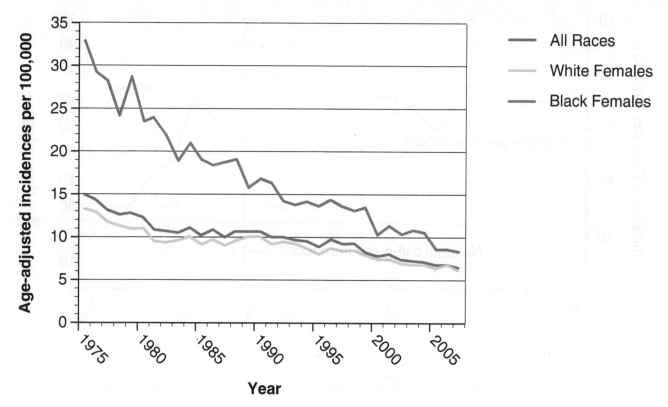

FIGURE 4.2. Age-adjusted incidence rates (ASIRs) of invasive cervical cancer in the United States based on the SEER database 1975 to 2008. ASIRs of invasive cervical cancer dropped from 1975 to 2008 for both blacks and whites, but due to the initial higher ASIR in blacks, they showed a greater reduction during this time period. (From SEER Cancer Statistics. *http://seer.cancer.gov/* 2008 [Accessed July 19, 2011].)

women developing invasive cervical cancers indicate that a considerable proportion of them have not been recently screened. For example, data from Kaiser Northern California indicate that 56% of women developing cervical cancer have not recently been screened.[13] Similarly, linkage between cytologic screening registries and cancer registries in Sweden have found that 64% of Swedish women diagnosed with cervical cancer have not been recently screened.[14]

The impact of nationwide screening programs is clearly demonstrated by the Scandinavian experience.[15–17] In Finland, a national screening program to prevent cervical cancer, begun in the 1950s, dramatically lowered rates of cervical cancer to 5.5 cases per 100,000 women, and the experience in Sweden was similar. In contrast, in Norway, which only developed a nationwide screening program in 1995, the reduction in cervical cancer rates has been much smaller, and the rate of cervical cancer is three times higher (15.6 per 100,000) than in Finland (Figure 4.3).

In contrast to the experience in the Nordic countries, cervical cancer screening in countries without organized screening programs that include a "call/recall" follow-up system have had mixed results. Cytologic screening started in England in 1964 but failed to achieve sufficient coverage and follow-up of women with positive results. As a result, the screening program had little impact on cervical cancer rates.[18] However, following the establishment of a national "call/recall" system in 1988, coverage for all women aged 25 to 64 rose from 45% in 1988 to 85% in 1994 and has remained steady since. Since 1990, this has resulted in a dramatic reduction in incidence and mortality from cervical cancer (Figure 4.4).

The high ASIRs for cervical cancer in countries late to enter organized screening, such as the United Kingdom and Denmark, when compared to countries beginning screening decades earlier, such as Finland, are demonstrated in Figure 4.5.

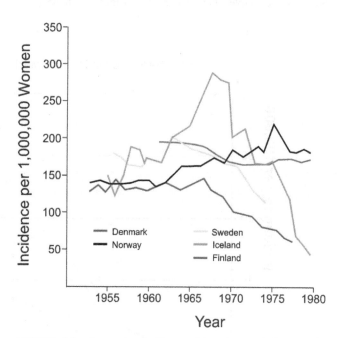

FIGURE 4.3. Decreasing incidence of invasive cervical cancer in those Scandinavian countries that introduced national call and recall screening programs (Sweden and Iceland) demonstrates a much steeper fall-off in cervical cancer rates than in those countries where organized screening was introduced recently or not at all (Denmark and Norway). Recent reductions in cervical cancer incidence occurring following the introduction of organized screening in these countries are not reflected here.

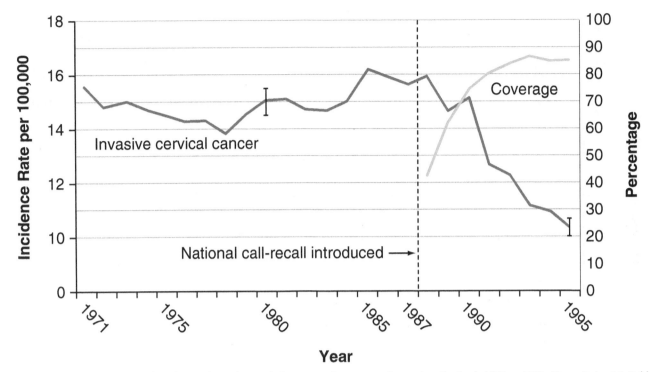

FIGURE 4.4.   Age-standardized incidence of invasive cervical cancer and coverage of screening, England, 1971 to 1995. (From Quinn M, Babb P, Jones J, Allen E. Effect of screening on incidence of and mortality from cancer of cervix in England: evaluation based on routinely collected statistics. *BMJ* 1999;318:904–8.)

In contrast to the reductions in invasive squamous cell carcinoma of the cervix observed over the last four decades in countries with screening, the ASIRs for invasive adenocarcinoma of the cervix have actually increased. In the United States, for example, there was a 29.1% increase in ASIR of

adenocarcinoma from 1976 to 2000 (from 1.23 to 1.76 per 100,000 white women).[19,20] Rapid increases in the incidence rate of invasive cervical adenocarcinoma also occurred in Europe between 1953 and 1997.[21] In England, the risk of cervical adenocarcinoma was estimated to be 14 times greater in

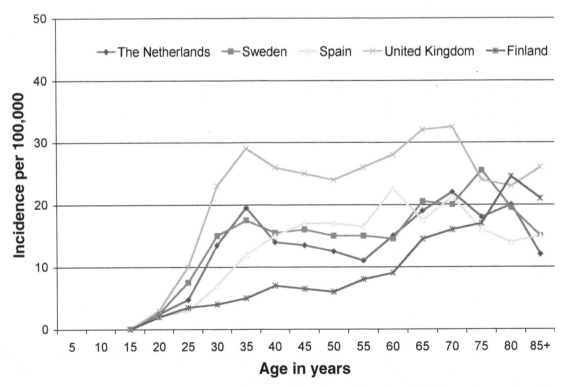

FIGURE 4.5.   Age-specific incidence rates of cervical cancer in five European countries reflect primarily differences in screening policy noted over time. (From Figure 2C: Bosch FX, De Sanjose S. Chapter 1: Human papillomavirus and cervical cancer-burden and assessment of causality. *J Natl Cancer Inst Monogr* 2003;31:3–13.)

women born in the early 1960s than in cohorts born before 1935.[22] The rate of increase was about 0.5% per year in Denmark, Sweden, and Switzerland. It was ≥3% per year in Slovakia and Slovenia.[21,23] For unknown reasons, no increase was observed in France.

Several theories have been proposed to explain the increasing rate of adenocarcinoma. Because abnormal cells from early glandular lesions are less easily detected by cytology than are squamous lesions, it is likely that part of the increase is due to the failure of cytology to adequately screen for adenocarcinoma *in situ*, the precursor lesion to adenocarcinoma.[24] However, an increase in the absolute numbers of cases of cervical adenocarcinoma has also occurred, and this may reflect new environmental influences on the columnar epithelium, such as oral contraceptive (OC) use, or the possibility that the prevalence of HPV 16 and HPV 18 infections, which account for the majority of adenocarcinomas, may be increasing.[22,24,25]

It is also important to note that screening appears to have very little effect on cervical cancer incidence before the age of 30 years as demonstrated by the nearly identical incidence curves for women of young age in a well-screened population (United Kingdom) and in a country with minimal screening (Brazil) (Figure 4.6).[24] In some developed countries, cervical cancer incidence is actually higher for young women aged 15 to 44 years than for age-matched women in less developed countries. Identical rates before age 30 years also indicate similar levels of exposure to HPV in screened and unscreened populations. However, for women aged >45 years living in less developed countries, cervical cancer incidence is more than double that found in more developed countries. After age 30 years, the shape of the incidence curve is highly dependent on the amount of screening that is taking place, as dramatically demonstrated by the divergence seen in cervical cancer incidence after 30 years of age in the United Kingdom (good screening program) and Brazil (minimal screening). Audits of the United Kingdom's screening system and in the United States also have shown no impact of cervical screening on cervical cancer incidence among young women.[26,27]

4.2.3 Other Factors Affecting Geographic Variations

In addition to the availability of cytologic screening, there are numerous other factors relating to sexual behavior, socioeconomic status, and biologic variables that influence geographic variations in the rate of invasive cervical cancer (Figure 4.7).

Low rates of cervical cancer are typically found in countries characterized by conservative sexual behavior, regardless of the widely varying levels of economic development.[28] The age-adjusted incidence rates of invasive cervical cancer in Spain, Italy, Ireland, Israel, China, and Kuwait are all under 10 cases per 100,000 women-years.[7] Because all of these countries are well known for their conservative sexual mores, their low rates reflect, in part, the fact that sexual behaviors play an important role in the pathogenesis of cervical cancer. Further support for the role of sexual behavior comes from the finding that an increase in cervical cancer incidence occurred among women who were in their early reproductive years during periods of social upheaval. This cohort effect has been best documented for women who were in their early reproductive years during either World War I or World War II.[29] These women had a higher risk for cervical cancer throughout their lives than did the cohorts of women who experienced their early reproductive years during the periods immediately before or after the wars. The increased risk of developing cervical cancer in these age cohorts may be attributable to a relaxation of sexual mores during the two wars. Similarly, the increase in cervical cancer mortality in young women observed in the United States and Europe starting in the 1980s is often attributed to changes in sexual behavior that began in the 1960s.[24]

Epidemiologic studies by Bosch and colleagues have clearly demonstrated that part of the geographic variation in cervical

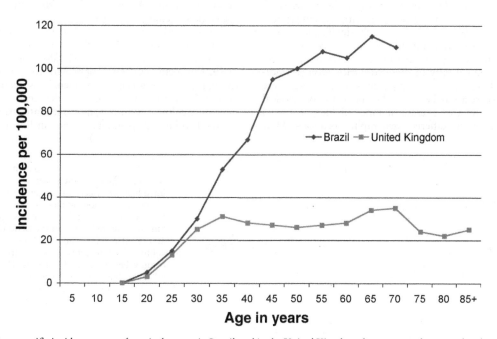

FIGURE 4.6.   Age-specific incidence rates of cervical cancer in Brazil and in the United Kingdom demonstrate the excess burden of invasive cervical cancer in developing countries and the apparent lack of impact of cervical screening on cervical cancer incidence among young women <30 but the dramatic decrease in incidence for women over 30 in the United Kingdom with substantial screening, but not seen in Brazil where screening was minimal. Compiled by IARC for the year 1985, 1990, and 2000. (Modified from Bosch FX, De Sanjose S. Chapter 1: Human papillomavirus and cervical cancer-burden and assessment of causality. *J Natl Cancer Inst Monogr* 2003;31:3–13, Figure 2.)

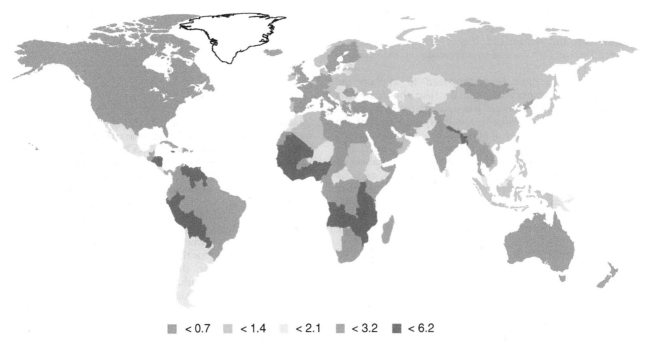

■ < 0.7   ■ < 1.4   ■ < 2.1   ■ < 3.2   ■ < 6.2

FIGURE 4.7. Cumulative incidence risk through age 74 years based on GLOBOCAN estimates. High ASIRs are seen in South America and much of sub-Saharan Africa. Low ASIRs are seen in much of Europe, North America, Australia, and the Middle East and parts of North Africa. (From Ferlay J, Shin HR, Bray F, Forman D, Mathers C, Parkin DM. Estimates of worldwide burden of cancer in 2008: GLOBOCAN 2008. *Int J Cancer* 2010;127:2893–917.)

cancer incidence is attributable to differences in the sexual behaviors of men and, potentially, rates of male circumcision.[30-33] These investigators conducted a series of analyses using population-based surveys to evaluate socioeconomic, medical, and sexual factors. The studies found that although there are marked variations in the average number of lifetime sexual partners of women in different areas, these variations were insufficient to explain the geographic variations in cervical cancer. Moreover, there was no statistically significant correlation between the age-adjusted incidence rate of invasive cervical cancer and the average number of lifetime sexual partners women had. In the majority of these countries, women traditionally had only one to very few partners. In contrast, there was a strong correlation between the incidence of cervical cancer and the estimated average number of lifetime sexual partners of men in the different geographic locations. Male

circumcision is associated with a lower prevalence of penile HPV infections and, in males with a history of multiple sexual partners, a reduction in invasive cervical cancer in their current female partners.[30]

Socioeconomic factors also appear to play a role as evidenced by the declining incidence of cervical cancer in many developed countries prior to the introduction of widespread cytologic screening (Figure 4.8).

For example, in the late 1940s, the incidence of invasive cervical cancer in the United States was 33 cases per 100,000 for white women and 70.4 per 100,000 for black women. By 1969, the incidence had dropped to 16.5 and 35.7, respectively, for the two groups of women. This decreased incidence occurred prior to the period of widespread cytologic screening.[29] In wealthier countries, mortality rates from cervical cancer tend to be higher among women in lower socioeconomic

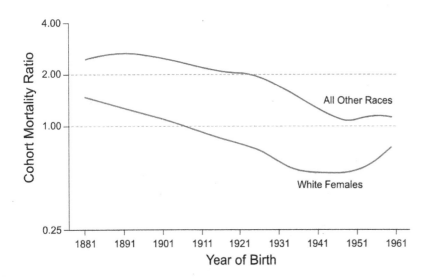

FIGURE 4.8. Mortality from invasive cervical cancer in the United States began to decline before the introduction of cervical screening with the Pap, indicating that socioeconomic forces also play a role in the cohort risk for this cancer. Also potentially important was the reduction in the denominator of women at risk of cervical cancer following the switch from subtotal hysterectomy (cervix sparing) to total hysterectomy beginning in the 1930s. Decline was seen in all races, but mortality was always lower with white females (Adapted from SEER Cancer Statistics. http://seer.cancer.gov, 2008 [Accessed July 19, 2011].).

groups. Although part of this difference is attributable to differences in access to cervical cancer screening, some of it may be related to differences in diet, cigarette smoking, or sexual exposures. For example, studies of women in Spain and Columbia have demonstrated a higher prevalence of genital HPV infections in women from lower, compared with higher, socioeconomic strata.[33,34] Similarly, black women in the United States have had up to a 2.7-fold higher risk for developing cervical cancer than white women.[9] This difference is associated with an increase of a similar magnitude in the prevalence of risk factors for cervical cancer, including multiple sexual partners, low income level, and multiparity.[35] In the United States, high rates of invasive cervical cancer are also observed in Vietnamese, Hispanic, Alaska Native, White women living in Appalachia, Haitian immigrants, and Korean women.[36]

4.3 RISK FACTORS FOR INVASIVE CERVICAL CANCER

Descriptive epidemiologic studies conducted prior to the realization that almost all cervical cancers are the direct result of a persistent infection with specific "oncogenic" HPV types identified numerous behavioral and environmental determinants of cervical cancer incidence (Table 4.2).[24,37,38]

These include demographic factors, such as a woman's age, place of residence, and socioeconomic status.[24,37] Sexual behaviors are important risk factors. These include both a woman's sexual behavior and the behavior of her partner(s), her history of sexually transmitted diseases (STDs), and her age at first sexual intercourse. For example, it has been shown that consistent use of condoms can reduce a woman's risk of acquiring HPV, although condom use has not yet been demonstrated to reduce a woman's risk for invasive cervical cancer.[39,40] Behavioral and medical factors, including tobacco smoking, access to medical care for screening, OC use, parity, and history of immunosuppression, are also important. Finally, a woman's nutritional status and genetic background may influence her risk for developing cervical cancer. However, almost all of these risk factors are either surrogates for exposure to an oncogenic HPV or confer relatively minor degrees of risk compared to infection with an oncogenic HPV. Epidemiologic studies have uniformly found that the overwhelmingly most important risk factor is a persistent anogenital infection with an oncogenic HPV.

4.3.1 Human Papillomavirus

Specific types of HPV have now been classified as human carcinogens.[41] Over 99% of invasive cervical cancers are associated with these specific "oncogenic" HPV types, indicating that HPV is a necessary cause of cervical cancer. The most recent assessment in 2007 by the International Agency for Research on Cancer (IARC is a cancer research arm of the World Health Organization [WHO]) concluded that there is strong epidemiologic evidence that HPV types 16 and 18 are carcinogenic in humans and cause invasive cervical cancer (Table 4.3).[41] In addition, the assessment concluded that case-control studies find a convincing association between HPV 31, 33, 35, 39, 45, 51, 52, 56, 58, and 66 and invasive cervical cancer, based largely on IARC studies conducted by Munoz and coworkers.[42,43] Thus all of these HPV types can be classified as "oncogenic" types. HPV types 26, 68, 73, and 82 were found to be associated with cervical cancer in some case-control studies, but were rarely found associated with cervical cancer in case series and were not found to be risk factors in prospective studies. Therefore, these HPV types should not be considered "oncogenic." Because HPV type-specific data analyses have largely failed to find an association between HPV 6 and 11 and cervical cancer, these types are not classified as "oncogenic." The IARC assessment also concluded that there is sufficient evidence to indicate a causal role for HPV 16 in the pathogenesis of basaloid and warty types of invasive vulvar cancers. The evidence for HPV 18 as causal agent for these cancers is "suggestive." There also is a strong association between HPV 16 and vaginal and anal cancer (see Chapters 14 and 17).[41]

The most comprehensive evaluation of the associations between oncogenic types of HPV and invasive cervical cancers was recently completed and included over 10,575 archival paraffin-embedded cervical cancer specimens studied using the sensitive polymerase chain reaction (PCR) method.[44] HPV DNA was identified in 85% of the specimens. Other studies have reported somewhat higher rates of HPV DNA in invasive cervical cancers. State-of-the-art molecular amplification techniques generally have detected oncogenic HPV DNA in 90% to 100% of invasive cervical cancers.[45] The lower rate reported in the recent study by de Sanjose and coworkers was attributed to technical difficulties with the PCR assay since the paraffin blocks were obtained from around the world, many were quite old, and the DNA was possibly degraded. This degraded

TABLE 4.2	RISK FACTORS FOR INVASIVE CERVICAL CANCER

Patient's age
Living in specific geographic regions such as sub-Saharan Africa
Low socioeconomic status
Lack of cytologic screening
Early age at sexual intercourse
Multiple sexual partners
Partners with multiple sexual partners
History of sexually transmitted infections, especially genital warts, HSV, *C. trachomatis*
High parity
Tobacco smoking
Use of OCs
Immunosuppression from any cause including HIV
Nutritional status
Genetic background

Risk Factors for cervical cancer identified in descriptive epidemiologic studies.
Adapted from Bosch FX, de Sanjose S. Chapter 1: Human papillomavirus and cervical cancer-burden and assessment of causality. *J Natl Cancer Inst Monogr* 2003;31:3–13; Munoz N, Castellsague X, de Gonzalez AB, Gissmann L. Chapter 1: HPV in the etiology of human cancer. *Vaccine* 2006;24(suppl 3):S1–S10.

TABLE 4.3   EVIDENCE FOR HUMAN CARCINOGENICITY OF SPECIFIC HPV GENOTYPES FOR CERVICAL CANCER

Strong epidemiologic evidence for carcinogenicity in humans
  HPV 16, 18
Convincing evidence for carcinogenicity, mainly from case-control series
  HPV 31, 33, 35, 39, 45, 51, 52, 56, 58, 59, 66
Data does not show a convincing association
  HPV 26, 68, 73, 82

Based on a comprehensive literature review, IARC has established the carcinogenicity of many of the anogenital HPV genotypes.
Adapted from *Human Papillomaviruses*. Lyon, France: IARC, 2007.

material makes molecular testing of archival material much more difficult. In the de Sanjose large global survey, the most common oncogenic HPV genotype was HPV 16, found in 61% of the HPV-positive cases. The second most common genotype was HPV 18, found in 10% of the HPV-positive cases. HPV 31, 33, and 45 were found in 4%, 4%, and 6% of the cases, respectively. The next most common types were HPV 35, 39, 52, and 58. All other types were identified in 1% or less of the cases. The distribution of types was similar for both squamous cell carcinomas and adenocarcinomas (Figure 4.9). This study also found that cancers associated with HPV 16, 18, and 45 occur at a much younger age than cancers associated with other types of oncogenic HPV. The average age of women with HPV 16-, 18-, and 45–associated cancers was 50, 48.2, and 46.8 years, respectively compared to 55.5 years for cancers associated with other oncogenic types of HPV.

The strength of the causality association of HPV with cervical cancer is based on an understanding of the molecular biology of HPV and its epidemiology. Epidemiologic proof of causality requires that the association does not conflict with what is known of the natural history and biology of the disease.[24,42] Criteria used to establish epidemiologic proof of causality for cancer and carcinogens in general are listed in Table 4.4.[24]

In brief: (1) exposure needs to precede development of the disease; (2) a reduction of disease should occur following reductions in exposure; (3) the links between agent and disease need to be strong and consistent; (4) there needs to be biologic plausibility; and (5) risk of disease needs to be related to level of exposure.

The specific evidence for a causal role of HPV in the induction of cervical cancer is based on both epidemiologic and laboratory studies and may be briefly summarized as (1) epidemiologic studies clearly indicate that persistent infection with an oncogenic HPV genotype is the single most important risk factor for the development of cervical cancer[38]; (2) oncogenic

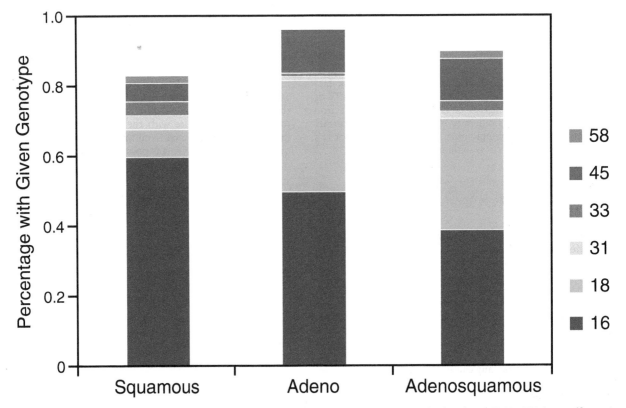

FIGURE 4.9. The distribution of HPV types in cervical cancers was determined by using PCR method to detect HPV DNA in paraffin sections from the tumors. The most commonly detected HPV types were HPV 16, 18, and 45 in squamous cell carcinomas, adenocarcinomas, and adenosquamous carcinomas of the cervix. (From de Sanjose S, Quint WG, Alemany L, et al. Human papillomavirus genotype attribution in invasive cervical cancer: a retrospective cross-sectional worldwide study. *Lancet Oncol* 2010;11:1048–56.)

TABLE 4.4	CRITERIA FOR PROOF OF CAUSALITY ARE ALL FULFILLED IN TERMS OF THE RELATIONSHIP OF HIGH-RISK HPV WITH CERVICAL CANCER	
■ CRITERIA	**■ CONCEPT**	**■ HPV AND CX CA**
Time sequence	Exposure must precede disease	+ + +
Experimental (prevention)	Reduction of disease following reductions in exposure	?
Strength and consistency	Highly associated with the disease in different settings	+ + +
Biologic plausibility and coherence	Mechanisms consistent with previous knowledge	+ + +
Dose-response	Risk of disease is related to level of exposure	+/−

From Bosch FX, De Sanjose S. Chapter 1: Human papillomavirus and cervical cancer-burden and assessment of causality. *J Natl Cancer Inst Monogr* 2003;31:3–13, Table 4.

HPV DNA can be detected in almost all cervical cancers[44,45]; (3) oncogenic genotypes have two oncogenes referred to as E6 and E7 capable of transforming a variety of cell types *in vitro*[46]; and (4) the E6 and E7 oncogenes are expressed in cervical cancers and blocking their expression in cultured cervical cancer cells causes the cells to revert to a nontransformed phenotype.[46] The HPV viral and host interactions leading to cell transformation and malignancy are described in several reviews, and in more detail in Chapter 5.[3,46,47]

4.3.2 Cofactors to HPV-Induced Oncogenesis

Although HPV is capable of transforming cells by itself, it has been hypothesized that cofactors may also play a role in cervical carcinogenesis. Cofactors to HPV in cervical carcinogenesis could potentially act in three ways: (1) by influencing the acquisition of HPV infection; (2) by increasing the risk of HPV persistence; and (3) by increasing the risk of progression from HPV infection to CIN 2,3 and cancer.[48] Nested case-control studies conducted in Denmark and the United Kingdom, as well as other epidemiologic studies, suggest that risk factors for HPV infection/CIN 1 are not necessarily the same as those for CIN 3 and cancer.[37,49,50]

4.3.2.1 Other STDs Including *Chlamydia trachomatis* and HSV-2

The specific role of other sexually transmitted agents including *C. trachomatis* and herpes simplex has been evaluated in numerous epidemiologic studies. It has been hypothesized that infection by sexually transmitted pathogens other than HPV could influence the natural history of HPV infection by altering the probability of persistence and progression of the infection.[51–53] In theory, any factor that increases epithelial turnover in the cervix and causes epithelial repair might promote viral persistence and transformation by altering the balance between a HPV infection and host immunity. Genital tract infections with *C. trachomatis* and HSV-2 may each cause intense cervical inflammation, and both have been associated with cervical cancer in large epidemiologic studies. After adjusting for race, marital status, parity, number of sexual partners, and history of other STDs, exposure to *C. trachomatis*, assessed by both serologic assays and direct detection of *Chlamydia* DNA in cervical cancers, has been found to be a significant and independent risk factor (2.0- to 2.5-fold increased risk) for cervical neoplasia in some studies.[54–58]

In the 1980s, it was shown that HSV-2 could transform cells in culture, and HSV RNA was identified in biopsies of CIN by *in situ* hybridization.[59] In addition, women with cervical cancer and women with high-grade CIN are more likely to have antibodies against HSV-2 than controls, as confirmed by a multicenter case-control study.[60] In the large IARC multicenter case-control study of risk factors for cervical cancer, HSV-2 seropositivity was associated with an increased risk of cervical cancer (odds ratio [OR] = 2.2) for squamous cell carcinoma among HPV-positive women with antibodies against *C. trachomatis*.[61] However, prospective serologic studies have found no significant association between exposure to HSV-2 and the subsequent development of cervical neoplastic disease.[62]

If infection with HSV-2 and *C. trachomatis* has a role as a cofactor, one likely mechanism involves cervical inflammation and repair resulting in the generation of free radicals that could lead to genetic damage and chromosomal alterations.[51] These infections could also act secondary to the effects of decreased mucosal immunity or reparative metaplasia induced by the acute and chronic cervicitis that frequently occurs in women with STDs. Coinfection with HSV-2 and *C. trachomatis* in cervical tissue may result in a more profound inflammatory state, as manifested by increased expression of proinflammatory cytokines over levels present during either infection alone[63] In fact, HPV infections alone do not induce an inflammatory state. It must be stressed, however, that because of the strong associations observed between infections with all STDs, it is difficult to rule out confounding when investigating the role of STDs other than HPV in cervical carcinogenesis.[37]

4.3.2.2 Cofactors and Variables Other than STDs

High parity, smoking, long-term OC use, and immunosuppression are cofactors that may modulate the risk of progression from HPV infection to CIN 2,3 and to cervical cancer. The strength of the evidence ranges from strong and consistent (smoking), to moderately high (parity) and less consistent (OC use).[48] Risk factors for CIN 3 and cervical cancer are similar for some of these cofactors.[64]

4.3.2.2.1 HIGH PARITY

High parity has been found in most case-control studies to be associated with cervical cancer, with risk rising with increasing number of pregnancies. The IARC-pooled reanalysis of data from 25 epidemiologic studies, including 16,563 women with cervical cancer and 33,542 women without cervical cancer, found that the relative risk (RR) for cervical cancer increases with the number of live births.[65] However, the actual increase in RR for invasive cancer associated with each full-term pregnancy was relatively low (RR = 1.10). The pooled analysis found that the effect of multiparity is independent of sexual behavior and socioeconomic variables.[37,38] Some have speculated that the reductions in cervical cancer rates seen in many developed countries prior to the introduction of widespread cervical cancer screening programs could be attributable, in large part, to the general reduction in the number of live births that occurred as living standards improved over the same period.[37] The mechanism by which multiparity increases risk of invasive cervical cancer is unknown, but a new dynamic phase of immature metaplasia occurs with pregnancy-induced eversion of columnar epithelium. Multiparity maintains this recurrent enhancement of the transformation zone on the exocervix for many years, thus facilitating the direct exposure to HPV, and possibly other cofactors.[48] Moreover, the similar levels of increased risk associated with both multiparity and with long-term OC use suggest that hormonal influences may be responsible for both. Exposure to progestational agents may be important in the promotion and persistence of HPV.[48]

4.3.2.2.2 Cigarette Smoking

Epidemiologic studies have clearly shown that smoking is an independent risk factor for invasive cervical cancer and is also a risk factor for the development of CIN 3. An IARC reanalysis of 23 epidemiologic studies from around the globe found that after adjusting for potential confounders, the risk of invasive squamous cell cervical carcinoma was increased in current smokers compared to never smokers (RR 1.60; 95% confidence interval [CI] = 1.48 to 1.73).[66] Other studies have shown that risk increases with increased intensity and duration of smoking (pack-years) and is more significantly associated with CIN 3 than CIN 1, suggesting that tobacco-containing carcinogens promote neoplastic progression in HPV-infected cells.[48,67] A more recent study utilized five large Nordic serum banks and evaluated serum levels of cotinine (a biomarker of tobacco exposure) and antibodies to HPV 16 and 18. Heavy smoking as evidenced by elevated levels of cotinine was found to be associated with an elevated risk of cervical cancer among HPV 16 and/or HPV 18 seropositive women (OR = 2.7; 95% CI = 1.7 to 4.3).[68] As a result of these studies, tobacco smoking is classified by IARC as a cause of cervical cancer.[69]

Several mechanisms have been postulated for the increased risk imposed by cigarette smoking. The secretion of smoke derivatives such as cotinine, nicotine, phenols, benzopyrene, and other hydrocarbons, at highly concentrated levels into the cervical mucus of women who smoke could have numerous effects[70,71] For example, the levels of nicotine and its major metabolite cotinine are increased 40- and 4-fold, respectively, in cervical mucus compared to the serum of smokers.[72] These agents may be directly carcinogenic to the cervical epithelium, as well as reduce local immune responses, possibly enhance HPV viral replication, and alter the HPV life cycle.[70]

4.3.2.2.3 Oral Contraceptive Pills

An increased incidence of squamous cell carcinoma of the cervix has been observed in women taking OCs in some, but not all, studies.[73] The strongest evidence comes from an IARC multicenter case-control study that found only a moderate association with cancer risk (OR = 1.4).[74] In this study there also was a strong dose-response relationship with duration of use. When compared with patients who never used OCs, those who used them for <5 years did not have increased risk of cervical cancer (OR = 0.73), but those who used them for a longer term and were HPV positive had increased odds of cervical cancer (OR = 2.82 for 5 to 9 years, and to 4.03 for 10 or more years). These risks did not vary by time since first or last use. Similarly, the U.K. National Case-Control Study of Cervical Cancer found that the risk of both squamous cell carcinoma and adenocarcinoma of the cervix increased with increasing duration of OC use.[75] Because of the public health significance of these findings, considerable effort has gone into confirming them. A meta-analysis of associations between OC use and cervical cancer concluded that there is a linear dose-response relationship and that the increased risk reverts within 5 to 10 years of OC cessation.[73] Therefore, it is now generally accepted that use of OC confers a measurable increase in risk for squamous cell carcinoma and perhaps an even greater risk of developing invasive adenocarcinoma of the cervix.[76]

OCs have several physiologic effects on cervical epithelium that might explain their association with cervical neoplasia. OCs produce an eversion of the columnar epithelium, thus activating HPV-vulnerable immature squamous metaplasia. Both HPV 16 and 18 have progesterone response elements that increase the expression of HPV E6 and E7 oncogenes, and increased expression of these oncogenes could explain the impact of OC use on the development of cervical cancer.[46]

4.3.2.2.4 Immunosuppression and HIV

Interactions between HIV and HPV were formally recognized in the early 1990s when cervical cancer was classified as one of the criteria for diagnosing acquired immunodeficiency syndrome (AIDS) in HIV-infected women. A strong association between HIV, HPV, and cervical neoplasia has now been clearly documented in multiple studies, and other studies have confirmed similarly increased risk for HPV and cervical neoplasia with both primary immunodeficiency and iatrogenic immunosuppression. The most likely mechanism for this association is the inability of immunocompromised women to clear HPV, increasing susceptibility to HPV and oncogenicity. Female renal transplant recipients have up to a 16-fold increased incidence of CIN, genital warts, and other lower genital tract and anal neoplasia.[77–80] For example, a recent report from the Netherlands found that renal transplant recipients have a 2- to 6-fold increase in CIN, a 3-fold increase in cervical carcinoma, and a 50-fold increase in vulvar carcinoma.[80] There is also evidence that the incidence of CIN is increased in women with systemic lupus erythematosus, and risk is further increased in those taking immunosuppressive drugs, especially cyclophosphamide.[81,82]

In HIV-infected women, the prevalence of cervical HPV infection has ranged from two to four times greater than that observed in HIV-uninfected control women.[83–86] These increases in prevalence are observed for all HPV types.[84] Additionally, HPV infections are significantly more likely to be persistent in HIV-infected women, and the prevalence and severity of HPV-associated lesions, including CIN, is higher.[83] The risk for developing both HPV infections and CIN increases as levels of immunosuppression increase.[87,88] However, this relationship is not as clear for HPV 16 as it is for other high-risk types of HPV.[89] In HIV-infected women, intraepithelial disease is typically multifocal, demonstrating high rates of persistence after standard therapy.[90] Although relationships between HIV and cervical cancer tend to be obscured by the intensive cytologic screening of HIV-infected women in developed countries and the relative short life expectancy of HIV-infected women living in developing countries, tumor registry data have documented increases in many forms of HPV-associated invasive cancers in HIV-infected individuals. For example, in the United States, the RR for invasive cervical cancer in women with HIV infection/AIDS compared to the women in the general population is 5.4 (95% CI = 3.9 to 7.2).[91] Similarly, an increased risk is also seen for vulvar/vaginal cancers (RR 5.8) and anal cancer (RR 6.8) in females.[91] Anal warts and other anal HPV-induced disease are also more common and persistent in men who are HIV infected than in men who do not have HIV, with the rate of anal disease varying inversely with the CD4 level (see Chapter 17).[92]

4.3.2.2.5 Genetic Factors

Some of the differences in rates of cervical cancer observed between Whites, Blacks, and Native Americans may be attributable to genetic differences.[93] The critical role of the human leukocyte antigen (HLA) system in presenting peptides to antigen-specific T-cell receptors may explain why only some HPV-infected women progress to cervical cancer.[93] An association between specific HLA haplotypes and cervical cancer has been demonstrated in a number of studies.[94–96] For example, increased risks of cervical squamous cell carcinoma have been shown to be associated with DRB1*1001, DRB1*1101, and DQB1*0301, and decreased risks have been associated with DRB1*0301 and DRB1*13.[93] These results add to the evidence that certain HLA class II alleles, allele combinations, or genes linked to them make some women more susceptible to progressing from oncogenic HPV infection to squamous cell carcinoma. Three large studies from the United States and Costa Rica noted an increased risk for cervical neoplasia among women with HLA-CW*0202.[97] These findings support the hypothesis that a single allele may be sufficient to confer protection against cervical neoplasia. Because natural killer cells are influenced by HLA-C and its receptors, the role played by HLA haplotypes in cervical neoplasia may reflect a direct effect on the efficiency of the immune response to HPV. Inherited genetic polymorphisms of immune response genes are also associated with risk for both CIN 3 and invasive cervical cancer.[97] One specific disease-liability allele is a protein that serves as a ligand for certain killer immunoglobulin-like receptors.[98]

A recent case-control study evaluated genetic polymorphisms in a large number of candidate genes using single nucleotide polymorphism analysis DNA in women who developed either CIN 3/cancer or had persistent infections with oncogenic HPV genotypes. Different genetic profiles were found that might be associated with both viral persistence and progression to CIN 3/cancer. Variations in genes influencing DNA repair, viral binding, and cell entry of viruses were associated with progression to CIN 3/cancer.[99]

4.4 SUMMARY: EPIDEMIOLOGIC EVIDENCE FOR THE ETIOLOGY OF CERVICAL CANCER

The evidence implicating specific HPV genotypes in the etiology of cervical cancer is now strong enough to establish a causative role for HPV.[41] Many of the other risk factors for cervical cancer, such as a history of other STDs, most likely represent surrogate markers for increased sexual exposure and risk of exposure to HPV. Immature squamous metaplasia within the cervical transformation zone appears to be the epithelium at greatest risk for cellular transformation by HPV. Metaplasia appears to be a maladaptive response to chronic irritation in many organs, but in the cervix, metaplasia is a ubiquitous finding among sexually active women. Risk for incident low-grade squamous intraepithelial lesion has been shown to be related to the rate of active metaplasia rather than to the size of the transformation zone. This suggests that dynamic changes in the transformation zone over time may facilitate the cellular manifestations of HPV infection. One mechanism proposed for the association between high parity and cervical cancer risk is the repeated eversion of endocervical cells onto the portio, increasing exposure of the transformation zone to carcinogenic influences. Exposure of this epithelium to HPV establishes its potential for subsequently developing into a cervical cancer precursor. The most active phases of metaplasia occur during fetal life, in the adolescent years immediately following puberty, and during pregnancy, which explains why both early age at first intercourse and high parity are risk factors for cervical neoplasia.

Cervical neoplasia originates as a complex interplay between HPV and the immature squamous metaplastic epithelium of the cervical transformation zone. Exposure to HPV is an extremely common event, especially in sexually active young women. However, despite the fact that HPV infections are common in young women who are at greatest risk for having immature squamous metaplasia, invasive cervical cancer occurs relatively uncommonly, even in unscreened women, suggesting that additional events or cofactors are required for the development of cervical cancer.

The role of cofactors in the development of cervical neoplasia is just beginning to be understood. As described in Chapter 5, the natural history of most HPV infections is exposure, followed by the development of a productive viral infection that is usually associated with a lesion (either a genital wart or CIN), followed by the induction of host-cell immunity against HPV, resolution of the lesion, and development of a latent infection. The eventual inability of even the most sensitive tests to detect HPV in most women indicates that clearance of the HPV infection may be a possibility. In contrast, the latter events do not occur in women who develop invasive cervical cancer. Instead, HPV infections become persistent, and other, probably random events occur that help promote malignancy. Cofactors such as cigarette smoking, nutritional factors, and infection with HIV appear to act by impairing the ability of mucosal cellular immunity to permanently suppress or eliminate HPV. Impaired immune surveillance may permit the long-term persistence of infection required for the development of invasive cancer. Other cofactors, such as OCs, may directly alter the natural history of HPV infections.

The commonness of this virus and the relative rarity of these cancers highlight the complexity of the natural history of HPV. The comprehensive understanding of HPV so recently established enables us to tell the story of the natural history of HPV, but as in the dialogue between the King and the white rabbit in Lewis Carroll's wonderful Alice in Wonderland, we might ask: "Where shall I begin, please, your majesties?" Like the King we will say, "Begin at the beginning and go until you come to the end. Then stop!"[100]

References

1. zur Hausen H. Human papillomaviruses and their possible role in squamous cell carcinomas. *Curr Top Microbiol Immunol* 1977;78:1–30.
2. *Human Papillomaviruses.* Lyon, France: IARC, 2005.
3. zur Hausen H. The search for infectious causes of human cancers: where and why (Nobel lecture). *Angew Chem Int Ed Engl* 2009;48:5798–808.
4. Burden of cervical cancer globally. WHO/ICO Information Center on HPV and Cervical Cancer 2011. http://www.who.int/hpvcentre/en/ (Accessed July 17, 2011).
5. Yang BH, Bray FI, Parkin DM, Sellors JW, Zhang ZF. Cervical cancer as a priority for prevention in different world regions: an evaluation using years of life lost. *Int J Cancer* 2004;109:418–24.
6. WHO/ICO Information Centre on HPV and Cervical Cancer. HPV and cervical cancer in the 2007 report. *Vaccine* 2007;25(suppl 3):C1–230.
7. Ferlay J, Shin H, Bray F, Forman D, Mathers C, Parkin D. *GLOBOCAN 2008 Cancer Incidence and Mortality Worldwide.* IARC CancerBase number 10. http://globocan.iarc.fr, 2008. Lyon, France: International Agency for Research on Cancer, 2010.
8. Ferlay J, Shin HR, Bray F, Forman D, Mathers C, Parkin DM. Estimates of worldwide burden of cancer in 2008: GLOBOCAN 2008. *Int J Cancer* 2010;127:2893–917.
9. SEER Cancer Statistics. http://seer.cancer.gov, 2008 (Accessed July 19, 2011).
10. Cancer Facts and Figures 2010. American Cancer Society, 2010. http://www.cancer.org/Research/CancerFactsFigures/CancerFactsFigures/cancer-facts-and-figures-2010 (Accessed May 31, 2011).
11. SEER Program—National Cancer Institute, USA. http://wwwseerimsncinihgov/ScientificSystems/1999.
12. Cox T. Management of cervical intraepithelial neoplasia. *Lancet* 1999;353:857–8.
13. Leyden WA, Manos MM, Geiger AM, et al. Cervical cancer in women with comprehensive health care access: attributable factors in the screening process. *J Natl Cancer Inst* 2005;97:675–83.

14. Andrae B, Kemetli L, Sparen P, et al. Screening-preventable cervical cancer risks: evidence from a nationwide audit in Sweden. *J Natl Cancer Inst* 2008;100:622–9.

15. Hakama M. Trends in the incidence of cervical cancer in the Nordic countries. In: Magnus K, ed. *Trends in Cancer Incidence Causes and Practical Implications.* New York: Hemisphere, 1982:279–92.

16. Hakama M. Screening for cervical cancer: experience of the Nordic countries. In: Franco E, Monsonego J, eds. *New Developments in Cervical Cancer Screening and Prevention.* London: Blackwell Science Ltd., 1997:190–9.

17. Hristova L, Hakama M. Effect of screening for cancer in the Nordic countries on deats, costs, and quality of life up to the year 2017. *Acta Oncol* 1997;36(suppl 9):1–60.

18. Quinn M, Babb P, Jones J, Allen E. Effect of screening on incidence of and mortality from cancer of cervix in England: evaluation based on routinely collected statistics. *BMJ* 1999;318:904–8.

19. Wang SS, Sherman ME, Hildesheim A, Lacey JV Jr, Devesa S. Cervical adenocarcinoma and squamous cell carcinoma incidence trends among white women and Black women in the United States for 1976–2000. *Cancer* 2004;100:1035–44.

20. Smith HO, Tiffany MF, Qualls CR, Key CR. The rising incidence of adenocarcinoma relative to squamous cell carcinoma of the uterine cervix in the United States—a 24-year population-based study. *Gynecol Oncol* 2000;78:97–105.

21. Bray F, Carstensen B, Moller H, et al. Incidence trends of adenocarcinoma of the cervix in 13 European countries. *Cancer Epidemiol Biomarkers Prev* 2005;14:2191–9.

22. Sasieni P, Adams J. Changing rates of adenocarcinoma and adenosquamous carcinoma of the cervix in England. *Lancet* 2001;357:1490–3.

23. Vizcaino AP, Moreno V, Bosch FX, Munoz N, Barros-Dios XM, Parkin DM. International trends in the incidence of cervical cancer: I. Adenocarcinoma and adenosquamous cell carcinomas. *Int J Cancer* 1998;75:536–45.

24. Bosch FX, de Sanjose S. Chapter 1: Human papillomavirus and cervical cancer-burden and assessment of causality. *J Natl Cancer Inst Monogr* 2003;31:3–13.

25. Castellsague X, Diaz M, de Sanjose S, et al. Worldwide human papillomavirus etiology of cervical adenocarcinoma and its cofactors: implications for screening and prevention. *J Natl Cancer Inst* 2006;98:303–15.

26. Sasieni P, Castanon A, Cuzick J. Effectiveness of cervical screening with age: population based case-control study of prospectively recorded data. *BMJ* 2009;339:b2968.

27. Chan PG, Sung HY, Sawaya GF. Changes in cervical cancer incidence after three decades of screening US women less than 30 years old. *Obstet Gynecol* 2003;102:765–73.

28. Beral V. Cancer of the cervix: a sexually-transmitted disease? *Lancet* 1974;i:1037–40.

29. Kessler II. Cervical cancer epidemiology in historical perspective. *J Reprod Med* 1974;12:173–85.

30. Castellsague X, Bosch FX, Munoz N, et al. Male circumcision, penile human papillomavirus infection, and cervical cancer in female partners. *N Engl J Med* 2002;346:1105–12.

31. Bosch FX, de Sanjose S, Castellsague X. Geographical and social patterns of cervical cancer incidence. In: Franco E, Monsonego J, eds. *New Developments in Cervical Cancer Screening and Prevention.* London: Blackwell Science Ltd., 1997:23–33.

32. Bosch FX, Castellsague X, Munoz N, et al. Male sexual behavior and human papillomavirus DNA: key risk factors for cervical cancer in Spain. *J Natl Cancer Inst* 1996;88:1060–7.

33. de Sanjose S, Bosch FX, Munoz N, et al. Socioeconomic differences in cervical cancer: two case-control studies in Colombia and Spain. *Am J Public Health* 1996;86:1532–8.

34. Cuello C, Correa P, Haenszel W. Socio-economic class differences in cancer incidence in Cali, Colombia. *Int J Cancer* 1982;29:637–43.

35. Schairer C, Brinton LA, Devesa SS, Ziegler RG, Fraumeni JF Jr. Racial differences in the incidence of invasive squamous-cell cervical cancer. *Cancer Causes Control* 1991;2:283–90.

36. Scarinci IC, Garcia FA, Kobetz E, et al. Cervical cancer prevention: new tools and old barriers. *Cancer* 2010;116:2531–42.

37. Bosch FX, de Sanjose S. The epidemiology of human papillomavirus infection and cervical cancer. *Dis Markers* 2007;23:213–27.

38. Munoz N, Castellsague X, de Gonzalez AB, Gissmann L. Chapter 1: HPV in the etiology of human cancer. *Vaccine* 2006;24(suppl 3):S1–S10.

39. Fukuchi E, Sawaya GF, Chirenje M, et al. Cervical human papillomavirus incidence and persistence in a cohort of HIV-negative women in Zimbabwe. *Sex Transm Dis* 2009;36:305–11.

40. Winer RL, Hughes JP, Feng Q, et al. Condom use and the risk of genital human papillomavirus infection in young women. *N Engl J Med* 2006;354:2645–54.

41. *Human Papillomaviruses.* Lyon, France: IARC, 2007.

42. Bosch FX, Lorincz A, Munoz N, Meijer CJ, Shah KV. The causal relation between human papillomavirus and cervical cancer. *J Clin Pathol* 2002;55:244–65.

43. Munoz N, Bosch FX, de Sanjose S, et al. Epidemiologic classification of human papillomavirus types associated with cervical cancer. *N Engl J Med* 2003;348:518–27.

44. de Sanjose S, Quint WG, Alemany L, et al. Human papillomavirus genotype attribution in invasive cervical cancer: a retrospective cross-sectional worldwide study. *Lancet Oncol* 2010;11:1048–56.

45. Walboomers JM, Jacobs MV, Manos MM, et al. Human papillomavirus is a necessary cause of invasive cervical cancer worldwide. *J Pathol* 1999;189:12–9.

46. Moody CA, Laimins LA. Human papillomavirus oncoproteins: pathways to transformation. *Nat Rev Cancer* 2010;10:550–60.

47. zur Hausen H. Papillomaviruses and cancer: from basic studies to clinical application. *Nat Rev Cancer* 2002;2:342–50.

48. Castellsague X, Munoz N. Chapter 3: Cofactors in human papillomavirus carcinogenesis—role of parity, oral contraceptives, and tobacco smoking. *J Natl Cancer Inst Monogr* 2003;31:20–8.

49. Kruger-Kjaer S, van den Brule AJ, Svare EI, et al. Different risk factor patterns for high-grade and low-grade intraepithelial lesions on the cervix among HPV-positive and HPV-negative young women. *Int J Cancer* 1998;76:613–9.

50. Deacon JM, Evans CD, Yule R, et al. Sexual behaviour and smoking as determinants of cervical HPV infection and of CIN 3 among those infected: a case-control study nested within the Manchester cohort. *Br J Cancer* 2000;83:1565–72.

51. Castle PE, Giuliano AR. Chapter 4: Genital tract infections, cervical inflammation, and antioxidant nutrients—assessing their roles as human papillomavirus cofactors. *J Natl Cancer Inst Monogr* 2003;31:29–34.

52. Schmauz R, Okong P, de Villiers EM, et al. Multiple infections in cases of cervical cancer from a high-incidence area in tropical Africa. *Int J Cancer* 1989;43:805–9.

53. Williams VM, Filippova M, Soto U, Duerksen-Hughes PJ. HPV-DNA integration and carcinogenesis: putative roles for inflammation and oxidative stress. *Future Virol* 2011;6:45–57.

54. Wallin KL, Wiklund F, Luostarinen T, et al. A population-based prospective study of *Chlamydia trachomatis* infection and cervical carcinoma. *Int J Cancer* 2002;101:371–4.

55. Smith JS, Munoz N, Herrero R, et al. Evidence for *Chlamydia trachomatis* as a human papillomavirus cofactor in the etiology of invasive cervical cancer in Brazil and the Philippines. *J Infect Dis* 2002;185:324–31.

56. Anttila T, Saikku P, Koskela P, et al. Serotypes of *Chlamydia trachomatis* and risk for development of cervical squamous cell carcinoma. *JAMA* 2001;285:47–51.

57. Koskela P, Anttila T, Bjorge T, et al. *Chlamydia trachomatis* infection as a risk factor for invasive cervical cancer. *Int J Cancer* 2000;85:35–9.

58. Paba P, Bonifacio D, Di Bonito L, et al. Co-expression of HSV2 and *Chlamydia trachomatis* in HPV-positive cervical cancer and cervical intraepithelial neoplasia lesions is associated with aberrations in key intracellular pathways. *Intervirology* 2008;51:230–4.

59. Galloway DA, McDougall JK. The oncogenic potential of herpes simplex viruses: evidence for a "hit and run" mechanism. *Nature* 1983;302:21–3.

60. Hildesheim A, Mann V, Brinton LA, Szklo M, Reeves WC, Rawls WE. Herpes simplex virus type 2: a possible interaction with human papillomavirus types 16/18 in the development of invasive cervical cancer. *Int J Cancer* 1991;49:335–40.

61. Smith JS, Herrero R, Bosetti C, et al. Herpes simplex virus-2 as a human papillomavirus cofactor in the etiology of invasive cervical cancer. *J Natl Cancer Inst* 2002;94:1604–13.

62. Lehtinen M, Koskela P, Jellum E, et al. Herpes simplex virus and risk of cervical cancer: a longitudinal, nested case-control study in the nordic countries. *Am J Epidemiol* 2002;156:687–92.

63. Rasmussen SJ, Eckmann L, Quayle AJ, et al. Secretion of proinflammatory cytokines by epithelial cells in response to *Chlamydia* infection suggests a central role for epithelial cells in chlamydial pathogenesis. *J Clin Invest* 1997;99:77–87.

64. Moreno V, Munoz N, Bosch FX, et al. Risk factors for progression of cervical intraepithelial neoplasm grade III to invasive cervical cancer. *Cancer Epidemiol Biomarkers Prev* 1995;4:459–67.

65. Cervical carcinoma and reproductive factors: collaborative reanalysis of individual data on 16,563 women with cervical carcinoma and 33,542 women without cervical carcinoma from 25 epidemiological studies. *Int J Cancer* 2006;119:1108–24.

66. Appleby P, Beral V, Berrington de Gonzalez A, et al. Carcinoma of the cervix and tobacco smoking: collaborative reanalysis of individual data on 13,541 women with carcinoma of the cervix and 23,017 women without carcinoma of the cervix from 23 epidemiological studies. *Int J Cancer* 2006;118:1481–95.

67. Szarewski A, Cuzick J. Smoking and cervical neoplasia; a review of the evidence. *J Epidemiol Biostat* 1998;3:229.

68. Kapeu AS, Luostarinen T, Jellum E, et al. Is smoking an independent risk factor for invasive cervical cancer? A nested case-control study within Nordic biobanks. *Am J Epidemiol* 2009;169:480–8.

69. *Tobacco Smoke and Involuntary Smoking.* Lyon, France: IARC Press, 2004.

70. Gadducci A, Barsotti C, Cosio S, Domenici L, Riccardo Genazzani A. Smoking habit, immune suppression, oral contraceptive use, and hormone replacement therapy use and cervical carcinogenesis: a review of the literature. *Gynecol Endocrinol* 2011;27(8):1–8.

71. Prokopczyk B, Cox JE, Hoffmann D, Waggoner SE. Identification of tobacco-specific carcinogen in the cervical mucus of smokers and nonsmokers. *J Natl Cancer Inst* 1997;89:868–73.

72. Hellberg D, Nilsson S, Haley NJ, Hoffman D, Wynder E. Smoking and cervical intraepithelial neoplasia: nicotine and cotinine in serum and cervical mucus in smokers and non-smokers. *Am J Obstet Gynecol* 1988;158:910–3.

73. Smith JS, Green J, Berrington de Gonzalez A, et al. Cervical cancer and use of hormonal contraceptives: a systematic review. *Lancet* 2003;361:1159–67.

74. Moreno V, Bosch FX, Munoz N, et al. Effect of oral contraceptives on risk of cervical cancer in women with human papillomavirus infection: the IARC multicentric case-control study. *Lancet* 2002;359:1085–92.

75. Green J, Berrington de Gonzalez A, Sweetland S, et al. Risk factors for adenocarcinoma and squamous cell carcinoma of the cervix in women aged 20–44 years: the UK National Case-Control Study of Cervical Cancer. *Br J Cancer* 2003;89:2078–86.

76. Chilvers C, Mant D, Pike MC. Cervical adenocarcinoma and oral contraceptives. *Br Med J* 1987;295:1446–7.

77. Penn I. Cancers of the anogenital region in renal transplant recipients. *Cancer* 1986;58:611–6.

78. Penn I. Tumors of the immunocompromised patient. *Ann Intern Med* 1988;39:63–73.

79. Harwood CA, Surentheran T, McGregor JM, et al. Human papillomavirus infection and non-melanoma skin cancer in immunosuppressed and immunocompetent individuals. *J Med Virol* 2000;61:289–97.

80. Meeuwis KA, van Rossum MM, van de Kerkhof PC, Hoitsma AJ, Massuger LF, de Hullu JA. Skin cancer and (pre)malignancies of the female genital tract in renal transplant recipients. *Transpl Int* 2010;23:191–9.

81. Klumb EM, Pinto AC, Jesus GR, et al. Are women with lupus at higher risk of HPV infection? *Lupus* 2010;19:1485–91.

82. Klumb EM, Araujo ML Jr, Jesus GR, et al. Is higher prevalence of cervical intraepithelial neoplasia in women with lupus due to immunosuppression? *J Clin Rheumatol* 2010;16:153–7.

83. Kojic EM, Cu-Uvin S. Update: human papillomavirus infection remains highly prevalent and persistent among HIV-infected individuals. *Curr Opin Oncol* 2007;19:464–9.

84. Clifford GM, Goncalves MA, Franceschi S. Human papillomavirus types among women infected with HIV: a meta-analysis. *AIDS* 2006;20:2337–44.

85. Sun XW, Kuhn L, Ellerbrock TV, Chiasson MA, Bush TJ, Wright TC Jr. Human papillomavirus infection in women infected with the human immunodeficiency virus. *N Engl J Med* 1997;337:1343–9.

86. Palefsky JM. Human papillomavirus infection and anogenital neoplasia in human immunodeficiency virus-positive men and women. *J Natl Cancer Inst* 1998;23:15–20.

87. Heard I. Prevention of cervical cancer in women with HIV. *Curr Opin HIV AIDS* 2009;4:68–73.

88. Ellerbrock TV, Chiasson MA, Bush TJ, et al. Incidence of cervical squamous intraepithelial lesions in HIV-infected women. *JAMA* 2000;283:1031–7.

89. Strickler HD, Palefsky JM, Shah KV, et al. Human papillomavirus type 16 and immune status in human immunodeficiency virus-seropositive women. *J Natl Cancer Inst* 2003;95:1062–71.

90. Einstein MH, Phaeton R. Issues in cervical cancer incidence and treatment in HIV. *Curr Opin Oncol* 2010;22:449–55.

91. Frisch M, Biggar RJ, Goedert JJ. Human papillomavirus-associated cancers in patients with human immunodeficiency virus infection and acquired immunodeficiency syndrome. *J Natl Cancer Inst* 2000;92:1500–10.

92. Palefsky J. Human papillomavirus-related disease in people with HIV. *Curr Opin HIV AIDS* 2009;4:52–6.

93. Madeleine MM, Brumback B, Cushing-Haugen KL, et al. Human leukocyte antigen class II and cervical cancer risk: a population-based study. *J Infect Dis* 2002;186:1565–74.

94. Wang SS, Wheeler CM, Hildesheim A, et al. Human leukocyte antigen class I and II alleles and risk of cervical neoplasia: results from a population-based study in Costa Rica. *J Infect Dis* 2001;184:1310–4.

95. Hildesheim A, Apple RJ, Chen CJ, et al. Association of HLA class I and II alleles and extended haplotypes with nasopharyngeal carcinoma in Taiwan. *J Natl Cancer Inst* 2002;94:1780–9.

96. Hildesheim A, Wang SS. Host and viral genetics and risk of cervical cancer: a review. *Virus Res* 2002;89:229–40.

97. Wang SS, Hildesheim A, Gao X, et al. Comprehensive analysis of human leukocyte antigen class I alleles and cervical neoplasia in 3 epidemiologic studies. *J Infect Dis* 2002;186:598–605.

98. Martin MP, Borecki IB, Zhang Z, et al. HLA-Cw group 1 ligands for KIR increase susceptibility to invasive cervical cancer. *Immunogenetics* 2010;62:761–5.

99. Wang SS, Gonzalez P, Yu K, et al. Common genetic variants and risk for HPV persistence and progression to cervical cancer. *PLoS One* 2010;5:e8667.

100. Wikiquotes "Alice's Adventures in Wonderland". http://en.wikiquote.org/wiki/Alice's_Adventures_in_Wonderland (Accessed July, 20, 2011).

The Biology and Importance of Human Papillomavirus Infection

5.1 INTRODUCTION
5.2 DESCRIPTION AND NATURE OF HUMAN PAPILLOMA-
VIRUS
   5.2.1 Low-Risk Viral Types
   5.2.2 High-Risk Viral Types
   5.2.3 Infections with Multiple HPV Types
   5.2.4 Functional Differences between Low-Risk and High-Risk
      HPV Types
5.3 NATURAL HISTORY OF GENITAL HPV INFECTION
   5.3.1 Transmission
5.4 LIFE CYCLE OF HPV
   5.4.1 Viral Entry

5.4.2 Productive Viral Infection
5.4.3 Host Containment
5.5 NATURAL HISTORY OF CERVICAL INTRAEPITHELIAL
NEOPLASIA
   5.5.1 Development of Low-Grade Disease
   5.5.2 Progression of Persistent HPV Infection to High-Grade
      CIN
   5.5.3 Progression to Invasion
5.6 DEVELOPMENT OF NEW BIOLOGIC MARKERS
5.7 SUMMARY

5.1 INTRODUCTION

The relationship between human papillomavirus (HPV) and cervical cancer is now well established.[1-5] HPV infection causes virtually all cases of CIN 3 and cervical cancer and approximately 40% to 50% of vaginal and vulvar cancers, 50% of penile cancers, and 90% of anal cancers.[1-6] By the mid-1990s, case-control studies had demonstrated that the great majority of women with cervical neoplasia have detectable levels of HPV DNA[7-10] and that the presence of high-risk HPV (hrHPV) predicted an increased risk of high-grade intraepithelial neoplasia.[10-15] On any given day, approximately 5% to 27% of healthy, otherwise asymptomatic women will test positive for hrHPV DNA[14,16-18]; in contrast, 90% to 100% of women with high-grade CIN will test positive.[19-23]

The study of the natural history and epidemiology of HPV infection was initially hampered by the inability to culture the virus and the relative insensitivity of early serologic tests to determine exposure. The first molecular probes for the detection of HPVs were developed in 1983,[24,25] and the number of high-risk genital HPV types detected has now grown to approximately 15, with 3 more listed as probable high risk.[26] In this short time, the DNA sequences have been mapped, RNA transcription and protein translations significantly described, and efficient, cost-effective tests developed. A clear understanding of the biology, morphologic expression, and natural history of cervical HPV infection is essential to the rational management of cervical neoplasia.

5.2 DESCRIPTION AND NATURE OF HUMAN PAPILLOMAVIRUS

Papillomaviruses are small, 8000 base-pair double-stranded DNA viruses that are species specific,[1] infect epithelial cells, and can induce a variety of benign and malignant tumors in humans and other species.[27] The virion is encased in a nonenveloped 72-sided icosahedral protein capsid (Figure 5.1.) The viral genome usually exists in an episomal (circular) configuration with only one strand transcriptionally active. The HPV genome is divided into three regions: the upper regulatory region (URR), the early (E) region, and the late (L) region (Figure 5.2). The URR is a noncoding region of the HPV genome that is responsible for regulation of viral replication and transcription of downstream sequences in the early region.[27,28] Functional papillomavirus genes are found only on the early (E) and late (L) regions and are referred to as open reading frames (ORFs). Each ORF is read as a specific unit by RNA polymerase.[27,28] The early region encodes predominantly for proteins important in viral replication, which occurs "early" in viral life cycle. The late region encodes for viral structural proteins necessary for capsid production, which occurs chronologically later in the viral life cycle.[1,27,28]

The URR activation of the early region is responsible for maintaining high viral copy number through promotion of viral replication.[28] In HPV types associated with cancer, the early region also encodes for proteins that promote cellular transformation. Eight different ORFs that can encode for proteins have been identified in the early region of HPV; these are designated E1 through E8 (Table 5.1).[28] The E1 ORF produces a protein helicase responsible for viral genomic replication. Transcript analyses of several HPV types have revealed that the viral E2 gene encodes both the E2 regulator protein and the E8∧E2C protein, a potent repressor of viral transcription and replication.[29] These proteins regulate transcription by exerting control over the expression of other early region ORFs, particularly E6 and E7.[27-29] Hence, they have an important function of suppressing the oncogenic potential of these two genetic loci. E2 is also required for proper plasmid partitioning in dividing cells to establish viral persistence.[30]

Integration of hrHPV types into the host-cell genome disrupts the HPV regulatory E2 protein, resulting in a loss

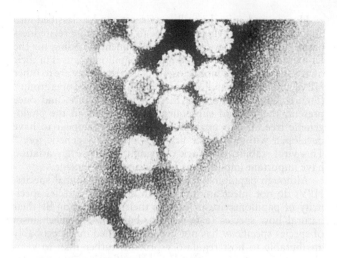

FIGURE 5.1. A highly magnified electron micrograph demonstrates the icosahedral structure of the HPV virion.

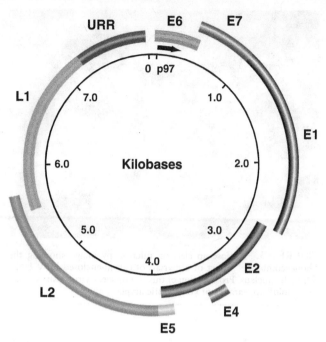

FIGURE 5.2. The nucleoside sequence of the HPV genome. The DNA exists in a double-stranded circular helix that can be divided into three regions: the upper regulatory region (URR), the early (E) region, and the late (L) region.

of negative feedback control of viral oncogene expression; this disruption has been considered a critical event in the pathogenesis of cervical neoplasia and a potential biomarker of progressive disease.[31]

The function of the E3 gene has been less clear, but E3 ubiquitin ligases may lead to the development and progression of various cancers.[32] The protein products from E4 are detected in large amounts in productive infections and may be important in altering the normal cytokeratin matrix of infected cells, allowing the release of viral particles from the cells.[27,28,33] Additionally, E4 messenger (m)RNA encoding transcripts are markedly down-regulated in high-grade lesions and cancer.[34] The E5 protein has been shown to cause binucleated cells as a result of cell-cell fusion, down-regulate host immune responses, and activate growth receptors, such as epidermal growth factor receptor and platelet-derived growth factor receptor.[27,28,35]

The varying carcinogenicity of HPV species, and types within species, is mainly related to the activity of two oncogenes, E6 and E7. Among other functions, their gene products interact with tumor suppressors p53 and pRb, respectively.[1] By disabling the most important antioncogenes, spontaneous mutations can accumulate over time, resulting eventually in cellular proliferation and immortalization.[36] The E8 protein appears to be complexed with the E2 regulator protein as E8∧E2C, as discussed above.[28,29]

The two late regions, L1 and L2, encode for proteins involved in construction of the capsid of the infective HPV genome (Figure 5.1). The L1 capsid protein—the major capsid protein—is structurally but not antigenically constant in all the HPV types, whereas the L2 produced minor capsid protein is much more variable among HPV types.[28,29] However, because the major antigenic determinates of L2 are usually conserved among types, the antigenic response to L2 is more cross-reactive. Without its surrounding capsid, HPV DNA is not infective (Figure 5.3). Hence, capsid production in terminal cells in the upper epithelial layers is critical if HPV is to pass from host to host. Transcription of L1 and L2 capsid proteins appears to be initiated by transcriptional regulators found only in differentiated host cells in the intermediate and superficial epithelial layers.[28,29] Large amounts of L1 and L2 encoded proteins can be detected in condyloma acuminata, but only small amounts are present in CIN 3 and cancer.[28]

TABLE 5.1	FUNCTIONS OF HPV GENES
■ **GENE DESIGNATION**	■ **FUNCTION**
E1	Initiation of viral DNA replication
E2	Regulation of viral transcription with an auxiliary role in DNA replication
E3	Less clear but E3 ubiquitin ligases may promote oncogenesis
E4	Disrupts cytokeratins
E5	Transformation (animals only)
E6	Transformation, targets degradation of p53 tumor supressor protein
E7	Transformation, binds to the pRB
E8	With E2, viral transcription and replication
L1	Major capsid protein
L2	Major capsid protein

Modified from Lowy DR, Howley PM. Papillomaviruses. In: Knipe DM, Howley PM, eds. *Fields Virology*. Philadelphia, PA: Lippincott Williams & Wilkins, 2001:2231–64, with permission.

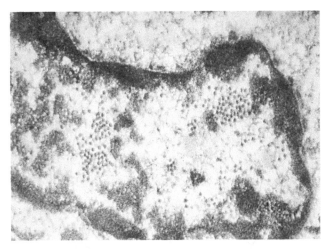

FIGURE 5.3.   A close-up electron microscopy image showing the "honeycomb-like" effect of a myriad of capsid-enclosed HPV DNA filling the nucleus. Proliferation of this intranuclear virus results in the "raisinoid" appearance of koilocytotic atypia.

Human and animal papillomaviruses can be classified into Supergroups in a phylogenetic tree to demonstrate relatedness based on comparison of nucleotide sequences coding for the L1 capsid protein. HPVs and animal papillomaviruses in their own Supergroup are more closely related than they are to other HPVs and animal papillomaviruses in a different Supergroup[37] (Figure 5.4). Mutations in these viruses are rare, and once present, they spread subsequently as markers in the phylogenetic tree.[38,39] For example, low-risk types appear to have developed within a single branch of the phylogenetic tree.[40] This viral stability and lack of significant genomic variation have important implications for vaccine development.

Although papillomaviruses occur in many animal species, HPVs do not infect any nonhuman hosts. The species specificity of papillomaviruses enables their classification by their natural host species (e.g., human, bovine). The mechanism of species specificity has not been determined but is probably attributable to host regulatory proteins rather than to virus absorption and penetration.[27] Subclassification into types is done according to nucleotide sequence. The most common HPV types are listed in Table 5.2.[27] Each papillomavirus type is highly tropic for a specific epithelium and has its own degree

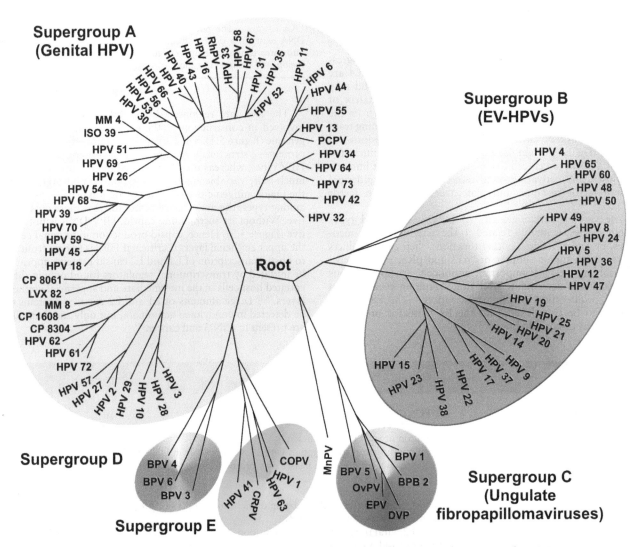

FIGURE 5.4.   Phylogenetic tree for 92 human (HPVs) and animal papillomaviruses demonstrates that HPVs are more closely related to animal papillomaviruses in their Supergroup than to HPVs in a different Supergroup. (Modified from Howley PM, Lowy DR. Papillomaviruses and their replication. In: Knipe DM, Howley PM, eds. *Fields' Virology*. Philadelphia, PA: Lippincott Williams & Wilkins, 2001:2197–229, with permission.)

TABLE 5.2	MAJOR CLINICAL ASSOCIATION OF GENITAL TRACT AND OTHER MUCOSAL HPVS

■ CLINICAL ASSOCIATION	■ HPV TYPE
Genital tract	
Subclinical infection	All genital HPVs
Exophytic condyloma	6, 11
Flat condyloma	6, 11, 16, 18, 31, others
Bowenoid papulosis	16
Giant condyloma (Bushke-Lowenstein tumor)	6, 11
Cervical cancer	
Strong or moderate association	16, 18, 31, 33, 35, 39, 45, 51, 52, 56, 58, 59, 68
Weak or no association	6, 11, 26, 42, 43, 44, 53, 54, 55, 62, 66
Vulvar cancer	16
Penile cancer	16
Respiratory papillomas	6, 11
Conjunctival papillomas	6, 11
Oral cavity	
Infection with genital tract HPVs	6, 11, 16

From Lowy DR, Howley, PM. Papillomaviruses. In: Knipe DM, Howley PM, eds. *Fields Virology*. Philadelphia, PA: Lippincott Williams & Wilkins, 2001:2231–64, with permission.

of oncogenicity, and variants within each type vary in oncogenicity within that type.[41] Although viral tropism is poorly understood, it is presumed to be secondary to differences in nucleotide structure and reflects interactions between viral- and host-encoded proteins at specific anatomic sites.

Papillomaviruses have developed over millions of years in specific hosts, and have differentiated within each host to infect specific sites.[38] Hence, the tropism of the alpha genus of HPV types for the anogenital and oral mucosa. Even within the mucosal HPV types, some types are more specific for infecting

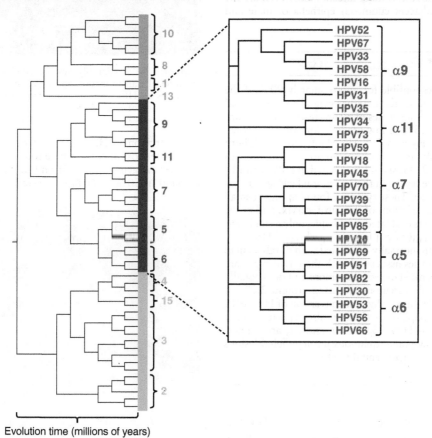

Evolution time (millions of years)

FIGURE 5.5. Phylogenetic tree of anogenital HPV types. The phylogenetic tree is based on the alignment of early and late ORFs. The carcinogenicity of HPV types reflects viral evolution. The most important HPV types in the *blue* section ([alpha] 1, 8, 10, 13) are associated with genital warts. HPV types in the *red* section ([alpha] 5, 6, 7, 9, 11) are associated with cervical cancers, CIN 2,3, and AIS (shown in detail). HPV types in the *green* section ([alpha] 2, 3, 4, 15) are commensal infections. (From Schiffman MH, Wentzensen N. From human papillomavirus to cervical cancer. *Obstet Gynecol* 2010;116(1):177–85, with permission.)

the cervix versus the vagina. More importantly, of the three main branches of the alpha genus, all established carcinogenic HPV types are in a single branch comprised of five groups ("species"): alpha-5, alpha-6, alpha-7, alpha-9, and alpha-11[38] (Figure 5.5). The five species in the high-risk group have different risk profiles. Alpha-9 is the most important species, consisting almost entirely of carcinogenic types.[41] HPV types are numbered in order of discovery. An HPV type is ≥10% different than all other characterized papillomavirus types in the L1 ORF.[42] More than 120 HPV types have now been described, more than 40 of which have a predilection for the anogenital tract. Of these, approximately 15 have been found in cervical cancers and have therefore been termed "high-risk" (HPVs 16, 18, 31, 33, 35, 39, 45, 51, 52, 56, 58, 59, 68, 73, and 82).[1,6,26,43] Three additional HPV types have been classified as "probable high-risk" (HPVs 26, 53, and 66), and 12 have been classified as low-risk types (HPVs 6, 11, 40, 42, 43, 44, 54, 61, 70, 72, 81, and CP6108).[26] For any given HPV type, viral isolates that differ by more than 2% in the coding regions and 5% in the noncoding regions of the viral genome with respect to the prototype isolates are designated variants. HPV-16 appears to have evolved along five major branches, two being present mainly in Africa, two in Asia, and one in Europe and India, and these variants are often named by these geographic regions. The most carcinogenic of the high-risk types are found in two clusters, one containing HPV 16 and one containing HPV 18.[27,38] Although genital HPV is a common term for this group, they may also infect several nongenital sites, including the upper airways, oral mucosa, conjunctiva, and periungual tissues.[28] The principle reservoirs of infection, however, are the moist mucosa and adjacent cutaneous epithelia of male and female genitalia.

5.2.1 Low-Risk Viral Types

HPV 6 and 11 are responsible for approximately 90% of the exophytic condylomata of the external genitalia, vagina, and cervix (Figure 5.6), for most cases of recurrent respiratory papillomatosis, and for <15% of low-grade lesions of the cervical transformation zone (Figure 5.7).[44] Mixed infections with both low-risk and high-risk viral types are common in women with CIN.[45,46] HPV types 42, 43, and 44 are related to HPV 6 and 11 on both the nucleotide level and their common lack of association with cervical cancer. These types are found in only a small proportion of low-grade lesions of the vulva, cervix, and penis. Of 1000 cervical cancers evaluated worldwide, only a single cervical cancer tested positive for a low-risk viral type.[3] However, although HPV 6/11 are normally associated with purely benign disease, rare malignancies associated with these two types are found, including Buschke-Lowenstein tumors and occasionally anal, vulvar, and penile carcinoma (causing around 2.5% to 5% of these lesions).[44] Rare malignant conversion of HPV 6/11 recurrent respiratory papillomas (RRP) is also reported. Other low-risk types, such as HPV 53, 61, 70, and 71, are primarily associated with low-grade squamous intraepithelial lesions (LSILs) throughout the lower genital tract.[37,47]

5.2.2 High-Risk Viral Types

The oncogenic risk of hrHPV types has been delineated by their close association with human tumors and by their ability to immortalize normal cells.[27] The relative risk of CIN 3 and cervical cancer associated with many of these genital HPV types has been well delineated.[26,43] Although 15 types have been classified as high risk, 8 cause most of the cervical cancers (In order of frequency: HPV 16, 18, 45, 33, 31, 52, 58, and 35). The majority belongs to species alpha-9 (HPV 16 related), but alpha-7 (HPV 18–related) types are disproportionately important for

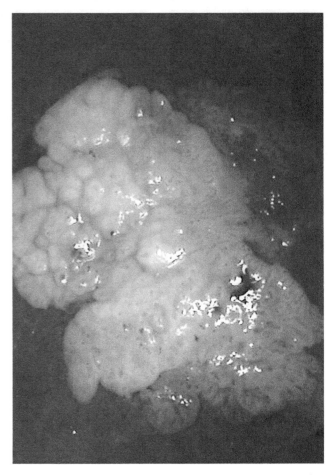

FIGURE 5.6. A clinically obvious condyloma acuminatum within the cervical transformation zone. Cervical condylomata are usually secondary to HPV 6 or 11, and are a relatively uncommon (3%) manifestation of cervical HPV.

adenocarcinoma.[1] HPV 16 is by far the most carcinogenic and is also the most important type found in HPV-induced cancers in other anogenital epithelia and in the oropharynx. HPV 16 is found in 50% to 60% of cervical cancers and HPV 18 in

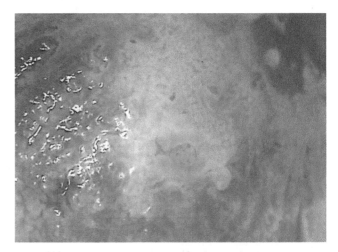

FIGURE 5.7. A low-grade HPV-associated lesion of the cervix that also tested positive for HPV 6. Although exophytic condylomas are virtually always secondary to low-risk HPV types, these same types also may present as flat lesions characterized by an irregular margin, indistinct acetowhitening, and a trivial vascular pattern. The differential for minor HPV changes, as demonstrated here, is with normal immature metaplasia.

Distribution of Human Papillomavirus Types Worldwide

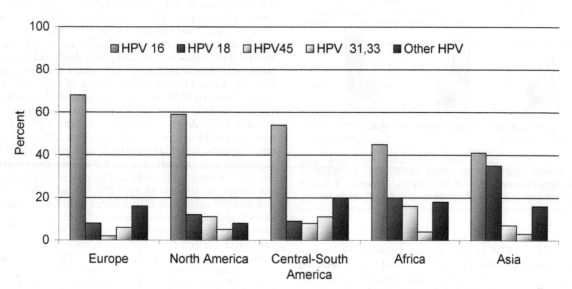

FIGURE 5.8.   HPV 16 is responsible for approximately 50% of invasive cervical cancers worldwide. Geographic variations do occur, with just over 40% of cancers in Asia testing positive for HPV 16 and almost 70% HPV 16 positive in Europe. (From Bosch FX, Manos MM, Munoz N, et al. Prevalence of human papillomavirus in cervical cancer: a worldwide perspective. *J Natl Cancer Inst* 1995;87:796–802, with permission.)

10% to 12% (Figure 5.8).[1,43] Data pooled from 11 case-control studies from nine countries documented that the most common HPV types in patients with squamous cell cervical cancer in descending order of frequency were 16, 18, 45, 31, 33, 52, 58, and 35 (Table 5.3).[26] The most common types among women in the control group not having cancer were types 16, 18, 45, 31, 6, 58, 35, and 33. Therefore, the four most common types in the population are also the four most common types in women with cervical cancer.

HPV 16 is uniquely likely to persist and to cause neoplastic progression when it persists, making it a remarkably powerful human carcinogen that merits separate clinical consideration.[38] HPV 16 is the most common type detected in CIN 3, and HPV 16 CIN 3 appears to occur at a younger age than CIN 3 positive for other carcinogenic HPV genotypes.[48,49] Among women ≥30 years with CIN 3, HPV 16 was found in 49%, HPV 31 in 9.2% and HPV 18 in 8.5%. There was a decrease at older ages in the fraction of CIN 3, AIS and CIN 3/AIS associated

TABLE 5.3   DISTRIBUTION OF HPV TYPES IN 1918 WOMEN WITH HISTOLOGICALLY CONFIRMED SQUAMOUS-CELL CERVICAL CANCER AND 1928 CONTROL WOMEN

HPV TYPE	CASES		CONTROLS		OR (95% CI)*	
	NO.	%	NO.	%	NO.	%
Negative	46	3.39	1091	84.44	1.00	
HPV 16	685	50.52	42	3.25	434.34	(278.30–677.87)
HPV 18	177	13.05	17	1.32	248.56	(138.37–446.48)
HPV 31	36	2.65	8	0.62	122.16	(52.87–282.26)
HPV 33	14	1.03	1	0.08	368.34	(46.15–2939.53)
HPV 35	15	1.11	6	0.46	74.99	(26.82–209.72)
HPV 39	8	0.59	0	0	—	
HPV 45	74	5.46	9	0.70	197.46	(91.69–425.26)
HPV 51	13	0.96	4	0.31	65.65	(19.76–218.12)
HPV 52	37	2.73	4	0.31	198.99	(67.49–586.72)
HPV 56	9	0.66	5	0.39	45.24	(14.05–145.63)
HPV 58	31	2.29	6	0.46	115.64	(45.40–294.57)
HPV 59	17	1.25	1	0.08	418.60	(54.15–3236.17)
HPV 73	5	0.37	1	0.08	107.28	(11.52–999.43)

Data pooled from 11 case-control studies in nine countries.
*OR adjusted for age and center.
Modified from Munoz N, Bosch FX, de Sanjose S, et al.; International Agency for Research on Cancer Multicenter Cervical Cancer Study Group. Epidemiologic classification of human papillomavirus types associated with cervical cancer. *N Engl J Med* 2003;348:518–27, with permission.

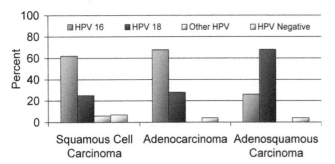

Distribution of Human Papillomavirus DNA in Invasive Cervical Carcinomas by Histologic Types

FIGURE 5.9. HPV 18 is more commonly associated with adenocarcinomas and adenosquamous carcinomas, in which it represents approximately 68% of the cancers. However, it is also found in approximately 25% of squamous cell cervical carcinomas.[3]

with HPV 16.[49] HPV 16 also causes approximately one-third of adenocarcinomas (Figure 5.9)[26] and is also detected in 40% to 90% of HPV-related intraepithelial neoplasias of the vulva (vulvar intraepithelial neoplasia [VIN]), vagina (vaginal intraepithelial neoplasia [VaIN]), penis (penile intraepithelial neoplasia [PIN]), head and neck, and anus (anal intraepithelial neoplasia [AIN]) (Figure 5.10).[50–53] Compared to the other carcinogenic HPV genotypes in aggregate, HPV 18 was strongly associated with CIN 3+ in women with a normal Pap.[49]

Although HPV 16 is a high-risk viral type, it is detected in at least 40% of minor low-grade lesions of the vulva and penis, 30% of minor-grade cervical lesions, 10% of external genital warts (EGWs), and up to 7% of cytologically normal younger women.[54] Most HPV infections are not associated with lesions, but the longer HPV 16 persists, the more likely CIN 3 will develop.[48] This wide clinical variability associated with HPV 16 indicates that women infected with this virus, although at greater risk for HPV-associated malignancies, most commonly remain asymptomatic or develop lesions that do not progress

to invasive cancer. It is still not entirely understood why some HPV 16–associated CIN may progress to invasion, whereas others do not. One possibility is that there may be individual differences in the genetic capability of the host immune response to suppress HPV expression.[55] Another is the existence of unique variants of specific HPV types that may have significant clinical implications.[41] HPV variants generally differ in risk of persistence, at least partly due to deletions in transcriptional silencer elements.[56] For some HPV types, especially HPV 16, variant lineages differ in risk of CIN 3+.[41] An association between HPV 16 variants, particularly non-European variants, and the development of cervical cancer has been well documented.[55] Asian American or African HPV 16 variants have a fivefold or greater risk of cancer compared to European variants, which are still very high risk.[41] There is some suggestion that variants of other HPV types also confer different risks of viral persistence and/or progression to precancer, but except for some work on HPV 18 and HPV 58 variants, and on HPV variants in HIV-infected individuals, there is little known about the natural history of variants of types other than HPV 16 among immunocompetent women.[41,57–59] Cervical cancer derived from HPV 16 harbors almost exclusively certain E6 variants (94%), whereas CIN 3 demonstrates a more uniform distribution of variants (56%) and prototype (44%) (Figure 5.11).[56] The underlying genetic details that make non-European variants of HPV 16 more carcinogenic are not well understood, but variations identified to date are in areas likely to be important for protein-protein interaction with p53, resulting in degradation and loss of DNA checking and apoptosis, or in areas of other immunologic significance. In contrast, E7 variations are rare. Such variation within HPV 16 may be partially responsible for the variability in risk noted for individuals infected with this viral type.[56,60–64]

HPV 18 is less frequently detected in any grade of CIN than would be expected, considering its place as the second most common (25%) viral type in invasive cervical cancers. This suggests that these cancers may arise *de novo* without traversing the intraepithelial spectrum or that they transit too rapidly to be detected by routine screening.[65] One possible explanation is that the E2 gene appears to be disrupted earlier in HPV 18 infections than with other HPV types, which may result in earlier integration of HPV 18, coupled

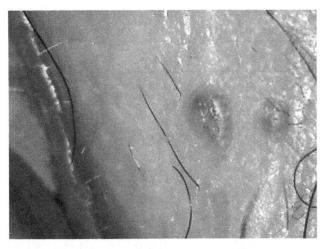

FIGURE 5.10. Two pigmented lesions on the left labium majus typed positive for HPV 16 and histologically interpreted as VIN 3. These lesions are relatively common in young women. Despite their association with a known oncogenic viral type and the high-grade morphologic appearance, these may occasionally be transient lesions with resolution occurring before treatment can be scheduled.

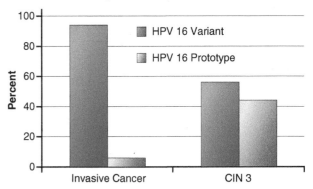

Distribution of Human Papillomavirus Type 16 and Variants in Cervical Intraepithelial Neoplasia and Invasive Carcinoma

FIGURE 5.11. HPV 16 variants have deletions in transcriptional silencer elements that may be responsible for the ability of some HPV 16 to persist. In contrast to the more uniform distribution of variants and prototype in CIN 3, demonstration of a virtual preponderance of HPV 16 variants in cervical cancer supports this significance. (Modified from Zehbe I, Wilander E, Delius H, Tommassino M. Human papillomavirus 16 E6 variants are more prevalent than the prototype. *Cancer Res* 1998;58:829–33, with permission.)

with a substantial reduction in viral load, potentially explaining why HPV 18–associated disease is often reported to be characterized by minor cytologic change that underestimates the severity of the underlying histologic abnormality.[31] Adenocarcinomas in young women are particularly suspect of fitting this model as they are most commonly associated with HPV 18 and often are not detected in a timely manner by cytologic screening.[49,66] Cancers associated with HPV 18 occur 2.6 times more frequently within 1 year of a negative Pap test than cancers associated with HPV 16.[65]

5.2.3 Infections with Multiple HPV Types

Women with long-term persistence of HPV infection appear to be generally more susceptible to other HPV infections, especially longer-lasting infections, than are women who cleared their HPV infections.[66] Therefore, women least likely to clear their HPV infections accumulate multiple HPV types. The large National Cancer Institute natural history study in Guanacaste, Costa Rica, found that 43% of HPV-positive women were infected with multiple types.[67] Compared with single infections, coinfection with multiple □9 species was associated with significantly increased risk of CIN 2+ (OR = 2.2). However, the risk appeared to be the sum of the estimated risk from individual types rather than evidence of synergistic interactions.[67] A large population study in the Netherlands documented multiple HPV types in 11.8% of HPV-positive cytology specimens with normal or atypical squamous cells of undetermined significance (ASC-US) cytology, 34.5% of HPV-positive cytology samples with CIN 1 and 2, and in 4.4% of the HPV-positive cancer cytology specimens.[68] The increasing number of types found in women with squamous intraepithelial lesions (SILs) compared with women who have normal cytologic specimens likely reflects tolerance and persistence of HPV infection in individuals developing CIN, whereas dominance of single type in cancers reflects the known monoclonal development of HPV-induced cancer.[69] Permissive immunity would allow accumulation of HPV infections upon exposure to different types because of an inability to clear each infection as it occurs. Therefore, the accumulation of multiple HPV types could serve as a surrogate marker for increased risk for cervical neoplasia that reflects decreased immunocompetence and subsequent viral persistence.[70]

In the rare cases in which multiple infections are found in carcinomas, additional CIN lesions within the specimen due to other type(s) may be the source.[68,70] In most studies, acquisition of multiple types was more likely in women with HPV 16.[68,69]

5.2.4 Functional Differences between Low-Risk and High-Risk HPV Types

All papillomaviruses share the need to induce DNA synthesis in host cells to replicate viral DNA. This is commonly achieved by the interaction of the E7 protein with members of the retinoblastoma (pRb) gene family of the host, which would normally lead to the induction of growth arrest or apoptosis in the infected cell (Figure 5.12).[71] Although both low-risk and high-risk HPV types have the capability of prohibiting apoptosis in the proliferating cells of low-grade cervical intraepithelial lesions (CIN 1) and condylomata, only the E5, E6, and E7 proteins of hrHPV types neutralize cell cycle regulators responsible for inhibiting malignant proliferation.[28,47,72] E5 may have several possible transforming functions, including a role in EGF-related signal transduction and a role in the disruption of cell-to-cell communication, which

is often observed in transformed cells.[27,28] HPV E6 and E7 proteins each have several individual effects on cell proliferation and genetic abnormalities, but both are necessary to initiate neoplastic transformation.[1,27,28] Their gene products are known to inactivate the major tumor suppressors, p53 and retinoblastoma protein (pRB), respectively. In addition, one function of E6 is to activate telomerase, and E6 and E7 cooperate to effectively immortalize human primary epithelial cells. Though expression of E6 and E7 is itself not sufficient for cancer development, it seems to be either directly or indirectly involved in every stage of multistep carcinogenesis.[36,73,74]

E6 proteins from low-risk HPV types cannot induce degradation of p53, nor can E7 from low-risk HPV inactivate pRB.[74] The result is that low-risk HPV types have minimal capability to promote cellular immortalization, transformation, and oncogenesis.[27] The E6 oncoprotein is necessary for oncogenesis to occur; degradation of p53 and subsequent blockage of the normal apoptotic response to inappropriate DNA replication depends entirely on the action of this protein.[75] Increased telomerase expression has been found in tissues infected with HPV 16 or 18 expressing HPV E6. Telomerase expression is significantly higher in cervical cancers (85%) and CIN 2 and 3 (61%) than in CIN 1 (10%) or normal histology (7%).[27]

HPV E7 from high-risk, but not from low-risk, HPV types also interacts with cellular growth regulatory proteins that may contribute to cell transformation.[76] The protein product of E7 binds the tumor suppressor protein of pRb (Figure 5.13).[27] The retinoblastoma tumor suppressor protein is a critical regulator of the DNA synthesis (S) phase of cell division.[27] Normal epithelial cells have terminally withdrawn from cellular replication, as only basal cells can replicate. Therefore, induction of epithelial proliferation by HPV requires that the pRb protein be suppressed.[28] hrHPV E7 proteins have a higher affinity for pRb proteins than low-risk HPV E7 proteins due to a single amino acid difference in the E7 protein of low-risk types.[77] This difference ensures that hrHPV E7 will increase cell proliferation, and thereby cellular transformation, by promoting transition from the G1 to the S phase.[28,78] Additionally, HPV E7 proteins can inactivate the cyclin-dependent kinase inhibitors p21[79] and p27,[80] which are important in inducing growth arrest in cells.[28]

Therefore, the function of E7 in the oncogenic process may be to (1) override cell cycle checkpoint controls, (2) modulate the expression of cellular proteins, (3) deregulate cellular carbohydrate metabolism, and (4) modulate apoptosis.[27] hrHPV E6 and E7 proteins are also individually able to induce genomic instability in normal human cells, with E6-inducing gene amplifications and deletions and E7-inducing aneuploidy.[81] E6 and E7 proteins also can cooperate to induce centrosome-associated defects of mitotic spindle formation that may result in aneuploidy and chromosomal instability.[82] Low-risk HPV E6 and E7 proteins do not induce genomic instability.[83] Thus E7 may act as a mitotic mutator, resulting in the abnormal mitoses and genomic instability demonstrated in the malignant progression of HPV-associated lesions.[84,85] The absence of molecular plausibility for low-risk HPV types in the oncogenic process explains the segregation of HPV types into those found in malignancies and those that are not. The mechanism by which rare low-risk HPV 6 or 11 cancers, such as Buschke-Lowenstein verrucous carcinomas, occur is not clear.

One function common to both low- and high-risk HPV types is their ability to evade host-immune recognition, which may be enhanced by HPV E7 suppression of the interferon signal.[86] This may be one mechanism by which expression of HPV E6 and E7 proteins may promote viral persistence and interruption of cellular growth pathways that normally would lead to growth arrest and cell death.[28] Apoptosis of DNA-damaged human keratinocytes is markedly reduced in cells expressing either HPV 16 E6 or E7 protein.[87] Such inhibition may render the cells susceptible to the accumulation of mutations

Physiologic

High Risk HPV

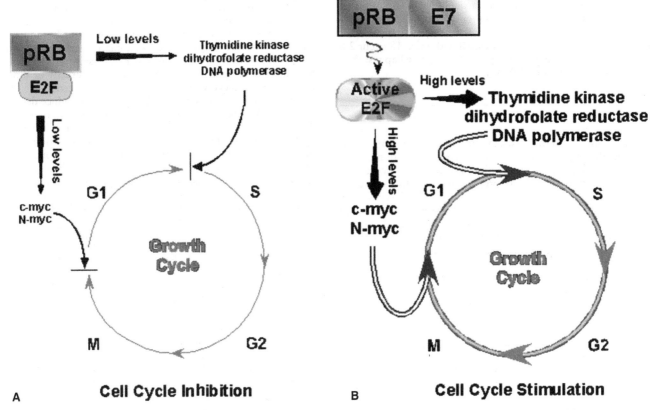

A   **Cell Cycle Inhibition**

B   **Cell Cycle Stimulation**

FIGURE 5.12.   Both low- and high-risk viral types need to replicate by inhibiting apoptosis (cell death) in proliferating cells that would normally follow any abnormal cell growth. One mechanism by which HPVs accomplish this is by interaction of the E7 protein with protein produced by the pRb family of host genes responsible for ordering cell destruction. Demonstrated here are the interactions between HPV-16 E7, pRb, and E2F-1: **(A)** Physiologic: G1 phase growth-arrested cell under physiologic conditions; **(B)** High-risk HPV: proliferating cell-infected high-oncogenic-risk HPV type. (Modified from Park TJ, Fujihara H, Wright TC. Molecular biology of cervical cancer and its precursors. *Cancer* 1995;76:1902, with permission.)

necessary for carcinogenesis. HPV oncogenesis likely requires long-term persistence of the virus for the process to have the time for exposure to random events that eventually lead to the accumulation of these mutations.

Viral integration appears to occur when poorly understood viral, host, and cofactor interactions result in loss of host-cellular control and persistence of hrHPV.[88] Integration of HPV DNA into the host genome is a rare irreversible genetic alteration that is likely to initiate a chain of events involving the impairment of the tumor suppressor genes p53 and pRb and subsequent genomic instability and cell immortalization.[61] When HPV integrates, viral DNA most frequently breaks in the HPV E1/E2 gene region.[89] Disruption of the E2 ORF results in loss of the function of E2,[89] which normally produces an important protein that regulates expression of the major E6 and E7 oncogenes (Figure 5.14). Since the E2 protein is essential for control over both transcription and replication, loss of E2 function can produce increased transcription of E6 and E7 oncogenes.[28,89] Keratinocytes containing integrated HPV 16 have been shown to have a growth advantage over those containing episomal HPV 16 because of the increased levels of HPV 16 E6 and E7 protein.[90] Expression of E6 and E7 is retained in cervical cancers, but E5 expression is commonly lost following viral integration.[2] The frequency of HPV integration increases with increasing disease severity and therefore is likely to be an important and

perhaps critical step in progression to invasion.[6] The discrepancy between the high rate of HPV infection and the low incidence of cervical cancer may be secondary to the relative infrequency of these interactions all occurring in an individual.

5.3 NATURAL HISTORY OF GENITAL HPV INFECTION

5.3.1 Transmission

Cancers caused by genital tract HPVs are associated with risk factors related to sexual practices, which are in large part surrogate measures for HPV exposure. It is likely that the transmission of viral infections to nongenital sites increases as a consequence of certain sexual behaviors, such as multiple sexual partners, oral-genital contact, or by autoinoculation from a genital infection, and therefore will be captured by use of standard sexual behavior measures. Sexual behaviors known to be associated with HPV exposure include high number of lifetime sexual partners, young age at first intercourse, shorter time between meeting a partner and having intercourse, and a history of sexually transmitted disease(s).[91] While other mechanisms of transmission are possible, they are

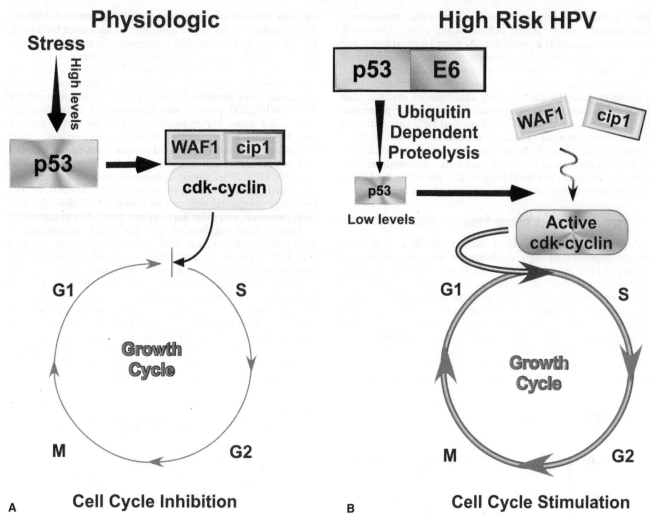

FIGURE 5.13. Interactions between HPV 16 E6 p53 and CDK-cyclin: **(A)** Physiologic: G1 phase growth-arrested cell that has been exposed to some form of cellular stress; **(B)** High risk HPV: proliferating cell-infected high-oncogenic-risk HPV type. (Modified from Park TJ, Fujihara H, Wright TC. Molecular biology of cervical cancer and its precursors. *Cancer* 1995;76:1902, with permission.)

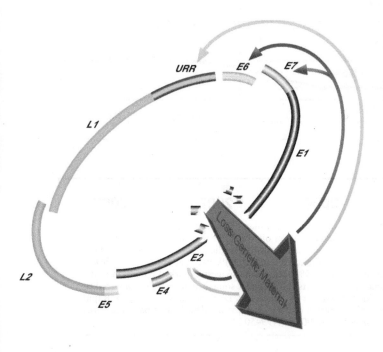

FIGURE 5.14. Loss of normal cell regulatory control occurs with integration of HPV DNA into the host chromosome. In the episomal state, E2 has regulatory control over E6 and E7 (*blue arrow*) and also regulates the upper regulatory region (URR) (*green arrow*). Breakage of the chromosome between E1 and E2 prior to integration interrupts this control.

likely to be less common sources of infection than intercourse. Interactions between sexual behaviors and other known risk factors for cancers at a particular site must be considered. For instance, in the case of oropharyngeal cancers, alcohol and tobacco use may confuse analysis of sexual behavior.

Postmarketing data from the use of the quadrivalent HPV vaccine in Australia provide early confirmatory evidence that HPV prevention in one sex provides some level of protection in the opposite sex (Figure 5.15). Universal HPV vaccination of girls and women aged 12 to 26 was initiated in 2007. In 2008, genital warts declined 25% per quarter in women under 28 years and by 5% per quarter in heterosexual men.[92] Although far from definitive evidence, this trend suggests that the widely held belief that vaccinating one sex will protect another may be valid.

5.3.1.1 Sexual Transmission

Evaluations of large cohorts of women initially seen prior to sexual exposure strongly confirms the sexually transmitted nature of HPV infections.[91,93–95] In a 2-year follow-up of nearly 100 women, virginal at enrollment, only virgins who initiated intercourse became HPV DNA positive on cervical HPV testing and/or developed HPV 16 antibodies.[94] The study also demonstrated the high transmission rate of HPV, with a third becoming positive for at least one HPV type, and the high rate of spontaneous resolution of recently acquired infections, as only 3% remained persistently positive. Similar findings have been demonstrated by others.[95,96] Cervical cancer is, therefore, the

ultimate outcome of a persistent sexually transmitted infection. Sexual activity is the most important risk factor for both penile HPV lesions and for cervical carcinogenesis; the sexual history of either partner is equally important in risk analysis. However, the contribution of "the male factor" has always been difficult to evaluate accurately.[97] An eightfold difference in cervical cancer rates between Colombia (48/100,000 women) and Spain (6/100,000 women) was demonstrated to be associated with a 3.3 times higher number of lifetime sexual partners and 1.6 times higher number of visits to prostitutes, among Colombian men when compared to men from Spain.[98] Consistent with this association was a 5.0-fold increased prevalence of penile HPV DNA among Colombian men.[99] Condom use is only partly protective, even when used conscientiously, because the entire anogenital skin can be infected, including the scrotum, perineum, and other surfaces not covered by condoms.[1,100]

Genital tract papillomaviruses are readily transmitted by genital-to-genital contact, and although exposure to multiple HPV types is common, there is no evidence of HPV-type interaction, as each infection appears to act separately.[101,102] The length of the average incubation period from HPV exposure to lesion expression varies greatly and may range from a few weeks to occasionally years or decades.[103] Transmission studies of visible EGWs show that lesions of recent origin are more likely to be infective than chronically present lesions.[103] Over 64% of women identified with incident HPV 6 or HPV 11 infection developed clinically identified genital warts within 36 months.[96] That up to 66% of sexual partners of persons with EGWs develop

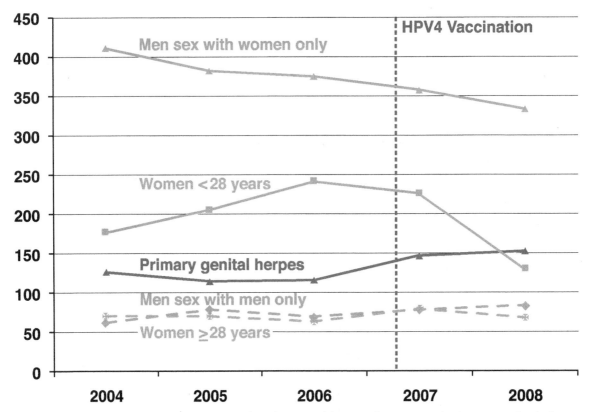

FIGURE 5.15.   Results of a retrospective study to determine if the Australian HPV vaccination program has had a population impact on presentations of genital warts. The proportion of women in the vaccine age group diagnosed with warts decreased by 25.1% per quarter in 2008 in comparison with a negligible quarterly increase in the same age-group prior to vaccination. Men were not provided the same access to HPV vaccination, but nevertheless demonstrated an average quarterly decrease in genital warts of 5%. These data suggest a marked reduction in the incidence of genital warts among vaccinated women and supports the idea that some benefit may be conferred to heterosexual men. (Adapted from Fairley CK, Hocking JS, Gurrin LC, Chen MY, Donovan B, Bradshaw CS. Rapid decline in presentations of genital warts after the implementation of a national quadrivalent human papillomavirus vaccination programme for young women. *Sex Transm Infect* 2009;85:499–502.)

similar lesions is evidence of how easily HPV is transmitted.[103–105] Presumably, the 40% not proven to have lesions either do not become infected, never express disease, or develop lesions so transiently that they remain undetected. Altered epithelial immunity with increasing age may be a factor when the period between exposure and the development of an identifiable lesion is long.[106] The potential for a protracted period between exposure and the presence of a specific lesion reduces the possibility for most individuals of determining when and where HPV exposure occurred. However, the strongest predictor of HPV detection and new disease expression is a history of recent exposure to a new sexual partner.[94,107]

5.3.1.2 Extragenital and Fomite Transmission

Although the primary route of HPV transmission is sexual, current evidence is strong enough to conclude HPV can also be transmitted nonsexually.[107] Several studies have explored whether HPVs can be transmitted horizontally through caring for the child with infected hands, bathing, towels, and fomites.[108] HPV infections can be transmitted horizontally to infants and children via saliva or other contacts,[107] and genital-oral transmission of specific HPV types is suggested by detection of HPV 6, 11, and 16 in oral specimens.[109] In one of the largest prospective studies on HPV detection during pregnancy, at birth, and 6 weeks postpartum, HPV detected at the postpartum visit in the mother was a stronger determinant of HPV infection in the child than HPV detected during pregnancy, suggesting that horizontal mother-to-child transmission may play a more important role than vertical transmission in determining HPV DNA detection in children.[110] Mothers, relatives, caregivers, and fomites harbor HPVs that likely can be horizontally transmitted to the child, in particular in the first weeks of life when there is a close caring physical contact relationship with the infant.

Genital warts found in children often raise the suspicion of sexual abuse despite the fact that the origin of anogenital HPV infection in children is often not apparent with no indication of sexual abuse documented.[111,112] Despite this, the development of genital condylomata in children is distressing because of its potential implications. HPV 6 and 11 are the most common genotypes in genital warts in children just as they are in adults, but HPV 16/18 has been reported in up to 4%.[107] As HPV 6, 11, and 16 are found in oral lesions in adults, it should be kept in mind that these types may also be transmitted by inoculation. Further, genital condyloma acuminata may occur in sexually naive girls, and perianal condyloma acuminata may occur in persons who deny heterosexual or homosexual contact. One large study demonstrated that most cases of anogenital warts in children (128/131) are likely to be the result of nonsexual transmission, particularly during the prenatal and perinatal period.[111]

hrHPV has consistently been identified in approximately 25% of cancers of the oral cavity, pharynx, and larynx, with about 50% found in the tonsils and at the base of the tongue.[113,114] HPV-associated oral cancers differ from similar non–HPV-related cancers by a lower frequency of p53 mutations, more basaloid cell type and better prognosis.[113–116] Although heavy alcohol use and tobacco use are the most common etiologic factors in head and neck cancers (HNCs), most studies show only alcohol to have a synergistic effect with HPV in the etiology of HPV-associated HNC.[114,117] The most common HPV types identified in HNC squamous cell carcinoma are HPV 16, 6, 11, 31, and 33, but HPV 16 accounts for the majority (86+%).[114] It is interesting to note that the classically LR HPV 6 and 11 subtypes have been found in some tonsillar and laryngeal carcinomas other than the rare benign laryngeal papillomas that undergo malignant transformation. HPV 6 and 11 have also been detected in Ackerman's tumor (verrucous carcinoma of the oral cavity). It is clear that low-risk HPV types 6 and 11 can play a role in certain rare malignancies of the oropharynx.[114]

As in cervical and other HPV-induced cancers, genetic alterations of the p16 INK4A gene leads to loss of control of the restriction point in the G1 phase of the cell cycle, thus favoring cellular transformation.[118] Because p16INK4A expression loss defines a subgroup of oral cancer patients with worse clinical outcome, the viral load of HPV in HNCs, as well as p16 expression, may be the most relevant prognostic markers in HPV-induced HNCs, more important than staging by the classical histopathologic parameters.[118] As further proof of the role of HPV in these cancers, the total number of lifetime sexual partners, young age at first intercourse, and a history of genital warts, even after adjustment for alcohol and tobacco exposure, are all documented as significant risk factors for oral cancer.[113,115]

Besides possible genital-oral transmission of HPV, HPV-induced extragenital skin lesions may occasionally serve as viral reservoirs. The potential for this is illustrated by the detection of HPV 16 in periungual warts, bowenoid papulosis and squamous cell carcinoma of the finger.[119,120] Nonsexual transmission of HPV types 6 and 11 to the conjunctiva and nose has also been reported.[121] Additionally, HPV 16 and HPV 18 E6 gene expression has been demonstrated in conjunctival cancers.[122] HPV infection of the conjunctiva most likely occurs by autoinoculation, although it has been speculated that intrapartum exposure of the fetus as it passes through an infected birth canal might be another possible route of exposure.[123] Additionally, fomite transmission may be responsible for some cases of nonsexual exposure. Transmission of nongenital HPV types to the genital area has been described from tanning beds and other fomite surfaces.[124] Transmission from medical examination tables and instruments has yet to be documented, although viral DNA can be detected in the medical office setting.[125]

5.3.1.3 Vertical Transmission

Vertical transmission can be divided into three categories according to the assumed time of HPV transmission: (1) periconceptual transmission (time around fertilization), (2) prenatal (during pregnancy), and (3) perinatal (during birth and immediately thereafter).[107] Prospective studies have demonstrated that infection of newborns with mucosal HPV is common, including high-risk types. HPV 16 the most prevalent, but HPV 6, 18, 54, and 61 also detected.[107] HPV DNA detection in amniotic fluid, fetal membranes, cord blood, and placental trophoblastic cells all suggest that HPV infection can occur in utero during the prenatal period.[107] The detection of HPV DNA in the endometrium, fallopian tube, and even ovary raises the possibility that HPV could be present in the endometrium at the time of conception and result in periconceptual vertical transmission.[107] The occasional finding of HPV-induced lesions in the infant at birth suggests either periconceptual or prenatal HPV transmission. Perinatal transmission directly from mother to infant during the birth process is thought to be the most common route of vertical transmission. A number of studies have demonstrated a median 39% (0.2% to 73%) concordance between cervical HPV detected in the mother and HPV detected soon after birth on the infant.[107] However, although a recent study showed concordance between newborn and mother in HPV detection (HPV+/+ and HPV−/−) to be 71%, vertical transmission of HPV to the baby was not common, as only 1.5% of newborns were found to be HPV positive despite a 30% detection rate in the mothers.[126] One large prospective study found a strong and statistically significant association between mother's and child's HPV status at the 6-week postpartum visit; children of mothers who were HPV positive at the postpartum visit were about five times more likely to test HPV positive than children of corresponding HPV-negative mothers.[110] Even in this study, transmission from mother to infant was low, and HPV persistence in infants was rare. Because HPV may be transmitted prior to delivery, cesarean section does not completely protect newborns against HPV. However, the largest meta-analysis of vertical transmission of HPV demonstrated the rate of HPV detection after vaginal delivery to be higher than after cesarean (18.3% vs. 8%).[127] Fortunately, most vertical HPV transmission appears to be transient, with persistent infections in oral and genital mucosa being found in <10% and 2%, respectively. HPV detection declines quickly over the first year, with most studies no longer finding HPV DNA in the infant's genital mucosa by 1 year after delivery. Persistent genital HPV infection was detected in one large Finnish study in only 1.5% of the infants during the follow-up.[128] Seroconversion to the HPV types initially detected indicates that such clearance is due to a successful immune response.

The most serious consequence of vertical transmission of HPV is juvenile-onset recurrent respiratory papillomatosis (JORRP), caused primarily by HPV 6 or HPV 11. Although a failure of innate and adaptive immunity in clearing HPV from the upper airway keratinocytes is likely primarily responsible for the rare cases of RRP, patients with this disorder appear to have normal responses to other pathogens.[129] Hence, RRP should be recognized as a complex, multigene disease manifesting as a tissue, and HPV-specific, immune deficiency that prevents effective clearance and/or control of HPV 6 and 11 infection.[129] When not cleared, HPV 11 is more likely to cause more severe disease and earlier onset.[107] RRP is classified as either juvenile-onset (JO) or adult-onset (AO), based upon the bimodal age distribution of this clinical finding.[107] JORRP presents in prepubertal children usually before 5 years of age, while in adult-onset RRP (AORRP) the typical age is 20 to 40 years.[130] The incidence of JORRP in the United States is 1.7 to 4.3 per 100,000.[130] Seven of every one thousand births with a maternal history of genital warts during pregnancy were subsequently found to result in the development of RRP in the child.[107] The median age of a child developing laryngeal papillomas following delivery to a mother with known genital warts at the time of delivery was 4.3 years. However, most children developing RRP have been born to mothers with no history of genital warts during pregnancy, and the median time to development of RRP in these children is 5.9 years. Typically, the most severe disease occurs in those with the youngest age of onset. Malignant transformation of RRP has been reported in 3% to 5% of the RRP patients, but nearly all cases are associated with previous irradiation of the papillomas or a history of heavy smoking.[107]

The virtual requirement of sexual intercourse as a prerequisite for cervical cancer indicates that either cervical colonization at the time of birth with oncogenic HPV types does not occur or, if it does, cofactors transmitted sexually may be necessary for viral promotion. Another possibility is that maternal antibodies circulating in the newborn and/or the unfavorable hormonal milieu present in the neonate after clearance of maternal estrogen and progesterone may limit HPV persistence in the neonate. If vertical transmission of HPV resulted in even transient infection, such exposure could potentially influence later immune response at the time of sexual exposure.[91,131]

5.4 LIFE CYCLE OF HPV

Since a large percentage of the population is exposed cumulatively over time to HPV, it is clear that the majority never develop detectable HPV-induced lesions. About 5% of

acute HPV infections persist past a few years.[1] An even smaller fraction of women infected with HPV develop persistent infection or cancer. Therefore, it would appear that clinically expressed disease is more often the exception than the rule.[1,132] Evaluation of newly diagnosed HPV in women with negative cytologic results suggests that only about 15% will have a subsequent abnormal Pap test within 5 years.[133] Most of these infections likely result in only transient expression, as a complex interplay of host, viral, and environmental factors triumph over the viral intruder. For a relative minority of individuals, however, this complex interplay has far different results; persistent expression may escape immune control and result in a variety of morphologic possibilities. The first step begins with viral entry.

5.4.1 Viral Entry

HPV is transmitted in desquamated genital epithelial cells (Figure 5.16) that degenerate, leaving HPV capsids free to bind to a receptor on the basal keratinocytes that are most likely exposed in sites of microtrauma or are already thin and immature, such as the transformation zones of the cervix, anal verge, or oropharynx (Figure 5.17).[1,134] It is these transformation zones where the two kinds of epithelium meet, columnar and squamous, that carcinogenic HPV is most likely to cause cancer. In contrast, areas lacking a transformation zone, but often affected by trauma, such as the posterior fourchette and inner aspect of the labia minora in females and the prepuce and frenulum in males, are areas most commonly found to have genital warts and least likely to undergo malignant transformation.

HPV has a unique way of selectively infecting epithelial cells that has not been observed with any other virus (Figure 5.18). The molecular mechanisms of viral binding and entry are an active area of research, and understanding is rapidly evolving. Once the virus is exposed to the basement membrane and basal layers of the epithelium, the HPV L1 protein binds a specific receptor in the basement membrane, causing a confirmation change in the viral structure that exposes the L2 proteins.[135] Once bound to this receptor, local enzymes cleave the now exposed L2 protein of the virus coat. This cleavage allows a previously hidden part of the L1 molecules to become exposed

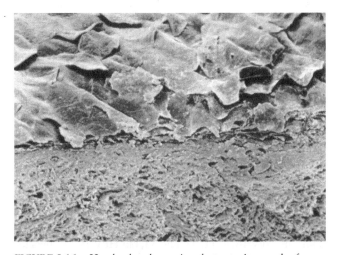

FIGURE 5.16.   Hand-colored scanning electron micrograph of squamous epithelium, demonstrating squamous cells about to be shed from the surface epithelium. These shed squames contain the formed and infectious HPV particles.

human
papillomavirus

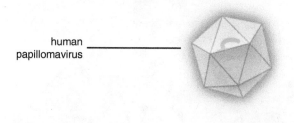

FIGURE 5.17. HPV DNA is released from the surrounding protein capsid and infects the basal epithelium in areas of microtrauma.

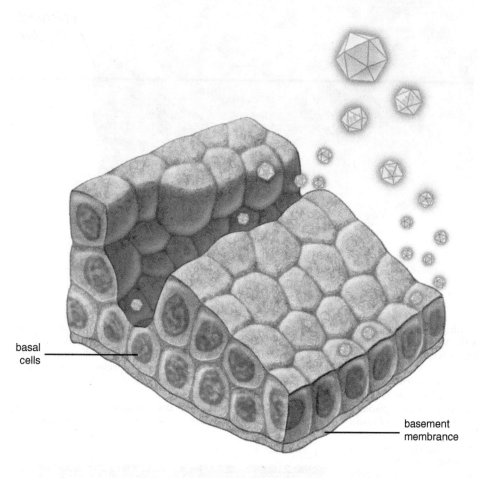

basal
cells

basement
membrance

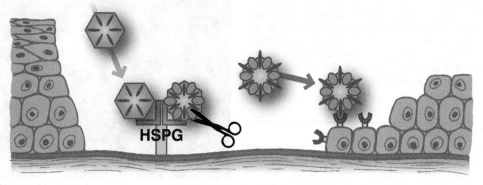

HSPG

FIGURE 5.18. HPV has a unique way of infecting basal epithelial cells unknown among other viruses. To infect cells, the L1 virus proteins must first bind the heparan sulfate proteoglycan (HSPG) receptor on the basement membrane that causes a confirmation change. This exposes the viral L2 proteins to cleavage by the local enzyme furin or PC 5/6. This cleavage allows a previously hidden epitope of the L1 molecules to become exposed and bind to a receptor on the newly forming basement layer of the epithelium. This mechanism gives the virus the advantage of only infecting the basement layers of the epithelium. (Modified from Schiller JT, Day PM, Kines RC. Current understanding of the mechanism of HPV infection. *Gynecol Oncol* 2010;118(1 suppl):S12–7, with permission.)

FIGURE 5.19. HPV begins to replicate in immature metaplasia.

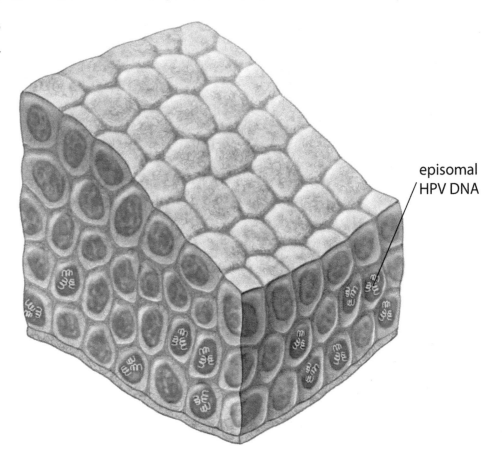

episomal HPV DNA

and bind to a receptor on the newly forming basement layer of the epithelium. This mechanism gives the virus the advantage of only infecting the metabolically active basement layers of the epithelium.[135]

The capsids are internalized via a keratinocyte-specific receptor. Once within the host cells, the viral genome is transported to the cell nucleus, where it establishes an episomal infection; that is, HPV DNA exists as a self-replicating plasmid that is not integrated into the human chromosome. To ensure a persistent infection of the basal stem cells, the genome is replicated once per cell cycle during S phase.[27] It is likely that HPV DNA may remain present but quiescent within cells either before or after active infection.[136] However, it is not clear whether this state of "quiescence" can be permanent or whether genomes involved in switching on viral replication typically do so soon after infection, with some resulting in expressed HPV disease and others suppressed by the host immune response too quickly to be detected. The traditional term for this state of quiescence is viral "latency," but it must be understood that this term indicates only that HPV cannot be detected by any conventional means, including molecular, cytologic, or visual methods.

5.4.2 Productive Viral Infection

A productive infection begins when HPV replicates independent of host chromosomal DNA synthesis (Figure 5.19). Since most HPV-induced cellular abnormalities are transient, it is still not known what proportion of infected individuals express HPV. Viral replication induces the host cells to proliferate abnormally, resulting in acanthosis, koilocytosis, nuclear atypia, and multinucleation. Lesional morphology may range from flat to papillary.[137] Although the exact factors that determine HPV expression are unknown, a complex interplay between host, viral, and environmental factors is most likely important.[137] Many individuals will never have detectable HPV-induced cellular changes, while others may manifest a wide range of disease expression, from transient minimally abnormal cytologic and colposcopic changes (Figure 5.20) to invasive cancer.

HPV DNA is present in low copy number in the basal cells of lesional tissue, but once DNA replication begins, approximately

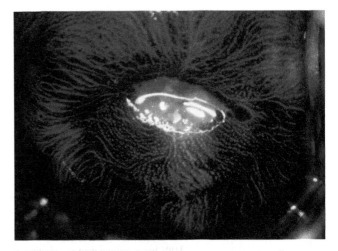

FIGURE 5.20. Minimal HPV expression may occasionally present as pinpoint acetowhite spots on the cervix and vagina, often called minimally expressed papillomavirus infection (MEPI). Here these spots (reverse punctation) are demonstrated after the application of aqueous iodine solution. The findings are nonspecific, as they may be found in other inflammatory conditions.

50 to 100 HPV genomes are generated per cell (Figure 5.21).[27] HPV replication involves E1 and E2 proteins.[28,37] E4 also plays a role in productive infection by contributing to DNA replication or by facilitating viral release through its role in the disruption of cytokeratin network.[27] Various growth factors and their receptors are also produced during HPV replication. These include the epidermal growth factor receptor EGFr[138] and proliferating cell nuclear antigen PCNA.[139] Once a productive lesion develops, viral replication produces increasing numbers of viral genomes in cells that are closest to the surface (Figure 5.22). Hence, infected cells most likely to be desquamated contain the highest viral load. In the upper epithelial layers, HPV L1 and L2 capsid proteins are expressed in increased amounts.[140] The accumulation of these proteins, and of complete HPV virions in the upper layers of lesions (Figure 5.23), produces the cytopathic effects of HPV, which include a hyperchromatic irregular "raisinoid"-shaped nucleus and vacuolated cytoplasm (Figure 5.24). These cytopathic effects are termed koilocytosis.

Wound healing in abrasions may stimulate basal cell division and vascular proliferation that may accelerate viral replication.[141] Clinically, the reoccurrence of genital warts along the healing margins of ablated epithelial areas (the Koebner reaction) is a demonstration of the effects of such viral promotion during cell replication.[142] Whatever initiates viral replication and a productive infection, once initiated, the rapid epithelial and capillary proliferation that ensues is initially uninhibited by immunity. Epithelial proliferation results in acanthosis, hyperchromasia, and increased mitotic activity. Extensive vascular overgrowth, most commonly induced by HPV 6 or 11, results in the stromal projections of exophytic papillomas (Figure 5.25). In contrast, high-risk viral types are more likely to produce flat or slightly raised lesions with capillary and stromal proliferation insufficient to produce the classic "cauliflower"-shaped wart (Figure 5.26). When HPV-induced epithelial alterations do occur, there is enormous variability in the sites involved, disease extent, lesion morphology, clinical course, therapeutic response, and risk of neoplastic transformation. The complexity of possible disease presentations complicates management decisions.

5.4.3 Host Containment

One significant aspect of our current understanding of the HPV life cycle is that infections, whether by high- or low-risk types, that are able to be cleared by the host immune system

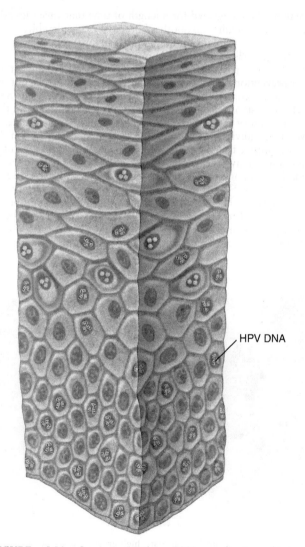

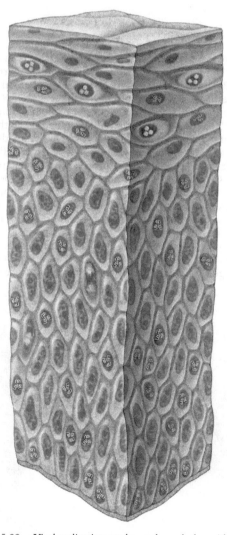

FIGURE 5.21. Once vegetative DNA replication begins, approximately 50 to 100 HPV genomes are generated per cell with only the bottom layer of cells demonstrating cytopathic effects initially. Histology is CIN 1.

FIGURE 5.22. Viral replication works up through the epithelium as cells mature, producing increasing numbers of viral genomes in cells that are closest to the surface. Here increasing numbers of abnormal cells with increased nuclear/cytoplasmic ratio extend two-thirds through the epithelium to produce a CIN 2.

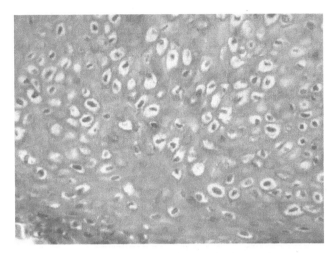

FIGURE 5.23. Histology of a low-grade lesion demonstrates koilocytes almost entirely in the upper layer of the epithelium where HPV replication occurs: histologic features of a productive low-grade infection are demonstrated here. These include acanthosis, cytoplasmic vacuolization, nuclear atypia, and multinucleation.

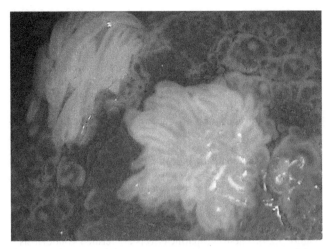

FIGURE 5.25. Exuberant stromal projections of exophytic papillomas dot this cervical ectopy in islands of metaplasia.

in a short period pose almost no risk of malignancy.[143] When HPV does not clear within a short period, defects in the host immune response may be a contributory factor. Fortunately, most HPV infections are transient, with the median time to clearance of incident cervical HPV being just over 9 months and nearly 91% of infections becoming undetectable within 2 years.[95] The longer an infection lasts, the higher the likelihood that it will continue to persist.[1,101,144] However, determining persistence is even more complex when multiple HPV types infect the cervix, potentially causing benign productive infection and CIN 3 at the same time.[1] Whether disease persists or regresses, the extent and severity of the lesions and the success of therapy ultimately depend primarily on the balance between the success of the host immune response and that of the virus to elude it. Emergence of a host immune response depends initially on recognition of the presence of HPV. Because HPV does not kill the epithelial cell that it infects and epithelial cells are not good antigen-presenting cells, the presence of HPV

may not be recognized for a length of time that varies greatly from one individual to another but may be considerable. Once detected, the primary immunologic response to HPV-infected epithelial cells is a cellular immune response. Antibodies are produced as part of the immune response and are important for prevention of new infection but do not appear to be important in effecting regression of established HPV infections and related lesions.[61,145] Mononuclear cells predominate in the inflammatory response observed in regressing condylomas,[146] whereas individuals with impaired T-lymphocyte function do not manifest this containment stage, suggesting that cellular immunity plays the major role in host defense against HPV infection. Langerhans cells are decreased in both CIN and in condylomas,[147] with the threshold for suppression varying by HPV type.[148] The activity of natural killer cells also appears to be related to HPV type, as HPV 6– and HPV 11–induced condylomas and verrucous carcinomas are associated with a decreased activity of natural killer cells and an increased

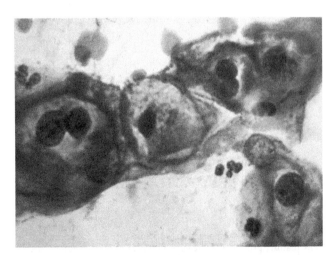

FIGURE 5.24. The cytopathic effects of HPV includes a hyperchromatic irregular "raisinoid"-shaped nucleus and vacuolated cytoplasm, producing the classic koilocyte.

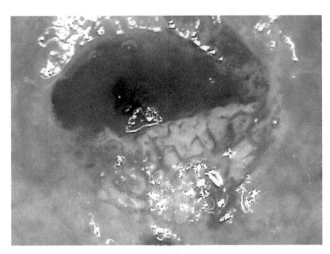

FIGURE 5.26. Subclinical, flat, high-grade lesion secondary to a hrHPV type. High-risk types generally do not produce stromal proliferation as is seen with low-risk types and, therefore, rarely have a papillary appearance. Vascular proliferation has resulted in both mosaic and punctation.

production of interferon gamma and interleukin-2, events not seen in HPV 16–induced lesions.[140,149]

Clinical condyloma will spontaneously regress in up to 20% of infected individuals during the first 3 months after clinical expression, marking the end of any clinically apparent episodes.[150] In another 60% of patients, localized destruction of obvious vulvar condylomas leads to a lasting clinical remission. In the remaining 10% to 20%, HPV-induced lesions linger, proving refractory to standard office treatments (Figure 5.27). Control of these lesions typically requires a more comprehensive treatment approach that may include expensive outpatient procedures, such as carbon dioxide laser, occasionally followed by immune-boosting regimens such as interferon, imiquimod, or sinecatechins.

Whether by spontaneous or treatment-aided remission, absence of recurrence is de facto evidence of type-specific immune memory. HPV antibody detection is a marker of current and/or past exposure to HPV.[61,151–153] Antibodies are likely to be protective against reinfection with the same type, particularly those antibodies that target the L1 and L2 proteins that comprise the virion capsid. The duration of antibody protection against infection from either natural infection or HPV vaccination is unclear. T-cell responses to HPV, however, have not been demonstrated to be type specific.[154,155] Therefore, T-cell responses generated postinfection may provide some protection from progression of HPV infection by new types into early lesions.[61] In a true state of sustained clinical remission, all disease expression ceases and the patient is no longer contagious, since viral capsid replication in the outer epithelial layers ends even though HPV genomes may remain in basal cells in a quiescent stage.[136] If HPV returns to a "latent" state, it may be found only in the basal cells, where only a limited number of viral genes are transcribed. The strong cell-mediated immunity that engenders regression of HPV-infected lesions prevents recurrence of HPV expression from the basal cells in the majority of immunocompetent individuals.[136] Since the late genes (L1 and L2) required for forming infectious viral particles are not actively transcribed, such HPV persistence is not likely to be contagious unless rare release from immune suppression results in new HPV expression. In contrast, patients with subclinical disease may continue to shed virus and may remain contagious to other sex partners despite the absence of visible lesions.

The 10% to 20% of patients with hrHPV types who either have persistent active disease or who "recur" after a lesion-free interval comprise the subset at risk for neoplastic progression. Presumably, most people in this subset have reduced immunocompetence to HPV of unknown etiology, although some "persistence" or "recurrence" will represent exposure to new HPV types.[129] For example, it has been demonstrated that individuals who recur within 6 months posttreatment usually harbor the same HPV type as their original lesion and probably represent an incomplete immune response, whereas those who recur after 6 months most often harbor a different HPV type.[156] Patients with ineffective responses to lesions caused by one HPV type may respond effectively to other HPVs. The rare hereditary skin disorder, epidermodysplasia verruciformis, provides important insight into the nature and extent of HPV infection and the importance of immunity. Almost one-half of the presently known HPV types have been isolated from the nongenital skin of these individuals, who have a disorder in local cellular immunity. The inability of immunity to clear these viruses permits the long-term persistence required for the malignant conversion of flat warts, which occurs in approximately 25% of patients with epidermodysplasia verruciformis and often at a young age.[61] The prevalence of numerous novel HPV types in individuals with this disorder indicates how ubiquitous HPV must be, since it is highly unlikely that these uncommon cutaneotropic viruses would persist in nature if they infected only immunocompromised hosts. That some individuals may be genetically more susceptible to HPV is also demonstrated by evidence that having a sister or mother with cervical cancer doubles the risk for cervical cancer.[157] Thus, heritability might explain some of the variation in cervical cancer risk (see Chapter 4).[61,158]

5.5 NATURAL HISTORY OF CERVICAL INTRAEPITHELIAL NEOPLASIA

5.5.1 Development of Low-Grade Disease

Exposure to HPV is very common in the teens and twenties soon after initiation of intercourse, yet easily detectable clinically expressed HPV disease is relatively uncommon. For instance, 38% of female university students tested positive for HPV DNA by PCR, yet, at any one time, only about 13% of these women developed SIL cytologic changes secondary to HPV.[95] However, very frequent screening would likely result in much higher rates. A 3-year follow-up of young women by cytologic evaluation and PCR showed a 60% cumulative rate of HPV infection, but most incident infection was transient as the median duration was only 8 months (Figure 5.28).[16,159] However, a study of women with a higher median age demonstrated a longer median duration of infection.[160] Additionally, as in other studies, HPV 16 was more likely to persist than other types (18.3 months mean duration from first detection, followed by HPV 31 and HPV 53 at 14.6 and 14.9 months, respectively). The transient nature of most HPV infections is also confirmed by data documenting that the lifetime number of sexual partners is not as strongly related to HPV positivity as is the number of partners in the last 5 years.[161]

Therefore, it appears that one of three clinical pathways may subsequently occur after HPV infection (Figure 5.29): (1) Most infections either remain permanently latent (undetectable by molecular, cytologic, and colposcopic means) or only transiently produce cytologic changes missed by

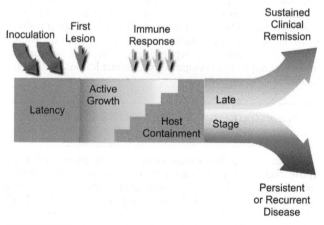

FIGURE 5.27. An overview of a typical expressed HPV infection: Following inoculation a period of nonexpression occurs, often termed "latency." Some individuals suppress or clear their HPV infection without ever having detectable HPV lesions, while others have HPV-induced cell proliferation that results in lesional development. "Host containment" follows immune recognition of the presence of HPV, resulting in sustained clinical remission for the majority. However, 10% to 20% will have lesions that do not clear due to the absence of an adequate immune response.

FIGURE 5.28. In one study, the probability of losing a newly acquired HPV infection was very high (70%) in the first 12 months after detection of HPV and then dropped off so that only another 11% not already cleared at 12 months became HPV negative within 18 months. Only 9% remained HPV positive at 24 months. (Adapted from Ho GYF, Bierman R, Beardsley L, Chang CJ, Burk RD. Natural history of cervicovaginal papillomavirus infection in young women. *N Engl J Med* 1998;338:423–8, with permission.)

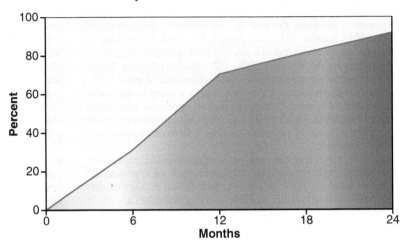

The Probability of Losing a Newly Acquired Human Papillomavirus Infection Over Time

infrequent screening. Whether such undetectable HPV infections persist indefinitely or are permanently cleared is not known, but the example of the high rate of HPV expression in immunosuppressed individuals argues that most immunocompetent individuals remain persistently infected with the virus held "in check" by their immune response.[162] (2) Other women will develop HPV-associated cervical or vaginal disease, detectable by cytologic changes diagnostic of HPV infection, including koilocytotic atypia.[163] It is not known whether this group represents the majority of HPV infections and is just underrepresented by the transient nature of expression and infrequent opportunity for detection. Some will shed cells that demonstrate some but not all of the features of a HPV infection (e.g., ASC-US).[164] Most women with only minor atypia or low-grade intraepithelial neoplasia have lesions that will either regress spontaneously or persist unchanged. (3) Those who develop high-grade CIN during follow-up remain persistently hrHPV DNA positive,[14,165] usually at high quantitative levels.[166] Intermittently HPV-positive women do not appear to be at risk for progression of disease, at least during short-term (24-month) follow-up.[1,167] Regression of CIN lesions is at least partly age dependent, as CIN has been shown to regress in about 80% of women under 34 years and in about 40% of women over 34 years.[168]

The most comprehensive review of the literature on progression, regression, and persistence rates for cervical disease comes from a compilation of all studies on the natural history of CIN from 1952 to 1992 (Table 5.4).[169] Rates were shown to vary greatly depending on study size, length of follow-up, and whether the diagnosis was established by histologic or only cytologic and colposcopic means. For low-grade lesions, the average rate of regression in all studies combined was approximately 60% and the average persistence rate approximately 30%. Progression to CIN 3 occurred in 11% and progression to invasion in 1%. Data from the ASC-US/LSIL Triage Study (ALTS) confirmed progression to CIN 2 or 3 over 2-year follow-up in 13.0% of women with CIN 1 detected after referral for the evaluation of a LSIL or a HPV-positive ASC-US Pap.[170] The findings were almost identical to the progression rate for women in the same study found to have either a completely normal cervix at colposcopy or an atypical transformation zone but normal findings on biopsy (11.2% and 11.6% subsequent detection of CIN 2 or 3 over 2-year follow-up, respectively).[170] These findings indicate that it is the

presence of hrHPV, and not the presence or absence of CIN 1, that determines risk for subsequent detection of CIN 2 or 3.

Because CIN was historically viewed as a progressive biologic continuum leading to cervical cancer,[171,172] older management protocols advocated aggressive treatment of all CIN lesions, including low-grade lesions. Recently, however, most have come to view CIN 1 as simply the acute manifestation of a usually transient HPV infection. In contrast, CIN 3 in adult women is considered a true precancer with biologic potential for progression. Some studies have questioned whether CIN 1 lesions ever progress or are simply self-limited productive infections that may only persist or subsequently regress. The theory that CIN 1 progresses to CIN 2, which then progresses to CIN 3, has been replaced by reports showing that patients who appear to progress actually have two adjacent concurrently established lesions with separate natural histories and different likelihoods of detection at given points in time.[173,174] These data could explain why developing high-grade lesions are almost always at the advancing new squamocolumnar junction and proximal to low-grade lesions. Additionally, Burghardt and Ostor[175] have shown that the abrupt transition between lesions of differing morphology, and the occasional finding of normal tissue separating such lesions, support the theory of adjacent development of distinct lesions of different clonal origins.

5.5.2 Progression of Persistent HPV Infection to High-Grade CIN

While the well-differentiated cytopathic effects of CIN 1 are those classic for a replicative viral infection, CIN 3 lesions are characterized by undifferentiated cells classic for the neoplastic process. CIN 2 lesions are likely a "mixed bag" of low-grade transient HPV lesions destined to regress and true undergraded CIN 3s that are likely to persist. Characteristic findings of CIN 3 lesions include nuclear crowding, substantial pleomorphism, loss of tissue organization and cellular polarity, and abnormal mitotic figures.[27] Additionally, abnormal cells extend past the lower third of the epithelium in CIN 2 and throughout the epithelium in CIN 3. High-grade CIN results from persistent hrHPV infection. One longitudinal study of the natural history of HPV infection did not detect a single CIN 2 or 3 among women whose infection had cleared

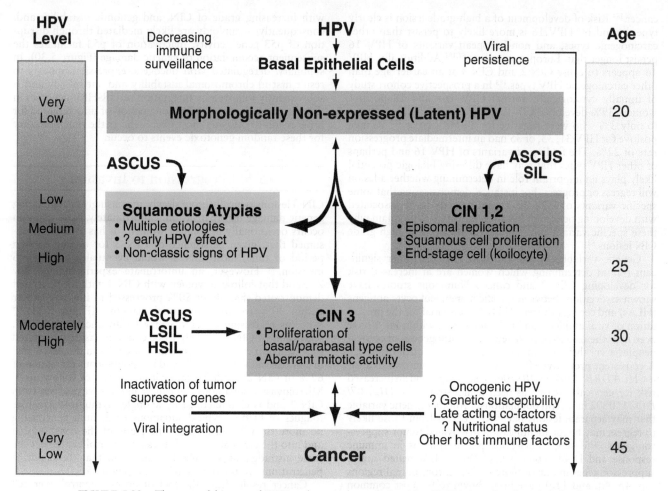

FIGURE 5.29.   The natural history of HPV and cervical neoplasia. After HPV infects basal epithelial cells, morphologic changes may occur after varying lengths of latency. Cytologic findings may clearly indicate HPV expression (LSIL, koilocytotic atypia) or may be more difficult to interpret (ASC-US). Histology may demonstrate morphologic changes ranging from atypia suggestive, but not definitive for HPV, to CIN 1. Given time, most of these minor manifestations will actually regress spontaneously following immune recognition of the presence of HPV. A minority will develop a high-grade lesion, probably from monoclonal cellular changes that develop either within, or outside of, previous low-grade lesion development. High-grade lesional development does not preclude an immune response, but it does significantly decrease the probability of spontaneous resolution. The factors that promote transit from high-grade CIN to invasion are not completely understood, but a combination of a hrHPV type, perhaps some genetic susceptibility, late-acting cofactors, and possibly nutritional factors may all be important. Genomic instability results in inactivation of tumor suppressor genes and in viral integration into the host DNA. (Modified from Cox JT. Epidemiology of CIN: what is the role of HPV? In: Jones HW, ed. *Cervical Intraepithelial Neoplasia. Baillieres Clinical Obstet Gynecol*. London, UK: Bailliere Tindall, 1995;9(1):1–37, with permission.)

by the third visit,[27,176] but CIN 2 and even CIN 3 has been detected within 1 to 3 years from incident infection,[177,178] and most CIN 3 is diagnosable within 10 years of the initial inciting HPV infection.[1] As HPV persists, the probability of clearance decreases as the probability of CIN 3 increases.[144] Risk of CIN 3 among persistent infections is highest between 25 and 35 years of age and then falls.[1] The least common outcome is long-term carcinogenic HPV persistence without the development of CIN 3, but occasionally this does occur.[179] In Ostor's[169] review of natural history studies, CIN 3 regressed in 32% and progressed to invasion in more than 12%. The rates for progression or regression of CIN 2 were squarely between those for CIN 1 and CIN 3 (Table 5.4).

Prevalence of CIN 3 decreases between the age of 35 and 65, with a second peak in prevalence demonstrated in some countries in women over age 65 years.[180] Although a majority of CIN 1 and CIN 2 lesions are associated with hrHPV types, only a small number will go on to develop CIN 3 or invasive

| TABLE 5.4 | COMPILED DATA FROM STUDIES PUBLISHED SINCE 1950 ON REGRESSION, PERSISTENCE, AND PROGRESSION OF CIN |

			PROGRESS	
REGRESS	PERSIST		TO CIN 3	TO CANCER
CIN 1	60%	30%	10%	1%
CIN 2	40%	40%	20%	5%
CIN 3	33%	<56%	—	>12%

From Ostor AG. Natural history of CIN: a critical review. *Int J Gynecol Pathol* 1993;12:186–92, with permission.

cancer.[181] Risk of development of a high-grade lesion is clearly type dependent. HPV 16 is more likely to persist than other carcinogenic types, and non-European variants of HPV 16 persist longer than European variants.[62,182] Additionally, HPV 16 appears to cause CIN 2 and CIN 3 at an earlier age than other carcinogenic HPV types.[183] In a prospective cohort study of initially cytologically normal HPV 16– and 18–positive women, 39% developed CIN 2 or 3 within 2 years, in contrast to only 3% who were negative for all HPV types.[173] Women positive for HPV 31, 33, or 35 had an intermediate progression rate of 22%. The finding of variants of HPV 16 and perhaps of other HPV types that may have differing biologic potential likely plays an important role in determining whether a lesion will regress or progress. For instance, demonstrating that some specific variants of HPV 16 are more likely to be associated with developing persistent infection may partially explain why these specific variants are more prone to produce high-grade CIN lesions.[62]

Genetic variables within the host have the other significant role in determining which women are at increased risk for developing CIN 3 and cancer. Numerous studies have shown associations between specific human leukocyte antigens (HLAs) and cervical cancer.[55,61] HLA is essential for the presentation of viral antigens, and polymorphisms within HLA have been hypothesized to be involved in the pathogenesis of cervical neoplasia via their role in the immunologic control of HPV.[64] A consistent protective effect has now been demonstrated for the *HLA DRB*1301-DQB1*0603* haplotype, and an increased risk for cervical disease has been demonstrated for *HLA* B7/*DQB1*0302* in several populations.[61] Another genetic variable that may separate lesions likely to progress from those likely to regress may be the identification inactivated tumor suppressor genes, and single nucleotide polymorphisms in immune response and DNA repair genes.[63,64,184,185] Inactivated tumor suppressor genes in one or more of four chromosomal regions (3p, 4p, 4q, and 11q) have been shown to be most common in invasive cervical cancers (88%), with declining presence in lesser grades of abnormality: CIN 3 (41%), CIN 2 (22%), and CIN 1 (0%).[184] This finding strongly suggests that CIN 3 arises from a single precursor cell infected with an oncogenic HPV type and destabilized by loss of specific tumor suppressor and immune response repair genes. Other cellular events that appear to be associated with progression are aneuploidy and HPV integration (see Chapter 4).[186]

A higher DNA index and aneuploidy are noted in CIN 3 than in CIN 1 and 2 lesions.[187] HPV integration increases

with increasing grade of CIN, and genomic instability and, consequently, aneuploidy are likely mediated through disruption of p53 gene activity. Inactivation of p53 facilitates the subsequent accumulation of genetic damage (Figure 5.30). In summary, deregulated viral oncogene expression appears to result first in chromosomal instability and aneuploidy and is subsequently followed by integration of HR-HPV genomes in the affected cell clones.[186] The long period of time required for progression to invasion most likely reflects the time necessary for these random genotoxic events to occur.

5.5.3 Progression to Invasion

CIN 3 lesions typically grow slowly, increasingly accumulating genetic damage before invasion. Unfortunately, early invasion occurs occasionally in younger women.[1] It has long been presumed that, given persistence of CIN 3 for a long enough period of time, most CIN 3 would eventually progress to invasion.[188] However, an unfortunate experiment in New Zealand that followed women with CIN 3 without treatment demonstrated that about 50% progressed to invasive cancer within 30 years after the initial diagnosis (Figure 5.31).[189] Whereas regression of CIN 3 may be an uncommon event, regression of CIN 2 is likely to be common, as demonstrated by a deficit in cumulative detection of CIN 2 in the ALTS trial in comparison with CIN 3[190] and by spontaneous regression of 62% of CIN 2 in adolescents within 2 years of follow-up.[181] Microinvasive squamous cell cancer likely always arises from CIN 3 and is characterized by a single or multiple irregular tongues of highly atypical squamous epithelium penetrating no more than 3 mm through the plane of the basal lamina and into the cervical stroma.[27] Invasive cervical cancer has the same histologic appearance but differs in that the depth of penetration into the stroma is >3 mm (Figure 5.32).

Cancer results from the loss of normal control over cell growth. Normal tissue maintenance is an orderly process of cell aging, cell death, and cell replacement. When this orderly process goes awry because of mutations in the cell DNA or other genotoxic stress, the normal cell response is either growth arrest or the induction of programmed cell death (apoptosis). Apoptosis is a strategy used by organisms to counter malignant progression or tumorigenesis. The two tumor suppressor proteins—p53 and the retinoblastoma susceptibility gene product, pRb—are produced when a cell experiences DNA damage, when growth factors are limiting, or when oncogenes force the cell into a replicative state.[28] In response to DNA damage, an increase in p53 protein levels is observed.[28] This increase leads to either arrest in cell-cycle progression or apoptosis, as described earlier in this chapter. While these events are well described, many molecular events required for progression to cervical cancer are yet to be determined. For instance, although the inactivation of p53 and Rb gene products by E6 and E7 proteins is well known, the role of additional genes targeted by hrHPVs, such as C-MYC, RAS, and telomerase/human telomerase reverse transcriptase (hTERT), still needs to be clarified.[61,191] Additionally, silencing of tumor suppressor genes via promoter hypermethylation in HPV-infected host cells has been demonstrated to be a frequent human epigenetic event.[61,192,193] In this process, a methyl group is attached to the promoter region of a gene, resulting in the suppression of gene expression. This process is common in human cancers and suggests another role played by HPV in the oncogenic pathway. Cancer progression is also characterized by a disruption of the normal cell cohesion with consequent breakdown of normal communication between neighboring cells. HPV E6 in oncogenic types has been shown to degrade cell adhesion proteins.[194,195]

The incidence of invasive cervical cancer plateaus in US women between the ages of 40 and 60 (Figure 5.33).[196] In most

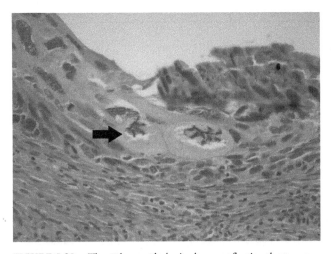

FIGURE 5.30. The only morphologic change reflecting the accumulation of genetic damage is aneuploidy, as demonstrated at the *arrow*.

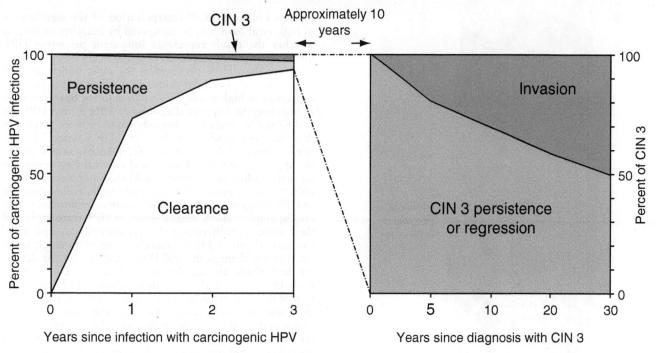

FIGURE 5.31.   Risk of HPV persistence and progression. Left graph: Proportion of carcinogenic HPV infections that clear, persist, or progress to cervical intraepithelial neoplasia grade 3 (CIN 3) in the first 3 years after incident infection. (Data from Rodriguez AC, Schiffman M, Herrero R, et al. Rapid clearance of human papillomavirus and implications for clinical focus on persistent infections. *J Natl Cancer Inst* 2008;100:513–7.) Right graph: Proportion of CIN 3s that invade to cancer when left untreated within 30 years after the initial diagnosis. (Data from McCredie MR, Sharples KJ, Paul C, et al. Natural history of cervical neoplasia and risk of invasive cancer in women with cervical intraepithelial neoplasia 3: a retrospective cohort study. *Lancet Oncol* 2008;9:425–34). Although regression of CIN 3 has been reported anecdotally, we have no data to estimate the magnitude and therefore assume for this graph that all noninvading CIN 3s persist. (From Schiffman MH, Wentzentsen N. From human papillomavirus to cervical cancer. *Obstet Gynecol* 2010;16:180, with permission.)

immunocompetent individuals, the complex steps involved in viral integration and cellular transformation must require this extended period of time from the earliest exposure to HPV to the development of invasive potential. Increasing time also permits the chance occurrence of secondary events that may be necessary for transformation (Figure 5.34). Such progression is most commonly monoclonal, usually involving integration of HPV DNA into the host genome.[197] However, HPV 16 DNA may not always be integrated in carcinomas, as it has been detected in episomal form or as a combination of episomal and integrated forms.

5.6 DEVELOPMENT OF NEW BIOLOGIC MARKERS

The low sensitivity and specificity of Pap testing for true precancerous lesions; interobserver variability in the interpretation of cytologic, colposcopic, and histologic images; the risk of pregnancy complications after treatment of CIN; and the trend toward expectant management of CIN 1 have increased the need for markers that more specifically separate women at true risk for progression from all others. Such risk stratification will be even more important if HPV testing is recommended as a primary cervical cancer screening test. Since only a small proportion of women with hrHPV infection are at risk of invasive cervical cancer, more

specific markers for risk of progression must be identified if molecular cervical cancer screening is to become more cost-effective.

Viral persistence is one marker that is established as a predictor of risk for progression and is the only marker other than hrHPV types presently included in clinical guidelines.[14,41,61–64,66,70,101,179,182,198] Unfortunately, testing for persistence to stratify risk necessarily delays triage of at-risk women to colposcopy, which may prolong anxiety for some women and occasionally may delay diagnosis of a high-grade or cancerous lesion. Clearly, other markers to clarify which women with positive screening tests have true cancer precursors need to be identified.

Although CIN 2 and 3 and cervical cancer have been shown in some cross-sectional studies to have a consistently higher viral load,[199,200] difficulties with sampling variability, controlling testing for cell count, and the existence of high viral load in some low-grade lesions detract from the potential utility of measuring viral load as a risk marker.[61,200,201] However, recent studies have demonstrated a clear association between HPV load and persistence of HPV 16 and 18 infections in young women at the early stages of their sexual life.[202] In the 2-year follow-up in the ALTS trial, HPV 16 viral load in newly detected infections, and changes in viral load over time, predicted persistence and progression.[203] The risk of CIN 3 increased with increasing HPV 16 DNA load at the follow-up visit. Even if viral load can be determined using new PCR methods,

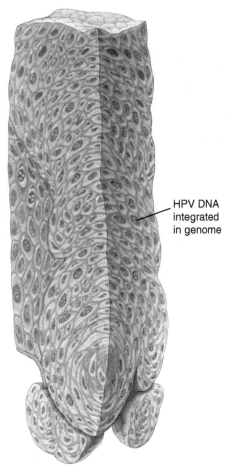

HPV DNA
integrated
in genome

FIGURE 5.32. Invasive cervical cancer has the same histologic appearance as microinvasive cancers in that single or multiple areas of invasion may occur but differs in that the depth of penetration into the stroma is >3 mm.

such as kinetic PCR,[204] interpretation of the significance of high viral load will be hampered by inability to predict whether the result represents long-term persistent HPV infection or recent infection.

Other than HPV persistence, the most widely studied marker is p16, a cellular tumor suppressor that is strongly expressed in high-grade CIN.[1] p16 staining has been used in histology to improve diagnosis of CIN 3, and HPV E6 and E7 mRNA tests have been shown to be more specific in detecting high-grade CIN than HPV DNA tests.[205] Immunohistochemical detection of p16INK4A has shown promise in the evaluation of equivocal cervical Pap testing in limited studies on diverse worldwide populations.[206–208] Other markers presently under study include identification of HPV integration into the host genome, telomerase markers, 3q amplification, measurement of HPV transcripts and their ratios, proliferation (Ki67), aneuploidy, and HPV variants (Figure 5.35).[1,209] Another area of research interest is using changes in viral DNA methylation for detecting high-grade cervical lesions and cancer. One current research focus is on the biologic significance of L1 methylation of the viral genome, since it is associated with minimal expression or complete loss of L1 seen with high-grade dysplasia and cancer.[210,211] Identification of host cellular gene methylation using a panel of four methylated genes yielded a sensitivity and specificity of 89% and 100%, respectively, for the detection of cervical adenocarcinoma.[212]

Telomerase activation and telomere maintenance are essential for cell immortalization and are activated by the E6 oncoprotein of hrHPVs. One study looking at immunohistochemical staining for hTERT (telomerase reverse transcriptase) found that expression of hTERT was increased in parallel with the grade of CIN, with major up-regulation upon transition to CIN 3 (OR 18.81).[213] Another study found that hTERT, Bcl-2, and S100A9 were overexpressed in CIN lesions, and the expression pattern changed during the progression toward CIN 3 lesions.[214]

A marker's clinical utility will likely depend on whether the marker is to be used for screening, diagnosis, or prognosis and

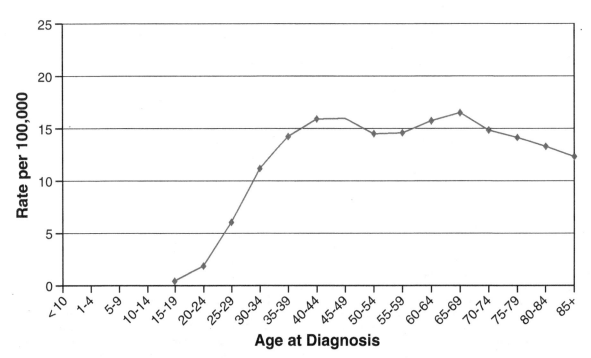

Age at Diagnosis

FIGURE 5.33. Cervical cancer incidence by age, all races from 13 SEER areas (San Francisco, Connecticut, Detroit, Hawaii, Iowa, New Mexico, Seattle, Utah, Atlanta, San Jose-Monterrey, Los Angeles, Alaska Native Registry, rural Georgia). Rates are per 100,000 women (From National Cancer Institute SEER Cancer Statistics Review 1975–2008 http://seer.cancer.gov/csr/1975_2008/index.html [Accessed August 20, 2011].)

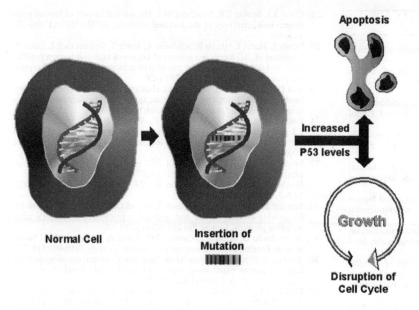

FIGURE 5.34. Schematic of a mutation arising in an otherwise normally functioning cell. Such mutations would normally result in increased p53 protein levels, which would lead to either cell death or arrest of cell division and replication.

whether the population is already screened heavily, rarely, or not at all. For instance, a marker will need to be highly specific in well-screened populations to prevent overtreatment of HPV-infected women, most of whose lesions will regress,[61] whereas screening in developing countries will require increased sensitivity even at the expense of specificity and will need to be inexpensive. At the present time, all potential markers are investigational.

5.7 SUMMARY

There is now no doubt about the role of specific oncogenic HPV types in the etiology of essentially all cervical cancers and of many neoplasias of the vulva, vagina, anus, and penis. Specific

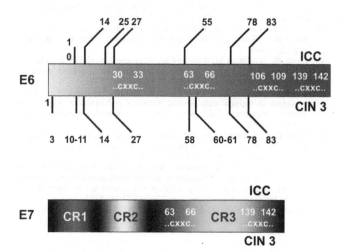

FIGURE 5.35. The location of gene loci variations between prototype HPV 16 and variant HPV 16. Such variations may be useful as molecular markers for risk for progression. (Modified from Zehbe I, Wilander E, Delius H, Tommassino M. Human papillomavirus 16 E6 variants are more prevalent than the prototype. *Cancer Res* 1998;58:829–33, with permission.)

high-risk types of HPV are found in association with nearly 100% of invasive cervical cancers. The interaction of hrHPV and immature metaplastic epithelium initiates the process that leads to the development of cervical neoplasia in some women. Mature squamous epithelium is at lower risk for development of cancer or its precursors. However, exposure to HPV is an extremely common event, whereas the development of cervical cancer is relatively rare. This indicates that other factors must be important to disease progression. The increase in high-grade CIN and cervical cancer observed in immunosuppressed patients suggests that immune surveillance plays a critical role in preventing persistent infections and the subsequent development of high-grade and invasive lesions. Other possible factors may include a genetic propensity, infection by other microbial agents, the use of tobacco products, specific dietary deficiencies, and the effect of hormonal contraceptives and pregnancy. The long period between exposure and the development of cancer supports the concept that cervical cancer develops by a multistage model of carcinogenesis. Events that are probably important include alterations at tumor suppressor gene loci, integration of HPV into the genome, hypermethylation products of HPV and possibly specific mutations. Therefore, malignant progression, when it does occur, commonly takes many years or decades. The term "progression" may be a misnomer, however, as "apparent" progression may really represent adjacent "de-novo" development of higher-grade CIN within an area of lower-grade disease.

Squamous epithelial cancers of the vulva, vagina, penis, anus, and oropharynx are often induced by HPV as well. However, only the anal verge and oropharynx have a transformation zone that is nearly equivalent to that of the cervix. The increased vulnerability of the transformation zones to oncogenic HPV, particularly in the cervix and anus, accounts for the significantly greater risk of HPV-induced cancers in these areas and for the similar virtually exclusive etiology. In contrast, malignancies of the vagina, vulva, and penis are among the rarest of cancers and are often not caused by HPV.

Because phylogenetic studies have provided evidence of minimal HPV genomic drift over the millennia, it may be assumed that HPV is a stable virus. The instigation of prophylactic HPV vaccination provides hope that a successful vaccination program may profoundly reduce cervical cancer worldwide during the 21st century.

References

1. Schiffman M, Wentzensen N. From human papillomavirus to cervical cancer. *Obstet Gynecol* 2010;116(1):177–85.
2. Bosch FX, Manos MM, Munoz N, et al. Prevalence of human papillomavirus in cervical cancer: a worldwide perspective. *J Natl Cancer Inst* 1995;87:796–802.
3. Walboomers JM, Jacobs MV, Manos MM, et al. Human papillomavirus is a necessary cause of invasive cervical cancer worldwide. *J Pathol* 1999;189:1–3.
4. Bosch FX, Lorincz A, Munoz N, Meijer CJLM, Shah KV. The causal relation between human papillomavirus and cervical cancer. *J Clin Pathol* 2002;55:244–65.
5. Bosch FX, Burchell AN, Schiffman M, et al. Epidemiology and natural history of human papillomavirus infections and type-specific implications in cervical neoplasia. *Vaccine* 2008;26(suppl 10):K1–16.
6. Schiffman M, Kjaer SK. Chapter 2: natural history of anogenital human papillomavirus infection and neoplasia. *J Natl Cancer Inst* (monograph) 2003;31:14–9.
7. Morrison EA, Ho GF, Vermund SH, et al. Human papillomavirus infection and other risk factors for cervical neoplasia: a case-control study. *Int J Cancer* 1991;49:6–13.
8. Munoz N, Bosch FX, Shah V, et al., eds. *The Epidemiology of Cervical Cancer and Human Papillomavirus*. Lyon, France: International Agency for Research on Cancer (WHO), l992. IARC Scientific Publications No. 119.
9. Peng HQ, Liu SL, Mann V, et al. HPV types 16 and 33, Herpes Simplex Type 2, and other risk factors in cervical cancer in Sichuan Province, China. *Int J Cancer* 1991;47:711–6.
10. Jones CJ, Brinton LA, Hamman RF, et al. Risk factors for in situ cervical cancer: results from a case-control study. *Cancer Res* 1990;50:3657–62.
11. Cuzick J, Terry G, Ho L, et al. Type specific HPV DNA as a predictor of high-grade cervical intraepithelial neoplasia. *Br J Cancer* l994;69:167–71.
12. Konno R, Sato S, Yajima A. Progression of squamous cell carcinoma of the uterine cervix from cervical intraepithelial neoplasia infected with human papillomavirus: a retrospective follow-up study by in situ hybridization and polymerase chain reaction. *Int J Gynecol Pathol* 1992;11:105–12.
13. Koutsky LA, Holmes KK, Critchlow CW, et al. Cohort study of risk of cervical intraepithelial neoplasia grade 2 or 3 associated with cervical papillomavirus infection. *N Engl J Med* 1992;327:127–78.
14. Nobbenhuis M, Walboomers, JM, Helmerhorst TI. Rozendaal, L. Relation of human papillomavirus status to cervical lesions and consequences for cervical-cancer screening: a prospective study. *Lancet* 1999;354:20.
15. Jacobs MV, Zielinski D, Meijer CJ, et al. A simplified and reliable HPV testing or archival Papanicolaou-stained cervical smears: application to cervical smears from cancer. *Br J Cancer* 2000;82:1421–6.
16. Ho GYF, Bierman R, Beardsley L, Chang CJ, Burk RD. Natural history of cervicovaginal papillomavirus infection in young women. *N Engl J Med* 1998;338:423–8.
17. Peyton CL, Gravitt PE, Hunt WC, et al. Determinants of genital human papillomavirus detection in a US population. *J Infect Dis* 2001;183:1554–64.
18. Dunn EF, Unger ER, Sternberg M, et al. Prevalence of HPV infection among females in the United States. *JAMA* 2007;297:813–19.
19. Cox JT, Lorincz AT, Schiffman MH, et al. HPV testing by hybrid capture appears to be useful in triaging women with a cytologic diagnosis of ASCUS. *Am J Obstet Gynecol* 1995;172:946–54.
20. Manos MM, Kinney WK, Hurley LB, et al. Identifying women with cervical neoplasia: using human papillomavirus DNA testing for equivocal Papanicolaou results. *JAMA* 1999;281:1605–10.
21. Solomon D, Schiffman MH, Tarone R. Comparison of three management strategies for patients with atypical squamous cells of undetermined significance: baseline results from a randomized trial. *J Natl Cancer Inst* 2001;93:293–9.
22. The Atypical Squamous cells of Undetermined Significance/Low-Grade Squamous Intraepithelial Lesions Triage Study (ALTS) Group. Human papillomavirus testing for triage of women with cytologic evidence of low-grade squamous intraepithelial lesions: baseline data from a randomized trial. *J Natl Cancer Inst* 2000;92:1014–8.
23. Castle PE, Schiffman M, Wheeler CM, Wentzensen N, Gravitt PE. Human papillomavirus genotypes in cervical intraepithelial neoplasia grade 3. *Cancer Epidemiol Biomarkers Prev* 2010;19(7):1675–81.
24. Durst M, Gissmann L, Ikenberg H, zur Hausen H. A papillomavirus DNA from a cervical carcinoma and its prevalence in cancer biopsy samples from different geographic regions. *Proc Natl Acad Sci USA* 1983;80:3812–5.
25. Gissman L, Wolnik L, Ikenberg H, et al. Human papillomavirus types 6 and ll DNA sequences in genital and laryngeal papillomas and in some cervical cancers. *Proc Natl Acad Sci USA* l983;80:560.
26. Munoz N, Bosch FX, de Sanjose S, et al.; International Agency for Research on Cancer Multicenter Cervical Cancer Study Group. Epidemiologic classification of human papillomavirus types associated with cervical cancer. *N Engl J Med* 2003;348:518–27.
27. Munger K, Howley PM. Human papillomavirus immortalization and transformation functions. *Virus Res* 2002;89(2):213–28.
28. Chow LT, Broker TR, Steinberg BM. The natural history of human papillomavirus infections of the mucosal epithelia. *APMIS* 2010;118(6–7):422–49.
29. Fertey J, Hurst J, Straub E, Schenker A, Iftner T, Stubenrauch F. Growth inhibition of HeLa cells is a conserved feature of high-risk human papillomavirus E8^E2C proteins and can also be achieved by an artificial repressor protein. *J Virol* 2011;85(6):2918–26.
30. Van Tine BA, Dao LD, Wu SY, et al. Human papillomavirus (HPV) origin-binding protein associates with mitotic spindles to enable viral DNA partitioning. *Proc Natl Acad Sci USA* 2004;101:4030–5.
31. Collins SI, Constandinou-Williams C, Wen K, et al. Disruption of the E2 gene is a common and early event in the natural history of cervical human papillomavirus infection: a longitudinal cohort study. *Cancer Res* 2009;69(9):3828–32.
32. Inoue Y, Imamura T. Regulation of TGF-beta family signaling by E3 ubiquitin ligases. *Cancer Sci* 2008;99(11):2107–12.
33. Doobar J. An emerging function for E4. *Papillomavirus Rep* 1991;2:145–7.
34. Schmitt M, Dalstein V, Waterboer T, Clavel C, Gissmann L, Pawlita M. Diagnosing cervical cancer and high-grade precursors by HPV16 transcription patterns. *Cancer Res* 2010;70(1):249–56.
35. Borzacchiello G, Roperto F, Campos MS, Venuti A. 1st International Workshop on Papillomavirus E5 oncogene—a report. *Virology* 2010;408:135–7.
36. Yugawa T, Kiyono T. Molecular mechanisms of cervical carcinogenesis by high-risk human papillomaviruses: novel functions of E6 and E7 oncoproteins. *Rev Med Virol* 2009;19(2):97–113.
37. Howley PM, Lowy DR. Papillomaviruses and their replication. In: Knipe DM, Howley PM, eds. *Fields' Virology*. Philadelphia, PA: Lippincott Williams & Wilkins, 2001:2197–229.
38. Schiffman M, Herrero R, Desalle R, et al. The carcinogenicity of human papillomavirus types reflects viral evolution. *Virology* 2005;337:76–84.
39. Ho L, Chan SY, Chow V, et al. Sequence variants of HPV type l6 in clinical samples permit verification and extension of epidemiological studies and construction of a phylogenic tree. *J Clin Microbiol* 1991;29:1765–72.
40. Chan S-Y, Chew S-H, Kiyafumi E, et al. Phylogenetic analysis of the human papillomavirus type 2 (HPV-2), HPV-27, and HPV-57 group, which is associated with common warts. *Virology* 1997;239:296–302.
41. Schiffman M, Rodriguez AC, Chen Z, et al. A population-based prospective study of carcinogenic human papillomavirus variant lineages, viral persistence, and cervical neoplasia. *Cancer Res* 2010;70(8):3159–69.
42. de Villiers EM, Fauquet C, Broker TR, Bernard HU, zur Hausen H. Classification of papillomaviruses. *Virology* 2004;324:17–27.
43. Bosch FX, De Sanjose S. Chapter 1: Human papillomavirus and cervical cancer-burden and assessment of causality. *J Natl Cancer Inst* (monograph) 2003;31:3–13.
44. Lacey CJN, Lowndes C, Shah KV. Chapter 4: Burden and management of non-cancerous HPV-related conditions: HPV-6/11 disease. *Vaccine* 2006;24(3):S3/35–41.
45. Nielsen A, Kjaer SK, Munk C, Iftner T. Type-specific HPV infection and multiple HPV types: prevalence and risk factor profile in nearly 12,000 younger and older Danish women. *Sex Transm Dis* 2008;35(3):276–82.
46. Chaturvedi AK, Katki HA, Hildesheim A, et al.; CVT Group. Human papillomavirus infection with multiple types: pattern of coinfection and risk of cervical disease. *J Infect Dis* 2011;203(7):910–20.
47. Lowy DR, Howley PM. Papillomaviruses. In: Knipe DM, Howley PM, eds. *Fields' Virology*. Philadelphia, PA: Lippincott Williams & Wilkins, 2001:2231–64.
48. Castle PE, Schiffman M, Wheeler CM, Wentzensen N, Gravitt PE. Human papillomavirus genotypes in cervical intraepithelial neoplasia grade 3. *Cancer Epidemiol Biomarkers Prev* 2011;19(7):1675–81.
49. Castle PE, Shaber R, Lamere BJ, et al. Human Papillomavirus (HPV) genotypes in women with cervical precancer and cancer at Kaiser Permanente Northern California. *Cancer Epidemiol Biomarkers Prev* 2011;20(5):946–53.
50. Smith JS, Backes DM, Hoots BE, Kurman RJ, Pimenta JM. Human papillomavirus type-distribution in vulvar and vaginal cancers and their associated precursors. *Obstet Gynecol* 2009;113(4):917–24.
51. Insinga RP, Liaw KL, Johnson LG, Madeleine MM. A systematic review of the prevalence and attribution of human papillomavirus types among cervical, vaginal, and vulvar precancers and cancers in the United States. *Cancer Epidemiol Biomarkers Prev* 2008;17(7):1611–22.
52. Blomberg M, Nielsen A, Munk C, Kjaer SK. Trends in head and neck cancer incidence in Denmark, 1978–2007: focus on human papillomavirus associated sites. *Int J Cancer* 2011;129(3):733–41.
53. Nielsen A, Munk C, Kjaer SK. Trends in incidence of anal cancer and high-grade anal intraepithelial neoplasia in Denmark, 1978–2008. *Int J Cancer* 2011;129(3):733–41. http://onlinelibrary.wiley.com/doi/10.1002/ijc.26115/full (Accessed August 20, 2011).
54. Schiffman MH, Burk RD. Human papillomaviruses. In: Evans AS, Kaslow R, eds. *Viral Infections of Humans* (4th ed.). New York, NY: Plenum Press, 1995:345–92.
55. Hildesheim A, Wang SS. Host and viral genetics and risk of cervical cancer: a review. *Virus Res* 2002;89:229–40.

56. Zehbe I, Wilander E, Delius H, Tommassino M. Human papillomavirus 16 E6 variants are more prevalent than the prototype. *Cancer Res* 1998;58:829–33.

57. Villa LL, Sichero L, Rahal P, et al. Molecular variants of human papillomavirus types 16 and 18 preferentially associated with cervical neoplasia. *J Gen Virol* 2000;81:2959–68.

58. Lizano M, Berumen J, Guido MC, Casas L, Garcia-Carranca A. Association between human papillomavirus type 18 variants and histopathology of cervical cancer. *J Natl Cancer Inst* 1997;89:1227–31.

59. Chan PK, Lam CW, Cheung TH, et al. Association of human papillomavirus type 58 variant with the risk of cervical cancer. *J Natl Cancer Inst* 2002;94:1249–53.

60. Xi LF, Koutsky LA, Galloway DA, et al. Genomic variation of human papillomavirus 16 and risk for high-grade cervical intraepithelial neoplasia. *J Natl Cancer Inst* 1997;89:796–802.

61. Wang SS, Hildesheim A. Chapter 5: Viral and host factors in human papillomavirus persistence and progression. *J Natl Cancer Inst Monogr* 2003;31:35–40.

62. Gheit T, Cornet I, Clifford GM, et al. Risks for persistence and progression by human papillomavirus type 16 variant lineages among a population-based sample of Danish women. *Cancer Epidemiol Biomarkers Prev* 2011;20(7):1315–21.

63. Wang SS, Gonzalez P, Yu K, et al. Common genetic variants and risk for HPV persistence and progression to cervical cancer. *PLoS One* 2010;5(1):e8667.

64. Wang SS, Bratti MC, Rodríguez AC, et al. Common variants in immune and DNA repair genes and risk for human papillomavirus persistence and progression to cervical cancer. *J Infect Dis* 2009;199(1):20–30.

65. Kurman RJ, Schiffman MH, Lancaster WD, et al. Analysis of individual human papillomavirus types in cervical neoplasia: a possible role for type 18 in rapid progression. *Am J Obstet Gynecol* 1988;159:293–6.

66. Castle PE, Rodríguez AC, Burk RD, et al.; Proyecto Epidemiológico Guanacaste Group. Long-term persistence of prevalently detected human papillomavirus infections in the absence of detectable cervical precancer and cancer. *J Infect Dis* 2011;203(6):814–22.

67. Chaturvedi AK, Katki HA, Hildesheim A, et al.; CVT Group. Human papillomavirus infection with multiple types: pattern of coinfection and risk of cervical disease. *J Infect Dis* 2011;203(7):910–20.

68. Kleter B, van Doorn LJ, Schrauwen L, et al. Development and clinical evaluation of a highly sensitive PCR-reverse hybridization line probe assay for detection and identification of anogenital human papillomavirus. *J Clin Microbiol* 1999;37:2508–17.

69. Iftner T, Villa LL. Chapter 12: Human papillomavirus technologies. *J Natl Cancer Inst* (monograph) 2003;31:80–8.

70. Wallin KL, Wiklund F, Angstrom T, et al. Type-specific persistence of human papillomavirus DNA before the development of invasive cervical cancer. *N Engl J Med* 1999;341:1633–8.

71. Elbel M, Carl S, Spaderna S, Iftnert T. A comparative analysis of the interactions of the E6 proteins from cutaneous and genital papillomaviruses with p53 and E6AP in correlation to their transforming potential. *Virology* 1997;239:132–49.

72. Armstrong DL, Roman A. The relative ability of human papillomavirus type 6 and human papillomavirus type 16 E7 proteins to transactivate E2F-responsive elements is promoter- and cell-dependent. *Virology* 1997;239:238–46.

73. zur Hausen H. Papillomaviruses and cancer: from basic studies to clinical application. *Nat Rev Cancer* 2002;2:342–50.

74. Munger K, Basile JR, Duensing S, et al. Biological activities and molecular targets of the human papillomavirus E7 oncoprotein. *Oncogene* 2001;20:7888–98.

75. Hengstermann A, Linares LK, Ciechanover A, Whitaker NJ, Scheffner M. Complete switch from Mdm2 to human papillomavirus E6-mediated degradation of p53 in cervical cancer cells. *Proc Natl Acad Sci USA* 2001;98:1218–23.

76. Zwerschke W, Jansen-Dürr P. Cell transformation by the E7 oncoprotein of human papillomavirus type 16: interactions with nuclear and cytoplasmic target proteins. *Adv Cancer Res* 2000;78:1–29.

77. Heck DV, Yee CL, Howley PM, Munger K. Efficiency of binding the retinoblastoma protein correlates with the transforming capacity of the E7 oncoproteins of the human papillomaviruses. *Proc Natl Acad Sci USA* 1992;89:4442–6.

78. Gonzalez SL, Stremlau M, He X, Basile JR, Munger K. Degradation of the retinoblastoma tumor suppressor by the human papillomavirus type 16 E7 oncoprotein is important for functional inactivation and is separable from proteasomal degradation of E7. *J Virol* 2001;75:7583–91.

79. Jones DL, Alani RM, Münger K. The human papillomavirus E7 oncoprotein can uncouple cellular differentiation and proliferation in human keratinocytes by abrogating p21Cip1-mediated inhibition of cdk2. *Genes Dev* 1997;11:2101–11.

80. Zerfass-Thome K, Zwerschke W, Mannhardt B, Tindle R, Botz JW, Jansen-Dürr P. Inactivation of the cdk inhibitor p27KIP1 by the human papillomavirus type 16 E7 oncoprotein. *Oncogene* 1996;13:2323–30.

81. Duensing S, Munger K. Centrosome abnormalities, genomic instability and carcinogenic progression. *Biochim Biophys Acta* 2001;1471:M81–8.

82. Duensing S, Lee LY, Duensing A, et al. The human papillomavirus type 16 E6 and E7 oncoproteins cooperate to induce mitotic defects and genomic instability by uncoupling centrosome duplication from the cell division cycle. *Proc Natl Acad Sci USA* 2000;97:10002–7.

83. Southern SA, Evans MF, Herrington CS. Basal cell tetrasomy in low-grade squamous intraepithelial lesions infected with high-risk human papillomaviruses. *Cancer Res* 1997;57:4210–3.

84. Duensing S, Duensing A, Crum CP, Munger K. Human papillomavirus type 16 E7 oncoprotein-induced abnormal centrosome synthesis is an early event in the evolving malignant phenotype. *Cancer Res* 2001;61:2356–60.

85. Skyldberg B, Fujioka K, Hellström AC, Sylvén L, Moberger B, Auer G. Human papillomavirus infection, centrosome aberration, and genetic stability in cervical lesions. *Mod Pathol* 2001;14:279–84.

86. Park JS, Kim EJ, Kwon HJ, Hwang ES, Namkoong SE, Um SJ. Inactivation of interferon regulatory factor-1 tumor suppressor protein by HPV E7 oncoprotein. Implication for the E7-mediated immune evasion mechanism in cervical carcinogenesis. *J Biol Chem* 2000;275:6764–9.

87. Magal SS, Jackman A, Pei XF, et al. Induction of apoptosis in human keratinocytes containing mutated p53 alleles and its inhibition by both the E6 an E7 oncoproteins. *Int J Cancer* 1998;75:96–104.

88. zur Hausen H. Human papillomaviruses in the pathogenesis of anogenital cancer. *Virology* 1991;184:9–13.

89. Sang BC, Barbosa MS. Increased E6/E7 in HPV-18 immortalized human keratinocytes results from inactivation of E2 and additional cellular events. *Virology* 1992;189:448–55.

90. Jeon S, Allen-Hoffman BL, Lambert PF. Integration of human papillomavirus type 16 into the human genome correlates with a selective growth advantage of cells. *J Virol* 1995;69:2989–97.

91. Schiffman M, Kjaer SK. Chapter 2: Natural history of anogenital human papillomavirus infection and neoplasia. *J Natl Cancer Inst* (monograph) 2003;31:14–9.

92. Fairley CK, Hocking JS, Gurrin LC, Chen MY, Donovan B, Bradshaw CS. Rapid decline in presentations of genital warts after the implementation of a national quadrivalent human papillomavirus vaccination programme for young women. *Sex Trans Infect* 2009;85:499–502.

93. Rylander E, Ruusuvaara L, Almstromer MW, Evander M, Wadell G. The absence of vaginal human papillomavirus 16 DNA in women who have not experienced sexual intercourse. *Obstet Gynecol* 1994;83(5, pt 1):735–7.

94. Kjaer SK, Chackerian B, van den Brule AJ, et al. High-risk human papillomavirus is sexually transmitted: evidence from a follow-up study of virgins starting sexual activity (intercourse). *Cancer Epidemiol Biomark Prev* 2001;10:101–6.

95. Winer RL, Hughes JP, Feng Q, et al. Early natural history of incident, type-specific human papillomavirus infections in newly sexually active young women. *Cancer Epidemiol Biomarkers Prev* 2011;20(4):699–707.

96. Winer RL, Kiviat NB, Hughes JP, et al. Development and duration of human papillomavirus lesions, after initial infection. *J Infect Dis* 2005;191(5):731–8.

97. Munoz N, Castellsague X, Bosch FX, et al. Difficulty in elucidating the male role in cervical cancer in Colombia, a high risk area for the disease. *J Natl Cancer Inst* 1996;88:1068–75.

98. Bosch FX, Castellsague X, Munoz N, et al. Male sexual behavior and human papillomavirus DNA: key risk factors for cervical cancer in Spain. *J Natl Cancer Inst* 1996;88:1060–7.

99. Castellsague X, Ghaffari A, Daniel RW, et al. Prevalence of penile human papillomavirus DNA in husbands of women with and without cervical neoplasia: a study in Spain and Colombia. *J Infect Dis* 1997;176:353–61.

100. Winer RL, Hughes JP, Feng Q, et al. Condom use and the risk of genital human papillomavirus infection in young women. *N Engl J Med* 2006;354:2645–54.

101. Plummer M, Schiffman M, Castle PE, Maucort-Boulch D, Wheeler CM. A 2-year prospective study of human papillomavirus persistence among women with a cytological diagnosis of atypical squamous cells of undetermined significance or low-grade squamous intraepithelial lesion. *J Infect Dis* 2007;195:1582–9.

102. Vaccarella S, Franceschi S, Snijders PJ, Herrero R, Meijer CJ, Plummer M. Concurrent infection with multiple human papillomavirus types: pooled analysis of the IARC HPV prevalence surveys. *Cancer Epidemiol Biomarkers Prev* 2010;19:503–10.

103. Oriel JD. Natural history of genital warts. *Br J Vener Dis* 1971;47:1–13.

104. Maymon R, Bekerman A, Werchow M, et al. Clinical and subclinical condyloma: rates among male sexual partners of women with genital human papillomavirus infection. *J Reprod Med* 1995;40:31–6.

105. Barasso R, de Brux, Croissant O, Orth G. High prevalence of papillomavirus-associated penile intraepithelial neoplasia in sexual partners of women with cervical intraepithelial neoplasia. *N Engl J Med* 1987;317:916–23.

106. Meanwell CA, Cox MF, Blackledge G, et al. HPV 16 DNA in normal and malignant cervical epithelium: implications for the aetiology and behavior of cervical neoplasia. *Lancet* 1987;1:703–7.

107. Syrjanen S. Current concepts on human papillomavirus infections in children. *APMIS* 2010;118(6–7):494–509.

108. Burchell AN, Winer RL, de Sanjose S, Franco EL. Chapter 6: Epidemiology and transmission dynamics of genital HPV infection. *Vaccine* 2006;24(suppl 3):S52–61.

109. Jenison SA, Yu XP, Valentine JM, et al. Evidence of prevalent human papillomavirus types in adults and children. *J Infect Dis* 1990;162:60–9.

110. Castellsagué X, Drudis T, Cañadas MP, et al. Human papillomavirus (HPV) infection in pregnant women and mother-to-child transmission of genital HPV genotypes: a prospective study in Spain. *BMC Infect Dis* 2009;9:74.

111. Jones V, Smith SJ, Omar HA. Nonsexual transmission of anogenital warts in children: a retrospective analysis. *Sci World J* 2007;7:1896–9.

112. Mammas IN, Sourvinos G, Spandidos DA. Human papilloma virus (HPV) infection in children and adolescents. *Eur J Pediatr* 2009;168:267–73.

113. Gillison ML, Shah KV. Chapter 9: Role of mucosal human papillomavirus in nongenital cancers. *J Natl Cancer Inst* (monograph) 2003;31:57–65.

114. Pannone G, Santoro A, Papagerakis S, Lo Muzio L, De Rosa G, Bufo P. The role of human papillomavirus in the pathogenesis of head & neck squamous cell carcinoma: an overview. *Infect Agent Cancer* 2011;6:4.

115. Schwartz S, Yueh B, McDougall J, Daling J, Schwartz S. Human papillomavirus infection and survival in oral squamous cell cancer: a population-based study. *Otolaryngol Head Neck Surg* 2001;125:1–9.

116. Wiest T, Schwarz E, Enders C, Flechtenmacher C, Bosch F. Involvement of intact HPV16 E6/E7 gene expression in head and neck cancers with unaltered p53 status and perturbed pRb cell cycle control. *Oncogene* 2002;21:1510–7.

117. Smith EM, Ritchie JM, Summersgill KF, et al. Human papillomavirus in oral exfoliated cells and risk of head and neck cancer. *J Natl Cancer Inst* 2004;96:449–55.

118. Fischer CA, Kampmann M, Zlobec I, et al. p16 expression in oropharyngeal cancer: its impact on staging and prognosis compared with the conventional clinical staging parameters. *Ann Oncol* 2010;21(10):1961–6.

119. Riddel C, Rashid R, Thomas V. Ungual and periungual human papillomavirus-associated squamous cell carcinoma: a review. *J Am Acad Dermatol* 2011;64(6):1147–53.

120. Sato T, Morimoto A, Ishida Y, Matsuo I. Human papillomavirus associated with Bowen's disease of the finger. *J Dermatol* 2004;31(11):927–30.

121. McDonnell PJ, McDonnell JM, Kessis T, et al. Detection of human papillomavirus type 6/11 DNA in conjunctival papillomas by in situ hybridization with radioactive probes. *Hum Pathol* 1987;18:115–9.

122. Scott I, Karp C, Nuovo G. Human papillomavirus 16 and 18 expression in conjunctival intraepithelial neoplasia. *Ophthalmology* 2002;109:542–7.

123. McDonnell J, Wagner D, Ng S, Bernstein G, Sun Y. Human papillomavirus type 16 DNA in ocular and cervical swabs of women with genital tract condylomata. *Am J Ophthalmol* 1991;112:61–6.

124. Perniciaro C, Kicker CH. Tanning bed warts. *J Am Acad Dermatol* 1988;18:586–7.

125. Ferenczy A, Bergnon C, Richart R. HPV DNA in fomites on objects used for the management of patients with genital HPV infections. *Obstet Gynecol* 1989;74:950–4.

126. Smith EM, Parker MA, Rubenstein LM, Haugen TH, Hamsikova E, Turek LP. Evidence for vertical transmission of HPV from mothers to infants. *Infect Dis Obstet Gynecol* 2010;32:63–9.

127. Medeiros LR, Ethur AB, Hilgert JB, et al. Vertical transmission of the human papillomavirus: a systematic quantitative review. *Cad Saude Publica* 2005;21:1006–15.

128. Rintala MA, Grenman SE, Jarvenkyla ME, Syrjanen KJ, Syrjanen SM. High-risk types of human papillomavirus (HPV) DNA in oral and genital mucosa of infants during their first 3 years of life: experience from the Finnish HPV Family Study. *Clin Infect Dis* 2005;41:1728–33.

129. Bongura VR, Hatam LJ, Rosenthal DW, et al. Recurrent respiratory papillomatosis: a complex defect in immune responsiveness to human papillomavirus-6 and -11. *APMIS* 2010;118:455–70.

130. Derkay C, Watrak B. Recurrent respiratory papillomatosis: review. *Laryngoscope* 2008;118:1236–47.

131. Mant C, Cason J, Rice P, Best JM. Non-sexual transmission of cervical cancer-associated papillomaviruses: an update. *Papillomavirus Rep* 2000;11:1–5.

132. Moscicki AB, Hills N, Shiboski S, et al. Risks for incident human papillomavirus infection and low-grade squamous intraepithelial lesion development in young females. *JAMA* 2001;285:2995–3002.

133. Castle PE, Wacholder S, Sherman ME, et al. Absolute risk of a subsequent abnormal Pap among oncogenic human papillomavirus DNA-positive, cytologically negative women. *Cancer* 2002;95:2145–51.

134. Schiffman M, Castle PE, Jeronimo J, Rodriguez AC, Wacholder S. Human papillomavirus and cervical cancer. *Lancet* 2007;370:890–907.

135. Schiller JT, Day PM, Kines RC. Current understanding of the mechanism of HPV infection. *Gynecol Oncol* 2010;118(1 suppl):S12–7.

136. Stanley M. Chapter 17: Genital human papillomavirus infections—current and prospective therapies. *J Natl Cancer Inst* (monograph) 2003;31:117–24.

137. Park TJ, Fujihara H, Wright TC. Molecular biology of cervical cancer and its precursors. *Cancer* 1995;76:1890–1907.

138. Chapman WB, Lorincz AT, Willett GD, et al. Epidermal growth factor receptor expression and presence of human papillomavirus in cervical squamous intraepithelial lesions. *Int J Gynecol Pathol* 1982;11:221–6.

139. Dollard SC, Wilson JL, Demeter LM, et al. Production of human papillomavirus and modulation of the infections program in epithelial raft cultures. *Genes Dev* 1992;6:1131–42.

140. Schneider A, Koutsky LA. Natural history and epidemiological features with genital HPV infection in the epidemiology of cervical cancer and human papillomavirus. In: Munoz N, Bosch FX, Shah KV, Meheus A, eds. *The Epidemiology of Human Papillomavirus and Cervical Cancer.* New York, NY: Oxford University Press, 1992:25–52.

141. Taichman LB, La Porta RF. The expression of papillomaviruses in epithelial cells. In: Salzman NP, Howley PM, eds. *The Papovaviridae.* Vol 2. New York, NY: Plenum Press, 1987:l09–39.

142. Papay F, Wood B, Coulson M. Squamous cell papilloma at the tracheo-esophageal puncture stoma. *Arch Otolaryngol Head Neck Surg* 1988;114:564–8.

143. Pim D, Banks L. Interaction of viral oncoproteins with cellular target molecules: infection with high-risk vs low-risk human papillomaviruses. *APMIS* 2010;118:471–93.

144. Rodriguez AC, Schiffman M, Herrero R, et al. Rapid clearance of human papillomavirus and implications for clinical focus on persistent infections. *J Natl Cancer Inst* 2008;100:513–7.

145. Sun Y, Eluf-Neto J, Bosch FX, et al. Serum antibodies to HPV16 proteins in women from Brazil with invasive cervical carcinoma. *Cancer Epidemiol Biomark Prev* 1999;8:935–40.

146. Rogozinski TT, Jablonska S, Jarzabek-Chorzelska M. Role of cell-mediated immunity in spontaneous regression of plane warts. *Int J Dermatol* 1988;27:322–6.

147. Tay SK, Jenkins D, Maddox P, et al. Lymphocyte phenotypes in cervical intraepithelial neoplasia and human papillomavirus infection. *Br J Obstet Gynaecol* 1987;94:16–21.

148. Hawthorn RJ, Murdoch JB, MacLean AB, MacKie RM. Langerhans' cells and subtypes of human papillomavirus in cervical intraepithelial neoplasia. *BMJ* 1988;297:643–6.

149. Cauda R, Tyring SK, Grossi CE, et al. Patients with condyloma acuminatum exhibit decreased interleukin-2 and interferon gamma production and depresses natural killer activity. *J Clin Immunol* 1987;7:304–11.

150. Eron LJ, Judson F, Tucker S, et al. Interferon therapy for condyloma acuminata. *N Engl J Med* 1986;315:1059–64.

151. Schiller JT, Hildesheim A. Developing HPV virus-like particle vaccines to prevent cervical cancer: a progress report. *J Clin Virol* 2000;19:67–74.

152. Lehtinen M, Dillner J, Knekt P, et al. Serologically diagnosed infection with human papillomavirus type 16 and risk of subsequent development of cervical carcinoma: nested case-control study. *BMJ* 1996;312:537–9.

153. De Sanjose S, Hamsikova E, Munoz N, et al. Serological response to HPV16 in CIN-III and cervical cancer patients. Case-control studies in Spain and Colombia. *Int J Cancer* 1996;66:70–4.

154. Tsukui T, Hildesheim A, Schiffman MH, et al. IL-2 production by peripheral lymphocytes in response to human papillomavirus-derived peptides: correlation with cervical pathology. *Cancer Res* 1996;56:3967–74.

155. Kadish AS, Timmins P, Wang Y, et al. Regression of CIN and loss of HPV infection is associated with cell-mediated immune responses to a HPV type 16 E7 peptide. *Cancer Epidemiol Biomark Prev* 2002;11:483–8.

156. Mitchell MF, Tortolero-Luna G, Cook E. A randomized clinical trial of cryotherapy, loop electrosurgical excision for treatment of squamous intraepithelial lesions of the cervix. *Obstet Gynecol* 1998;92:737–44.

157. Hemminki K, Li X, Mutanen P. Familial risks in invasive and in situ cervical cancer by histological type. *Eur J Cancer Prev* 2001;10:83–9.

158. Magnusson PK, Lichtenstein P, Gyllensten UB. Heritability of cervical tumours. *Int J Cancer* 2000;88:698–701.

159. Einstein MH, Burk RD. Persistent human papillomavirus infection: definitions and clinical implications. *Papillomavirus Rep* 2001;12:119–23.

160. Richardson H, Kelsall G, Tellier P, et al. The natural history of type-specific human papillomavirus infections in female university students. *Cancer Epidemiol Biomarkers Prev* 2003;12:485–90.

161. Svare EI, Kjaer SK, Worm AM, et al. Risk factors for HPV infection in women from sexually transmitted disease clinics: comparison between two areas with different cervical cancer incidence. *Int J Cancer* 1998;75:1–8.

162. Palefsky JM, Minkoff H, Kalish LA, et al. Cervicovaginal human papillomavirus infection in human immunodeficiency virus-1 (HIV)-positive and high-risk HIV-negative women. *J Natl Cancer Inst* 1999;91:226–36.

163. Meisels A. The story of a cell. *Acta Cytol* 1983;27:584–96.

164. Schneider A. Sensitivity of the cytological diagnosis of cervical condylomata in comparison with HPV DNA hybridization studies. *Diagn Cytopathol* 1987;3:250–5.

165. Meijer CJLM, van den Brule AJC, Snijders PJF, et al. Detection of human papillomavirus in cervical scrapes by the polymerase chain reaction in relation to cytology: possible implications for cervical cancer screening. In: Munoz N, Bosch FX, Shah KV, Meheus A, eds. *The Epidemiology of Human Papillomavirus and Cervical Cancer.* Lyon, France: IARC Scientific Publications, 1992:271–81.

166. Ylitalo N, Sorensen P, Josefsson AM, et al. Consistent high viral load of human papillomavirus 16 and risk of cervical carcinoma in situ: a nested case-control study. *Lancet* 2000;355:2194–8.

167. Moscicki AB, Palefsky J, Smith G, et al. Variability of human papillomavirus DNA testing in a longitudinal cohort of young women. *Obstet Gynecol* 1993;82:578–85.

168. Herrero R, Muñoz N. Human papillomavirus and cancer. *Cancer Surv* 1999;33:75–98.

169. Ostor AG. Natural history of CIN: a critical review. *Int J Gynecol Pathol* 1993;12:186–92.

170. Cox JT, Schiffman M, Solomon D; ASCUS-LSIL Triage Study (ALTS) Group. Prospective follow-up suggests similar risk of subsequent cervical intraepithelial neoplasia grade 2 or 3 among women with cervical intraepithelial neoplasia grade 1 or negative colposcopy and directed biopsy. *Am J Obstet Gynecol* 2003;188:1406–12.

171. Richart RM. Natural history of cervical intraepithelial neoplasia. *Clin Obstet Gynecol* 1968;10:748–84.

172. Kiviat NB, Koutsky LA. Do our current cervical cancer control strategies still make sense? *J Natl Cancer Inst* 1996;88:317–8.

173. Koutsky LA, Holmes KK, Critchlow CW, et al. Cohort study of risk of cervical intraepithelial neoplasia grade 2 or 3 associated with cervical papillomavirus infection. *N Engl J Med* 1992;327:1272–8.

174. Ferenczy A, Franco E. Persistent human papillomavirus infection and cervical neoplasia. *Lancet Oncol* 2002;3:11–6.

175. Burghardt E, Ostor AG. Site and origin of squamous cervical cancer: a histomorphologic study. *Obstet Gynecol* 1983;62:117–26.

176. Schlecht NF, Kulaga S, Robitaille J, et al. Persistent human papillomavirus infection as a predictor of cervical intraepithelial neoplasia. *JAMA* 2001;286:3106–14.

177. Garland SM, Hernandez-Avila M, Wheeler CM, et al.; Females United to Unilaterally Reduce Endo/Ectocervical Disease (FUTURE) I Investigators. Quadrivalent vaccine against human papillomavirus to prevent anogenital diseases. *N Engl J Med* 2007;356(19):1928–43.

178. Woodman CB, Collins S, Winter H, et al. Natural history of cervical human papillomavirus infection in young women: a longitudinal cohort study. *Lancet* 2001;357:1831–6.

179. Rodriguez AC, Schiffman M, Herrero R, et al. Longitudinal study of human papillomavirus persistence and cervical intraepithelial neoplasia grade 2/3: critical role of duration of infection. *J Natl Cancer Inst* 2010;102:315–24.

180. Herrero R, Hildesheim A, Bratti C, et al. Population-based study of human papillomavirus infection and cervical neoplasia in rural Costa Rica. *J Natl Cancer Inst* 2000;92:464–74.

181. Moscicki AB, Ma Y, Wibbelsman C, et al. Rate of and risks for regression of cervical intraepithelial neoplasia 2 in adolescents and young women. *Obstet Gynecol* 2010;116(6):1373–80.

182. Louvanto K, Rintala MA, Syrjänen KJ, Grénman SE, Syrjänen SM. Genotype-specific persistence of genital human papillomavirus (HPV) infections in women followed for 6 years in the Finnish Family HPV Study. *J Infect Dis* 2010;202(3):436–44.

183. Castle PE, Schiffman M, Wheeler CM, Wentzensen N, Gravitt PE. Human papillomavirus genotypes in cervical intraepithelial neoplasia grade 3. *Cancer Epidemiol Biomarkers Prev* 2011;19(7):1675–81.

184. Larson AA, Liao S-Y, Stanbridge EJ, et al. Genetic alterations accumulate during cervical tumorigenesis and indicate a common origin for multifocal lesions. *Cancer Res* 1997;57:4171–6.

185. Lazo PA. The molecular genetics of cervical carcinoma. *Br J Cancer* 1999;80:2008–18.

186. Melsheimer P, Vinokurova S, Wentzensen N, Bastert G, von Knebel Doeberitz M. DNA aneuploidy and integration of human papillomavirus type 16 e6/e7 oncogenes in intraepithelial neoplasia and invasive squamous cell carcinoma of the cervix uteri. *Clin Cancer Res* 2004;10(9):3059–63.

187. Watanabe T. Flow cytometric evaluation of DNA ploidy pattern and cell heterogeneity in cervical dysplasia and carcinoma in situ. *Nippon Sanka Fujinka Gakkai Zasshi* 1993;45:1381–8.

188. Garnett GP, Waddell HC. Public health paradoxes and the epidemiological impact of a HPV vaccine. *J Clin Virol* 2000;19:101–11.

189. McCredie MR, Sharples KJ, Paul C, et al. Natural history of cervical neoplasia and risk of invasive cancer in women with cervical intraepithelial neoplasia 3: a retrospective cohort study. *Lancet Oncol* 2008;9:425–34.

190. ASCUS-LSIL Triage Study (ALTS) Group. Results of a randomized trial on the management of cytology interpretations of atypical squamous cells of undetermined significance. *Am J Obstet Gynecol* 2003;188:1383–92.

191. Levine AJ. P53, cellular gatekeeper for growth and division. *Cell* 1997;88:323–31.

192. Sartor MA, Dolinoy DC, Jones TR, et al. Genome-wide methylation and expression differences in HPV(+) and HPV(−) squamous cell carcinoma cell lines are consistent with divergent mechanisms of carcinogenesis. *Epigenetics* 2011;6(6):777–87.

193. Virmani AK, Muller C, Rathi A, et al. Aberrant methylation during cervical carcinogenesis. *Clin Cancer Res* 2001;7:584–9.

194. Takizawa S, Nagasaka K, Nakagawa S, et al. Human scribble, a novel tumor suppressor identified as a target of high-risk HPV E6 for ubiquitin-mediated degradation, interacts with adenomatous polyposis coli. *Genes Cells* 2006;11:453–64.

195. Lee C, Laimins LA. Role of the PDZ domain-binding motif of the oncoprotein E6 in the pathogenesis of human papillomavirus type 31. *J Virol* 2004;78:12366–77.

196. National Cancer Institute SEER Cancer Statistics Review 1975–2008 http://seer.cancer.gov/csr/1975_2008/index.html (Accessed August 20, 2011).

197. Doorbar J. Papillomavirus life cycle organization and biomarker selection. *Dis Markers* 2007;23:297–313.

198. Wright TC Jr, Massad LS, Dunton CJ, Spitzer M, Wilkinson EJ, Solomon D; 2006 American Society for Colposcopy and Cervical Pathology-sponsored Consensus Conference. 2006 consensus guidelines for the management of women with abnormal cervical cancer screening tests. *Am J Obstet Gynecol* 2007;197(4):346–55.

199. Schiffman M, Herrero R, Hildesheim A, et al. HPV DNA testing in cervical cancer screening: results from women in a high-risk province of Costa Rica. *JAMA* 2000;283:87–93.

200. Sherman ME, Schiffman M, Cox JT. Effects of age and HPV viral load on colposcopy triage: data from the randomized atypical squamous cells of undetermined significance/low-grade squamous intraepithelial lesion triage study (ALTS). *J Natl Cancer Inst* 2002;94:102–7.

201. Gravitt PE, Burk RD, Lorincz A, et al. A comparison between real-time polymerase chain reaction and hybrid capture 2 for human papillomavirus DNA quantitation. *Cancer Epidemiol Biomark Prev* 2003;12:477–84.

202. Ramanakumar AV, Goncalves O, Richardson H, et al. Human papillomavirus (HPV) types 16, 18, 31, 45 DNA loads and HPV-16 integration in persistent and transient infections in young women. *BMC Infect Dis* 2010;10:326.

203. Xi LF, Hughes JP, Castle PE, et al. Viral load in the natural history of human papillomavirus type 16 infection: a nested case-control study. *J Infect Dis* 2011;203(10):1425–33.

204. Gravitt PE, Peyton C, Wheeler C, Apple R, Higuchi R, Shah KV. Reproducibility of HPV 16 and HPV 18 viral load quantitation using TaqMan real-time PCR assays. *J Virol Methods* 2003;112:23–33.

205. Cuschieri K, Wentzensen N. Human papillomavirus mRNA and p16 detection as biomarkers for the improved diagnosis of cervical neoplasia. *Cancer Epidemiol Biomarkers Prev* 2008;17:2536–45.

206. Eleuterio J Jr, Giraldo PC, Goncalves AK, et al. Prognostic markers of high-grade squamous intraepithelial lesions: the role of p16INK4a and high-risk human papillomavirus. *Acta Obstet Gynecol Scand* 2007;86:94–8.

207. Meyer JL, Hanlon DW, Andersen BT, Rasmussen OF, Bisgaard K. Evaluation of p16INK4a expression in ThinPrep cervical specimens with the CINtec p16INK4a assay: correlation with biopsy follow-up results. *Cancer* 2007;111:83–92.

208. Wentzensen N, von Knebel Doeberitz M. Biomarkers in cervical cancer screening. *Dis Markers* 2007;23:315–30.

209. Sherman ME. Chapter 11: Future directions in cervical pathology. *J Natl Cancer Inst* (monograph) 2003;31:72–9.

210. Turan T, Kalantari M, Calleja-Macias IE, et al. Methylation of the human papillomavirus-18 L1 gene: a biomarker of neoplastic progression? *Virology* 2006;349:175–83.

211. Doorbar J, Cubie H. Molecular basis for the advances in cervical screening. *Mol Diagn* 2005;9:129–142.

212. Wisman GB, Nijhuis ER, Hoque MO, et al. Assessment of gene promoter hypermethylation for detection of cervical neoplasia. *Int J Cancer* 2006;119:1908–14.

213. Branca M, Giorgi C, Santini D, et al. Upregulation of telomerase (hTERT) is related to the grade of cervical intraepithelial neoplasia, but is not an independent predictor of high-risk human papillomavirus, virus persistence, or disease outcome in cervical cancer. *Diagn Cytopathol* 2006;34:739–48.

214. Koskimaa H, Kurvinen K, Costa S, Syrjänen K, Syrjänen S. Molecular markers implicating early malignant events in cervical carcinogenesis. *Cancer Epidemiol Biomarkers Prev* 2010;19(8):2003–12.

CHAPTER 6

DARON G. FERRIS
EDWARD J. MAYEAUX, JR.

Colposcopic Equipment, Supplies, and Data Management

6.1 INTRODUCTION
6.2 COLPOSCOPES
  6.2.1 Overview
  6.2.2 Objective Lenses and Focal Length
  6.2.3 Illumination and Filters
  6.2.4 Magnification
  6.2.5 Oculars, Video, and Monocular Observation Tubes
  6.2.6 Mounting
  6.2.7 Focus Controls
  6.2.8 Cost
  6.2.9 Colposcope Care
6.3 VIDEO COLPOSCOPE
6.4 EXAMINATION TABLE AND INSTRUMENT STAND
6.5 COLPOSCOPIC INSTRUMENTS
  6.5.1 Vaginal Specula
  6.5.2 Lateral Sidewall Retractors
  6.5.3 Endocervical Specula
  6.5.4 Biopsy Forceps

  6.5.5 Endocervical Curette
  6.5.6 Other Instruments
6.6 CHEMICAL AGENTS AND SUPPLIES
  6.6.1 Saline
  6.6.2 Acetic Acid Solution
  6.6.3 Lugol's Solution
  6.6.4 Monsel's Solution
  6.6.5 Silver Nitrate Sticks
  6.6.6 Topical and Local Anesthetics
  6.6.7 Bactericidal Solutions for Instrument Care
  6.6.8 Disposable Supplies
6.7 VIDEO AND PHOTOGRAPHIC SYSTEMS FOR OPTICAL COLPOSCOPES
  6.7.1 Video Systems
  6.7.2 Colpophotography
6.8 IMAGE, DATA MANAGEMENT, AND PATIENT TRACKING SYSTEMS
6.9 SUMMARY

6.1 INTRODUCTION

Colposcopy requires properly maintained equipment and the supplies needed to facilitate adequate patient examination. Colposcopists should ensure that the examination room is fully stocked with all necessary instruments, supplies, and properly functioning equipment prior to each scheduled colposcopic visit (Table 6.1). Appropriate care and routine maintenance of colposcopic equipment and instruments are critical for optimum performance. This chapter includes a discussion of basic colposcopic equipment, instruments, chemical agents, and colposcopy supplies needed for routine colposcopy. Additionally, an overview of supplemental equipment such as cameras, video equipment, digital imaging systems, and colposcopic image and data management systems that might be useful to clinicians with academic or busy colposcopic practices is provided.

6.2 COLPOSCOPES

6.2.1 Overview

A colposcope is an optical instrument that permits illuminated and magnified examination of the lower genital tract. The intense light transilluminates the epithelium, and magnification allows for close examination of the surface epithelium and subepithelial blood vessels. There are two major types of colposcopes: the traditional optical colposcope[1] and the newer video colposcope (Figures 6.1 and 6.2).[2] The video colposcope with monitor, which completely replaces the standard binocular optics of the traditional colposcope, enables colposcopists to view the cervix on a video monitor rather than directly through the eyepiece. There are several factors to consider when using or purchasing a colposcope.

6.2.2 Objective Lenses and Focal Length

Colposcopes have either a single or a double objective lens positioned in the front of the instrument. While colposcopes made with a single objective lens are adequate, colposcopes designed with double objective lenses provide true stereoscopic images since each eyepiece is linked visually to a separate complex of lenses. Objective lenses have a fixed focal length derived from the curvature of the lens. Focal length determines the distance between the objective lens and the cervix or, from a practical perspective, the *working distance* between the colposcope and the vaginal speculum when the cervix is in focus (Figure 6.3). Focal length corresponds to the space available between the colposcope and speculum for introducing and working with biopsy and treatment instruments. The shorter the focal length, the smaller the available working space. Most colposcopes have lenses with a 300-mm focal length. This focal length provides the greatest versatility and operator comfort when using biopsy instruments, without compromising colposcopic detail. A 240-mm objective lens, although excellent for colpophotography, does not allow sufficient room between the colposcope and speculum to accommodate most biopsy instruments and hinders colposcopically directed laser surgery and electrosurgical loop excision procedures. One colposcope has an adjustable focal length of 200 to 350 mm. This allows focusing using a knob instead of moving the colposcope (Figure 6.4).

TABLE 6.1   COLPOSCOPY EQUIPMENT, MATERIALS AND SUPPLIES

Colposcope—Binocular or video, 300-mm focal length, variable magnification, red-free (green or blue) filter
Vaginal specula in various sizes
3%–5% acetic acid
Lugol's iodine solution
Cotton-tipped applicators and large cotton swabs and/or cotton balls
Endocervical specula in various sizes
Biopsy forceps such as Tischler, baby Tischler, or Kevorkian forceps
Endocervical curette and/or endocervical brushes
Ring forceps or tissue forceps
Biopsy specimen containers with fixative and labels
Hemostatic agent such as silver nitrate sticks or Monsel's paste (ferric subsulfate)

6.2.3 Illumination and Filters

A colposcope should have a powerful light source capable of incremental adjustments to provide the desired amount of illumination. Some newer colposcopes automatically adjust the level of illumination. There are many types of light sources, including incandescent bulbs, arc lamps, tungsten and halogen lamps, and light-emitting diode (LED) sources. Tungsten, halogen and arc lamps, and LEDs provide brighter lighting and are superior for colpophotography, videocolposcopy, and computer-based digitized image capture (Figure 6.5). Different types of lamps provide different color hues. Incandescent bulbs provide a warm, reddish color and halogen bulbs, LEDs, and arc lamps emit a very white color, whereas other types of bulbs produce a cool, bluish hue.

A colposcope should provide illumination of the entire field of view at low magnification. In general, the intensity of illumination decreases as the level of magnification increases; however, very intense light sources on newer colposcopes provide ample illumination at high magnification levels.[2] The position of the light source is also relevant because the bulb may generate considerable heat. If the light source is in the head of the colposcope, the heat can be uncomfortable for both the colposcopist and the patient. Several colposcopes have a small fan to direct heat away from the colposcope and patient. Newer LED-type illumination sources produce very little heat. On other colposcopes, the bulb is placed away from the head of the scope, and fiber-optic cable is used to deliver light to the colposcope head. The fiber-optic cable should be enclosed within a protective sheath of flexible plastic or metal to protect it from potential damage (Figure 6.6). Otherwise, if twisted or bent, the small glass fibers within the cable may break, resulting in nonilluminated dark "spots" and overall reduced illumination. Spare light bulbs and fuses should be available and readily accessible during procedures.

A red-free (green or blue) filter is a desirable feature because it increases contrast in the colposcopic image while only slightly reducing the overall illumination. Red-free filters block red light transmission, making blood vessels appear black. They also may modify contrast between acetowhite and

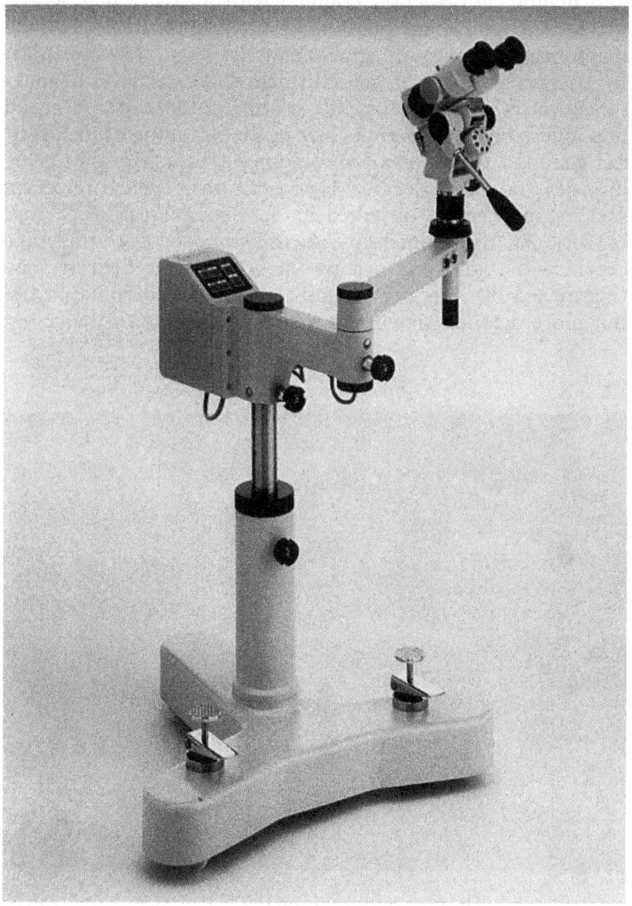

FIGURE 6.1.   An optical or traditional colposcope. The colposcopist views the examination directly through the oculars, which gives true binocular vision.

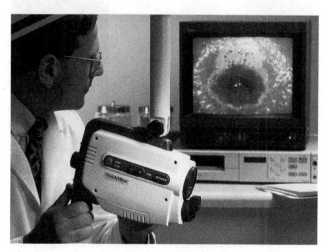

FIGURE 6.2.   A video colposcope and high-resolution video monitor. The colposcopist views the examination indirectly on the monitor.

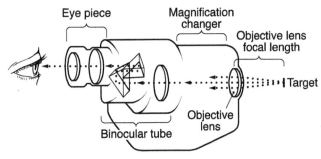

FIGURE 6.3. Diagram of the focal length of an objective lens. The eyepieces, binocular tubes, and magnification complex are the other components of the optical colposcope. (From Ferris DG, Willner WA, Ho JJ. *The Journal of Family Practice* 1991;(33):506–51. Reprinted with permission, Dowden Health Media.)

nonacetowhite epithelium. It is easy to interpose filters between the light source or optics and the area viewed on both optical and video colposcopes. On optical colposcopes, a knob, lever, or sliding mechanism activates the red-free filter (Figure 6.7). On video colposcopes, a small touch button on the sides of the scope electronically activates the filter (Figure 6.8). Green filters, which are standard on most modern colposcopes, ideally should be encased within the colposcope to prevent dust accumulation. The polarized light filter on the video colposcope eliminates glare that may interfere with the examination.

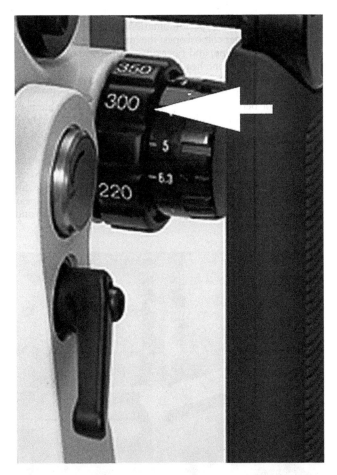

FIGURE 6.4. This colposcope has an adjustable focal length of 200 to 350 mm. This knob (*arrow*) is used to focus instead of moving the colposcope.

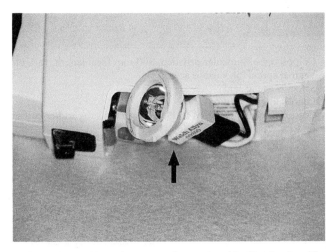

FIGURE 6.5. This arc lamp provides intense white illumination. The bulb (*arrow*) can be easily replaced.

6.2.4 Magnification

Colposcopic magnification is determined not only by the magnification lens but also by the objective lens and the oculars (Figure 6.9).[3] For example, if a single objective lens and magnification lens coupled with 10× oculars (eyepieces) produce a final magnification of 7.5×, the same objective and magnification lenses coupled with a 20× ocular would produce a final magnification of 15×. Colposcopes with a magnification range of approximately 2× to 15× are ideal for assessing the lower genital tract. A greater level of magnification is not necessary for routine colposcopy. A broad magnification range permits low-power scanning of the external genitalia and allows for colposcopic visualization during biopsies and electrosurgical loop excisions. The entire cervix and vagina can be observed at 3.5× magnification (Figure 6.10A). At approximately 7.5× magnification, the average cervix will completely occupy the colposcopic field of view (Figure 6.10B). Greater magnification (15×) permits partial but more detailed viewing of a smaller portion of the cervix

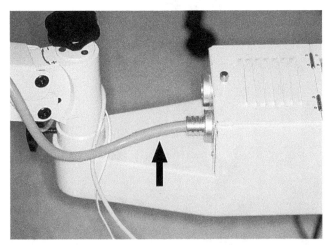

FIGURE 6.6. The fiber-optic cable on this colposcope (*arrow*) can be plugged into one of two separate lamp receptacles. Such engineering allows a quick change to a new bulb if the other fails during a colposcopic examination.

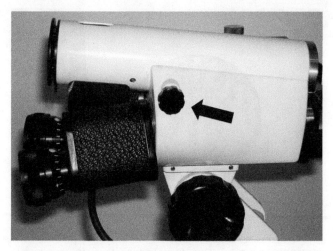

FIGURE 6.7. The green filter is selected by a small knob (*arrow*) centrally positioned on this colposcope.

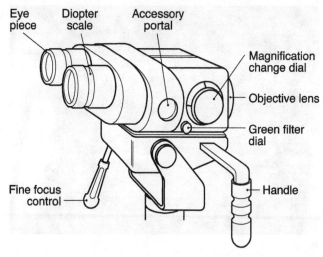

FIGURE 6.9. Components of an optical colposcope. (From Ferris DG, Willner WA, Ho JJ. *The Journal of Family Practice* 1991;(33): 506–51. Reprinted with permission, Dowden Health Media.)

(Figure 6.10C). Hence, as magnification is increased, the field of view (what is seen using the colposcope) decreases. Colposcopic examination of the cervix generally requires 7.5× to 15× magnification. Higher magnification, such as 20× to 30×, is less useful clinically but allows closer inspection of fine vascular detail (Figure 6.10C).

Colposcopes with only a single level of magnification (high or low) are not ideal because they severely restrict detailed examinations and are cumbersome to use. Colposcopes with either multiple fixed magnification or zoom magnification are preferable. Adjusting a knob usually achieves the desired level of magnification on colposcopes with multiple fixed magnification (Figure 6.11). Zoom magnification provides a continuous range of magnification from lowest to highest levels. Although the optical quality of the image obtained from zoom magnification colposcopes may be somewhat lower than that of fixed magnification colposcopes, the difference in image quality is not sufficient to impair clinical accuracy. Electronic or motorized zoom magnification operated by a button is a standard feature of the video colposcope and is available as an option on some zoom magnification optical colposcopes.

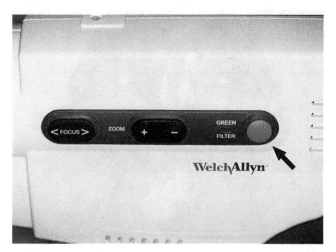

FIGURE 6.8. The video colposcope's electronic green filter is activated by depressing the small button at the rear of the operations panel.

6.2.5 Oculars, Video, and Monocular Observation Tubes

Interchangeable or fixed oculars (eyepieces) of various magnification permit adjustments in magnification and individual eyepiece focusing. The binocular tubes containing the oculars can be adjusted to accommodate the colposcopist's interpupillary distance and vision. Diopter settings, which are present on some oculars, indicate the unique focus setting of each ocular (Figure 6.12). The midpoint, or "0" setting, is the default for colposcopists with normal or normal-corrected vision. For colposcopists who wear eyeglasses but choose not to use them during colposcopy, twisting the eyepieces toward the negative or positive diopter settings allows proper focus for colposcopists with myopia or hyperopia, respectively. However, if video colposcopy via a beam splitter is used, ocular hoods or eyepiece cups may be extended for colposcopists who wear contact lenses or have normal uncorrected vision (Figure 6.13). These may be inverted (flattened or removed) if the colposcopist prefers to wear glasses during the examination (Figure 6.12). One advantage to the use of eyepiece cups is that they reduce ambient light, which may be distracting.

The angle of the oculars or binocular tubes in relation to the direct line of sight from the eye to the cervix varies from inclined (45 degrees) (Figure 6.14) to straight in-line tubes (180 degrees) (Figure 6.14B). Straight in-line oculars permit viewing directly toward the target. Thereby, a casual glance away from the oculars allows a nonmagnified observation of the same target. Clinicians who have difficulty focusing with binoculars may prefer a videocolposcope, which has no oculars.

Video may be added to many standard colposcopes through two common additions. The first involves attaching a completely separate lens system (Figure 6.15) that allows the monitor to show the same general view as the colposcopist but not exactly what is viewed through the eyepiece. Most of these have only one magnification regardless of the levels of magnification of the colposcope. The second method involves adding a beam splitter between the objective lenses and the eyepieces. This system has the advantage that the viewer sees exactly what the colposcopist sees, but has the disadvantage that overall illumination may be decreased. The port of both systems can be attached to a charged coupled device (CCD) camera and high-resolution video monitor.

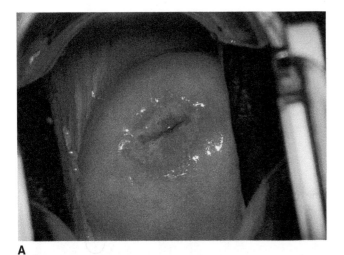

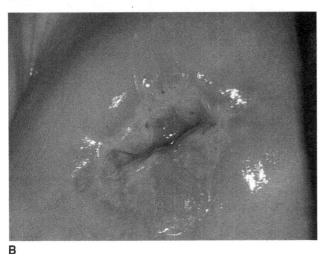

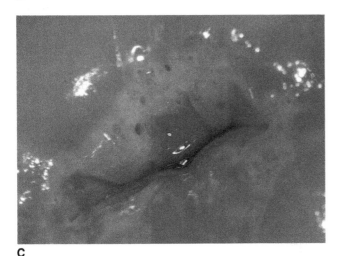

FIGURE 6.10.   The cervix at (**A**) 3.5×, (**B**) 7.5×, and (**C**) 15× magnification. Note how the area of the cervix in view shrinks as the magnification increases.

A monocular observation tube attached to a colposcope portal also permits viewing by a second person (Figure 6.16). In the teaching setting, the capacity for simultaneous observation by an inexperienced colposcopist has instructional value. However, in the nonteaching clinical setting, where this capacity is rarely needed, the monocular observation tube has limited usefulness. Since the monocular observation tube is awkward

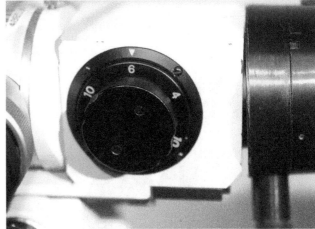

FIGURE 6.11.   Colposcope with multiple fixed magnification changer.

to use, offers no depth perception, and can be expensive, a video colposcopy system with a monitor might be a better investment in settings where the capacity for joint observation by students, nursing assistants, and patients is useful.

6.2.6 Mounting

Colposcopes can be affixed to an examination table, mounted on a stand, or fitted to a swivel arm attached to the wall or ceiling. Mobile colposcopes are usually the most practical since they permit easy transfer from room to room or within a room. Some colposcopes are mounted by a universal joint to a small, flat platform on a wheelless base that is stabilized by the colposcopist's feet (Figure 6.17). A weighted or wide colposcope base prevents inadvertent tipping of the scope and potential injury to the delicate optics. Since colposcopes mounted on wheels often depend on mobility for coarse focusing, wheel locks designed to prevent accidental rolling are rarely activated (Figure 6.18).

Types of supports available for the colposcope head include center-post, flexible articulating arm, or overhead boom-type (Figures 6.19A–C). Of these three, center-post and flexible articulating arm scopes provide better stationary viewing. Overhead boom scopes often have unintended play, even

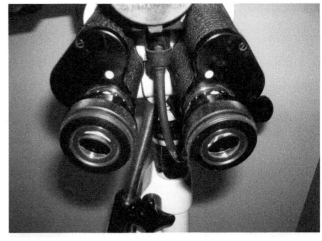

FIGURE 6.12.   The diopter scales on each eyepiece are set to the 0 position when the dots on the eyepieces and colposcope are aligned.

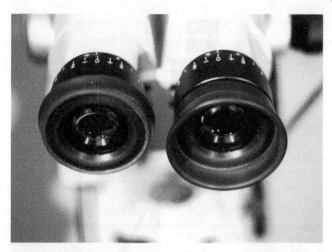

FIGURE 6.13. Ocular hoods. The right hood is extended to help prevent obscuring ambient light.

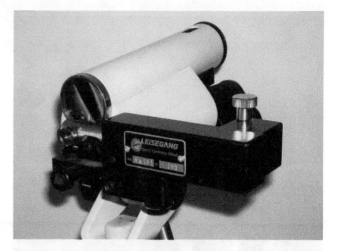

FIGURE 6.15. Optical colposcopes with an externally attached separate lens system for video colposcopy.

though the tension at each joint is adjustable. When selecting a type of colposcope support, it is important to consider individual preference, available examination room space, frequency of colposcope transportation, and cost. Colposcopic head and platform stability are particularly important for laser-adapted colposcopes.

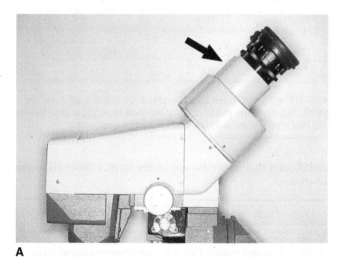

A

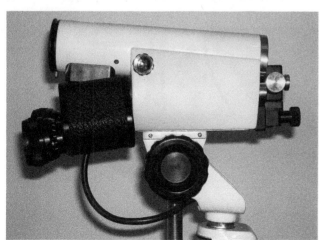

B

FIGURE 6.14. **A:** Inclined eyepieces (*arrow*) are preferred by some colposcopists. **B:** Colposcope with straight in-line oculars.

6.2.7 Focus Controls

Colposcopes can be focused by both coarse and fine movement methods. When using an optical or video colposcope, moving the colposcope head in relation to the patient accomplishes coarse focus. If the colposcope is mounted on a center-post and wheels, coarse focus usually requires the entire unit to move. If the colposcope head is mounted on a flexible articulating arm or an overhead boom, the base remains stationary, and the articulated arm and head are placed in the roughly correct position, only the head moves.

At low magnification, simply moving the head of the colposcope toward or away from the target or anatomical organ being examined achieves rapid coarse focus. Fine focus may be achieved with smaller, more precise movements of the scope or its head, or by manipulating a fine focus handle, knob, or lever on the colposcope that moves only the colposcope head in relation to the remainder of the colposcope (Figure 6.20). This minor adjustment allows for fine focus at both low and high magnification levels. Additionally, gentle manipulation of the vaginal speculum may be used for focusing at high magnification since most colposcopes have a narrow depth of field. Depth of field refers to the area in focus as measured in a line along the observation path at a particular level of magnification. At low-level magnification, the depth of field is quite wide. At a high level of magnification, the depth of field is limited, and therefore, only several millimeters of movement brings an object into or out of focus. The video colposcope provides a bidirectional, button-activated, motorized fine focus similar to the same feature found on video camcorders. This fine-focus mechanism allows the external video colposcope to remain stable, with focus achieved solely by the movement of the internally positioned optics. Some motorized optical colposcopes have foot switch-activated, motorized fine focus that smoothly moves the head of the colposcope.

6.2.8 Cost

The cost of a colposcope varies from $5000 to more than $20,000 depending on optical quality, sophistication of design, components, mounting system, and photographic and video capabilities. A higher purchase cost usually reflects better quality in colposcopes. Although most colposcopes are well constructed, it is important to have access to good, prompt service for problems with lighting, optics, video, or

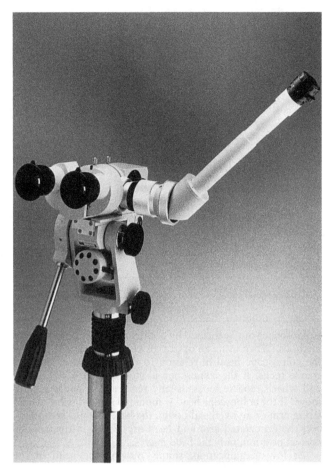

FIGURE 6.16. A monocular co-observation tube permits simultaneous observation of colposcopy by a single learner.

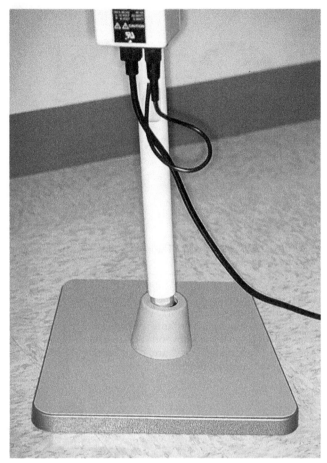

FIGURE 6.17. A colposcope mounted on a universal joint on a small, flat, wheelless platform. Colposcopists must place their feet on the foot platform for stability when using this colposcope.

colpophotographic quality. Accessible customer support is particularly important until the colposcope user becomes familiar with this relatively costly piece of equipment. Used colposcopes are available from resellers and individuals, but care must be taken to ensure the quality of such scopes and that lamps and parts are readily available.

6.2.9 Colposcope Care

Colposcopes require care and maintenance. When moving the scope a considerable distance, be careful not to bump or jar the optics out of alignment to avoid seriously compromising the colposcopic image. Cover the colposcope at the end of each day to prevent dust from accumulating on oculars and lenses. When the oculars or lens(es) become dusty, clean with lens paper, not with cloths, paper towels, or sponges that may scratch the lenses. Adjust the tension of the support mechanism as needed. Protect fiber-optic light cables from trauma, twisting, or bending to avoid breaking the encased glass strands. Replace light bulbs and fuses as necessary, making sure to disconnect the electrical supply first. Make sure to have extra bulbs immediately available to prevent disruption of a procedure when a bulb fails. All tools necessary to change a failed bulb should also be immediately available. To remove potentially infectious bodily secretions and blood, routinely use a disinfectant to wipe portions of the colposcope that come in regular contact with clinicians. Optics should only be cleaned with cleaners rated for optics. Be sure to choose a

disinfectant that is safe for use on the surface materials of the instrument.

6.3 VIDEO COLPOSCOPE

Video colposcopy is a relatively newer method for examining the lower genital tract.[2] The video colposcope system includes

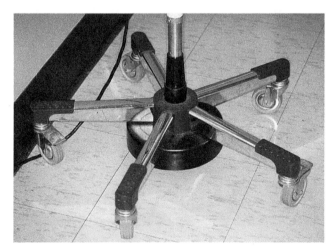

FIGURE 6.18. A wide, weighted base helps prevent accidental tipping of the colposcope.

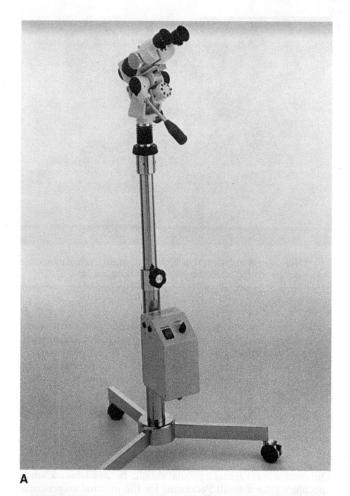

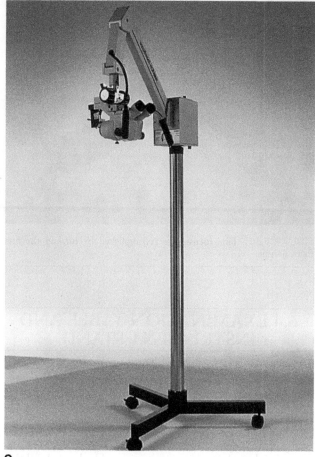

FIGURE 6.19. Colposcopes mounted on a (**A**) center post, (**B**) flexible articulating arm, and (**C**) overhead boom.

a video colposcope (a video camcorder-type device) and a high-resolution video monitor. The video colposcope is mounted on either a center pole stand or an overhead boom (Figure 6.21). Because the video colposcope has no eyepieces, the technique differs from traditional optical colposcopy in that the colposcopist does not view the target area directly through the eyepiece. Instead, observation by the colposcopist is directed to the image shown on the video monitor. The video colposcope has an excellent light source, electronic green filter, polarized light filter, and motorized, touch-activated controls for fine focus and zoom magnification. Touch-activated buttons on the handle electronically capture colposcopic images that are digitally saved in a computer or printed using a color video printer.

A modified colposcopy technique enhances depth perception. Observed shadows and light reflections create an apparent three-dimensional image on the two-dimensional video monitor. "Point and see" is the best way to describe this visualization process. The colposcopist uses the handle to move the scope to the correct focal length and parallel with the axis of the vagina. The fine focus button allows the operator to further sharpen the video image, if necessary. The colposcopist accomplishes assessment and sampling by observing the image displayed on the video monitor. The video colposcope costs about the same as a good optical colposcope that does not include video or photographic capability (i.e., beam splitter, adaptor, CCD, camera, and video monitor).

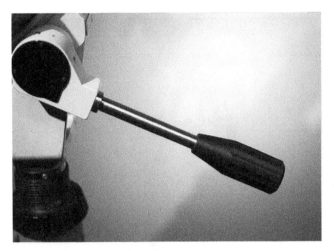

FIGURE 6.20. Fine focusing is accomplished by turning the fine focus handle.

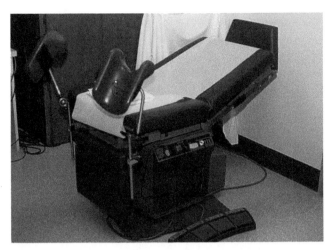

FIGURE 6.22. A mechanical or hydraulic patient examination table with leg supports facilitates the colposcopy examination.

6.4 EXAMINATION TABLE AND INSTRUMENT STAND

Although a standard nonhydraulic gynecologic table is suitable for colposcopic examinations, the foot of the table may be too low for some examiners. Raising it slightly often provides a better view of the cervix. Raising the head of the table slightly may be more comfortable for the patient while allowing the colposcopist to optimize communication. Either padded heel supports or behind-the-knee leg supports are adequate for the colposcopic examination table, but behind-the-knee leg supports can reduce patient fatigue during prolonged examinations or procedures. Some women, however, may prefer the sense of control foot stirrups provide. A mechanical or hydraulic table offers distinct advantages (Figure 6.22). Adjustment of the examination table height and angle to better align with the angle of the patient's vagina in relation to the colposcope light source allows for better visualization of the cervix and vagina.

The colposcopist should have convenient access to a stable instrument stand, cart, or counter space for the instruments, supplies, and solutions required for a colposcopic examination. Figure 6.23 shows a standard setup of instruments, solutions, and supplies used by many colposcopists.

6.5 COLPOSCOPIC INSTRUMENTS

6.5.1 Vaginal Specula

Different-sized vaginal specula should be available: a small speculum (like a small Pederson) for the unusual colposcopic examination of young girls and virginal women, a medium Pederson speculum for women with a narrow vagina, and medium and large Graves specula for most women. A short Cusco or Collins' speculum is ideal for examining the vaginal vault in posthysterectomy patients. A large metal Graves speculum is required for patients with vaginal wall laxity or prolapse, obesity, or pregnancy. Use of the widest speculum tolerated by the patient usually provides the best cervical visualization. An extended or long Graves or Pederson speculum is the best choice for an extremely long vagina.

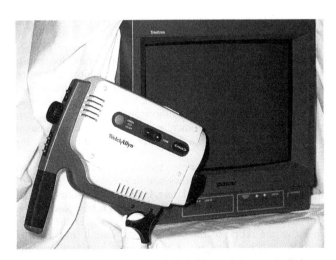

FIGURE 6.21. Components of the video colposcope include an electronic green filter, motorized zoom magnification changer, motorized fine focus control, light source, and handle-mounted image management buttons.

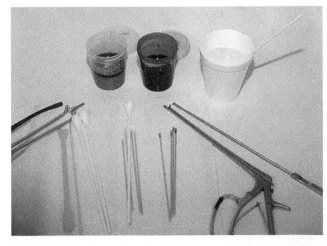

FIGURE 6.23. Setup for colposcopic instruments, chemicals, and supplies.

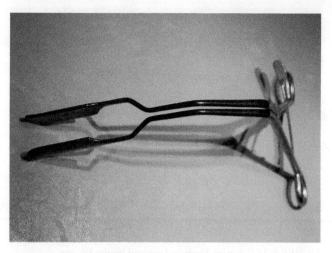

FIGURE 6.24. A lateral vaginal sidewall retractor. The instrument retracts prolapsing vaginal sidewalls that hinder colposcopic visualization. Note the offset blades that allow for wider visualization.

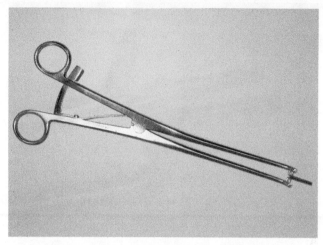

FIGURE 6.25. An endocervical speculum permits visualization of components of the transformation zone or cervical lesions positioned within the canal.

Metal and disposable plastic specula are both appropriate for colposcopy. When using plastic specula with independent light sources, an additional speculum light source is not necessary. However, the speculum light source must usually be extinguished for effective use of the colposcope's red-free filter. Blackened specula are designed specifically for CO_2 laser surgery but are also ideal for colpophotography because they reduce reflection. Specula with an electrically resistant coating that are designed to hold smoke evacuation tubing are the best choice for electrosurgical loop excision procedures.

6.5.2 Lateral Sidewall Retractors

Lateral vaginal sidewall retractors may be helpful when examining patients who have lax vaginal walls that block the view of the cervix through the vaginal speculum (Figure 6.24). Vaginal sidewall retractors have long, narrow, rounded blades designed to be placed between the blades of a vaginal speculum. Instruments with blades that are offset to the handles allow greater retraction of the sidewalls and better visualization. Use of these instruments requires caution to avoid pinching the wall of the vagina between the blades of the lateral sidewall retractor and the blades of the speculum. A large Graves speculum or a specially designed speculum with a wide introital opening is preferable because it allows the vaginal sidewall retractor to open fully. Another approach to retract the vaginal sidewalls is to cut off the distal end of either a condom or the middle finger or thumb of a rubber glove and place it over the vaginal speculum blades before insertion into the vagina. Be sure to confirm that the patient does not have a latex allergy, and have latex-free options for such occasions. Finally, some specially designed speculums have built-in blades that open to retract the lateral vaginal walls.

6.5.3 Endocervical Specula

Use of an endocervical speculum will improves visualization of the squamocolumnar junction or cervical lesion extending into the endocervical canal (Figure 6.25). The endocervical speculum has narrow opposing blades that extend into the endocervical canal and open to gently retract the tissue for better visualization (Figure 6.26). Although the blades of most endocervical specula are 1.5 to 2 cm long, it is difficult to see to this depth within the

canal. Endocervical specula generally allow good visualization of the first 5 to 10 mm of the endocervical canal. Many colposcopists have several different sizes of endocervical specula on hand to accommodate varying diameters of the os. Specula with wide blades are best for a patulous or average-sized cervical os, and specula with narrow blades are preferable for a narrow or stenotic os (Figure 6.27A,B). Modified de Jardin gallbladder forceps, Campion endocervical forceps, long pickups, Kelly clamps, or even ring forceps also can be used to examine the distal part of the endocervical canal. These types of forceps are used to separate the opposing walls of the endocervix to permit easy, relatively atraumatic access to the canal.

6.5.4 Biopsy Forceps

Cervical biopsy forceps are designed specifically to permit relatively small (~2-mm to 5-mm) tissue specimens to be obtained from the cervix (Figure 6.28). The many types of biopsy forceps all have their proponents. A few of the most commonly used types include the Tischler, baby Tischler, Tischler-Morgan, Eppendorfer, Burke, Kevorkian, Townsend,

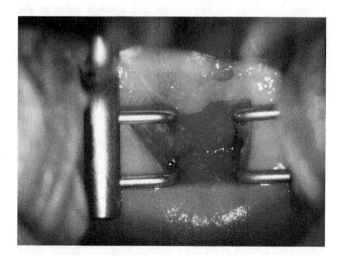

FIGURE 6.26. Endocervical speculum used in an examination of the squamocolumnar junction or proximal extent of neoplasia within the endocervical canal.

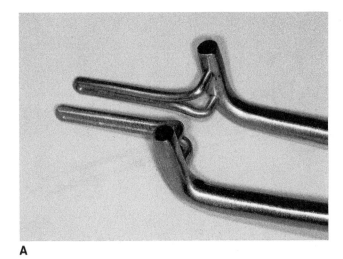

A

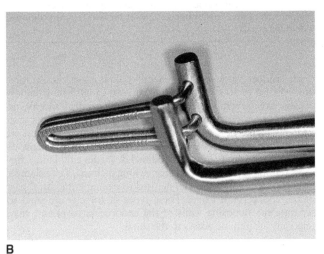

B

FIGURE 6.27. Endocervical specula of two different sizes, (**A**) a narrow blade for a stenotic os and (**B**) a wider blade for a parous os.

and the mini-Townsend biopsy forceps. Because the different types of biopsy forceps remove varying amounts of cervical tissue, they have a range of clinical uses.

The standard Tischler-Morgan biopsy forceps has an oval cutting "cup" on the upper edge and a single tooth at the front to fix the cervix during the biopsy (Figure 6.29). The oval configuration and cutting cup make these forceps excellent for taking large biopsies of up to 5 mm in diameter and up to 4 mm in depth. Although the diagnosis of intraepithelial lesions seldom requires such large biopsies, they are useful when cancer is clinically suspected. Because the cutting surface is completely oval, small biopsies obtained with Tischler-Morgan biopsy forceps are somewhat difficult to orient in the pathology laboratory. Specimen orientation is important so that the histologic sections can be cut perpendicular to the epithelial surface.

Biopsy forceps with square jaws or half-oval, half-square "bites" are designed to produce a biopsy specimen that is easy to orient correctly. There are numerous types of square-jawed biopsy forceps, including the Kevorkian, Tischler-Kevorkian, and Coppleson styles. Specimens obtained using these forceps have straight edges, allowing for easier orientation. Kevorkian forceps also have a distal row of teeth on the lower jaw designed to fix the cervix and facilitate tissue excision (Figure 6.30). One drawback of this design is that the four teeth make it difficult to obtain a deep biopsy.

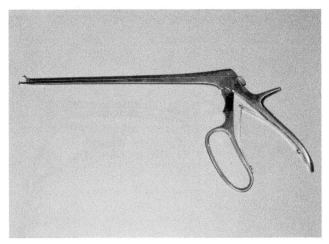

FIGURE 6.28.   A mini-Townsend cervical biopsy forceps.

Burke, baby Tischler, and mini-Townsend biopsy forceps have smaller heads and remove less tissue than do the Tischler-Morgan or standard Kevorkian biopsy forceps (Figure 6.31). Since 1-mm to 2-mm biopsy depth is usually adequate, these smaller biopsy forceps are commonly used in routine practice. Smaller biopsies are generally preferable to larger biopsies, except when cancer is suspected, because they produce less bleeding and pain. Smaller biopsy forceps are also easier to use for biopsies of lesions within the distal endocervical canal. The jaws of the Burke forceps open widely to facilitate biopsies of lesions in difficult-to-access regions (Figure 6.32). For difficult endocervical biopsies, consider the Eppendorfer forceps (without teeth), which can also be used on the vulva and vagina.

Some biopsy forceps have a thumb-activated locking mechanism above the handle to close the forceps jaws securely once a biopsy has been taken (Figure 6.33A,B). This device locks the jaws in a closed position to prevent the specimens from being lost as the biopsy forceps is withdrawn from the vagina. The locking mechanism also helps protect the sharp cutting surfaces during sterilization. Since no single instrument is ideal for all situations, experienced colposcopists usually have different types of biopsy forceps available. Additionally, many clinicians use small, round dermal (Keyes) biopsy punches to sample vulvar lesions (Figure 6.34).

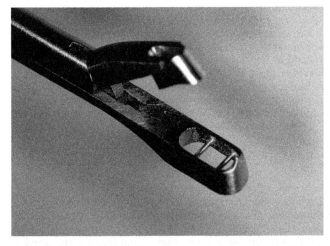

FIGURE 6.29.   A Tischler-Morgan biopsy forceps with a single tooth and oval cutting interface.

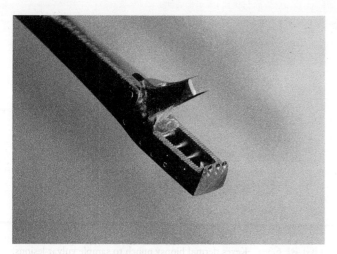

FIGURE 6.30.   Kevorkian biopsy forceps with four teeth along the lower jaw. These teeth may impede biopsy collection.

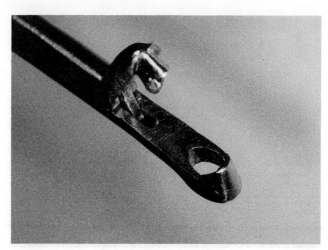

FIGURE 6.32.   The Burke biopsy forceps with jaws that open widely.

Biopsy instruments eventually become blunt with use, particularly if autoclaved in metal trays and not wrapped individually before sterilization. Because dull instruments increase crush artifact in the specimen and cause more pain,[4] instruments should always be sharp and well maintained. A good test of instrument sharpness is to biopsy a piece of thin plastic or Mylar sheet. A sharp instrument cuts cleanly through the material without fraying edges. Some instruments come with a lifetime resharpening service. If not, sharpening services for surgical instruments are available in most areas. Use caution when considering utilizing an inexperienced person or service to sharpen biopsy forceps since improper sharpening can render a forceps unusable.

6.5.5 Endocervical Curette

Endocervical curettes are used to obtain tissue samples from the endocervical canal. A cutting edge at the end of the long handle is scraped over the epithelium of the endocervix to remove tissue (Figure 6.35). A small depression in the handle denotes instrument alignment with the distal cutting edge. There are numerous different styles of endocervical curettes,

the most common of which is the rectangular-shaped Kevorkian curette. Kevorkian curettes are available either with or without a specimen-retention grid, or "basket" (Figure 6.36A,B). The basket consists of metal wires or a perforated cage that traps mucus and tissue. Some clinicians prefer instruments with a basket because it increases the amount of material retained in the curette, while others prefer those without baskets since trapped material may be difficult to remove, and additional tissue may be retrieved from the cervical os with ring, or smaller Singley forceps or an endocervical brush. As with cervical biopsy forceps, a sharp instrument yields more tissue and causes less discomfort than a dull curette.

Additional styles of endocervical curettes include rounded rather than square cutting heads and small-diameter instruments that are useful for women with a partially stenotic os. A Cytobrush® or if the os is too stenotic, a saline-moistened, small, calcium alginate swab rotated in the endocervical canal may provide a suitable specimen. Some clinicians routinely use cytobrushes instead of a metal curette to sample the endocervical canal. Chapter 7 includes a discussion of different approaches to sampling the endocervical canal.

6.5.6 Other Instruments

Ring forceps, long-nosed forceps, and long pick-up forceps are useful for applying soaked cotton balls to the mucosal surfaces, removing tissue, mucus, and endocervical polyps. A skin hook is a small, curved hook with one or more sharp projections at the end of a long handle that can be used to stabilize or lift tissue. Several different types of skin hooks are available. Although seldom needed for routine cervical colposcopy, skin hooks are useful in special circumstances, such as everting the lateral corners of the proximal vaginal cuff in women who have had a prior hysterectomy, fixing a vaginal lesion for biopsy, or retrieving tissue that has slipped away from a biopsy instrument.

Long-handled scissors, needle drivers, medium-caliber absorbable suture on a cutting needle, and pickups are rarely needed, except when rare persistent bleeding at biopsy or surgical sites requires suturing (Figure 6.37). A thin sound or narrow round probe with a bulbous head is occasionally useful for identifying or gaining access to the endocervical canal. A set of small cervical dilators is also quite useful for dilating the endocervical canal in women with stenosis. Some clinicians

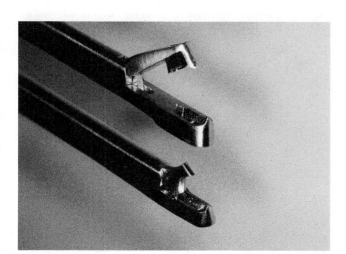

FIGURE 6.31.   Comparison of cervical biopsy bite sizes, a large Tischler-Morgan bite (**above**), and the smaller mini-Townsend bite.

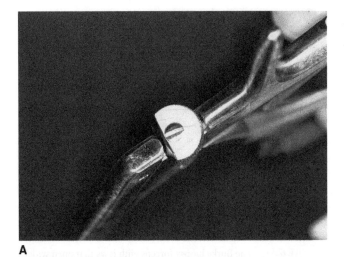

A

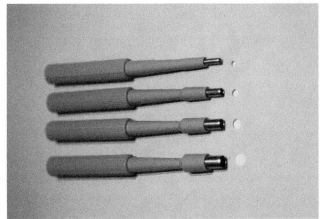

FIGURE 6.34.   Keyes dermal biopsy punch to sample vulvar lesions.

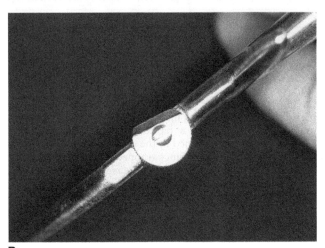

B

FIGURE 6.33.   A thumb-activated locking mechanism on biopsy forceps seen in the (**A**) open and (**B**) locked position.

use a spray bottle to apply 5% acetic acid, although care must be taken to avoid "splash-back." A tenaculum is usually not required to perform colposcopy or cervix biopsy.

6.6 CHEMICAL AGENTS AND SUPPLIES

6.6.1 Saline

Normal saline (Figure 6.38) is a commonly used moistening and cleansing solution. It does not modify the appearance of the cervical epithelium and is useful for cleaning the cervix when evaluating abnormal blood vessels and leukoplakia prior to the application of 5% acetic acid solution. Saline solution poured from a large stock bottle into smaller disposable cups or containers can be used for individual procedures.

6.6.2 Acetic Acid Solution

Application of acetic acid solution (Figure 6.38) enhances the detection of anogenital neoplasia during colposcopy. Acetic acid in a 3% to 5% solution is available either as white

vinegar, purchased from a grocery store, or as a prepared solution from the pharmacy. It is important to know that the acid content of the vinegar purchased from a consumer outlet, such as a grocery store, is usually 5%. Brands with <3% acidity are not suitable for colposcopy. Most colposcopists prefer 5% acetic acid solutions to 3% because the higher concentration produces a more rapid and longer-lasting tissue response. On the other hand, a 3% solution of acetic acid is less irritating and may be a better option when there is a possibility of vulvovaginitis and for examining the vulva of women with fair skin. When using acetic acid provided by a pharmacy, it is important to ensure that it is a 3% to 5% solution, as 0.5% solutions are sometimes used in wound dressings. It is very important to ensure that 85% trichloroacetic acid or glacial acetic acid not be mistakenly used during colposcopy since either could result in severe burns, especially if liberally applied in the amount typical of acetic acid application. Approximately 10 to 20 mL of 5% acetic acid solution poured into a separate small container or cup from a larger stock bottle is typically used for each patient and disposed of at the end of the procedure. Some practitioners add a small amount of food coloring to either the normal saline or the acetic acid in order to be able to easily identify the solution by sight from the other.

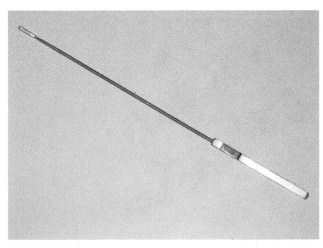

FIGURE 6.35.   An endocervical curette used to obtain a histological sample from the endocervical canal. The distal cutting edge is aligned with the depression located in the handle.

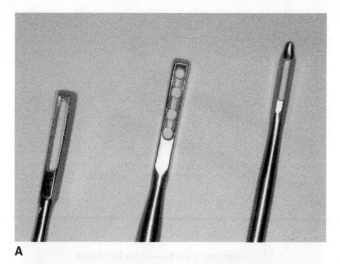

A

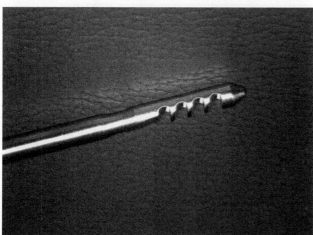

B

FIGURE 6.36.   **A,B:** An endocervical curette without a specimen retention grid (basket, **left**), with a specimen retention grid (**center**), and with a rounded end (**right**). A London curette with four cutting surfaces is seen in (**B**).

6.6.3 Lugol's Solution

Aqueous Lugol's solution (Figure 6.39) is an iodine-based contrast solution (iodine and potassium iodide). It is essential for properly evaluating the vagina and is sometimes used for cervical evaluation (see Chapter 14, Colposcopy of the Vagina). The iodine in Lugol's solution transiently stains the glycogen in squamous cells, imparting a dark, mahogany brown color to normal glycogenated epithelium. In contrast, most neoplastic tissues do not contain glycogen and, thus, do not stain. Lugol's iodine is commonly diluted with tap water or normal saline to a half-strength solution. The diluted solution is easier to apply, provides a better staining reaction, and causes minimal mucosal irritation. Full-strength Lugol's solution can be useful when examining postmenopausal women not on estrogen replacement therapy, as reduced vaginal epithelial glycogen usually stains poorly with the half-strength solution. Patients should *always* be asked if they have an iodine allergy before Lugol's solution is applied. Since patients may not know if they are allergic to iodine, it is important to ask about shellfish allergies. When using Lugol's solution, be careful to avoid staining the patient's clothing or your own, as iodine is difficult to remove. Be aware that topical benzocaine works effectively to quickly remove Lugol's iodine from epithelium.

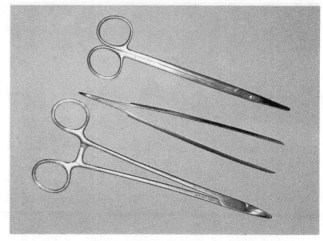

FIGURE 6.37.   Long scissors, needle driver, and pickups are rarely required to achieve hemostasis.

6.6.4 Monsel's Solution

Monsel's (ferric subsulfate) paste or solution (Figure 6.40) is a hemostatic agent that can be used after biopsy or surgical excisions. When mixed according to USP formulary, Monsel's solution is a thin, brown-colored liquid that is commonly used for dermatologic applications. Monsel's performs best for colposcopic procedures when it is dehydrated to a thick, mustard-colored, paste-like consistency. Monsel's paste may be purchased in single patient use containers, or it may be produced by thickening the thinner dermatologic solution. Do this by placing the standard solution in a small open container where it is exposed to the air, and after several days, a precipitate forms on the bottom of the container with an overlying thin, dark brown fluid. The dark-brown solution should be poured off the top and discarded. Once prepared, the paste should be stored in a closed container. Left alone, the Monsel's paste texture will slowly harden over time, but adding and mixing in small amounts of fresh Monsel's solution whenever the paste becomes excessively thick will maintain a proper paste-like consistency.

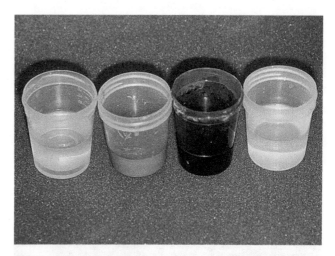

FIGURE 6.38.   Chemical solutions used as epithelial contrast agents and hemostatics during colposcopy: normal saline, Monsel's paste, Lugol's iodine solution, and 3% to 5% acetic acid (from left to right).

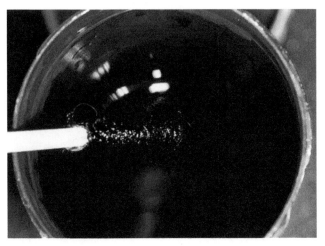

FIGURE 6.39.   Lugol's solution used for colposcopic examination of the cervix and vagina.

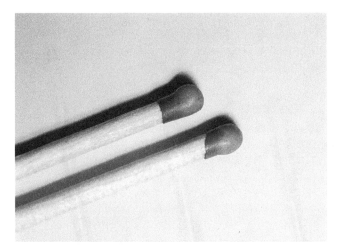

FIGURE 6.41.   Silver nitrate sticks used for hemostasis.

Because Monsel's paste is highly acidic (pH = 1), avoid excessive or inadvertent application to tissues not requiring hemostasis. Monsel's solution causes severe tissue artifacts that can preclude histologic evaluation; therefore, it is important to keep the solution away from tissues that are yet to be biopsied. This is particularly an issue for endocervical curettage since adverse histologic effects of Monsel's solution can persist for several weeks.

6.6.5 Silver Nitrate Sticks

Silver nitrate sticks provide hemostasis by chemical cautery. To stop bleeding, the head of the stick is applied to the biopsy site (Figure 6.41). Some women will experience a mild burning or cramping sensation when the stick is applied to the cervix. Because silver nitrate cauterizes tissue and produces an opaque white color, minimize contact with the surrounding epithelium. Excessive application may obscure adjacent acetowhite lesions. Subsequent histologic assessment of tissue obtained through an area of silver nitrate cautery will demonstrate a black precipitation of silver near the basement membrane, but this discoloration will not adversely affect the pathologic interpretation.

6.6.6 Topical and Local Anesthetics

Cervical biopsy and endocervical curettage causes pain in some women. Although some colposcopists use topical anesthetics prior to cervical biopsy and endocervical curettage to minimize patient discomfort,[5] placebo-controlled trials have not demonstrated that topical applications of xylocaine and benzocaine to be superior to placebo in reducing pain in women undergoing colposcopy or endocervical curettage.[4,6,7] Therefore, the routine use of topical anesthetics during colposcopy is not recommended.

Injectable local anesthetics, such as 1% or 2% xylocaine or lidocaine with or without epinephrine, are an effective pain-relief measure for electrosurgical loop excisions and biopsies of the vagina, vulva, and penis. Many colposcopists use dental syringes to inject local anesthetics because the prefilled cartridges are convenient. A Campion syringe is also useful for injecting anesthetics into the cervix or proximal vagina (Figure 6.42). Other providers use needle extenders or spinal needles on standard syringes to inject anesthesia into the cervix. A topical mixed 5% lidocaine/prilocaine anesthetic cream (EMLA or ELA-Max-eutectic mixture of local anesthetics) reduces the discomfort associated with injecting xylocaine or lidocaine into the vulva or penis, but in order to maximize

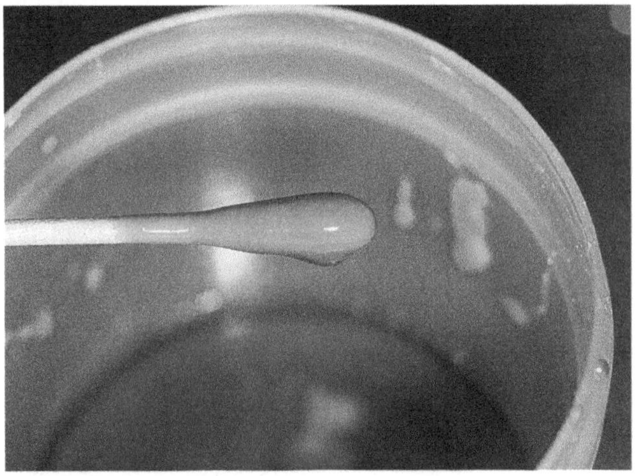

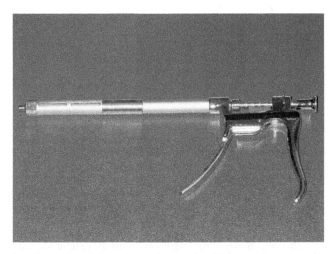

FIGURE 6.42.   A Campion syringe used to inject anesthetics into the cervix or proximal vagina.

FIGURE 6.40.   Monsel's paste used for hemostasis.

effectiveness to the depth of 2 mm, it is ideal to cover the area of application under a nonbreathable barrier for at least 20 to 60 minutes.[8,9] While useful to minimize discomfort on the external genitalia, it is not used on the cervix.

6.6.7 Bactericidal Solutions for Instrument Care

Commercial bactericidal solutions containing glutaraldehyde may be used to sterilize instruments. These solutions should be used only in well-ventilated areas. A 70% alcohol solution or a 10% solution of bleach may be used to clean surfaces not amenable to sterilization techniques, keeping in mind that bleach solutions are quite damaging to biopsy forceps and other instruments, including colposcopes. Instruments may also be sterilized using a gas or steam autoclave.

6.6.8 Disposable Supplies

Large and small cotton swabs and cotton balls are useful to apply solutions, to tamponade a bleeding site, to remove debris, solutions, or blood from the cervix or vagina, and to maneuver the cervix to obtain proper visualization. One-inch squares of brown paper, filter paper, or index cards are useful to put biopsies on before submersion in fixative. Disposable protector pads placed beneath the patient's buttocks absorb dripping acetic acid and blood. Gauze pads (4″ × 4″) are useful for applying acetic acid solution to the introitus, vulvar, and perirectal areas, but because they are abrasive, they are not appropriate for the cervix. Sanitary napkins and tampons should be available, along with vaginal packs of tightly rolled gauze pads to tamponade bleeding sites.

6.7 VIDEO AND PHOTOGRAPHIC SYSTEMS FOR OPTICAL COLPOSCOPES

6.7.1 Video Systems

Video systems for optical colposcopes allow the patient and others to simultaneously view the procedure while the colposcopist looks through the colposcope. This capacity is particularly useful when training residents and students in colposcopy. Even in the nonteaching setting, video capacity helps patients better understand their cervical findings and aids in communicating with them about cervical disease. Additionally, video systems permit colposcopists to document their examination using color video prints, CDs, or DVDs. There is no difference in reimbursement with the addition of video.

Not all colposcopes adapt easily for image acquisition. Optical colposcopes that have a beam splitter (image diverter) and accessory portals permitting the attachment of different types of cameras provide the best video images and photographs (Figure 6.43).[10] The beam splitter ensures that the image viewed by the colposcopist is identical to the one appearing on the monitor. For colposcopes without beam splitters, attaching a small CCD video camera to the side of the colposcope allows image acquisition. Since this type of system operates independently of the colposcope, however, it requires separate magnification and focus-control adjustments.

Most video systems consist of a small CCD video camera attached to the colposcope's beam splitter by means of an adapter. Images captured by the CCD video camera are transmitted to a high-resolution video monitor. Video images can be printed easily by dedicated color video printers, or the image can be captured by the computer's frame-grabber card and then printed using a standard color computer printer or electronically stored. Because of their ease of use, these methods of capturing video images have largely replaced 35-mm colpophotography, even though resolution of images on video monitors or video color print images is not as detailed as those obtained using colpophotography. However, video technology is changing rapidly and cameras are constantly improving. If the budget for purchase of a colposcope does not permit a video camera and monitor, it may be wise to purchase a colposcope capable of accommodating a beam splitter so that video can be added later.

6.7.2 Colpophotography

Some colposcopists like to document their examinations using colpophotography.[10] The availability of cervical images as either photographs or color video prints allows the clinician to reconcile clinical findings with the biopsy report, provides

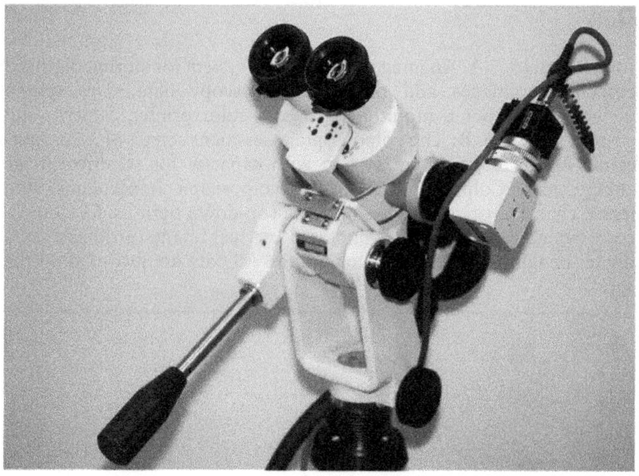

FIGURE 6.43.   Optical colposcope with a beam splitter, adapter, and CCD video camera.

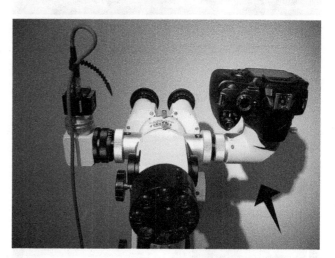

FIGURE 6.44.   A 35-mm camera (*arrow*) system for colposcopic photography.

an excellent form of self-education and quality control, documents pertinent findings and possible adverse events during clinical trials, and aids during the ongoing follow-up of patients referred for the management of abnormal cervical screening results who were not treated for high-grade CIN or AIS. Most colpophotography is now done with a digital camera, as 35-mm film is more costly and increasingly difficult to obtain. Cameras are attached to the colposcope's beam splitter (Figure 6.44). When in focus and correctly illuminated, colpophotographs obtained with digital and 35-mm cameras provide excellent resolution. Good colpophotography can be extremely challenging, and many colposcopists question whether the extra expense for photographic capabilities is justified outside referral centers or academic units.

6.8 IMAGE, DATA MANAGEMENT, AND PATIENT TRACKING SYSTEMS

Current computer-based systems are designed specifically to capture and store digitized colposcopic images, archive pertinent patient information, print visit information and color images for

A

B

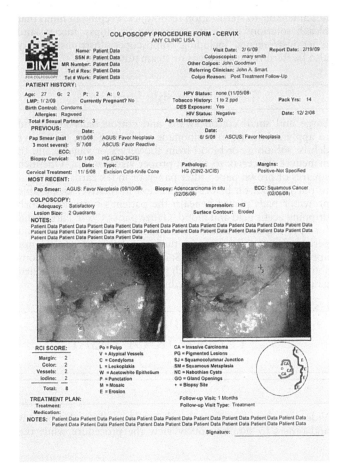

C

FIGURE 6.45. **A:** An image management system for storing digitized colposcopic images and pertinent colposcopy data. The system includes a computer, monitor, keyboard, color printer, camera, and custom software. **B:** The colposcopic assessment screen of a computerized image management system with capacity for selective image enlargement. Colposcopic adequacy, colposcopic impressions, and lesion characteristics are accessible as drop-down options. **C:** Colposcopy evaluation form with annotated cervical images produced by a digital imaging system and color printer. All data are recorded on the form.

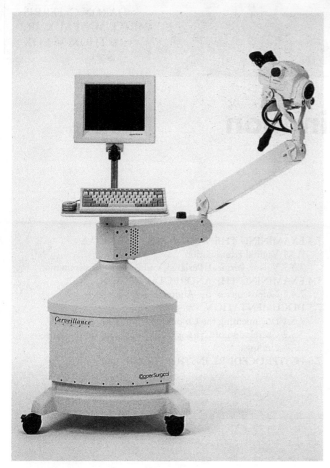

FIGURE 6.46. A colposcope and image management system combined as a single unit.

hard-copy documentation, provide patient tracking and recall services, and produce template or customized consultation letters (Figure 6.45A–C). A colposcope and computer are combined as a single unit in one model (Figure. 6.46). Immediate or delayed colposcopic consultation features are available. Linked colposcopy computer systems provide interactive distant telemedicine consultation by modem for less experienced clinicians and those who are geographically isolated.[11,12] These computer systems also enable procedure documentation and rapid retrieval of images obtained during colposcopic examinations. The ability to annotate images directly on the captured video image obviates the need for hand-drawn cervical findings (Figure 6.45C). Computerized image management systems also permit documentation of changes in lesion location, size, and volume. They provide objective outcomes in response to treatment or nontreatment, as well as monitor remote colposcopy practice for quality control purposes in clinical trials.[13]

6.9 SUMMARY

The quality of colposcopic equipment and supplies strongly influences the ease, efficiency, and safety of colposcopic examinations. The correct equipment, tools, and supplies should always be available. Inappropriate, outmoded equipment and improperly maintained instruments significantly increase patient discomfort, place an undue burden on the colposcopist, and compromise the safety of the procedure.

References

1. Ferris DG, Willner WA, Ho JJ. Colposcopes: a critical review. *J Fam Pract* 1991;33:506–15.
2. Ferris DG. Video colposcopy. *J Low Genit Tract Dis* 1997;1:15–8.
3. Wright VC. Understanding the colposcope optics, light path, magnification and field of view. In: Wright VC, ed. *Obstetrics and Gynecology Clinics of North America, Contemporary Colposcopy*. Philadelphia, PA: Saunders, 1993.
4. Ferris DG, Harper DM, Callahan B, et al. The efficacy of topical benzocaine gel in providing anesthesia prior to cervical biopsy and endocervical curettage. *J Low Genit Tract Dis* 1997;1:221–7.
5. Rabin JM, Spitzer M, Dwyer AT, Kaiser IH. Topical anesthesia for gynecologic procedures. *Obstet Gynecol* 1989;73:1040–4.
6. Prefontaine M, Fung-Kee-Fung M, Moher D. Comparison of topical xylocaine with placebo as a local anesthetic in colposcopic biopsies. *Can J Surg* 1991;34:163–5.
7. Clifton PA, Shaughnessy AF, Andrews S. Ineffectiveness of topical benzocaine spray during colposcopy. *J Fam Pract* 1998;6:242–6.
8. Wahlgren CF, Quiding H. Depth of cutaneous analgesia after application of a eutectic mixture of local anasthetics lidocaine and prilocaine (EMLA cream). *J Am Acad Dermatol* 2000;42:584–8.
9. Friedman PM, Fogelman JP, Nouri K, Levine VJ, Ashinoff R. Comparative study of the efficacy of four topical anesthetics. *Dermatol Surg* 1999;25:950–4.
10. Ferris DG, Willner WA, Ho JJ. Colophotography systems: a review. *J Fam Pract* 1991;33:633–9.
11. Ferris DG, Macfee MS, Miller JA, Litaker MS, Crawley D, Watson D. The efficacy of telecolposcopy compared with traditional colposcopy. *Obstet Gynecol* 2002;99:248–54.
12. Ferris DG, Litaker MS, Miller JA, Macfee MS, Crawley D, Watson D. Qualitative assessment of telemedicine network and computer-based telecolposcopy. *J Low Genit Tract Dis* 2002;6:145–9.
13. Ferris DG, Litaker M, ASCUS/LSIL Triage Study (ALTS) Group. Colposcopy quality control by remote review of digitized colposcopic images. *Am J Obstet Gynecol* 2004;191:1934–41.

The Colposcopic Examination

7.1 OVERVIEW AND PREPARATION FOR COLPOSCOPY
 7.1.1 Purpose of Colposcopy
 7.1.2 Objectives of the Colposcopic Examination
 7.1.3 Indications and Contraindications
 7.1.4 Patient Preparation for Colposcopy
 7.1.5 Initial Clinical Workup
7.2 COLPOSCOPIC TECHNIQUE
 7.2.1 Visualization
 7.2.2 Assessment
 7.2.3 Sampling
 7.2.4 Complications during Colposcopy

7.3 EXAMINING THE VAGINA AND THE VULVA
 7.3.1 Vaginal Examination
 7.3.2 Vulvar, Perineal, Perianal, and Bimanual Examinations
7.4 EXAMINING THE ANORECTAL REGION
 7.4.1 Colposcopy of the Anorectal Region
7.5 DOCUMENTATION
 7.5.1 Documenting the Colposcopic Findings
 7.5.2 Correlation of Cytology, Histology, and Colposcopy Findings
7.6 POSTPROCEDURE INSTRUCTIONS

7.1 OVERVIEW AND PREPARATION FOR COLPOSCOPY

7.1.1 Purpose of Colposcopy

Colposcopy is used predominately to evaluate women with abnormal Papanicolaou (Pap) test results. The purposes of the colposcopic examination are to identify the source of abnormal cells identified in the Pap test; to diagnose, in conjunction with a colposcopically directed biopsy, the type and grade of lesions present; and to delineate the extent of cervical lesions to determine the appropriate approach to treatment. The colposcope is a magnifying instrument used to examine the epithelium and vasculature of the uterine cervix, lower genital tract, and anogenital area to detect neoplasia by identifying abnormal tissue for biopsy, or affirming normality. Utilization of chemical solutions, such 3% to 5% acetic acid and Lugol's iodine, further enhances the procedure by aiding in discrimination between normal tissue and abnormal lesions. The goal of colposcopic examination is to direct biopsies to the most abnormal-appearing areas, and when none are found, to randomly sample the transformation zone in order to maximize histologic evaluation. Collectively, the results from the cytologic test, the histologic evaluation of biopsied epithelium, and the colposcopic impression of cervical abnormalities derive the final diagnosis to determine appropriate patient management. Although individual colposcopic techniques vary somewhat, a systematic approach ensures inclusion of all critical steps. To become a competent colposcopist, a clinician needs to understand how to conduct a colposcopic examination, be knowledgeable about the visual features of cervical disease, and master the necessary psychomotor skills. This chapter includes background that will allow clinicians to perform a comprehensive colposcopic examination of female patients.

7.1.2 Objectives of the Colposcopic Examination

Specific objectives for colposcopy ensure a proper and complete colposcopic examination (Table 7.1). Prior to insertion of the speculum, the vulva should be visually inspected. During each colposcopic examination, the colposcopist must (1) inspect the cervix and vagina; (2) identify the squamocolumnar junction (SCJ) along its entire circumference (i.e., 360 degrees) and the encompassing transformation zone; (3) determine whether the colposcopic examination is adequate or inadequate; (4) identify and assess suspected neoplastic lesions with respect to size, extent, and severity of disease; (5) when appropriate, sample the endocervical canal by curettage or brush; (6) identify the most severe lesion(s) and obtain biopsies; and (7) correlate the results of the Pap test, cervical biopsies, and the colposcopic impression to determine appropriate patient management. Achieving these objectives maximizes diagnostic accuracy. Communicating the clinical findings and their significance to the patient is critical and an integral part of every colposcopic examination. Finally, clear documentation of the indications, procedure, findings, and plan is necessary to complete the procedure.

7.1.3 Indications and Contraindications

There are numerous indications for colposcopy (Table 7.2). The most common indication for colposcopy is an abnormal Pap test. Colposcopy is indicated for women with a Pap test interpretation of atypical squamous cells favor high-grade (ASC-H), low-grade squamous intraepithelial lesion (LSIL), high-grade squamous intraepithelial lesion (HSIL), cancer, and for women with cytology suspicious for glandular neoplasia (atypical glandular cells [AGC] and adenocarcinoma *in situ* [AIS]).[1] Colposcopy is also indicated for adult women with atypical squamous cells of undetermined significance

TABLE 7.1	OBJECTIVES OF COLPOSCOPY

- Visualize the cervix, vagina, vulva, and perianal area
- Identify the SCJ and transformation zone
- Determine whether the exam is adequate or inadequate
- Identify and assess size, shape, contour, location, and extent of neoplastic lesions
- Sample the endocervical canal (unless patient is pregnant)
- Identify and biopsy most severe lesions
- Correlate the Pap test, biopsy report, and colposcopic impression
- Plan appropriate treatment plan
- Communicate findings to patient

(ASC-US), particularly if found on repeat to continue to be interpreted as ASC-US, or to have a concomitant positive high-risk human papillomavirus (HPV) test.[1] Colposcopy is also acceptable, along with cytology and/or HPV testing, for the follow-up of women referred for evaluation of high-grade or abnormal glandular cytology and not found to have a significant lesion in their colposcopy/biopsy or treated for cervical intraepithelial neoplasia grade 2,3 (CIN 2,3) or followed without initial treatment (with CIN 1 or CIN 2).[2] Chapters 19 and 20 include in-depth descriptions of the guidelines for managing patients with an abnormal Pap test or cervical histology result.

Colposcopy is also useful in enhancing the assessment of cervical or vaginal lesions, ulcers, masses, or growths. Other possible indications for colposcopy include positive findings on a visual naked eye examination following acetic acid wash or on a spectroscopic examination. Women with recurrent "unsatisfactory" or "satisfactory with severe inflammation" Pap test results may be candidates for colposcopy, particularly if they have increased risk factors for cervical neoplasia. Women with a history of *in utero* diethylstilbestrol (DES) exposure, women whose sexual partners have genital condylomata or neoplasias, women who have been treated previously for cervical neoplasia, and patients with vulvar or vaginal neoplasia are also candidates for colposcopy. A history of unexplained abnormal vaginal bleeding or recurring unexplained postcoital bleeding should prompt a careful colposcopic examination.

TABLE 7.2	COLPOSCOPY INDICATIONS

Cytologic abnormality* (ASC-US with a +HR-HPV test or repetitive ASC-US, and all ASC-H, LSIL, HSIL, AGC, AIS, cancer)
Gross or palpable cervical ulcer, mass, or growth
Concern for cancer on visual or spectroscopic examination
Unexplained lower genital tract bleeding
History of *in utero* DES exposure
Patient concern over partner with lower genital tract neoplasia or condyloma
Postsurgical follow-up examination*
Vulvar or vaginal HPV-associated lesion

*See Chapter 19.
ASC-US, atypical squamous cells of undetermined significance; ASC-H, atypical squamous cells, cannot exclude HSIL; LSIL, low-grade squamous intraepithelial lesion; HSIL, high-grade squamous intraepithelial lesion; AGC, atypical glandular cells; AIS, adenocarcinoma *in situ*; HPV, human papillomavirus.

There are no absolute contraindications for colposcopy. Colposcopic examination with biopsy is safe for women taking anticoagulant medication. Endocervical sampling (ECS), but not colposcopy, is contraindicated in pregnant women. In most cases, women with acute cervicitis or severe vaginitis should be evaluated and treated for specific infections prior to colposcopy since tissue fragility associated with infection, bleeding, and inflammatory changes may compromise visibility and thus the accuracy of the colposcopic evaluation. It is preferable not to perform colposcopy on women actively menstruating, but a successful examination is possible in women with minimal flow. If concern exists that the patient will not return for examination after the condition clears, colposcopy should be performed even under these visually obscuring conditions (Figure 7.1A,B).

7.1.4 Patient Preparation for Colposcopy

Women are usually told that they should undergo colposcopy when they are notified of an abnormal Pap test result. At that time, it is important to briefly describe colposcopy in order to prepare the patient and allay her anxiety. Explain that the examination takes approximately 15 to 20 minutes and may

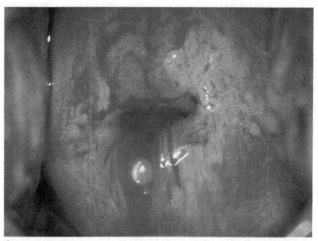

A

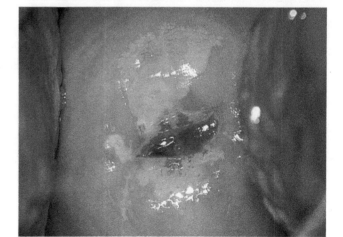

B

FIGURE 7.1.   The cervix of a nonadherent woman who is menstruating and has a history of a HSIL on Pap test (**A**). Colposcopy was conducted regardless of her menses, and high-grade acetowhite lesions of the anterior and posterior cervix can now be seen easily (**B**).

determine whether the results of the Pap test are correct and, if so, may also identify the origin of the abnormal cells. A colposcopy education pamphlet may help clarify the procedure and serve as a resource for later reference. Although premedication is usually not required, selected women may benefit from a nonsteroidal anti-inflammatory drug (NSAID) or, more rarely, an anxiolytic agent prior to the procedure. However, ibuprofen has been shown to only be equivalent to placebo for pain prevention during colposcopy.[3] If a benzodiazepine is used to treat anxiety, informed consent must be obtained before the patient is under the influence of the medication.

Colposcopy can be performed any time during the menstrual cycle, excepting days of heavy menstrual blood flow, but the best time to perform this procedure is during days 8 to 12 of the menstrual cycle, when the cervical mucus is clear and less viscous. Since such precise scheduling is not possible, colposcopic examinations are most often done randomly throughout the menstrual cycle. Postmenopausal women and other women with atrophic epithelial changes (Figure 7.2) may benefit from a limited 2- to 3-week course of topical estrogen prior to their examination. A prior history of estrogen receptor–positive breast cancer is not an absolute contraindication for a short course of estrogen; however, it is probably prudent to consult with her oncologist.

Instructions to patients should include avoiding intravaginal products, medications, douching, or sexual intercourse for 24 hours prior to colposcopy. Patients should have the option to have a friend or relative with them during the examination. This may be particularly helpful for consenting adolescents, highly anxious women, and handicapped patients.

Ideally, the colposcopist should explain the procedure in depth to the patient prior to performing the examination and inquire about allergies. Explain that a speculum will be inserted in a similar manner as is done for her Pap test, following which a microscope-like device, or colposcope, positioned outside her body, will be used to look closely at the surface of the cervix and vagina. Vinegar, and sometimes iodine, will then be applied to the cervix using soft cotton-tipped applicators or cotton balls. Application of the 3% to 5% acetic acid or vinegar may cause a mild external burning sensation, particularly when vulvovaginal inflammation is present. Any abnormal lesions that may be present will temporarily appear white. The magnification of the colposcope and the changes brought about by acetic acid help identify the source of the abnormal cells found on the Pap test. If a potentially abnormal

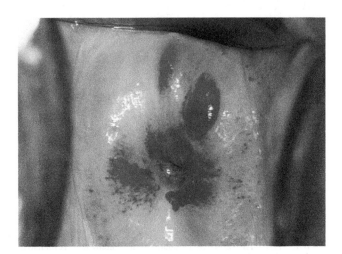

FIGURE 7.2. Atrophic changes of the cervix may complicate the colposcopic examination.

area is identified, typically more than one biopsy should be obtained. Reassure the patient that many women (~50%) feel no, or very minimal, sensation. Others may note a mild-to-moderate, transient pinch-like discomfort during the biopsy. Severe pain is quite unusual.[3] The examination might also necessitate another procedure known as endocervical sampling. ECS usually causes a brief menstrual-like cramping pain. An examination of the vagina and vulva may also be necessary, but biopsies from these areas are seldom required. Be sure that the patient understands that simply taking a biopsy does not imply that she has cervical cancer, or even a precancerous lesion. Explain the association of HPV and cervical cancer/precancer and that often, no treatment is necessary.

It may be advisable to obtain informed consent during a consultation prior to the examination or immediately preceding colposcopy, cervical biopsy, and possible ECS. As with informed consent for any medical procedure, informed consent for colposcopy should be in writing, following a thorough explanation by the clinician and an opportunity for the patient to ask questions and receive understandable answers.

7.1.5 Initial Clinical Workup

Prior to performing a colposcopic examination, it is important to obtain a gynecologic history focusing on several key areas, including a history of *in utero* DES exposure, method of contraception, age of sexual debut, pregnancy history, history of pelvic inflammatory disease, and current symptoms of vaginitis or acute cervicitis. Get the date of the most recent menstrual period, and if pregnant, estimated gestational age. The clinician should inquire about a prior history of sexually transmitted disease, particularly HPV infection, and premalignant or malignant cervical disease and treatment. It is also important to specifically elicit any history of abnormal vaginal bleeding or postcoital bleeding, since these entities indicate the possibility of occult invasive disease. Discuss possible sources of immunosuppression, such as from steroid medication, posttransplantation medication, diabetes mellitus, or infection with the human immunodeficiency virus (HIV). Ask the patient about possible hemorrhagic diathesis or use of anticoagulants or antiplatelet drugs which might increase the risk of excessive bleeding. Remember to encourage cessation of tobacco use postprocedure, if applicable.

7.2 COLPOSCOPIC TECHNIQUE

A systematic approach to colposcopy is essential. The colposcopic examination consists of four distinct and orderly tasks: visualization, assessment, sampling, and correlation. Colposcopists initially obtain proper visualization of the cervix and lower genital tract, assess the normal landmarks and any abnormal epithelium, and selectively sample areas of possible neoplasia, as indicated. Finally, colposcopists must correlate their colposcopic impression with the referring Pap test report and the results of their histologic sampling to determine appropriate management.

7.2.1 Visualization

7.2.1.1 Visualizing the Cervix

Adequate visualization of the cervix is essential during colposcopy. The widest speculum that does not cause patient discomfort should be used to maximize visualization. On initial insertion of the speculum, the ectocervical portion of the cervix is the main area visible (Figure 7.3). As the blades of the

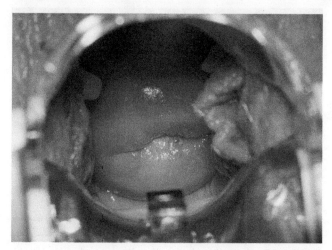

FIGURE 7.3. Only the ectocervix is visible on initial insertion of the speculum. Notice the slightly prolapsing vaginal sidewalls and the lack of complete illumination of the cervix.

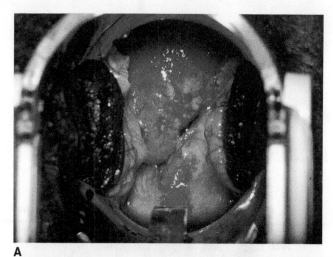

A

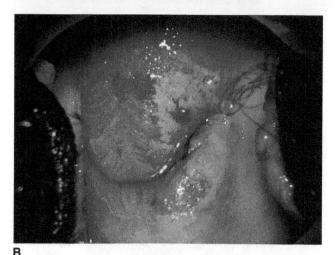

B

FIGURE 7.5. Use of a latex glove finger "tube" placed over the vaginal speculum blades limits vaginal sidewall prolapse. Colposcopic view without use of "tube" (**A**) and with use of tube (**B**).

speculum are opened, the anterior and posterior lips of the cervix separate, and the external os and part of the endocervical canal become visible (Figure 7.4). Therefore, it is important to open the speculum blades as widely as possible without producing discomfort. Increasing the speculum aperture at the yoke enlarges the introitus, allowing a greater amount of colposcopic illumination of the cervix and maximum visualization, especially in patients with vaginal redundancy.

Prolapsing vaginal walls, common in obese, pregnant, or elderly women, may hinder proper visualization of the cervix. A latex glove finger "tube," condom, or lateral sidewall retractor may be helpful in such patients to keep the vaginal sidewalls from obscuring visualization of the cervix (Figure 7.5A,B). Visualization is greatly facilitated by the combination of a hydraulic or mechanical examination table and an adjustable stool (see Figure 6.11). The hydraulic table and adjustable stool allow colposcopists to adjust the height of the patient and their position relative to the cervix. Proper patient/colposcopist positioning minimizes posturally induced back strain for the colposcopist.

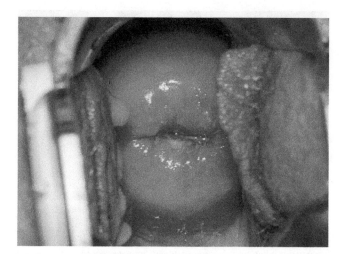

FIGURE 7.4. Once the speculum blades are opened with tolerance, the external os and distal endocervical canal are visible. The ectocervix is also well illuminated.

The position of the cervix relative to the examiner can be changed by placing a large moistened cotton swab in the proximal fornix (alongside the cervix) and then applying gentle cephalad pressure (Figure 7.6A,B). This action moves the cervix toward the swab, permitting better visualization of both an eccentrically oriented cervix and the vaginal fornix. This approach reduces the risk of the cotton swab causing abrasion-induced bleeding of the surface of the transformation zone when pressure is applied there. Another method of atraumatically maneuvering the cervix in the anterior and posterior directions is to gently move the speculum blades up or down. A moistened swab placed gently on the ectocervix outside the transformation zone can also be used to reposition the cervix (Figure 7.7).

7.2.1.2 Focusing the Colposcope

The colposcopic examination begins by initially viewing the entire cervix through the colposcope at low-power (2× to 4×) magnification (Figure 7.8). At low magnification, coarse focus can be achieved by simply moving the colposcope head closer or farther away from the cervix. The distance between the colposcope objective lens and the cervix in focus equates to the focal length of the objective lens. A 300-mm objective

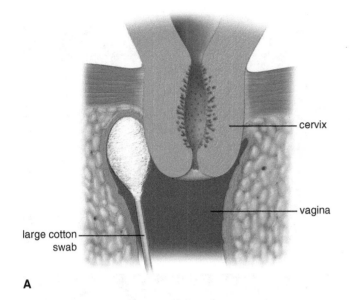

A

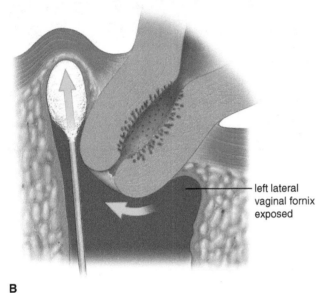

B

FIGURE 7.6. To move a cervix deviated toward the left fornix to the patient's right side or center vaginal position, place the moistened cotton swab in the right proximal vaginal fornix (at 9 o'clock position), and push forward gently toward the patient's head (**A**). The cervix will move toward the swab (patient's right side) without actually touching the cervix, permitting visualization of the left side of the cervix and left proximal vaginal fornix (**B**).

lens, available on most modern colposcopes, enables sufficient space between the patient and colposcope for instrument manipulation. Once coarse focus is achieved, minor adjustments can be made by manipulating a fine focus handle or lever that moves only the optical colposcope head. In the case of a video colposcope, a bidirectional button accomplishes fine focus while the colposcope remains stationary. The entire cervix is visible at approximately 7× to 8× magnification. More detailed examination of small colposcopic features may be facilitated by incremental increases to a higher power magnification (~10× to ~15×) (Figure 7.9). Magnification >15× is generally not required for colposcopy, but may further accentuate delicate vascular changes.

Novice colposcopists occasionally have difficulty focusing. The problem may be attributable to the eyepieces of an optical

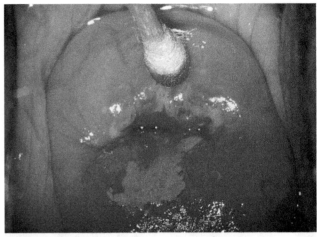

FIGURE 7.7. A small swab placed on the ectocervix to assist with positioning. An acetowhite CIN 2 is noted on the ectocervix. The examination is adequate because the entire SCJ and lesion are clearly seen.

colposcope being set at diopter settings that do not conform to focus for both eyes. Alternatively, one interchangeable eyepiece may not be seated fully within the eyepiece-housing receptacle (binocular tubes), hence contributing to a blurred image. Reliance solely on the fine focus handle or button when the target is either too close or too far away from an optical or video colposcope may cause focusing problems. Setting both eyepiece diopter settings at "0" or a central mark (dot) may correct diopter problems for a colposcopist having 20/20 vision and when performing colposcopy with corrective glasses or contact lenses. If not, another method is to first focus the colposcope using only one eye and eyepiece. Then look through only the opposite eyepiece with the other eye open and focus by turning the diopter ring for only the other eyepiece. Make sure that both eyepieces are completely seated within their respective eyepiece receptacles.

Focusing is best accomplished by first looking at the lateral field of view to see what is in focus. If the speculum or vaginal wall is clearly visible, use coarse-focus positioning to move the colposcope forward, closer to the cervix. If the image is

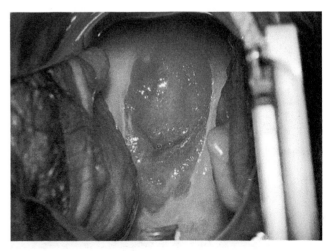

FIGURE 7.8. Low-power magnification of the cervix and proximal vagina. A normal ectropion is present, viewed as the central reddish portion of the cervix.

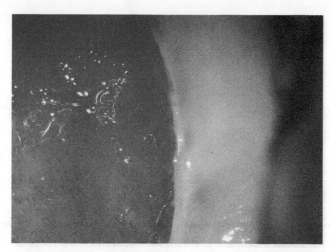

FIGURE 7.9.   A high-power magnification of the cervix from Figure 7.8 demonstrating a highly magnified view of the squamous and columnar epithelium and the SCJ.

completely blurred, the colposcope is too close to the target, and it should be pulled back. If withdrawing the colposcope does not correct the problem, be sure that the oculars are set at your interpupillary distance to avoid seeing a double image. When both hands are occupied, colposcopes on a wheel base can be focused easily by placing the feet atop the base and using them to adjust the position of the entire scope. Fine focus at a high-power magnification level can be achieved by gently pulling or pushing the vaginal speculum to obtain a clear view of the cervix.

7.2.1.3 Papanicolaou and Microbiologic Test Collection

When indicated, specimens for viral and bacterial testing should be obtained prior to application of saline or 3% to 5% acetic acid. Excessive vaginal or endocervical canal discharge should be noted and in such cases appropriate specimens obtained for culture, Gram stain, saline and potassium hydroxide (KOH) wet mount preparation, whiff test, pH determination, and other relevant microbiologic tests (e.g., *Neisseria gonorrhoeae, Chlamydia trachomatis*), as indicated. Colposcopy should be rescheduled following treatment if a severe cervical or vaginal infection is present, since these infections can appreciably complicate the examination.

Repeating the Pap test at the time of colposcopy typically provides little additional clinical information and can occasionally strip away the epithelium from the stroma and precipitate bleeding. If it is necessary to perform a Pap test, it should be obtained before applying any solutions to the cervix.

7.2.1.4 Removing Obscuring Blood and Mucus

Blood and mucus may obscure the cervix, particularly when located within the endocervical canal. A small cotton-tipped applicator soaked in 3% to 5% acetic acid and placed within the endocervical canal will frequently stop bleeding from this area. A larger, acetic acid–soaked swab placed on the ectocervix also works well to control bleeding on the portio. Hemostatic agents should not be used prior to colposcopic assessment since they distort the appearance of the epithelium. Dry cotton swabs should be avoided except for absorbing and removing obscuring blood, pooling contrast solutions, or applying Monsel's paste because they can be abrasive when rubbed across or rotated on columnar epithelium. Mucus

protruding from the os and obscuring a portion of the ectocervix can often be moved from side to side with a small, moistened swab, allowing the underlying epithelium to be viewed. In other cases, mucus can be removed using a small forceps or a cytobrush. Otherwise, it may be simply pushed into the endocervical canal with a small, moistened cotton swab or a moistened calcium alginate swab at the end of a thin wire shaft.

7.2.1.5 Application of Normal Saline

Once the cervix is positioned, normal saline is used to moisten the epithelium and remove obscuring mucus and cellular debris. The examination should focus on two important findings at this point: leukoplakia and abnormal blood vessels. Leukoplakia (Figure 7.10A–F) is a white, thickened area of epithelium that is visible before the application of acetic acid (Chapter 8). Leukoplakia may be difficult to differentiate from acetowhite changes after the application of acetic acid, or thin sheets of loosely adhering superficial epithelium in leukoplakia may be dislodged from the underlying thickened white patch when acetic acid is applied. Leukoplakia should always be biopsied, but not until after the colposcopic assessment has been completed.

Small abnormal vessels are best visualized after the application of normal saline and prior to acetic acid application. Acetic acid causes tissue edema that exerts a mild, transient, vasoconstrictive effect on fine-caliber blood vessels, which can frequently cause tiny abnormal vessels to become invisible. A red-free (green) filter (Figure 7.11A,B), which enhances angioarchitecture, is often used during the saline examination of the cervix. The green filter absorbs red light, causing blood vessels to appear black, making them easier to discern against a green background. Many colposcopists omit the normal saline assessment of the cervix. When saline is not used, approximately 5 minutes may be required following acetic acid application to fully appreciate the unmodified vasculature.

7.2.1.6 Application of 3% to 5% Acetic Acid

Acetic acid (3% to 5%) is then applied to the cervix to help discriminate normal from abnormal epithelium. This weak acid is applied liberally and frequently to the cervix using cotton balls and ring forceps, large cotton swabs, or a spray technique (Figure 7.12A,B). Gauze pads (4' × 4') should not be used to apply solutions to the cervix because of their abrasive properties. Some clinicians find that the use of a spray bottle to apply acetic acid onto the cervix limits epithelial abrasion, particularly during pregnancy, but care must be taken to prevent "splash-back." Irrespective of how the acetic acid is applied, the amount must be sufficient to elicit an optimal acetowhite reaction. Less experienced colposcopists commonly make the mistake of applying too little acetic acid or not waiting long enough for the full effect to take place. These errors can cause important lesions to escape detection. Saturated cotton balls held with sponge-holding ring forceps apply a large volume of acetic acid to the cervix and help insure a good acetic acid effect. If cotton-tipped applicators are used, they must be large and fully soaked with acetic acid. Twirling a large cotton-tipped applicator in the container of acetic acid will cause partial unraveling of the cotton, producing a mop-like applicator similar to that of a well-soaked cotton ball. A second application of acetic acid ensures that sufficient time has elapsed (a total of 1 to 2 minutes) for the acetic acid reaction to occur. Since the effects of acetic acid are transitory, frequent repeated applications are necessary to retain an acetowhite effect. A red color in columnar epithelium indicates the need for additional acetic acid application (Figure 7.13A,B). Normally, columnar epithelium blanches slightly white following acetic acid application,

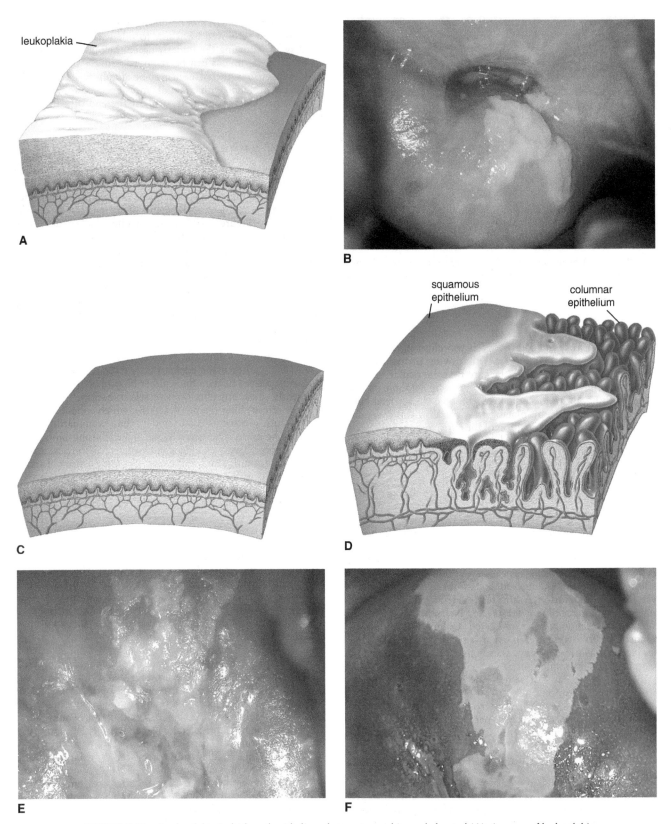

leukoplakia

squamous
epithelium

columnar
epithelium

A

B

C

D

E

F

FIGURE 7.10.   Leukoplakia is thickened epithelium that appears white and elevated (A). An area of leukoplakia noted on the cervix following the application of normal saline, but prior to use of acetic acid (B). The thickened epithelium appears white during initial inspection. Leukoplakia can be contrasted with normal squamous epithelium that has a pink color and is macular in topography (C), and immature metaplasia (D) that is very thin and translucent. The next case demonstrates leukoplakia before acetic acid application (E) and after Lugol's iodine application (F).

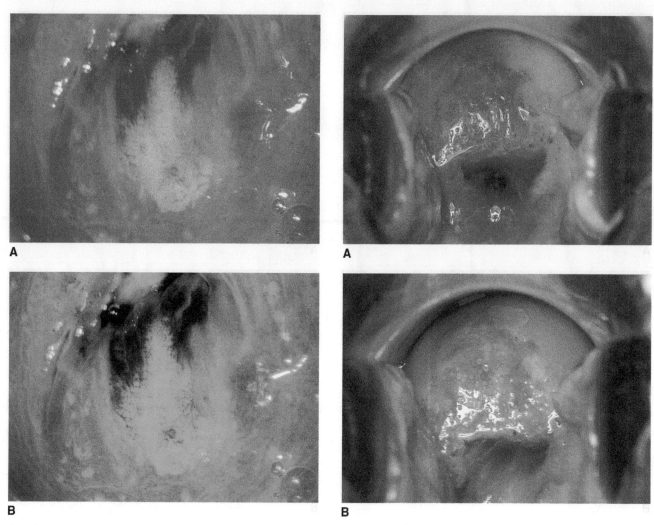

FIGURE 7.11. A green-filter examination of the cervix enhances recognition of the cervical vasculature. The green filter absorbs red light, causing the blood vessels to appear black. A cervical lesion of the posterior cervical lip after 3% to 5% acetic acid application (A) and as seen with the green filter (B).

FIGURE 7.12. The cervix before (A) and after (B) application of 3% to 5% acetic acid demonstrating an easily observed acetowhite CIN 3 lesion on the anterior cervix noted only following acetic acid application.

but this effect is quite brief. Once the blanched white color reverts to red, acetic acid should be reapplied. When applying acetic acid, avoid rotating or scouring motions that might cause bleeding. Steady direct application or gentle dabbing of acetic acid on the transformation zone is more effective.

Acetic acid interacts with both normal and neoplastic epithelia, causing them to swell and change color. Following acetic acid application, both normal and abnormal tissues composed of cells with an increased nuclear-to-cytoplasmic ratio appear transiently white (acetowhite). The surrounding normal squamous epithelium retains its usual pink color. The rate of appearance and disappearance of the acetic acid effect varies with different types of lesions. Therefore, it is important to view the cervix through the colposcope while applying acetic acid. An adequate acetic acid response is indicated by faint acetowhite blanching of the normally red columnar epithelium (when visible). Fine vascular patterns initially become less distinct after the application of acetic acid. However, as the acetic acid reaction begins to subside, the capillary patterns become more distinct against a white background (Figure 7.14A–C). At this time, the vascular patterns of cervical neoplasia are most vivid. In general, the acetowhite color develops faster and persists longer in more severe grades of neoplasia.

Following application of acetic acid, the cervix and vaginal fornices should be systematically examined at low-power magnification (2× to 5×) to allow any acetowhite lesions to be identified. When areas of acetowhite epithelium are identified, the colposcopist should be careful to complete the systematic low-magnification inspection of the entire cervix and vaginal fornices before proceeding to higher-power magnification (Figure 7.15A–H) to ensure that additional lesions are not overlooked. After this low-magnification examination, all abnormal areas should be examined at high power (10× to 15×). The site and extent of all abnormal epithelia must be noted carefully.

7.2.1.7 Application of Diluted Lugol's Iodine Solution

Half-strength Lugol's iodine is another contrast solution often used during colposcopy. Provided the patient is not allergic to iodine, Lugol's solution is applied in the same fashion as 3% to 5% acetic acid. Lugol's iodine stains intracellular glycogen dark brown (see Chapter 6). Except in estrogen-deficient postmenopausal women, original squamous epithelium of postpubertal women and areas of mature metaplasia are heavily glycogenated and will appear mahogany brown following the

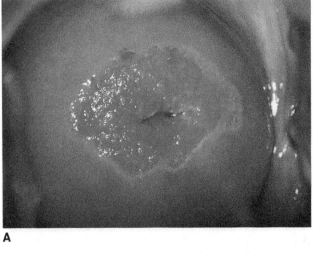

A

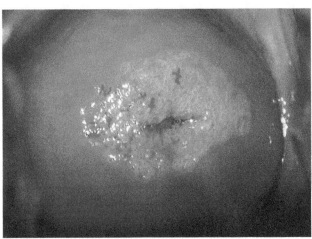

B

FIGURE 7.13.   Columnar epithelium is red prior to 3% to 5% acetic acid application (**A**) and blanches faintly white after 3% to 5% acetic acid application (**B**).

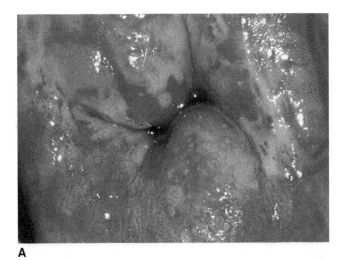

A

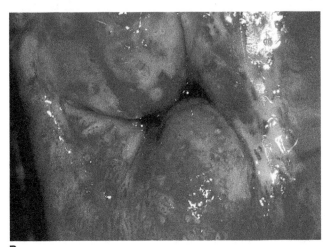

B

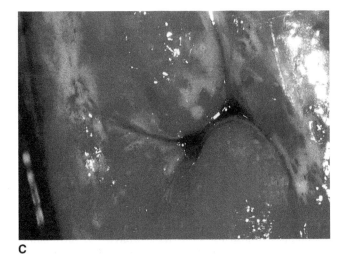

C

FIGURE 7.14.   Time-lapsed colpophotography of a cervical lesion (CIN 3) immediately following (**A**), 3 minutes after (**B**), and more than 5 minutes after 3% to 5% acetic acid application (**C**). Dense acetowhite epithelium and coarse punctation are visible. The vessels become more prominent as the acetic acid effect fades (**B**).

application of Lugol's solution. In estrogen-deficient women, there is less glycogenization of the squamous epithelium, and the epithelium stains a tan or light-brown color. Schiller's iodine solution is 1/15 the concentration of Lugol's solution, and therefore, it is rarely used during colposcopy.

Neoplastic epithelium, normal columnar epithelium, immature squamous metaplastic epithelium, and leukoplakia contain little or no glycogen and do not stain with Lugol's solution (Figure 7.16A–D). Columnar or immature metaplastic epithelium appears reddish pink or light yellow. Neoplastic epithelium can have a range of staining patterns. Usually, cervical intraepithelial neoplasia 2,3 (CIN 2,3) will appear as either a white-yellow or a mustard-yellow color, and CIN 1 will appear a brighter orange-yellow color. This color difference may assist in differentiating low-grade from high-grade lesions. Some squamous intraepithelial lesions, particularly those that are low grade, have small, randomly dispersed areas of glycogen within larger areas of neoplastic epithelium lacking glycogen, which produces a variegated yellow-brown ("tortoise-shell") staining pattern. Inflammatory lesions, including acute ectocervical and vaginal infections such as trichomoniasis, produce small, diffuse patches of glycogen-free epithelium that also do not stain after application of aqueous iodine. When inflammation is severe and the epithelium

is denuded, the underlying stroma appears pink. Otherwise, inflammation produces patchy mustard-yellow areas.

Iodine staining is an optional colposcopy procedure for examining the cervix. It is not used by all colposcopists, and even those who use it do not do so for all patients. However, iodine staining is an essential step in assessing the severity of cervical disease if using the Reid Colposcopic Index (see Chapter 9).[4,5] It also may be helpful for detecting small high-grade lesions (CIN 2,3) that can otherwise be missed. For example, inexperienced colposcopists commonly overlook CIN 2,3 within a larger low-grade lesion (CIN 1). In these cases, iodine staining may make the high-grade disease more visible by highlighting the internal margin between the mustard-yellow, high-grade lesion and the variegated, partially stained low-grade lesion (Figure 7.17A,B). Sometimes a faint acetowhite lesion on the ectocervix or vagina is not obvious until Lugol's iodine is applied, producing a more vivid yellow/brown contrast. Therefore, the iodine examination may be

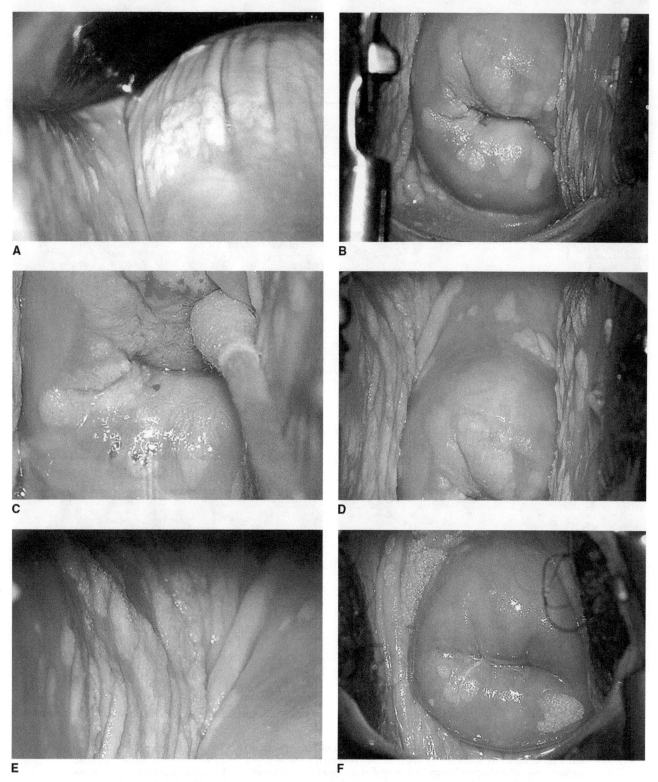

FIGURE 7.15.   Vaginal neoplasia located in the proximal vaginal fornix in a woman with an abnormal Pap test result (A). The next two cases demonstrate condyloma present on the cervix and within the vagina (B–E) and (F–H).

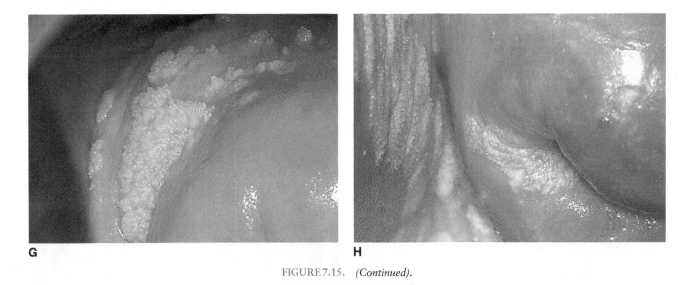

G

H

FIGURE 7.15.   *(Continued).*

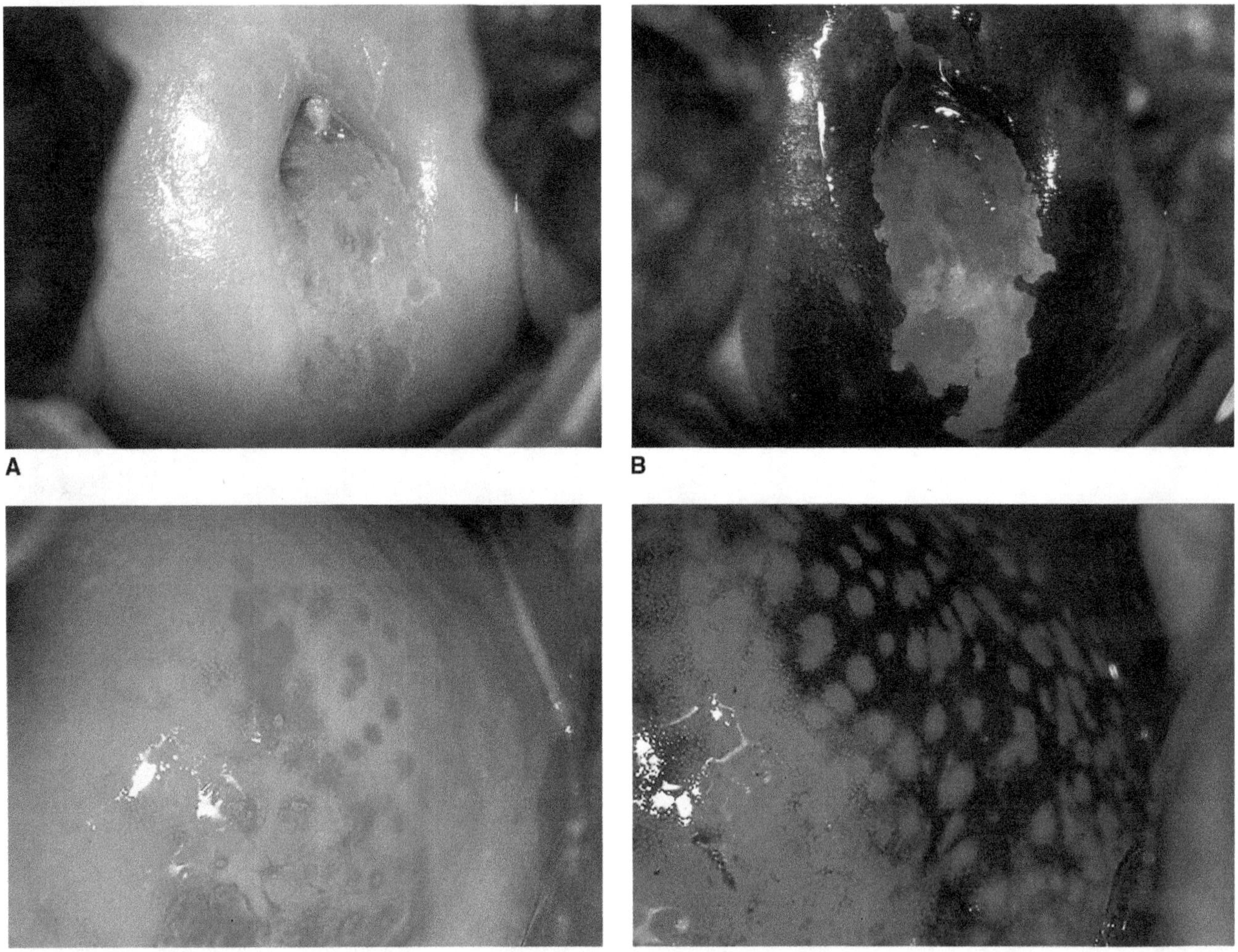

A

B

C

D

FIGURE 7.16.   The cervix before (**A**) and after Lugol's iodine application (**B**). The acetowhite lesion on the posterior lip of the cervix is not readily apparent (**A**). However, a yellow-appearing cervical lesion is easily contrasted against a normal mahogany brown background of squamous epithelium (**B**). In the next case of trichomonas cervicitis, multiple discrete red spots are seen on the cervix before Lugol's application (**C**). After Lugol's, the red areas of inflammation appear yellow (**D**) against the brown normal noninflamed epithelium.

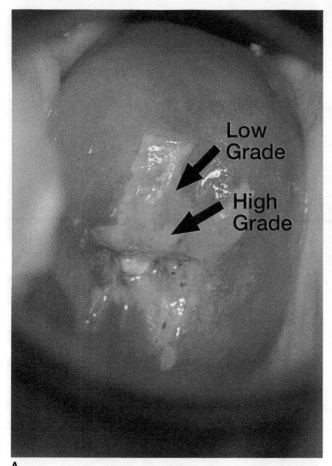

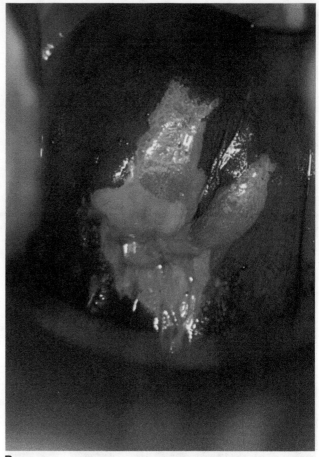

A   **B**

FIGURE 7.17.   An acetowhite lesion is seen on the anterior lip of the cervix (**A**). A high-grade yellow lesion (*arrow*) positioned within a larger variegated low-grade lesion is better appreciated following Lugol's iodine application (**B**). The lesions are seen at the 12 o'clock position. The iodine provides a more distinct contrast between the centrally positioned high-grade lesion and the low-grade lesion in the periphery.

beneficial when the source of a woman's abnormal cytology cannot be ascertained following the acetic acid examination. In the colposcopic examination of the vagina, iodine staining of the mucosa is invaluable because vaginal lesions are usually more difficult to see than cervical following the use of acetic acid. Vaginal intraepithelial neoplasia (VaIN) assumes a mustard-yellow color against a surrounding brown color of normal vaginal epithelium when estrogenized (Figure 7.18A,B).

There are numerous issues to consider with the routine use of iodine staining. It must be stressed that both normal immature epithelium and high-grade precursor lesions reject iodine and stain mustard-yellow. Thus, iodine-staining patterns are relatively nonspecific. Iodine application prevents assessment of the underlying vasculature and other colposcopic signs. Therefore, colposcopic examination with 3% to 5% acetic acid must be done before applying iodine. Additionally, areas selected for biopsy prior to the application of iodine may be difficult to relocate after staining because iodine staining hides vascular changes and subtle acetowhite differences necessary for accurate biopsy placement. Therefore, colposcopists need to maintain a mental image of how the cervix appeared after the application of acetic acid to biopsy the correct areas. When Lugol's iodine staining complicates the remainder of the examination and histologic sampling process, topical benzocaine solution works well to quickly "erase" unwanted iodine staining.

7.2.2 Assessment

Following colposcopic visualization of the cervix, colposcopists must assess their visual findings. Assessment includes identification of squamous and columnar epithelium, the SCJ, and transformation zone; recognition of neoplastic lesions; and estimation of the linear extent, size, and degree of severity of neoplastic lesions, if present.

7.2.2.1 Concept of the "Adequate" Colposcopic Examination

Prior to the introduction of colposcopy, women with abnormal Pap tests required cold-knife conizations to rule out invasive cancer (see Chapter 1). Colposcopy provided a less traumatic and more cost-efficient method of ruling out invasive cancer based on the colposcopic appearance and one or more small selective biopsies, but it has limitations. Invasion can only be ruled out if the entire transformation zone, and all lesions, are colposcopically visible in their entirety and sampled. Therefore, early in the history of colposcopy, the concept of the "adequate" colposcopic examination developed to identify patients who were candidates for outpatient conservative management.

When an examination is classified as "adequate," the entire transformation zone has been visualized with the

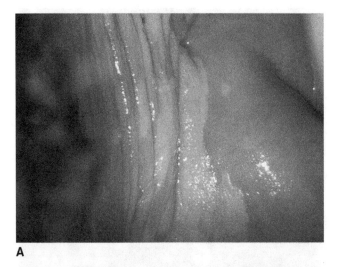

A

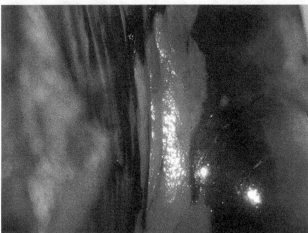

B

FIGURE 7.18.   An acetowhite vaginal intraepithelial neoplasia 3 (VaIN 3) lesion of the proximal fornix (**A**), and the same VaIN 3 noted following Lugol's iodine solution application (**B**). Note the mustard-yellow lesion surrounded by mahogany brown normal squamous epithelium.

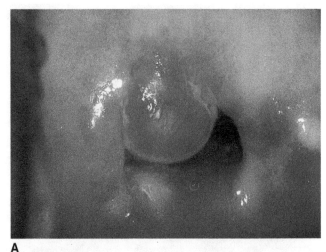

A

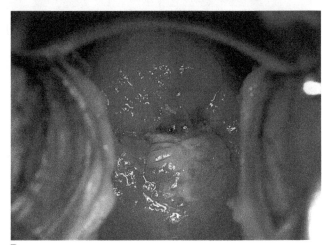

B

FIGURE 7.19.   An inadequate examination because the SCJ cannot be seen (**A**). A large nabothian cyst is seen on the right anterior cervical lip. Its presence obscures viewing the entire SCJ. A cervical lesion extends up the endocervical canal beyond full view (**B**). The examination is inadequate because the proximal extent of the lesion cannot be identified.

colposcope. In practice, this means that 360 degrees of columnar epithelium, 360 degrees of squamous epithelium, and consequently, 360 degrees of the current SCJ can be seen. Additionally, if a cervical lesion is present, the entire lesion, including both the distal and proximal margins, must be colposcopically visible in order for the examination to be classified as "adequate" (Figure 7.7). When 360 degrees of columnar epithelium and the SCJ, or lesion, cannot be visualized in their entirety, the examination is classified as "inadequate" and an excisional procedure may be necessary (Figure 7.19A,B).

7.2.2.2 Identification of the Transformation Zone

The first step during colposcopic assessment is to try to identify the limits of the transformation zone. This requires identification of the SCJ. The approximate area of the original SCJ can sometimes be identified in younger women in whom gland openings and nabothian cysts often remain visible in areas of squamous metaplasia. However, the original junction can be difficult, if not impossible, to identify in older women. Although it is helpful to identify the original SCJ, it

is important to remember that the region immediately adjacent to the new, or current, SCJ is the region most likely to contain cervical neoplasia (Figure 7.20). Because complete visualization of the SCJ and columnar epithelium are necessary to have a adequate colposcopic examination, colposcopists should always observe and then document in the clinical record whether or not the entire SCJ and transformation zone were observed or whether the examination was adequate or inadequate.

In many young women and in women of any age who currently are, or have recently been pregnant, the current or new SCJ is positioned in full colposcopic view on the ectocervix (Figure 7.21A). The thin SCJ appears transiently white following acetic acid application. In postmenopausal women, women who receive progestin-only contraception for an extended time, and those who have previously received cervical ablative or excisional therapy, the junction and columnar epithelium are more commonly located at the external os or deep within the endocervical canal (Figure 7.21B). Colposcopic assessment of postmenopausal women was inadequate for only 57% in one study,[6] whereas the experience of many colposcopists is that nearly all postmenopausal women will have an

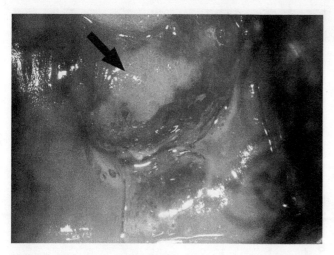

FIGURE 7.20.   An acetowhite low-grade cervical lesion (*arrow*) adjoining the SCJ.

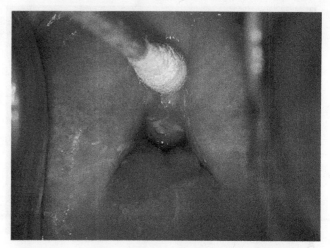

FIGURE 7.22.   A high-grade cervical lesion with the SCJ visible at the external os. The proximal limit of the lesion is seen clearly using a cotton-tipped applicator to evert the endocervix. The examination is adequate.

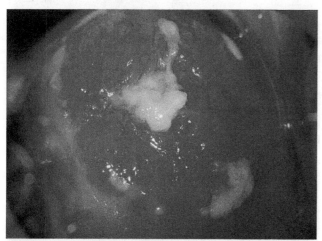

A

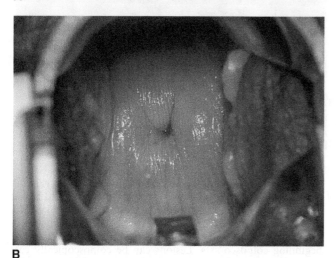

B

FIGURE 7.21.   A low-grade cervical lesion seen in a young woman with a cervical ectropion (**A**). The entire SCJ is visible. The SCJ is not seen following electrosurgical loop excision of the cervix (**B**).

inadequate examination. If the SCJ is in the endocervical canal and not easily visualized, gentle manipulation may facilitate complete evaluation without inducing bleeding. This can be accomplished in any one of several ways. To evert a patulous cervix, open the vaginal speculum blades as wide as the patient will tolerate; push large, moistened cotton-tipped applicators cephalad in the anterior and posterior vaginal fornices; or lift or push the tissue near the cervical os with small moistened cotton-tipped applicators (Figure 7.22). Another method is to gently open the external os and inspect the distal endocervical canal using an endocervical speculum (Figure 7.23A–E). For estrogen-deficient women, 3 to 4 weeks of estrogen therapy may result in a adequate examination at subsequent colposcopy. Be sure to have the patient stop the therapy several days before the colposcopy so that obscuring cream is not present in the vagina during the examination. In other women, the endocervical margin of cervical neoplasia cannot be identified (Figure 7.23A). Some colposcopists dilate the external os using laminaria, but this approach often strips the epithelium from the stroma, making the subsequent colposcopic assessment impossible. In one study, a compressed polyvinyl alcohol sponge impregnated with magnesium sulfate was used in women with inadequate colposcopic examinations. Twenty-nine, of forty-one women whose entire SCJ could not be seen initially, had adequate colposcopy examinations 4 hours after the sponge was placed in the endocervical canal.[7] However, this approach has not generally been adopted.

7.2.2.3 Identification of Epithelial Abnormalities

The second step during colposcopic assessment is to identify the source of the abnormal cells present on the Pap test. A lesion that accounts for the Pap test findings will often, but not always, be readily apparent. When a cervical lesion is not seen, or if the lesion that is identified does not appear to explain the cytologic abnormality, a systematic colposcopic assessment with biopsies will usually identify the source of the abnormal Pap result. Following application of acetic acid or Lugol's iodine solution, neoplastic lesions most commonly exhibit typical features as described above that allow them to be identified. These features are derived from alterations in (1) color, (2) vascular caliber and pattern, (3) margins, and (4) surface

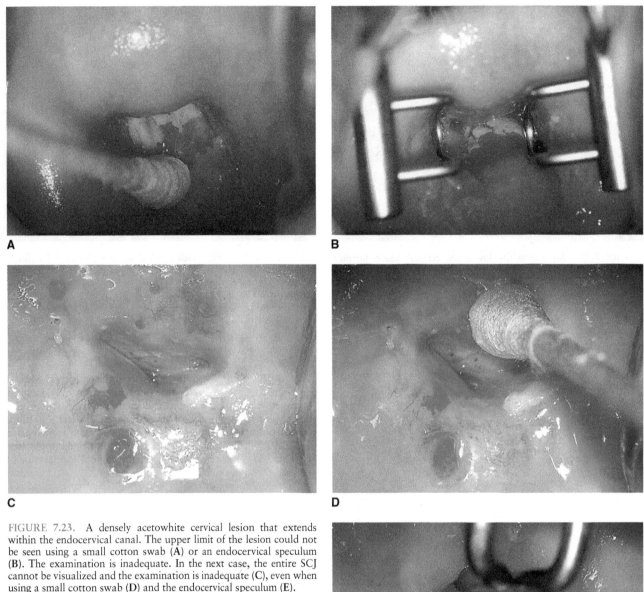

FIGURE 7.23. A densely acetowhite cervical lesion that extends within the endocervical canal. The upper limit of the lesion could not be seen using a small cotton swab (A) or an endocervical speculum (B). The examination is inadequate. In the next case, the entire SCJ cannot be visualized and the examination is inadequate (C), even when using a small cotton swab (D) and the endocervical speculum (E).

contour. Chapters 8 and 9 provide a detailed description of these alterations. Colposcopic assessment involves carefully visualizing the transformation zone to identify abnormal-appearing areas and evaluating these areas for each of these four parameters listed above. Following evaluation of these parameters, the colposcopist then formulates a colposcopic impression that equates to the expected histologic composition of a given area. Colposcopic assessment also involves looking for the warning signs of invasive cervical cancer. Chapter 10 includes a description of these signs.

Some colposcopists use a colposcopic index or grading system to predict the severity of squamous disease and to aid in formulating their colposcopic impression.[4,5] These systems provide a structured appraisal directed at minimizing subjectivity and are useful in assessing cervical lesions, especially for beginning colposcopists. Lesions can be colposcopically categorized as normal, or nonneoplastic, low-grade disease (CIN 1, HPV), high-grade disease (CIN 2, CIN 3, AIS), or cancer (squamous or adenocarcinoma). The results of the ASCCP/ NIH Research Group showed that colposcopic assessments in the ASCUS LSIL Triage Study (ALTS) were significantly correlated with CIN grade but insufficient to conclusively determine diagnosis.[8] In ALTS, the initial colposcopy to an ASCUS or LSIL Pap result only found 53% of the CIN3 ultimately detected during 2-year follow-up.[9] Undoubtedly, some of these lesions developed subsequent to the initial colposcopy, some were likely so small or thin to not be initially colposcopically identifiable, and some were missed.[10] In order to maximize sensitivity for detection of high-grade squamous and glandular precancer and cancer, it is important to biopsy more than just the most abnormal-appearing area. A minimum of two or more biopsies significantly reduces the risk of missing important lesions.[11] Chapter 9 addresses colposcopic grading.

7.2.2.4 Determining the Size, Shape, Contour, Location, and Extent of Cervical Lesions

Once the colposcopic impression is formulated, the next step is to determine the size, shape, contour, location, and extent of cervical lesions. Cervical lesions range from very small (only several millimeters in diameter) (Figure 7.22) to large (four quadrant) (Figure 7.14B). Generally speaking, the larger the size and linear length of the neoplasia, the greater the severity. However, four-quadrant condylomata and other low-grade

lesions, most frequently seen in immunocompromised women, do not conform to this adage, and women with immature metaplasia may have acetowhite epithelium with a fine mosaic vascular pattern around the circumference of the cervix without having associated CIN. The shape or borders of a cervical lesion may indicate the severity of disease (see Chapter 9). Lesions with irregular margins generally represent low-grade disease, while lesions with more regular or smooth edges are likely to be high grade. Similarly, lesion contour may reflect the level of neoplasia. For example, raised, exophytic lesions may be either condyloma or cancer. The source of the abnormal Pap test may be located in the vagina and/or in variable positions on the cervix or within the canal (Figure 7.24A,B). Lesions may be focal (solitary) or multifocal (diffusely distributed). Size, shape, contour, and location of cervical neoplasia influence the selection of the most appropriate treatment; therefore, colposcopists should appraise these lesions' characteristics before selecting a type of treatment.

Determining the peripheral margin of a cervical lesion is usually easy, especially after staining the cervix with Lugol's iodine solution. Occasionally, transformation zones and lesions extend beyond the portio and into the vaginal fornices (especially in DES-exposed patients). Isolated vaginal lesions are sometimes of a higher grade than are the lesions on the cervix. Identifying a cervical lesion's proximal margin is one of the most important tasks for a colposcopist. Careful attention to the endocervical margin ensures that excisional procedures rather than ablative modalities are used to manage lesions extending beyond colposcopic view within the endocervical canal. In young women, the SCJ is located usually on the portio, distal or peripheral to the external os. In these patients, identifying the proximal or endocervical margins of cervical neoplasia is quite easy (Figure 7.25). In older patients (Figure 7.26), or in those treated previously for cervical neoplasia, the SCJ can be located at or proximal to the external os. In these women, identifying the proximal or endocervical margin of a lesion can be difficult. For estrogen-deficient women with atrophic changes, a short course of therapy with estrogen may alter the anatomy sufficiently to permit a adequate examination on a subsequent colposcopy. In some cases, use of a cotton-tipped applicator or endocervical speculum allows the inner margin of a lesion to be identified (Figure 7.22). In other women, simple approaches are inadequate to identify the endocervical margin of cervical neoplasia (Figure 7.23A–E).

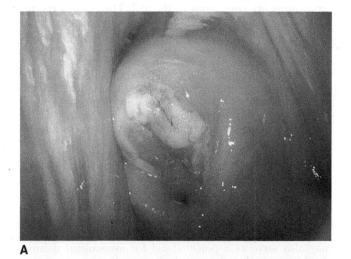

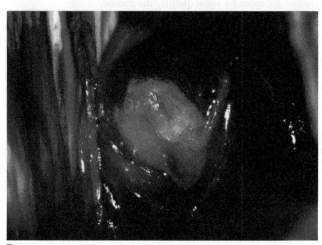

FIGURE 7.24. Lesions of both the cervix (CIN 1) and vagina (VaIN 1) in this woman following application of 3% to 5% acetic acid (**A**) and Lugol's iodine (**B**).

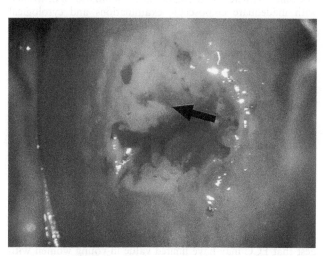

FIGURE 7.25. A CIN 2 on the ectocervix. The proximal lesion margin is seen easily (*arrow*). The colposcopic examination is adequate.

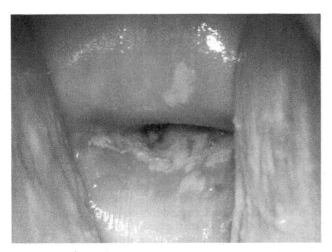

FIGURE 7.26.   A low-grade lesion is seen on the posterior lip of the cervix in this older woman. The upper extent of the lesion and the SCJ are not visualized. The examination is inadequate.

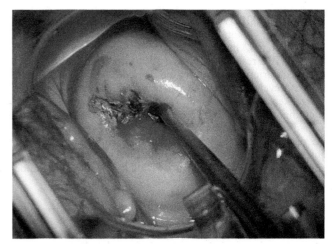

FIGURE 7.27.   Endocervical curettage with a metal curette requires a representative sampling of the endocervical canal.

7.2.3 Sampling

Colposcopists must collect an adequate and representative histologic sample of the most severe disease located on the ectocervix, within the endocervical canal, or elsewhere in the lower genital tract, when indicated. Additionally, biopsy of areas of even normal-appearing transformation zone at the SCJ may improve the sensitivity of colposcopy for high-grade lesions.[11] Histologic sampling is necessary to confirm the colposcopic assessment and the grade of neoplasia (if present). Besides biopsy, histologic sampling may include endocervical curettage (ECC) or endocervical brushing.

7.2.3.1 Endocervical Sampling

The term endocervical sampling includes ECC and endocervical brushing; either is performed to evaluate nonvisualized areas of the endocervical canal, as indicated (Figure 7.27). In women with adequate colposcopic examinations, an ECS allows for detection of glandular neoplasia (sometimes multifocal) and rare "skip lesions" (isolated areas of squamous neoplasia, not contiguous with the SCJ found primarily in women who have had prior cervical treatment or surgery) in women with adequate colposcopic examinations. In women with inadequate colposcopic examinations and cytological abnormalities, an ECC can help detect neoplastic lesions that are beyond colposcopic view within the endocervical canal. ECS is recommended in the evaluation of women with an AGC or HSIL Pap test result.

7.2.3.1.1 SELECTIVE USE OF ECS IN COLPOSCOPIC PRACTICE

Many colposcopists today are reconsidering the role of ECS. In the 1970s, ECC was considered an essential component of the colposcopic examination. The necessity for an ECS was based on Townsend's and Richart's report of women who developed invasive cervical cancer after undergoing colposcopic evaluation and cryosurgery.[12] Their analysis showed that the omission of ECS was the most common potential error in this series. This finding led to the following recommendation: before being considered eligible for ablative therapy, a woman should have not only a adequate colposcopic examination but also a negative ECS. However, findings from the ALTS suggest that ECC may have limited value in young women with equivocal or mildly abnormal cytologic results.[13]

The potential distribution of cervical lesions must be understood when considering collecting an ECS. Isolated areas of squamous neoplasia within the endocervical canal (e.g., "skip lesions") are extremely uncommon in women who have not been previously treated for cervical neoplasia, and glandular (AIS) skip lesions are uncommon in the absence of glandular abnormality contiguous to the SCJ. Therefore, a routine ECS in a woman with a adequate colposcopy examination is unlikely to detect an unsuspected lesion unless a rare occult glandular neoplasia is discovered. A routinely collected ECS may also inadvertently sample an ectocervical lesion when no neoplasia resides in the endocervical canal. Such an error would prompt a potentially unnecessary conization. According to the 2006 ASCCP guidelines, ECS is preferred for nonpregnant women referred for the evaluation of an AGC or HSIL Pap, for women referred for LSIL cytology in whom no lesion is identified, and those with an inadequate colposcopy. ECS is acceptable for those referred for an ASC-US or ASC-H Pap result and found to have a adequate colposcopy but no identifiable lesion. It is also necessary prior to any cervical ablation.[1] Since an ECS is usually uncomfortable and increases the cost of histologic evaluation, it is not routinely used outside these parameters. An ECS may detect glandular lesions that are difficult to recognize colposcopically. A negative ECS may also serve as a potential aid for medicolegal defense, should a cancer be subsequently diagnosed.

ECS is also an essential part of the colposcopic examination for women being evaluated for an abnormal Pap test who have a previous history of treatment for cervical neoplasia.[2] Novice colposcopists should probably perform an ECS on all nonpregnant patients referred for colposcopy. Experienced colposcopists may be more selective in their use of ECS as per the ASCCP Guidelines. An ECS is contraindicated in pregnant women.[1]

7.2.3.1.2 OBTAINING AN ECS

Debate exists on whether or not to obtain the ECS prior to, or after, the cervical biopsy. Traditionally, an ECS was obtained prior to cervical biopsies. One reason this sequence is followed is hypothetically to reduce the risk of obtaining a false-positive ECS. Once a cervical biopsy is taken, CIN 2,3 at the edge of the biopsied area may peel away or fragment from the underlying stroma and possibly slide to the external os and mix with endocervical tissue fragments as they are collected from the external os. However, the majority of false-positive ECSs result from accidentally nicking an ectocervical CIN adjacent to the external os. Another reason some colposcopists obtain the ECS first is that after a cervical biopsy, bleeding is sometimes great enough to either obscure the colposcopist's view or make it difficult to collect the endocervical curettings. However, bleeding following biopsy that obscures remaining procedures is rarely an important factor, if hemostasis at the biopsy sites is secured. Nevertheless, some colposcopists advocate taking the cervical biopsy before the ECC because they believe the first priority is to sample the most severe lesion, which is usually on the ectocervix and occasionally may be obscured by bleeding after ECS.

There are two options for sampling the endocervical canal: an endocervical curette or a cervical brush (Cytobrush®). A conventional endocervical curette captures sheets or strips of epithelium that provide greater test specificity than specimens obtained in a Cytobrush® sample.[14,15] In contrast, a vigorous Cytobrush® sampling of the endocervical canal followed by cytologic assessment of the exfoliated cells is more sensitive for detecting CIN, but less specific, than is a conventional ECC (Figure 7.28A,B). The Cytobrush-obtained sample is also less likely to provide a sufficient specimen.[16]

Prior to performing the ECS, the examiner should inform the woman that it will produce brief uterine cramping pain. Topical anesthetics are ineffective in reducing the pain associated with endocervical curettage,[3,17,18] but use of sharp curettes may reduce the discomfort.[17] Consider obtaining the ECS while looking through the colposcope at low magnification to

carefully guide the sampling device into the endocervical canal and through the back-and-forth motion. Holding the sampling device like a pencil, advance it at least 15 mm into the endocervical canal or just short of the internal os.

When performing an ECC, press the distal cutting tip firmly against the tissue and move the curette using short "to and fro" strokes, rotating the tip of the curette simultaneously in a circular motion so that the entire canal is sampled in a "corkscrew" fashion (Figure 7.29). An alternative sampling technique is to draw the curette repeatedly toward the external os along the canal while rotating the curette radially after each withdrawal until the entire canal circumference is sampled (Figure 7.30). Satisfactory sampling has been accomplished when mucus, tissue, and blood appear at the external os and within the basket or open chamber of the curette (Figure 7.31). When removing the curette, it is important to avoid inadvertently sampling ectocervical lesions that extend close to the external os. Whenever possible, withdraw the curette so that the cutting edge faces an area of normal epithelium. Avoid sampling endometrial tissue located above the internal os, typically over 25 to 30 mm from the external os. Prior to removing the open chamber curette, rotate it rapidly to trap cellular elements, mucus, and blood within it. If the curette is removed straight from the canal, mucus and cellular material may be pulled out of each side of the curette, leaving the specimen within the canal and the curette chamber empty. Specimen retrieval is usually less of a problem when a curette with a retention grid is used. Frequently, much of the endocervical tissue remains entrapped in blood at the external os. Forceps, a cervical brush, or both can be used to maximize retrieval of this material from the os (Figure 7.32). Use of a cervical brush following curette sampling may increase cellular yield of the sample.[19] A Cytobrush can also be used to retrieve material trapped in the curette basket.

As mentioned earlier, some clinicians prefer to use a cervical brush instead of a curette. When using this method, introduce the cervical brush into the canal and rotate vigorously. When

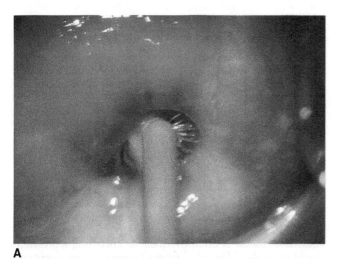

A

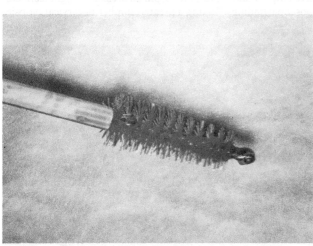

B

FIGURE 7.28.   A Cytobrush used (**A**) to take an endocervical histologic specimen (**B**).

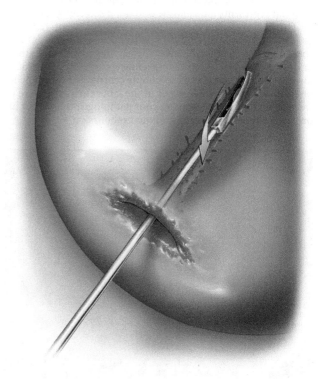

FIGURE 7.29.   Screw-type ECS performed with "to and fro" scraping motions while rotating the curette.

FIGURE 7.30. Hoeing-type ECS by withdrawing the curette along the canal, then replacing the curette near the internal os, rotating slightly, and then withdrawing until all of the canal is sampled.

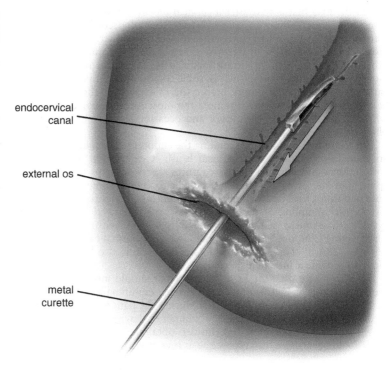

endocervical canal

external os

metal curette

withdrawn, place the specimen into a container of formalin for histologic interpretation (Figure 7.33). The cellular material and mucus can also be stripped from the bristles into formalin using an Ayre's spatula or filter paper. Other options include rolling the cervical brush specimen across a glass slide with immediate fixation with a 95% ethanol solution, or placing it in a liquid cytology medium followed by submission for histologic interpretation. If a slide or a liquid-based specimen is submitted, it is important to note on the requisition form that the material represents a diagnostic and not a screening specimen.

The ECS specimen may be placed on a square of Telfa, tea bag, or brown paper, and dropped into a separately labeled specimen container of fixative. Depending upon the pathologist's preference, the ECC specimen may also be placed directly into formalin and the sample centrifuged into a pellet or strained through filter paper in the laboratory. If unsure of the best method to use, contact your pathologist to find out his or her preferred method of specimen submission.

7.2.3.2 Cervical Biopsy

In a majority of cases, cervical biopsy begins with the selection of the most abnormal-appearing areas for sampling, regardless of cervical location. The exception is when multiple biopsies will be taken, and there is concern that bleeding may obscure one or more important areas requiring biopsy because of biopsy location and inability to secure hemostasis as the biopsies are taken. Under these circumstances, it may be preferable to obtain biopsies from the posterior cervical portio first to keep blood from an anterior portio biopsy from obscuring biopsy sites posteriorly. Since the most prominent areas of colposcopic change do not necessarily coincide with the areas of greatest histological abnormality, colposcopists are always at risk of not selecting the most abnormal sites for biopsy. Large peripheral acetowhite areas are readily recognized, but focal, more severe coexisting disease is often overlooked. Therefore, representative biopsies should be taken from all areas with significant colposcopic findings. Taking a greater number of cervical biopsies

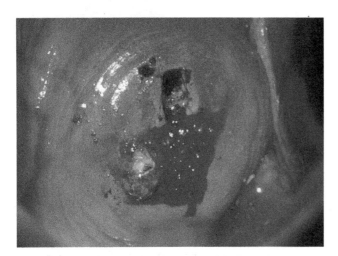

FIGURE 7.31. The endocervical specimen at the cervical os following curettage.

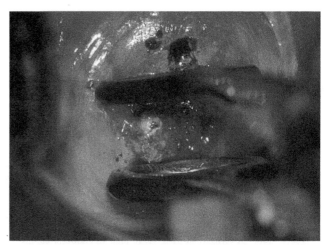

FIGURE 7.32. Retrieving the endocervical specimen using ring forceps.

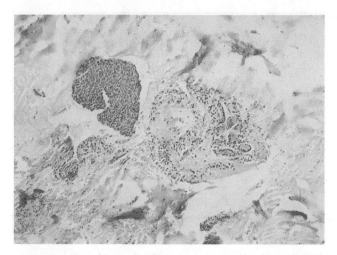

FIGURE 7.33. A positive endocervical curettage specimen demonstrating neoplasia. (Hematoxylin-eosin stain; medium-power magnification.)

greatly improves the detection of cancer precursor lesions.[20] Usually, the abnormal area closest to the SCJ is preferentially biopsied since this is the region most likely to have maximum disease severity. The number of biopsies taken from an individual patient depends on the size, severity, and number of lesions present, but in general, taking more than one biopsy is recommended. Cervical biopsies are best obtained while looking through the colposcope at low-power magnification.

After selecting the biopsy site, orient the opened biopsy forceps so that the fixed jaw end of the biopsy forceps is positioned closer to, or within, the os (Figure 7.34). The biopsy forceps should be positioned directly over the lesion to be biopsied. It is unnecessary to obtain normal adjoining epithelium with biopsy of a neoplasm. However, if an ulcer is being biopsied, it is important to include tissue adjacent to the ulcer with the specimen. Necrotic, nondiagnostic material may occupy the center of an ulcer, hence the necessity for supplying surrounding tissue that may contain abnormal histology for review. When biopsying a lesion on the posterior portio, hold the biopsy instrument handles upside down. Lifting the biopsy handles upward prior to biopsying an anterior portio lesion places the lesion in the center of the jaws, reducing the risk of slippage. Pushing the cervix backward with the opened

biopsy forceps until the support structures of the uterus prevent further cephalad uterine motion also helps keep the forceps from slipping off the biopsy site. A sharp biopsy forceps minimizes slippage. A specimen is obtained by quickly squeezing the forceps handles together and then locking the jaws (if so equipped) prior to passing the forceps to an assistant. In most instances, biopsies need to be only 2 mm deep. Deeper biopsies are only needed when invasion is suspected.

After taking a biopsy, it is best to confirm colposcopically that the intended area was adequately sampled. If an adequate or representative sample was not obtained, another biopsy should be attempted immediately. Hemostasis can then be accomplished by pressing a cotton swab against the biopsy site or applying silver nitrate or Monsel's paste (ferric subsulfate) (Figure 7.35A,B). Monsel's paste or silver nitrate must directly contact the actual biopsy site to be effective. If applied to a bloody surface, these agents only coagulate extravasated blood and do not produce hemostasis. The entire base and sides of the biopsy site must be cauterized, including the epithelial wound edges, which tend to bleed moderately. Monsel's paste or silver nitrate sticks must be applied precisely and only to the biopsy site(s). Usually, application of these hemostatic agents is only required after all biopsies have been obtained. However, when hemostasis is necessary to prevent bleeding from obscuring sites not yet biopsied, imprecise application of these agents can also be similarly problematic. Furthermore, improper use of these hemostatic agents can

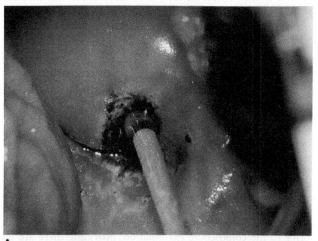

A

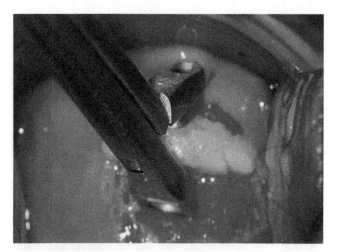

FIGURE 7.34. Obtaining a cervical biopsy from the ectocervix using sharp cervical biopsy forceps. The fixed jaw of the biopsy forceps is usually positioned closer to the cervical os.

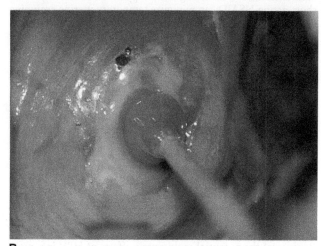

B

FIGURE 7.35. Hemostasis is achieved following cervical biopsy using silver nitrate sticks (A) or Monsel's paste (B).

ruin the histology of subsequent biopsy specimens, including ECS collected within the next 3 weeks. Sutures are rarely required following biopsy, but in the event they are, the necessary supplies and instruments should be readily available. However, in performing a biopsy on the cervix of a pregnant patient or one with invasive cancer, excessive bleeding can be prevented by placing a cotton-tipped applicator soaked in Monsel's paste against the site immediately following removal of the biopsy forceps. When hemostatic agents are not sufficient to stop bleeding or when hemostatic agents are not available, a single strand of gauze packing may be inserted against the cervix after the procedure and removed by the patient several hours later. After all biopsies are obtained and hemostasis achieved, excessive blood, acetic acid, and hemostatic agents should be removed from the distal vagina with care taken to not interfere with hemostasis at the biopsy sites.

Biopsy specimens are placed into a bottle containing fixative. Specimens mounted on paper prior to fixation are more likely to be optimally oriented, have a preserved SCJ, and have intact surface epithelium than are specimens placed directly into fixative.[21] Some pathologists, however, accept biopsy samples submitted directly in fixative. Ideally, clinicians learning colposcopy should place each cervical biopsy in a separate container, allowing the colposcopist to compare each specific histologic result with his/her colposcopic impression at each biopsy site. More experienced colposcopists often elect to place multiple specimens in one bottle since pathologists often charge the patient by the bottle and the patient is always treated based on the worse biopsy. Cervical biopsies should always be separated from the ECS specimen.

7.2.4 Complications during Colposcopy

The most common minor complication of colposcopy is excessive bleeding following cervical biopsy. Brief, mild-to-moderate bleeding should always be anticipated following collection of a histologic specimen. Significant bleeding is likely when a biopsy is taken from pregnant patients and those with acute cervicitis or cervical cancer. Since pressure and rapid application of silver nitrate or Monsel's paste work effectively, hemostasis rarely requires sutures. Thin epithelium in women with atrophic changes due to estrogen deficiency is easily traumatized, resulting in ecchymosis, superficial lacerations, avulsions and pain. These complications and discomfort can be prevented easily by prescribing a short course of topical estrogen for several weeks prior to the colposcopic examination, providing there are no contraindications to estrogen therapy. Premedication with a short-acting NSAID can minimize temporary uterine cramping discomfort caused by cervical biopsy and ECC. Proven, specific medications for each woman's dysmenorrhea may work best for pain prophylaxis. Inadvertent irritation due to cauterization of sensitive introital mucosa may occur when hemostatic agents are applied imprecisely. Common management errors result from inability or failure to visualize the entire SCJ or proximal extent of a lesion, failure to sample the endocervical canal, or failure to formulate a colposcopic impression. Chapter 21 includes a discussion of common management errors.

7.3 EXAMINING THE VAGINA AND THE VULVA

7.3.1 Vaginal Examination

Because of the potential multicentric effects of HPV infection, the colposcopic examination should include the entire lower genital tract. All patients should have a brief colposcopic vaginal inspection. A more comprehensive vaginal examination is

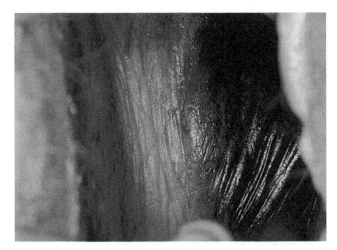

FIGURE 7.36. Vaginal lesion noted following Lugol's iodine solution application. The lesion is yellow and the surrounding brown epithelium is normal.

necessary when a woman presents with an abnormal Pap test, especially a high-grade result, and no cervical lesion is found to explain the cytologic findings. A careful colposcopic examination of the vagina is also indicated for women with an abnormal Pap test and a previous hysterectomy or a history of DES exposure. Prior to cervical conization or hysterectomy, it may be prudent to conduct a comprehensive vaginal examination to detect coexisting or even primary occult vaginal neoplasia.

With proper visualization, a comprehensive colposcopic examination of the vagina is fairly straightforward (see also Chapter 13). The colposcopic examination should also include inspection of the entire vagina, including the fornices and cul-de-sac, following application of 3% to 5% acetic acid. The vagina should be reexamined after applying half-strength Lugol's iodine solution (Figure 7.36). The lateral walls of the vagina may be difficult to visualize because of rugae and the parallel orientation to the light source. Opening the speculum widely tends to flatten rugae in nulliparous women. Small, moistened cotton-tipped applicators may also be used to manipulate these vaginal folds (Figure 7.37). Gentle lateral displacement of the speculum handle to the same side and slight repositioning of the colposcope to the opposite side will make it easier to view the sidewall. The examination should also include the anterior and posterior vaginal walls

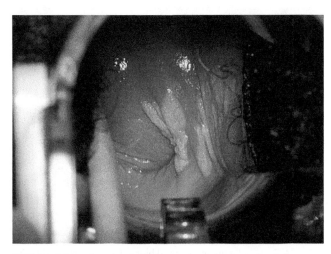

FIGURE 7.37. A moistened, large cotton swab is used to help examine an acetowhite lesion of the left lateral vaginal fornix.

obscured by the blades of the speculum. For a brief inspection with routine colpo, this can be done by inspecting them as the speculum is withdrawn slowly in the anterior/posterior plane. Alternatively, the vaginal speculum blades may be rotated to a lateral alignment to observe the anterior and posterior walls. Warn the patient that she may experience some discomfort as the speculum is rotated to be opened about 90 degrees from the previous position. To prevent unnecessary discomfort (urethral trauma and superficial lacerations), the speculum blades should be relaxed prior to rotation. Colposcopic changes with acetowhitening are more subtle and often take longer to develop after application of acetic acid than for cervical lesions. Mosaic changes are very rare, but punctation is often seen and must be considered to be a strong indicator of high-grade VaIN. Lugol's solution should be applied to the entire vagina when an abnormality is not identified colposcopically following 5% acetic acid application.

Vaginal biopsies should be obtained from all significant acetowhite or iodine-negative colposcopic lesions, including vaginal ulcerations or grossly exophytic lesions. A vaginal biopsy is obtained in a manner similar to that of a cervical biopsy, except that deep biopsies should not be taken and local anesthesia (i.e., subcutaneous lidocaine) is required if the lesion is located in the distal two-third of the vagina adjacent to the introitus. Consider buffering the lidocaine with a 1:10 ratio of sodium bicarbonate to reduce the stinging from the anesthetic. Grasping the biopsy site gently with forceps will identify women with inadequate anesthesia and those with upper vaginal lesions who require local anesthetic. If the biopsy forceps are unable to grasp the stretched vaginal mucosa, relax the vaginal speculum blades to reduce sidewall tautness and facilitate biopsy. Skin hooks are usually not needed, but they can facilitate eversion of the lateral corners of the vaginal cuff in women who have undergone a hysterectomy. The biopsy forceps are aligned as closely as possible to perpendicular to the mucosa with the movable jaw more distally positioned. This orientation permits the colposcopist to observe where the biopsy will actually be taken. Vaginal biopsy rarely causes significant bleeding. Monsel's paste or silver nitrate may be used as necessary for hemostasis. Vaginal biopsies are submitted separately in a fashion similar to that for cervical histologic interpretation and labeled appropriately (e.g., proximal right lateral vagina).

7.3.2 Vulvar, Perineal, Perianal, and Bimanual Examinations

A careful inspection of the vulva and perianal areas should be performed after the speculum is removed. The vulva, perineum, and perianal areas may be examined using the naked eye, a handheld low-power magnification device, or the colposcope (at 2× to 4×) (discussed in detail in Chapter 15). Although colposcopy of the vulva with acetic acid application is not required in most women referred for colposcopy, in some instances, use of this solution and magnification facilitates the identification of small lesions. If acetic acid is used, it should be applied to the external genitalia using cotton balls, 4″ × 4″ gauze pads, or a spray mist for 3 to 5 minutes (see Chapter 15). Because the epithelium external to Hart's line on the vulva is keratinized, it takes longer for acetowhitening to occur. Lesions around or beneath the clitoral hood, within the distal urethra, in the minor vestibular glands, beneath hymenal remnants, and in the perianal region are frequently overlooked (Figure 7.38A–K). Lesions identified that are significantly acetowhite, nonacetowhite, red, or pigmented lesions, as described in Chapter 15, are biopsied as indicated using a cervical biopsy forceps, a knife for superficial "shave" excision, or a Keyes punch following administration of an anesthetic. Specimens are then submitted for pathologic interpretation in separately labeled bottles. Other indications for biopsy of vulvar lesions are listed in Chapter 15.

Because a majority of women will have had a recent pelvic examination performed when the Pap test was obtained, the bimanual examination may not be necessary at the time of colposcopy, although some colposcopists perform a bimanual examination after each colposcopic examination. This is particularly true when the patient has been referred and not previously seen by that colposcopist. Occasionally, a patient will present with negative colposcopic findings but have a palpable cancer of the endocervix, vagina, or lower bowel. Colposcopic evidence of invasive cancer of either the cervix or vagina should mandate a careful bimanual examination. When a bimanual examination follows a cervical biopsy, the examination should be gentle enough not to precipitate bleeding.

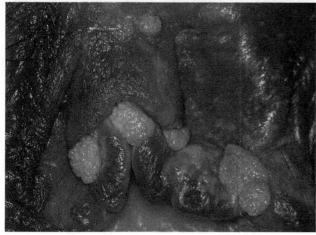

A

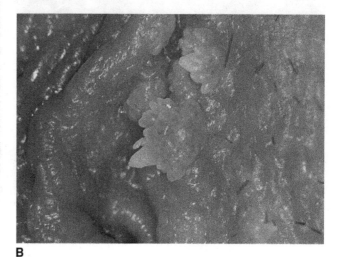

B

FIGURE 7.38. Examination of the vulva and perirectal areas showing condylomata of the clitoral hood (**A**), vulva (**B**), posterior fourchette (**C**), and the perirectal (**D**) regions induced by HPV. Condyloma frequently arise at hair follicles (**E**), particularly following minor trauma from shaving. Some condyloma are more readily detected (**F,G**). Examination of the vulva may detect severe vulvar precancer lesions (VIN 3) (**H,I**). Condyloma should not be confused with micropapillomatosis labialis, a normal anatomic finding (**J,K**).

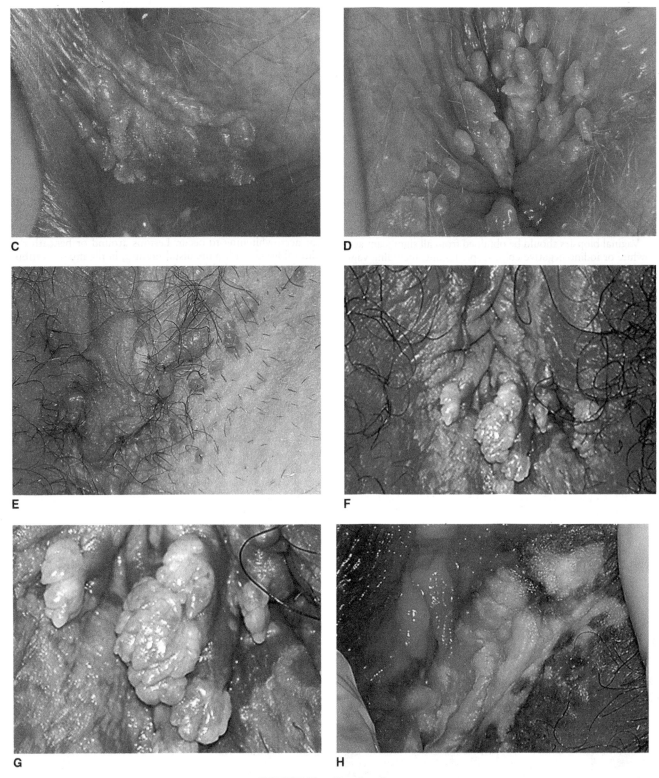

FIGURE 7.38.   *(Continued)*.

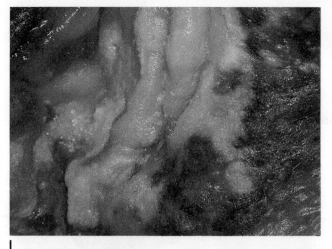

I

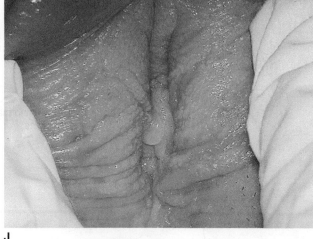

J

FIGURE 7.38.   *(Continued)*

K

7.4 EXAMINING THE ANORECTAL REGION

Colposcopy is also used to examine the anorectal region, or anorectal transformation zone, (discussed in detail in Chapter 17) in women and men for the presence of anal intraepithelial neoplasia (AIN) and squamous cell cancer (Figure 7.39A,B).[22] The procedure called high-resolution anoscopy (HRA) has been advocated particularly for HIV-positive patients, who have a higher prevalence of anorectal oncogenic HPV, AIN, and cancer than do HIV-negative patients.[23] In concert with the follow-up recommendations for abnormal cervical cytology, abnormal anal cytology prompts appropriate management.

Patients considered at risk can be screened for anorectal neoplasia using an anorectal cytologic specimen. This is particularly important for women with immune deficiency. A history of anal intercourse and/or cervical, vaginal, or vulvar HPV-related neoplasia also increases risk for anal neoplasia, even in women with no known immune suppression. To collect a cytologic specimen, a moistened Dacron swab is inserted deeply within the anal canal to sample the anal transformation zone, which is a squamous (anal)/columnar (rectal) cellular interface, analogous to the cervical transformation zone. The specimen is submitted, processed, and examined like a Pap test of the cervix. Be sure the pathologist is clearly informed that this specimen is from an anal Pap test, not a cervical Pap test. Patients with abnormal cellular changes consistent with high-risk HPV-positive ASC-US, ASC-H, SIL, or cancer are then examined by HRA. Those with high-grade AIN should be referred for treatment. Since evaluation and treatment for AIN is not available in some communities, clinicians should define referral systems for therapy before initiating screening for AIN.

7.4.1 Colposcopy of the Anorectal Region

Colposcopy of the anal transformation zone is quite similar to colposcopy of the lower genital tract, except for minor procedural differences. A 3% acetic acid–soaked gauze-wrapped Dacron swab is inserted through an anoscope to the anal canal and the anoscope is withdrawn. After several minutes, the swab is removed, and the anoscope is reinserted to begin the colposcopic examination. Alternatively, the anoscope can be inserted and left in place for the duration of the procedure. Acetic acid is then applied to the anal transformation zone using large cotton swabs. The anal transformation zone is first inspected. Anal low- and high-grade lesions resemble comparable lesions of the cervix except that fine mosaic and punctation are not commonly found (Figure 7.40A–C).[24] Lesions are typically flat and acetowhite and have coarsely dilated vessels. Papillary and exophytic condylomata may also be encountered. Shallow biopsies are collected and submitted in the usual fashion for histologic interpretation. See Chapter 17 for a more complete description of the procedure.

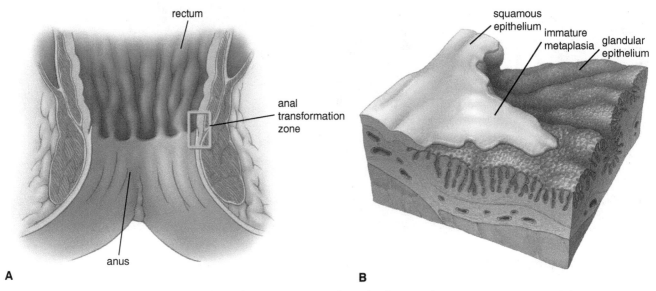

FIGURE 7.39.   The anorectal transformation zone is similar to that found on the cervix (**A**). Squamous epithelium from the anus adjoins columnar epithelium from the rectum (**B**).

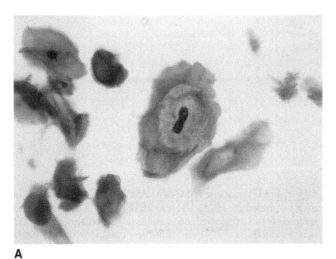

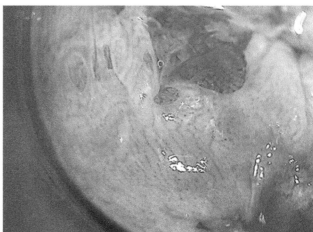

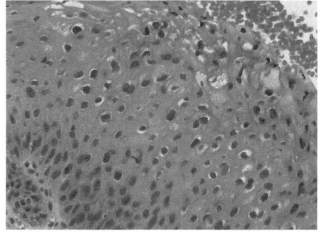

FIGURE 7.40.   Anal Pap test that demonstrates LSIL (**A**) (Papanicolaou stain, high-power magnification). The anal colposcopic exam reveals an acetowhite lesion along the SCJ. Diffuse punctation is observed (**B**). Histology (**C**) from a biopsy of this lesion that demonstrates AIN 1 (Hematoxylin-eosin stain; medium-power magnification). Photos courtesy of Drs. Teresa Darragh and Joel Palefsky.

7.5 DOCUMENTATION

7.5.1 Documenting the Colposcopic Findings

The findings of the colposcopic examination should be fully documented. A standardized reporting form is an essential part of that documentation (Figure 7.41A). The form should include pertinent history, clinical findings, colposcopic impression, and management plans. A diagrammatic representation of the colposcopic findings that can be understood by other clinicians is an essential part of documentation. A large circle typically represents the cervix with the external os indicated in the center as a smaller circle. A stamp or preprinted form facilitates documentation. The current SCJ should be indicated as a solid line. The clinician should draw the colposcopic lesions to scale and describe key features such as color, margin, contour, and vascular pattern. Symbols can be used to indicate specific features and biopsy sites (Figure 7.41B). The written documentation should also clearly state whether or not the colposcopic examination was adequate.

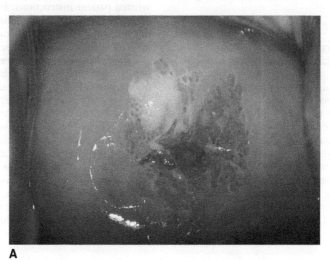

A

B

FIGURE 7.41. An example of proper documentation of colposcopic examination findings (A). The cervical findings are documented in (B).

Photodocumentation (video print, 35 mm, and digital image) assists patient education, management, clinician education, and follow-up monitoring. Colposcopic documentation may also be accomplished using a computer-based data/image management system (see Figure 6.33A). A patient/laboratory/management-tracking log should be maintained to ensure appropriate care and follow-up. Computerized colposcopy tracking software programs facilitate appropriate recall, communication, and education. Photographic documentation of colposcopic findings may also provide valuable medicolegal documentation, if necessary.

7.5.2 Correlation of Cytology, Histology, and Colposcopy Findings

Colposcopy, cervical cytology, and histology are collectively useful in diagnosing and determining the appropriate management of women with cervical neoplasia. The results of all three should agree within one degree of severity (Figure 7.42A–C). The first step in resolving discrepancies is a review of the cytology and histology by one pathologist, preferably an individual with an interest in lower genital tract abnormalities (Figure 7.43A–C). If review confirms the original diagnoses and the discrepancies, reexamination of the patient with additional histological sampling may be necessary. In difficult cases, it may be prudent to refer the patient to an expert colposcopist. On reexamination of the patient, the endocervical canal and proximal vagina require particular attention. If the second examination does not resolve the discrepancy, other procedures, such as cervical conization, may be indicated when the unexplained cytologic finding is high grade.[2]

7.6 POSTPROCEDURE INSTRUCTIONS

After undergoing colposcopy and cervical biopsy (Figure 7.44A–G), women should receive specific verbal and written patient instructions. Patients occasionally need to take NSAIDs for transient cramping or discomfort. Vaginal bleeding heavier than a normal menstrual period is rare following cervical biopsy and should be evaluated and treated. Reapplication of Monsel's paste or silver nitrate will usually restore hemostasis. Patients should be told to expect a slight serous, mildly blood-tinged, vaginal discharge with a brown or black (Monsel's paste, silver nitrate) color for several days following cervical biopsy. It is generally best for women to refrain from sexual activity for a day or two after a biopsy to prevent bleeding from the biopsy site. Explain that the histology report may not return for several days, or weeks, and that you will notify the patient of the results as soon as they are available. Finally, tell your patient what you have found or expect to find based on the colposcopic examination. When appropriate, reassure the patient that she does not have evidence of a cervical cancer. This helps to relieve her anxiety while awaiting the pathology results.

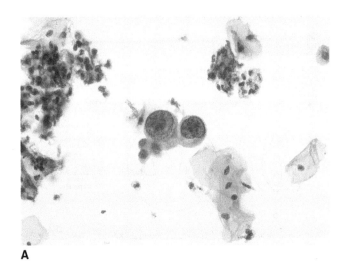

A

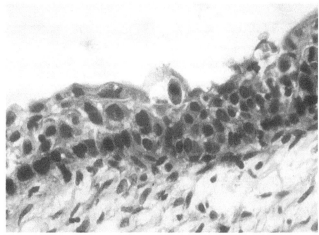

B

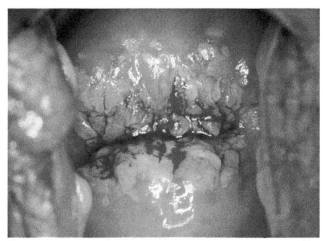

C

FIGURE 7.42. Agreement of the cytology (HSIL) (A) (Papanicolaou stain, high-power magnification), histology (CIN 3) (hematoxylin-eosin stain; high-power magnification) (B) and colposcopic impression (high-grade lesion/CIN 3) (C) permits conservative therapy.

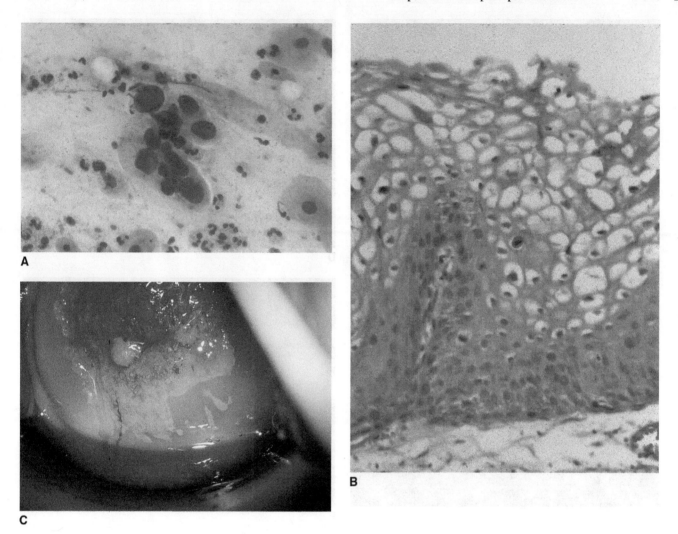

FIGURE 7.43.   Lack of agreement of the cytology (cancer) (Papanicolaou stain, high-power magnification), histology (hematoxylin-eosin stain; medium-power magnification) (CIN 1) and colposcopic impression (low-grade lesion/CIN 1) mandate review of the laboratory results, endocervical curettage, inspection of the proximal vagina, and further evaluation by conization, if otherwise unexplained.

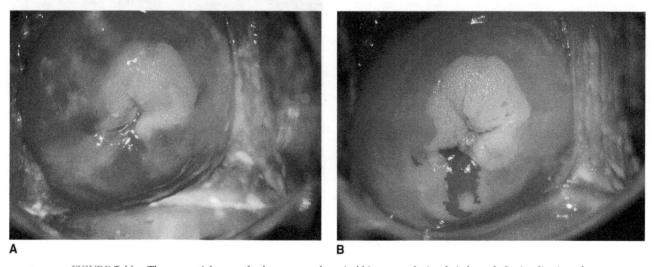

FIGURE 7.44.   The sequential steps of colposcopy and cervical biopsy are depicted: A through G: visualization of the cervix following normal saline application (A), assessment of a large three-quadrant acetowhite lesion following application of 3% to 5% acetic acid (B), sampling the lesion with biopsy forceps (C), the cervix immediately after cervical biopsy (this important step confirms proper histologic sampling) (D), sampling of the endocervical canal using an endocervical curette (E), and securing hemostasis with a silver nitrate stick (F), and/or Monsel's paste (G).

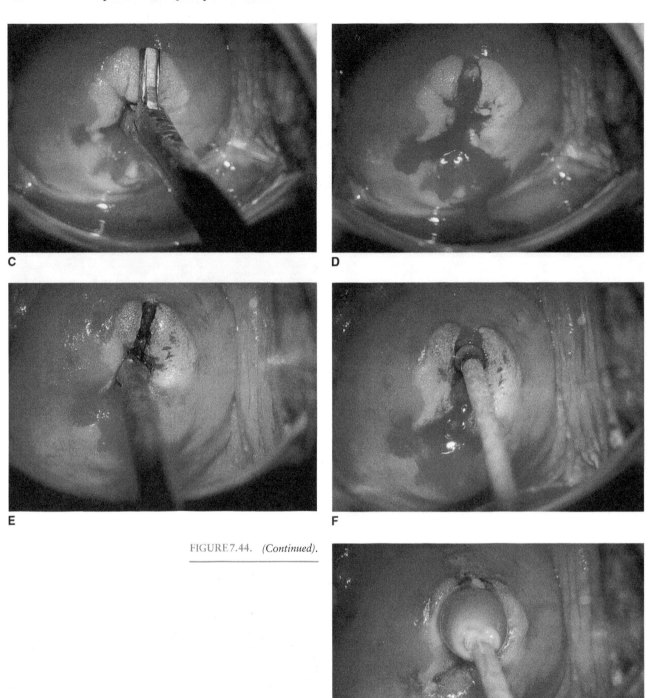

C

D

E

F

FIGURE 7.44.   *(Continued).*

G

References

1. Wright TC Jr, Massad LS, Dunton CJ, Spitzer M, Wilkinson EJ, Solomon D. 2006 consensus guidelines for the management of women with abnormal cervical screening tests. *J Low Genit Tract Dis* 2007;11:201–222.
2. Wright TC Jr, Massad LS, Dunton CJ, Spitzer M, Wilkinson EJ. 2006 consensus guidelines for the management of women with cervical intraepithelial neoplasia or adenocarcinoma in situ. *J Low Genit Tract Dis* 2007;11:223–39.
3. Church L, Oliver L, Dobie S, Madigan D, Ellsworth A. Analgesia for colposcopy: double-masked, randomized comparison of ibuprofen and benzocaine gel. *Obstet Gynecol* 2001;97:5–10.
4. Ferris DG, Greenberg NM. Reid's colposcopic index. *J Fam Pract* 1994;39: 65–70.
5. Reid R, Scalzi P. Genital warts and cervical cancer. VII. An improved colposcopic index for differentiating benign papillomaviral infections from high-grade cervical intraepithelial neoplasia. *Am J Obstet Gynecol* 1985;153:611–8.
6. Toplis PJ, Casemore V, Hallam N, Charnock M. Evaluation of colposcopy in the postmenopausal woman. *Br J Obstet Gynaecol* 1986;93: 843–51.
7. Johnson N, Crompton AC, Wyatt J, Buchan PC, Jarvis GJ. Using Lamicel to expose high grade cervical lesions during colposcopic examinations. *Br J Obstet Gynaecol* 1990;97:46–52.
8. Massad LS, Jeronimo J, Schiffman M, National Institutes of Health/American Society for Colposcopy and Cervical Pathology (NIH/ASCCP) Research Group. Interobserver agreement in the assessment of components of colposcopic grading. *Obstet Gynecol* 2008;111: 1279–84.
9. The ASCUS-LSIL Triage Study (ALTS) Group. Results of a randomized trial on the management of cytology interpretations of atypical squamous cells of undetermined significance. *Am J Obstet Gynecol* 2003; 188:1383–92.
10. Yang B, Pretorius RG, Belinson JL, Zhang X, Burchette R, Qiao YL. False negative colposcopy is associated with thinner cervical intraepithelial neoplasia 2 and 3. *Gynecol Oncol* 2008;110:32–6.
11. Cox JT. More questions about the accuracy of colposcopy: what does this mean for cervical cancer prevention? *Obstet Gynecol* 2008;111: 1266–7.
12. Townsend DE, Richart RM, Marks E, Nielsen J. Invasive cancer following outpatient evaluation and therapy for cervical cancer. *Obstet Gynecol* 1981;57:145–9.
13. Solomon D, Stoler M, Jeronimo J, Khan M, Castle P, Schiffman M. Diagnostic utility of endocervical curettage in women undergoing colposcopy for equivocal or low-grade cytologic abnormalities. *Obstet Gynecol* 2007;110:288–95.
14. Anderson W, Frierson H, Barber S, Tabbarah S, Taylor P, Underwood P. Sensitivity and specificity of endocervical curettage and the endocervical brush for the evaluation of the endocervical canal. *Am J Obstet Gynecol* 1988;159:702–7.
15. Hoffman MS, Sterghos S Jr, Gordy LW, Gunasekaran S, Cavanagh D. Evaluation of the cervical canal with endocervical brush. *Obstet Gynecol* 1993;82:573–7.
16. Gibson CA, Trask CE, House P, Smith SF, Foley M, Nicholas C. Endocervical sampling: a comparison of endocervical brush, endocervical curette and combined brush with curette technique. *J Low Genit Tract Dis* 2001;5:1–6.
17. Ferris DG, Harper DM, Callahan B, et al. The efficacy of topical benzocaine gel in providing anesthesia prior to cervical biopsy and endocervical curettage. *J Low Genit Tract Dis* 1997;1:221–7.
18. Clifton PA, Shaughnessy AF, Andrew S. Ineffectiveness of topical benzocaine spray during colposcopy. *J Fam Pract* 1998;46:242–6.
19. Tate KM, Strickland JL. A randomized controlled trial to evaluate the use of the endocervical brush after endocervical curettage. *Obstet Gynecol* 1997;90:715–7.
20. Gage JC, Hanson VW, Abbey K, et al. Number of cervical biopsies and sensitivity of colposcopy. *Obstet Gynecol* 2006;108:264–72.
21. Heatley MK. A comparison of three methods of orienting cervical punch biopsies. *J Clin Pathol* 1999;52:149–50.
22. Sonnex C, Scholefield JH, Kocjan G, et al. Anal human papillomavirus infection: a comparative study of cytology, colposcopy and DNA hybridization as a method of detection. *Genitourin Med* 1991;67:21–5.
23. Sobhani I, Vuagnat A, Walker F, et al. Prevalence of high-grade dysplasia and cancer in the canal in human papillomavirus-infected individuals. *Gastroenterology* 2001;120:857–66.
24. Jay N, Berry M, Hogeboorn CJ, Holly EA, Darragh TM, Palefsky JM. Colposcopic appearance of anal squamous intraepithelial lesions. *Dis Colon Rectum* 1997;40:919–28.

CHAPTER 8

DARON G. FERRIS
EDWARD J. MAYEAUX, JR.
J. THOMAS COX

Normal and Abnormal Colposcopic Features

8.1 INTRODUCTION
8.2 THE NORMAL TRANSFORMATION ZONE
    8.2.1 Neoplastic Alteration of the Normal Transformation Zone
8.3 THE "ABNORMAL" TRANSFORMATION ZONE
8.4 COLPOSCOPIC FINDINGS
    8.4.1 Critical Colposcopic Considerations
    8.4.2 Identification of Colposcopic Signs

8.5 NORMAL AND ABNORMAL COLPOSCOPIC SIGNS
    8.5.1 Epithelial Color
    8.5.2 Vasculature
    8.5.3 Surface Topography
    8.5.4 Margin Characteristics of Abnormal Cervical Epithelium

8.1 INTRODUCTION

Once the cervix can be visualized clearly through the colposcope, attention is directed to identifying the squamocolumnar junction (SCJ) and the surrounding transformation zone (Figure 8.1). When the examination follows an abnormal cytologic finding, the colposcopic mission becomes one of detecting the source of the abnormal screening test result. Assuming a cervical etiology, the abnormal cells most likely evolved from an alteration within the epithelium of the transformation zone. Thus, recognition of abnormalities within the transformation zone is the most critical objective of colposcopy. The key value of colposcopy is in the ability of the experienced colposcopist to recognize a variety of different morphologic appearances consistent with either normal epithelium or specific abnormal histologic diagnoses. Within the cervical epithelium, neoplasia can produce visibly striking changes, which can be assessed colposcopically according to severity, size, and location providing the basis for planning a therapeutic approach.

In addition to cytologic and histologic findings, proper patient management depends upon the colposcopic impression, which evolves directly from critical assessment of unique characteristics of the epithelium and vasculature. Discriminating normal from abnormal colposcopic findings is not always simple. Although some solitary colposcopic signs can be interpreted as normal or abnormal, the combination of multiple signs or appearances may be confusing. Only ample training and sufficient experience permit colposcopists to discern subtle differences, like those between normal variants and low-grade lesions and those between low-grade lesions and high-grade lesions. Even with experience, definitive discrimination usually requires biopsy and histologic assessment. This chapter describes the colposcopic features that enable discrimination of normal from abnormal and various levels of abnormality.

8.2 THE NORMAL TRANSFORMATION ZONE

A detailed description of the development and histology of the normal transformation zone is in Chapter 2. For the colposcopist to better discriminate normal from abnormal colposcopic findings, a brief review is given here. A detailed description of epithelial and vascular colposcopic findings of the normal transformation zone is presented later in the chapter.

The cervix is covered by three different types of epithelium: squamous, columnar, and immature and mature metaplasia (Figure 8.2A,B). The junction of squamous and columnar epithelia forms the boundary of the transformation zone. Nonkeratinized stratified squamous epithelium extends from Hart's line (the embryologic junction between the vagina and vulva) (Figure 8.3) to the SCJ on the cervix at the woman's birth. Histologically, squamous epithelium contains four types of cells: basal, parabasal, intermediate, and superficial (Figure 8.4A,B). Basal cells differentiate and mature through the other three cellular stages as they ascend from the basement membrane to the surface. Columnar epithelium is a single cell layer of tall mucus-secreting cells. Cervical columnar epithelium courses proximally from the SCJ and within the endocervical canal to the internal os. Columnar epithelium covers villi, small polypoid projections that contain central loop capillaries (Figure 8.5A–J). Metaplastic epithelium lies between the squamous and columnar epithelium. Metaplastic epithelium is formed when metaplastic cells replace columnar cells. These cells eventually differentiate to become squamous epithelium. Metaplasia is a normal process that occurs naturally in all women.

The position of the SCJ on the ectocervix at birth is known as the original SCJ. The SCJ noted at colposcopy in any postmenarchal female is called the new SCJ or simply "SCJ" (Figure 8.6A–D). In reproductive-age women, the SCJ is

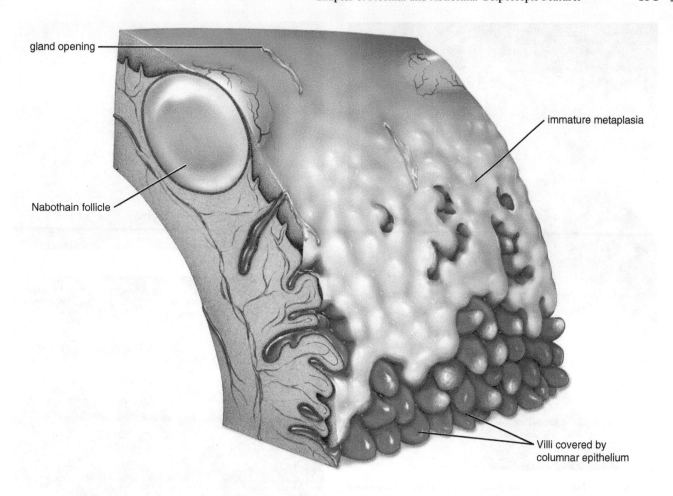

gland opening

immature metaplasia

Nabothain follicle

Villi covered by
columnar epithelium

FIGURE 8.1.   The normal transformation zone includes immature and mature metaplastic epithelium, nabothian follicles, and gland openings.

variably positioned on the ectocervix or may be slightly within the endocervical canal. Later in life, the SCJ may not be easily identified colposcopically since the cellular interface may be hidden deeply within the endocervical canal (Figure 8.7). Between the original SCJ and the advancing new SCJ lies an area of continuously changing epithelium.

This area has been termed the transformation zone in recognition of the apparent transformation of columnar cells to squamous cells. The dynamic nature of this process results in a mix of immature and then mature metaplastic epithelium. These metaplastic cells comprise the transformation zone.

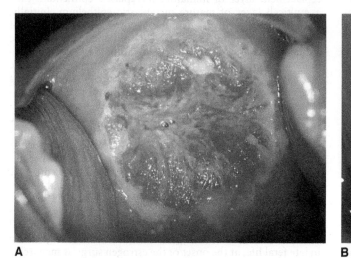

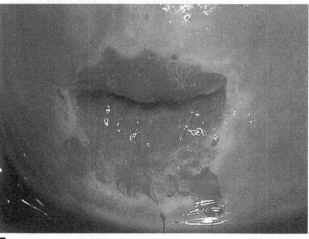

A

B

FIGURE 8.2.   A,B: The normal cervix and transformation zone with pink squamous epithelium, white immature metaplasia, and red columnar epithelium. (Courtesy of, and approved for reproduction by, the International Cervical Cancer (INCCA) foundation.)

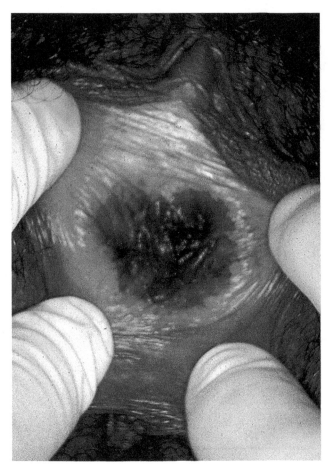

FIGURE 8.3.   Hart's line, or the junction between the glycogenated vaginal epithelium darkly stained with Lugol's and the yellow staining of keratinized vulvar squamous epithelium. This interface represents the most distal portion of the vagina.

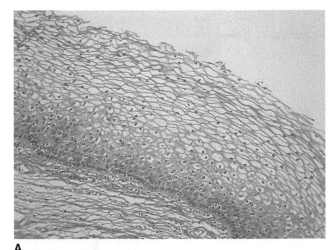

A

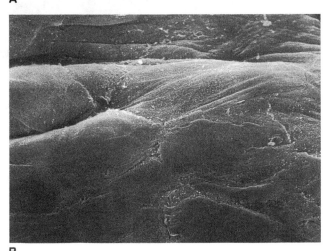

B

FIGURE 8.4.   **A:** Squamous epithelium contains basal, parabasal, intermediate, and superficial cells that differentiate from the basement membrane in that order (hematoxylin-eosin stain; medium-power magnification). **B:** A surface scanning electron micrograph of squamous epithelium. Notice the overlapping of cells creating an impenetrable surface.

Although some transformation begins during fetal life as a consequence of exposure to maternal estrogen, the estrogen surge that begins at puberty and lasts until menopause is responsible for the changes noted during a woman's reproductive life. This estrogen surge at puberty initiates glycogen storage in epithelial cells and subsequent colonization of *Lactobacillus acidophilus* within the vagina. In addition to producing hydrogen peroxide to limit opportunistic pathogens, the lactobacilli produce lactic acid that reduces the vaginal pH to <4.7. This highly acidic environment may minimally damage superficial squamous cells, which are continuously replaced within the multilayered squamous epithelium. Mucus secretion by columnar epithelium serves both reproductive and vaginal hygienic purposes. However, the mucus is an inefficient protective shield from the acidic environment. Because the columnar epithelium is thin and fragile, it is easily traumatized by the acid. In contrast to squamous epithelium, columnar epithelium is without multiple underlying replacement cell layers. Consequently, the cellular injury from lactic acid may help stimulate a defensive transformation of the susceptible single-cell layer columnar epithelium to a more resilient multicell-layer metaplastic epithelium. However, it is not known whether the acidic environment actually causes metaplasia.

Transformation may occur by means of one of two mechanisms. With the first, the traumatized acid-irritated columnar epithelium is replaced by small, round, nuclear dense reserve cells positioned beneath the columnar epithelium. These cells eventually proliferate and differentiate to form a thin

replacement layer of immature metaplastic epithelium, then a multicell layer of mature metaplastic epithelium. Initially, this metaplastic cellular change appears on the exposed tips of columnar villi (Figure 8.8A–E). Next, the immature metaplastic epithelium fuses or bridges with immature metaplastic epithelium on adjoining villi. Finally, opalescent sheets of immature metaplasia are formed that extend as tongue-like projections toward the os. The second method of transformation (squamous epithelialization) involves an advancing immature metaplastic epithelium that undermines columnar epithelium. As the columnar epithelium is lifted from the underlying stroma, it is replaced by a thin metaplastic layer. The epithelial transformation process is episodic but progressive, starting in the periphery of the transformation zone and advancing concentrically toward the os and extending up the endocervical canal in later life. Noncontiguous islands of immature metaplasia may be seen proximal to the advancing SCJ. These eventually coalesce with broad sheets of immature metaplasia along the SCJ (Figure 8.9A–F). Maximal transformation zone activity is seen in late fetal life, at the onset of the estrogen surge at menarche, during the first pregnancy, and in women using combined hormonal contraceptive methods. Cellular alterations secondary to infection with human papillomavirus (HPV) can arise in

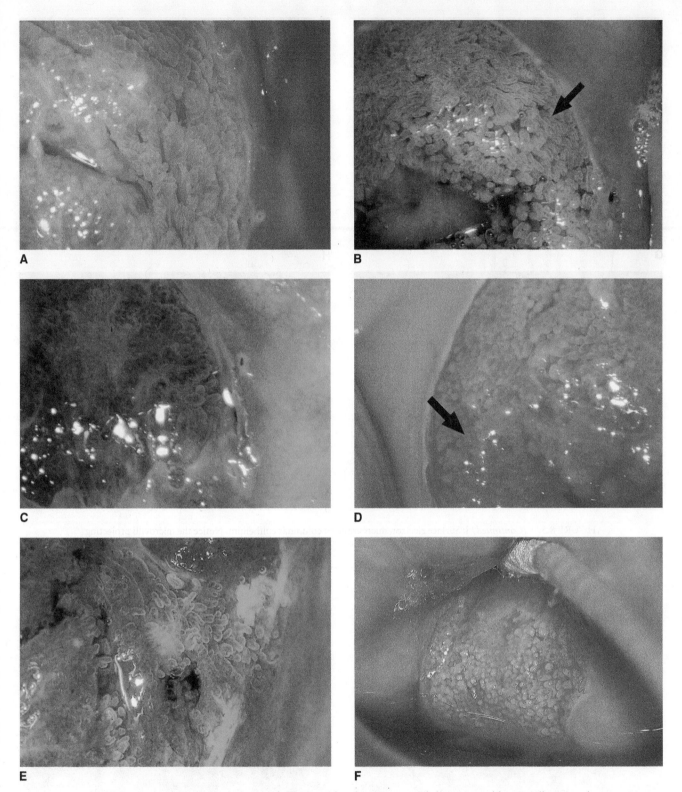

FIGURE 8.5. **A–J:** High-power images of villi covered with columnar epithelium. Central loop capillaries can be seen (*arrows*).

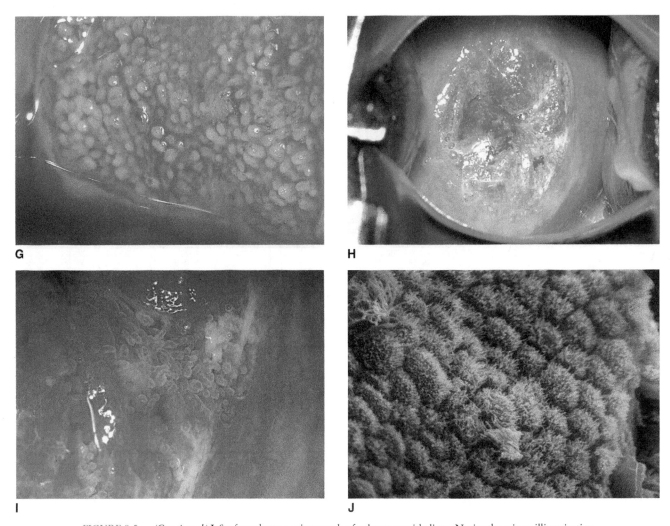

FIGURE 8.5.   *(Continued)* **J:** Surface electron micrograph of columnar epithelium. Notice the microvilli projecting from the cell's surfaces. (Courtesy of, and approved for reproduction by, the International Cervical Cancer (INCCA) foundation.)

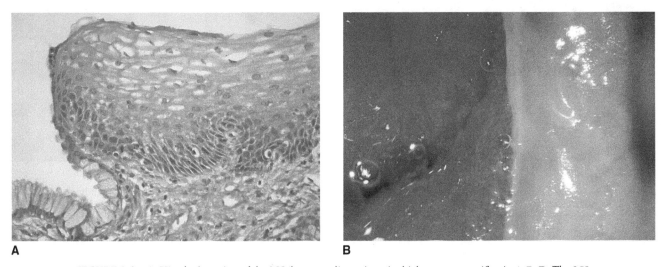

FIGURE 8.6.   **A:** Histologic section of the SCJ (hematoxylin-eosin stain; high-power magnification). **B–D:** The SCJ separates pink squamous epithelium from red columnar epithelium. The SCJ *(arrow)* appears as a thin white line after 3% to 5% acetic acid application to the cervix.

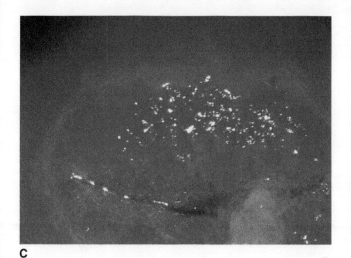

C

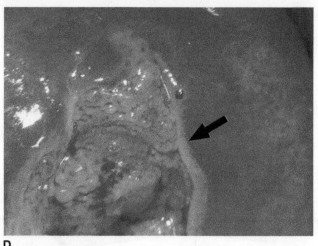

D

FIGURE 8.6. (Continued)

this immature metaplasia, resulting in cervical squamous neoplasia. Consequently, colposcopy focuses on examination of this susceptible tissue.

Mature metaplasia lies between immature metaplasia and the original SCJ. Mature metaplastic epithelium is a multicell layer of fully differentiated squamous epithelium. This epithelium differs from immature metaplasia in that the latter contains only a few layers of mainly undifferentiated cells. However, mature metaplasia has two unique features (gland openings and nabothian cysts) not found in original squamous epithelium but often apparent by histologic and colposcopic examination. If advancing metaplastic epithelium surrounds a cleft between columnar villi on the surface but does not completely replace all the columnar epithelium and fill the space between columnar villi, a gland opening results (Figure 8.10A–F). Mucus produced by the deeply confined, remaining columnar cells protrudes to the surface through this opening. Should the cleft become occluded by metaplastic epithelium at the surface, the mucus produced by the retained

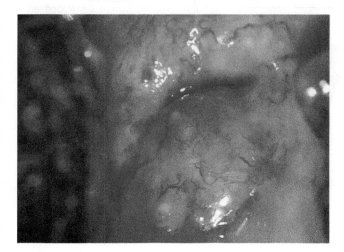

FIGURE 8.7. The SCJ is located within the endocervical canal and cannot be seen in this postmenopausal patient. However, remnants of the transformation process, including nabothian follicles, are apparent. The epithelium is thin and, therefore, prominent blood vessels can be easily seen. This epithelium is mature metaplasia.

columnar cells becomes trapped beneath, resulting in a nabothian cyst or follicle (Figure 8.11A–I). The normal transformation zone is recognized colposcopically and histologically by the presence of mature and immature metaplastic epithelium, along with nabothian follicles and gland openings, both remnants of the transformation process.

8.2.1 Neoplastic Alteration of the Normal Transformation Zone

The normal transformation zone, a dynamic region of epithelium, consists of both mature and immature metaplastic epithelium. Immature metaplasia is more susceptible to cellular insult that may divert it from the normal maturation process. Infection of these immature cells by HPV is the cellular insult that appears to be uniquely necessary in the process of neoplastic transformation. A complex series of cellular events (Chapter 5) may ensue, leading to various degrees of cellular abnormality. As lesions evolve, epithelial and vascular morphologic characteristics of the normal transformation zone assume a wide range of abnormal colposcopic features.[1–5] However, progressive cellular and vascular evolution is neither universal nor unidirectional, as certain low-grade lesions may persist unaltered or, more commonly, may regress to normal tissue. A complicated interaction involving immature metaplastic epithelium infected by oncogenic HPV, local immunity, viral persistence, and clonal progression of the persistently infected epithelium to cervical precancer, may eventually lead to invasion.[6] The process for deviation to an abnormality occurs in very immature, unstable metaplastic epithelium of the normal transformation zone.

8.3 THE "ABNORMAL" TRANSFORMATION ZONE

The term " 'abnormal' transformation zone" (ATZ) is not recognized officially as an international colposcopic term, but is useful to indicate colposcopic findings in the transformation zone that deviate from findings most consistent with normal developing metaplasia. The colposcopic characteristics that will be discussed as most consistent with alteration of the normal transformation zone are typically initiated in immature

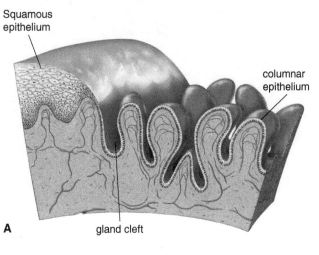

A

Squamous epithelium

columnar epithelium

gland cleft

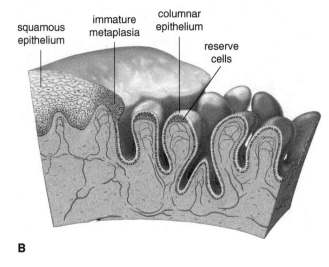

B

squamous epithelium

immature metaplasia

columnar epithelium

reserve cells

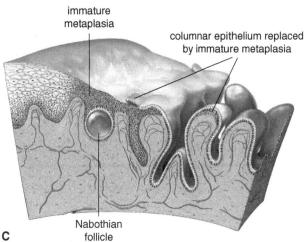

C

immature metaplasia

columnar epithelium replaced by immature metaplasia

Nabothian follicle

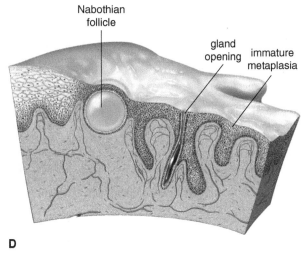

D

Nabothian follicle

gland opening

immature metaplasia

FIGURE 8.8. The transformation process is depicted in these five figures. **A:** Normal squamous and columnar epithelium are seen. **B:** Reserve cells are now noted beneath some columnar cells on the tips of the villi. These villi tips blanch white following 3% to 5% acetic acid application. **C:** Columnar epithelium trapped beneath advancing metaplasia results in trapped mucous producing a nabothian follicle. **D:** Advancing maturing metaplasia. **E:** Eventually the columnar epithelium is replaced by metaplastic epithelium.

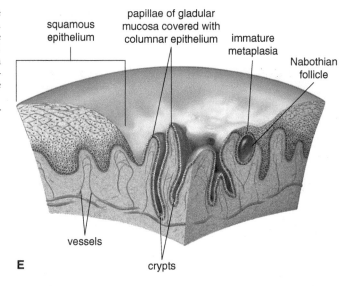

E

squamous epithelium

papillae of gladular mucosa covered with columnar epithelium

immature metaplasia

Nabothian follicle

vessels

crypts

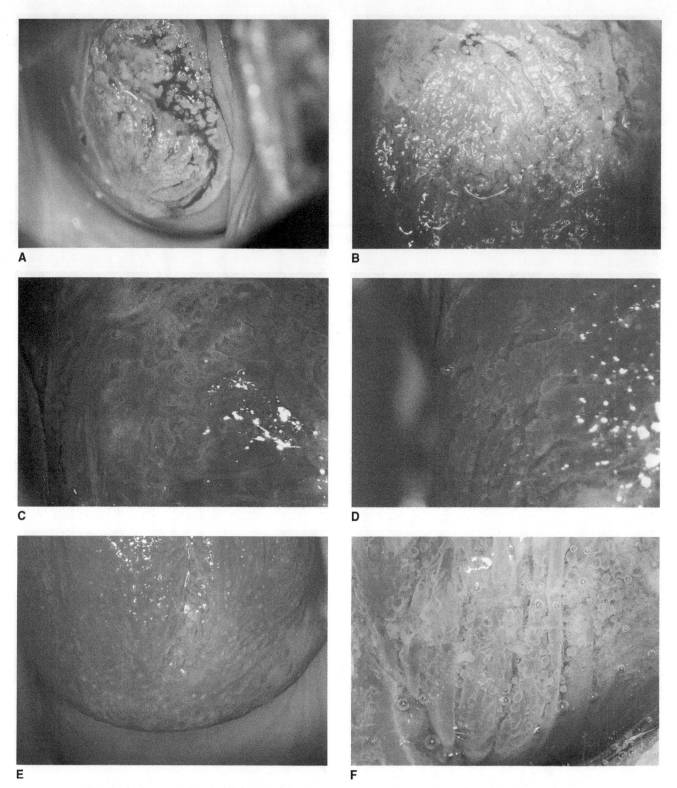

FIGURE 8.9.   A–F: Various stages of the metaplastic process are seen from blanching of the villi tips to bridging across villi and finally to opalescent sheets of metaplasia. (Courtesy of, and approved for reproduction by, the International Cervical Cancer (INCCA) foundation.)

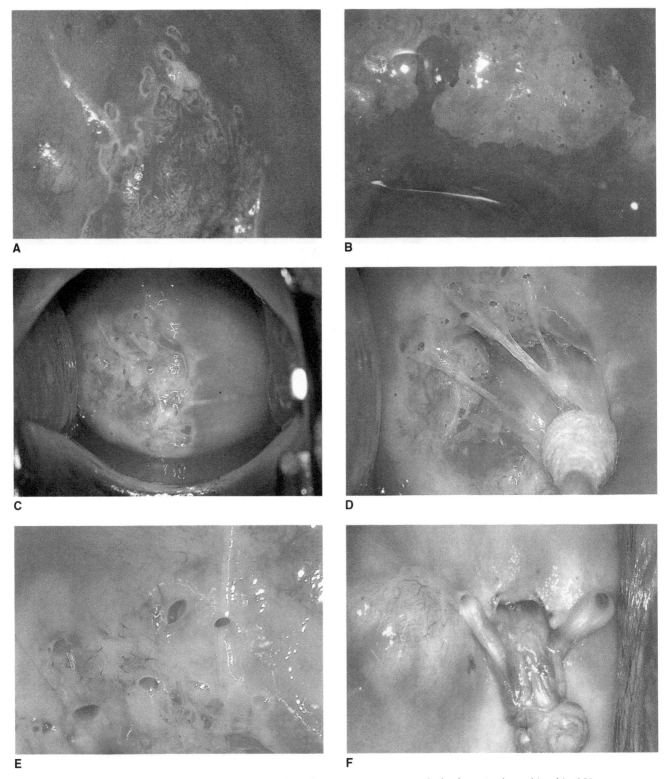

FIGURE 8.10.   Gland openings can be seen above the contiguous SCJ. **A:** Each gland opening has a thin white SCJ with a central reddish color indicating retained columnar epithelium. **B:** Small gland openings are seen in this area of immature metaplasia. Mucus can be seen protruding from the gland openings in (**C–F**).

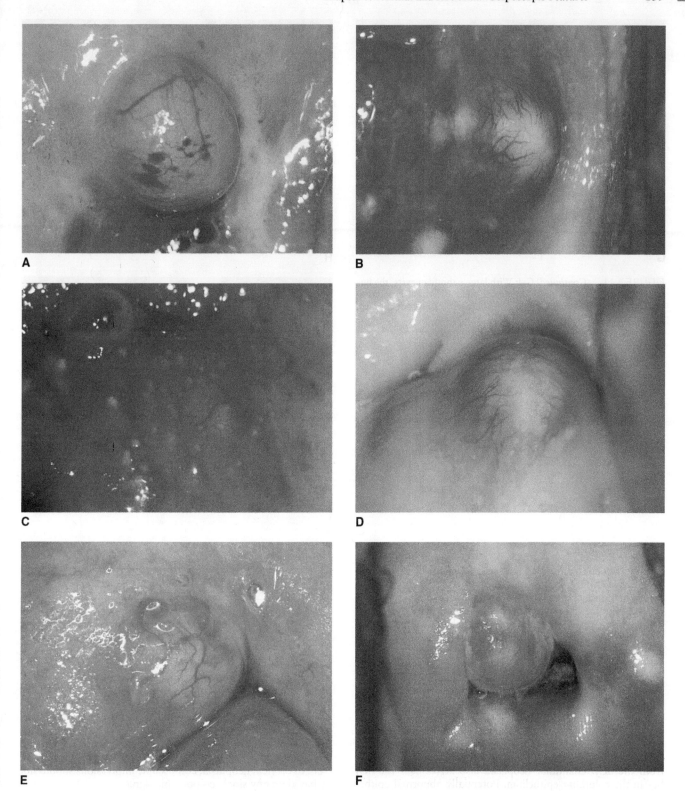

FIGURE 8.11.   **A–F:** Amber-yellow round nabothian cysts with overlying dilated, but normal branching blood vessels.

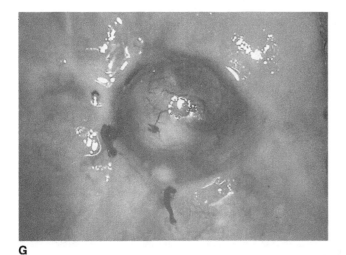

G

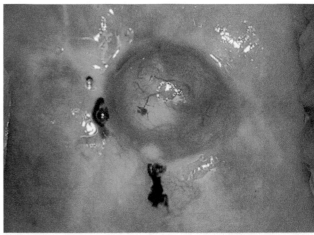

H

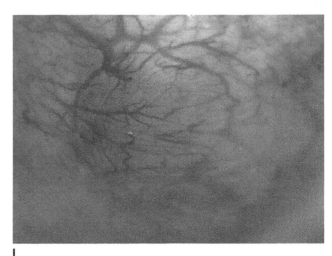

I

FIGURE 8.11. *(Continued)* **G–I:** With large nabothian cysts, the hue within the cyst is often bluish due to the effect of a large amount of clear mucus within. (Courtesy of, and approved for reproduction by, the International Cervical Cancer (INCCA) foundation.)

metaplastic epithelium, whereby the normal uniform and progressive differentiation of squamous cells is modified to an epithelium lacking cell maturation. Increasingly abnormal cells and the accompanying involvement of more of the epithelial thickness results in the colposcopic changes that encompass the ATZ. When a malignancy evolves, the abnormal cells break through the basement membrane and may extend beyond. Diverse modifications of the normal supporting vasculature also emerge. These vascular changes result from interaction with the dynamic epithelium or from proliferation stimulated by angiogenic factors associated with viral infection or neoplasia.[7–12]

The most significant neoplastic lesions initiate near the new or current SCJ. Squamous neoplasia originates in metaplastic epithelium along the SCJ and typically extends distally from the SCJ. Glandular neoplasia also arises near the SCJ but in the columnar epithelium. Potentially abnormal epithelial features include leukoplakia, acetowhite epithelium, and iodine-negative epithelium. Epithelial absence, in the form of an ulceration or erosion, is abnormal. Epithelial proliferation that causes a raised contour with respect to the normal adjoining surface also may represent an abnormality. Punctation, mosaic, and atypical blood vessels are all potentially abnormal vascular colposcopic signs. All of these epithelial and vascular colposcopic features associated with the ATZ also may be seen in the normal transformation zone.

8.4 COLPOSCOPIC FINDINGS

8.4.1 Critical Colposcopic Considerations

There is no single colposcopic sign or anatomical feature detected within the cervical transformation zone that differentiates disease from normality or provides definitive evidence of the presence or degree of premalignant or early invasive neoplasia. Any condition that causes increased cellular division, decreased cellular maturation, increased or decreased thickness of epithelium, abnormal cellular metabolism, or increased vascularization can produce atypical colposcopic findings. Because no solitary colposcopic sign permits independent differentiation of the normal transformation zone from the spectrum of cervical neoplasia, colposcopic impressions should not be based on any single colposcopic sign.

Abnormal colposcopic features may occur in normal variants seen during the early estrogen surge, during pregnancy, with use of combined hormonal contraceptive methods, after *in utero* exposure to diethylstilbestrol (DES), and with estrogen withdrawal. Benign conditions such as squamous metaplasia, regeneration, repair, inflammation, and infection also may produce dramatic vascular and epithelial colposcopic changes. To minimize the risk of interpreting benign conditions as abnormal, the full complement of colposcopic signs must be considered collectively in deriving a colposcopic impression with the highest degree possible of reliability and validity. For example, the same colposcopic features noted in areas of immature squamous metaplasia may also be seen in women with inflammation, repair, low-grade cervical lesions, and cervical cancer.

8.4.2 Identification of Colposcopic Signs

Normal and abnormal colposcopic findings may involve all or part of the transformation zone. These findings can extend distal to the original SCJ to affect the peripheral cervix and vagina. Alternatively, the colposcopic findings may involve epithelium of the endocervical canal. Shifting of the transformation zone over time means that normal and abnormal colposcopic findings do not need to be site specific or location dependent.

The intense illumination and magnification of the colposcope permit assessment and differentiation of normal and abnormal colposcopic features. Except for leukoplakia, the more common abnormal colposcopic signs are not apparent with naked-eye observation. Certainly, grossly nodular malignancies or large exophytic condylomas of the cervix may be clearly visible and readily palpable. However, proper recognition of less apparent and less severe degrees of neoplasia is necessary to identify cervical intraepithelial neoplasia (CIN). Tiny capillary anomalies can be more fully appreciated using the visual enhancements provided by a modern colposcope. Contemporary management of women with lower genital tract neoplasia requires expertise in the recognition of these subtle abnormal colposcopic features.

The chemical solutions used during colposcopy permit visualization, identification, and discrimination between certain normal and abnormal areas of the transformation zone. Saline may be used initially to moisten the cervix and to permit the nontraumatic removal of obscuring debris. Additionally, saline facilitates visualization of the vasculature prior to the application of acetic acid. Acetic acid (3% to 5%) permits a transient observation of immature portions of the normal transformation zone and detection of more persistent acetowhite changes noted with epithelial abnormalities. Lugol's iodine solution contrasts normal glycogenated epithelium from nonglycogenated immature normal or abnormal epithelium. The red free (green) filter, which blocks red light transmission, enhances the recognition of blood vessels, and is most important in the identification of abnormal vessels associated with severe neoplastic transformation. By filtering out the red color, vessels appear black against a light green epithelial background. The surface contour of the cervix varies vastly. Normal and abnormal topography may be smooth or flat, papillary, nodular, papular, uneven, raised, or ulcerated. The edges of normal epithelia or abnormal lesions can also assume a multitude of patterns. Margins may be extremely irregular, delicately feathered, nearly indistinct, almost straight, rounded, curved, complex, or visibly peeling.

8.5 NORMAL AND ABNORMAL COLPOSCOPIC SIGNS

Leukoplakia, acetowhite epithelium, ulceration, punctation, mosaic, and atypical vessels are the colposcopic signs seen in both normal and abnormal epithelium of the lower genital tract. Colposcopic signs that collectively, in whole, in part, singly, or in combination, represent normal and abnormal epithelium are shown in Table 8.1, which also includes the theoretical reasons for the colposcopic signs.

The colposcopic features considered most important for differentiating normal from abnormal conditions and discriminating levels of abnormality may be grouped systematically as follows:

TABLE 8.1	NORMAL AND ABNORMAL COLPOSCOPIC SIGNS	
■ **TYPE OF TISSUE**	■ **COLPOSCOPIC SIGN**	■ **ETIOLOGY**
Epithelial	Acetowhite epithelium	Increased cellular and nuclear density Intracellular protein agglutination Abnormal intracellular keratins
	Leukoplakia	Traumatically induced, thickened superficial epithelium Abnormal keratin production from a viral or neoplastic process
	Ulceration	Absence of epithelium caused by trauma, infection, medications, or neoplasia
Vascular	Punctation and mosaic	Alterations in epithelial capillaries due to (a) proliferative effect of the normal immature metaplastic process (b) capillary proliferative effect of HPV (c) intraepithelial pressures exerted by expanding blocks of neoplastic epithelium
	Atypical blood vessels	Very immature metaplastic epithelium The proliferative effect of vascular endothelial growth factor and angiogenin, tumor angiogenesis factors noted in invasive cancer Catabolic oxygen demands of invasive cancer Random invading directions of cancer Postradiation angiogenesis Granulation tissue

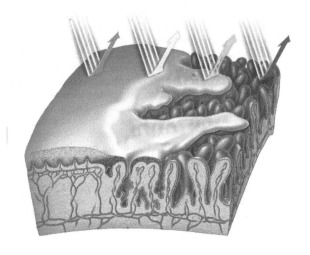

A

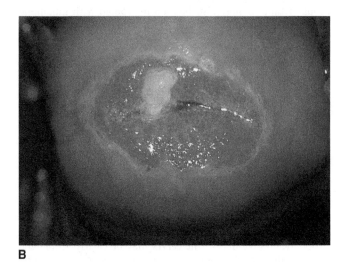

B

FIGURE 8.12.   **A:** The color of the normal cervix is derived from the interaction of the colposcope light with the tissue. **B:** squamous epithelium is pink and columnar epithelium red prior to the application of 3% to 5% acetic acid.

- *Epithelial color:* before and after the application of normal saline, 3% to 5% acetic acid, or Lugol's iodine solution
- *Vasculature:* type of vessel, vessel pattern, vessel caliber, and intercapillary distances
- *Surface topography:* flat, ulcerated, or raised surfaces
- *Margin characteristics:* border shape of discrete epithelial lesions

8.5.1 Epithelial Color

8.5.1.1 Before Application of 3% to 5% Acetic Acid and Lugol's Iodine Solution

8.5.1.1.1 NORMAL CERVIX

As described in Chapter 2, healthy mature squamous epithelium can be distinguished easily from columnar epithelium or immature squamous epithelium based on color tone. This is accomplished following normal saline application but before the application of 3% to 5% acetic acid or Lugol's iodine solution. Color is derived colposcopically by the interaction of transmitted colposcopic light with the epithelium and stroma (Figure 8.12A,B). Certain wavelengths of the colposcope's white light are either reflected back to the observer immediately or absorbed, then emitted as specific wavelengths of light that convey a unique color. The nuclear-to-cytoplasmic ratio of epithelial cells and epithelial thickness affect the intensity of reflected white light. As each increases, the amount of white light returned to the colposcopist increases, and the amount of red color emitted from transilluminated blood vessels decreases.

Healthy mature nonkeratinized stratified squamous epithelium (whether original squamous epithelium or mature metaplastic epithelium) has a pink color (Figure 8.13). The epithelium appears pink because a network of capillaries underlies stratified squamous epithelium, which may be 10 to 15 cell layers thick. A majority of the white light from the colposcope, combined with a small amount of red color from deeply positioned capillaries, blends to emit a pink tone (Figure 8.14). A more pale pink color may be seen in postmenopausal women not receiving estrogen replacement therapy because of a thinner epithelium (Figure 8.15A,B). When observed through the

colposcope at high-power magnification, tiny, wispy, superficially located dark red blood vessels can be detected against the homogeneous pink background (Figure 8.16A,B). These loop capillaries in stromal papillae penetrate into the lower one-third of the squamous epithelium to nourish the maturing cells. The reduced epithelial thickness over the loop capillaries allows greater transmission of a focal red color.

Both columnar epithelium and immature metaplastic epithelium appear red (Figure 8.17A,B) at initial inspection. Columnar epithelium may be "beefy" red or dull red, depending on the amount, turbidity, and viscosity of overlying mucus, and vascular prominence secondary to inflammation. The red color is derived from the interaction of the colposcope light with the thin tissue. The close proximity of the underlying loop capillaries, which are covered by only a single cell layer of columnar epithelium, emits a predominant red hue from the transilluminated light. The color of immature metaplastic epithelium varies depending on its stage of maturation. Very immature metaplasia is quite thin, composed of only a few cell layers; consequently, prior to acetic acid application, this

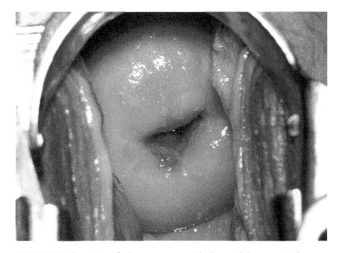

FIGURE 8.13.   Stratified squamous epithelium of the cervix, demonstrating a pink color.

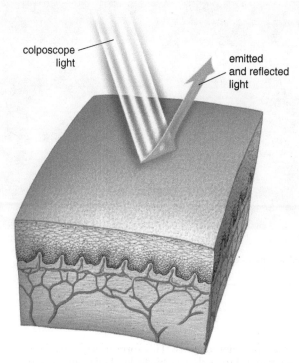

FIGURE 8.14. Squamous epithelium appears pink because the white light of the colposcope combined with a small amount of red color from the deeply residing capillaries blend to produce a light pink color.

epithelium appears a moderate red color (Figure 8.18A–D). The red color is not as intense as that seen with columnar epithelium because the capillaries lie slightly deeper beneath the thin maturing epithelium. As the epithelium matures and thickens, less red color can be appreciated. With complete metaplastic differentiation, the epithelium assumes a characteristic pink color similar to that observed in original squamous epithelium.

Amber yellow, round nabothian cysts may be observed in metaplastic epithelium (Figure 8.11A–I). Nabothian cysts evolve from the transformation process when advancing metaplastic epithelium seals a gland cleft opening, thereby trapping mucus secreted from columnar epithelium recessed

deeply within the gland cleft. An abundance of retained mucus slowly stretches the overlying epithelium and stroma. The epithelium becomes compressed and thinned as the trapped mucus accumulates. The bulging, gently rounded amber protrusion conveys a translucent quality upon colposcopic illumination. Prominent, readily transilluminated blood vessels will usually be apparent in the epithelium overlying the cysts. Although these vessels appear dilated, they exhibit normal arboreal branching. Because these large-caliber vessels are associated with a contour change, they may be mistaken for atypical blood vessels seen with invasive cancer. However, the smooth, yellow, translucent contour and the dichotomously branching vessels are characteristic of nabothian cysts. Rarely, bleeding may occur into the cyst producing a dark red or black color.

During pregnancy, the normal cervix assumes a bluish hue (Figure 8.19). This discoloration results from hormonally mediated vascular congestion. Cervical changes during pregnancy are discussed further in Chapter 12.

8.5.1.1.2 Abnormal Cervix
8.5.1.1.2.1 Leukoplakia

8.5.1.1.2.1.1 Definition   The term *leukoplakia* means "white patch" and is defined as an epithelium that appears white when viewed with the naked eye or with the colposcope prior to the application of 3% to 5% acetic acid (Figure 8.20). When considering leukoplakia, it is necessary to remember that a variety of histologic processes can appear as white areas on the cervix. Most commonly, regions of leukoplakia are associated with an increase in the amount of keratin at the surface of the epithelium. This histologic process is referred to as "hyperkeratosis" (Figure 8.21). When the hyperkeratotic material retains pyknotic cell nuclei, it is referred to as "parakeratosis" (Figure 8.22). Thus, the term keratosis has been used to refer to areas of leukoplakia. However, not all leukoplakias demonstrate benign hyperkeratosis or parakeratosis. Some represent neoplastic or acanthotic (thickening of the intermediate and superficial layers of the squamous epithelium) processes and appear white because of the increased nuclear density of underlying neoplastic cells and the thickened epithelium, which reflects a substantial amount of white light back to the colposcopist (Figure 8.20). The current International Federation of Cervical Pathology and Colposcopy

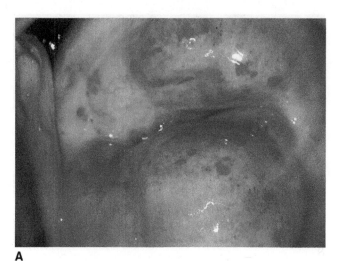

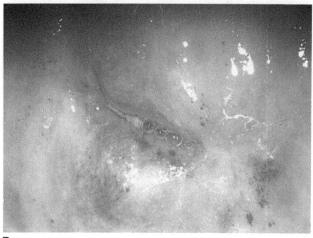

A   **B**

FIGURE 8.15.   A, B: An atrophic cervix is pale pink. The epithelium is thin. Consequently, small subcutaneous hemorrhages induced by minor contact trauma are seen. (Courtesy of, and approved for reproduction by, the International Cervical Cancer (INCCA) foundation.)

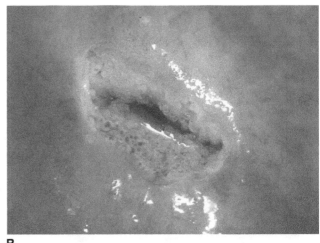

A   B

FIGURE 8.16.   **A, B:** Tiny, small network capillaries of normal squamous epithelium. (Photograph [A] courtesy of Dr. Kenneth L. Noller.)

colposcopic terminology (Table 8.2) uses the term *keratosis* instead of *leukoplakia* even though not all white lesions of the cervix demonstrate hyperkeratosis or parakeratosis on histologic examination.[13]

8.5.1.1.2.1.2 Etiology   Leukoplakia results from a variety of noxious stimuli, including HPV infection, trauma (particularly chronic irritation), and neoplasia (both preinvasive and invasive). However, many cases are idiopathic, especially those occurring in young women. When associated with chronic trauma, leukoplakia may be thought of simply as an epithelial response to irritation, such as might occur with use of a diaphragm, retained tampon, or pessary. Normal epithelium must protect underlying structures from external injury, penetration, and hence, infection. By defensively thickening the epithelium, either through hyperkeratosis or acanthosis, leukoplakia provides a protective barrier that can better withstand insult and

protect epithelial integrity. This form of leukoplakia is sometimes referred to as dystrophic leukoplakia, since it represents a dystrophic process. It is usually associated with hyperkeratosis and mild or minimal acanthosis.

8.5.1.1.2.1.3 Colposcopic Appearance   Leukoplakia appears as a white, thickened, raised epithelium observed prior to the application of 3% to 5% acetic acid (Figure 8.23A,B). It may be seen with the naked eye but is better appreciated after saline application and using the colposcope. Leukoplakia occurs on the cervix, both within and outside the transformation zone. Leukoplakia may also be seen elsewhere in the lower genital tract. The location of leukoplakia is important since it may reflect the underlying etiology. When leukoplakia occurs in original squamous epithelium, it usually represents a benign condition (Figure 8.24A,B). When leukoplakia occurs within the transformation zone, severe

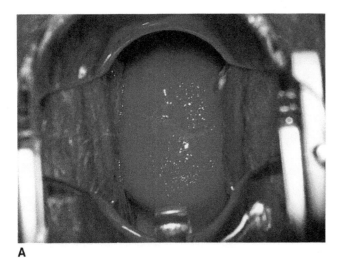

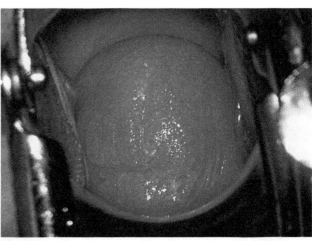

A   B

FIGURE 8.17.   **A, B:** Columnar epithelium of an ectropion of the cervix, demonstrating a red color. The red color of columnar epithelium prior to the application of 3% to 5% acetic acid is derived from the interaction of the colposcope light with the tissue and underlying vessels.

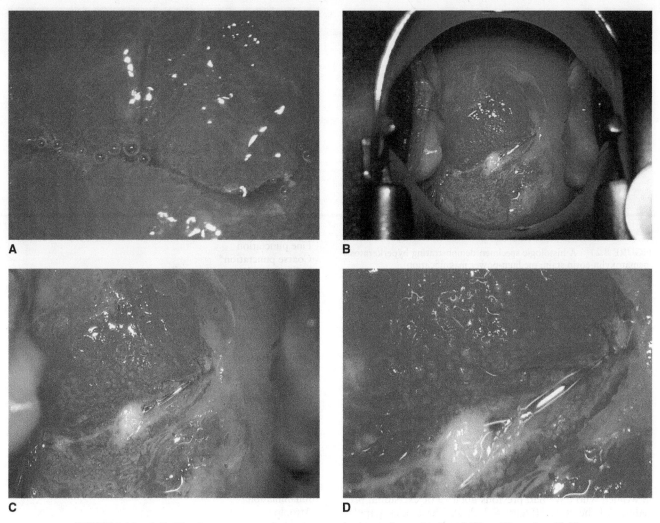

FIGURE 8.18. A–D: Very immature metaplasia appears red prior to the application of 3% to 5% acetic acid. The color results from the interaction of the white light of the colposcope with the epithelium and underlying blood vessels.

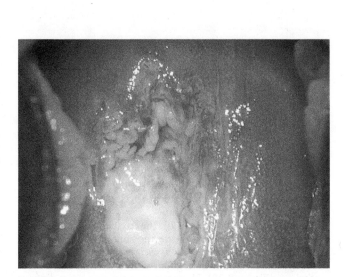

FIGURE 8.19.   The cervix during pregnancy, demonstrating a bluish hue, thick mucus, and eversion of columnar epithelium.

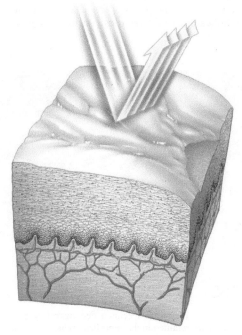

FIGURE 8.20.   The white color of leukoplakia results from the reflection of the white colposcope light back to the colposcopist.

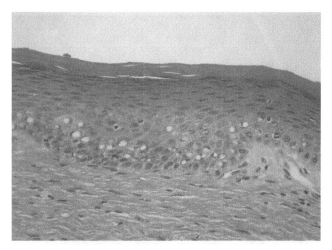

FIGURE 8.21. A histologic specimen demonstrating hyperkeratosis (hematoxylin-eosin stain; medium-power magnification).

TABLE 8.2	INTERNATIONAL FEDERATION OF CERVICAL PATHOLOGY AND COLPOSCOPY (IFCPC) COLPOSCOPIC TERMINOLOGY

I. NORMAL COLPOSCOPIC FINDINGS

Original squamous epithelium
Columnar epithelium
Transformation zone

II. ABNORMAL COLPOSCOPIC FINDINGS

Flat acetowhite epithelium
Dense acetowhite epithelium*
Fine mosaic
Coarse mosaic
Fine punctation
Coarse punctation*
Iodine partial positivity
Iodine negativity*
Atypical vessels*

III. COLPOSCOPIC FEATURES SUGGESTIVE OF INVASIVE CARCINOMA

IV. INADEQUATE COLPOSCOPY

Squamocolumnar junction not visible
Severe inflammation, severe atrophy, trauma
Cervix not visible

V. MISCELLANEOUS FINDINGS

Condylomata
Keratosis
Erosion
Inflammation
Atrophy
Deciduosis
Polyps

* Major change.
Walker P, Dexeus S, DePalo G, Barrasso R, Campion M, Girardi F, et al. International terminology of colposcopy: An updated report from the International Federation for Cervical Pathology and Colposcopy. *Obstet Gynecol* 2003;101:175–177.

underlying neoplastic conditions, including cancer, should be considered.

Leukoplakia varies in color, size, distribution, and contour (Figure 8.25). Leukoplakia is snow-white to silver-white in color. Areas of leukoplakia are frequently well demarcated and can appear as multiple small areas, focal lesions, or as large confluent patches with smooth or irregular borders. Leukoplakia may be macular or raised, but it typically has an elevated smooth or mildly irregular contour. The surface may have a waxy or shiny texture. Consequently, saline and acetic acid solutions may be repelled from the surface much like how water interacts on the surface of a newly waxed automobile. Tiny pinpoint white elevations are commonly noted in women who have had previous ablative or excisional procedures of the cervix (Figure 8.26A,B). These micropapular projections may assume an intermittent linear pattern, radiating from the os much like spokes of a bicycle wheel. Each small elevation represents focal benign parakeratosis overlying a loop capillary. Large elevated patches of keratosis that are referred to as "iceberg leukoplakia" are occasionally seen and may indicate chronic irritation, such as occurs in women

using pessaries to prevent uterine prolapse through the vagina (Figure 8.27A–E)

Usually, no vascular pattern is observed on the surface of leukoplakia. It is important to stress that it is impossible to predict the nature of the epithelium underlying leukoplakia with any degree of certainty by colposcopic visualization. Highly abnormal vascular patterns can be hidden if located sufficiently deep beneath an overlying thickened keratin layer. Peeling away the keratotic tissue frequently produces bleeding that obscures the underlying tissue. In cases of leukoplakia associated with chronic irritation, peeling away the keratotic layer may reveal an underlying fine red punctation.

Colposcopic examination of the tissue surrounding an area of leukoplakia may indicate the source of the keratotic area. For instance, leukoplakia associated with neoplasia may partially cover or abut a large area of abnormal acetowhite epithelium (Figure 8.28). However, an adjoining premalignant epithelium is usually visible only following 3% to 5% acetic

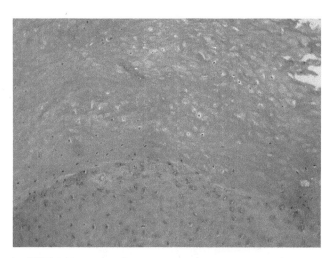

FIGURE 8.22. A histologic specimen demonstrating parakeratosis in which nuclei are retained in the superficial cells (hematoxylin-eosin stain; high-power magnification).

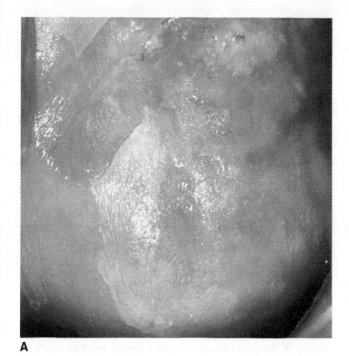

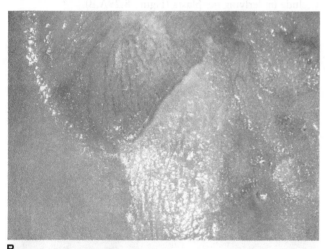

FIGURE 8.23. **A, B:** Leukoplakia of the cervix, demonstrating white, thickened, raised epithelium prior to the application of 3% to 5% acetic acid.

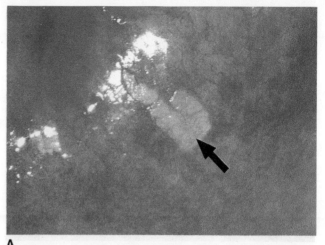

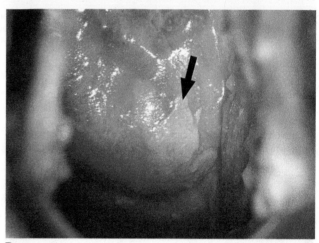

FIGURE 8.24. **A, B:** Leukoplakia noted outside the cervical transformation zone (*arrow*). Such lesions are not likely to be associated with a neoplastic process.

acid application. In many cases, it is possible to detect cancers with leukoplakia prior to acetic acid application.

8.5.1.1.2.1.4 Clinical Significance Leukoplakia is generally thought to be a benign epithelial process, but it is possible for areas of leukoplakia to completely cover and obscure underlying neoplastic lesions. Clinicians should consider all the probable causes of leukoplakia to derive a satisfactory explanation. Colposcopists may initially confuse leukoplakia with cervical candidiasis. However, gentle swabbing will not remove leukoplakia entirely—only perhaps the most superficial layers. Trauma, viral effects, neoplasia, or idiopathic processes must be entertained as possible etiologies for leukoplakia. Leukoplakia is a clinical diagnosis. While a cervical cytologic report of hyperkeratosis or parakeratosis might suggest the presence of lower genital tract leukoplakia, it is not considered an indication for colposcopy in the absence of other cellular abnormalities. However, leukoplakia, observed

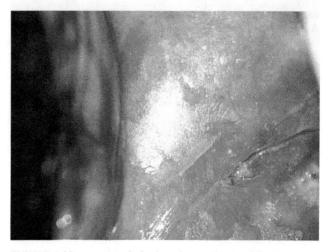

FIGURE 8.25. An irregularly shaped area of leukoplakia located at the 10 o'clock position.

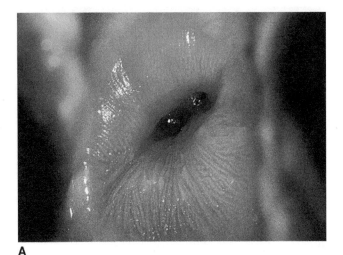

A

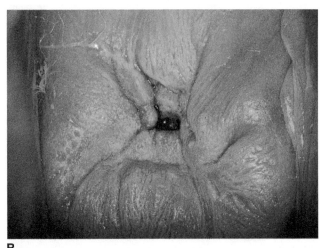

B

FIGURE 8.26.   **A, B:** Parakeratosis noted after loop excision of the cervix. Pinpoint, white elevations of the epithelium are noted. The normally flat squamous epithelium assumes a "grainy," pebbled texture.

during clinical examination of the cervix or when obtaining a Pap test, is an indication for a colposcopic examination. Although most cases of leukoplakia represent a benign process, even lesions presenting in the original squamous epithelium can occasionally indicate a serious neoplastic condition, such as a keratinizing invasive squamous cell carcinoma. Leukoplakia obscures meaningful colposcopic evaluation of other abnormal colposcopic signs. Therefore, regardless of the localization of the area of leukoplakia, a biopsy must be taken to exclude underlying neoplasia (Figure 8.29A,B).

8.5.1.1.2.2 Neoplasia

Unless accompanied by leukoplakia, most premalignant lesions of the cervix cannot be discriminated from normal epithelium

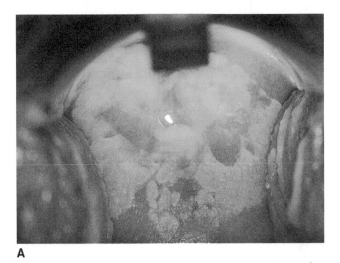

A

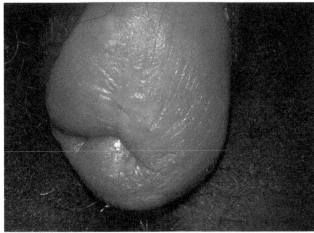

B

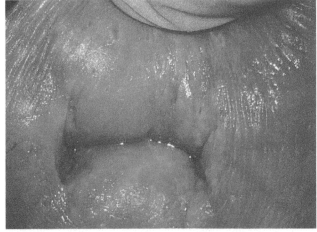

C

FIGURE 8.27.   **A:** Leukoplakia seen in a woman who wore a pessary to prevent uterine prolapse. **B, C:** Hyperkeratosis of the cervix is seen in another woman with uterine prolapse. The tissue thickened in response to the chronic irritation caused by the continual trauma.

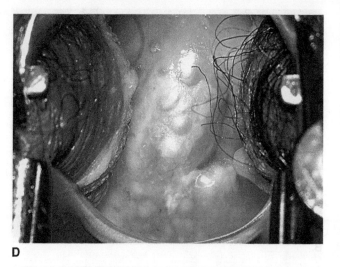

D

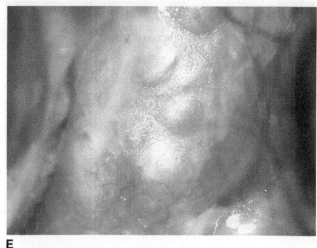

E

FIGURE 8.27.   *(Contined)* In the next case (**D, E**), an area of hyperkeratosis is seen along with prominent nabothian follicles. (Courtesy of, and approved for reproduction by, the International Cervical Cancer (INCCA) foundation.)

based solely on color. Epithelial contrast solutions are generally required to provide sufficient recognition. In contrast, many invasive cancers are recognized by their color following saline application. Advanced cancers may be yellow or red with varying shades of either color. Cancers may also exhibit a "glassy" or gelatinous appearance. Areas of necrotic epithelium may appear brown or black. However, many early cervical cancers appear pink prior to the application of contrast solutions. Cancers may have coexisting areas of leukoplakia that will impart a white color before application of 3% to 5% acetic acid.

8.5.1.2 After Application of 3% to 5% Acetic Acid

8.5.1.2.1 BACKGROUND

The use of 3% to 5% acetic acid during colposcopy was introduced to remove the thin film of mucus that adheres to and may obscure the cervical epithelium. We now recognize its most important role as a contrast agent used to help identify neoplasias of the lower genital tract.

8.5.1.2.2 NORMAL AND ABNORMAL CERVIX

The appearance of mature nonkeratinized squamous epithelium does not change after the application of 3% to 5% acetic acid. Healthy, mature stratified epithelium, whether

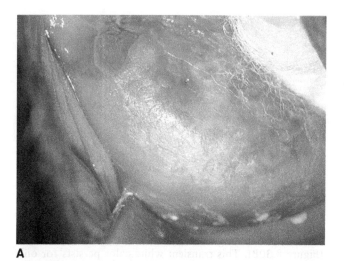

A

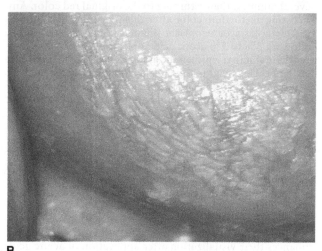

B

FIGURE 8.29.   **A, B:** This area of leukoplakia was associated with an abnormal Pap test. Therefore, biopsy is mandatory to exclude an underlying occult neoplasia.

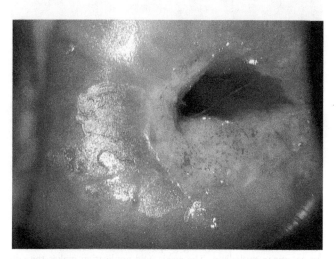

FIGURE 8.28.   Leukoplakia associated with neoplasia abutting against an area of abnormal acetowhite epithelium.

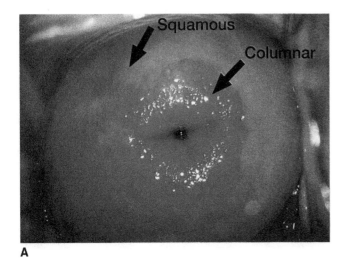

A

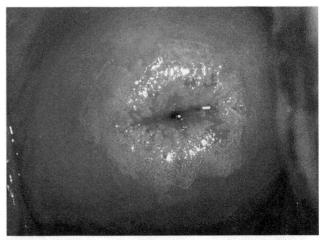

B

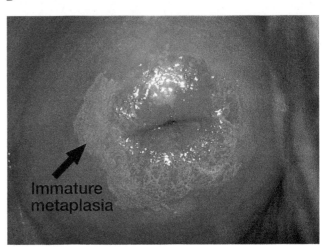

C

FIGURE 8.30. **A:** Before acetic acid application, the squamous epithelium is pink (*arrow*), and columnar and immature metaplasia are red (*arrow*). **B:** Immediately following acetic acid application, squamous epithelium remains pink, columnar epithelium blanches a faint white color, and immature metaplasia becomes translucent white. **C:** The columnar epithelium returns quickly to a red color, while the area of immature metaplasia remains white (*arrow*).

it is original squamous epithelium or mature metaplastic epithelium, retains its pink-tan color after the application of 3% to 5% acetic acid (Figure 8.30A). In contrast, the dark red color of columnar epithelium becomes somewhat blanched, assuming a transient, translucent white color (Figure 8.30B). This transient white color persists for only several minutes, then returning to the original red color. Any persisting acetowhite color after this time represents immature metaplasia or neoplasia (Figure 8.30C). Furthermore, following 3% to 5% acetic acid application, each villus covered by columnar epithelium assumes a more distinct outline, appearing as grape-like or narrow polypoid structures (Figure 8.31). Normal fine caliber capillaries, spaced uniformly about 0.1 mm apart, may not be as readily apparent immediately following 3% to 5% acetic acid application. Slowly, the tiny vessels will become visible at high-power magnification of the colposcope once the acetic acid reaction begins to fade. Nabothian cysts do not change color after acetic acid application (Figure 8.11A–I). They retain their amber yellow color. Prominent branching vessels may be seen overlying the transilluminated thinned epithelium. Gland openings may be seen near the SCJ as round openings in immature metaplasia. The openings are surrounded by a thin rim of acetowhite epithelium (Figure 8.10), which enhances their visualization after application of acetic acid. As will be discussed in Chapter 11, enlarged gland (crypt) openings may be seen in adenocarcinoma *in situ* (AIS). A red color is seen in the center of the gland openings because columnar epithelium remains in the deep gland clefts.

8.5.1.2.2.1 Acetowhite Epithelium

8.5.1.2.2.1.1 Definition Acetowhite epithelium refers to epithelium that transiently changes color from pink or red to white after the application of 3% to 5% acetic acid. The temporary reaction is noted in immature metaplastic,

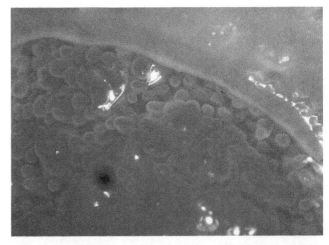

FIGURE 8.31. A high-magnification colpophotograph of columnar epithelium demonstrating grape-like villous structures covered by columnar epithelium. The acetic acid application makes the villi appear more distinct.

reparative, and neoplastic epithelium. The changes may be seen on the cervix, vagina, vulva, or anorectal areas. Acetowhite epithelium is the most common colposcopic feature observed. Although acetowhite epithelium is seen in all cases of CIN, it is also seen in 57% of normal cervices.[14] Prior to the application of acetic acid, immature metaplasia and many neoplastic lesions appear a reddish-pink or normal color. However, seconds to minutes after 3% to 5% acetic acid is applied, these epithelia assume a variably white color (Figure 8.32A–C). The acetowhite effect is transitory and disappears relatively rapidly (2 to 10 minutes) after discontinuing the application of acetic acid.

The acetowhite color can present with different shades of white. Furthermore, the opacity or translucency of the acetowhite response varies across the spectrum of CIN. Normal immature metaplasia and low-grade cervical lesions (CIN 1) usually appear faintly acetowhite or slightly translucent (Figure 8.32B,C). The acetowhite response of high-grade lesions appears more opaque. The amount of whiteness has been shown to be proportional to severity of disease.[15] For example, immature metaplasia and low-grade lesions are frequently described as having a "snow-white" or faintly white appearance that is quite transparent after the application of acetic acid (Figure 8.33A–C). In contrast, high-grade colposcopic lesions (CIN 2,3) may have a "dirty" white appearance that is quite opaque to transillumination of the colposcope light (Figure 8.34A,B). These findings vary depending on patient age. Women older than 35 years of age have CIN lesions that are typically thinner than those in women aged 35 and younger.[16] Consequently, the lesions of women

over 35 may not be as acetowhite as those in younger women. Evaluating the cervix for acetowhite color is a critical part of every colposcopic examination since it allows identification of the presence and distribution of cervical lesions.

8.5.1.2.2.1.2 Etiology

Tissues that reflect the majority of the projected white light from the colposcope back to the colposcopist or temporarily absorb the white light but emit most of the white light back appear acetowhite (Figure 8.35A–C). The exact mechanism responsible for the transient acetic acid–induced color change is unknown and, therefore, continues to be debated. However, there are several potential mechanisms for the acetowhite color. Acetic acid may produce osmotic changes in the tissue that cause a diffusion of intracellular fluid to the extracellular space. The transient transfer of fluid from within the cells to the extracellular space causes tissues to temporarily assume a greater nuclear-to-cytoplasmic ratio. Consequently, the intracellular cytoplasm becomes concentrated, less free water is present, and the cells become more reflective to white light. Increasing nuclear density results in less absorption and more reflection of light. Another postulated explanation is that acetic acid may induce conformational changes in either intracellular proteins (especially intermediate filaments such as cytokeratin proteins) or the nuclear matrix that render selective tissues more reflective to white light.

8.5.1.2.2.1.3 Colposcopic Appearance

Acetowhite areas are visualized colposcopically as transient but colposcopically distinct regions of white epithelium within normal surrounding pink or red epithelium. It is important to visualize the cervix as the 3% to 5% acetic acid is applied and the acetowhitening

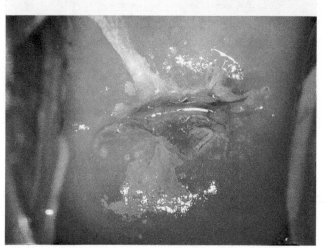

A

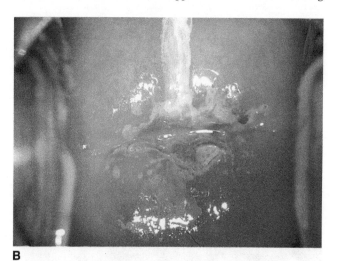

B

FIGURE 8.32. The cervix (A) before and (B, C) after acetic acid application. An acetowhite low-grade lesion gradually appears on the posterior lip of the cervix. Mucus (seen in [B] and [C]) can obstruct complete visualization if it cannot be removed. Manipulation from side to side, as demonstrated here, can resolve this problem.

C

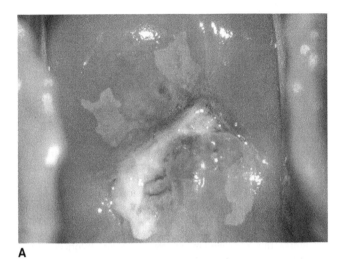

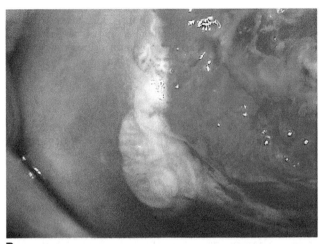

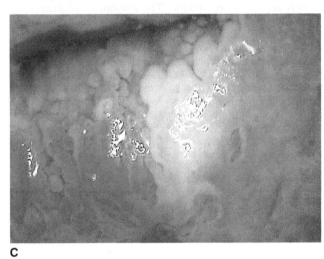

FIGURE 8.33.   **A:** Geographic areas of CIN 1, demonstrating a transparent acetowhite color. **B, C:** CIN 1 can also be snowy white in color.

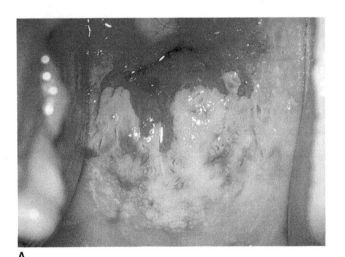

FIGURE 8.34.   Acetowhite epithelium associated with CIN 3 that demonstrates an opaque acetowhite color in both (**A**) and (**B**).

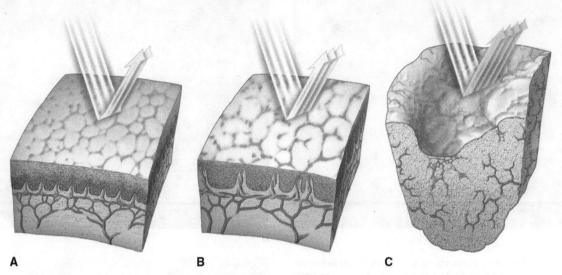

A   **B**   **C**

FIGURE 8.35.   **A–C:** After 3% to 5% acetic acid has been applied to the cervix, the resulting acetowhite color is determined by the interaction of the colposcope light with the epithelium and blood vessels. The white color of CIN 1 is (**A**) more translucent white and not as opaque as that seen with (**B**) CIN 3 or (**C**) invasive cancer.

attains its maximum affect (Figure 8.36A–C). Acetowhite epithelium may be unifocal or multifocal, positioned within or outside the cervical transformation zone. The shade of white can include translucent white, snow-white, off-white, gray, and yellow, with varying degrees of luster and opacity. Color depends on the cellular nuclear-to-cytoplasmic ratio; thickness and type of epithelium; underlying type, caliber, and spacing of the vasculature; and duration, concentration, and coverage of acetic acid.

The rates of development and persistence of acetowhite color vary depending on whether the tissue is normal or abnormal, and whether 3% or 5% acetic acid is used. The acetowhite effect observed in normal immature metaplastic epithelium develops most rapidly. Since more time is required for abnormal epithelium to turn acetowhite, colposcopists must always observe the cervix for several minutes to ensure that the maximum acetowhite effect is observed. A second acetic acid application aids and hastens the onset of the acetowhite color. On second application, one should usually allow 1 to 2 minutes for the full development of an acetowhite color to occur. High-grade lesions (especially regions of CIN 3 retain the acetowhite effect for a longer time (5 to 10 minutes) than do less-severe grades of neoplasia.[15] To maintain the acetowhite effect, many clinicians reapply acetic acid continuously during the entire colposcopic examination. A quicker, perhaps more pronounced, acetowhite response is noted with 5% acetic acid compared with the less concentrated 3% acetic acid. The transient color change persists for a greater duration when using 5% acetic acid, but the more concentrated solution may cause a slightly greater burning sensation when applied to women with fair complexions or women suffering from a lower genital tract inflammatory process, such as vaginitis or vulvitis.

Evaluation of specific colposcopic features of acetowhite epithelium—degree and opacity of whiteness, lesion edges or margin, size, and surface contour—facilitates the differentiation of acetowhite epithelium associated with normal tissue from acetowhite epithelium associated with pathologic conditions (Figure 8.37A,B). For example, most neoplastic lesions have a distinct margin with a

greater degree of acetowhite color than seen in immature metaplasia. Moreover, the surface epithelium of neoplastic lesions may appear thicker, raised, and more opaque or "dense." Lesion size is useful in determining the nature of observed acetowhite changes. Except for large cervical condyloma, in general, as lesion surface area increases, so does lesion severity.[17] The linear extent of CIN 3 typically does not exceed 15 mm.[18] Furthermore, larger and more severe lesions usually have greater depth of extension into the gland clefts. Specific colors, degree of surface luster or shine, and duration of the acetic acid reaction all reflect the severity of the underlying disease process. Although it is traditionally taught that degree of whiteness correlates with severity of underlying disease, many low-grade HPV-induced lesions will produce a prominent, vivid, snow-white acetic acid reaction (Figure 8.38A–C). Yet, the surface of these opaque lesions appears shiny in contrast with a duller or flat appearance of more severe lesions.

The acetowhite color of normal immature metaplastic epithelium develops rapidly and fades rapidly. It may be difficult to reestablish the same level of acetowhitening by reapplying more acetic acid once the initial acetowhite color has faded. The white color appears translucent, especially in regions of very immature metaplasia (Figure 8.39A,B). As these regions mature, the epithelium may retain the distinctive appearance and contour of the early phases of metaplasia until late in the process. Hence, a gently pebbled texture reflecting the underlying villous remnants may be observed. Frequently, the margins of immature metaplasia are indistinct, as the acetowhite epithelium tends to blend gradually with the adjacent squamous epithelium or mature metaplastic epithelium.

The acetowhite effect observed in regions of low-grade lesions is frequently similar or identical to that observed in regions of immature metaplasia (Figure 8.40A). In other instances, the acetowhite effect observed in low-grade lesions appears more opaque white (Figure 8.40B,C). Reliable discrimination between low-grade lesions and immature metaplasia based on acetowhite color alone is not guaranteed for

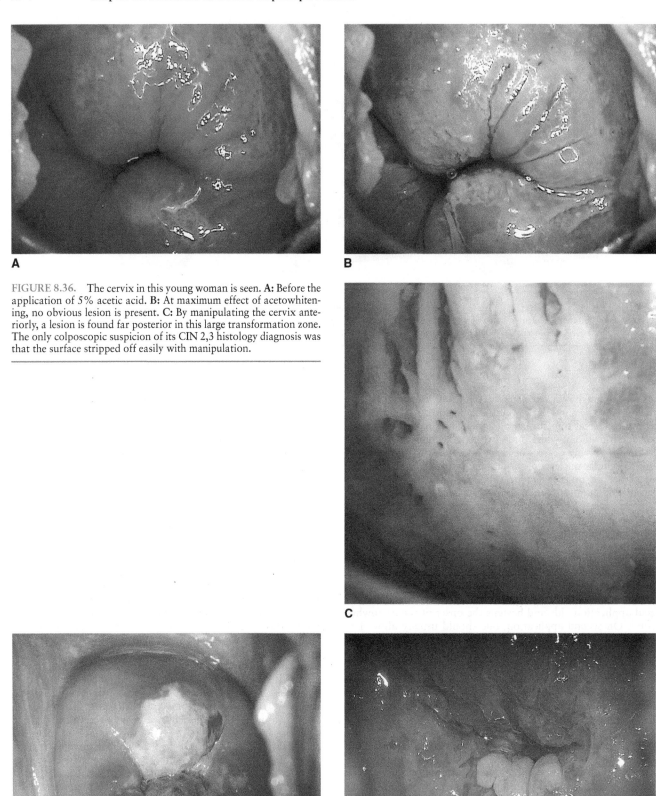

FIGURE 8.36.   The cervix in this young woman is seen. **A:** Before the application of 5% acetic acid. **B:** At maximum effect of acetowhitening, no obvious lesion is present. **C:** By manipulating the cervix anteriorly, a lesion is found far posterior in this large transformation zone. The only colposcopic suspicion of its CIN 2,3 histology diagnosis was that the surface stripped off easily with manipulation.

FIGURE 8.37.   **A:** CIN 3 on the anterior cervical lip and an area of translucent acetowhite immature metaplasia is seen on the posterior lip. The more opaque acetowhite color indicates the area that should be biopsied. Excellent opacity differences are also seen in the second case (**B**). The translucent immature metaplasia on the posterior cervix contrasts with the opaque acetowhite color of the CIN 3. (Courtesy of, and approved for reproduction by, the International Cervical Cancer (INCCA) foundation.)

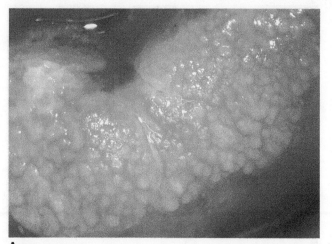

A

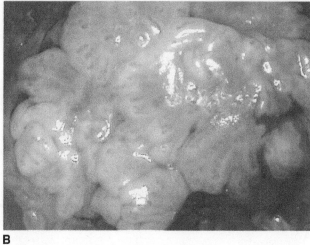

B

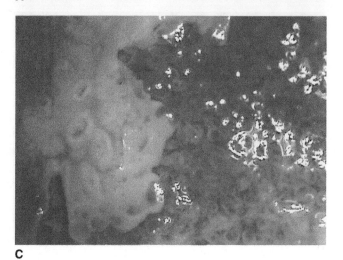

C

FIGURE 8.38. **A:** A snowy-white lesion within a field of normal pink surrounding squamous epithelium. The lesion is characteristic of cervical condyloma. **B:** A classic snowy-white condyloma at the SCJ. **C:** A snowy-white lesion histologically CIN 1 with cupping around gland openings.

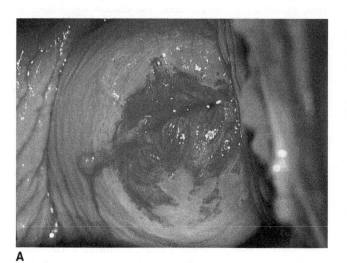

A

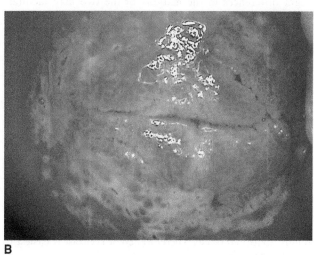

B

FIGURE 8.39.   A translucent acetowhite color on the anterior and posterior cervix, depicting very immature metaplasia. **B:** The translucent acetowhite surrounds many gland openings.

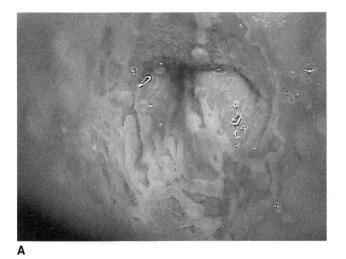

A

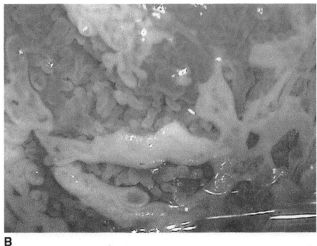

B

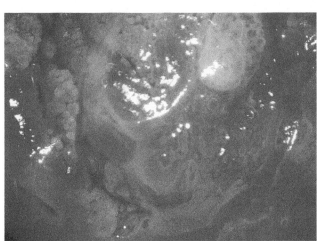

C

FIGURE 8.40. **A:** LSIL Pap referral with areas of translucent and slightly denser acetowhitening in a large transformation zone undergoing metaplastic evolution. **B:** Bridges of different degrees of acetowhitening over the tips of columnar villi probably indicate that the denser acetowhite bridges are CIN 1 and the more translucent are immature metaplasia. However, biopsy is necessary to confirm. **C:** In this colpophotograph, the acetowhite area in the upper right corner of the photograph is more striking than the acetowhitening scattered throughout in the rest of the transformation zone. The more striking acetowhite is a low-grade lesion (CIN 1), while the more translucent acetowhitening is immature metaplasia.

even an expert colposcopist (Figure 8.41A–C). Recognizing slight differences in the margins of the two may facilitate differentiation. The margins of low-grade lesions, compared with those of metaplasia, are usually more clearly demarcated from the adjacent normal epithelium. An asymmetrical, focal acetowhite distribution along the SCJ is more likely indicative of low-grade lesions than of immature metaplasia, but the latter can also have feathery margins (Figure 8.42A–C).

The acetowhite color observed in regions of high-grade lesions (Figure 8.43) and cancer (Figure 8.44) is usually more intense and more persistent than color seen in regions of low-grade lesions or metaplasia. With increasing disease severity, the acetowhite color tends to be more opaque than that seen in lower-grade lesions.[15] A dull appearance, sometimes referred to as "dirty" or "oyster" white, may be noted in the highest-grade lesions. The margins of high-grade acetowhite lesions are almost always well defined, often raised and "rolled," and distinct from surrounding normal and sometimes adjacent mildly abnormal tissue. Therefore, color contrast is easiest to detect in these lesions.

8.5.1.2.2.1.4 Clinical Significance Acetowhite epithelium may represent a wide histologic spectrum from simply normal

epithelium (i.e., immature squamous metaplasia, inflammation, repair) to invasive cancer. The clinical significance of acetowhite epithelium in a particular patient depends on various factors, including patient age, associated cytologic findings and, perhaps most importantly, other colposcopic features. An easily visualized active, normal, immature transformation zone in a young woman may be confused with a low-grade neoplastic process, particularly when the Pap test that prompted the examination indicated atypical squamous cells (ASC) or low-grade squamous intraepithelial lesion (LSIL). Since an active metaplastic process is rarely seen in postmenopausal women because the active transformation zone is typically not present on the ectocervix, acetowhite epithelium noted in older women may more commonly represent a neoplastic process. Similarly, regions of acetowhite color in women with an atypical glandular cells (AGC), AIS, or high-grade squamous intraepithelial lesion (HSIL) Pap test result should be viewed carefully. In general, large prominent acetowhite areas are more likely to represent clinically significant lesions than are small, nonconfluent acetowhite regions.[17] However, large, symmetrical, circumferential acetowhite areas of the cervix in young women may represent simply a normal "congenital" transformation zone or a very large active transformation zone with widespread immature metaplasia (Figure 8.45A,B) (see Chapters 2 and 14).

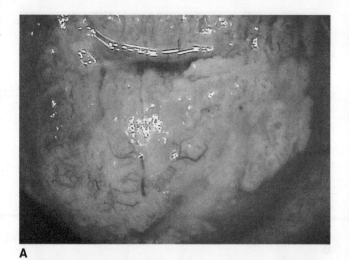

A

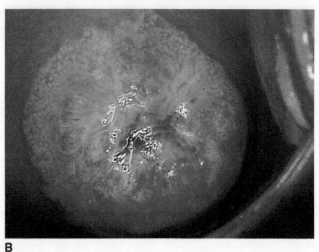

B

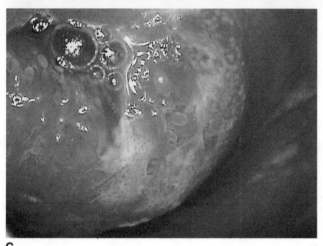

C

FIGURE 8.41.   These areas of acetowhite immature metaplasia cannot reliably be differentiated from CIN without histologic confirmation. **A:** Translucent and denser acetowhite over branching blood vessels. **B, C:** Large symmetrical transformation zone with some areas more densely acetowhite and fading slower in acetowhite effect than other areas.

Although acetowhite epithelium, even in normal processes, can be quite dramatic, its presence alone remains a nondiagnostic entity. Determining indications for biopsy based solely on the presence of acetowhite epithelium promotes nonspecific sampling of many regions of entirely normal epithelium. This is particularly true for adolescent and young women with a cervical ectropion and active immature transformation zone clearly visualized on the ectocervix.[14]

8.5.1.3 After Application of Lugol's Iodine Solution

8.5.1.3.1 BACKGROUND

Iodine solutions temporarily stain different epithelial types to assist colposcopic identification and discrimination. Lugol's iodine solution is a stain for glycogen.[2] For clinical use, Lugol's solution is generally diluted to one-half to one-quarter strength to avoid possible skin and mucus membrane irritation.

8.5.1.3.2 NORMAL CERVIX

8.5.1.3.2.1 Lugol's Iodine–negative and Iodine-positive Epithelium

8.5.1.3.2.1.1   Definition   Iodine-negative or Lugol's-negative epithelium does not contain glycogen. Hence,

nonglycogen-containing normal immature metaplasia appears yellow and normal columnar epithelium appears pink following Lugol's iodine application. In contrast, iodine-positive epithelium contains glycogen and, therefore, normal original vaginal and cervical mucosal squamous epithelium and mature metaplastic epithelium assume a transient mahogany-brown color following Lugol's iodine application. Although maximum glycogen deposition in squamous epithelium is seen in the late follicular phase, immediately prior to ovulation,[19] the brown color response varies little in fully estrogenized women. When positive, the iodine color changes persist for a longer duration than does the more abbreviated white color modification noted following application of 3% to 5% acetic acid to other epithelia.

8.5.1.3.2.1.2   Etiology   The presence of intracellular glycogen determines iodine absorption within tissues. Iodine has an affinity for glycogen. Normal, fully mature metaplastic cells and original squamous cells contain sufficient stores of glycogen and, hence, stain brown, indicating the benign nature of the tissues. Immature metaplastic cells, although benign, reject iodine uptake and consequently appear yellow. Since most neoplastic epithelia have no glycogen, they also stain yellow instead of brown. Just as acetowhite epithelium may denote

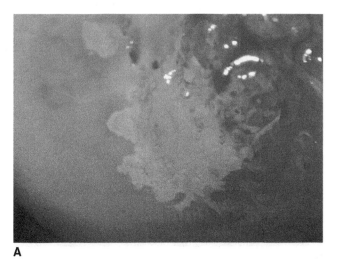

A

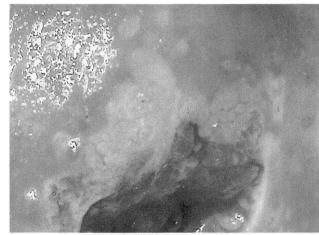

B

FIGURE 8.42. **A:** A low-grade lesion with an irregular "geographic" margin. **B:** A low-grade lesion with an irregular margin is seen in this cervix at the SCJ at 12 to 2 o'clock. **C:** An area of immature metaplasia with a straighter margin and more translucent acetowhitening is seen on the same cervix from 6 to 8 o'clock.

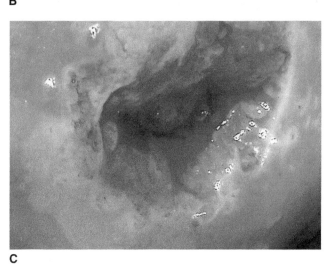

C

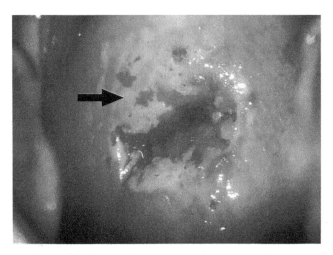

FIGURE 8.43. A HSIL of the cervix following 3% to 5% acetic acid application. The area of CIN 2 (*arrow*) can be contrasted with the less opaque areas of immature metaplasia.

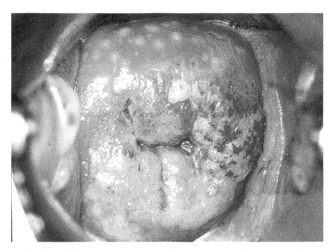

FIGURE 8.44. Acetowhite epithelium of cervical cancer. (Photo courtesy of Dr. Vesna Kesic.)

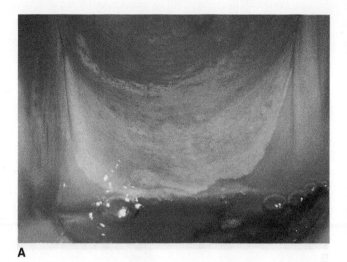

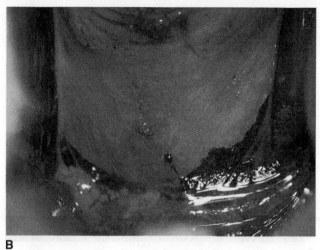

A

B

FIGURE 8.45. **A:** A congenital transformation zone extends into the posterior vaginal fornix. This area may mimic a LSIL or areas of immature metaplasia. **B:** The same area as noted in (**A**) is also seen following the application of Lugol's iodine solution.

either benign or neoplastic tissue, Lugol's iodine–negative epithelium may indicate benign or neoplastic tissue.

8.5.1.3.2.1.3 Colposcopic Appearance During the reproductive years, the original squamous epithelium of the cervix and vagina, as well as areas of mature metaplastic epithelium, are well glycogenated and stain dark brown after the application of Lugol's iodine solution. In contrast, endocervical columnar epithelium and immature metaplastic epithelium do not contain significant amounts of intracellular glycogen and, therefore, appear red or slightly yellow after Lugol's iodine solution is applied (Figure 8.46A,B).

8.5.1.3.2.1.4 Clinical Significance Because Lugol's iodine solution evokes a transient, nonspecific, iodine-negative response, it is not possible to discriminate normal from neoplastic epithelium based only on absence of staining with Lugol's solution alone. Because a yellow color may indicate immature metaplasia, leukoplakia, or neoplasia, other colposcopic signs must be considered to formulate an accurate colposcopic impression. A mahogany-brown color response indicating iodine uptake, however, denotes an invariably benign epithelium, suggesting to the colposcopist that epithelium previously expected to be suspicious for neoplasia is of little concern.

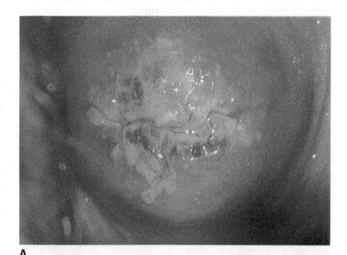

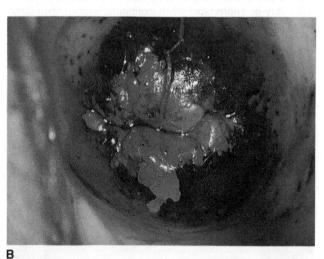

A

B

FIGURE 8.46. **A:** Mature metaplastic epithelium appears pink following 3% to 5% acetic acid application, and a very active transformation zone with numerous shades of acetowhite is seen. **B:** Since it contains glycogen, it stains a rich mahogany brown color. The iodine-negative areas that are yellow represent immature metaplastic epithelium following Lugol's iodine solution application. However, without histologic evaluation it would be difficult to accurately predict whether this is all an entirely normal process or has one or more areas of neoplastic change.

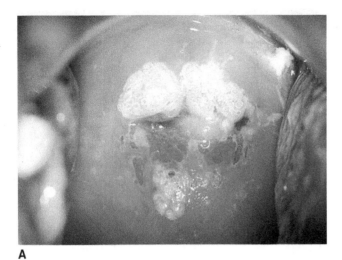

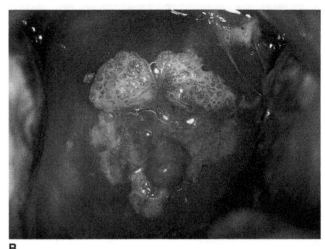

A   **B**

FIGURE 8.47.   An iodine-negative color corresponding to the acetowhite lesions is noted. CIN 1 (**A**) after 3% to 5% acetic acid application and (**B**) following Lugol's iodine application.

8.5.1.3.3 ABNORMAL CERVIX

8.5.1.3.3.1 Lugol's Iodine–negative and Iodine-positive Epithelium

8.5.1.3.3.1.1 Colposcopic Appearance   Neoplastic epithelium always appears yellow (iodine negative) following application of Lugol's iodine solution unless it is eroded, ulcerated, or a glandular neoplasia. Some large low-grade lesions display a variegated yellow/brown patchy uptake, sometimes termed "tortoise-shell" (Figure 8.47A,B), denoting areas of CIN 1 intermingled with areas of normal epithelium. Otherwise, low-grade lesions tend to appear uniformly more orange or darker yellow. In comparison, high-grade lesions can assume a blanched, whitish-yellow color (Figure 8.48A,B). This variation in yellow color may be appreciated when examining women with large, complex, or mixed lesions. Some neoplasias also have a large amount of hyperkeratotic material at the epithelial surface, which turns a characteristic bright yellow color after Lugol's staining. However, attempting to differentiate low-grade CIN

from high-grade CIN simply on the basis of variations in the color of iodine-negative epithelium is not productive, as normal immature metaplastic epithelium also appears yellow or iodine negative following Lugol's iodine application.

While iodine-positive epithelium (mahogany brown) is never considered abnormal, normal-appearing brown epithelium may infrequently obscure dysplastic epithelium residing deeply within gland clefts. Iodine-positive epithelium may also cover the entire ectocervix, falsely conveying a "normal" examination to the colposcopist, while iodine-negative abnormal epithelium may be hidden within the endocervical canal or in the vagina.

8.5.1.3.3.1.2 Clinical Significance   When Lugol's iodine staining is used, iodine-negative epithelium should be considered along with other colposcopic findings, to derive a meaningful colposcopic impression. Even though the contrast agents are complementary, not all colposcopists use Lugol's iodine solution routinely, and some use it only for evaluation of the vagina when colposcopic evaluation of the cervix does

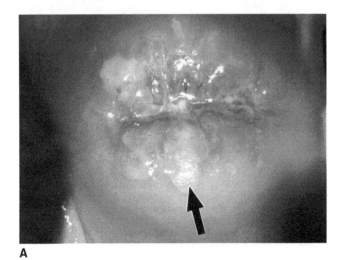

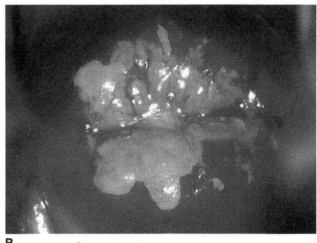

A   **B**

FIGURE 8.48.   A high-grade cervical lesion following (**A**) acetic acid (*arrow*) and (**B**) Lugol's iodine application. A bland whitish-yellow color indicates the absence of glycogen.

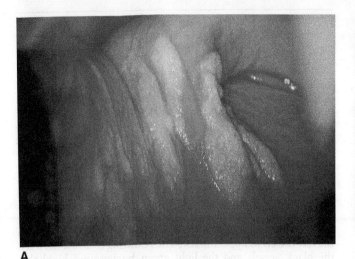 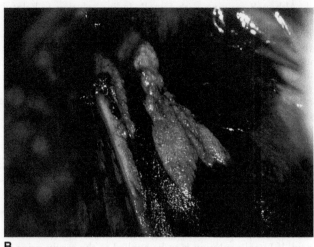

FIGURE 8.49. This woman's cervix appeared normal with colposcopic examination. However, her Pap test was reported as LSIL. Examination of the vagina using (A) 3% to 5% acetic acid and (B) Lugol's solution detected the source of the abnormal cytologic findings.

not appear to identify a source of a significantly abnormal cytology result. Additionally, postmenopausal women and some premenopausal women who use progestin-only contraceptives and are estrogen deficient have little glycogen in the thinner original squamous epithelium and mature metaplastic epithelium. Hence, the atrophic epithelial response to iodine staining will be a light brown to tan color instead of a positive dark mahogany brown. This limited uptake can initially be confused with an iodine-negative response. The sharp contrast between iodine-negative and iodine-positive epithelium, consequently, is diminished. When evaluation with Lugol's iodine is considered important in a woman with estrogen deficiency, a 2- to 3-week course of daily vaginal estrogen therapy prior to colposcopy will augment glycogen deposition in normal epithelium, facilitating the use of this colposcopic aid.

Iodine-negative epithelium seen during colposcopy, although not independently predictive of neoplasia, should be considered suspicious in women with abnormal cervical cytologic findings. This is particularly true for older women and women who have had prior therapy for cervical neoplasia and in whom the SCJ is located within the endocervical canal. Typically, neoplastic

iodine-negative epithelium will correspond to areas of acetowhite epithelium (Figures 8.47A,B and 8.48A,B).

Use of Lugol's iodine solution may be useful when the findings of the colposcopic examination are discordant (i.e., the Pap test indicates significant dysplasia, but the colposcopic examination using 3% to 5% acetic acid is unable to detect similar disease). For example, occasionally, a noteworthy iodine-negative lesion is observed colposcopically on the cervix when no acetowhite lesion can be appreciated. In these rare cases, the source of cytologic abnormality is identified only by use of Lugol's iodine solution.

Since acetowhite effects in the vaginal mucosa are generally more difficult to appreciate, Lugol's iodine solution is also particularly helpful in evaluating the vagina (Figure 8.49A,B). A careful Lugol's iodine examination of the vagina may identify lesions that explain discordance between a positive cytologic finding and a negative cervical examination. Therefore, Lugol's iodine examinations of the vagina are critical prior to conization for discordant pathology/colposcopy findings. Lugol's iodine is also frequently used to demarcate the outer margins requiring ablation or excision just prior to therapy (Figure 8.50A,B).

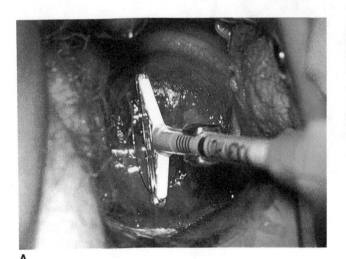 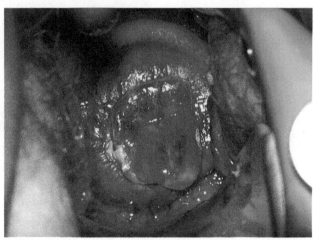

FIGURE 8.50. All yellow iodine-negative areas of the cervix (A) are excised using the loop electrode. After removing the specimen (B), no iodine-negative areas are seen, indicating that all immature metaplasia and neoplasia have been removed from the ectocervix.

Although staining with Lugol's iodine solution is helpful in delineating the size and distribution of many lesions and invasive cancers, iodine staining has a number of drawbacks that limit its usefulness. One limitation, as noted earlier is that a number of nonneoplastic conditions produce nonstaining areas—immature metaplasia, hyperkeratosis, inflammation, scar tissue, congenital transformation zones (CTZs), and atrophy. Sometimes, the thinly stretched normal mature metaplastic epithelium overlying a nabothian follicle will appear as an iodine-negative round area with indistinct margins. The same area will not appear white following 3% to 5% acetic acid application. The most serious limitation is that iodine staining will mask most other colposcopic signs, including the vascular pattern and variations in acetowhite color. Vascular patterns are critical to the recognition of invasive cancers and important in evaluation for CIN. Therefore, Lugol's iodine staining should be performed only after a careful colposcopic assessment has been performed using saline and 3% to 5% acetic acid. If Lugol's solution is to be applied to the cervix prior to biopsy, colposcopists must visually remember the most abnormal area to direct biopsy placement. If necessary, topical benzocaine solution or gel can be used to quickly reverse iodine effects on glycogen-containing epithelium.

8.5.2 Vasculature

8.5.2.1 Background

Blood vessels of various types can be observed easily through high-power magnification (10× to 15×) of the colposcope (Figure 8.51). The specific vessel pattern, vessel caliber, and intercapillary distance between these vessels help differentiate normal from abnormal vessels.[20] Because of the vasoconstrictive effects of 3% to 5% acetic acid, vessels are best studied after the application of normal saline and before 3% to 5% acetic acid is applied. Although a 3% to 5% acetic acid application may transiently diminish the vascular pattern, the ensuing vessel contrast against a white background often enhances colposcopic inspection of vessels, particularly when there is punctation or mosaic. Vessel visualization may be accentuated by use of the colposcope's red free (green) filter, which causes the red vessels to appear black. The resulting contrast between the black vessels and the light green background highlights small delicate vessels that might otherwise blend into the pink background. At times, abnormal vessels resemble normal vessels. Normal vessels may also mimic abnormal vessels. To identify alterations in blood vessels and vascular patterns most

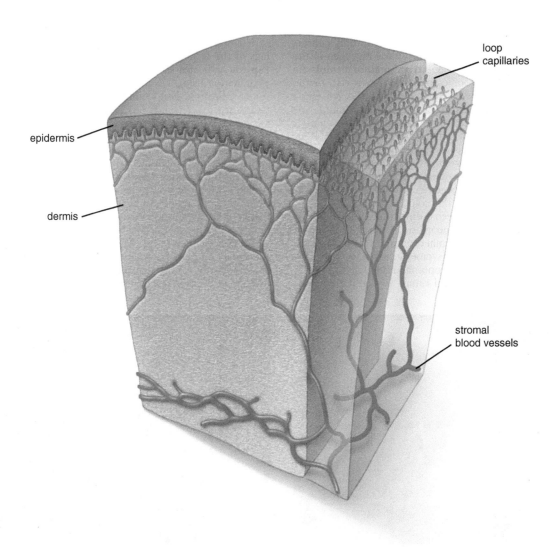

FIGURE 8.51. The vascular supply to the cervical epithelium. Small loop capillaries terminate in the lower one-third of squamous epithelium.

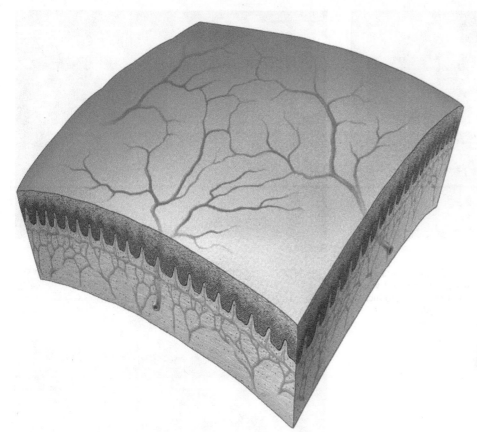

FIGURE 8.52. Network vessels forming a vascular plexus.

indicative of disease, colposcopists must recognize normally appearing vascular patterns.

8.5.2.2 Vasculature of the Normal Cervix

As outlined in Chapter 2 (Anatomy and Histology of the Normal Female Lower Genital Tract), the original squamous epithelium has two types of blood vessels, referred to as network and hairpin capillaries.[3,4] Network vessels form a vascular plexus that lies in the submucosal stroma beneath the basement membrane (Figure 8.52). When viewed through the colposcope, the vascular plexus appears as a fine reticular network of small terminal vessels that are haphazardly arranged (Figure 8.53). The network vessels underlying the original squamous epithelium are most prominent when they become hyperemic and dilated during pregnancy or as a result of cervicovaginal infections. Additionally, these vessels are seen readily in patients who take oral contraceptives and when connective tissue papillae extending into the squamous epithelium decrease in height, as in postmenopausal women. Under these conditions, the vessels appear to form vascular pseudoanastomoses, which can be seen under the squamous epithelium (Figure 8.54A–C). The second type of vessels, hairpin terminal vessels, extends toward the epithelial surface in the connective tissue papillae. These vessels have both afferent (arterial) and efferent (venous) branches (Figure 8.55). When viewed along the vessel axis, they appear as fine red dots or punctation. When viewed obliquely, the afferent and efferent capillaries resemble hairpins or fine loops. Capillaries in normal epithelium are closely spaced and uniformly distributed. The intercapillary distance ranges from 50 to 250 μm with an average distance of 100 μm.[20]

The vessels underlying the metaplastic epithelium of the transformation zone vary depending on the degree of maturation of the transformation zone. In zones of immature metaplasia, prominent long parallel vessels or branched vessels oriented radially to the external os are often seen (Figure 8.56A–G).

Parallel vessels are somewhat dilated and course horizontally for rather long distances near the surface of the epithelium. Branched vessels taper along their course and have a regular or orderly appearance. Branches from the long terminal vessels usually emerge at an acute angle, much like branches projecting from a tree trunk. These branches have a smaller diameter than the parent vessel. Each succeeding branching vessel is of a smaller caliber (Figure 8.57). At the end of the long terminal vessels, a network of fine capillaries that have a normal intercapillary distance can be seen. These tree-like branched vessels can be observed, greatly dilated, overlying nabothian cysts or cervical polyps (Figure 8.58A–G). In addition to long terminal vessels, the transformation zone also has network vessels

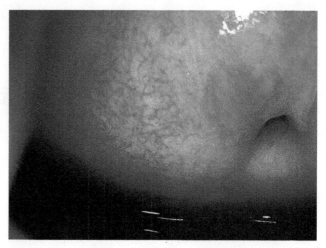

FIGURE 8.53. Network vessels of the normal cervix, demonstrating a fine reticular network of small terminal vessels that are haphazardly arranged. (Photo courtesy of Dr. Kenneth L. Noller.)

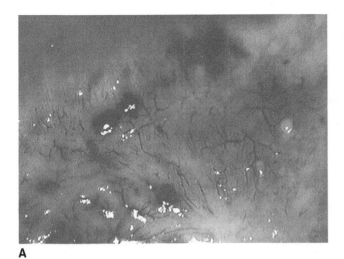

A

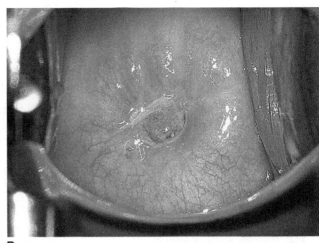

B

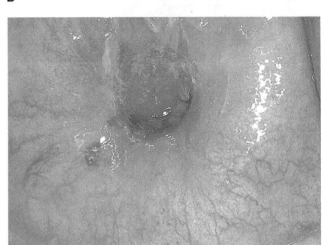

C

FIGURE 8.54. **A:** Network vessels demonstrating pseudoanastamoses beneath the squamous epithelium. Larger network blood vessels are seen in (**B**) and (**C**). (Courtesy of, and approved for reproduction by, the International Cervical Cancer (INCCA) foundation.)

FIGURE 8.55. Hairpin terminal vessels obliquely oriented toward the surface of the epithelium, demonstrating afferent and efferent capillary loops.

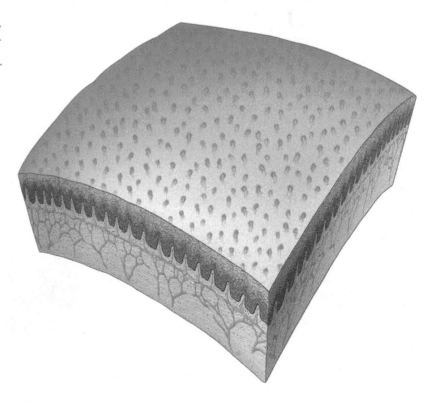

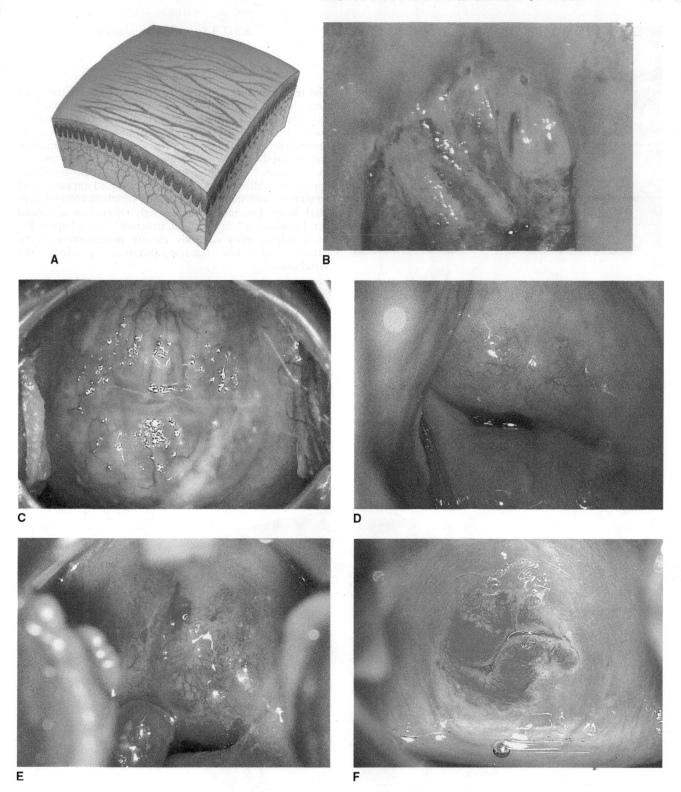

FIGURE 8.56. **A:** Long parallel blood vessels usually seen in (**B, C**) immature metaplasia. **C–E:** Branched vessels are also more commonly seen in immature metaplasia. Large parallel blood vessels (**F**) are seen easily using the red free (green) filter (**G**). (**A** [illustration]: copyright © 2004, 2011. ASCCP. All rights reserved. **B–G** [Colpophotographs]: courtesy of, and approved for reproduction by, the International Cervical Cancer (INCCA) foundation.)

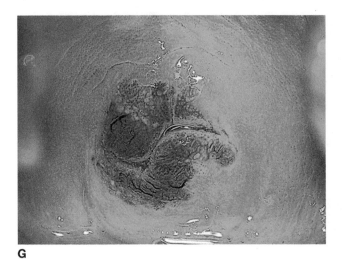

G

FIGURE 8.56.   *(Continued)*

8.5.2.3 Specific Vasculature

8.5.2.3.1 PUNCTATION

8.5.2.3.1.1 Definition

The term *punctation* is used to refer to the appearance of single-looped terminal capillaries within stromal papillae of either the original squamous epithelium or the transformation zone. These twisted vessels run perpendicularly or obliquely toward the epithelial surface. The vessels are a variation of hairpin capillaries. When viewed end-on vertically through the attenuated epithelium overlying them, these capillaries appear as reddish points or dots. The stippled appearance of punctation corresponds to the tops of simple or complex capillary loops. Punctation was formerly referred to as "grund der Leukoplakie" or "ground structure" (see Chapter 1).[5] Most colposcopists currently classify punctation as being either fine punctation or coarse punctation, depending on the vessel caliber.

8.5.2.3.1.2 Etiology

Punctation is a nondiagnostic colposcopic finding, since it may represent either a normal vascular pattern or an abnormal modification of existing vascular architecture. All normal cervices have stromal papillae containing single-looped capillaries, both within the original squamous epithelium, and within the metaplastic epithelium of the transformation zone. Vessels within the stromal papillae extend within the lower third of the epithelium to perfuse differentiating cells. The stromal papillae observed in the original squamous epithelium are formed during embryogenesis and remain throughout life. When cervicitis is present, especially when it is associated with *Trichomonas vaginalis* infection, the hairpin capillaries become dilated and appear to extend higher into the connective tissue papillae, immediately underneath the surface. Marked inflammation,

under the surface epithelium, and hairpin capillaries that can project into stromal papillae of the maturing metaplastic epithelium in a manner similar to that seen in the original squamous epithelium.

The vessels of the endocervix consist of afferent and efferent loops of terminal vessels that extend toward the surface in the lamina propria of each of the columnar cell–covered endocervical villi. When viewed tangentially at high magnification, these vessels also appear as hairpin loops (Figure 8.5A,B). Endocervical vessels are not easily discerned by casual colposcopic inspection, however, especially if viewed end-on.

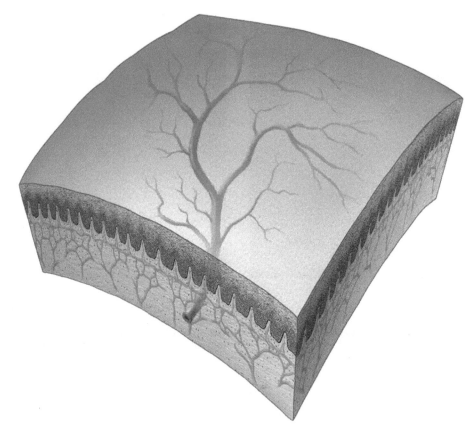

FIGURE 8.57.   A branched vessel appears much like a tree with a trunk, branches, and twigs. The caliber of the vessels gradually constrict towards the terminal vessels.

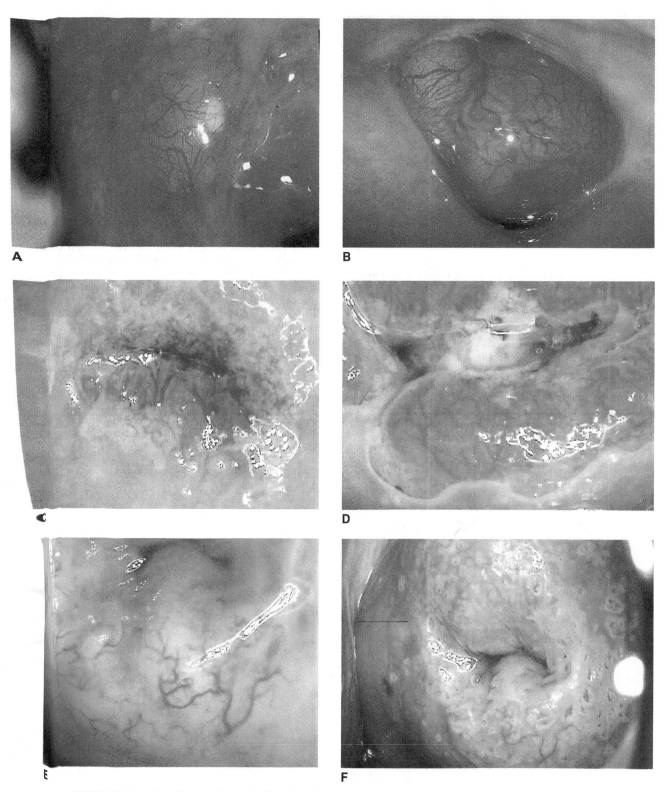

FIGURE 8.58.   Tree-like vessels greatly dilated overlying (**A**) a nabothian cyst and (**B**) a cervical polyp. C, D: Branching blood vessels under columnar epithelium with adjacent immature metaplasia. **E:** Prominent branching vessels in large transformation zone can occasionally look alarming, but (**F**) after the application of 5% acetic acid, these clearly lie under immature and maturing metaplasia. However, a dense acetowhite area is noted at 6 o'clock extending into the canal.

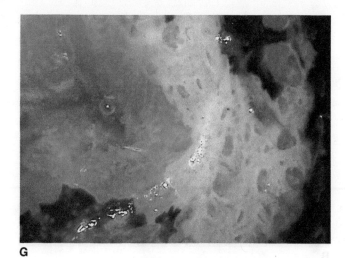

G

FIGURE 8.58. *(Continued)* **G:** Following Lugol's application, the top of the area of matured metaplasia overlying much of the area with branching blood vessels stains dark mahogany brown, whereas adjacent immature metaplasia does not stain.

Punctation occurring in the transformation zone is derived from hairpin capillaries in stromal papillae that invaginate perpendicular to the epithelial surface. In the transformation zone, these papillae arise during the development of squamous metaplasia. Prior to the development of squamous metaplasia, the region that will become the transformation zone is covered by columnar villi, each of which have a central afferent and efferent loop capillary. During the transformation process, the clefts or folds between the villi become filled by immature metaplastic epithelium (Figure 8.8C,D). Initially, the original afferent and efferent capillary loop remains central within each villus. As the clefts fill with metaplastic epithelium, the vessels and encompassing stroma develop into stromal papillae, similar to those of the original squamous epithelium. The vessels in the stromal papillae adjacent to the blocks of immature metaplastic squamous epithelium can appear as a fine vascular punctation pattern when viewed through the colposcope. When examined histologically, the epithelium usually demonstrates "epithelial pegs" with adjacent prominent stromal papillae that are elongated and extend almost to the epithelial surface. The "epithelial pegs" are of a variable width and often branch. The immature metaplastic epithelium usually forms a sharp histologic junction with mature metaplastic epithelium. This explains why regions of punctation, even when associated with normal evolving metaplastic epithelium, are usually sharply delineated colposcopically within contrasting acetowhite epithelium. As regions of metaplastic epithelium mature, the stromal papillae become less prominent and more flattened, and extend for a shorter distance toward the epithelial surface. These alterations eliminate the punctation vascular pattern seen in mature metaplastic epithelium.

The punctation that occurs in regions of neoplasia can be thought of as an accentuation of the process by which

such as that induced by *T. vaginalis*, will often result in hairpin capillaries with two or more loops at the top. This particular manifestation of hairpin capillaries has been referred to as staghorn or double capillaries (Figure 8.59). When present on the cervix, the appearance is often called the "strawberry" cervix. Punctation secondary to inflammation is diffuse or clustered in distribution and usually not confined within sharply bordered areas (Figure 8.60A–E). However, it should be noted that double capillaries can also be observed in regions of high-grade lesions (CIN 2,3).

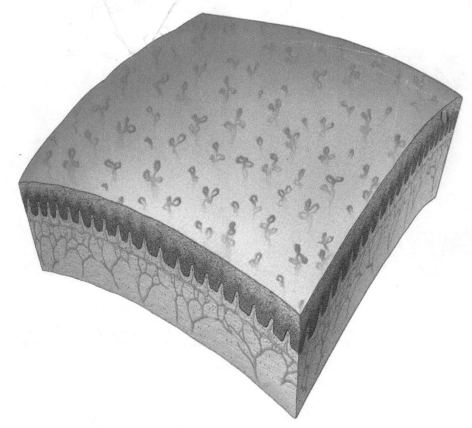

FIGURE 8.59. Double-loop capillaries seen with Trichomonas cervicitis.

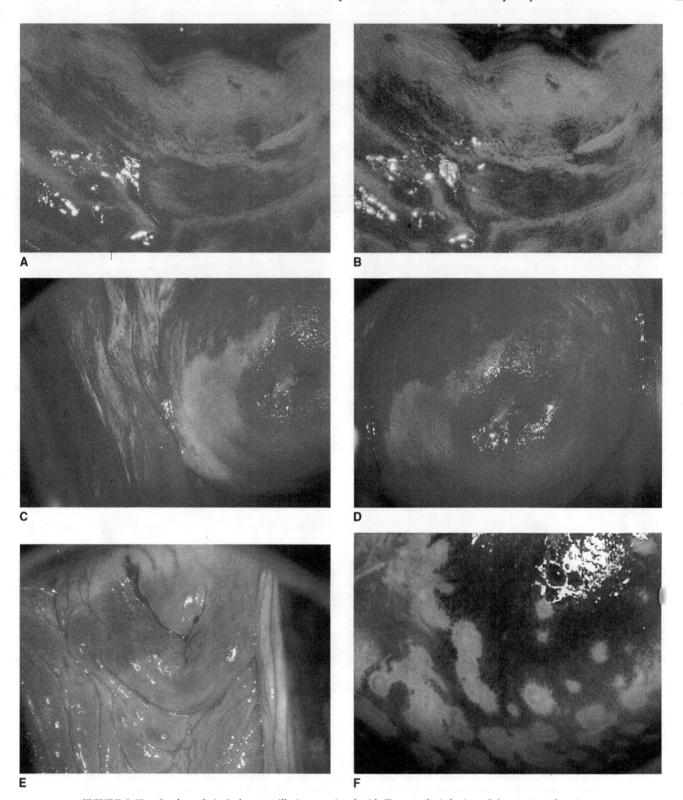

FIGURE 8.60. Staghorn hairpin loop capillaries associated with *T. vaginalis* infection of the cervix and vagina. These diffuse punctate vessels are seen (**A**) without and (**B**) with use of the red free (green) filter. In another patient, diffuse punctation is noted in the vagina (**C**) and on the cervix (**D**) caused by an inflammatory process. **E:** The last patient also has a diffuse vascular inflammatory response on the cervix and in the vagina. **F:** A "strawberry cervix" following Lugol's application demonstrates larger erosions that do not take up any Lugol's, and are therefore pink, and tiny yellow-staining dots that overlie nonconfluent staghorn loop capillaries.

fine punctation arises in the transformation zone during the development of squamous metaplasia (Figure 8.61A). Proliferating blocks of neoplastic epithelium may cause compression of these vessels. Initially, laterally expanding epithelial compressive forces may impede venous return and cause

a dilatation of the loop capillaries (Figure 8.61B). Further growth and epithelial expansion cause complete arterial occlusion of some of the capillaries, now surrounded by expanding cellular blocks of neoplasia, and lateral displacement of remaining loop capillaries. The resulting obliteration

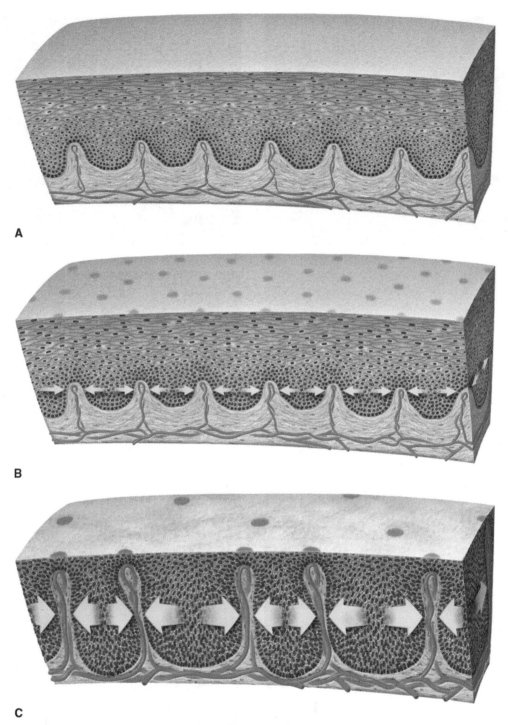

FIGURE 8.61.   A: Loop capillaries are of normal fine caliber, with uniform distribution and narrow intercapillary spacing prior to any neoplastic process. **B:** Once neoplastic cells develop, they expand to perhaps exert pressure on these capillaries. Venous occlusion causes the vessels to dilate. With CIN 1, the intercapillary spacing and distribution remain similar to that seen in normal epithelium. However, with CIN 3, the vessels dilate further because of greater venous occlusion. **C:** As the blocks of neoplastic tissue grow, the vessels are displaced outwards and some arterioles become occluded. Now the intercapillary distance is increased and randomly distributed.

and displacement of some of the central capillaries creates a greater intercapillary distance, or space, between adjoining vessels (Figure 8.61C). The surrounding vessels also dilate more and are referred to as coarse punctation. Histologically, the neoplastic epithelium forms epithelial pegs that are wider and more irregular than those formed by immature metaplastic epithelium. Between these nests of neoplastic epithelium, tall stromal papillae containing the loop capillaries extend to just beneath the surface.

Punctation occurring in regions of neoplasia can evolve independently of the underlying villous angioarchitecture. For example, it has been suggested that changes of the stroma and blood vessels producing epithelial pegs almost invariably accompany the neoplastic process.[5] This suggestion is based on the fact that punctation is often observed in high-grade neoplastic lesions of the vulva, penis, and vagina, which lack a preexisting papillary endocervical configuration. Furthermore, HPV-induced condylomas at mucosal sites other than the cervix frequently contain punctation. Although controversial, evidence suggests that subepithelial angiogenesis may occur in premalignant as well as malignant lesions.[7]

8.5.2.3.1.3 Colposcopic Appearance

Punctation appears as tiny red dots of variable dimensions usually present within an area of acetowhite epithelium. The acetowhite effect that occurs after the application of acetic acid provides an excellent background against which red punctation is seen. However, when there is a strong acetowhite effect in the surface epithelium, the acetowhite epithelium can reflect so much light that the underlying vascular pattern is obscured. Additionally, 3% to 5% acetic acid causes temporary vasoconstriction. Hence, it is easier to initially overlook fine punctation than coarse punctation. In cases wherein the acetowhite effect obscures the vascular pattern, the underlying red vascular pattern will reappear as the acetowhite effects begin to fade, enabling visualization of coarse and particularly fine punctation (Figure 8.62A,B).

In some instances, however, punctation is better seen prior to the application of acetic acid. Although punctation can also be observed after normal saline is applied to the cervix, novice colposcopists may have difficulty observing fine punctation prior to applying acetic acid because of the lack of contrast provided by an acetowhite background. Coarse punctation is more readily apparent following saline

application to the cervix. The red free (green) filter makes it easier to recognize the punctation, which appears as small black dots (Figure 8.63A–D).

Both the size or diameter of punctation (caliber of the loop vessels) and the distance between punctation (intercapillary distance) vary depending on the severity of underlying disease. Usually, as the caliber of the loop capillaries forming punctation increases, so does the intercapillary distance and the severity of the underlying disease.[20,21] Fine punctation is a regular pattern of looped capillaries of narrow diameter, usually closely and uniformly spaced (Figure 8.64). In fine punctation, the intercapillary distance more closely resembles the distances found between villi of the original columnar epithelium, and for this reason, fine punctation is commonly found in immature metaplasia (Figure 8.65A–D). Since the distance between each capillary is minimal, fine punctation appears as a delicate stippling when present in a circumscribed acetowhite lesion (Figure 8.66A–D). Fine punctation often occurs together with a fine mosaic vascular pattern (Figures 8.66A–D and 8.67A,B).

In coarse punctation, the capillaries appear more pronounced because the loop capillaries are dilated and the intercapillary distance is greater. Furthermore, coarse punctation is more irregularly or chaotically spaced (Figure 8.68A–D). The intercapillary distances in normal epithelium rarely (1.8%) measure more than 300 µm.[20] With increasing severity of neoplasia, the percentage of capillaries found to be separated by >300 µm increases significantly. In CIN 3 lesions with punctation, 57% exhibit intercapillary distances of more than 300 µm.[20] These coarse, dilated capillary loops are usually evident to experienced colposcopists prior to acetic acid application. After acetic acid application, very dilated capillaries (papillary punctation) may appear to project above the surface of the surrounding, densely acetowhite epithelium. The dilated capillaries are separated from each other by randomly wide intercapillary distances (Figure 8.69). Microinvasive cervical cancer should be considered when these large diameter vessels also visibly dilate above the surface of the epithelium, rendering the appearance of a pincushion-like surface. These vessels individually reflect the tangential colposcope light to resemble a field of tiny white stars. Evaluation of this papillary punctation at higher colposcopic magnification may show tiny corkscrew-shaped capillaries, which should not be confused with atypical blood vessels. Coarse punctation often occurs together with a coarse mosaic vascular pattern (Figure 8.70).

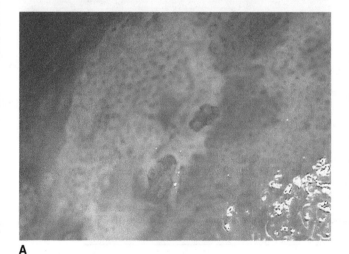

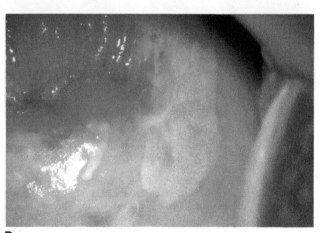

A   B

FIGURE 8.62.   **A, B:** Fine punctation seen against faintly acetowhite epithelium. (Courtesy of, and approved for reproduction by, the International Cervical Cancer (INCCA) foundation.)

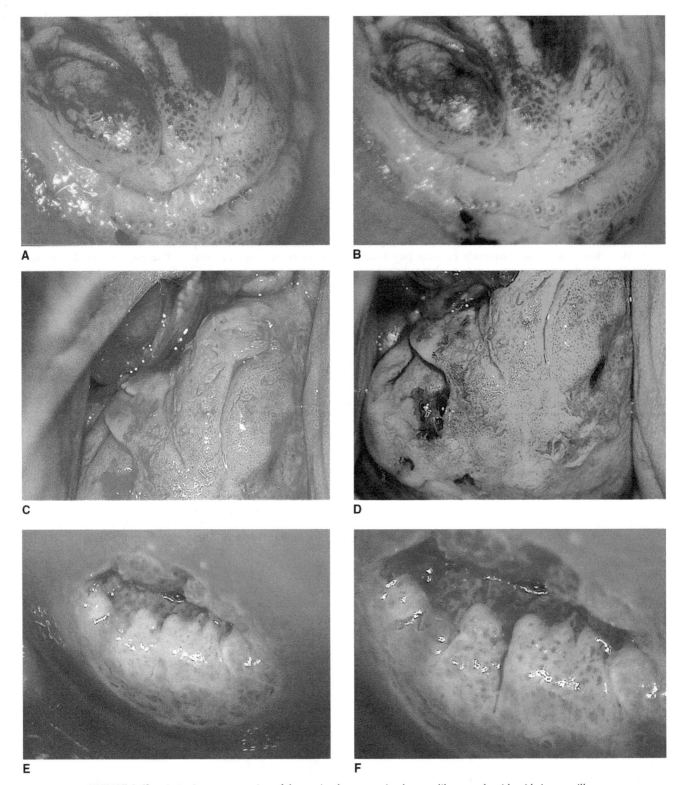

FIGURE 8.63.   **A, B:** Coarse punctation of the cervix, demonstrating large-caliber vessels with wide intercapillary distances. These vessels are prominent both after acetic acid (**A**) and (**B**) when viewed using the red free (green) filter. **C, D:** The second case also demonstrates coarse punctation visualized following the application of acetic acid, without (**C**) and with (**D**) use of the red free (green) filter. **E, F:** Coarse punctation in a CIN 2,3 lesion. Note the location of the high-grade lesion central near the os, with normal metaplasia adjacent posterior to the lesion and most distant from the os. (Courtesy of, and approved for reproduction by, the International Cervical Cancer (INCCA) foundation.)

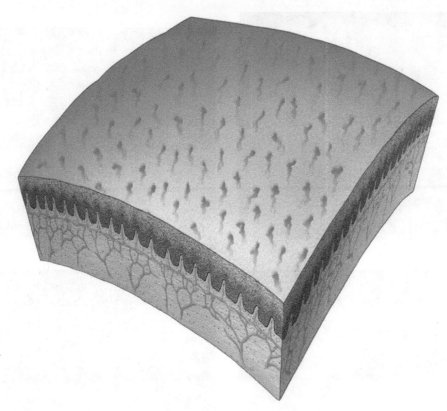

FIGURE 8.64. Fine-caliber punctation demonstrating a uniformly spaced pattern in CIN 1. (Copyright © 2004, 2011. ASCCP. All rights reserved.)

8.5.2.3.1.4 Clinical Significance

Punctation was originally described by Hinselmann[22] when he noted vascular changes following removal of the keratin layer overlying invasive cancer. Therefore, early colposcopists equated punctation with the "matrix of cancer." Punctation became a key criterion for defining the atypical transformation zone, which was erroneously considered to be a unique entity with malignant potential. Today, most colposcopists recognize that the vascular changes of punctation can occur in normal epithelium, inflammatory epithelium, and the full spectrum of squamous neoplasia. Therefore, it is not simply the presence or absence of punctation but rather vessel caliber, uniformity of distribution, and intercapillary distance of punctation that predict disease severity.

Fine punctation can occur in a variety of conditions, including immature metaplasia, CTZs, infections, and CIN 1 lesions. When fine punctation is caused by inflammation, the punctation is diffuse without borders, and the application of neither 3% to 5% acetic acid nor Lugol's iodine will demonstrate a well-defined lesion (Figure 8.60A,B). Biopsy may be required to exclude low-grade lesions, particularly if the patient has been referred for the evaluation of an abnormal Pap test. When fine punctation is confined to an area of increased acetowhitening within a field of immature metaplasia, it is usually indicative of CIN 1 (Figure 8.71). When fine punctation is confined to an abnormal acetowhite lesion on the original squamous epithelium, it may represent either a HPV-induced lesion or a variation of the normal metaplastic process.

A vascular pattern of coarse punctation usually indicates a high-grade lesion/CIN 2,3 (Figures 8.72 and 8.73A–C), and possibly early invasion. Microinvasion should always be considered when the capillaries of coarse punctation visibly dilate at the surface of a high-grade CIN or sprout a small side vessel resembling a tadpole or comma. Frequently, a complex vessel pattern may be seen in CIN 3 lesions in which coarse punctation is intermingled with areas with a coarse mosaic pattern or without vessels. Figure 8.73C. However, most CIN 2,3 demonstrates neither coarse punctation nor coarse mosaic. Instead, most high-grade lesions have no colposcopically apparent vessels. In fact, the absence of vessels noted within a densely opaque acetowhite lesion generally denotes the presence of CIN 3 (see Chapter 9).

8.5.2.3.2 Mosaic

8.5.2.3.2.1 Definition

The term *mosaic* refers to a vascular pattern produced when capillaries in stromal papillae are arranged parallel to the epithelial surface and form a basket-like structure around blocks or pegs of epithelium. When viewed through the surface epithelium overlying the stromal papillae, the vessels form a chicken-wire or honeycomb pattern encompassing blocks of acetowhite epithelium, resulting in a mosaic tile or cobblestone-like appearance (Figure 8.74A–C). Mosaic (*felderung* in German) was initially considered to be a pathologic finding. However, it is now realized that although mosaic is an important attribute of neoplastic epithelium, it may also be seen in normal immature squamous metaplastic epithelium. In current colposcopic terminology, mosaic is subdivided into fine mosaic and coarse mosaic, depending on vessel caliber and intercapillary spacing.

8.5.2.3.2.2 Etiology

Like punctation, mosaic may occur either in the normal process of metaplastic transformation or as an abnormal modification of preexisting, normal vascular architecture in the development

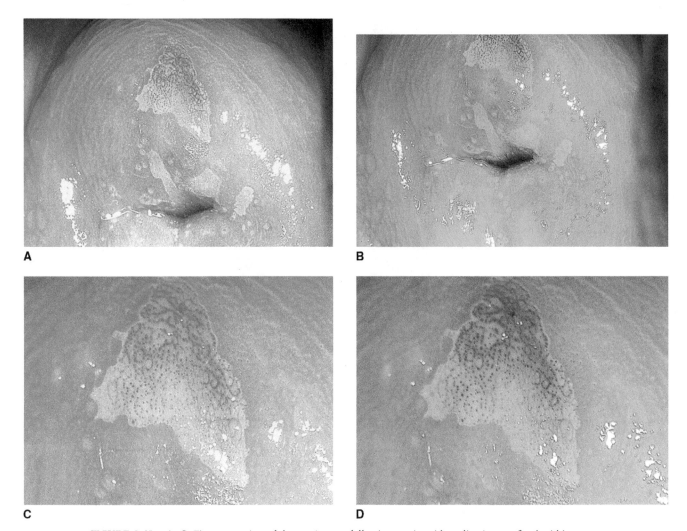

A   **B**

C   **D**

FIGURE 8.65.   **A, C:** Fine punctation of the cervix seen following acetic acid application confined within a geographic satellite lesion. **B, D:** Fine punctation enhanced by use of the red free (green) filter. The intercapillary space is regular, and the distance between each vessel is considered narrow with regular spacing. The intercapillary distances of fine punctation are narrow (**A–D**). (Courtesy of, and approved for reproduction by, the International Cervical Cancer (INCCA) foundation.)

of CIN. The etiology of punctation and mosaic are similar. Both develop from single-looped hairpin capillaries within stromal papillae adjacent to epithelial pegs of immature squamous metaplasia or neoplastic squamous epithelium in the transformation zone. As mosaic develops, the epithelial pegs remain discrete; it is the stromal papillae encompassing the loop capillaries that interconnect to form a peripheral vascular rim around the isolated pegs. When the epithelium is cut parallel to the surface of epithelium, the connected vessels can be observed histologically as separated from each other by plates of stroma.

The formation of mosaic has been studied extensively by Kolstad and Stafl,[4] who described three different patterns of mosaic, each of which represents a variation in the way stromal vessels encompass the adjacent avascular epithelial fields. One pattern arises when rows of hairpin capillaries coursing perpendicular to the epithelial surface form avascular epithelial fields (Figure 8.75). This pattern typically produces a fine mosaic

and is most commonly associated with immature metaplasia or CIN 1. Another pattern is formed when relatively thin-caliber terminal vessels run parallel to the surface and surround endocervical gland openings in large areas of normal immature metaplasia. The third pattern, which is associated with neoplasia, is formed when terminal vessels in the stromal papillae produce a "basket-like" network around epithelial pegs. The terminal vessels tend to be dilated and irregular in caliber and the epithelial pegs composed of neoplastic epithelium are typically large and irregular in shape. The process produces the coarse mosaic that is associated with high-grade lesions (CIN 2,3) and microinvasive carcinoma (Figure 8.76A–C). It is possible that enlarging epithelial pegs exert compressive and occlusive forces on the surrounding vessels. Pronounced compressive forces from expanding blocks of dysplasia may obliterate some small arterioles and laterally displace others. Vessels may also dilate when low-level venous capillary compression occludes

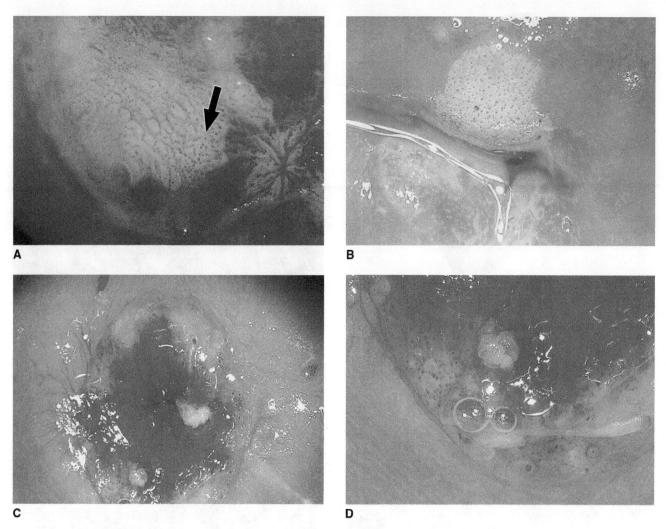

FIGURE 8.66.   **A:** Fine punctation (*arrow*) of the cervix following acetic acid application. In some areas, a mosaic pattern is forming. **B:** Acetowhite epithelium makes a good background to contrast the vessel changes. **C, D:** Fine punctation in a cervix following an excisional procedure. Also note the globular acetowhite columnar epithelial finding. (Courtesy of, and approved for reproduction by, the International Cervical Cancer (INCCA) foundation.)

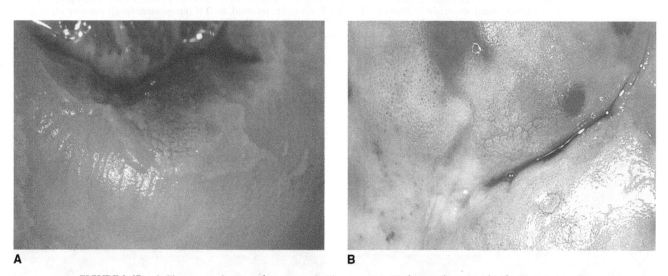

FIGURE 8.67.   **A:** Fine punctation vascular pattern. **B:** Fine punctation is frequently seen with a fine mosaic vascular pattern. (Courtesy of, and approved for reproduction by, the International Cervical Cancer (INCCA) foundation.)

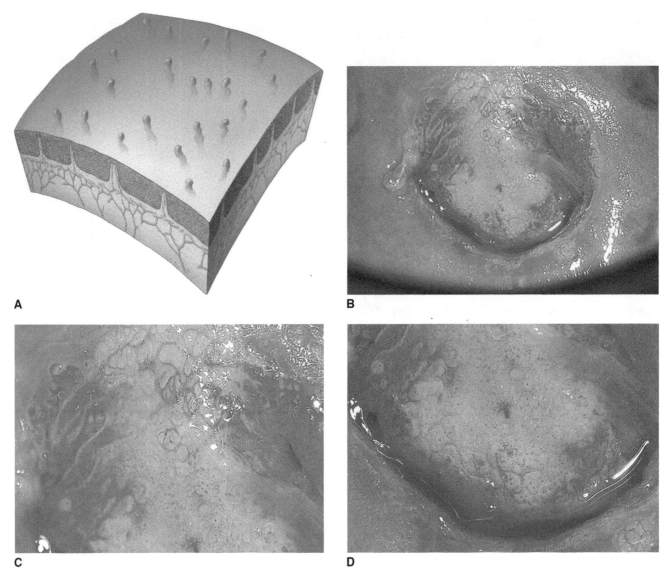

FIGURE 8.68.   A: Coarse punctation with dilated loop capillaries, randomly distributed vessels and a wide intercapillary distance. **B–D:** Coarse punctation irregularly spaced in a lesion on the anterior cervix. Mosaic is also present. (**A** [illustration]: copyright © 2004, 2011. ASCCP. All rights reserved. **B–D** [Colpophotographs]: courtesy of, and approved for reproduction by, the International Cervical Cancer (INCCA) foundation.)

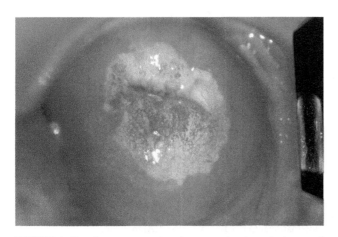

FIGURE 8.69.   Coarse punctation demonstrating irregularly spaced vessels.

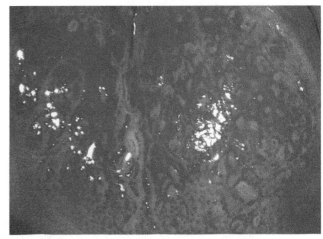

FIGURE 8.70.   A coarse punctation and coarse mosaic vessel pattern in a patient with CIN 3.

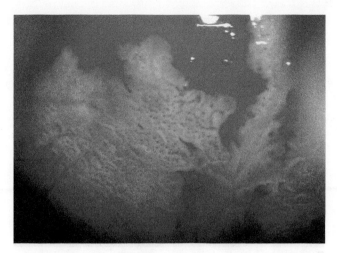

FIGURE 8.71. Fine punctation observed in an area of immature metaplasia that colposcopically is suspect for at least a LSIL.

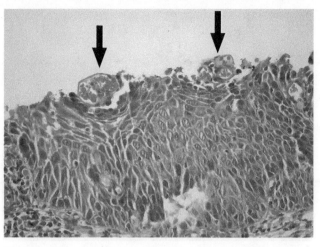

FIGURE 8.72. Histophotograph of punctation (*arrow*) within a cervical neoplasm (hematoxylin-eosin stain; medium-power magnification). These vessels appear very dilated.

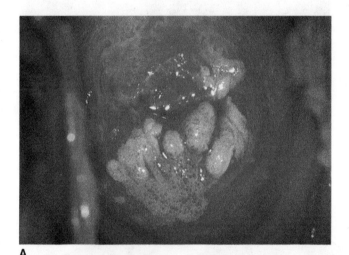

A

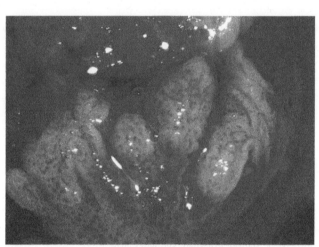

B

FIGURE 8.73. **A:** Coarse punctation associated with a HSIL. **B:** With closer inspection, these vessels are randomly distributed and have a wide intercapillary distance. **C:** Two large knobby punctations in the upper right of this CIN 3 lesion, and other punctations within mosaic patterns. Also note the atypical vessel. No invasion found in entire excisional specimen.

C

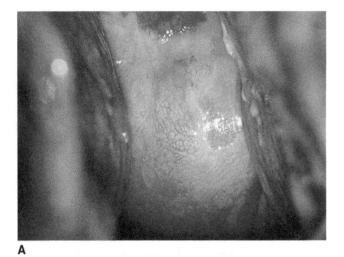

A

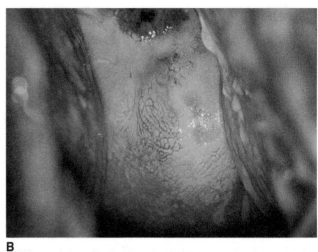

B

FIGURE 8.74.   **A:** Mosaic vessels of the cervix, demonstrating blocks of acetowhite epithelium surrounded by blood vessels in a honeycomb or chicken-wire pattern. **B, C:** This vascular pattern is readily seen by use of a red free (green) filter.

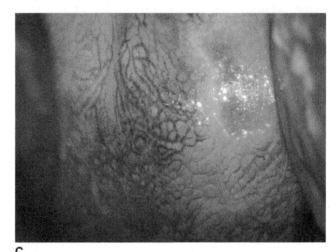

C

FIGURE 8.75.   One example of a fine mosaic pattern wherein rows of hairpin capillaries coursing perpendicular to the epithelial surface produce a central avascular epithelial field. This pattern is seen in immature metaplasia and CIN 1. The intercapillary distance is narrow, and the vascular distribution is uniform. (Copyright © 2001, 2011. ASCCP. All rights reserved.)

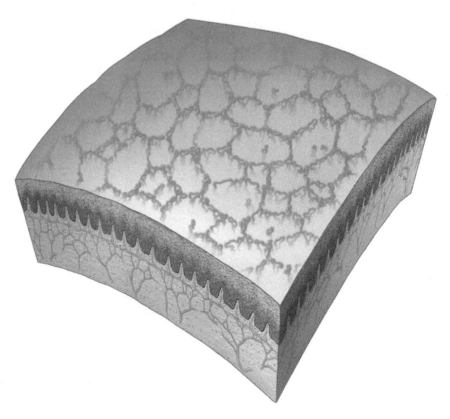

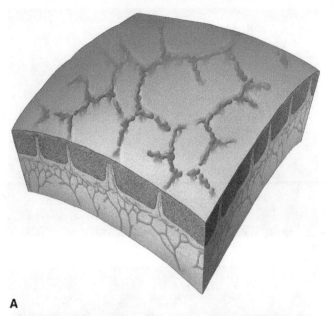

A

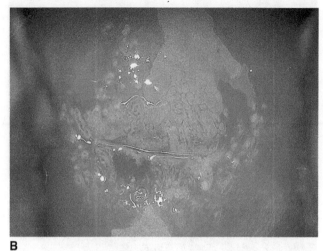

B

FIGURE 8.76. **A:** Schematic of an irregular mosaic vascular pattern as seen in CIN 3. The vessels are dilated, the intercapillary distance is increased, and the vascular distribution is quite random. **B, C:** Irregularly shaped mosaic tiles are noted in these colpophotos. (**A** [illustration]: copyright © 2004, 2011. ASCCP. All rights reserved. **B,C** [Colpophotographs]: courtesy of, and approved for reproduction by, the International Cervical Cancer (INCCA) foundation.)

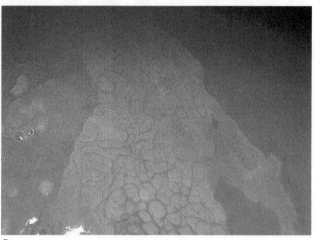

C

blood flow return. Therefore, vessels may dilate, occlude, or be displaced depending on how the venous or arterial capillaries are affected by varying levels of pressure and forces exerted by the expanding blocks of neoplastic epithelium.

8.5.2.3.2.3 Colposcopic Appearance
Mosaic vasculature appears colposcopically as a red bordered tile-like, polygonal grid viewed within an area of acetowhite epithelium (Figure 8.77A–D). The small blocks of epithelium, or epithelial pegs, encompassed by the mosaic vessels vary in size, shape, and uniformity. The intercapillary distances between mosaic vessels vary depending on the severity of neoplasia. In general, as vessel caliber and intercapillary distance increase, the severity of neoplasia also increases. Also, as neoplasia becomes increasingly more severe, more nonuniformly shaped epithelial blocks surrounded by mosaic vessels appear. Although definitive diagnosis requires biopsy, the type of mosaic pattern, when considered with other abnormal colposcopic signs, assists in clinically predicting the state of disease (Figure 8.78A–D). As with other vascular signs, mosaic vessels are present in both normal and abnormal epithelium—normal

CTZ; normal immature squamous metaplasia, or any level of neoplasia. The categories of fine and coarse mosaic vessels are based on their diameter. Because 3% to 5% acetic acid exerts a vasoconstrictive response soon after application, vessel caliber classification is made prior to its application or as the acetic acid effects wane (Figure 8.79A–C).

A fine mosaic pattern appears as a closely interwoven, lacy, delicate network of capillaries of nearly normal caliber, dispersed perpendicularly in stromal ridges resembling red grout between small white ceramic tiles. A uniformly consistent small intercapillary distance may be seen with immature metaplasia, a CTZ (Figure 8.45A,B), and CIN 1 lesions (Figure 8.80A–E). These narrow-diameter vessels are usually not apparent by colposcopic examination prior to acetic acid application. The network of pale, narrow red lines confined within an area of acetowhite epithelium may not display a mosaic pattern throughout, and thus, the pattern may be interrupted and scattered. Coexisting areas of punctation may be found among the mosaic patterns. A solitary punctate capillary is sometimes seen surrounded by a mosaic vessel pattern. Colposcopists use the term *umbilication* to describe this appearance.

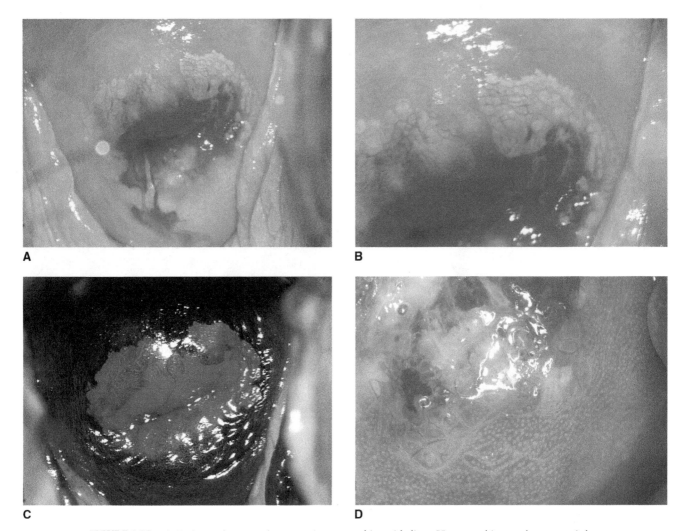

FIGURE 8.77. **A, B:** A mosaic pattern is seen against acetowhite epithelium. However, this vascular pattern is lost following the application of Lugol's iodine solution **(C)**. The developmental stages of a mosaic pattern can be seen in **(D)**. A translucent acetowhite low-grade lesion with a fine mosaic pattern lies along the SCJ. In the periphery, a fine mosaic can be seen but no acetowhite epithelium. Beyond this area, small fine punctate vessels associated with a subclinical HPV infection are noted. Some of these vessels are arranged in a linear pattern that will start the development of a mosaic. The other vessels appear diffusely and randomly arranged.

A coarse mosaic vascular pattern is characterized by dilated, varicose vessels that enclose larger diameter, irregularly shaped mosaic epithelial blocks (Figure 8.76A–C). The abnormal coarse vascular pattern is also confined invariably to a well-demarcated, dense acetowhite lesion. This mosaic network of capillaries is more pronounced and is an intense red color; it may be seen readily during some colposcopic examinations using saline (Figure 8.81A,B). The epithelial pegs between the vessels are larger and more varied in shape, reflecting irregularity and an increase in intercapillary distance (Figure 8.82A,B). A wide, irregular, nonuniform intercapillary distance and coarse-caliber vessels would be typical of a mosaic pattern seen with CIN 3 (Figure 8.83). Mosaic vessels associated with CIN 3 are occasionally dilated above the surface plane of surrounding epithelium. When this occurs, a surface topography that appears "pockmarked" can be seen.

Mosaic vessels are generally not seen in invasive cancers but may be present in surrounding CIN. Yet, a focal area of microinvasive cancer may occur within a field of coarse mosaic vessels associated with a high-grade lesion. Careful colposcopic inspection may identify a microinvasive cancer interrupting the pattern of coarse irregular mosaic.

Mosaic vessels are primarily restricted to the cervix and not usually found in vaginal intraepithelial neoplasia. However, a mosaic pattern may be observed in the vagina in women whose CTZ extends into the vaginal fornices or cul de sac (Figure 8.45A,B). A mosaic may also be seen in vaginal adenosis undergoing metaplasia; and, a mosaic pattern observed in the vagina may indicate prior *in utero* exposure to DES (Chapter 14).

8.5.2.3.2.4 Clinical Significance

Mosaic blood vessels are recognized quickly by colposcopists because of the unique capillary arrangement, but the pattern alone has no specific meaning. Critically analyzing capillary diameter, intercapillary distance, and uniformity of spacing, however, provides insight into the nature of the epithelium being inspected. For example, the mean intercapillary distance between mosaic vessels in CIN 2 is significantly less than that seen in CIN 3 (0.06 vs. 0.12 mm).[23] The distribution of a mosaic vessel pattern also helps to determine the type of

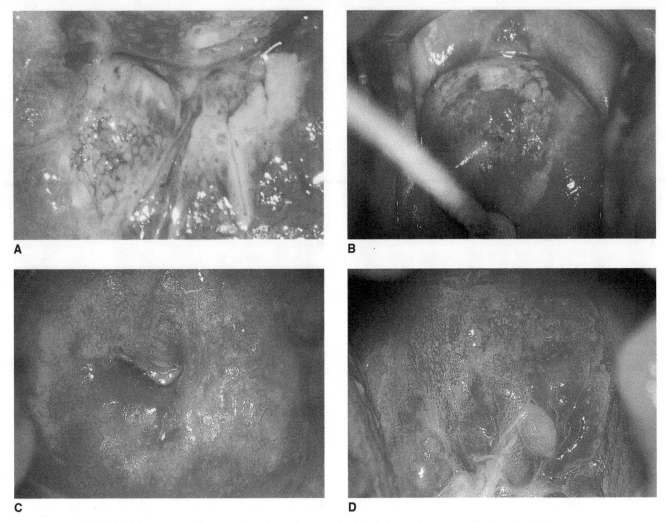

FIGURE 8.78.   **A:** Several areas of mosaic on the posterior lip of the cervix are seen. **B:** A very small but coarse mosaic vessel pattern is seen in the lesion at 1 to 2 o'clock. **C, D:** Two other large acetowhite lesions with mosaic and punctation are seen. (Courtesy of, and approved for reproduction by, the International Cervical Cancer (INCCA) foundation.)

epithelium observed. In a study of intercapillary distances measured by computer, the mean perimeter of a mosaic was 0.25 mm for CIN 2 and 0.44 mm for CIN 3.[23] The mosaic network also may be incomplete and patchy, as segments of the mosaic appear to be missing. In areas of CIN 3 and early microinvasive cancer, large fields of dense acetowhite epithelium may be interposed between sections of a rather loose mosaic arcade.

8.5.2.3.3 ATYPICAL BLOOD VESSELS

8.5.2.3.3.1 Definition

Atypical blood vessels are superficial vessels that exhibit bizarre variations in diameter, course, spacing, and branching patterns compared with normal blood vessels (Figure 8.84). These vessels are generally very dilated compared with other typical capillaries on the cervix. They traverse superficially within the epithelium, often oriented parallel to the surface. Although normal variants may be seen, atypical vessels are most commonly associated with invasive cancer and should be assumed so until confirmed otherwise by biopsy diagnosis (Figure 8.85A–G).

8.5.2.3.3.2 Etiology

Atypical vessels associated with malignancies develop in response to vascular endothelial growth factor (VEGF) and angiogenin (AGN), tumor angiogenesis factors, or substances secreted by cancers.[11,12] These agents promote endothelial proliferation and capillary formation by stimulating the growth of new vessels necessary to support an enlarging tumor.[9] Elevated levels of VEGF and AGN are seen in tissues only after premalignant lesions have been transformed into cancer.[11,12] Moreover, levels of VEGF are significantly greater in tumors larger than 4 cm, and those with deep stromal invasion, lymphovascular emboli, parametrial invasion, and pelvic lymph node metastasis.[11] Rapid and uncontrolled growth of solid tumors requires neovascularization.[8] As evidence of neovascularization in the early stages of cancer, histologic specimens from microinvasive cancer contain more stromal microvessels than normal or dysplastic tissue.[9] Cancer spreads in chaotic, unpredictable and random directions, in contrast with normal epithelium. In abnormal epithelium, the supporting vessels must assume abnormally novel routes (Figure 8.86). The rapid cancer growth and accompanying vascular response

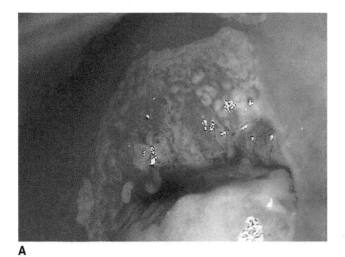

A

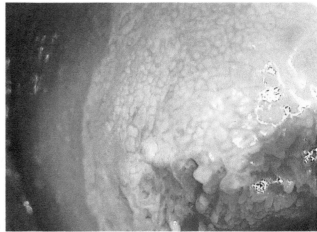

B

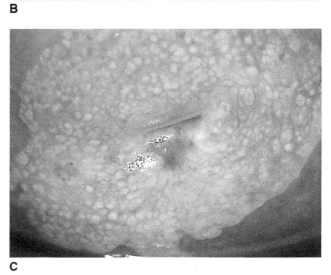

C

FIGURE 8.79. **A:** As the acetic acid effect begins to wane first in the anterior portio lesion, a prominent mosaic can be seen. Also seen extending into the canal posteriorly is a densely acetowhite CIN 3 lesion that has not yet begun to fade. **B, C:** Fine to moderately coarse and irregular mosaic is seen in (**B**) a large area of immature metaplasia with a small CIN 1 at the SCJ at the center of the photo and (**C**) with punctation in a symmetrical CTZ.

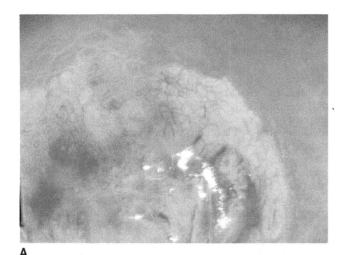

A

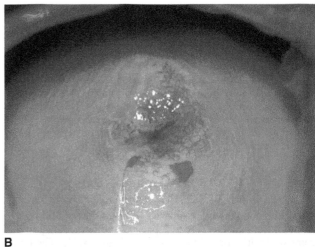

B

FIGURE 8.80.   **A, B:** A fine mosaic pattern is seen against an acetowhite background in these two patients.

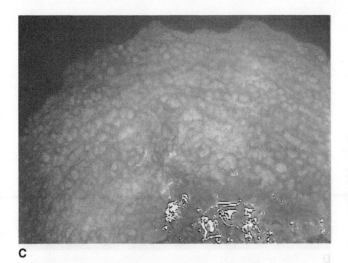

C

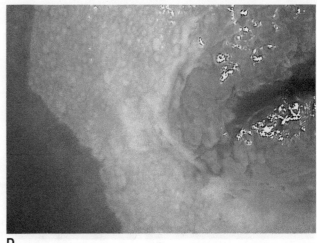

D

FIGURE 8.80.   *(Continued)* **C, D:** A fine symmetrical mosaic pattern is also seen in this CTZ, **(E)** but a more prominent area posteriorly that faded slower in acetowhite effect was documented on biopsy to be CIN 1.

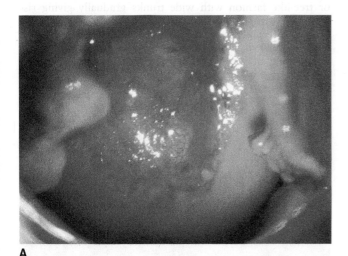

E

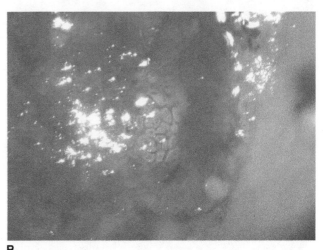

A

B

FIGURE 8.81.   **A, B:** A mosaic vascular pattern of the cervix seen at low and high magnification following saline application.

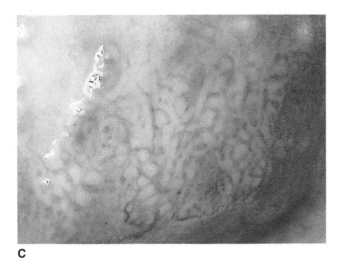

C

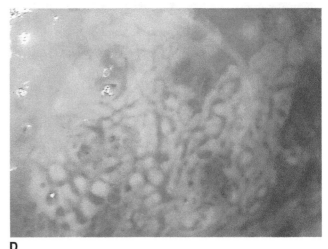

D

FIGURE 8.81. *(Continued)* **C, D:** Faint mosaic is also seen in another patient's cervix after saline application, with the dramatic effect of 5% acetic acid on the same area in (**D**).

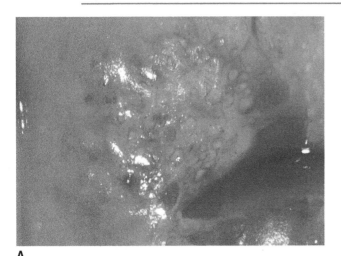

A

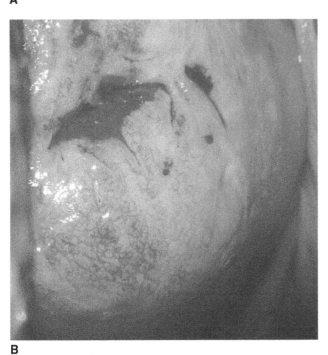

B

FIGURE 8.82. A coarse mosaic pattern with a variably wide intra-capillary distance and dilated vessels is seen. Both patients had CIN 3.

supercede the usual orderly deposition of blood vessels in normal cervical tissue. Both the development of new vessels and enlargement of existing capillaries characterize the vascular modifications associated with cancer. When cancer growth exceeds the distribution of the existing normal vasculature, neovascularization follows. Consequently, new vessels may be seen within the nodular contour of an exophytic cancer. Deep atypical vessels within an endophytic tumor are not usually transilluminated. In addition, large-bore vessels develop to deliver more blood to rapidly proliferating neoplastic tissue. The focal catabolic demand of cancer stimulates creation of pipeline-like vessels in an attempt to supply sufficient oxygen and energy to maintain the rapidly expanding tissue. Failure to deliver leads to anoxia and subsequent tissue necrosis. These extremely large-diameter vessels can make abrupt direction changes or traverse straight, prolonged distances.

8.5.2.3.3.3 Colposcopic Appearance

Blood vessels in benign epithelia branch in a dichotomous or tree-like fashion with wide trunks gradually giving rise to large, then smaller branches, followed by tiny twig-like branches. Terminal branches of atypical vessels often show no uniform taper or gradual decrease in diameter. While usually maintaining an overall varicosity, atypical vessels may display

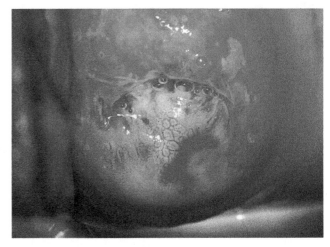

FIGURE 8.83. A coarse mosaic pattern on the posterior lip of the cervix in this woman with CIN 3.

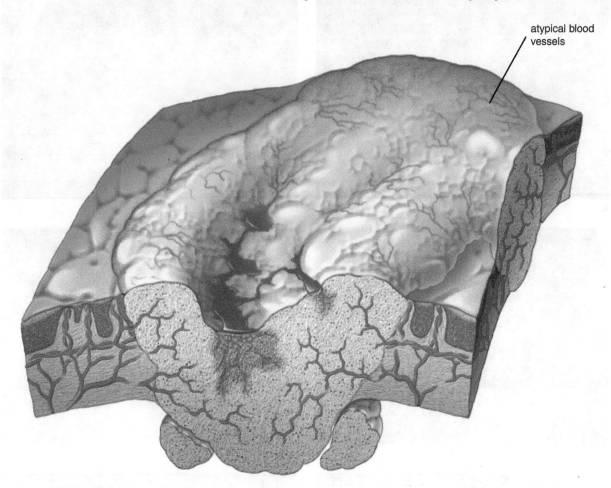

atypical blood vessels

FIGURE 8.84.   Atypical blood vessels associated with a cervical cancer. The cancer depicted has contour changes, with both exophytic growth and ulceration due to tissue necrosis.

an abrupt change in diameter or irregularly varied caliber. These vessels also exhibit a noticeably random course, changing direction suddenly. Moreover, atypical vessels are characteristically unique. In exophytic tumors, atypical vessels are superficially positioned and covered by very few cell layers of epithelium (Figure 8.87A,B). As such, these large blood vessels transilluminate readily and may be appreciated at low-power magnification. The vessels remain horizontal to the surface, are frequently elongated, and exhibit minimal branching. When present, the branching is irregularly spaced and varied in branching angle. Intercapillary distances are greater, leaving large avascular epithelial spaces between vessels. Early cancers may demonstrate normal to slightly increased vessel spacing (decreased overall vascularity),[4] whereas advanced cancers usually favor larger avascular areas.[20,24] In fact, in invasive cancer, most capillaries (85.5%) are spaced more than 300 μm apart.[20] Furthermore, as the stage of invasive cancer increases, the percentage of cancers with intercapillary distances >450 μm increases proportionally (stage I—23.1%, stage II—36.4%, and stages III/IV—54.5%).[1,25] In addition to very wide intercapillary spacing, atypical vessels are distributed randomly or nonuniformly.

The number of atypical blood vessels increases as the severity of cancer increases. In early-stage ectocervical cancers, only a few atypical vessels may be noted. Kolstad demonstrated that atypical blood vessels are rare (0.7%) in low-grade dysplasia (CIN 1), but more common in CIN 3 (16.7%), microinvasive

carcinoma (76.9%), and invasive carcinoma (96.6%).[20] In another study, atypical blood vessels were detected in 2.8% of women with CIN 3, 50% of women with microinvasion, and 92% of women with invasive cancer.[26] Sugimori et al.[27] detected atypical blood vessels in 9% of women with CIN 3. A meta-analysis by Hopman et al.[14] found atypical blood vessels in 44% of women with microinvasion and 84% of women with invasive cancer. Sillman[26] determined that 82% of women with atypical vessels had invasion, although some may not demonstrate atypical vessels because their location may prohibit colposcopic visualization.

Atypical blood vessels associated with cancer have been categorized as resembling corkscrews, tadpoles, hairpins, spaghetti, and other unusual configurations (Figure 8.88). The atypical blood vessels of adenocarcinoma are described (Chapter 11) as resembling tendrils, roots, willow branches, and waste threads.[3,28] Atypical blood vessels, particularly those associated with adenocarcinoma, may arise from alterations of central loop capillaries within columnar villi. Single corkscrew vessels with sharp, tortuous, irregular bends may be associated with squamous cancers. Branching, network and hairpin atypical vessels, considered variants of normal, are also seen in squamous cancers. Branching vessels may exhibit a fairly prolonged, gently curved or straight course. However, abrupt vessel constriction can occur followed by immediate dilation. Extremely varicose atypical vessels may terminate suddenly without the gradual narrowing seen

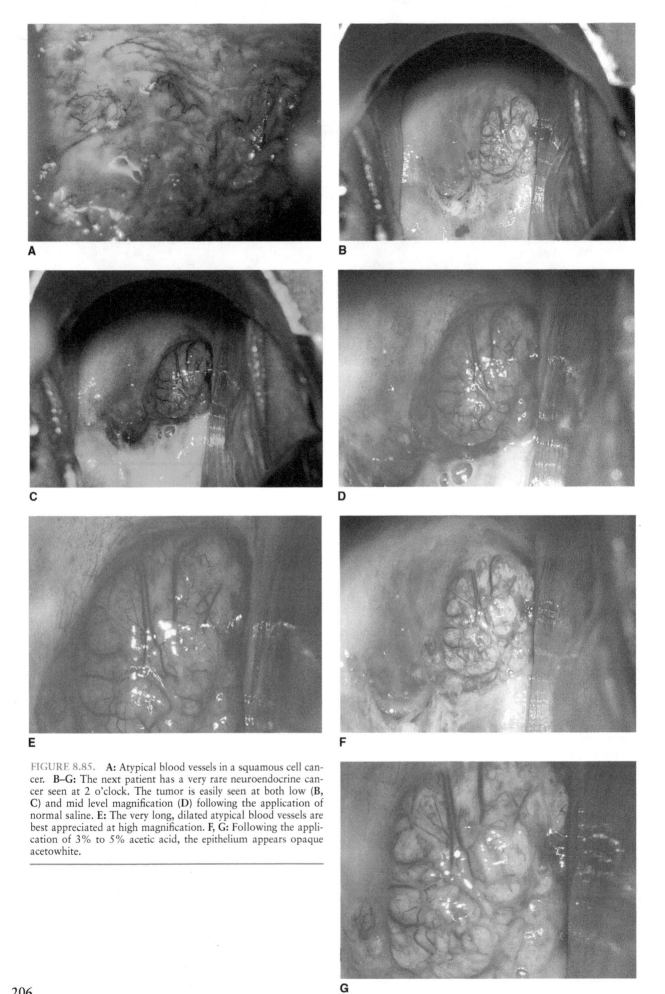

FIGURE 8.85.   **A:** Atypical blood vessels in a squamous cell cancer. **B–G:** The next patient has a very rare neuroendocrine cancer seen at 2 o'clock. The tumor is easily seen at both low (**B, C**) and mid level magnification (**D**) following the application of normal saline. **E:** The very long, dilated atypical blood vessels are best appreciated at high magnification. **F, G:** Following the application of 3% to 5% acetic acid, the epithelium appears opaque acetowhite.

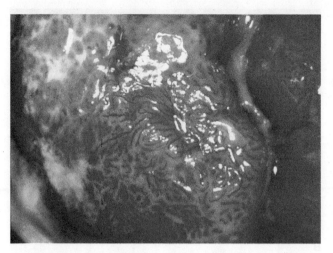

FIGURE 8.86. Atypical blood vessels are dilated and do not demonstrate normal branching patterns in an almost spaghetti-like arrangement.

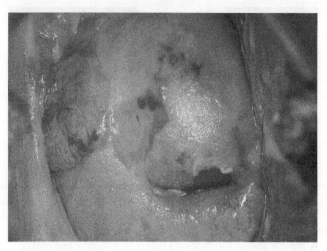

FIGURE 8.88. Elongated spaghetti-like atypical vessels are seen on the right side of the patient's cervix. An opaque CIN 3 lesion without visible vessels covers the majority of the ectocervix. (Photograph courtesy of Dr. Vesna Kesic.)

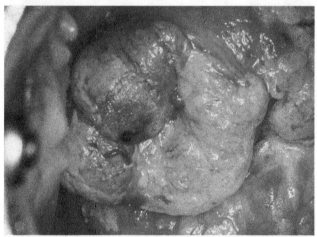

in normal vessels (Figure 8.89). These vessels may encircle large areas of otherwise avascular-appearing epithelium. Network atypical vessels demonstrate variable caliber changes and abrupt side branching of much smaller-caliber vessels (Figure 8.90A–C). A coarse interlaced pattern with large intercapillary distances, various constrictions, and dilations may be seen. Hairpin atypical vessels are dilated, rounded hairpin capillaries. They are usually widely spaced. Depending on their orientation to the surface of the epithelium (vertical, horizontal, or tangential), the entire loop, or only portions thereof, may be seen.

Atypical vessels are described by some as a variance of the normal network, hairpin, and branching blood vessels.[25] However, the pattern of atypical vessels is completely chaotic, without the order of normal vasculature.[29] Succinctly stated, atypical vessels display an unlimited spectrum of expression, encompassing a lack of symmetry and uniformity in caliber, branching, and spacing. Chapters 10 and 11

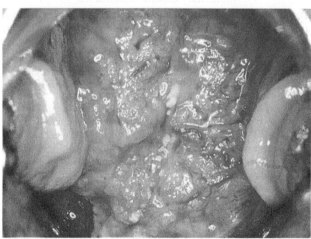

FIGURE 8.87. A,B: Very dilated atypical blood vessels located superficially on large exophytic cervical cancers. (Photos courtesy of Dr. Vesna Kesic.)

FIGURE 8.89. Very dilated atypical blood vessels are seen to abruptly terminate without tapering or branching in this woman with adenocarcinoma. (Photo courtesy of Dr. Vesna Kesic.)

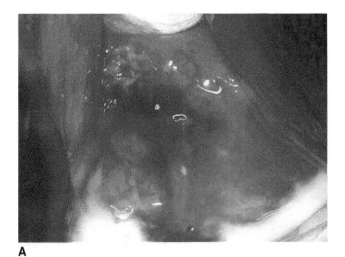

A

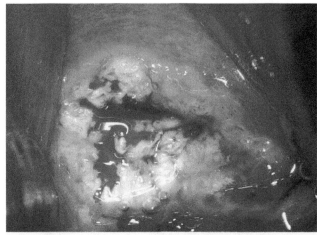

B

FIGURE 8.90. Atypical blood vessels are seen in this patient following (**A**) saline, (**B, C**) 3% to 5% acetic acid application.

C

include further discussion of atypical vessels as a warning sign for invasive cancer.

8.5.2.3.3.4 Clinical Significance

Atypical vessels must be considered as a sign of cancer until proven otherwise by biopsy. This is particularly true if observed in women with abnormal cervical cytology or a history of cervical neoplasia. The presence of other associated abnormal colposcopic signs; opaque, dull, thickened acetowhite epithelium; ulceration; yellow friable necrotic epithelium; and an exophytic mass strongly imply the malignant nature of observed atypical blood vessels. Novice colposcopists, fearful of uncontrollable bleeding, frequently question whether atypical vessels should be biopsied. Contrary to this concern, atypical vessels and the surrounding epithelium should be sampled without reservation and to a sufficient depth to allow an accurate histologic diagnosis. Bleeding is not usually increased and can be controlled with simple pressure and Monsel's paste.

There are several causes for atypical vessels to be present in the absence of a malignancy. Occasionally, atypical vessels may be observed in areas of very early normal immature metaplasia (Figure 8.91A–E). These vessels are covered by a thin layer of very translucent epithelium. The vessels exhibit an increased caliber compared with other normal surrounding vessels and may extend parallel to the epithelial surface for rather long distances. Their course is usually fairly straight with minor variation of direction. Tiny vessels may diverge

from the main vessel, displaying normal branching of decreasing-caliber capillaries. Absence of other colposcopic warning signs of cancer, along with a faint, translucent, extremely transient acetowhite background and young patient age, would suggest a benign mimic (Figure 8.92A–D). In addition, atypical vessels are frequently encountered in women who previously received local radiation therapy of the lower genital tract (Figure 8.93A,B). Because the epithelium is usually atrophic and thin, these rather bizarre vessels are readily apparent. Since these women also have a history of local cancer, it can be extremely challenging to discriminate postradiation atypical vessels from recurrent cancer-associated atypical vessels. Again, no evidence of other warning signs for invasive cancer suggests the benign nature of postradiation therapy atypical vessels, but histologic sampling usually is required for confirmation of etiology. Atypical blood vessels may also be seen in decidual tissue associated with pregnancy (Chapter 12). Atypical blood vessels may be seen in tissue undergoing active reparative change, such as that seen during the healing phase following surgery of the cervix (Figure 8.94A–C). Finally, very bizarre vessels may be seen in granulation tissue. The reddish tissue color, tissue friability, and raised contour of granulation tissue may make discrimination from cancer difficult. Most granulation tissue is seen in the proximal vaginal cuff in women following hysterectomy (Chapter 14). Histologic confirmation may be particularly warranted in women posthysterectomy for neoplastic indications.

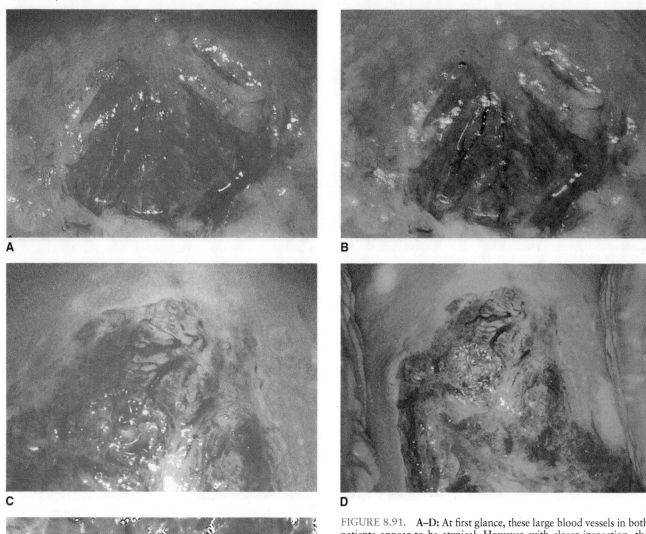

FIGURE 8.91.   **A–D:** At first glance, these large blood vessels in both patients appear to be atypical. However, with closer inspection, the vessels lie in immature metaplastic epithelium and do taper with some branching. **E:** Atypical vessels in a large ectopy in a very young woman with extensive immature metaplasia, proven to be normal on multiple biopsies.

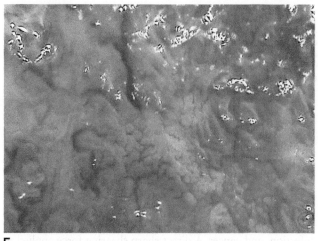

8.5.3 Surface Topography

8.5.3.1 Ulceration, Erosion

8.5.3.1.1 Definition

An ulceration or erosion of the cervix is defined as a focal or multifocal absence of epithelium (Figure 8.84). A well-defined, circumscribed area void of cervical epithelium is noted, and only the underlying papillary or reticular stroma remains visible. Because the term *ulceration* is nearly synonymous with erosion, clinicians often use the terms interchangeably even though an ulceration is anatomically deeper than a more superficial erosion. The term *erosion* is also commonly confused with ectropion even though each denotes a distinctly different colposcopic finding, with the latter representing the normal eversion of columnar epithelium on the ectocervix. The two terms may be interchanged mistakenly because both appear colposcopically as red areas of the cervix displaying

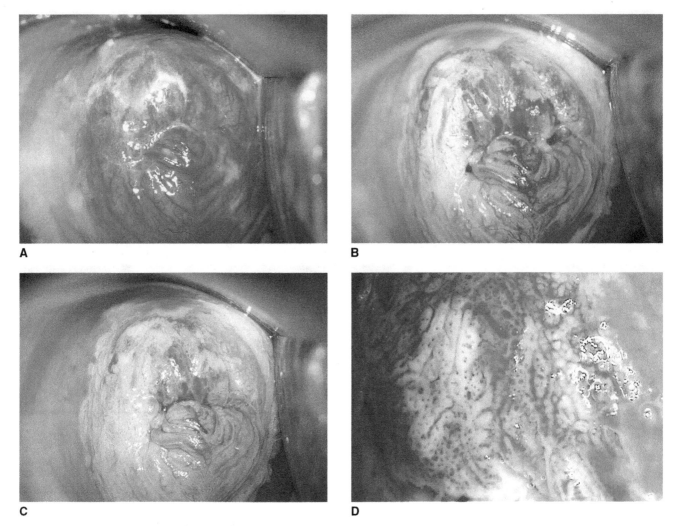

FIGURE 8.92.   **A:** Very dilated nonbranching blood vessels are seen on the posterior lip of the cervix during the saline examination. These appear to be atypical vessels. **B, C:** Following 3% to 5% acetic acid application, a large area of acetowhite epithelium is noted. The epithelium of the posterior cervix is translucent white especially in the area of the large vessels. This represents immature metaplasia. It is easy to overlook the opaque acetowhite epithelium at 9 o'clock with coarse punctation that represents CIN 3. **D:** A prominent straight vessel in a young woman within extensive mosaic and punctation in a large area of immature metaplasia.

mildly irregular contours (Figure 8.95A–C). The red villous projections of an ectropion are rounded, uniform in distribution, and assume a faint acetowhite blush following 3% to 5% acetic acid application. The surface is pebbled and has a slightly depressed relationship to the elevated surrounding squamous and metaplastic epithelium.

The base of a true erosion may be friable, variably irregular in contour, and nonacetowhite following application of 3% to 5% acetic acid. The demarcation between a superficial erosion and surrounding epithelium may be gradual and somewhat imperceptible. In contrast, ulcerations exhibit a rather distinct, recessed, steep interface with the surrounding normal or neoplastic epithelium (Figure 8.96). Both erosions and ectropions may bleed easily following even gentle contact with moistened cotton applicators. This is especially true when an inflammatory process is present. While an ectropion is a normal finding mainly in young women, and especially among those using oral contraceptive pills, an erosion is abnormal, but not necessarily associated with a neoplastic process. If, however, an erosion is observed in a woman with prior abnormal cervical cytology or a history or risk of cervical neoplasia, the erosion

and surrounding epithelium could represent a potential severe neoplasia or malignancy. All erosions should be assessed by colposcopic examination and histologic sampling to confirm or refute neoplasia (Figure 8.97).

8.5.3.1.2 ETIOLOGY

Ulcerations develop for a variety of reasons, including trauma, infection, and cancer. A direct sharp shearing force applied to healthy epithelium may cause an acute abrasion or erosion. Chronic pressure on the epithelium, like that of a tampon retained for a prolonged time in the vagina, may produce an ulceration. Ulcerations may also result from other intravaginal devices or from an adverse response to intravaginal medications. The probability of inadvertent epithelial injury is greater when epithelium becomes thin, as in estrogen-deficient women with atrophic change. Cervicitis promotes tissue fragility, increasing the likelihood of traumatic ulceration which is usually benign. Focal cytopathic effects from viral or bacterial infections may cause ulcerations. Herpes simplex virus (HSV) produces multiple clusters of small, irregular ulcerations (Figure 8.98A,B). Syphilis and chancroid ulcerations are more likely

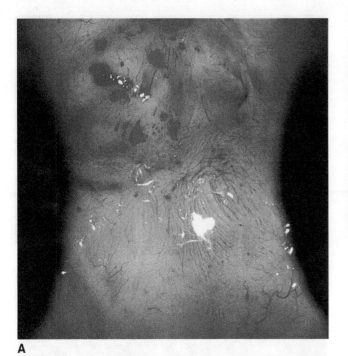

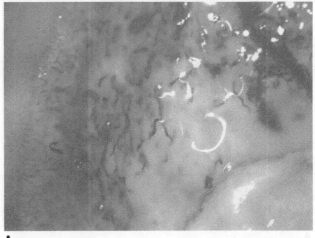

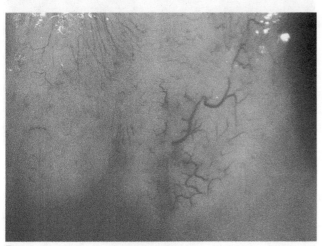

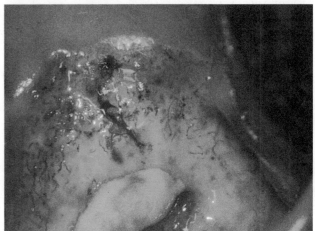

A

B

FIGURE 8.93.   **A, B:** Atypical blood vessels seen in a woman following radiation therapy of the lower genital tract. The epithelium is atrophic and subcutaneous hemorrhages can be seen. There was no recurrence of cancer.

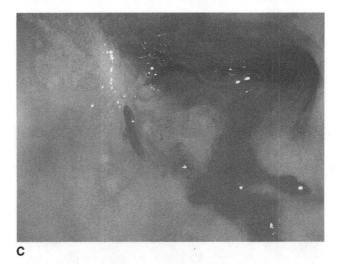

C

FIGURE 8.94.   **A, B:** These bizarre corkscrew-like blood vessels were seen in a patient approximately 2 weeks following a loop excision procedure. The vessels lie in reparative tissue along the wound margin. The next patient (C) has a straight dilated atypical-appearing vessel at 8 o'clock. She also has an area of recurrent CIN 1 at 9 o'clock.

to be larger, well circumscribed, and solitary. Abnormal vaginal discharge may accompany ulcerations caused by infectious organisms as well as by malignancy.

However, an ulcer may be induced unintentionally in previously intact, severely neoplastic epithelium because of the propensity of hemidesmosomes (tiny papillary structures that bind the basal cells and cytoskeleton to the underlying stroma)[30] to lose their adhesive properties in the neoplastic process. Consequently, one should never assume that all epithelial trauma associated with the introduction of the vaginal speculum blades is benign.

More importantly, ulcerations may evolve in epithelial areas invaded by rapidly proliferating cancers (Figure 8.99A,B). Under these circumstances, the rate of tumor growth may exceed oxygen delivery capacity by the enlarged but widely

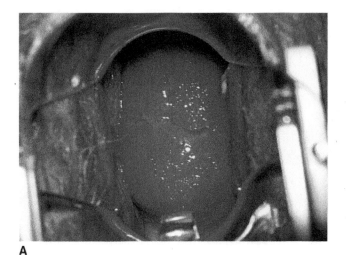

A

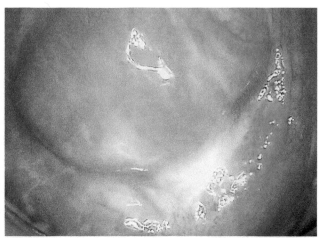

B

FIGURE 8.95.   **A:** An ectropion of the cervix or eversion of columnar epithelium onto the ectocervix that is mistaken as an erosion. **B:** A huge irregular ectopy with columnar epithelium creating a red appearance out to the cervicovaginal junction. **C:** Application of 3% to 5% acetic acid to the ectopy shown in (**B**) clarifies the benign nature of the ectopy by creating a faint acetowhite blush to the columnar villi present throughout the ectopy. Such large red ectopies were once termed "erosions."

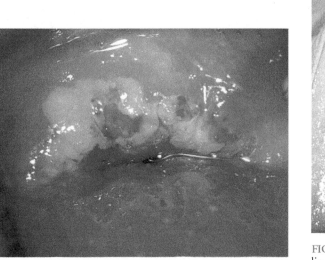

C

FIGURE 8.96.   Ulceration of the cervix demonstrating a well-demarcated area without visible surface epithelium. The ulceration lies within a CIN 3 on the anterior lip of the cervix.

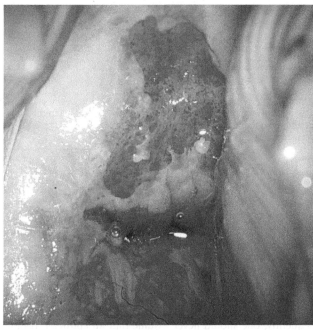

FIGURE 8.97.   A large red recessed erosion is seen on the anterior lip of the cervix. The surrounding acetowhite epithelium was diagnosed histologically as CIN 2. It is important that the biopsy contains epithelium adjacent to an ulceration, particularly when the ulceration adjoins colposcopically suspect abnormal tissue.

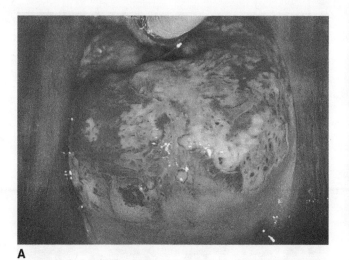 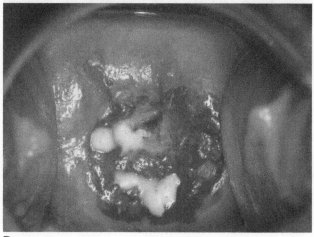

FIGURE 8.98. **A:** Herpes cervicitis can mimic invasive cancer. **B:** Both are erythematous and friable. An associated exudate is also seen in each case. (Photo [B] courtesy of Dr. Vesna Kesic.)

spaced blood vessels. Focal hypoxic ischemia and tissue necrosis ensue when intercapillary distance exceeds 350 μm.[25] As intercapillary distances of invasive cancer surpass 450 μm, superficial necrosis of the cervical epithelium occurs in 94.1% of women.[25] Intravascular pressure also determines tissue viability. For example, the oxygen tension of capillary blood in normal tissue measures 66 mm Hg, but is reduced to a mean of 58.6 mm Hg in invasive cancer.[25]

8.5.3.1.3 COLPOSCOPIC APPEARANCE

When viewed through the colposcope, ulcerations appear as well-demarcated, recessed, red, raw areas without visible surface epithelium. They may be encompassed by normal or neoplastic epithelium (Figures 8.96 and 8.99). The type of surrounding epithelium indicates whether the ulceration is likely to be associated with a benign or neoplastic process. A raised margin, elevated above the surrounding epithelial surface, or an adjoining dense acetowhite epithelium may indicate neoplasia. A well-defined, rolled ulcer margin or edge may be seen with infection caused by *Treponema pallidum* (syphilis), or in

a patient with a retained vaginal tampon. An irregular border may indicate HSV infection or cancer. A tear of colposcopically normal-appearing tissue may simply indicate benign trauma.

A dull, thickened, adjoining epithelium suggests neoplasia. Tissue friability is suspicious for infection or neoplasia. Associated hemorrhage, blood clots, and serous drainage may fill and obscure an underlying ulceration. If the ulceration is benign and due to trauma, ecchymosis may be observed in adjoining, otherwise normal epithelium and a flap of freshly avulsed, normal-appearing epithelium may remain at the ulcer margin. When ulceration is associated with infection, tiny vesicles or pustules may be seen in the periphery.

The shape and depth of ulcerations may also offer etiologic clues. Round ulcers may indicate infection, and irregularly shaped ulcers may suggest neoplasia. Trauma may produce frayed or sharply demarcated edges, depending on the health of the epithelium and source of injury (see Chapter 14 for traumatic vaginal ulcer). Deep, necrotic ulcerations are more likely to be observed secondary to cancer, while shallow ulcers are more often a result of minor trauma or infection.

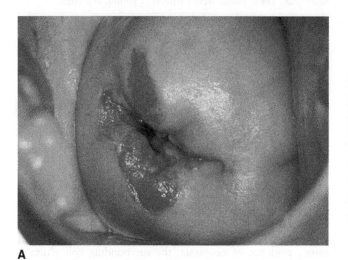 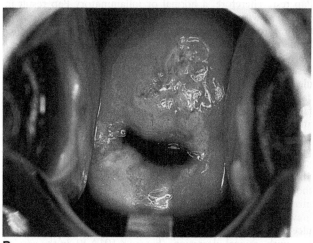

FIGURE 8.99. **A, B:** Ulcerations are also frequently seen in conjunction with invasive cervical cancers. (Photo [A] courtesy of Dr. Vesna Kesic.)

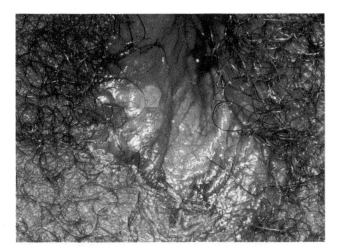

FIGURE 8.100.   A cluster of herpetic vesicles on the vulva.

Ulcerations may occur as small or large solitary ulcers, or as multifocal ulcers of various sizes. The number of ulcerations and size are determined by the etiology. Diffuse ulcerations may be caused by viral agents or adverse reactions to intravaginal products or medications. Solitary ulcers may result from bacterial infection, neoplasia, or trauma. The size of ulcerations can vary for specific infections, trauma, and neoplasia.

Healing ulcerations may exhibit various stages of metaplasia and repair. An intense, flame-shaped erythematous band of inflammatory tissue may be noted in the epithelium that borders a healing ulcer. This red area surrounding an ulcer actually represents tiny closely spaced capillaries and sometimes extravasation of erythrocytes into the stroma.[29] Because of the abundant neovascularization in a healing ulcer, solitary capillaries may not be appreciable.

8.5.3.1.4 Clinical Significance

Definitive diagnosis of ulcerations is best made in conjunction with patient history and laboratory testing. Because the primary objective of colposcopy is to identify lower genital tract neoplasia, all ulcerations must be assessed. While previous abnormal cervical cytology increases the probability of neoplasia, an intense inflammatory process may accompany a cancer to the extent that the cancer cells are obscured on the Pap test. Therefore, a normal or inflammatory Pap result in a woman with a cervical ulceration does not exclude malignancy. Large, deep biopsies of the ulcer *and* adjoining epithelium are necessary to diagnose neoplasia.

Swab sampling of a fresh ulcer base or adjoining intact vesicles for culture or dark-field examination helps to confirm ulcers caused by HSV and syphilis, respectively. Often cervical herpes will be accompanied by vulvar herpetic lesions. Herpetic lesions start as a cluster of vesicles or pustules with an erythematous base, but unlike vulvar herpetic lesions that bring the patient in for evaluation of symptoms, cervical herpetic lesions are usually asymptomatic (Figures 8.100 and 8.101A,B). Identifying this transient asymptomatic vesicular phase when solely on the cervix is unusual. When present on the cervix, the vesicles rupture, producing small, superficial ulcerations. An abnormal serous, watery vaginal discharge may ensue, which sometimes can be quite heavy. Coexisting ulcers of the vulva and buttock regions may be seen in conjunction with cervical ulcerations (Figure 8.101A,B). In the case of externally located ulcerations, the woman may be aware that she has previously had a herpes infection. Unfortunately, some women experience only herpes cervicitis and remain virtually

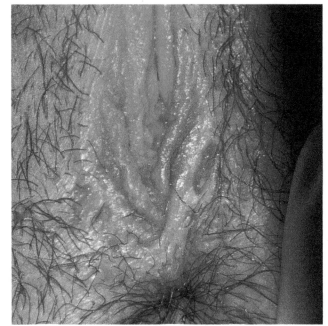

A

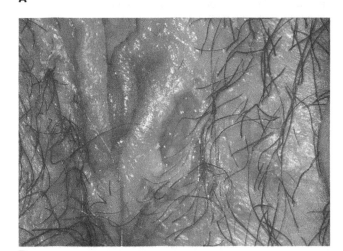

B

FIGURE 8.101.   **A, B:** Primary herpetic ulcerations in the posterior fourchette. These lesions were particularly painful and large.

asymptomatic, increasing the likelihood that she will transmit the infection to sexual partners. Since detecting infection by means of dark-field examination is difficult from an access and interpretive perspective, serologic testing may be essential to confirm a diagnosis of syphilis.

Trauma may be the source of ulcerations. Ulcerations from use of intravaginal medication are suspected by history and distribution. While trauma is likely to occur in atrophic epithelium, cancers are also more prevalent in older women. Finally, trauma produced during insertion of a vaginal speculum may cause an acute "false" ulceration with fresh bleeding. An iatrogenic ulcer usually involves normal, thin, or atrophic epithelium. Biopsy is not necessary if the colposcopist is certain that the patient has no risk factors or clinical and laboratory evidence of neoplasia, the surrounding epithelium is clearly normal in appearance, and the loss of epithelium was observed to be secondary to trauma during introduction of the speculum. However, if any doubt exists about the possibility of neoplasia, a biopsy must be obtained. One must remember that iatrogenic ulcers are more likely to occur in friable epithelium susceptible to trauma (atrophic or neoplastic epithelia).

8.5.3.2 Epithelial Elevations

8.5.3.2.1 DEFINITION

Variation of surface contour may be found in normal cervical epithelium of the ectocervix. While native squamous and mature metaplastic epithelia are generally flat or macular, columnar epithelium is distinctly villiform (Figure 8.5A–I). Nabothian follicles may project above the epithelial surface as gently rounded, yellow mounds (Figure 8.11A–I). These cysts may enlarge enough to be mistaken for tumors by clinicians unfamiliar with normal cervical anatomy. Immature metaplasia assumes a continuum of topography, initially adopting a villiform, then a pebbled, undulating, or papular, and finally a macular contour. The contour of the normal endocervical canal is irregular. When the SCJ is located near the external os, deep radial recesses from gland clefts may be seen to fold 5 mm beneath the surface. When the SCJ is positioned above the external os, the visible portion of the distal canal may appear smooth. A small percentage of women have papillary projections from tissue of the medial labia minora and introitus region known as micropapillomatosis labialis (MPL) (Chapter 15). The filiform surface can be confused with a vulvar condyloma (Figure 8.102A,B). A symmetrical distribution, absence of a coalesced base for the papillary projections, and minimal translucent acetowhitening favor MPL. Similar, normal papillary projections (Figure 8.103A–F) can be found in the normal vagina and cervix. These projections will stain with Lugol's to the same degree as the adjacent nonpapillary mucosa, adding to the reassurance of normalcy. Vesicular eruptions associated with infection or allergy result from the accumulation of a transudate beneath the superficial epithelium. Small, transient vesicular eruptions of the cervix or vagina caused by HSV, bullous or emphysematous cervicitis and vaginitis (Figure 8.104), or allergic reactions should not be confused with benign cysts of the vagina (see Chapter 14).

More profound epithelial contour changes may be observed in the abnormal cervix. Some of the greatest morphologic variation is seen with HPV lesions or CIN 1 of the cervix. Micropapillary, papillary, cerebriform, papular, plaque-like, and grossly exophytic lesions are all possible raised presentations of cervical HPV (Figure 8.105A–K). Some CIN 3 lesions are raised and plaque-like. Greater elevation may be seen if coexisting leukoplakia is present. The morphologic expression of cervical cancer varies depending on cell type, location, and whether the invasion is primarily endophytic or exophytic. Exophytic tumors are nodular, raised, or papular (Figure 8.106A–D). Advanced, large tumors may be readily seen without a colposcope and are easily palpated during bimanual examination. Because the ectocervix is predominately flat, particularly for most women older than 40 years of age, epithelial elevations of the ectocervix in these women should be suspect for neoplasia. Contour changes emanating from the endocervical canal may be benign or associated with a malignancy. Microglandular hyperplasia, papillary AIS, polyps, fibroids, decidua, and adenocarcinoma can produce striking contour changes within columnar epithelium.

8.5.3.2.2 ETIOLOGY

Elevations of the epithelium are caused by many factors, including trauma, infection, and benign and malignant tumors. Chronic, focal trauma to the cervix may produce circumscribed, plaque-like elevations of keratosis or leukoplakia (Figure 8.107). Tiny, diffuse, multiple pinpoint elevations may be seen after cervical surgery (Figure 8.108A–D).

HPV types 6 and 11 cause papillary or exophytic epithelial elevations (Figure 8.105A–K). The virus may stimulate capillary proliferation and growth whereby the afferent and efferent loop capillaries, normally restricted within the lower one-third of the squamous epithelium, expand within elongated rete pegs. Tiny, narrow, finger-like papillary projections are called asperities or micropapillae (Figure 8.109A–H). When present, asperities impart a mildly irregular surface contour that can be appreciated only with colposcopic magnification.

In addition to HPV-induced condylomas, nodular, papular, exophytic, or raised lesions may represent severe grades of cervical neoplasia. Raised plaque-like epithelial contour is suggestive of CIN 3 or cancer (Figure 8.110A–C). Once cells become malignant, their normal feedback mechanism to inhibit uncontrolled growth is lost. When one normal cell abuts against an adjoining cell, normal tactile intercellular feedback dictates recognition of the occupied space. Cancer cells do not retain this important feedback control and, thus, continue to divide and proliferate without regard to the adjoining cells. Such rampant growth causes nodular, exophytic lesions that extend above the surface of the epithelium and invade deeply within and below the epithelium as endophytic tumors. VEGF and AGN present in cancer cause

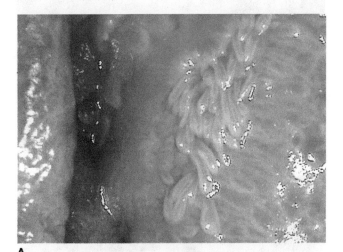

A

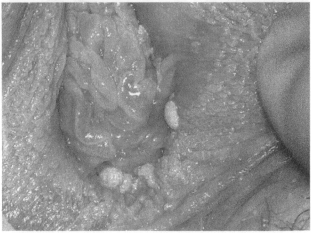

B

FIGURE 8.102.   **A:** The normal papillary projections of MPL should not be confused with (**B**) introital condyloma as seen in the posterior fourchette of this patient.

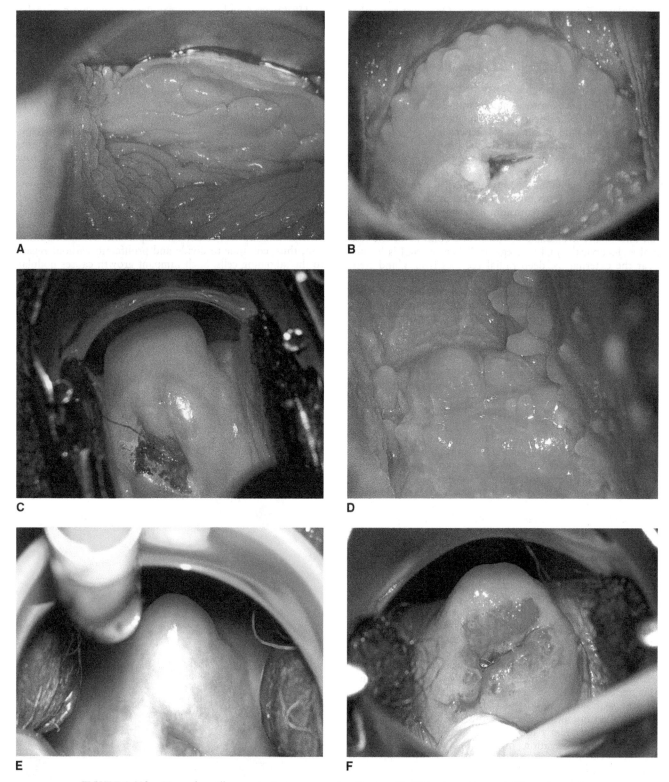

FIGURE 8.103.   Normal papillary projections are occasionally seen (**A, D**) in the vagina and (**B**) on the cervix. These papillary projections in the vagina (**D**) and on the cervix (**B**) are not warts, but normal anatomical variants. The projection from the anterior cervix (**C–F**) is called a cock's comb deformity. Although most commonly associated with exposure *in utero* to DES, in these cases the findings represent a variant from the normal round shape of the cervix in women without a history of prior DES exposure. (Courtesy of, and approved for reproduction by, the International Cervical Cancer (INCCA) foundation.)

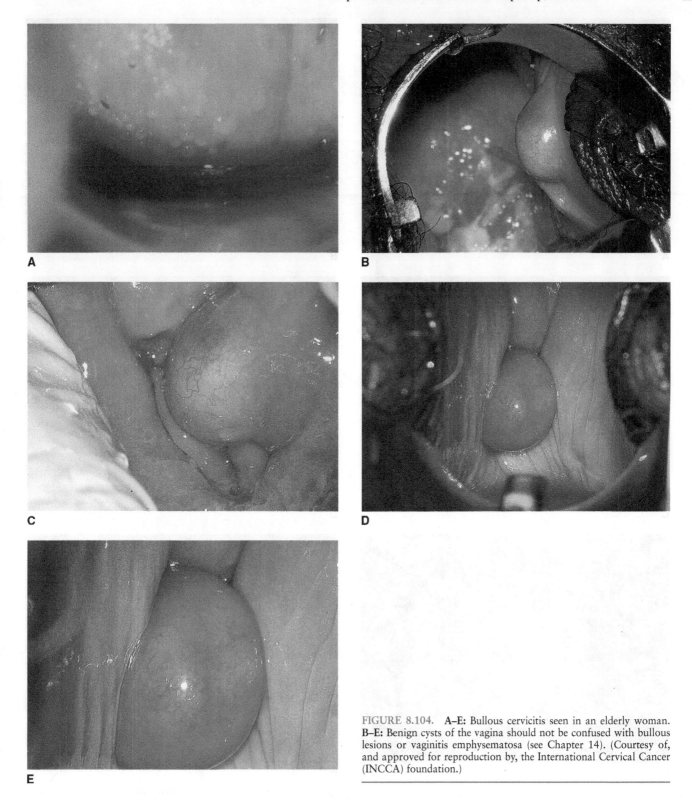

FIGURE 8.104. **A–E:** Bullous cervicitis seen in an elderly woman. **B–E:** Benign cysts of the vagina should not be confused with bullous lesions or vaginitis emphysematosa (see Chapter 14). (Courtesy of, and approved for reproduction by, the International Cervical Cancer (INCCA) foundation.)

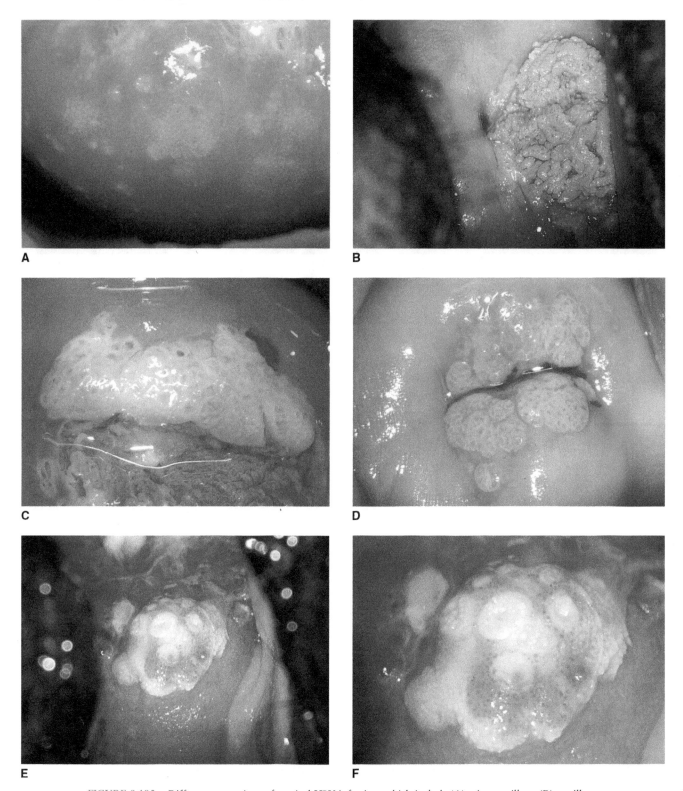

FIGURE 8.105.   Different expressions of cervical HPV infection, which include (A) micropapillary, (B) papillary, (C, D) cerebriform, (E, F) "cupping" or inverted,

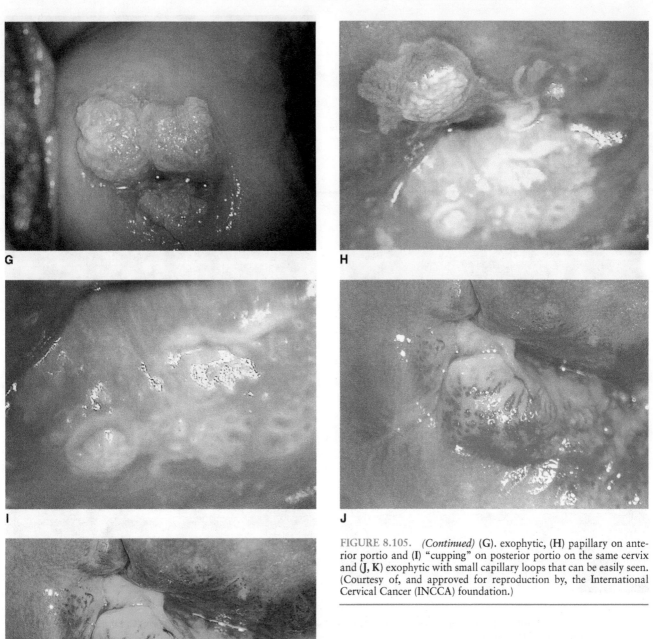

FIGURE 8.105.   *(Continued)* (G). exophytic, (H) papillary on anterior portio and (I) "cupping" on posterior portio on the same cervix and (J, K) exophytic with small capillary loops that can be easily seen. (Courtesy of, and approved for reproduction by, the International Cervical Cancer (INCCA) foundation.)

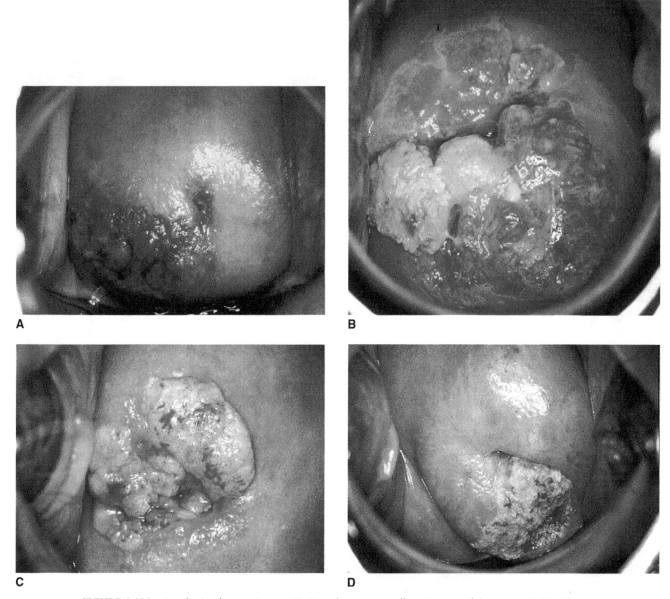

A

B

C

D

FIGURE 8.106.   Exophytic adenocarcinomas (**A, B**) and squamous cell carcinomas of the cervix (**C, D**). (Photos courtesy of Dr. Vesna Kesic.)

proliferation of new and large-caliber blood vessels that permit cellular expansion beyond the normal integrity of the epithelium. If the cancer exceeds its necessary vascular supply, ulcerations develop and the exophytic mass may assume an even more irregular contour.

8.5.3.2.3 COLPOSCOPIC APPEARANCE

Elevations are best observed colposcopically when using a stereoscopic colposcope. Because many colposcopes do not permit stereoscopic viewing, associated shadows, contrasting tangential light reflections, and color hue and shades can be used to determine contour changes. Light reflection from surface irregularity is perhaps the best indication of contour elevation. Gentle manipulation of the cervix also helps the colposcopist discern subtle surface variations. Elevations of the cervix may be unifocal or multifocal, confined to the cervix, or present diffusely within the lower genital tract. Large, focal lesions or tiny, dispersed elevations may indicate HPV infection. The causative agent determines the contour, height, surface area, number, shape, and color of epithelial elevations.

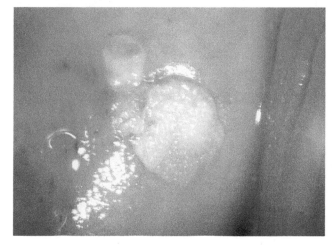

FIGURE 8.107.   Leukoplakia or a plaque-like white patch on the cervix prior to 3% to 5% acetic acid application.

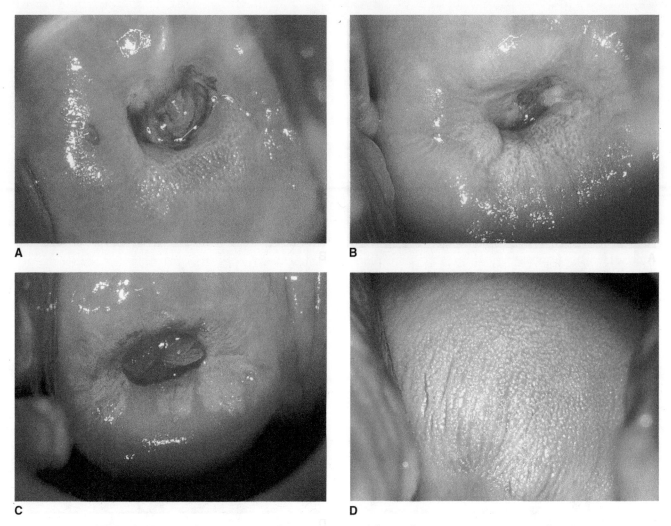

FIGURE 8.108.   **A:** Parakeratosis seen on the posterior cervix following loop excision. Tiny nonacetowhite elevations are noted. **B:** Parakeratosis is also seen in another patient following cryotherapy. This should be contrasted with parakeratosis seen following loop excision (**C**) but with acetowhite recurrent CIN 1 confirmed on biopsy. **D:** Occasionally an irregular surface with diffuse parakeratotic projections will be found in the absence of a history of prior cervical surgery. (Courtesy of, and approved for reproduction by, the International Cervical Cancer (INCCA) foundation.)

Following 3% to 5% acetic acid application, micropapillae or asperities caused by HPV produce a pebbled, acetowhite epithelial appearance much like sand imbedded in paint (Figure 8.109A–H). Small-loop capillaries may be seen in these tiny epithelial projections when viewed at high-level magnification. Application of Lugol's iodine greatly assists the identification of asperities, which appear as tiny yellow surface elevations (peaks) against a mahogany brown background. The colposcopic appearance resembles a "starry night" pattern unique to subclinical HPV infection (Figure 8.109H).

Although similar tiny iodine-negative dots, streaks, and patches may be seen with other inflammatory conditions, they are usually flat or macular. Trichomonas cervicitis or vaginitis is characterized grossly by small red patches that, with closer inspection, appear as randomly diffuse clusters of fine punctation (Figure 8.111A,B). These clusters may be mildly elevated as a gradually rounded tapered mound. Following application of Lugol's iodine, multiple well-circumscribed clusters of small yellow irregular patches or dots that conform to the previous diffuse red patches may be seen colposcopically. Vaginal candidiasis can also create Lugol's negative spots and patches, but does not typically completely denude the mucosa, hence the yellow hue (Figure 8.111C,D).

Papillary projections that appear as long, filiform acetowhite clusters are caused primarily by HPV types 6 and 11. Central afferent and efferent loop capillaries may be noted, especially as the acetic acid reaction fades. A brain-like surface contour may be seen, although it is rarely associated with HPV infection. This distinctive cerebriform contour change, however, may also represent invasive cancer. Similarly, cauliflower-like growths may indicate either condylomas or cancer. Papular lesions can represent either extreme of the neoplastic spectrum, HPV infection or cancer, but the former etiology by far the most common. Although cervical dysplasia normally retains a macular contour, sometimes CIN 3 lesions may be elevated slightly or plaque-like. Leukoplakic plaques, with sharply defined margins rising abruptly from the surrounding epithelium, may be associated with a neoplastic process.

Because cervical cancer may appear papillary, it may be difficult to discriminate it colposcopically from a large condyloma (Figure 8.112A–D). Cancer is typically more compact and focal than the long, finger-like papillae seen more commonly with HPV-associated lesions. Verrucous carcinoma can mimic a benign condyloma. However, recognition of this similar morphology always demands histologic sampling to

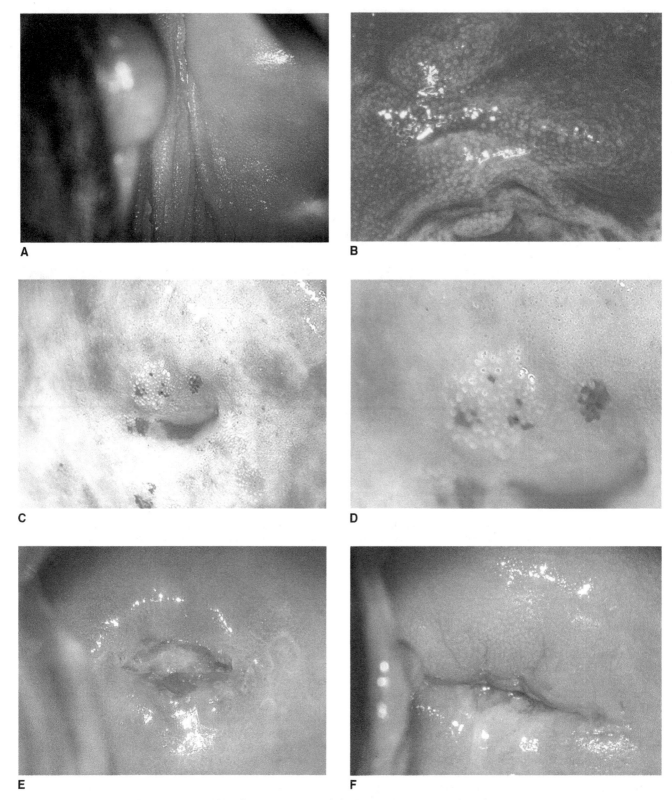

FIGURE 8.109.   A–H: Micropapillae, or asperities, of the vagina produced by HPV infection. **B–D:** Tiny raised capillaries associated with HPV infection are also seen. **H:** "Starry night" pattern of nonstaining asperities on a dark mahogany brown background are seen in the left vaginal fornix in this young woman referred for evaluation of a LSIL Pap and found to have CIN 1. (Courtesy of, and approved for reproduction by, the International Cervical Cancer (INCCA) foundation.)

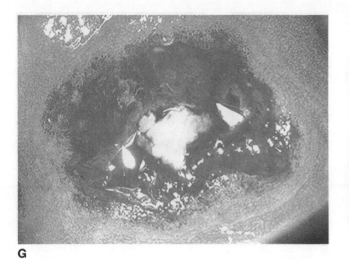

G

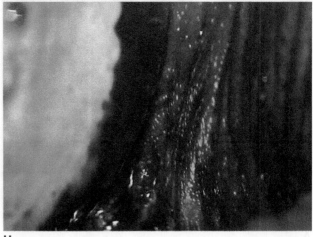

H

FIGURE 8.109. *(Continued)*

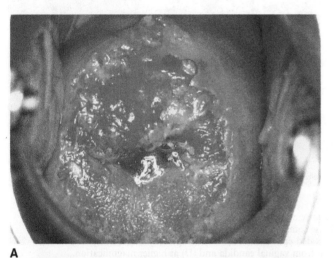

A

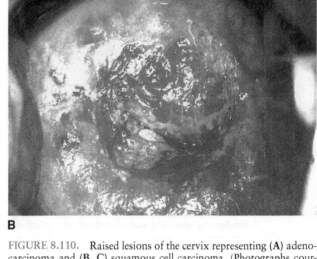

B

FIGURE 8.110. Raised lesions of the cervix representing (**A**) adeno-carcinoma and (**B, C**) squamous cell carcinoma. (Photographs courtesy of Dr. Vesna Kesic.)

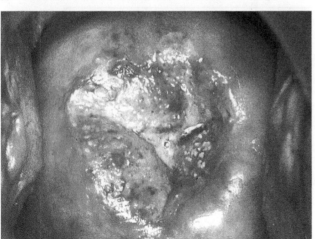

C

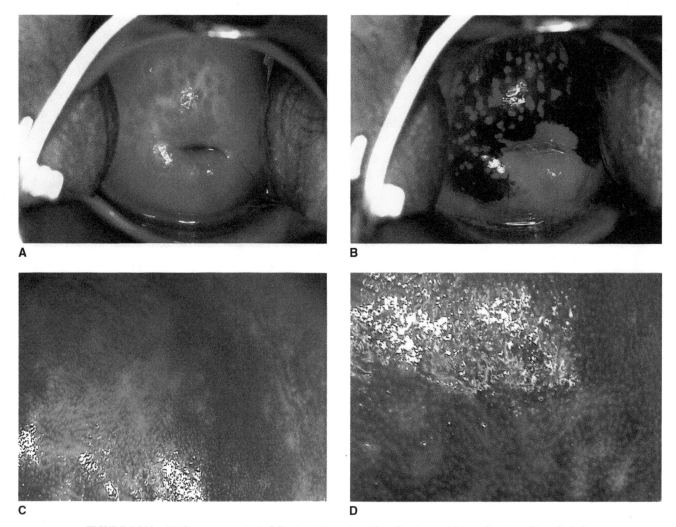

FIGURE 8.111. Trichomonas cervicitis following (**A**) acetic acid application and (**B**) application of Lugol's iodine application. Note that the red dots in (**A**) correspond with the completely nonstaining red dots in (**B**) that stand out after the dark staining of Lugol's in the surrounding noneroded epithelium (**C**). Classic splotchy Lugol's negative patches and spots in a woman with significant inflammation from vaginal candida and (**D**) at higher magnification.

establish the correct diagnosis. Cancers more commonly present as nodular, papular, or raised exophytic growths of the cervix. Coexisting atypical blood vessels, yellow epithelium, ulcerations, bleeding, and friable, erythematous epithelium suggest cancer (Figure 8.113A,B).

An elevated surface contour is never a normal colposcopic finding, provided the normal villiform pattern of columnar epithelium and nabothian cysts are excluded. However, benign nonneoplastic elevations may be seen secondary to congenital contour irregularities, large nabothian cysts, and protruding endocervical or endometrial polyps and fibroids (Figure 8.114A–M). Mass-like protuberances from the external cervical os usually represent benign endocervical polyps, occasionally prolapsing fibroids (Figure 8.115), and rarely neoplasia or products of conception. Polyps may be covered by columnar epithelium that imparts a pebbled, red surface. Otherwise, polyps are covered by varying degrees of smooth metaplasia. Surface irregularities or projections may be seen as a cock's comb or cervical collar in women exposed to DES *in utero*. These changes are discussed in greater detail in Chapter 13. A red, fleshy protrusion covered by columnar epithelium surrounding the external os following excisional surgery of the cervix is known as a cervical

button (Figure 8.116A–D). The protuberance results from either an accelerated growth of columnar epithelium arising from the base of the surgical wound or contraction of the scar around the excisional margin. This benign change may appear in conjunction with a fine radial punctation vessel pattern that extends centrally toward the os from the surgical excision margins. A slightly thickened, pebbled epithelial texture may be observed in the area of excision secondary to parakeratosis. The tiny surface projections usually correspond to and overlie the radial punctation vessels. A lack of surrounding acetowhite epithelium helps to distinguish this normal postoperative finding from neoplasia (Figure 8.117A–G).

8.5.3.2.4 CLINICAL SIGNIFICANCE

Contour elevations of the cervix may be normal congenital variations (Figure 8.114K–M), abnormal benign conditions, or may be caused by neoplasia. In the majority of cases, surface elevations should be considered abnormal. Neoplasia must be suspected, particularly when accompanied by abnormal cervical cytologic findings. A good colposcopist will also look for other abnormal colposcopic signs to assist the derivation of a clinically based colposcopic impression.

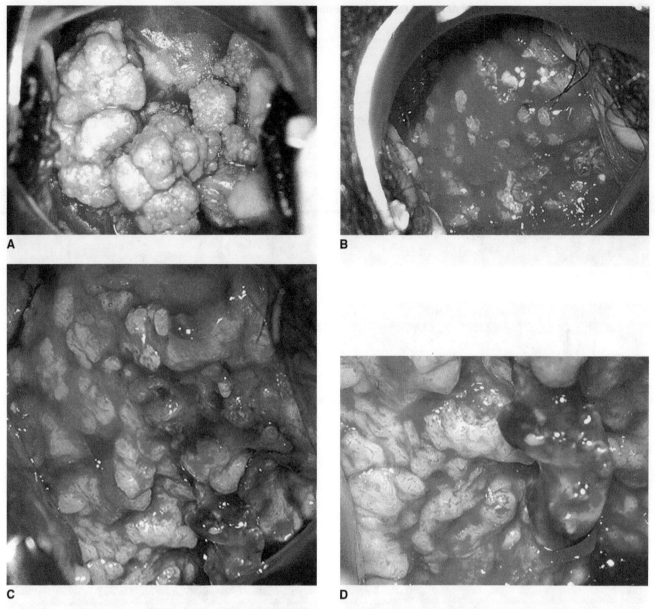

FIGURE 8.112.   **A:** A large exophytic condyloma covers an occult cervical cancer hidden beneath it. **B–D:** A small opaque acetowhite high-grade lesion is seen on the anterior cervix. A large exophytic cervical cancer is seen for comparative purposes. (Courtesy of, and approved for reproduction by, the International Cervical Cancer (INCCA) foundation.)

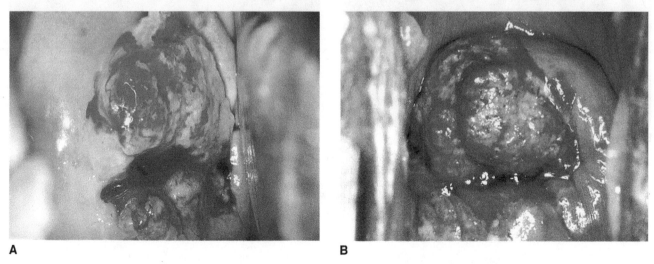

FIGURE 8.113.   A large yellow cervical cancer can be seen eroding beneath the epithelium on the anterior cervix. **A:** The normal epithelium is buckled forming a curved ridge secondary to the undermining. **B:** A necrotic, friable exophytic cervical cancer.

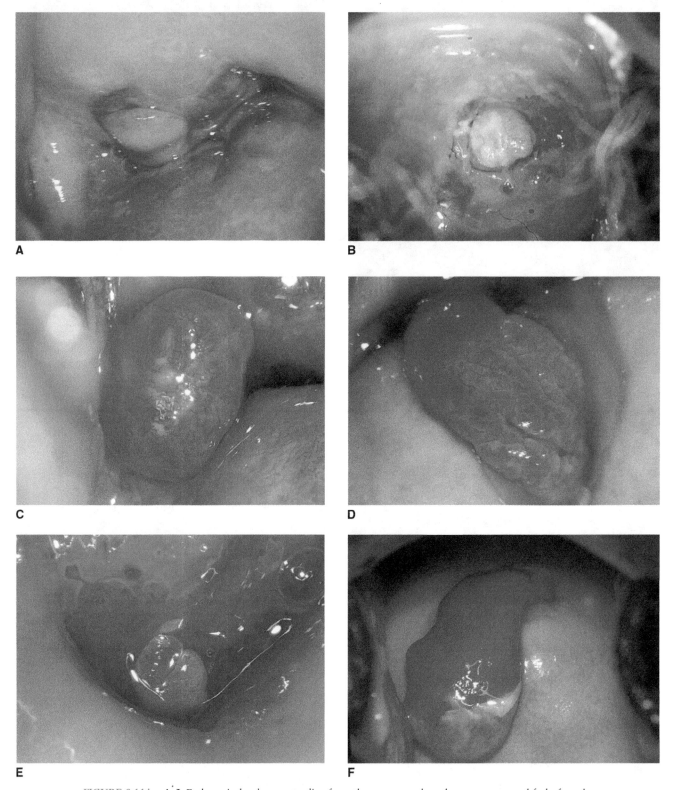

FIGURE 8.114. **A–J:** Endocervical polyps protruding from the os can produce the appearance and feel of an elevated or irregular surface. **D:** A red polyp protruding from the os is seen following acetic acid application. **E:** A small endocervical polyp was noted during evaluation of an ASC-US Pap test report. **F:** A large tongue-like endocervical polyp protrudes from the os. This polyp in a 17-year-old woman was diagnosed as botryoid rhabdomyosarcoma, a malignant tumor.

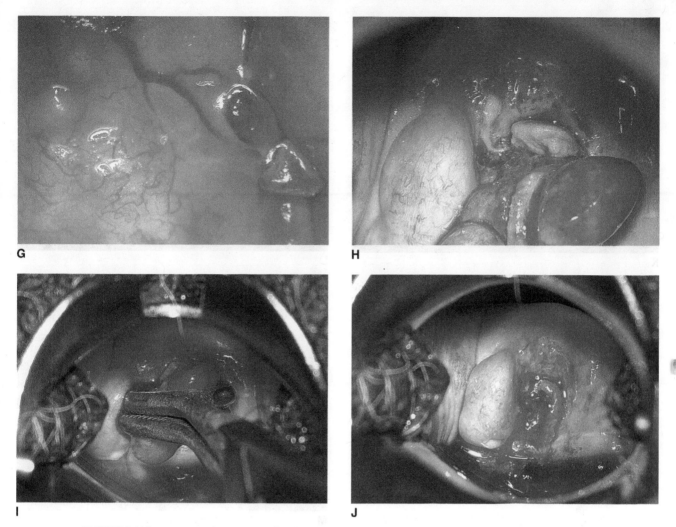

FIGURE 8.114.   *(Continued)* **G:** Two small polyps are seen at the os adjacent to a large nabothian follicle accentuating overlying branching blood vessels. **H:** A polyp adjacent to a large nabothian cyst. **I, J:** Protruding endocervical polyps can usually be easily removed with a ring forceps, as demonstrated. The cervix in **(H)** and **(I)** following removal of the polyp.

8.5.4 Margin Characteristics of Abnormal Cervical Epithelium

8.5.4.1 Abnormal Cervix

8.5.4.1.1 BEFORE APPLICATION OF 3% TO 5% ACETIC ACID AND LUGOL'S IODINE SOLUTION

8.5.4.1.1.1 Colposcopic Appearance

Sometimes, cervical lesions may be noted before epithelial contrast agents are applied to the cervix. In this circumstance, a raised margin or outline of the lesion will help determine the etiology. White areas of leukoplakia, pink condyloma, decidua, and exophytic cancers may be noted during the initial colposcopic inspection. Compared with the normal surrounding epithelium, leukoplakia is variably raised. The extent of elevation is determined by the amount of keratin accumulation. The raised interface or margin of leukoplakia may slope gradually or rise abruptly. A steep margin gives an impression that the area might be peeled off easily. The margins of leukoplakia are generally irregular or jagged, and rarely smooth or straight. Smaller surrounding satellite patches of leukoplakia may also be observed. Diffuse pinpoint areas of leukoplakia with steep margins can be best appreciated at high-power colposcopic magnification. These tiny areas may represent leukoplakia atop asperities or parakeratosis seen following surgery. Papillary or protuberant condyloma may be seen during cytologic sampling. These lesions with distinctive margins should be distinguished from decidual reaction of pregnancy, microglandular hyperplasia, and invasive cancer. Cervical cancers, especially when more advanced, can usually be seen without contrast solutions and colposcopy. A multitude of various abrupt or gradual margins can be encountered with cancer. The margins of all these abnormal entities are also defined by their unusual elevated contour. It is the elevated contour, not necessarily margins, that most likely captures the attention of a colposcopist prior to the application of epithelial contrast solutions.

8.5.4.1.2 AFTER APPLICATION OF 3% TO 5% ACETIC ACID OR LUGOL'S IODINE SOLUTION

8.5.4.1.2.1 Colposcopic Appearance

The margins of most abnormal flat cervical lesions can be better appreciated following the application of both 3% to 5% acetic acid and Lugol's iodine (Figure 8.118). This

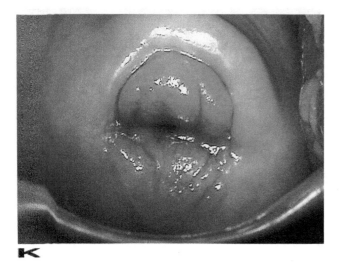

K

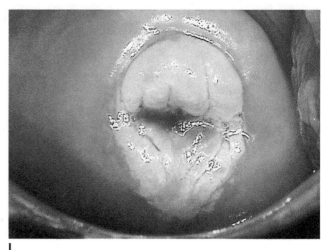

L

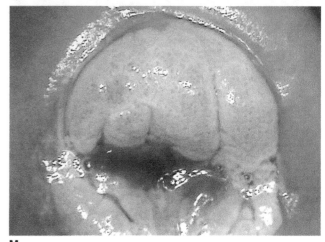

M

FIGURE 8.114.   *(Continued)* K–M: Protruding ectopy of congenital origin (K) before and (L, M) after the application of 5% acetic acid, which confirms the villiform pattern of columnar epithelium, and the metaplastic fusing evident on higher power (M). (Courtesy of, and approved for reproduction by, the International Cervical Cancer (INCCA) foundation.)

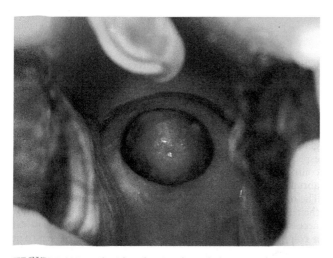

FIGURE 8.115.   Fibroid prolapsing through the external os.

demarcation allows appraisal of the margin characteristics. In most instances, acetowhite lesions of the cervix will exhibit the same margin as that seen following Lugol's iodine application (Figure 8.119A–C). In the case of macular, faintly acetowhite changes, Lugol's iodine will generally provide a more vivid and distinct contrast between different epithelial types. The observed margins between pink and white epithelium or between yellow and brown epithelium may vary tremendously. Occasionally, the margin interface may also exhibit a contour change, rendering them more easily detectable based on a color, margin, and topographic contrast.

Margins or staining interfaces may be noted between two different normal epithelia, between normal and abnormal epithelia, and between two different types of abnormal epithelium. Acetowhite or Lugol's iodine–negative immature metaplasia will generally form an irregular margin with mature metaplasia and columnar epithelium (Figure 8.120). An exception is the smooth margin between the epithelium of a CTZ and squamous epithelium. Normally, no visible margin between mature metaplasia and original squamous epithelium can be seen, even after application of contrast solutions. However, a faintly visible margin between normal epithelia may be appreciated in women following surgical excision procedures of the cervix. In this case, a slight variation in epithelial color, along with normal radial punctation and

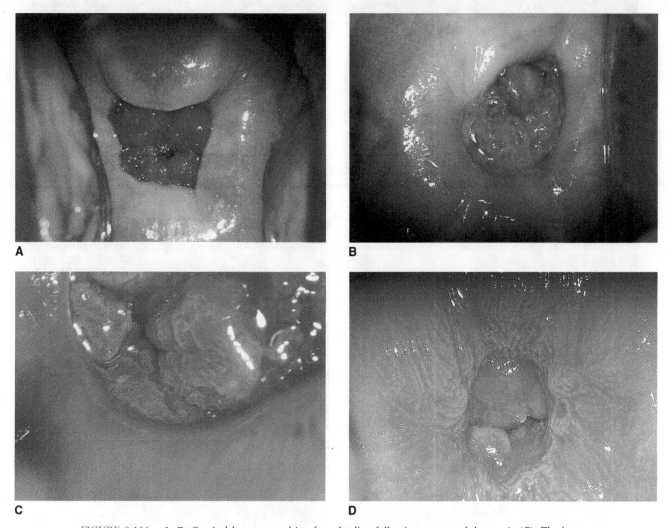

FIGURE 8.116.   **A, B:** Cervical buttons resulting from healing following surgery of the cervix (**C**). The button initially is covered with columnar epithelium, but eventually (**D**) exposure to the vaginal environment induces metaplastic transformation over the exposed "button." (Courtesy of, and approved for reproduction by, the International Cervical Cancer (INCCA) foundation.)

parakeratosis, may be noted. The excision line is not accentuated by contrast solutions, provided normal epithelium occupies each side of the line. The margins between normal and abnormal epithelia assume a greater variation, from irregular to smooth, indistinct to sharp, and macular to elevated. Both immature metaplasia and CIN 1 lesions of the cervix exhibit similar margin types. Irregular, jagged, feathered, flocculated, or indistinct borders may be seen with either entity (Figure 8.121). The vague nature of these margins may be attributable to the effect of a poorly circumscribed viral infection in the case of CIN 1, or to the diffuse, varied reaction to acid-induced epithelial trauma noted with evolving immature metaplasia. Small satellite areas positioned in the periphery, away from large central lesions, also may be seen with immature metaplasia or CIN 1. These margin types are generally associated with macular epithelial areas and, therefore, no surface contour change can be appreciated. However, papillary condyloma, equivalent to CIN 1, should not be confused with immature metaplasia. Although very immature metaplasia may overlie a villus, which is normally covered by columnar epithelium, the villi and condyloma are not usually confused. The margins associated with CIN 2 and CIN 3 are more uniform, typically straight or gently rounded (Figure 8.122A,B). An abrupt histologic border between a severe

dysplasia and normal epithelium conveys the sharp contrast seen colposcopically. These well-delineated high-grade lesion margins contrast readily with the sometimes diffuse, ill-defined margins of CIN 1 or immature metaplasia. The blocks of neoplastic epithelium are well circumscribed and segregated from dissimilar epithelium. With these grades of neoplasia, severely abnormal epithelium may appear slightly raised. The thickened epithelium may appear to be peeled from the stroma. An AIS may be less distinct with respect to colposcopic margins. These acetowhite lesions are more apt to blend with the surrounding acetowhite blanched normal columnar epithelium or immature metaplasia. However, some adenocarcinomas are quite distinct (Figure 8.123).

The margins of advanced cancer are usually well delineated from the surrounding normal epithelium. The margins are perhaps less well defined from nonmalignant areas of neoplasia if microinvasive cancer or an endophytic cancer coexists. However, this is not always the case (Figure 8.124A,B). Exophytic cancers have readily discerned margins that are very abrupt in relief. When palpated, the tumor may feel firm or hard when compared with the softer adjoining normal tissue. The margins demonstrate slight to moderate irregularity if the tumor is friable and necrotic. Otherwise, the margins of cancer are more discrete and smooth. Early adenocarcinoma margins

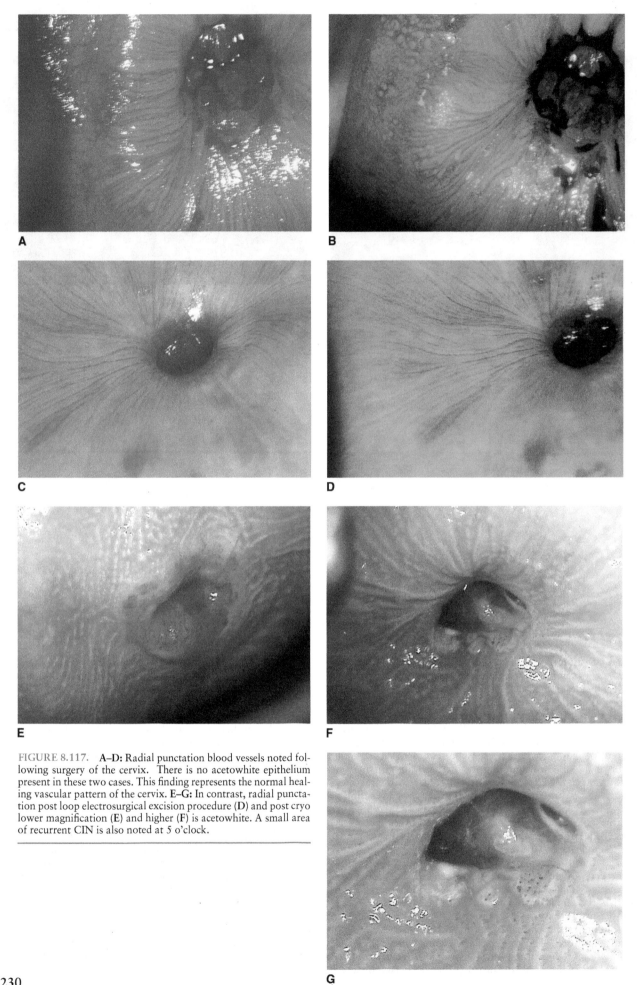

FIGURE 8.117. **A–D:** Radial punctation blood vessels noted following surgery of the cervix. There is no acetowhite epithelium present in these two cases. This finding represents the normal healing vascular pattern of the cervix. **E–G:** In contrast, radial punctation post loop electrosurgical excision procedure (**D**) and post cryo lower magnification (**E**) and higher (**F**) is acetowhite. A small area of recurrent CIN is also noted at 5 o'clock.

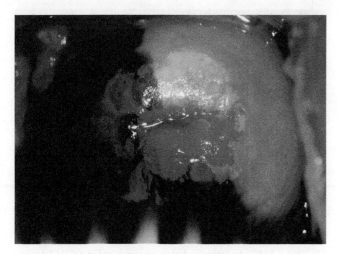

FIGURE 8.118. A large low-grade lesion is seen simultaneously after acetic acid and Lugol's iodine solution applications.

may not be as readily recognized or distinguished from normal columnar epithelium as squamous cancer is from adjoining squamous epithelium.

Unique margins between two different types of abnormal epithelium may be noted during the colposcopic examination. In this case, an acetowhite opaque, proximally positioned lesion may be distinguished from a more translucent peripherally located lesion. Sometimes a larger variegated lesion

stained with Lugol's iodine will encompass a smaller, pale, iodine-negative lesion. Usually, the margin between these two areas is smooth or straight. Because both areas may be of similar color, the margin between abnormal epithelium may not be as well defined. Also, the more centrally positioned lesion may be quite small compared with the larger surrounding lesion. When a CIN 2 or CIN 3 is positioned within a larger CIN 1 lesion or area of immature metaplasia, an internal margin may be noted (Figure 8.125). This interface is an abnormal/abnormal margin. Moreover, an internal margin also may be noted between CIN 3 and an invasive cancer. At times, a surface contour change may help to further delineate the junction. If one area is raised (usually the central lesion) the demarcation should be more easily recognized. An associated surface ulceration also may be present. Coexisting squamous and glandular neoplasias may adjoin each other. Provided the glandular lesions are seen on the surface and are not confined to gland clefts, colposcopists may discern a colposcopically visible interface. However, because early glandular neoplasias can mimic immature metaplasia, the glandular lesion is likely to be less apparent.

8.5.4.1.2.2   Clinical Significance

Unique attributes of lesion margins should be noted during colposcopy. The margin characteristics of acetowhite or Lugol's iodine–negative epithelium help the colposcopist define normality and varying levels of abnormality. As such, lesion margin is considered a valuable colposcopic sign. Margin characteristics of neoplastic epithelium are discussed in greater detail in Chapter 9.

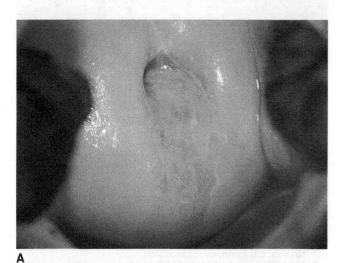

A

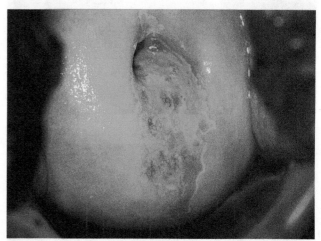

B

FIGURE 8.119. A: An acetowhite lesion with an irregular margin is seen on the posterior cervix. B: A fine mosaic vascular pattern is best seen using the red free (green) filter of the colposcope. C: The iodine-negative yellow epithelium corresponds to the acetowhite epithelium. The lesion also extends into the endocervical canal beyond colposcopic visualization.

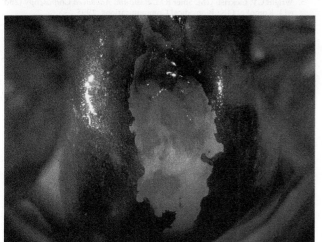

C

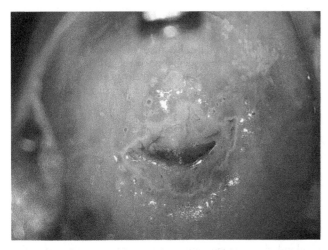

FIGURE 8.120. An irregular margin noted with immature metaplasia following acetic acid application.

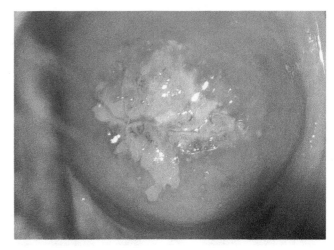

FIGURE 8.121. An irregular lesion margin noted in a CIN 1 lesion.

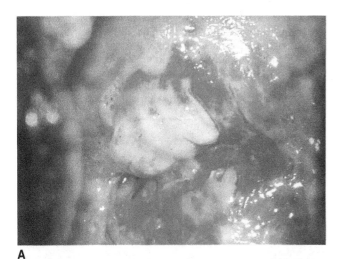

A

B

FIGURE 8.122. **A, B:** A fairly uniform straight lesion margin observed in both patients with CIN 3.

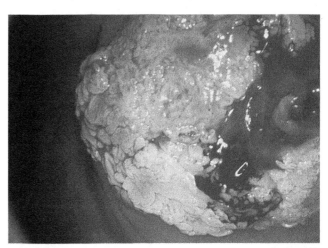

FIGURE 8.123. An obvious AIS with a distinct margin.

References

1. Coppelson M, Pixley EC, Reid B. *Colposcopy: A Scientific and Practical Approach to the Cervix, Vagina, and Vulva in Health and Disease* (3rd ed.). Springfield, IL: Charles C. Thomas, 1987.
2. Burke L, Antonioli DA, Ducatman BS. *Colposcopy Text and Atlas.* Norwalk, CT: Appleton and Lange, 1991.
3. Wright CV, Lickrish GM, Shier RM. *Basic and Advanced Colposcopy* (2nd ed.). Komoka, ON: Biomedical Communications, 1995.
4. Kolstad P, Stafl A. *Atlas of Colposcopy* (3rd ed.). Oslo, Norway: Scandinavian University Books, 1982.
5. Burghardt E, Ostor AG. *Colposcopy, Cervical Pathology. Textbook and Atlas.* New York: Thieme Stratton, 1984.
6. Moscicki AB, Schiffman M, Kjaer S, Villa LL. Chapter 5: Updating the natural history of HPV and anogenital cancer. *Vaccine* 2006;24(suppl 3): S3/42–51.
7. Maxwell GL, Sosson AP, Oster C, Miles P, Webb J, Carlson J. Subepithelial angiogenesis in cervical intraepithelial neoplasia. *J Lower Genital Tract Dis* 1998;2:191–4.
8. Folkman J. Anti-angiogenesis: new concept for therapy of solid tumors. *Ann Surg* 1972;175:409–16.
9. Abulafia O, Triest WE, Sherer DM. Angiogenesis in squamous cell carcinoma in situ and microinvasive carcinoma of the uterine cervix. *Obstet Gynecol* 1996;88:927–32.
10. Stafl A, Mattingly RF. Angiogenesis of cervical neoplasia. *Am J Obstet Gynecol* 1975;121:845–52.
11. Cheng WF, Chen CA, Lee CN, Chen TM, Hseik FJ, Hseih CY. Vascular endothelial growth factor in cervical carcinoma. *Obstet Gynecol* 1999;93:761–5.
12. Bodnev-Adler B, Hefler L, Bodner K, Levdolter S, Frischmuth K, Kainz C, et al. Serum levels of angiogenin (ANG) in invasive cancer and in cervical intraepithelial neoplasia (CIN). *Anticancer Res* 2001;21:809–12.

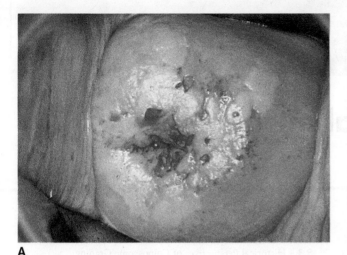 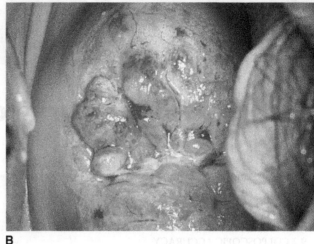

FIGURE 8.124. **A, B:** Two examples of microinvasive cervical cancer. These microinvasive lesions are associated with very large, high-grade lesions. (Photos courtesy of Dr. Vesna Kesic.)

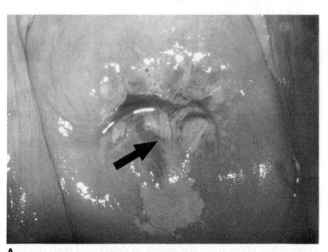 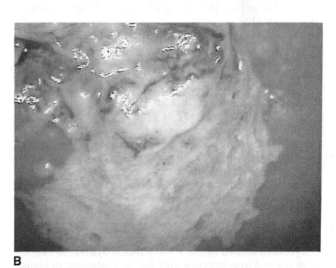

FIGURE 8.125. **A:** An internal margin or border located closer to the SCJ (*arrow*), demarcating a high-grade cervical lesion near the os and a lower-grade lesion in the periphery. **B:** Internal margin of a CIN 2 near the os with immature metaplasia distally.

13. Walker P, Dexeus S, DePalo G, Barrasso R, Campion M, Girardi F, et al. International terminology of colposcopy: an updated report from the International Federation for Cervical Pathology and Colposcopy. *Obstet Gynecol* 2003;101:175–7.

14. Hopman EH, Kenemans P, Helmerhorst TJM. Positive predictive rate of colposcopic examination of the cervix uteri: an overview of the literature. *Obstet Gynecol Survey* 1998;53:97–106.

15. Sakuma T, Hasegawa T, Tsutsui F, Kurihara S. Quantitative analysis of the whiteness of the atypical cervical transformation zone. *J Reprod Med* 1985;30:773–6.

16. Zahm DM, Nidl I, Greinke C, Hoyer H, Schneider A. Colposcopic appearance of cervical intraepithelial neoplasia is age dependent. *Am J Obstet Gynecol* 1998;178:1298–304.

17. Tidbury P, Singer A, Jenkins D. CIN3: the role of lesion size in invasion. *Br J Obstet Gynecol* 1992;99:583–6.

18. Boonstra H, Aalders JG, Koudstaal J, et al. Minimum extension and appropriate topographic position of tissue destruction for treatment of cervical intraepithelial neoplasia. *Obstet Gynecol* 1990;75:227–31.

19. Difiore MSH. *Atlas of Human Histology* (4th ed.). Philadelphia, PA: Lea and Febiger, 1975.

20. Kolstad P. The colposcopic diagnosis of dysplasia, carcinoma in situ, and early invasive cancer of the cervix. *Acta Obstet Gynec Scand* 1964;43:105–8.

21. Follen MM, Lavine RU, Carillo E, Richart RM, Nuovo G, Crum CP. Colposcopic correlates of cervical papillomavirus infection. *Am J Obstet Gynecol* 1987;157:809–14.

22. Hinselmann H. *Einfurung in die Kolposkopie*. Hamburg, Germany: Hartung, 1933.

23. Mikhail MS, Romney SL. Computerized measurement of intercapillary distance using image analysis in women with cervical intraepithelial neoplasia: correlation with severity. *Obstet Gynecol* 2000; 95(suppl):S2–3.

24. Kolstad P. The development of the vascular bed in tumors as seen in squamous-cell carcinoma of the cervix uteri. *Br J Radiol* 1965; 38:216–23.

25. Kolstad P. Intercapillary distance, oxygen tension and local recurrence in cervix cancer. *Scand J Clin Lab Invest* 1968;106:145–57.

26. Sillman F, Boyce J, Fruchter R. The significance of atypical vessels and neovascularization in cervical neoplasia. *Am J Obstet Gynecol* 1981;139:154–9.

27. Sugimori H, Matsuyama T, Kashimura M, et al. Colposcopic findings in microinvasive carcinoma of the uterine cervix. *Obstet Gynecol Surv* 1979;34:804.

28. Wright VC. Colposcopy of adenocarcinoma in situ and adenocarcinoma of the uterine cervix: differentiation from other cervical lesions. *J Lower Genital Tract Dis* 1999;3:83–97.

29. Johannison E, Kolstad P, Soderberg G. Cytologic, vascular, and histologic patterns of dysplasia, carcinoma in situ, and early invasive carcinoma of the cervix. *Acta Radiol* 1966;258(suppl):1–136.

30. Bloom W, Fawcett DW. *A Textbook of Histology* (10th ed.). Philadelphia, PA: W.B. Saunders, 1975.

CHAPTER 9

DARON G. FERRIS
J. THOMAS COX
EDWARD J. MAYEAUX, JR.

Colposcopy of Cervical Intraepithelial Neoplasia

9.1 INTRODUCTION
9.2 COLPOSCOPIC ACCURACY
    9.2.1 Sensitivity and Specificity
    9.2.2 Lesion Size, Thickness of the Epithelium, Age, HPV Type, and Other Variables
    9.2.3 Improving Sensitivity by Taking More Biopsies
    9.2.4 What Does This All Mean for the Practicing Colposcopist?
9.3 COLPOSCOPIC GRADING OF CERVICAL NEOPLASIA
    9.3.1 Rationale for Colposcopic Grading
    9.3.2 Importance of Grading Systems for Colposcopy

9.3.3 The Colposcopic Impression
9.3.4 Historical Perspectives of Colposcopic Grading Systems
9.4 COLPOSCOPIC FEATURES OF CERVICAL INTRAEPITHELIAL NEOPLASIA
    9.4.1 Colposcopy of CIN 1
    9.4.2 Colposcopy of CIN 2
    9.4.3 Colposcopy of CIN 3

9.1 INTRODUCTION

During the first few decades of colposcopy practice, cervical screening was also in its early decades. The result was that many women referred to colposcopy for the evaluation of abnormal cervical cytology had large prevalent high-grade lesions.[1] Colposcopic triage guidelines based on the old Papanicolaou Classification System also contributed to the majority of lesions seen by colposcopists being high grade, as atypical squamous cells of undetermined significance (ASC-US) had not yet been created by the 1988 Bethesda System, so patients were referred to colposcopy only for the evaluation of higher-grade Pap results.[2] Additionally, few studies compared the results of histology derived from same-patient colposcopically directed biopsy and conization specimens, instead of comparing colposcopic impression to biopsy results, usually within one grade. Hence, in the early years of colposcopic practice, the sensitivity and specificity of colposcopy were reported to be much higher than reported in more recent studies. Large high-grade lesions were usually easier to identify, and most women coming to colposcopy had cervical intraepithelial neoplasia (CIN). A 1998 meta-analysis of real-time colposcopy studies from the early decades of colposcopic practice (1960 to 1996) confirmed this impression, reporting the estimated sensitivity of colposcopy for detection of CIN 3 to be 85%.[3] Hopman et al.[4] in a review the same year found colposcopically directed biopsies, when compared to same-patient cone specimens derived by large loop excision of the transformation zone, to be undercalled on average in only 20% of cases. A 2003 review of correlation of colposcopic impression and biopsy diagnosis by highly trained colposcopists in the British Columbia cytology-colposcopy program also demonstrated high rates of agreement (Table 9.1).[5]

However, other than the British Columbia evaluation, nearly all more recent studies of the accuracy of both real-time colposcopy, and retrospective reviews of static colposcopic images, have demonstrated colposcopy to be far less sensitive and specific than previously reported.[6–18] While reasonable

questions can be raised about the accuracy of studies based on review of static images[9,10,14,16,17] when compared to studies based on real-time colposcopy,[3–8,11–13,15,18–20] the results are fairly comparable. Although our understanding of the accuracy of colposcopy has changed, it does not negate the value or importance of the procedure to cervical cancer prevention. Until a test or procedure emerges that is more predictive of risk and location of cervical neoplasia, colposcopy will continue to be the one vital link that binds the success of the screening program and detection of histologic cervical precancer requiring treatment.[1,21,22] The unparalleled success in cervical cancer prevention has come from the ability to detect and treat the precursor lesion to squamous cell cervical cancer (CIN 3) before it gains the capacity to invade,[23] and it is widely accepted to have occurred secondary to the partnership between cervical cytology screening and treatment of colposcopically detected lesions.[1,24] Therefore, our understanding that the colposcopic impression is less precise and reproducible than previously taught does not take away from its vital role in determining where to biopsy within a large lesion or in selecting which two to three areas among many should be biopsied. This role is even more challenging with the addition of human papillomavirus (HPV) testing to screening and management because its high sensitivity, but mediocre specificity and positive predictive value, has almost doubled nonspecific referral to colposcopy that was previously due mainly to ASC-US cytology.[21] Colposcopic evaluation and guided biopsy remain the critical tools in distinguishing which women require destruction of the cervical transformation zone among a majority that do not. This makes optimizing the accuracy of colposcopy and biopsy more critical than ever.[21]

In order to guide colposcopists in the quest to be as accurate as possible, Chapter 9 begins with an overview of recent studies on the accuracy of colposcopy and the importance of taking more than one biopsy. Colposcopic grading systems and recent reviews of the accuracy and role of grading systems follow. The bulk of the chapter then reviews the colposcopic findings of classic CIN 1, CIN 2, and CIN 3, with the

TABLE 9.1   CORRELATION BETWEEN COLPOSCOPIC IMPRESSION AND FINAL COLPOBIOPSY HISTOLOGY

BIOPSY RESULT	COLPOSCOPIC IMPRESSION (%)				
	BENIGN*	CIN I	CIN II	CIN III	COLPOSCOPIC OVERT CANCER
Benign or within normal limits	75.5	33.7	17.2	7.9	11.5
CIN I	15.9	41.4	22.4	9.5	4.2
CIN II/III	8.6	25.0	60.5	82.4	35.5
Invasive cancer	0.06	0.02	0.04	0.14	48.8
Satisfactory correlation[b]	91.4	91.8	82.8	82.6	84.2

The British Columbia Colposcopy-Cytology Program has colposcopy referral centers staffed by highly trained colposcopists required to have very high cyto-colpo-histo correlation and to undergo certification and recertification in colposcopy on a regular basis. Correlations between colposcopic impression and final colpobiopsy histology is highest for CIN 3, followed by "within normal limits." Lowest correlation was for CIN 1, followed by "colposcopic overt cancer," which was histologic cancer in just under 50% of cases.
*Benign includes negative and reactive changes.
[†]One step difference or less.
**Gold boxes denote exact correlation (%) between colposcopic impression and final histology.
From Benedet JL, Matisic JP, Bertrand MA. An analysis of 84,244 patients from the British Columbia cytology-colposcopy program. *Gynecol Oncol* 2004;92(1):127–34, with permission.

understanding that many histologic lesions of each grade will not conform to all, or even any, of these colposcopic features.

9.2 COLPOSCOPIC ACCURACY

9.2.1 Sensitivity and Specificity

In estimating the sensitivity and specificity of colposcopy, CIN 3 is the best disease endpoint because CIN 2 is poorly reproducible and often regresses.[21] Additionally, as the true precursor to cervical cancer, it is the endpoint, other than invasive cancer itself, that is most critical for detection. One of the early studies comparing the severest finding on colpobiopsy to that found on paired loop excision demonstrated that 41% of CIN 3+ detected in the loop specimen was not present in the paired punch biopsy.[25] Over half of these had only CIN 1 or normal in the biopsy, and three did not have the adenocarcinoma *in situ* (AIS), nor an invasive cancer, found in the cone. However, when the CIN 3 was small, the punch biopsy was more likely to be of greater severity than the loop specimen, indicating that even some small CIN 3s could be colposcopically detected.[25] Of concern was that even when lesions were large (>2 quadrants), undercall by biopsy of CIN 3+ occurred in nearly a third. In a later study, the same group evaluated the colposcopic impression and management decisions of 30 well-trained colposcopists made after video viewing of transformation zones from normal through varying abnormalities up to CIN 3.[26] They reported considerable interobserver variability and variation in diagnostic accuracy in scoring cervical images, particularly at the lower end of the spectrum of abnormality, which can lead to overtreatment. Knowledge of the cytology result improved the accuracy of the colposcopic impression.

Massad et al.[7] evaluated the strength of the correlation between colposcopic impression and biopsy histology in a large urban colposcopy referral clinic. Exact agreement was found in only 37%, but results agreed within one grade in 75%. Of concern was that the negative predictive value of a benign colposcopic impression was only 68% and sensitivity for CIN 2,3 was only 56%. Similar results for sensitivity for CIN 2,3 was also found in the ASC-US/LSIL (low-grade

squamous intraepithelial lesion) Triage Study (ALTS), a multicenter randomized trial that included nationally recognized expert "quality control" colposcopists and more than 40 experienced clinical-site colposcopists. Only 54.8% of women with a cumulative final histologic diagnosis of CIN 3 that included enrollment and 2-year follow-up had a positive colposcopic biopsy (≥CIN 2) at enrollment.[6,21] While the estimated sensitivity of the initial colposcopy for CIN 3 in ALTS did not account for the likelihood that some of the CIN 3 subsequently detected during 2-year follow-up may have been either newly incident or so small as to not be discernible at the initial colposcopically, numerous other studies have demonstrated similar sensitivity for CIN 3.[1]

ALTS clinician-investigators have performed many ancillary analyses concentrating on the enrollment colposcopic examination of women with eventual diagnosis of CIN 3.[21] Because most of these studies were retrospective, many employed blinded review of digitized colpophotos or Cervigrams taken at the time of the enrollment colposcopy. While this might be expected to show inferior results than obtained from real-time colposcopy, in most studies the results are basically consistent between real-time and static image evaluations; the data from ALTS have consistently shown that real-time colposcopy and evaluations from digitized colposcopic images from the same examinations and from Cervigrams all perform suboptimally in detecting CIN 3.[6,9,10,13,27–29] Poor sensitivity was reported for the enrollment colposcopic impression[28] and equally poor sensitivity of a modified Reid Index grading system with its component scores of color, margin, and vessels.[10] When CIN 2 or worse was not found, subtler distinctions, including CIN 1 and normal, were not very reliable or predictive, partly because of either variability in histologic interpretation or inaccurate biopsy placement.[21,29,30] This interpretation was made as the result of data demonstrating that among women with an enrollment colposcopic examination not detecting CIN 2 or worse, the risk of subsequent diagnosis of CIN 3 was equivalent during the 2-year follow-up of women regardless of whether the initial colposcopy result was CIN 1 or was negative on colposcopically directed biopsy or no biopsy was done because the colposcopy looked normal.[27] As mentioned above, subsequent development of CIN 3 during the 2-year course of the trial may have accounted for some of these.

A 2008 study of 1850 patients presenting to M.D. Anderson Cancer Center (Houston, TX) demonstrated that the specificity of colposcopy is low, even in a high-risk colposcopy clinic (29% had CIN 2,3 or cancer).[22,31] Although a colposcopic impression of LSIL or greater performed well in terms of identifying high-grade lesions with a low number of false-negative results, the ability of the colposcopic impression to avoid false-positive results was low (specificity 45%).[22,31] Specifically, colposcopy had a sensitivity for CIN 2,3 of 98.3% and a specificity of 45.1% when the colposcopic impression threshold was low-grade (LSIL/CIN 1). Sensitivity fell to 71.4%, while specificity improved to 81.3% when the colposcopic impression threshold was CIN 2,3.[31] The higher sensitivity of colposcopy reported in this study was at least partially due to the departure from the "standard" of only taking one or two colposcopically directed biopsies from the area with the worst colposcopic impression by adding one or two biopsies of squamous and columnar epithelium from an area of normal appearance. Additionally, if the overall colposcopic impression was normal, biopsies were obtained from one or two normal sites and included both types of cervical epithelium. Problematic, however, is the possibility that taking biopsies in normal-appearing areas will increase misclassification of normal mimics of high-grade lesions, such as immature metaplasia, as CIN 2,3.[30]

9.2.2 Lesion Size, Thickness of the Epithelium, Age, HPV Type, and Other Variables

Most of the recent data on accuracy of colposcopy come from ALTS,[6,9,10,13,16,17,27–29] or from the large primary screening studies in China (SPOCCS I and SPOCCS II).[8,11,15] In ALTS, all women were initially referred because of ASC-US or LSIL cytology. Both interobserver agreement on assessing the components of colposcopic grading and the accuracy and reproducibility of colposcopic grading in the detection of CIN 2,3 were only fair to poor when assessed by ALTS experts from static images (Cervigrams) (Table 9.2).[16] Accuracy of colposcopic impression and biopsy site placement may be better for women referred to colposcopy with high-grade squamous intraepithelial lesion (HSIL) cytology. Benedet et al.[5] demonstrated that as the degree of cytologic abnormality worsened, the predictive accuracy of colposcopic diagnosis increased.[5] Since HSIL cytology is known to more frequently reflect larger CIN 2,3 lesions, it is not surprising that lesions initially missed colposcopically in ALTS were smaller the CIN 2,3 lesions identified at the initial colposcopic examination.[16,32] In addition, the reproducibility of components of colposcopic assessment may be greater for larger lesions.[16] In the SPOCCS studies from China, the high-grade lesions diagnosed by random biopsy, or solely by positive endocervical curettage (ECC), were smaller, thinner, and of lower grade than those diagnosed by colposcopic-directed biopsy.[8,33] Similarly, Sherman observed that the cases of CIN 3 missed by enrollment colposcopy in ALTS were very small.[32] A recent collaboration between the National Cancer Institute (NCI) and the University of Oklahoma (SUCCEED) provided further confirmation that the size of the CIN 3 matters in the success of colposcopy to correctly identify the most abnormal area for biopsy.[34] Loop electrosurgical excision procedure (LEEP) cone specimens obtained immediately after biopsy of the most abnormal-appearing area demonstrated that accurately targeting the worst lesion for biopsy, even when it was CIN 3, was challenging. However, those correctly targeted by biopsy were more likely to be the larger CIN 3s that may have a higher risk of progression to cancer.[32] Most invasive cancers are readily identified by colposcopy (Figure 9.1).

Another characteristic of high-grade lesions missed at colposcopy is that some CIN 2,3 is associated with thinner epithelium.[33,35] Zahm et al.[35] in 1998 showed that CIN found in women ≥35 years old was thinner and less colposcopically conspicuous than CIN in women <35 years. A 2008 study by Yang et al. showed the mean average epithelial thickness of CIN 2,3 from cervical quadrants with a colposcopic impression of normal to be 184 μm, in comparison to the 321 μm epithelial thickness found in biopsies from quadrants with colposcopic impressions of low grade, high grade, or cancer (Table 9.3).[33] As would be expected, CIN 2,3 had higher mean average nuclear density, but missed CIN 2,3 was thinner than normal/CIN 1 (Table 9.4).[33] The authors suggested that the failure to detect CIN 2 and CIN 3 at colposcopy does not necessarily represent a lack of expertise or a failure of technique on the part of the colposcopist, but rather reflects a measurable physical characteristic of the dysplastic epithelium that causes some lesions to be invisible to experts.[33]

TABLE 9.2	INTEROBSERVER AGREEMENT BETWEEN TWO RANDOMLY DESIGNATED EVALUATORS ON THE IDENTIFICATION OF VARIOUS COMPONENTS OF COLPOSCOPIC GRADING
Color	0.12 (0.06–0.19)
Margins	0.17 (0.10–0.24)
Mosaicism	0.16 (0.08–0.23)
Punctation	0.08 (0.02–0.15)
Atypical vessels	0.11 (0.00–0.22)

Digitized cervical images from 862 women enrolled in the ASCUS-LSIL Triage Study (ALTS) were assessed online by two randomly assigned evaluators from a pool of 20 experienced colposcopists. The results show that experienced colposcopists' ability to reproducibly grade the components of a modified Reid Index using static cervical images is only fair to poor.
From Massad LS, Jeronimo J, Schiffman M; National Institutes of Health/American Society for Colposcopy and Cervical Pathology (NIH/ASCCP) Research Group. Interobserver agreement in the assessment of components of colposcopic grading. *Obstet Gynecol* 2008;111(6):1279–84, with permission.

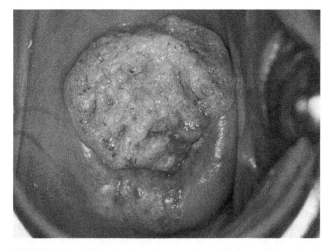

FIGURE 9.1. This microinvasive cancer could be easily confused with a large exophytic condyloma. (Photo courtesy of Dr. Vesna Kesic.)

TABLE 9.3	SENSITIVITY OF COLPOSCOPY FOR CIN 2,3 IN RELATION TO EPITHELIAL THICKNESS OF THE LESION

■ EPITHELIAL THICKNESS (μM)	■ SENSITIVITY OF COLPOSCOPY FOR CIN 2,3
0–139	31.3% (5/16)
140–290	75.8% (50/66)
291–441	88.6% (39/44)
>441	94.4% (17/18)
TOTAL	77.1% (111/144)

Yang et al. demonstrated that the sensitivity of colposcopy for CIN 2,3 varied with the mean average epithelial thickness of the lesion from only 31.3% when the epithelial thickness was 0–139 μm, to a high of 94.4% when the epithelial thickness was 291–441 μm.

CIN, cervical intraepithelial neoplasia.

Source: From Yang B, Pretorius RG, Belinson JL, Zhang X, Burchette R, Qiao YL. False negative colposcopy is associated with thinner cervical intraepithelial neoplasia 2 and 3. *Gynecol Oncol* 2008;110(1):32–6, with permission.

HPV type may play a role in determining colposcopic characteristics and accuracy of biopsy placement in detecting CIN 2,3.[21,22,36] Evaluation of a subset of women in the ALTS trial found that HPV 16 infection was associated with the worst colposcopically appearing lesions, regardless of grade of CIN on biopsy, that is, whether CIN 1 or CIN 2,3. Additionally, CIN 3 was more likely to be found at initial colposcopy rather than at follow-up biopsy or exit LEEP when it was due to HPV 16 than when due to other oncogenic HPV types.[36]

9.2.3 Improving Sensitivity by Taking More Biopsies

Hearp et al.[37] attributed close to 50% of missed high-grade CIN to sampling error, that is, biopsy placement. Clearly, the choice of whether, and where, to biopsy is more important than assigning a colposcopic impression.[21] Fortunately, a number of studies now document that the sensitivity of colposcopy

for CIN 3 can be improved significantly by taking two or more biopsies.[1,8,11,13,15,21,22,33] On the basis of review of static images, ALTS quality-control colposcopists demonstrated only mediocre agreement in biopsy placement among themselves and compared with clinical center colposcopists.[9] However, 72 colposcopists from 5 countries reviewed 50 Cervigrams blinded to the consensus diagnosis on the most colposcopically abnormal area for biopsy made previously by 6 experienced colposcopists.[38] The international colposcopists agreed with the consensus biopsy placement in 70%, indicating reasonably good interobserver agreement among colposcopists on the location of the most severe lesions in cervical images. Agreement was not significantly associated with country, duration of practice (less than or greater than 1 year), professional group (nurse, family doctor, pathologist, gynecologist, gynecologic oncologist), expert status (recognized national/international expert vs. colposcopist), and gender.

Guido et al.[28] evaluated biopsy placement in ALTS in relation to the geography of the cervix, observing that more biopsies were taken from the anterior (12 o'clock) and posterior (6 o'clock) positions than from 3 o'clock and 9 o'clock. However, the proportion of abnormal histology per biopsy, and the grade of neoplasia, did not vary significantly by position. Photographs taken at colposcopy (Cervigrams) demonstrated more acetowhitening anterior and posterior than the lateral locations and biopsy demonstrated acetowhitening to be more common even when the biopsies in the anterior/posterior locations were normal. Importantly, at each location the more colposcopists biopsied, the more CIN they found.[21,28] In fact, the sensitivity of enrollment colposcopy was shown to increase steadily with additional biopsy specimens, as was reported in another ALTS analysis that also demonstrated increased accuracy with additional biopsies regardless of the level of colposcopic training.[13] Independent of the severity of the colposcopic impression, the frequency with which colposcopists took two or more biopsies instead of one varied (in descending order) from nurse practitioners to general gynecologists to gynecologic oncology fellows to gynecologic oncologists. In fact, gynecologic oncologists and gynecologic oncology fellows did have a relatively higher sensitivity on the first biopsy sample, although this did not translate into higher sensitivity of the colposcopy procedure as a whole because general gynecologists and nurse practitioners took more biopsies resulting in comparable overall sensitivities.[13] Pretorius et al.[8] in the China screening study (SPOCCS) determined

TABLE 9.4	THE MEAN AVERAGE THICKNESS OF SQUAMOUS EPITHELIUM AND MEAN NUCLEAR DENSITY AS FUNCTIONS OF HISTOLOGY AND COLPOSCOPIC IMPRESSION

■ HISTOLOGY (μM)* (MEAN NUCLEAR DENSITY[†] [NUCLEI PER 2,500 μM^2])	■ COLPOSCOPY IMPRESSION			
	■ NORMAL	■ LOW GRADE	■ HIGH GRADE	■ CANCER
Normal	378 [7.5]	370 [9.0]	482 [6.8]	No slides
CIN 1	355 [7.4]	346 [8.5]	418 [8.7]	310 [17.5]
CIN 2	185 [14.7]	258 [12.5]	334 [12.8]	346 [14.6]
CIN 3	181 [15.5]	230 [13.4]	372 [13.1]	426 [16.0]

Colposcopic impression was clearly underestimated for CIN 2, CIN3 and cancer when the epithelial thickness of the high grade lesion measured <258 μm, irrespective of nuclear density, which was denser with higher grade lesions.

*Histology (μm) in **BLACK**.

[†]Mean nuclear density in RED.

CIN, cervical intraepithelial neoplasia; Colpo, colposcopic impression.

Source: Adapted from Yang B, Pretorius RG, Belinson JL, Zhang X, Burchette R, Qiao YL. False negative colposcopy is associated with thinner cervical intraepithelial neoplasia 2 and 3. *Gynecol Oncol* 2008;110(1):32–6, with permission.

that only 57% of CIN 2,3 was detected when biopsies were guided to only the most abnormal-appearing area. The addition of a random biopsy improved the percentage of detection by 37.4% and by another 5.5% with the addition of an ECC. SPOCCS also provided information on added sensitivity for CIN 3 of taking four biopsies and an ECC on every patient. When gynecologic oncologists performed colposcopic evaluations of each quadrant of the cervix separately, sensitivity for detection of CIN 3+ increased with each biopsy.[15] A directed biopsy was taken from any abnormality, but for quadrants in which there was no abnormality seen, a random biopsy specimen was taken from the squamocolumnar junction (SCJ) at 2, 4, 8, or 10 o'clock. An ECC was then obtained. Random biopsy in quadrants without colposcopic abnormality detected 37.1% of all the CIN 2+ detected in the trial. Sellors et al.[39] also demonstrated a 19% increase in detection of CIN 2+ by taking random biopsies from quadrants without visual abnormalities. Clearly, taking more biopsies is very important for maximizing colposcopic accuracy (Table 9.5).

Whether adding an ECC to every colposcopy, as advocated by Pretorius, is cost-effective is controversial. Although the China SPOCCS study demonstrated a 5.5% increase in sensitivity for CIN 2,3 by adding an ECC to every colposcopy, in ALTS the ECC was positive in <1% of women with otherwise negative colposcopy and cervical biopsy, and in only 3.7% overall.[40] The nearly three times increase in sensitivity by ECC in SPOCCS II compared to ALTS is likely to be at least partly secondary to the older age of participants in SPOCCS II (median age 40.9 years) in comparison to ALTS where only 5.2% of the patients having ECC were ≥40 years. In ALTS, the sensitivity of biopsy and the sensitivity of ECC for cumulative CIN 2 (detected at enrollment colposcopy and over the 2-year follow-up) varied by age: biopsy was more sensitive in younger than in older women, whereas the reverse was found for ECC.[40] Therefore, the marginal contribution of ECC (i.e., in addition to the biopsy) was accentuated in older women. In women <40 years of age, ECC yielded only 2% increased detection of cumulative CIN 2+ over the biopsy findings. In contrast, in women 40 and older, ECC increased sensitivity for cumulative CIN 2+ by 13%.[13] ASCCP consensus guidelines advise endocervical sampling for all women referred with HSIL and atypical glandular cell (AGC) cytology and when the colposcopic examination is inadequate and colposcopy is being performed for any abnormal screening test. The guidelines also state that ECC is preferred for women with ASC-US, ASC-H, or LSIL cytology when no lesion is identified on colposcopic examination.[41] Endocervical sampling is considered "acceptable" in the context of a adequate colposcopic examination, ASC-US, ASC-H or LSIL referral, and an identified lesion. Solomon et al.[40] asked whether it worth performing ECCs in women under 40 to increase detection of CIN 2+ by only 2%. In their discussion, they acknowledged that although performing an additional test will always increase sensitivity, the marginal gain in sensitivity must be balanced against the costs in terms of patient discomfort and the costs of testing. The question raises broader medical and societal issues regarding cost-effectiveness and what is acceptable risk. For the time being, it is likely that this decision will need to remain between the clinicians and the patient.

9.2.4 What Does This All Mean for the Practicing Colposcopist?

In summary, there are extensive new data showing that colposcopy and guided biopsies as typically practiced are missing a fair percentage of (mostly small) CIN 2 and CIN 3 lesions.[21] Studies in the earlier decades demonstrating higher sensitivity of colposcopy predated the demand on colposcopists to find these early, small, high-grade lesions that are most commonly found in women with HPV-positive normal or ASC-US Pap interpretations and with LSIL cytology.[1] These changes have placed colposcopists in the difficult position of finding lesions that may be at the limits of detection by virtue of being too small or too thin to detect. CIN 3 lesions associated with invasion are usually very much larger than CIN 3 not

TABLE 9.5	QUALITY IMPROVEMENT IN THE ABILITY TO DETECT HIGH-GRADE DYSPLASIA BY INCREASED NUMBER OF BIOPSIES		
STUDY	**TECHNIQUE**	**SENSITIVITY**	**SPECIFICITY**
Hearp et al.	Regular colposcopy-directed Bx	56%	49%
Gage et al.	Acetic acid, Bx taken of worst area, and any additional suspicious areas	Sensitivity only: 1 Bx _ 68.3% 2 Bx _ 81.8% 3 Bx _ 83.3%	
Colposcopy based on positive HPV or HSIL: 79.5% Colposcopy based on HSIL: 80.5%			
Pretorius et al.	Acetic acid, cervix divided into 4 quadrants; if lesion not seen in each, then random Bx taken along SCJ, fifth Bx was when ECC done	Sensitivity 0–2 Bx: 52.6% 3–4 Bx: 85.2% 4 Bx plus ECC: 91.5%	Specificity 4 Bx plus ECC 56.9%

These three studies clearly demonstrate that the sensitivity of colposcopy increases with increasing number of biopsies.
Bx, biopsies; ECC, endocervical curettage; HPV, human papillomavirus; HSIL, high-grade squamous intraepithelial lesions.
Source: From Chase DM, Kalouyan M, DiSaia PJ. Colposcopy to evaluate abnormal cervical cytology in 2008. *Am J Obstet Gynecol* 2009;200: 472–80, with permission.

associated with invasion.[42] The finding of extensive CIN 3 in the referral colposcopy for an ASC-US or LSIL Pap is unusual and rarely the size of a CIN 3 lesion with associated invasion that is, on average, seven times larger than that without invasion.[1,32,42] The median length of CIN 3 in ALTS was only 6.5 mm, and lesions in one-third were so small that colpobiopsy did not leave any residual CIN 3 to be detected in the LEEP specimen.[32] Sherman et al.[32] concluded from these data that aggressive follow-up of women with ASC-US and LSIL cytology that identifies tiny CIN 3 lesions lacking immediate potential for invasion might be of little importance if delayed detection yielded similar outcomes. Fortunately, the median time between age of peak detection of CIN 3 (29 years) and of microinvasive cervical cancer (42 years) gives reassurance that the oncogenic process typically spans many years.[24] Given the rarity of cervical cancer detected in follow-up to colposcopy not initially showing CIN 3, the increased sensitivity of colposcopy for larger high-grade lesions, and the association of lesion size with risk of invasion, pushing the limits of detection of small lesions by colposcopy may have little effect on the overall cervical cancer rate.[1] But this remains to be proven.

The accumulated data suggest very strongly that the heart of colposcopic practice is the identification of the most abnormal area(s) for biopsy.[21,22] Because colposcopic appearance is often complex, and the most abnormal area may be small, the sensitivity of the procedure will depend on taking more than a single biopsy in most cases. A number of studies now document that the sensitivity of colposcopy for CIN 3 can be improved significantly by taking two or more biopsies regardless of whether the colposcopist is a novice or experienced.[8,13,21] Clearly, taking more biopsies is the most important safeguard that colposcopists can take. More difficult is the question as to whether random biopsies should be obtained in colposcopically normal areas.[21] This approach has been proven to pick up more CIN 3,[8,11,13,15] but whether picking up these often small, thin, and likely early CIN 2,3 lesions[32,33] will decrease cervical cancer rates in screened women, or predominantly increase cost, anxiety, and morbidity, cannot be determined at this time. Considering that CIN 2 is a poorly defined entity with a high rate of spontaneous resolution,[43] and that larger CIN 3 lesions are of significantly greater risk than smaller CIN 3 for invasion,[32,42] this may be a reasonable concern.

Variability in the accuracy of colposcopy is secondary to issues discussed and likely also to issues not yet understood. We understand that accuracy depends in part on size and thickness of the lesion, HPV type, referral cytology, and number of biopsies taken. How much variability in accuracy is due to variability in expertise is less clear. All ALTS studies demonstrated only small differences in accuracy based on level of training, years of colposcopic practice, and definition of "expert," although all colposcopists in ALTS fell within a certain latitude of expertise. Recent review of biopsy placement in ALTS revealed less variability in biopsy placement among experts reviewing static ALTS images than in the colposcopists performing real-time colposcopy on the same patients.[29] This was despite the disadvantage of the experts in having to choose biopsy site location on static images. Additionally, the data from the British Columbia cytology-colposcopy program[5] and the MD Anderson Colposcopy clinic[31] tend to support the notion that increasing experience and skill with colposcopy increases accuracy. However, the data on the importance of expertise in colposcopic accuracy are certainly not as definitive as was once thought.[9,12,13,16,17]

Eventually molecular tests more specific for risk of progression of a lesion to cervical cancer may help differentiate which small, thin CIN 3 lesions are best detected and treated and which may not be as important. Additionally, computer-assisted optical devices may eventually be a good adjunct to colposcopy in improving the accuracy of each, and might possibly replace standard light colposcopy if accuracy is considerably improved.[22,44]

In the meantime, it is most prudent to increase the number of biopsies targeting any area with colposcopic abnormality, and when risk is highest, that is, for women referred for cytology reported as AGC or HSIL, and older women with any abnormal cytology, taking biopsies from normal areas may also be advisable. Taking five biopsies, as recommended by Pretorius et al., one from each quadrant to include the most abnormal areas and a random biopsy from the SCJ in normal quadrants, as well as an ECC, is an alternative option.[8,15]

9.3 COLPOSCOPIC GRADING OF CERVICAL NEOPLASIA

Colposcopy is the standard diagnostic procedure for evaluating abnormal cervical cytology and abnormal-appearing cervices. To manage cervical disease in patients properly, colposcopists must form a clinically based colposcopic impression to identify sites for biopsy within colposcopic findings that are commonly seen in the normal as well as the abnormal cervix. Before describing the colposcopic features of CIN, one must understand how colposcopists derive a clinical colposcopic impression. Although a final diagnosis is ultimately based largely on the histologic interpretation of a colposcopically directed biopsy, the colposcopist's clinical impression may help avoid missing a severe lesion through incomplete or imprecise sampling.

Admittedly, much subjectivity remains in forming a colposcopic impression, just as some subjectivity exists in arriving at cytologic and histologic diagnoses (Figure 9.2). In ALTS, interobserver reproducibility for cervical cytologic reports among pathologists was equivalent to the interobserver reproducibility for cervical histologic diagnoses (Kappa 0.46 and 0.46, respectively).[30] At best, this represents a moderate level of interobserver agreement. In other words, what one pathologist called CIN 2 may be diagnosed as CIN 1 or CIN 3 by another pathologist. Therefore it is not surprising that the interobserver reproducibility of colposcopy is far from perfect as well.[10,16,17] To systematically categorize a multitude of colposcopic appearances that vary across the spectrum of disease states from normal to neoplasia, colposcopists have developed clinical indices called colposcopic grading systems to estimate disease severity as closely as possible.

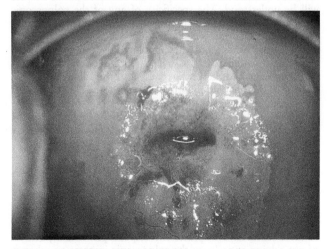

FIGURE 9.2.   The acetowhite lesion may be called CIN 1 by one colposcopist and immature metaplasia by another. This is the most difficult discrimination for a colposcopist.

9.3.1 Rationale for Colposcopic Grading

Pathologists evaluate certain cellular and epithelial criteria to reach cytologic and histologic interpretations. For example, whether reviewing cytologic or histologic samples, pathologists consider unique nuclear features, nuclear to cytoplasmic ratio, epithelial differentiation and maturation, and the extent of epithelial and stromal involvement by cellular atypia. This enables them to derive diagnoses that are more accurate and reproducible. Similarly, colposcopists must form colposcopic impressions based on macroscopically visible epithelial and vascular features within the tissue observed. These colposcopic features include the color and opacity of the cervical lesion both before and following use of epithelial contrast solutions; the shape and character of lesion margins; the presence of blood vessels and their diameter, pattern, and branching characteristics; distances between adjoining capillaries; surface contour or topography; the size of the lesion; and duration of physiologic response to a 3% to 5% acetic acid solution. These are the tools to form a colposcopic impression, but despite the interobserver variability in the diagnosis of histology, histology is still the arbiter of final diagnosis. Of course, if the histology diagnosis is significantly at odds with the colposcopic impression, it is important for the colposcopist to review the cytology, histology, and colposcopy.

Grading systems for colposcopy are systematic methods for estimating colposcopically the severity of cervical neoplasia by empirical analysis of unique colposcopic signs. Certain specific colposcopic signs reflect characteristics of abnormal epithelium within the transformation zone, but to various degrees may also be seen in normal cell transformation events as part of maturation of immature metaplasia. Aggregate colposcopic signs of the atypical transformation zone have been shown to be more accurately predictive of the clinical severity of cervical disease than individual signs in some, but not all studies.[10,45] For instance, the clinical consideration of only a single colposcopic sign, such as acetowhite epithelium, is typically very nonspecific in differentiating disease from normal, yet acetowhitening was the most predictive colposcopic finding in the study by Shaw et al.[45] Normal immature metaplasia and areas of inflammation appear transiently acetowhite following the application of 5% acetic acid solution. In addition most, but not all, CIN lesions appear acetowhite depending on the thickness of the epithelium. In contrast, if the colposcopist understands that acetowhitening is one of the colposcopic findings that helps in determining the best biopsy site(s) but does not alone provide a diagnosis, then the value of all of the colposcopic signs discussed in this chapter will be understood. The specificity of any of the colposcopic findings of acetowhite, margins, contour, mosaic, punctation and even atypical vessels is challenged by the common finding of any, and sometimes all, of these findings in young women with extensive immature metaplasia. The importance of learning colposcopic signs and the various methods of grading these signs for degree of apparent abnormality is not to be able to make a colposcopic "diagnosis" from the findings but to increase the colposcopist's likelihood of finding the most important areas for biopsy and to provide a basis for concern when biopsy results are significantly different from expected.

As discussed previously, studies on interobserver variability in colposcopic impression and biopsy site placement, even among experienced colposcopists, verify the subjectivity of colposcopy and support the importance of not only learning the classic colposcopic signs for neoplasia but also understanding that sometimes high-grade lesions do not display any of these features. This places the colposcopist in the position of not relying entirely on the colposcopic impression when it does not correlate with the cytologic and histologic findings. In turn, it is also important for the colposcopist to understand that cytology and histology also have been shown to be subjective and to therefore have only a moderate degree of interobserver variability. Hence, the colposcopist must question and

review the results of all cytology, colposcopy, and histology findings when there is a significant discrepancy in findings.

To form a clinically based colposcopic impression, many colposcopists use a colposcopic index or grading system. Colposcopic scoring systems were once thought to be consistently accurate, even for different population groups (e.g., HIV positive or pregnant patients) that may pose varied colposcopic challenges,[46] but as discussed in Section 9.2 a number of studies have recently demonstrated that while grading systems are helpful, they are still based on a subjective process.[6–18] Demonstration that colposcopic grading scores correlate better among colposcopists when diagnosing lesions associated with HPV 16 and with HSIL referral cytology reflects the fact that the colposcopic signs are generally more identifiable in larger high-grade lesions.[32,36,47] In the era of an effective HPV vaccine against HPV 16,[48,49] colposcopists in the future may be challenged even more to detect significant neoplastic lesions.

9.3.2 Importance of Grading Systems for Colposcopy

Colposcopic grading systems are important because they provide a structured, systematic method to critically analyze cervical findings. Adherence to a structured evaluation method helps to prevent overlooking pertinent colposcopic features and allow colposcopists to attain more accurate and consistent colposcopic impressions. A systematic approach, once learned and mastered, becomes routine and of benefit to all colposcopists. After receiving histologic results, a colposcopic impression based on systematic criteria can be analyzed retrospectively to determine any specific reasons for diagnostic discordance and may facilitate improving a colposcopist's ability to reach more accurate colposcopic impressions in the future. Well-designed colposcopic grading systems enhance colposcopic reproducibility. Colposcopic grading systems are helpful when selecting the most appropriate biopsy sites, particularly when large, complex lesions of the cervix are encountered. In these cases, colposcopists can evaluate multiple atypical-appearing areas of the cervix to determine which areas are likely to contain the most severe histologic changes. Because it is now clear that taking a biopsy from the single most abnormal-appearing area misses many high-grade lesions, as demonstrated by the studies in ALTS and SPOCCS, grading each area of the cervix with any atypical colposcopic finding and taking more than one biopsy should help determine the most potentially abnormal areas for biopsy.[8,13,15]

9.3.3 The Colposcopic Impression

By using a grading system, clinicians can form colposcopic impressions that can be compared with the pathologists' cytologic and histologic reports. A clinical colposcopic impression can enable the colposcopist to determine whether discordance exists between the colposcopic findings and the laboratory diagnosis. Because cytologic, histologic, and colposcopic interpretations can vary between observers,[10,30,50] a check and balance system to govern clinical and pathologic interpretation is essential. Notable disagreement between laboratory and colposcopic impression may indicate errors by either party or both. Serious histology/colposcopy discordance necessitates a review of the cytology and histology by the same or a different expert gynecologic pathologist, a repeat colposcopy examination and/or additional histologic sampling by the same or a more experienced colposcopist, or further diagnostic evaluation.

Routinely forming and documenting a colposcopic impression allows for procedural quality control. A unique quality control program in British Columbia monitors colposcopists by comparing their colposcopic impressions recorded on their histology requisition forms, with the histologic diagnosis for each patient.[5,51] If a colposcopist's clinical impressions do not agree

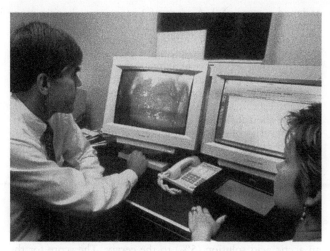

FIGURE 9.3.   Remotely monitoring the quality of colposcopy practice using a computer image/data management system.

with the histologic interpretations at least 80% of the time, the colposcopist receives remedial colposcopic training directed at improving clinical assessment of cervical lesions. More sophisticated quality control systems have been used for monitoring colposcopists in multisite studies, such as the NCI-funded ALTS trial.[10,52,53] In this study,[53] the colposcopic impressions, biopsy intent, biopsy site selection, and cervical image adequacy of participating colposcopists were monitored by quality control colposcopy experts who remotely reviewed digitized cervical images from each patient, that were transferred by computer modem (Figure 9.3). A colposcopist unable to adequately assess the severity of cervical lesions risks not obtaining the most abnormal tissue for pathologic interpretation. In ALTS, colposcopists and quality control reviewers underdiagnosed 16% and 25% of subjects and overdiagnosed 45% and 20% of subjects compared with histology, respectively.[53] The sensitivity and specificity for detecting ≥CIN 2 were 35% and 23%, and 90% and 95%, respectively. These disturbingly poor performance outcomes for colposcopy indicate that while colposcopic grading can be important in selecting biopsy sites in complex lesions, multiple biopsies are important to obtain adequate sensitivity for CIN 2,3 among women with abnormal Pap results. Additionally, at least part of the poor performance of the colposcopy QC review was the two-dimensional aspect of the digital images and the poor quality of many.[53]

9.3.4 Historical Perspectives of Colposcopic Grading Systems

9.3.4.1   Hinselmann Colposcopic Grading System

The importance of a colposcopic grading system was apparent to the inventor of the first colposcope, Dr. Hans Hinselmann. Like any scientist exploring new frontiers, Dr. Hinselmann saw the need to methodically categorize his newly documented observations on the first colposcopic findings. Although crude when compared to later developed systems, the two-part colposcopic grading system was divided into categories of "Simple Atypical Epithelium I and II," and "Highly Atypical Epithelium III and IV." While no one colposcopic grading system is necessarily superior, this early colposcopic grading system was the foundation on which latter colposcopists developed more sophisticated systems based on their increased understanding of abnormalities within the transformation zone.

9.3.4.2 Coppleson Grading System

Dr. Malcolm Coppleson, an Australian colposcopy pioneer, devised another grading system in the 1960s.[54] The Coppleson system underwent much revision, primarily as a result of the increasing recognition of low-grade CIN. The classification system is outlined in Table 9.6.

In clinical practice, the majority of women with abnormal Pap tests have colposcopic grade I and II lesions. Few have grade III. The difficulty with the Coppleson grading system is that much attention became focused on color and density of acetowhitening, and the terms "grade I to III acetowhitening" became colposcopic jargon. However, CIN 1 may appear at times as a dense, shiny acetowhite lesion with a prominent vascular pattern. Thus, the severity of many low-grade lesions can be overestimated using the system. The Coppleson system also failed to address the importance of findings involving the internal margins within an area of atypia, which usually indicate more severe disease within a larger lesion. A coexisting, more severe lesion that was not observed is a common explanation of a histologic diagnosis that is more severe than anticipated based on colposcopic findings. Most importantly, subjectivity and reproducibility of the Coppleson grading system was not assessed in a prospective study.

9.3.4.3 Stafl Grading System

In 1975, Dr. Adolph Stafl described a system for colposcopic grading based on four factors: surface pattern, color tone, intercapillary distance, and margin contour of the lesion with normal tissue.[55] His grading system was divided into normal, nonsignificant (inflammation), significant (CIN 1,2,3), and highly significant. Much emphasis was placed on the intercapillary distance within lesions, and a method was developed to objectively measure these very small distances. The original work of Kolstad[56] showed that increased intercapillary distance correlates with higher-grade histopathologic changes. The Stafl grading system had four important weaknesses. First, it relies on coarse punctation and mosaic that are relatively uncommon. Most CIN 3 lesions do not have prominent vascular patterns. Second, the epithelial and vascular proliferations associated with HPV infection can result in flat HPV/CIN 1 lesions, both of which can have prominent, although usually fine-caliber, vascular patterns. It is usually not difficult for the experienced colposcopist to distinguish these patterns, but the emphasis on surface capillary patterns weakened the reproducibility of results using the Stafl grading system. Third, the Stafl system did not consider certain margin characteristics

TABLE 9.6	THE COPPLESON GRADING SYSTEM

Grade I (insignificant, or suspicious)—Flat, acetowhite epithelium—borders not necessarily sharp; usually semitransparent with or without fine-caliber, regularly shaped vessels, often with ill-defined patterns; absence of atypical vessels; small intercapillary distance.
Grade II (significant, suspicious)—Flat, white epithelium of greater opacity with sharp borders; with or without dilated-caliber, regularly shaped vessels; defined patterns; absence of atypical vessels; usually increased intercapillary distance.
Grade III (highly significant, highly suspicious)—very white or gray opaque epithelium; sharply bordered; dilated-caliber, irregularly shaped, often coiled, often atypical vessels; increased but variable intercapillary distance; and sometimes irregular surface, micro-exophytic epithelium.

of lesions or the use of Lugol's iodine solution, which is occasionally helpful in visualizing these characteristics. Finally, most colposcopists are unable to measure the very small intercapillary distances, which are one of the four criteria used in the Stafl grading system.

9.2.4.4 Burke Grading System

Dr. Louis Burke, further refined the approach to grading cervical lesions by expanding the existing tripartite system.[57] The Burke grading system designated grades 1, 2, and 3 for each colposcopic finding of lesion surface, margin, color, duration of acetowhite changes, and vessel characteristics (Table 9.7). Like Stafl, Burke realized the importance of surface contour. Furthermore, the Burke system superseded the Coppleson index by considering the duration of acetowhite change that occurs in a lesion, which has now been proven to help predict the severity of cervical disease. The Burke system also considers maximum intercapillary distance and the caliber of vessels when diagnosing CIN 3. As stated earlier, many of these lesions are characterized by a relative paucity of coarse vessels.

9.3.4.5 Reid Colposcopic Index

In 1985, Dr. Richard Reid described the use of a new colposcopic index to differentiate low-grade cervical disease from high-grade disease.[58-60] Consequently, the Reid Colposcopic Index (RCI) is not designed to discriminate premalignant from malignant cervical neoplasia. The Reid Index defined and standardized specific aspects of certain colposcopic signs to more accurately grade lesions. Because the RCI has undergone considerable evaluation, this index will be described in greater detail, as it is used by colposcopists more than other grading systems.

9.3.4.5.1 RCI Design

The RCI considers four colposcopic signs, which are margin or border of lesion, color of lesion following application of 3% to 5% acetic acid solution, blood vessel characteristics within the lesion, and response of the lesion to the application of Lugol's iodine solution (Table 9.8). Each colposcopic sign is subdivided into three hierarchically distinct categories, each featuring characteristics seen in many women at specific stages of premalignant disease. Each category is assigned a numerical value from 0 to 2. Changes most consistent with HPV infection, CIN 1, and immature metaplasia are

assigned a score of 0. A score of 1 represents changes more consistent with the presence of CIN 1 to CIN 2, and a score of 2 reflects colposcopic findings most predictive of CIN 3. Each of the four colposcopic signs is considered separately, and numerical scores are assigned respectively, depending on the severity of that characteristic within the detected cervical lesion. The scores for each of four colposcopic signs are added to establish a total RCI score (Table 9.8). The numeric value of the total score is then used to determine the estimated severity of disease, or clinical colposcopic impression (Table 9.9). The accuracy of the RCI depends on deriving an aggregate diagnosis instead of considering only a solitary colposcopic sign.

9.3.4.5.2 The Four RCI Colposcopic Signs

The RCI considers morphologic and physiologic features common in premalignant cervical lesions. The first three colposcopic signs are evaluated following proper application of an acetic acid solution (5%) to the cervix. The score for the final colposcopic sign is dependent on a preliminary subtotal score of the first three signs. The score for the fourth sign can only be determined after application of Lugol's iodine solution (one-half strength) to the cervix.

9.3.4.5.2.1 Margin

The nature of a lesion margin, edge, or border varies depending on the severity of cervical neoplasia, making evaluation of the margin an important part of the colposcopic assessment. Low-grade lesion (CIN 1 or HPV) margins may be irregular, flocculated, feathered (Figure 9.4A–D), angular or "geographic" (Figure 9.5), indistinct (Figure 9.6A,B), exophytic or micropapillary (condyloma-like) in contour (Figure 9.7A–D), or surrounded by small "satellite" lesions (Figure 9.8). A score of 0 points is assigned to the lesion if these attributes are present. In contrast, smooth and fairly straight margins are more characteristic of an intermediate lesion (CIN 1,2). A score of 1 point is assigned to the lesion when these margin characteristics are noted (Figure 9.9). High-grade lesions (CIN 3) often have raised, peeling epithelial edges (Figure 9.10A–C). Distinct lesions encompassed within a larger lower-grade lesion and located closer to the SCJ may have an internal border that demarcates the area from the surrounding low-grade change (Figure 9.11A–I). Lesions with peeling edges or internal margins are more likely to be CIN 3 and thus receive 2 points for their margin score. All cervical lesion margins are assigned a score prior to addressing the next colposcopic sign.

TABLE 9.7	BURKE COLPOSCOPIC GRADING SYSTEM					
▪ GRADE	▪ SURFACE*	▪ MARGIN	▪ COLOR†	▪ TIME‡	▪ VESSELS§	▪ PATHOLOGY
I	Flat	Indistinct	White	Slow/short	Fine, normal intercapillary distance	Insignificant infection, repair HPV
II	Flat	Distinct	Whiter	Average/average	Dilated punctation, mosaic, slight ↑ intercapillary distance	Significant HPV, CIN 1, CIN 2
III	Raised	Sharp	Whitest	Fast/long	Coarse, marked ↑ intercapillary distance, atypical vessels	Highly significant CIN 3, microinvasion or invasive cancer

*Contour of lesion.
†Color following application of 3% to 5% acetic acid.
‡Onset of acetic acid effect/duration of acetic acid effect.
§Vessel caliber, intercapillary distance.
Histology.
Modified from Burke L, Antonioli DA, Ducatman BS, *Colposcopy Text and Atlas.* Norwalk, Connecticut: Appleton and Lange, 1991.

TABLE 9.8 REID COLPOSCOPIC INDEX

COLPOSCOPIC SIGN	ZERO POINTS	ONE POINT	TWO POINTS
Margin	Condylomatous or micropapillary contour Indistinct borders Flocculated or feathered margins Jagged, angular lesions Satellite lesions, acetowhite lesions outside the transformation zone	Regular lesions with smooth, straight outlines Sharp peripheral margins	Rolled, peeling edges Internal borders between lesions of different severity
Color	Shiny, snow white Transient, indistinct acetowhite, semitransparent	Shiny, off-white Intermediate white	Dull, oyster grey Persistent, dense acetowhite
Vessels	Fine punctation or fine mosaic. Uniform, fine-caliber, nondilated capillary loops	Absence of surface vessels following acetic acid application	Coarse punctation or coarse mosaic Individual vessels dilated Wide intercapillary distance
Iodine staining	Positive iodine uptake, producing a mahogany brown color Negative iodine uptake (mustard yellow) of a lesion recognized as low grade by above criteria ($\leq2/6$)	Partial iodine uptake Variegated, tortoise-shell appearance	Negative iodine uptake (mustard yellow) of a lesion considered high grade by above criteria ($\geq3/6$)
Total RCI score	0–2 = Normal or CIN 1	3–5 = CIN 1 or CIN 2	6–8 = CIN 2 or CIN 3

TABLE 9.9 FLOW SHEET TO DETERMINE RCI SCORE

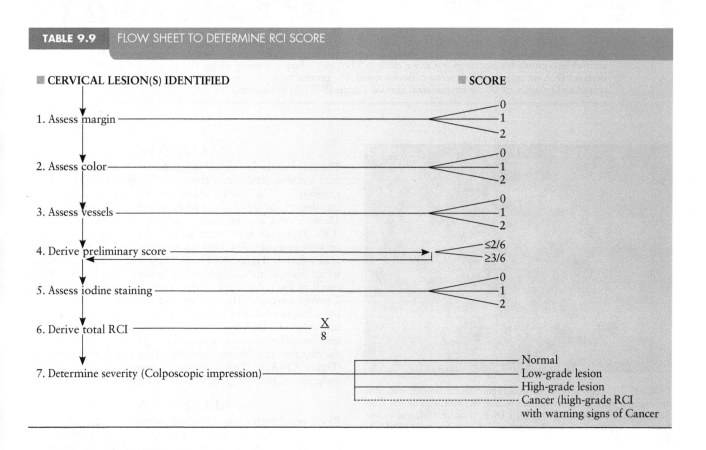

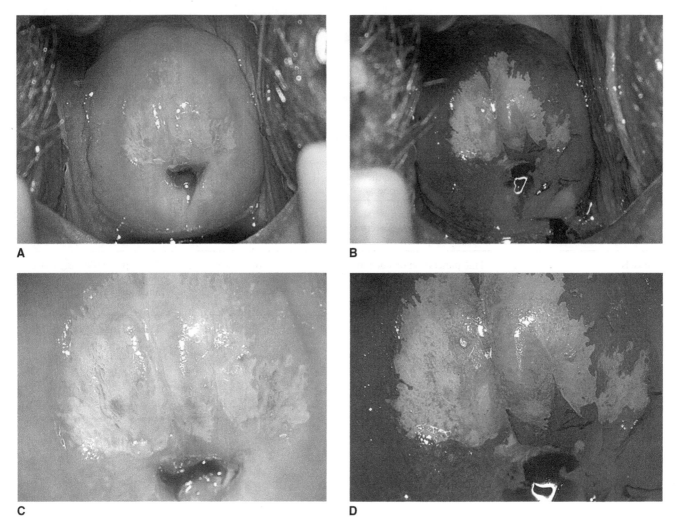

FIGURE 9.4. **A,B:** A large flame-shaped lesion is seen on the anterior cervix in this low-power image. **C:** The acetowhite is mostly translucent except at 9 o'clock to 10 o'clock where it is snowy white. The margins are clearly irregular. **D:** A variegated iodine staining pattern is noted. The cervical biopsy was read as CIN 1. (Courtesy of, and reproduced by approval of, the International Cervical Cancer [INCCA] foundation.)

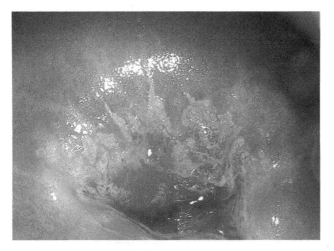

FIGURE 9.5. An angular or geographic lesion border with fine mosaic in a moderately translucent acetowhite area seen on the anterior cervix. They represent typical CIN 1. (Courtesy of, and reproduced by approval of, the International Cervical Cancer [INCCA] foundation.)

9.3.4.5.2.2 Color

The color of the lesion following the application of 5% acetic acid solution determines the second colposcopic sign. Low-grade (CIN 1 or HPV) lesions are semitransparent, nearly translucent, or shiny snow-white in color (Figure 9.12A–C). These lesions are assigned 0 points for color. High-grade (CIN 3) lesions most often have a denser, dirty oyster-gray or very opaque color after application of 3% to 5% acetic acid solution (Figure 9.13A,B). These lesions appear opaque white because the nuclear dense tissue of the lesion reflects much of the colposcope's light. They are assigned a score of 2 points for color. The opaque acetowhite color also persists for a longer period of time than does the translucent acetowhite color of CIN 1 lesions. An intermediate (CIN 1, 2) lesion may be off-white and moderately opaque in color, usually varying between the two extremes of the white color spectrum (Figure 9.14A, B). This is the most common category for color assignment, and it is given a score of 1 point.

9.3.4.5.2.3 Vessels

Blood vessel features are the third colposcopic sign considered in the RCI. Fine, narrow-caliber capillaries with small inter-capillary distances are most common in immature metaplasia

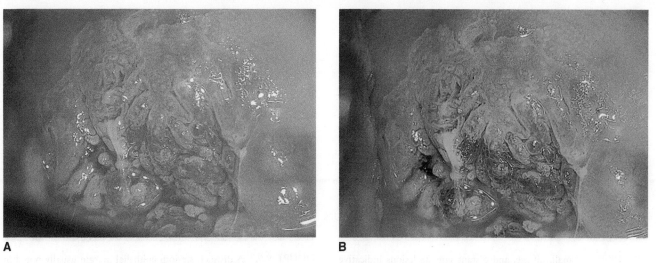

FIGURE 9.6.   **A,B:** A very subtle translucent acetowhite lesion is noted on the anterior cervix. The margin is irregular and (**B**) there are no prominent vessels seen with the green filter. The biopsy was CIN 1. (Courtesy of, and reproduced by approval of, the International Cervical Cancer [INCCA] foundation.)

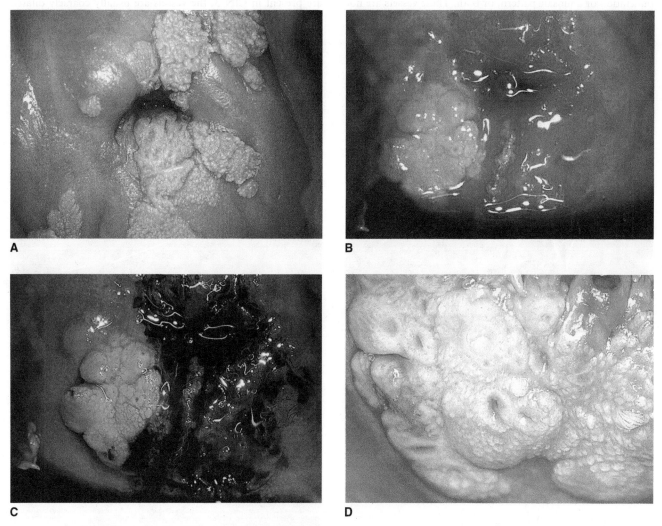

FIGURE 9.7.   **A:** A papillary margin caused by HPV. This margin is given a score of 0 points. **B,C:** In another patient, a fairly large exophytic lesion is seen at 7 o'clock to 8 o'clock. There is moderate bleeding noted, so a biopsy is essential to exclude cancer. **C:** The green filter exam does not disclose atypical blood vessels. The biopsy was condyloma. **D:** A large exophytic lesion with no visible vessels, an irregular surface contour, and classic cervical condylomatous appearance. Notice the condylomatous "cupping" around gland openings, which is different than the cupping seen in high-grade lesions. (Figure 9.7A–C courtesy of, and reproduced by approval of, the International Cervical Cancer [INCCA] foundation.)

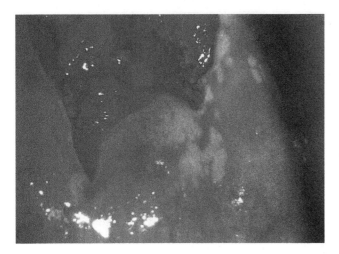

FIGURE 9.8. Small, diffuse, and distant satellite lesions indicative of a low-grade CIN. Satellite lesions give a margin score of 0 points.

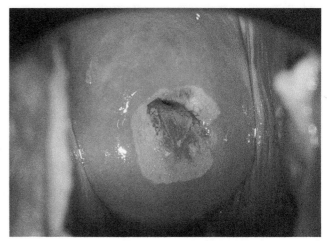

FIGURE 9.9. A distinct, smooth epithelial margin usually noted in CIN 2 or CIN 3. A straight margin is scored as 1 point.

or low-grade lesions. The small vessels may have either a punctation or a mosaic pattern, or both. These vessels are not coarsely dilated and are configured in fairly loose, uniformly spaced arcades (Figure 9.15A–G). Zero points are assigned to lesions with these vessel characteristics. Lesions with no visible vessels receive a score of 1 point, because the majority of both low- and high-grade CIN lesions do not have any vessels.

(Figure 9.16A–D). However, when mosaic and punctation are present in CIN 3, the vessels are usually coarsely dilated (Figure 9.17A–F). Therefore, mosaic and punctation with a wide, irregular capillary pattern are assigned a score of 2 points. The RCI pertains only to premalignant disease; thus, it does not include characteristics that may indicate more serious disease. Identifying coarsely dilated atypical blood vessels

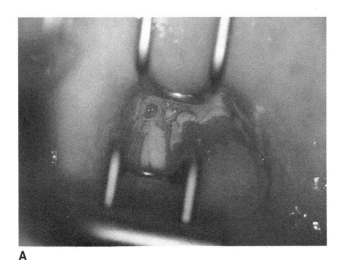

A

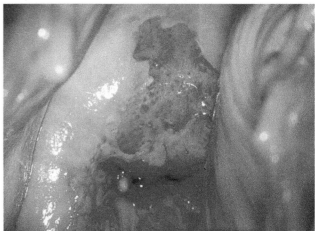

B

FIGURE 9.10. **A:** A raised, peeling lesion margin found in a woman with CIN 3. The acetowhite epithelium is very opaque and no vessels are apparent. The lesion extends into the endocervical canal beyond colposcopic view, and thus, the examination is inadequate. **B:** Peeling epithelium and a large erosion are seen. The biopsy indicated CIN 2. **C:** In another patient an acetowhite lesion is noted at 12 o'clock. The lesion appears thick and is peeling. We see no vessels in this CIN 3. (Figure 9.10C courtesy of, and reproduced by approval of, the International Cervical Cancer [INCCA] foundation.)

C

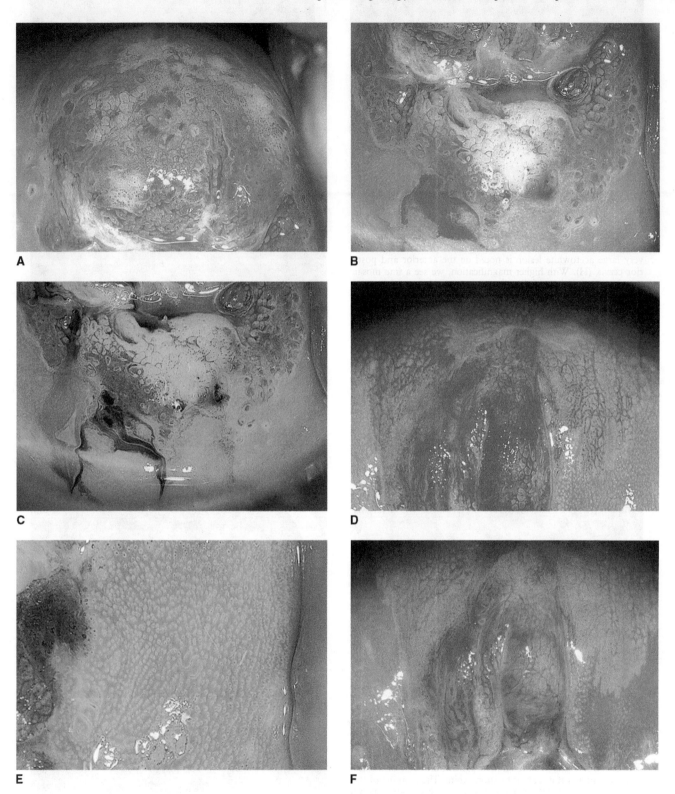

FIGURE 9.11.   A: In this large ectropion, a subtle acetowhite change may be easily overlooked. A small acetowhite lesion with a coarse mosaic is seen at 11 o'clock, and a snowy white lesion with punctation is seen directly more centrally. **B,C:** However, an even larger dense acetowhite lesion with coarsely dilated vessels is seen on the posterior cervix. The cervical biopsy in this area was diagnosed as CIN 3. **D:** In another patient, at first glance, a large acetowhite lesion with irregular margins and a fine mosaic is seen. On the green filter, exam (**E**) of the periphery identifies the tiny uniform papillary projections of a subclinical HPV infection. Yet, nearer the SCJ we see coarse vessels in white light (**F**), and with the green filter (**G**, next page), better appreciated at this higher magnification as a centrally positioned CIN 3 surrounded by CIN 1.

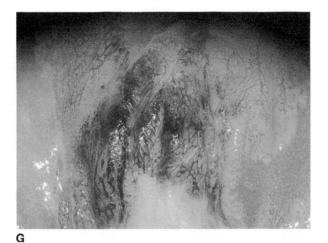

G

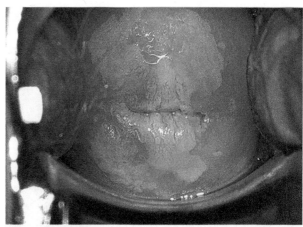

H

FIGURE 9.11. *(Continued)* **H,I:** In this third patient, an internal border can be seen between low-grade CIN and a CIN 3. A very large acetowhite lesion is noted on the anterior and posterior cervix (**H**). With higher magnification, we see a fine mosaic vessel pattern in the periphery but coarse vessels nearer the os. **I:** Biopsy confirmed CIN 3. (Figure 9.11A–D courtesy of, and reproduced by approval of, the International Cervical Cancer [INCCA] foundation.)

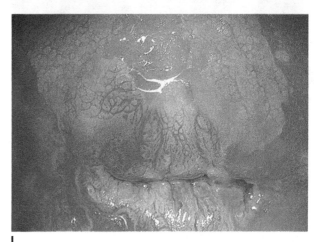

I

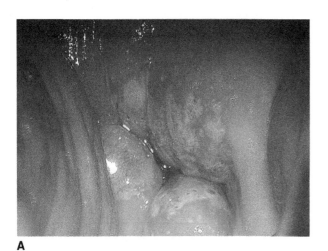

A

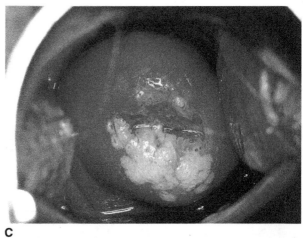

C

FIGURE 9.12. **A:** A large 3-quadrant lesion with irregular borders is seen. The vessels are fine caliber, and the color is translucent to medium opacity. The colposcopic examination is inadequate. This lesion is a CIN 1. **B:** In another patient, the color of the acetowhite lesion is transparent to snow-white. The margins of this lesion vary from irregular to more straight. **C:** This condylomatous lesion is snow white. Snow-white and indistinct white are scored as 0 points. (Courtesy of, and reproduced by approval of, the International Cervical Cancer [INCCA] foundation.)

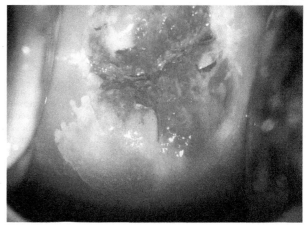

B

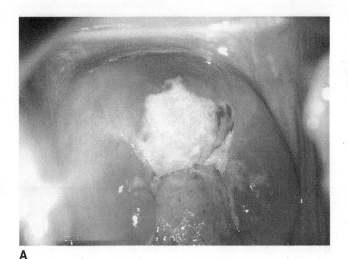
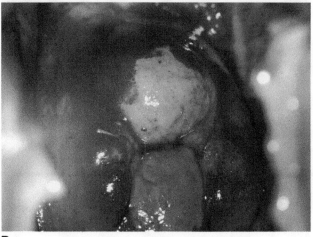

A   **B**

FIGURE 9.13.   An opaque acetowhite lesion indicating CIN 3 on the anterior lip of the cervix (**A**). Faint acetowhite epithelium representing immature metaplasia is noted on the posterior lip. The areas of CIN 3 and immature metaplasia are also noted following application of Lugol's iodine solution (**B**). Following application of Lugol's the CIN 3 lesion is seen to have a brighter yellow color than the immature metaplasia.

during a colposcopic examination, a finding not listed in the RCI, suggests the presence of invasive cancer.

9.3.4.5.2.4 Iodine

The final colposcopic sign must be evaluated following staining of the cervix with Lugol's solution, provided the patient has no known allergy to iodine. Following application of 3% to 5% acetic acid solution to the cervix, the first three colposcopic signs are assessed and scored separately (Table 9.9). A preliminary subtotal score for these first three signs is summed before scoring the fourth sign. Lesions that reject iodine (turn mustard yellow) are assigned a score of 0 if the preliminary subtotal score of the first three colposcopic signs is 2 or less.[58,60] Formerly acetowhite lesions that reject iodine and have a preliminary subtotal score of 3 or more receive 2 points. Lesions that turn a variegated color upon application of iodine receive a score of 1 point. The total RCI score is then determined by adding the number of points scored for the fourth individual sign to the subtotal of the first three signs. The rationale for varying the

number of points on the basis of the same iodine staining characteristics follows.

Normal original squamous epithelium and mature metaplastic epithelium contain glycogen, which has an affinity for iodine. Thus, these tissues transiently appear mahogany brown when stained with Lugol's iodine solution. Infrequently, low-grade (CIN 1 or HPV) lesions may also absorb iodine and appear a mahogany brown color, or they may totally reject the iodine and appear a mustard-yellow color (Figure 9.18A–E). More commonly, intermediate-grade CIN 1, 2 lesions have a variegated yellow/brown or "tortoise-shell" appearance resulting from partial or inconsistent iodine uptake. Hence, tortoise-shell variegated lesions are assigned a score of 1 point (Figure 9.19A–D). Because both immature metaplasia and CIN 3 (Figure 9.20A–D) do not have glycogen and, therefore, do not stain with Lugol's iodine, the number of points assigned for completely mustard color nonstaining depends on the number of points previously assigned on the basis of margins, color, and vessels in the lesion. Hence the assignment of 0 points if the score of the first three colposcopic findings

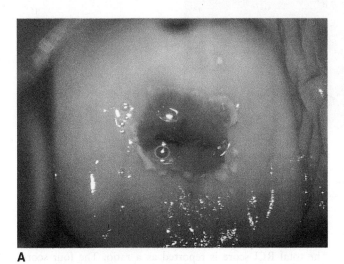
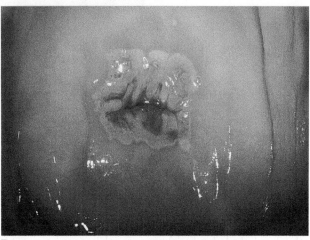

A   **B**

FIGURE 9.14.   An intermediate acetowhite lesion of the cervix indicating CIN 2. The cervix is seen before acetic acid application (**A**) and after (**B**). This color receives a score of 1 point.

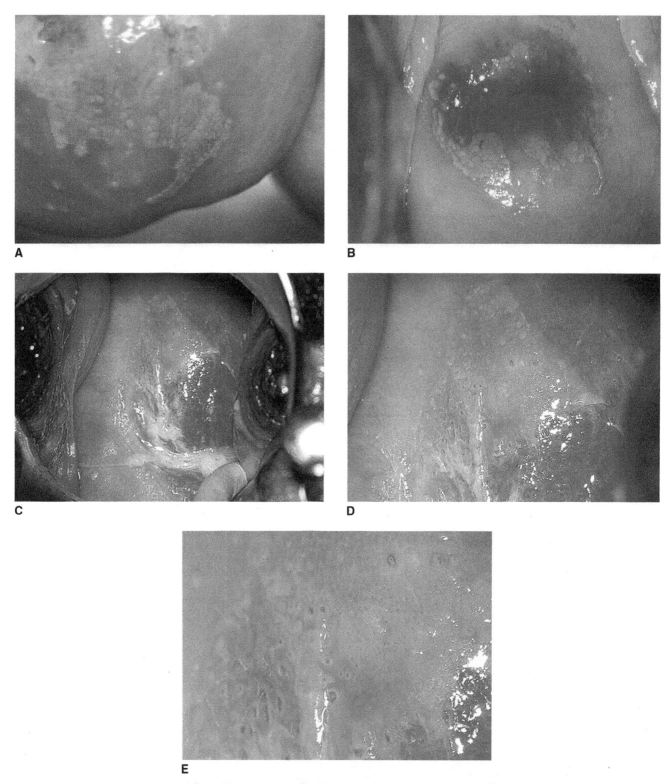

FIGURE 9.15.   **A,B:** A fine-caliber mosaic vessel pattern is seen with geographic and irregular margins in both lesions. The vessels are uniformly spaced with a narrow intercapillary distance. **C–E:** In another patient, at low power, this cervix appears nearly normal. However, there is a lesion at 11 o'clock **C,D:** With higher magnification (**E**), we see a translucent lesion with fine punctation and indistinct borders, a CIN 1.

is 0 to 2 points and the lesion is nonstaining.[58,60] If, on the other hand, the lesion has already scored 3 or more points on the basis of these factors, and is nonstaining, it gets assigned 2 points. Columnar cells reject iodine uptake and retain their reddish-pink color.

9.3.4.5.3 Scoring the Lesion

The total RCI score is reported as a ratio. The four scores derived from evaluation of the four colposcopic signs are added to define the RCI numerator. The RCI denominator always remains constant at 8, but the numerator or total score

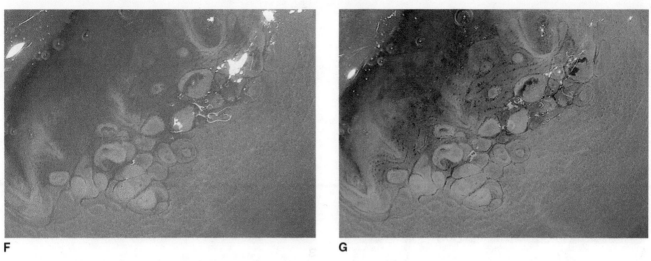

F   G

FIGURE 9.15. *(Continued)* **F:** In another patient, we note focal areas of opaque acetowhite in adjacent areas more translucent between 4 o'clock and 6 o'clock. Punctation within large mosaic plates can also be seen (umbilicated mosaic) and is almost always associated with CIN 3. **G:** With the green filter, some coarse punctation and mosaic with periglandular cuffing is seen in this indistinct CIN 3. (Figure 9.15C–G courtesy of, and reproduced by approval of, the International Cervical Cancer [INCCA] foundation.)

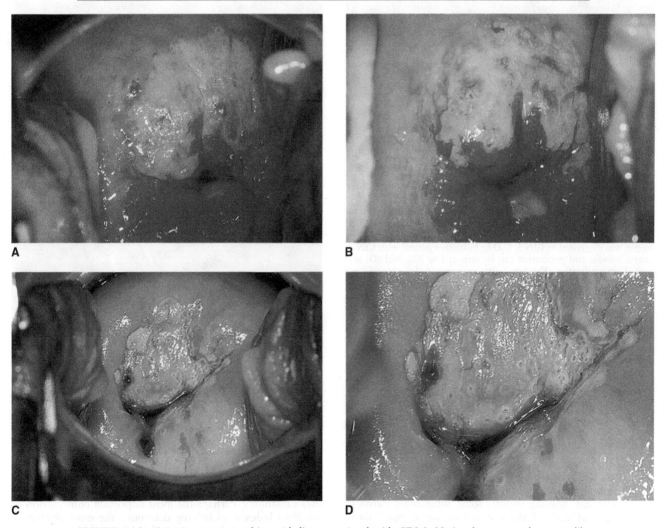

A   B
C   D

FIGURE 9.16. **A,B:** Opaque acetowhite epithelium associated with CIN 3. Notice that no vessels are readily apparent in the dense areas of acetowhite, but at 11 o'clock and 1–2 o'clock short non-branching (atypical) vessels can be seen. **C,D:** Another CIN 3 with opaque acetowhite is seen in (**C**) and (**D**). This lesion does not have any visible vessels. When scoring for vessels, a score of 1 point is assigned if no vessels are apparent. **D:** The lesion extends into the endocervical canal, and periglandular cuffing is prominently observed, increasing concern that this is a high-grade lesion. Histology was CIN 3. (Figure 9.16C,D courtesy of, and reproduced by approval of, the International Cervical Cancer [INCCA] foundation.)

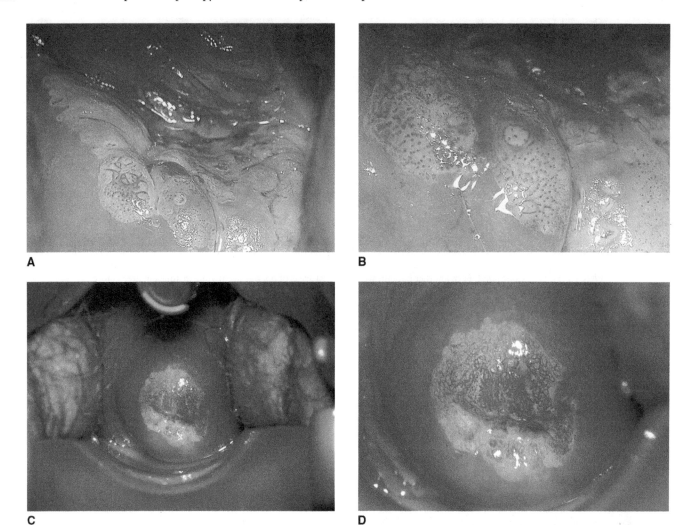

A

B

C

D

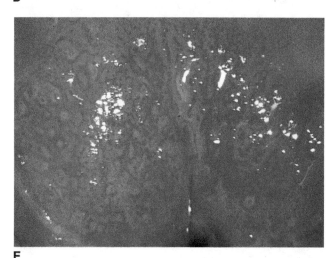

E

FIGURE 9.17. **A:** We see a very large lesion on the posterior cervix with smooth margins and an opaque color. **B:** Very coarsely dilated punctation and mosaic vessels are seen at 6 o'clock to 7 o'clock. The biopsy was diagnosed as CIN 3. **C,D,E:** In another patient with CIN 3, coarse mosaic and punctation can be seen at low (**C**), mid (**D**) and high (**E**) magnification. The very course appearance of the mosaic and punctation can be most appreciated at this high-power magnification (**E**). (Figure 9.17A,B courtesy of, and reproduced by approval of, the International Cervical Cancer [INCCA] foundation.)

fluctuates. The maximum possible total RCI score would be 8, and the minimum score would be 0.

As with any grading system, some subjectivity exists in the scoring of each of the colposcopic signs, particularly for color. For example, one observer may examine a lesion and attribute it 0 points for color, while another observer may give the same lesion 1 point for color. Therefore, of any of the grading systems discussed, the Reid Index provides the most detailed evaluation of important colposcopic findings, yet subjectivity of all the grading systems requires that

they be considered a helpful guide in forming a colposcopic impression, but not a final diagnosis. The final diagnosis must await histology. Perhaps the most important contribution of the Reid Index is in helping determine the most abnormal-appearing areas to biopsy, as will be discussed below.

At first, scoring is a tedious exercise. However, with practice, the scoring of these four criteria will take no more than 15 to 30 seconds. Colposcopists who consistently use the RCI should notice improvement in the accuracy of their colposcopic impression.

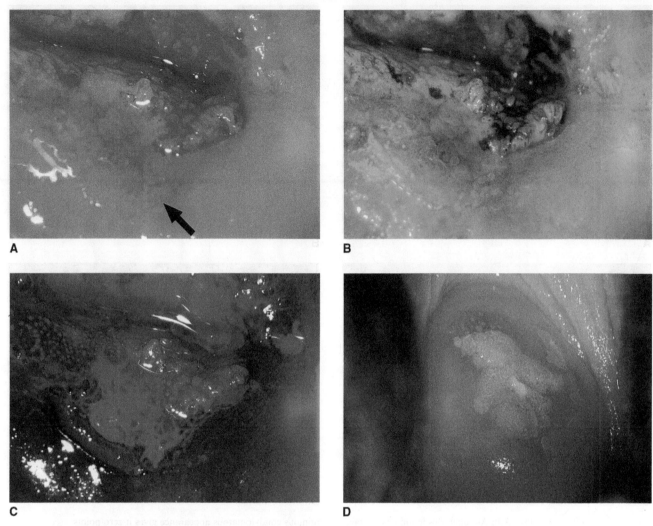

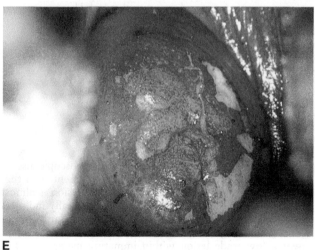

FIGURE 9.18.   **A:** The lesion on the posterior cervix (**A**) (*arrow*) has a moderately indistinct irregular margin (0 points), a translucent acetowhite color (0 points), and (**B**) a fine-caliber mosaic seen in the green filter (0 points). The preliminary score is 0/6. **C:** The same lesion totally rejects Lugol's iodine solution, and this is assigned 0 points for iodine. This patient's cervical biopsy was diagnosed as CIN 1. **D,E:** The other lesion (**D**) has an irregular margin with satellite lesions (0 points), an indistinct acetowhite color (0 points), and a fine mosaic pattern (0 points). The preliminary score is 0/6. **E:** The lesion picks up the iodine and appears brown (0 points). The total score of 0/8 suggests a low-grade lesion. The cervical biopsy was interpreted as CIN 1.

9.3.4.5.4 THE RCI CLINICAL CORRELATION

The RCI represents a weighted scoring system that helps form a colposcopic impression based on a structured analysis of the characteristics of premalignant cervical lesions. As such, a low RCI score implies less serious cervical disease and a high RCI score more severe disease (Table 9.10). Numerator scores from 0 to 2 are suggestive of CIN 1, HPV lesions such as condyloma, or normal immature metaplasia. Total RCI scores from 3 to 5 are suggestive of CIN 1 or CIN 2, with a score of

3 being more suggestive of CIN 1 and a score of 5 more suggestive of CIN 2. An RCI score from 6 to 8 is suggestive of CIN 2 to CIN 3. An RCI score of 8 for a cervical lesion demonstrating additional features considered to be warning signs for cervical cancer should be upgraded to a colposcopic impression of "rule-out" microinvasive or invasive cancer.

The index does not result in scores that are 100% in agreement with histologic findings, but 100% correlation is not the aim. Colposcopic findings that are discordant with histologic

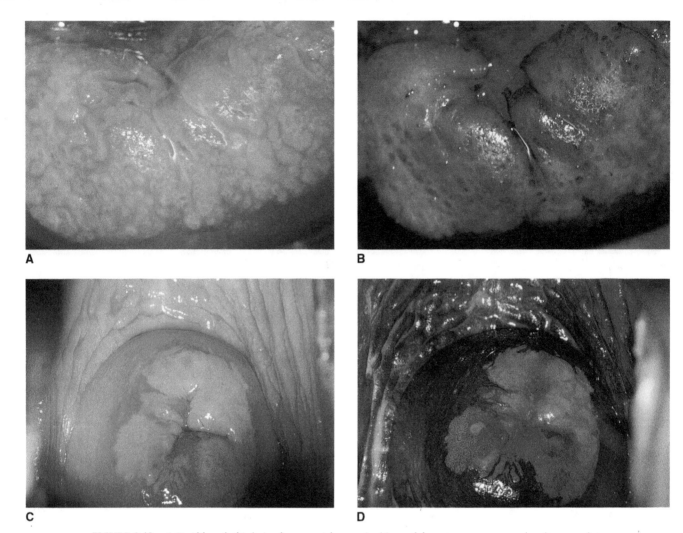

FIGURE 9.19. **A,B:** Although this lesion has a straight margin, it's condylomatous appearance gives it zero points for margin and 1 point for intermediate white color. A condylomatous surface pattern has aspects that look like mosaic plates, but on closer inspection no vessels can be seen (1 point). There is variegated iodine uptake (1 point), resulting in a total score of 3/8. The biopsy indicated CIN 1. **C,D:** A large acetowhite low-grade lesion is seen at 6 o'clock to 9 o'clock and a high-grade lesion is seen at 11 o'clock to 3 o'clock adjacent to the SCJ and cervical os. The posterior lesion has an irregular margin (0 points), a faint acetowhite color (1 point), and a fine mosaic (0 points). A variegated pattern of iodine uptake can be seen (1 point), earning the lesion a total score of 2/8 using the Reid's Colposcopic Index. A biopsy was diagnosed as CIN 1. The lesion at 11 o'clock to 3 o'clock has a smooth margin (1 point), an opaque acetowhite color (2 points), and no visible vessels (1 point), resulting in a preliminary score of 4/6. Because it totally rejects the iodine, it is assigned 2 points for iodine staining. The total score of 6/8 indicates that it is likely to be a high-grade lesion. The cervical biopsy was interpreted as CIN 3. C and D illustrate how the RCI helps direct biopsy placement within a large lesion.

findings occur even when the most experienced colposcopist performs the examination. Nevertheless, it would reasonable to expect that use of a structured approach, such as the Reid Index, would more accurately predict final histology than would be achieved by a less systematic approach. A number of studies have looked at both interobserver variability and colposcopic accuracy when the Reid Index is used, and will be discussed in the following sections.

9.3.4.5.5 SPECIAL CONSIDERATIONS CONCERNING THE RCI

Clinically obvious condylomas exhibiting a micropapillary or "cerebriform" (Figure 9.21) appearance automatically score 0 points for peripheral margin, even though the margin is in fact raised above the surrounding epithelium. Although raised, these lesions do not appear as if they could easily be peeled away from the underlying stroma. Their margins are also still primarily irregular and not smooth in shape.

One of the most valuable aspects of the index is the concept of an internal margin within a larger lesion (Figure 9.22A–G).

If in assessing a lesion colposcopically, the colposcopic disease pattern seen distally on the ectocervix is different than that seen proximally nearer the SCJ, the internal lesion is almost invariably more severe. An internal margin usually indicates evolution of a new high-grade lesion within a larger, more stable, preexisting low-grade lesion, although it also can represent a low-grade lesion within immature metaplasia. The point is that an internal margin represents an area that is more abnormal than that adjacent but peripheral. The higher-grade lesion should adjoin the SCJ. Therefore, the internal margin between the two lesions is a marker for a centrally positioned higher-grade lesion and scores 2 points for margin. Two exceptions are when the internal lesion is a clinically obvious condyloma acuminata, within a larger subclinical HPV-induced lesion or immature metaplasia, or when CIN 1 is present within immature metaplasia (Figure 9.23). Often, this exception is also characterized by the position of the internal lesion near, but not on, the SCJ. In this scenario, the low-grade lesion or immature metaplastic epithelium actually adjoins the SCJ.

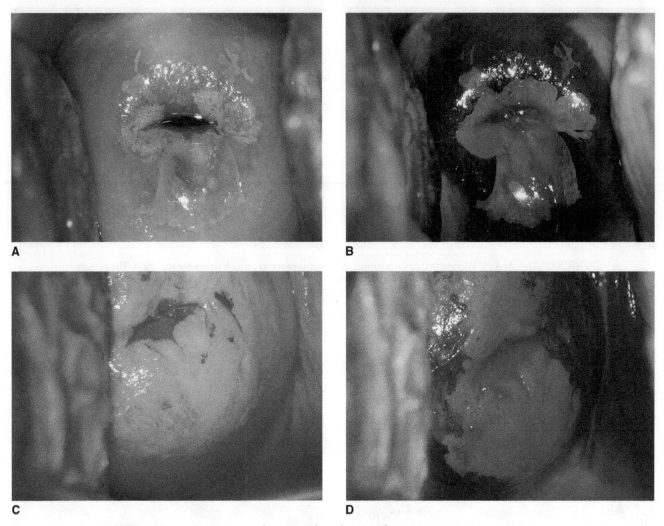

FIGURE 9.20. An opaque acetowhite, 3-quadrant lesion with a coarse punctation is seen in (**A**). An internal margin separates this CIN 3 from a low-grade lesion at 6 o'clock. The low-grade lesion has an irregular margin, translucent white color, and fine mosaic vessel pattern. The high-grade lesion's preliminary score is (2, 2, 2) 6/6. It completely rejects iodine (**B**), so its total score is 8/8. The low-grade lesion is scored as 0, 0, 0 for a preliminary score of 0/6. The pattern of iodine uptake is variegated; therefore, 1 point is assigned for iodine staining. The total score is 1/8, and this lesion is diagnosed as CIN 1. The large opaque acetowhite lesion (**C**), with smooth margins and no visible blood vessels scores 1, 2, 1, for a preliminary score of 4/6. It completely rejects iodine and turns yellow (**D**), so 2 points are assigned for iodine staining (**D**). The total score is 6/8, indicating a high-grade lesion. The biopsy was interpreted as CIN 3.

Both indistinct and snow-white HPV-induced lesions occur, as well as the dull oyster-grey color predictive of a high-grade lesion. These represent the two extremes and score 0 or 2 for color, respectively. However, most lesions exhibit a color in between, and score 1 point for color.

Many lesions have no colposcopically apparent capillary pattern within the acetowhite lesion. A lesion with no visible blood vessels or absent vessels scores 1 point for vessels (Figure 9.24). If a vascular pattern is present, it is necessary to determine whether it represents a fine vascular pattern (score 0) or a coarse vascular pattern (score 2). The coarse vascular pattern is uncommon. Sometimes when vessels are moderately dilated, it is difficult to determine whether vessels should be considered fine or coarse caliber. For instance, pregnancy or cervicitis may cause normally small blood vessels of a low-grade lesion to dilate. Lesions in which the vessel pattern is difficult to score almost invariably occur within immature elements of the transformation zone. Lesions in the immature components of the transformation zone occasionally have an unexpected histologic diagnosis of CIN 2 when a low-grade morphology was expected based on colposcopic findings. For this reason, if there is difficulty ascribing a score for vessel pattern, some colposcopists choose to overestimate and assign the lesion a score of 2 points. If the lesion is in fact low grade, it will receive lower scores for

TABLE 9.10	RCI CLINICAL CORRELATION
■ TOTAL COLPOSCOPIC SIGN SCORE	■ COLPOSCOPIC IMPRESSION
0–2	Normal or CIN 1 (low grade)
3–5	CIN 1 or CIN 2 (intermediate grade)*
6–8	CIN 2 or CIN 3 (high grade)†

*Total colposcopic score of 3 likely represents a low-grade lesion and a score of 5 predicts a high-grade lesion.
†Maximum scores accompanied by colposcopic warning signs of cancer should invoke a colposcopic impression of cancer.

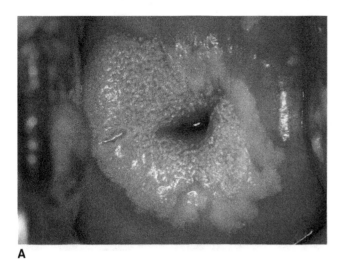

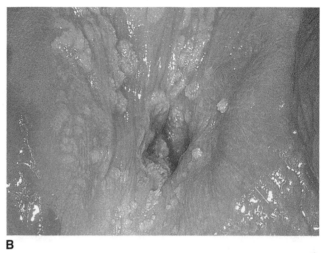

A   **B**

FIGURE 9.21.   **A:** A HPV lesion that has a micropapilliferous appearance, which scores the margin 0. The margin is scored 0. **B:** In a second patient, small, papular lesions are seen diffusely on the ectocervix of this woman following surgery. They represent condyloma in this immunocompromised patient. Margins would also be scored 0 here. (Figure 9.21B courtesy of, and reproduced by approval of, the International Cervical Cancer [INCCA] foundation.)

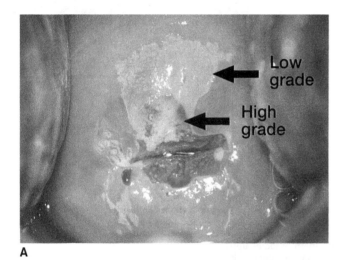

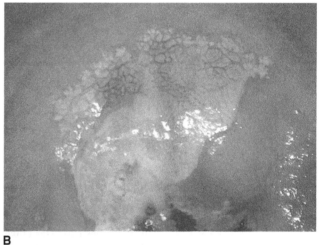

A   **B**

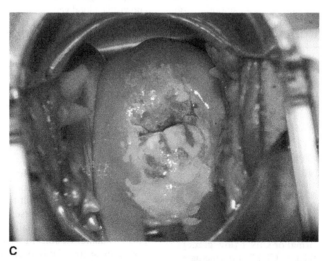

C

FIGURE 9.22.   A large low-grade lesion (*top arrow*) with a smaller high-grade lesion (*bottom arrow*) positioned along the SCJ is seen in (**A**). In this higher power magnification (**B**) the high-grade lesion with coarse punctation is separated from the low-grade lesion by an internal margin. The low-grade lesion in the periphery has a feathered margin, translucent white epithelium with a fine mosaic, and a punctation vessel pattern. **C:** In another woman there is a small high-grade lesion on the posterior cervix that is separated from the larger low-grade lesion by an internal margin.

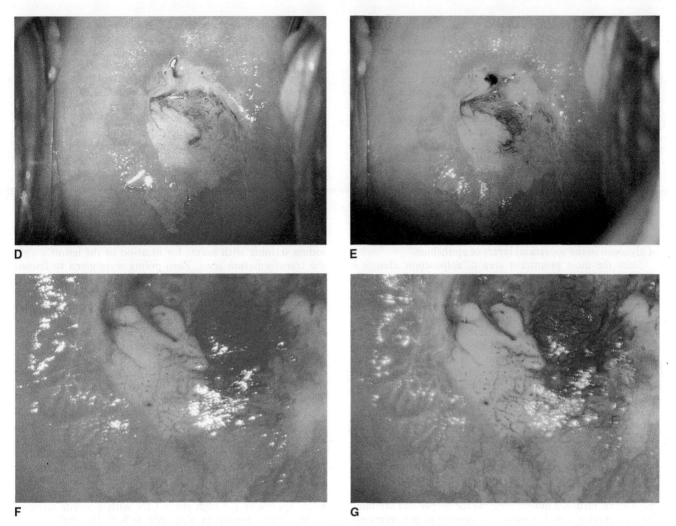

FIGURE 9.22. *(Continued)* **D–G:** A very opaque acetowhite lesion is separated from a large, translucent acetowhite lesion on the posterior cervix. The larger low-grade lesion (**D,E**) has a geographic margin (0 points), a translucent color (0 points), and fine-caliber vessels (0 points). The high-grade lesion (seen best in **F,G**) has a coarse vessel pattern, opaque epithelium, and internal margin, which all score 2 points each.

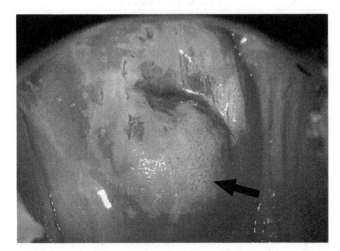

FIGURE 9.23. The exception to an internal margin identifying a high-grade lesion is demonstrated by this condyloma (*arrow*) positioned within a field of immature metaplasia, yet not adjoining the SCJ.

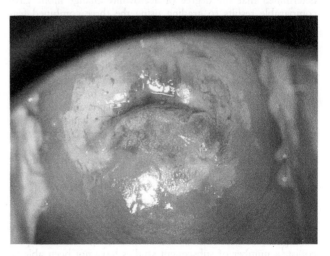

FIGURE 9.24. The lesion between 9 o'clock and 11 o'clock has no visible vessels and scores 1 point. The lesion at 6 o'clock has coarse vessels and scores 2 points for vessels.

the other signs. Thus, the impression made based on the total RCI score may still be consistent with the histology results.

As stated previously, it is important to assess and score the first three characteristics of the lesion using a 3% to 5% acetic acid solution before assessing the last score using Lugol's iodine solution. If the lesion scores 2 or fewer points for the first three signs, but rejects iodine staining and appears mustard yellow, the lesion will be downgraded and scored 0 points for iodine staining (Figure 9.18A–E). The explanation for the negative iodine staining is that low-grade lesions occur within poorly or nonglycogenated, immature elements of the transformation zone. On the other hand, if the lesion has scored a total of 3 or more points on the previously assessed characteristics, and then stains mustard yellow after application of Lugol's iodine solution, a score of 2 points is given for the iodine staining test (Figure 9.19C,D). In that lesion, the negative staining reflects a poorly differentiated high-grade lesion and a complete absence of glycogen in the superficial layers of epithelium.

Since the most prominent area of colposcopic change is not necessarily the area of greatest histologic abnormality, multiple biopsies are important. Peripheral areas of prominent acetowhite epithelium are often overinterpreted, while centrally the subtle acetowhite of a high-grade lesion or AIS may be easily overlooked. Epithelial thickness has been shown to impact detection of high-grade lesions.[33,35] Colposcopically undetected CIN 2,3 lesions found only on LEEP cone specimens were demonstrated to be nearly half as thick as CIN 2,3 detected on colposcopically directed biopsy, and they were much smaller.[33,61] Women who have atrophic epithelium from use of progestin-only contraception, oophorectomy, or menopause pose a special challenge to colposcopists, for these lesions will not appear as opaque as in well-estrogenized epithelium. Moreover, the sensitivity of colposcopy to detect high-grade lesions is lower in previously treated women compared with women never treated.[20] Women previously treated are more likely to have smaller, less easily detectable lesions, often in the endocervix. Hence, a lower threshold for biopsy and sampling the endocervical canal is most appropriate in posttreatment evaluation following an abnormal Pap. When in doubt, multiple biopsies increase diagnostic detection rates.[8,11,13]

9.3.4.5.6 REPRODUCIBILITY OF THE REID COLPOSCOPIC INDEX

A 2003 study prospectively evaluating the contribution of the three colposcopic features in diagnosing CIN of degree of acetowhite change, blood vessel pattern, and lesion margin determined that the degree of acetowhite change alone gave comparable results to grading using the three combined features.[45] However, the finding in the China study by Yang et al.[33] that some CIN 2,3 is thinner than normal or CIN 1 lesions questions the conventional wisdom that the most abnormal lesions are typically thicker and more densely acetowhite. While epithelial thickness affected the accuracy of colposcopic impression of CIN 2,3, it was not shown to do so for CIN 1 cases.[22] This brings into question whether the current standard of associating colposcopic impression of acetowhite changes with different grades of dysplasia may be inherently flawed secondary to differences in the histologic architecture of certain CIN 2 or CIN 3 lesions.[22] These conflicting findings make it even more important to not depend on any single colposcopic finding in interpretation of colposcopic signs of preinvasive cervical lesions.

The original study establishing the criteria used in the Reid Index was small and the correlation with final histology (97%) was higher than for any subsequent study.[58] While this may have partly reflected the skills of a most experienced colposcopist, a number of subsequent studies have not been able to document this degree of accuracy. Ferris et al.[50] used the RCI to achieve close to this degree of accuracy (92% correlation of colposcopic impression with histology) in a colposcopy residency training program. However, as discussed in Section 9.2, more recent studies have demonstrated much wider variability both in the accuracy of the colposcopic impression, and in the choice of biopsy site and number of biopsies taken. Results from the ALTS study have shown only fair to poor interobserver agreement in colposcopic impression using the Reid Index. Additionally, the sensitivity for ≥CIN 3 of a modified RCI (not using Lugol's) of ≥3/6 was only 37%.[10,53] The three colposcopic signs were also shown to not be individually sensitive in detecting CIN 3, thereby supporting the requirement in the Reid Index to evaluate margins, color, and vessels as each contributing to the final impression. However, one recent study comparing the strength of the correlation between colposcopy impression and biopsy histology in approximately 350 women evaluated at colposcopy by the Reid Index, and a similar number evaluated without using the RCI, demonstrated much higher correlation (74% vs. 45%) with the use of the Reid Index.[62]

In 2010, Hong et al.[63] used a modified RCI that replaced iodine staining with points for location of the lesion within the transformation zone. Zero points were given to lesions located only in the outer one-half of the transformation zone, whereas one point was given when most of the lesion was in the inner one-half of the T-zone and two points if the lesion extended into the endocervical canal. Using this system, the sensitivity and specificity of a colposcopic impression for CIN 2,3 were 91% and 93% respectively. The authors concluded that the accuracy of the RCI could be maximized by only making this one change, and leaving the point system for margins, color and vessels as originally described by Reid. This approach to modifying the RCI is encouraging and should be studied further. The Swede scoring system, which includes lesion size as a variable, has also been evaluated with encouraging, but somewhat mixed results.[64,65] Five variables were scored on a scale of 0, 1 or 2: acetowhiteness, margins and surface, vessels, lesion size, and iodine staining. A score of ≥5 points identified all (100%) CIN 2,3 and ≥8 points had a specificity of 90%. However, a 2010 study showed that while specificity for high-grade CIN with a Swede score of ≥8 was 95%, sensitivity was only 38%.[65] The authors suggested that the very high specificity might allow dropping the threshold to <8 points to increase sensitivity for CIN 2,3.

9.4 COLPOSCOPIC FEATURES OF CERVICAL INTRAEPITHELIAL NEOPLASIA

The spectrum of variation in colposcopic signs is a nondistinct continuum that spans the three levels of CIN. Even at the ends of the CIN continuum, discrimination between normal immature metaplasia and CIN 1 or between CIN 3 and microinvasive cancer may still present a diagnostic challenge. Use of a colposcopic grading system enhances the colposcopist's ability to form colposcopic impressions. Only years of colposcopic experience, supplemented by feedback from histologic sampling, refines a colposcopist's skill in estimating the severity of a cervical lesion. At the end of the day, all grading systems are likely most helpful in providing a structure in guiding biopsy placement. And do not forget that multiple biopsies reduce the risk of missed CIN 2,3+.[8,11,13,21,22]

The colposcopic appearance is determined by the architecture of the tissue being examined. Consequently, numerous combinations and various expressions of normal and abnormal tissue are possible within the transformation zone (leukoplakia, acetowhite epithelium, mosaic or punctation, and atypical blood vessels) [see Chapter 8]. Because variation will occur, the colposcopic impression may differ with the cytologic and histologic interpretations within one degree of severity, or more. In the next three sections, the colposcopic features of CIN will be discussed.

9.4.1 Colposcopy of CIN 1

9.4.1.1 Location of CIN 1

One of the greatest challenges in colposcopy is discriminating between immature metaplasia and the most minor level of cervical HPV expression, CIN 1 (Figure 19.25A–C). The colposcopic prediction of ectocervical CIN 1 tends to be much easier in women with fully mature transformation zones. This problem in differentiating between low-grade cervical HPV expression and immature metaplasia is further compounded by the extent of the transformation zone in many young women, which often occupies much of the portio.

Satellite CIN 1 lesions outside the active transformation zone may be recognized against the normal, pink squamous epithelium (Figure 9.26A,B). CIN 1 may be found anywhere on the ectocervix, in the endocervical canal (Figure 9.27), or in both locations (Figure 9.28A,B). Most CIN adjoins the SCJ (Figure 9.29A,B). However, in contrast to CIN 2,3, which is almost always adjacent to the SCJ, the location of CIN 1 is more variable, although usually found along the SCJ. As with higher-grade CIN, it is mainly the position of the SCJ that determines the location of CIN 1.

9.4.1.2 Contour of CIN 1

In addition to location, the contour of CIN 1 lesions can vary tremendously. Cervical condylomas are also classified histologically as CIN 1. Hence, CIN 1 has a range of morphologic expression, including micropapillary, papillary, papular, flat and raised contour. Less commonly, cerebriform or "brain-like" topography may be seen. Large exophytic condyloma occupying 4 quadrants of the cervix must be distinguished from invasive cancer by cervical biopsy (Figure 9.30A,B). These large HPV lesions normally have more distinct uniform papillary projections with centralized fine-caliber capillaries than the papillary projections in exophytic cervical cancer (Figure 9.31).

In contrast with elevated lesions, endophytic CIN 1 may be seen if the neoplastic epithelium extends within gland crypts. If the lesion is isolated to a gland crypt, a broad, slightly opaque acetowhite band of epithelium will be observed surrounding the gland opening (Figure 9.32). This periglandular cuffing is in contrast to the thin rim of acetowhite epithelium that surrounds normal, uninvolved gland openings. However, these occasionally occult endophytic lesions are usually associated with more apparent ectocervical lesions.

The majority of CIN 1 is macular in contour (Figure 9.33). In some cases, it may be maculopapular (Figure 9.34). Because macular CIN 1 lesions are most often flat to the surrounding normal squamous epithelium, they are not generally apparent without the use of contrast solutions (Figure 9.35A,B). The exceptions are condyloma and when a slightly elevated area of leukoplakia overlies a CIN 1 lesion. A fine micropapillary surface may be seen with subclinical low-grade HPV expression of the cervix or vagina (Figure 9.36A,B). Tiny light reflections give the surface a slightly pebbled appearance. With close inspection, small capillaries may be observed inside the finger-like projections. This

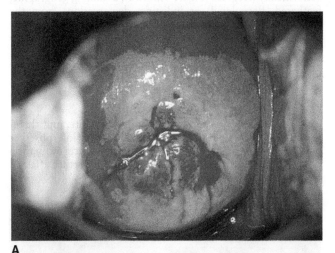

A

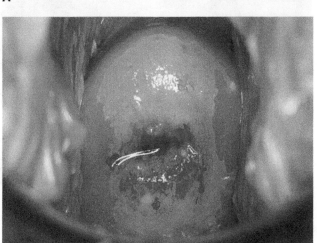

C

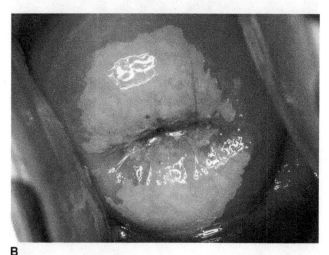

B

FIGURE 9.25.   **A–C:** The large acetowhite areas on these three cervices were diagnosed as immature metaplasia by biopsy. Each one could be easily interpreted colposcopically as CIN. Especially note the opaque acetowhite in (C), but the feathery margins look low grade.

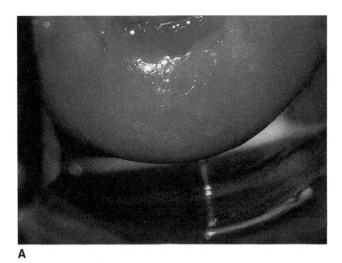
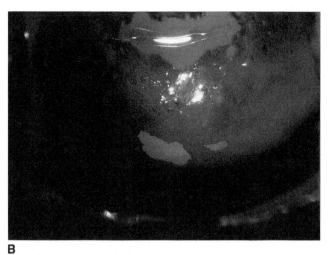

A   **B**

FIGURE 9.26. A small CIN 1 located outside the transformation zone is barely visible following application of 3% to 5% acetic acid solution (**A**) and clearly visible after Lugol's iodine (**B**).

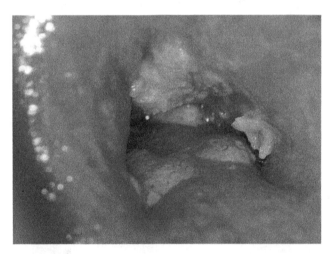

FIGURE 9.27. An exophytic condyloma within the endocervical canal. Fine vessels are seen on the posterior cervix.

presentation is frequently seen in women with a LSIL Pap test result and no discrete acetowhite lesion.

9.4.1.3 Margin of CIN 1

CIN 1 lesions tend to be diffuse and asymmetrical in shape (Figure 9.37A,B). The edges or borders of CIN 1 are characteristically irregular (Figure 9.38A,B), assuming geographic, feathered, flocculated, or indistinct demarcations from the surrounding normal epithelium (Figure 9.39A,B). Multiple or solitary satellite lesions in the periphery of a central lesion also support a colposcopic impression of CIN 1. Therefore, most CIN 1 margins are very uneven and irregular, reflecting the biologic nature of the lesion.

9.4.1.4 Color of CIN 1

Color is subjective, especially variations of white, and therefore is the colposcopic feature with the most interobserver variability in grading. Glare also may influence evaluation of color. The dilemma of color description is further affected

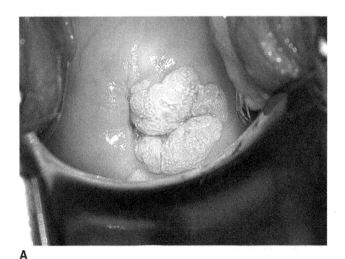
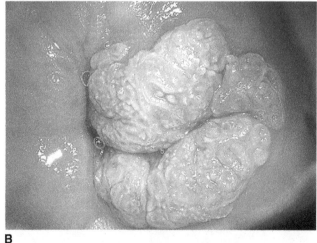

A   **B**

FIGURE 9.28. **A:** A 4-quadrant exophytic lesion is noted in this inadequate colposcopic examination. **B:** Higher-power magnification. The surface is irregular raising the suspicion of cancer versus condyloma. The biopsy was diagnosed as condyloma.

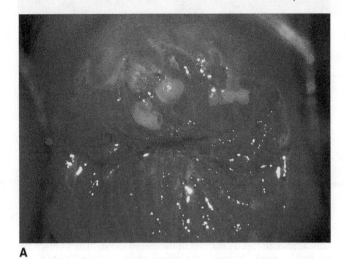
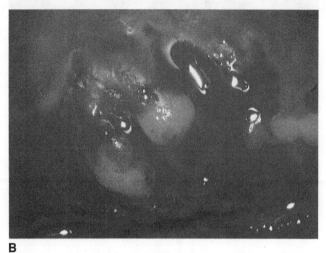

A

B

FIGURE 9.29. **A,B:** These CIN 1 lesions are located at the SCJ. These lesions would be considered at greater risk for subsequent detection of a high-grade lesion than the lesion seen in Figure 9.26 A,B.

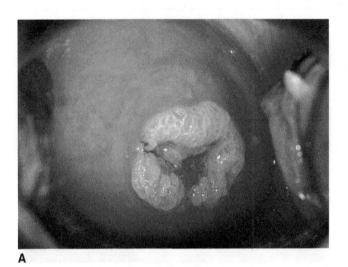
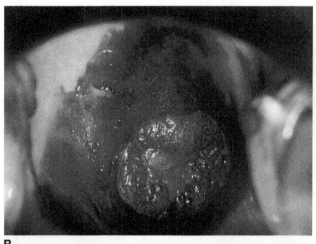

A

B

FIGURE 9.30. This large 4-quadrant acetowhite lesion of the cervix could be invasive cancer or an exophytic condyloma (**A**). The lesion absorbs iodine and turns mahogany brown. Hence, the latter diagnosis is favored pending a histologic diagnosis (**B**).

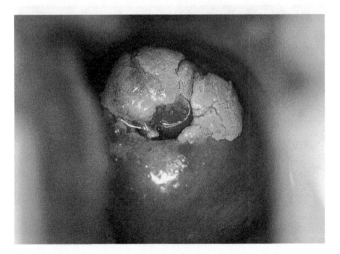
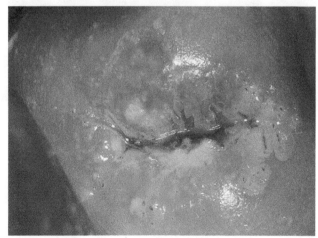

FIGURE 9.31. Fine vessels are noted in the papillary projections of this cervical condyloma.

FIGURE 9.32. CIN 1 is seen within gland crypts at 5 o'clock. The normally thin translucent acetowhite rim around gland openings is broader and more opaque.

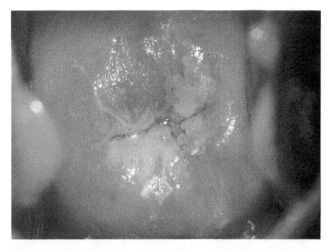

FIGURE 9.33. A macular CIN 1 on the anterior and posterior cervix.

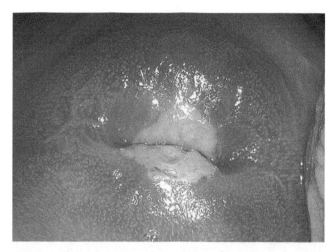

FIGURE 9.34. Dense acetowhite maculopapular lesions are noted on the anterior and posterior cervix with diffuse subclinical HPV changes outside smooth regular margins of the central lesions. The lesions have no visible vessels. Although the diffuse white "speckles" outside the main lesions would be low grade, the central lesion could easily be interpreted colposcopically as a CIN 2. However, the biopsies at 12 o'clock and 6 o'clock were interpreted as CIN 1. Courtesy of, and reproduced by approval of, the International Cervical Cancer (INCCA) foundation.

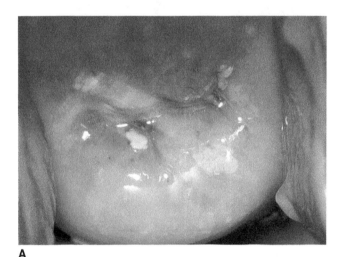

A

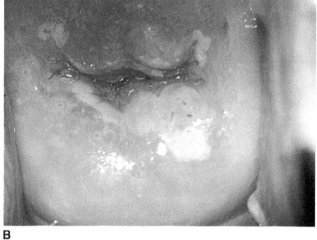

B

FIGURE 9.35. Only a small area of leukoplakia is noted at 4 o'clock prior to the application of 3% to 5% acetic acid solution (A). Following acetic acid application, a much larger acetowhite lesion is seen (B).

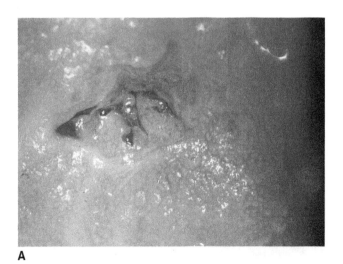

A

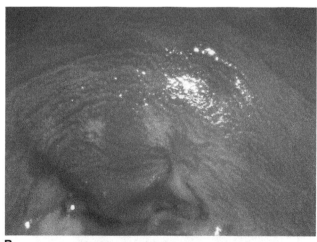

B

FIGURE 9.36. **A,B:** Subclinical HPV infection can cause a fine micropapillary surface contour. Central loop capillaries may be observed within these tiny projections extending above the surface of the epithelium.

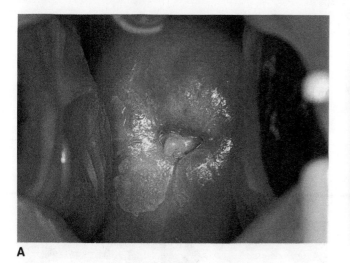

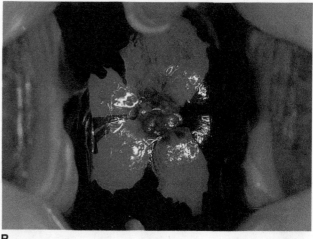

A   B

FIGURE 9.37.   Diffuse, asymmetrical CIN 1 after application of 3% to 5% acetic acid solution (**A**) and Lugol's iodine solution (**B**).

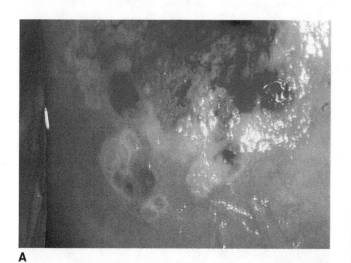

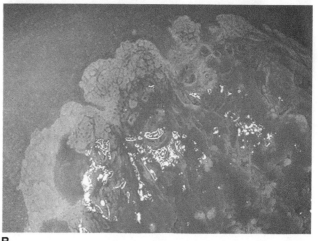

A   B

FIGURE 9.38.   **A,B:** Irregular margins in two cases of CIN 1. **B:** Also shows a fine mosaic pattern. Biopsies were only CIN 1 in each. Figure 9.38B courtesy of, and reproduced by approval of, the International Cervical Cancer (INCCA) foundation.

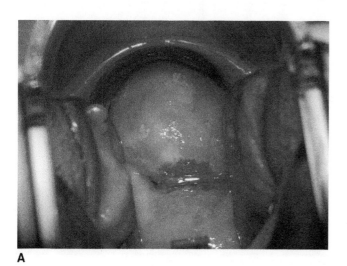

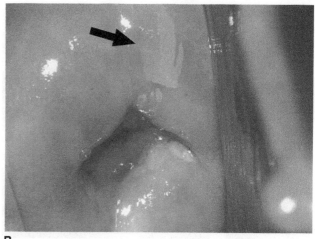

A   B

FIGURE 9.39.   **A:** Geographic margin and (**B**) feathered margins (*arrow*) both suggest CIN 1.

by the varied illumination sources for colposcopes, which emit slightly different wavelengths, or shades, of white light. Regardless, most CIN 1 lesions change from the pink color of surrounding normal mucosa to a transiently light or snowy white color following application of 3% to 5% acetic acid solution (Figure 9.40A–C). After the application of the 3%

to 5% acetic acid, some CIN 1 are almost translucent white or faint white, but generally not as translucent as immature metaplasia or the transient white blush appearance of columnar villi (Figure 9.41A,B). Conversely, condylomas may be shiny white, conveying an opaque quality more typically seen in high-grade CIN. When HPV induces leukoplakia, the white

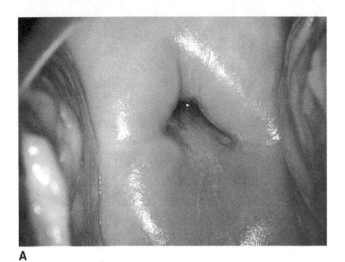

A

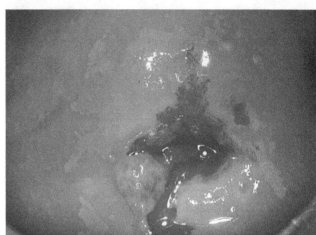

B

FIGURE 9.40.   Denser acetowhitening is seen on the posterior cervix in both (**A**) and (**B**). The latter cervix also has an anterior translucent area of acetowhite with a geographic margin and fine-caliber vessels. Biopsy of both at 6 o'clock is required to rule out a lesion of higher grade than CIN 1. **C:** A translucent acetowhite area with geographic margins and fine punctation is seen anteriorly.

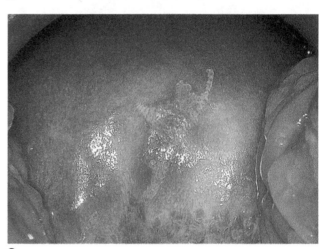

C

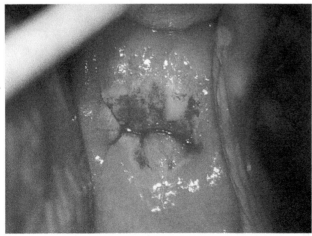

A

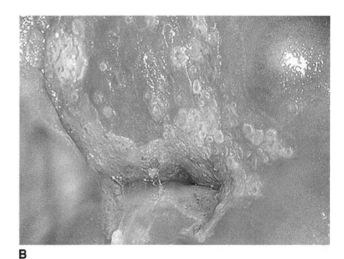

B

FIGURE 9.41.   **A:** An opaque acetowhite lesion is seen at 1 o'clock. **B:** The irregular margin, color, and satellite lesions seen here are typical of CIN 1. Figure 9.41B courtesy of, and reproduced by approval of, the International Cervical Cancer (INCCA) foundation.

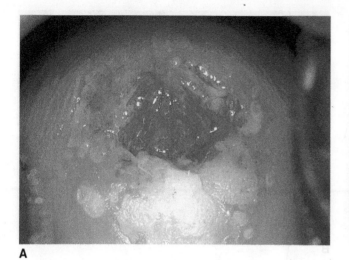

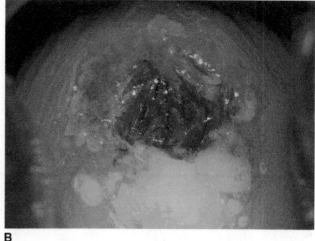

A   **B**

FIGURE 9.42.   An area of leukoplakia within the central area of this CIN 1 (**A**). The green filter does not enhance the colposcopic examination when vessels are not apparent (**B**).

color is more opaque than would be anticipated for the level of disease, and is present before the application of acetic acid (Figure 9.42A,B).

The duration and degree of acetowhitening of cervical lesions following the application of acetic acid has been quantitated previously.[66] Notable differences between the acetowhiteness of the three grades of CIN were detected, with CIN 1 having the lowest values and CIN 3 the highest. Moreover, the resolution rates of acetowhite color 4 minutes after the application of acetic acid were 65% for CIN 1, 41% for CIN 2, and 29% for CIN 3. The progressively diminishing duration of acetowhitening with decreasing lesion grade documents the tendency of CIN 1 to be more transiently acetowhite. Only the acetowhite color of squamous metaplasia resolved at a greater rate (78%) than CIN 1 within this time period.[66] Of course, as previously discussed, not all high-grade lesions are acetowhite, and some low-grade lesions appear densely acetowhite.[33]

9.4.1.5 Vessels of CIN 1

When blood vessels are noted colposcopically in CIN 1 lesions, they are invariably of a fine, narrow caliber (Figure 9.43A–C). If present, these vessels are typically more apparent than the small, wispy loop capillaries often seen in native squamous epithelium (Figure 9.44A,B). The vessels of CIN 1 are usually arranged uniformly. Consequently, a mosaic vascular pattern associated with CIN 1 is primarily homogeneous in distribution and appears delicate and lacy (Figures 9.45A,B, 9.46A,B, and 9.47A,B). Punctation is observed as tiny red dots closely and uniformly distributed (Figure 9.48A,B). Fine-caliber vessels may not be seen immediately following the application of 3% to 5% acetic acid solution. Although the tiny vessels contrast nicely against an acetowhite background, extremely narrow-caliber vessels may not be visualized until the full acetowhite effect begins to diminish.

Atypical blood vessels are not seen in CIN 1. However, superficial, parallel atypical blood vessels not associated with cancer may be seen in areas of very immature metaplasia (Figures 8.91 and 8.92), causing these areas to be easily confused with CIN 1 or cancer. These vessels are usually moderately coarse, are horizontally positioned, and have few branching vessels. Their position in a surrounding translucent acetowhite change provides reassurance that they are not likely to be within cervical cancer. However, presence of atypical vessels always warrants biopsy.

9.4.1.6 Iodine Staining of CIN 1

CIN 1 lesions may be either iodine negative with a mustard-yellow color after the application of dilute Lugol's iodine or tortoise-shell spotty iodine staining (Figure 9.49A–H). Superficial keratin sometimes associated with CIN 1 also rejects iodine in areas that were white prior to application of 3% to 5% acetic acid solution (Figure 9.50A,B). Because CIN 1 is frequently positioned in a field of immature metaplasia, if it is not tortoise-shell staining, both the CIN 1 and the immature metaplasia will appear yellow following application of Lugol's iodine solution, and thus may blend together, making differentiation challenging. Because glycogen is usually found in intermediate and superficial layers of squamous epithelium and the atypical cellular changes of CIN 1 are found primarily in the basal and parabasal layers, it is not uncommon to see some degree of partial or even full iodine uptake in isolated areas of CIN 1 (Figures 9.51A,B and 9.52A,B).

9.4.1.7 Size and Distribution of CIN 1

CIN 1 lesions are often relatively small (Figure 9.53A–C) with a mean length of approximately 2.8 mm.[66] Although CIN 1 lesions can span a much larger area,[67] colposcopically detectable CIN 2 and CIN 3 lesions are typically larger. The mean reported length of CIN 2 and CIN 3 are 5.8 and 7.6 mm, respectively, and the maximum length 18.2 and 20.6 mm, respectively.[67] Low-grade lesions may occupy only 1 quadrant or less of the cervix (Figure 9.54A–F) or occasionally, may involve multiple quadrants of the cervix, particularly in immunocompromised women (Figure 9.55A,B). However, when what appears to be CIN 1 is present in all 4 quadrants of the cervix, it must be discriminated from a large congenital transformation zone (CTZ), which may be similar in appearance (see Chapter 13). In the latter, acetowhite areas are usually more symmetrical than CIN 1 lesions, with less irregular margins, and the development of the acetowhitening effect of a CTZ typically is slower and lasts longer than CIN 1.

The distribution of CIN 1 varies from unifocal to multifocal (Figure 9.56A–C). Multiple, distinct, small, randomly scattered lesions are characteristic of CIN 1. These may be located within or outside of the transformation zone (Figure 9.57). It is not uncommon to see coexisting HPV-related disease extending into the vagina in the form of condyloma or low-grade vaginal HPV lesions (Figure 9.58). CIN 1 lesions tend to be relatively shallow, and therefore rarely extend deeper than

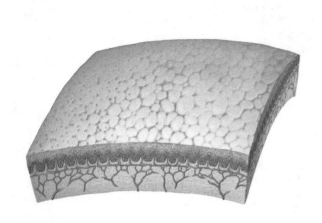

A

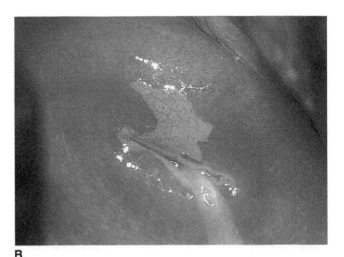

B

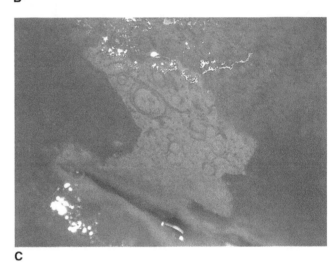

C

FIGURE 9.43.   **A:** An illustration of fine mosaic and fine punctation **B:** A small acetowhite lesion is seen on the anterior cervix. **C:** With greater magnification, we can appreciate the irregular margin and fine punctation and mosaic vessel pattern. The biopsy was CIN 1. (**A** [illustration]: copyright © 2004, 2011. ASCCP. All rights reserved. **B,C** [Colpophotographs]: courtesy of, and approved for reproduction by, the International Cervical Cancer (INCCA) foundation.)

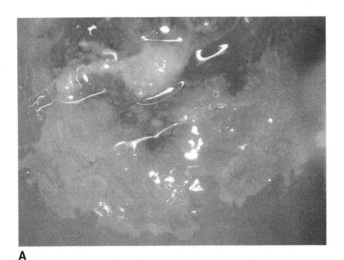

A

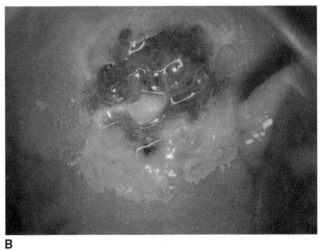

B

FIGURE 9.44.   **A,B:** These fine vessels associated with CIN 1 are much larger than the small network capillaries of native squamous epithelium.

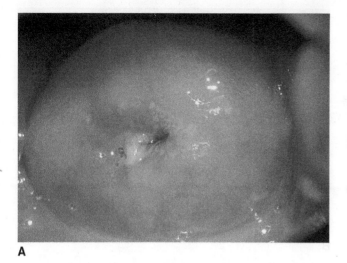
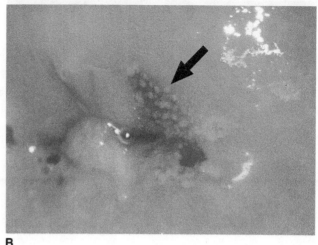

A   **B**

FIGURE 9.45.   At low magnification, an acetowhite lesion is seen at 9 o'clock (**A**). The mosaic pattern (*arrow*) is better appreciated at higher magnification (**B**).

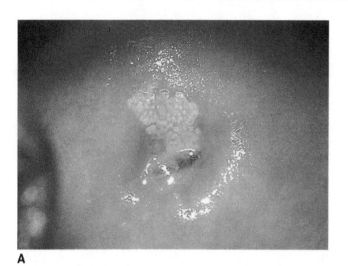
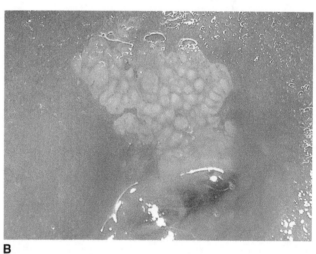

A   **B**

FIGURE 9.46.   A fairly opaque lesion is noted at 12 o'clock (**A**). Although opaque, there is a shiny, glossy appearance to this lesion. With greater magnification (**B**), we see a fine, somewhat irregular mosaic pattern with an irregular margin. The histology was CIN 1. Courtesy of, and reproduced by approval of, the International Cervical Cancer (INCCA) foundation.

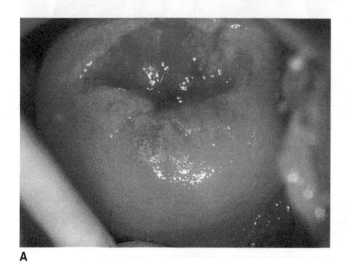
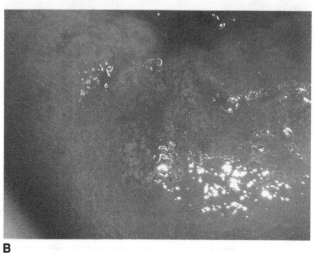

A   **B**

FIGURE 9.47.   A small CIN 1 can be seen on the posterior cervix (**A**). A fine mosaic pattern is noted in (**B**). Also of interest, small HPV-induced papillary projections with central loop capillaries are observed surrounding the lesion.

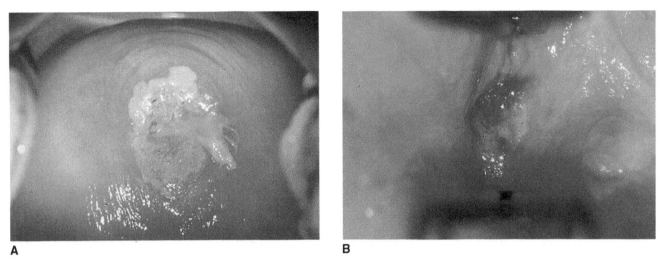

FIGURE 9.48.   **A:** A fine punctation is seen in this CIN 1. **B:** Another fine-to-moderate punctation is noted in this CIN 1 seen following loop excision, which may have accentuated the vessels.

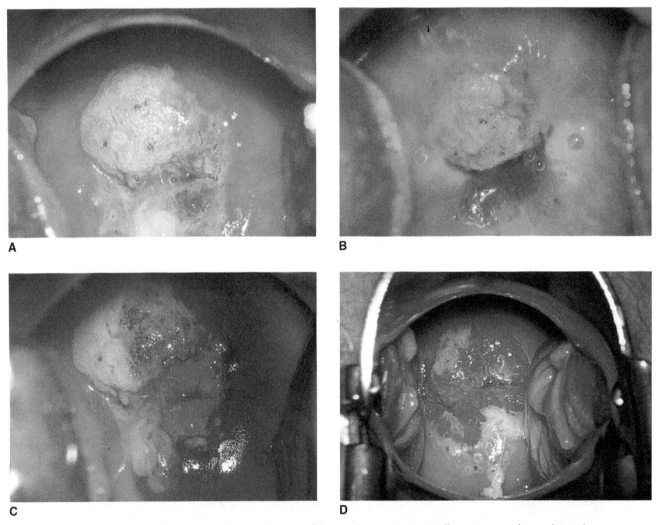

FIGURE 9.49.   A large condyloma occupies most of the anterior cervix (**A**). Small punctate vessels are observed using the green filter (**B**). Half of the lesion has been coated with application of Lugol's iodine solution (**C**). The lesion rejects the iodine and appears yellow against the brown-staining, normal squamous epithelium. In another patient (**D–H**), an acetowhite lesion can be seen at 4 o'clock along the SCJ (**D**).

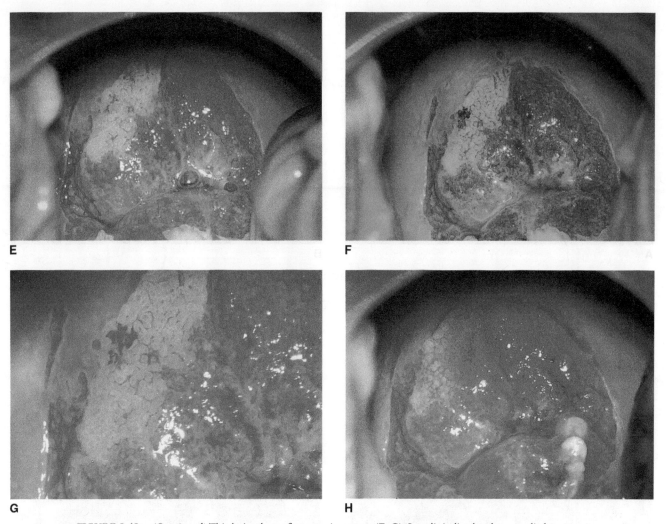

FIGURE 9.49. *(Continued)* This lesion has a fine mosaic pattern (**E–G**). Lugol's iodine has been applied to a portion of the lesion (**H**), and the former acetowhite area now appears yellow. Note the fading acetowhitening in the area not stained with Lugol's.

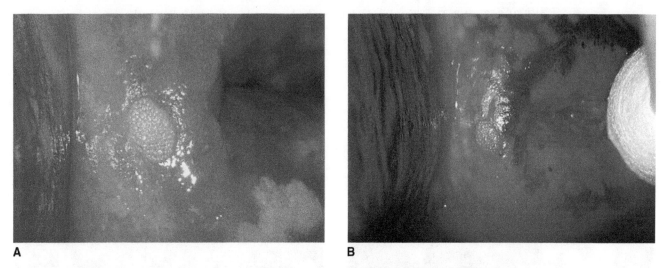

FIGURE 9.50. Leukoplakia covers this CIN 1 (**A**). Consequently, the condylomatous lesion appears yellow following application of Lugol's iodine solution (**B**).

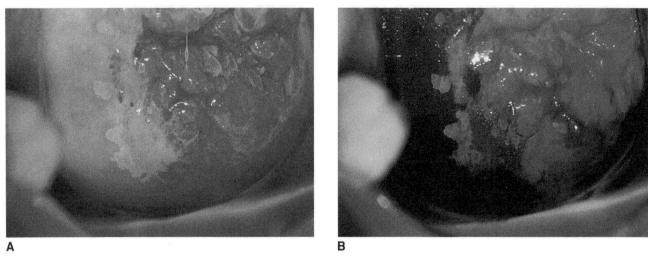

A   **B**

FIGURE 9.51.   **A,B:** The low-grade lesion with an irregular margin at 8 o'clock (**A**) has a variegated iodine-staining pattern. Some glycogen is present within the lesion.

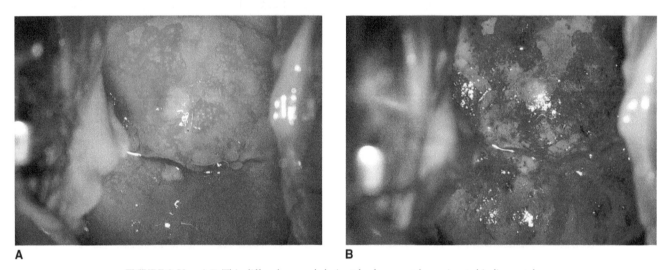

A   **B**

FIGURE 9.52.   **A,B:** This diffuse low-grade lesion also has a patchy variegated iodine uptake.

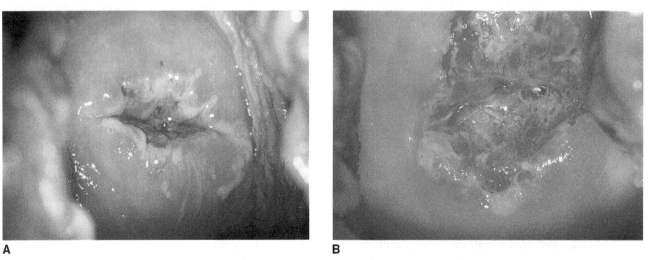

A   **B**

FIGURE 9.53.   Small CIN 1 lesions extend along much of the SCJ and at 3–5 o'clock, well out on the portio. **A:** Another small CIN 1 located along the SCJ. **B:** A small CIN 1 is seen at 6 o'clock.

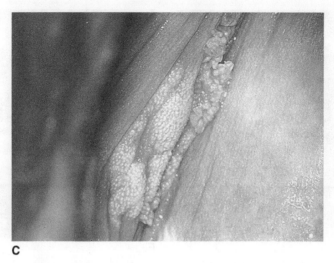

FIGURE 9.53. *(Continued)* **C:** Don't forget to look in the vagina with the colposcope. In another patient, we see exophytic lesions in the right proximal vagina. Figure 9.53C courtesy of, and reproduced by approval of, the International Cervical Cancer (INCCA) foundation.

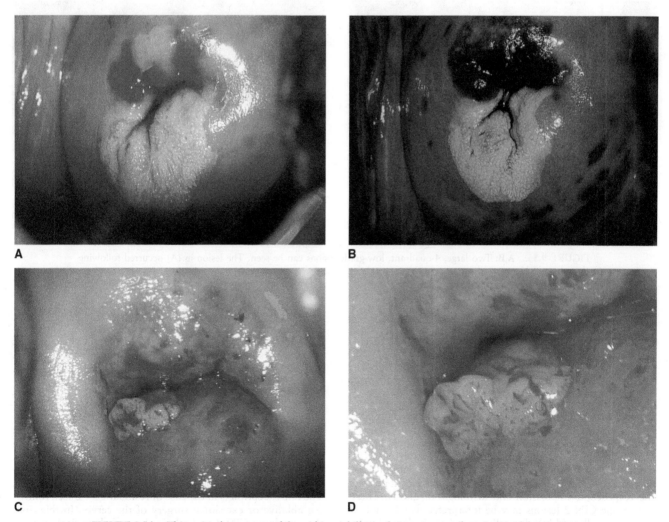

FIGURE 9.54. This series shows some of the wide variability in the appearance of cervical condylomas. **A:** A condyloma is seen occupying 1 quadrant of the posterior cervix. This woman also has Trichomonas cervicitis, as seen both with (**B**) and without (**A**) the green filter. **C,D:** Otherwise, some lesions are quite small, as the one seen at 6–9 o'clock. **D:** The fine capillaries of this condyloma are readily apparent.

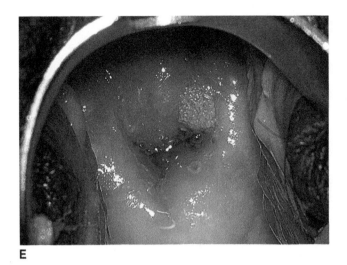

E

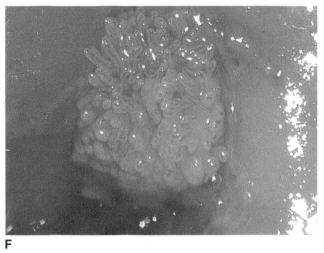

F

FIGURE 9.54. *(Continued)* **E,F:** A papillary lesion is seen on the anterior cervix. **F:** Tiny afferent and efferent capillaries are noted in this typical condyloma. Figure 9.54E,F courtesy of, and reproduced by approval of, the International Cervical Cancer (INCCA) foundation.

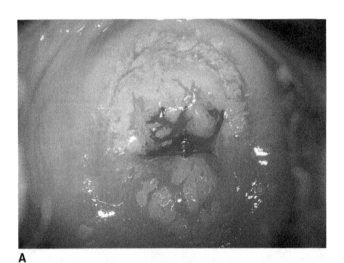

A

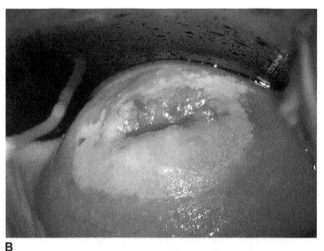

B

FIGURE 9.55. **A,B:** Two large, 4-quadrant, low-grade lesions can be seen. The lesion in (**A**) occurred following electrosurgical loop excision.

2 mm into gland crypts.[67] The mean depth of CIN 1 gland crypt involvement is approximately 0.4 mm.[67]

9.4.2 Colposcopy of CIN 2

Correctly correlating histologic CIN 2 with a colposcopic impression of CIN 2 is difficult (Figure 9.59A–C). For one reason, interobserver variability in both the colposcopic impression and the histologic diagnosis of CIN 2 is more than for CIN 3 and nearly as poor as for CIN 1.[30] This lack of interobserver agreement within each discipline influences agreement between the colposcopic impression and histologic diagnosis. Therefore, some CIN 2 lesions may be interpreted as CIN 1 both colposcopically and histologically, or as CIN 3, depending on overinterpretation or underintrepretation by either the colposcopist or the pathologist. The colposcopic characteristics of CIN

2 should appear more like those of CIN 3 than CIN 1, but this is not always the case because CIN 2 is not a reliable diagnosis. A small CIN 2 lesion may also blend into a larger field of CIN 1.

9.4.2.1 Location of CIN 2

Most CIN 2 lesions are located centrally on the cervix (Figure 9.60). Solitary CIN 2 lesions separated from the SCJ are not typical. Almost always, CIN 2 will be found near or adjoining the SCJ (Figure 9.61A,B), whether positioned on the ectocervix or within the endocervical canal (Figure 9.62A,B). The one exception is in the case of residual CIN 2 seen following ablative or excisional surgery of the cervix. In this case, the remaining CIN 2 will adjoin the healed surgical excision line, but may be separated from the new SCJ by immature and mature metaplastic epithelium.

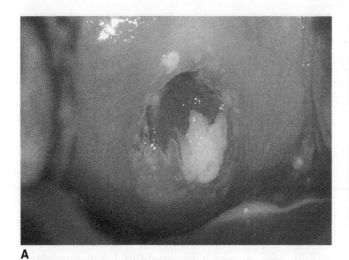

A

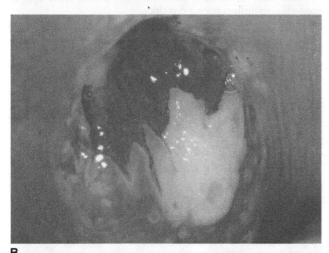

B

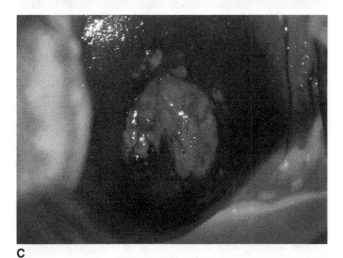

C

FIGURE 9.56. A unifocal CIN 1 is seen on the posterior cervix (**A,B**). The lesion mostly rejects Lugol's iodine solution and assumes a transient yellow color, but with some variegation (**C**).

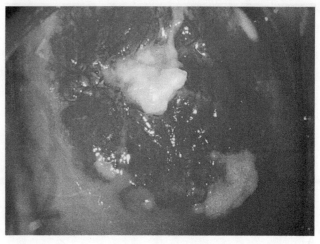

FIGURE 9.57. A CIN 1 along the SCJ and within the active transformation zone. This patient also has a large ectropion.

9.4.2.2 Contour of CIN 2

CIN 2 lesions tend to be macular, although some are slightly thickened (Figure 9.63). As such, their contour may not help discriminate CIN 2 from CIN 1 or CIN 3. Irregular surface contour may be expected with HPV-related CIN 1 lesions that may be overrated histologically as CIN 2 lesions. Coexisting leukoplakia will also cause epithelial elevation, but this is generally an exception for CIN 2 (Figure 9.64A–D).

9.4.2.3 Margins of CIN 2

The margins of CIN 2 lesions tend to be less irregular or geographic in shape than in CIN 1 lesions. Therefore, the margins are generally smooth, rounded, or straight with minor

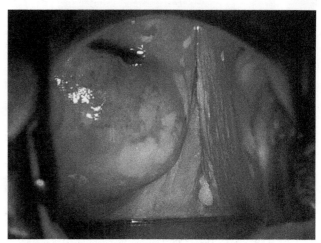

FIGURE 9.58. CIN 1 and low-grade vaginal HPV lesions in this immunocompromised woman with both HIV and hepatitis B.

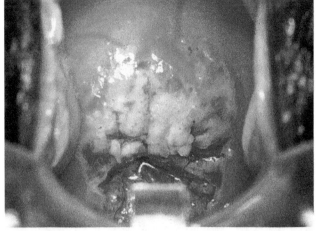

A

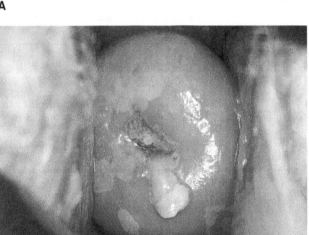

B

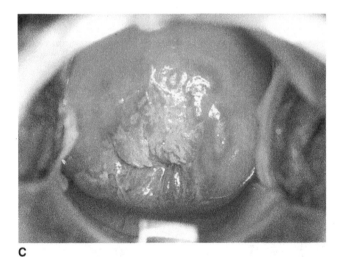

C

FIGURE 9.59.   **A–C:** Three CIN 2 lesions that demonstrate some features of CIN 1 and some of CIN 3.

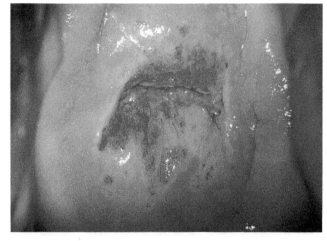

FIGURE 9.60.   A centrally positioned CIN 2 with dense opaque acetowhite epithelium from 3–5 o'clock.

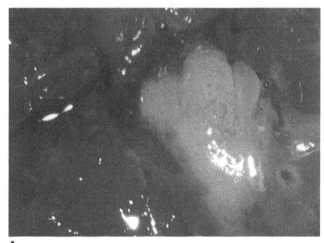

A

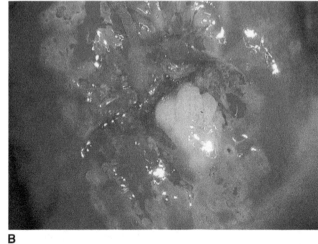

B

FIGURE 9.61.   **A,B:** A CIN 2 located along the SCJ seen at high and low magnification.

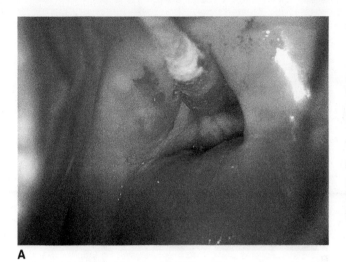
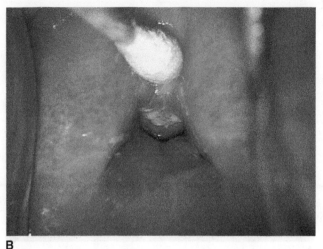

A   **B**

FIGURE 9.62.   A CIN 2 lesion located within the endocervical canal. The first examination was inadequate (**A**), but the upper extent of the lesion in (**B**) can be seen with elevation of the anterior canal with a cotton-tipped swab. Therefore, the colposcopic examination was adequate.

fine undulation (Figure 9.65A,B). The apparent external margin may resemble that of CIN 1 when a small focal area of CIN 2 is positioned adjacent to the SCJ within a larger CIN 1 lesion (Figure 9.66A,B). In this case, a distinct internal margin may not be seen clearly. CIN 2 may also form the peripheral rim around a more centrally positioned CIN 3. In this case, the margin is usually fairly straight with only minor variation.

9.4.2.4 Color of CIN 2

Basic white is the most common color seen in CIN 2 lesions following application of 3% to 5% acetic acid solution (Figure 9.67A,B). This color can vary from off-white to medium white. CIN 2 lesions are typically not shiny or snow-white. CIN 2 can be described as having an acetowhite color that is generally less translucent than that seen with CIN 1 lesions, but less opaque than with CIN 3, reflecting different degrees of nuclear density in each (Figure 9.68).[66] Typically, CIN 2 lesions remain acetowhite for a longer time than the more transient acetowhite effect seen with CIN 1 and are more transient than that seen in CIN 3.[66]

9.4.2.5 Vessels of CIN 2

When vessels are present in CIN 2, they tend to be of fine to medium caliber, and not nearly as prominent as when vessels are present in CIN 3 (Figure 9.69A, B). Intercapillary distances may be similar or slightly greater than those in CIN 1, or they may infrequently approach the wider spacing noted with CIN 3. The vessels are also less uniformly spaced than in CIN 1 (Figure 9.70A, B) and may assume a more random, heterogeneous distribution. Blood vessels may not be apparent in CIN 2, and even when present may require longer observation after application of acetic acid than would be the case with vessels in CIN 3 (Figure 9.71A–C). However, these vessels will become apparent once the acetic acid effect begins to diminish. Atypical blood vessels are not seen in CIN 2 lesions. Therefore the presence of atypical vessels is a concern for invasive cervical cancer coexisting with a high-grade lesion.

9.3.2.6 Iodine Staining of CIN 2

There is very little to no glycogen in the epithelium of CIN 2 lesions. Hence, a yellow iodine-negative color will invariably be present following application of Lugol's iodine solution (Figure 9.72A–E). The outline of the iodine-negative area should match the acetowhite area seen initially. A mahogany brown color never will be seen in a CIN 2 lesion but on rare occasions, a variegated yellow-brown iodine-stained pattern may be seen, probably reflecting the interobserver variability in differentiating histologic CIN 1 from CIN 2. Because both CIN 2 and CIN 3 are iodine negative, Lugol's iodine solution does little to help discriminate CIN 2 from CIN 3.

9.4.2.7 Size and Distribution of CIN 2

In general, CIN 2 lesions are larger (mean 5.8 mm) than CIN 1 (mean 4.1 mm), but not as large as CIN 3 (mean 7.6 mm) (Figure 9.73).[67] CIN 2 lesions rarely exceed 18.2 mm in length. CIN 2 lesions can extend more deeply into gland crypts than CIN 1 (maximum depths 3 and 2 mm, respectively). CIN 2 is invariably seen within the transformation zone (Figure 9.74), in contrast to CIN 1, which may be found outside the transformation zone. CIN 2 may be multifocal (Figure 9.75), but a unifocal lesion is more common. Satellite lesions are not usually representative of CIN 2. Colposcopists will usually find CIN 2 along the SCJ, located either on the ectocervix or within the endocervical canal (Figure 9.76).

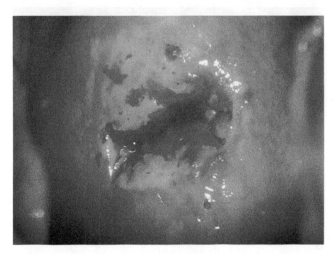

FIGURE 9.63.   A macular CIN 2 extending from 6–9 o'clock. Less dense acetowhitening is seen on the anterior portio.

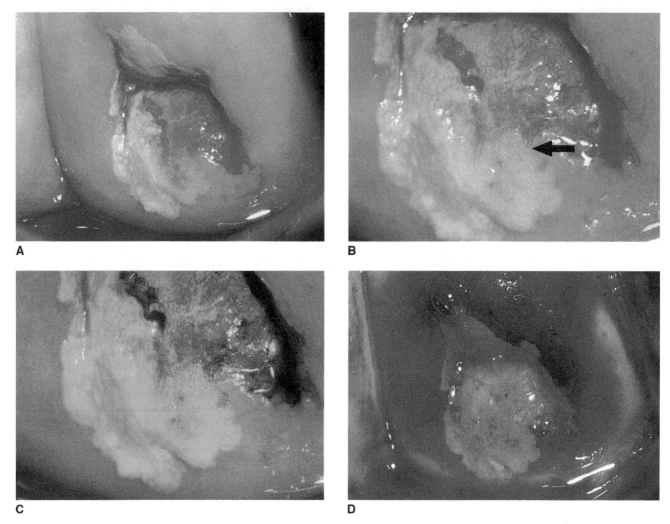

FIGURE 9.64.   **A:** A macular CIN 2 with leukoplakia is seen between 6 o'clock and 8 o'clock. However, an area of acetowhite epithelium is also seen between 11 o'clock and 12 o'clock. **B:** An area of punctation (*arrow*) is noted alongside the area of leukoplakia. The area of leukoplakia has an irregular contour. **C:** The punctation can be better seen using the green filter. All areas of acetowhite epithelium and leukoplakia reject Lugol's iodine solution and appear yellow (**D**).

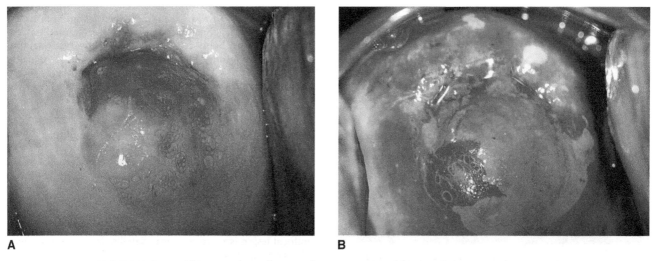

FIGURE 9.65.   **A:** This CIN 2 lesion has an indistinct margin and fine vessels. However, the margin is clearly smooth and not irregular as seen following application of Lugol's iodine solution (**B**).

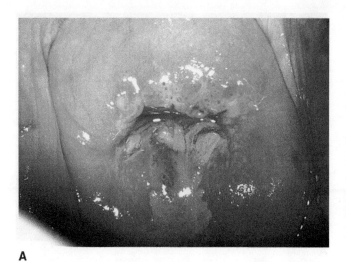

A

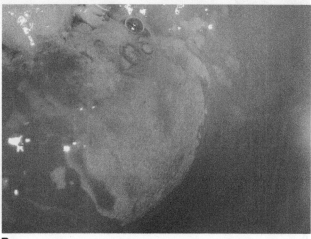

B

FIGURE 9.66.   An internal margin is seen in the lesion on the posterior cervix (**A**). A larger low-grade lesion is observed in the periphery. More opaque acetowhite epithelium of the CIN 2 demarcates the lesion from the less severe, more translucent CIN 1. In another patient (**B**), fine vessels and translucent acetowhite epithelium indicate CIN 1 in the periphery. However, a more opaque acetowhite lesion with coarse vessels can be seen closer to the SCJ.

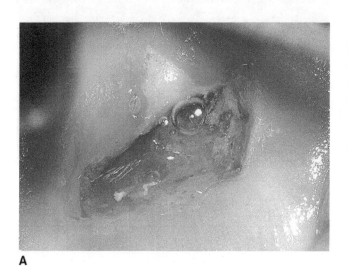

A

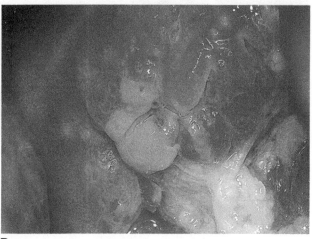

B

FIGURE 9.67.   **A:** A straight margin moderately opaque lesion without visible blood vessels. Biopsy was interpreted as CIN 2. **B:** The small medium opacity lesion with smooth margins and no visible vessels was confirmed to be CIN 2 by biopsy. Courtesy of, and reproduced by approval of, the International Cervical Cancer foundation.

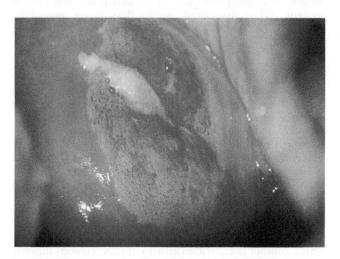

FIGURE 9.68.   This acetowhite color of the CIN 2 is less translucent than CIN 1 and less opaque than CIN 3.

Colposcopists should not be discouraged when their colposcopic impression of a lesion was CIN 1, but the histologic diagnosis is CIN 2, as this is not uncommon. Special attention to the lesion color (opacity) and vessel patterns may offer clues for rendering a more accurate colposcopic impression. Knowledge of a screening Pap test result may bias colposcopic grading.[61] Hence, referral on the basis of an ASC-US or LSIL Pap may result in downgrading of the colposcopic impression, as much as a HSIL Pap referral may upgrade it. Colposcopic differentiation of CIN 2 from CIN 1 or from CIN 3 (Figure 9.77 A–C) is often be beyond the limits of colposcopic differentiation.

9.4.3 Colposcopy of CIN 3

Once educated in the recognition of its classic colposcopic findings, colposcopists should be able to easily recognize moderate-to large-sized CIN 3 (Figure 9.78 A–D). Small CIN 3 lesions are more difficult to detect, and some really thin CIN 3s may

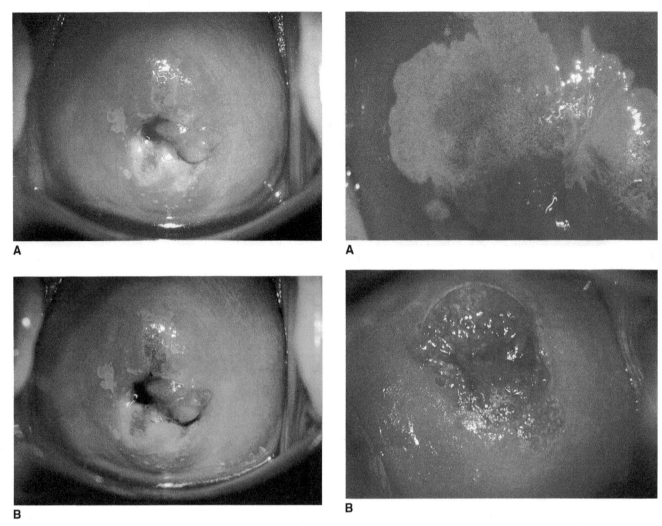

FIGURE 9.69.   A,B: Medium-caliber vessels seen in a CIN 2 lesion.

FIGURE 9.70.   Medium-caliber punctation (**A**) and mosaic (**B**) suggestive of CIN 2.

not be colposcopically visible.[33] However, not all that appears to be CIN 3 is in fact CIN 3. For example, a small area of microinvasion within a large CIN 3 may be overlooked. It is extremely difficult to diagnose microinvasive cancer clinically, particularly when it is small and focal. Overlooking a microinvasive cancer is particularly likely to occur when no coexisting warning signs of cancer (Chapter 10) are observed. During a busy colposcopist's career, not detecting a microinvasion might be anticipated. When present, a focus of microinvasion is typically hidden within a large, especially severe, CIN 3 lesion. Hence, before choosing an ablative treatment to treat CIN 3, it is important to take multiple biopsies and to excise, rather than ablate, large CIN 3 lesions. Moderate- to large-sized CIN 3 lesions should rarely, if ever, be misclassified as normal. Nevertheless, while learning colposcopy, and even occasionally after years of experience, some colposcopists will misidentify a CIN 3 lesion as lower grade, or even as normal. Also, a small CIN 3 lesion positioned within a larger CIN 1 lesion may be overlooked, even if careful colposcopy is performed.

9.4.3.1 Location of CIN 3

CIN 3 is invariably positioned along the SCJ, whether on the ectocervix or within the endocervical canal (Figures 9.79A–D,

9.80A–C, and 9.81A–E). The one possible exception is in women who have residual CIN 3 following surgery of the cervix (Figure 9.82A,B). Such postsurgical "skip" lesions may not adjoin the new SCJ, but may instead lie proximally within the endocervical canal at the extent of the treatment margin. When associated with a less severe neoplastic change, CIN 3 lesions are most proximal to the SCJ. Rarely, large CIN 3 lesions may also extend into the vaginal fornices.

9.4.3.2 Contour of CIN 3

The topography of CIN 3 lesions varies from macular (Figure 9.83A,B) to a generalized epithelial thickening that appears as if the intact abnormal epithelium could be peeled away from the underlying stroma (Figures 9.84A–D and 9.85A,B). Although a slightly elevated epithelium may be seen (Figures 9.86A,B and 9.87A–D), most CIN 3 is flat. Some severe CIN 3 lesions demonstrate topographic elevations seen simply as blood vessel protrusion above the surface of the epithelium. In these cases, the light of the colposcope will reflect tangentially from the edges of dilated vessels. If a similar, extremely dilated mosaic pattern is present, a scalloped, pockmarked epithelial surface will be seen. A nodular, papillary, papular, or exophytic contour noted within an area of CIN 3 lesions suggests the presence of cancer.

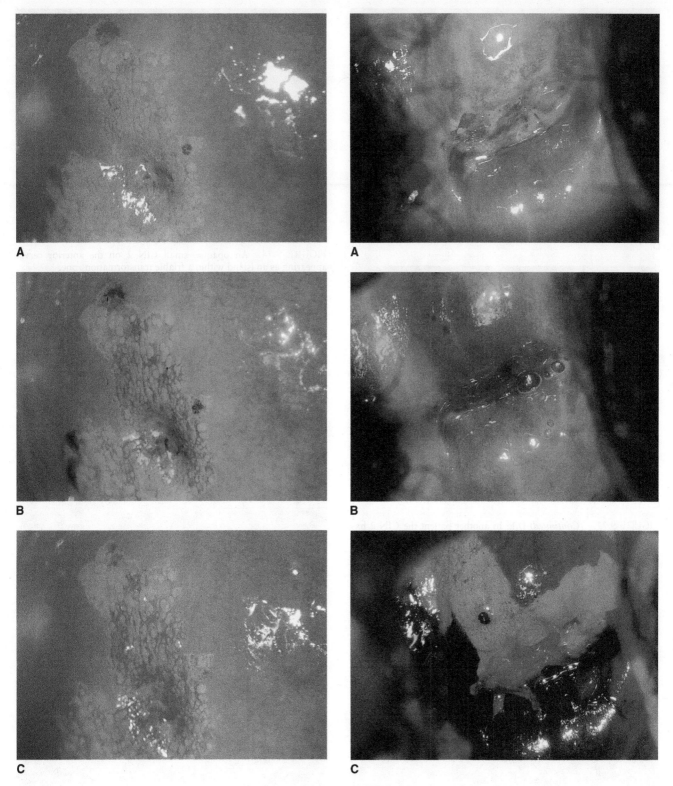

FIGURE 9.71.   Immediately after acetic acid application, the mosaic pattern of this CIN 2 appears of narrow caliber (A). This is better seen using the green filter (B). After several minutes, the vessels dilate slightly (C).

FIGURE 9.72.   An indistinct lesion on the anterior cervix (A). Punctation is noted with use of the green filter (B). However, the lesion is more easily seen following application of Lugol's iodine solution (C). The margins are smooth. The lesion rejects iodine and assumes a yellow color. The surrounding normal squamous epithelium is mahogany brown.

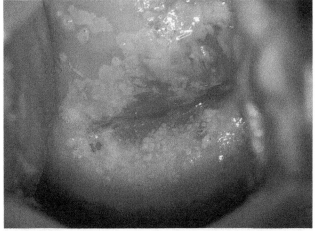

D

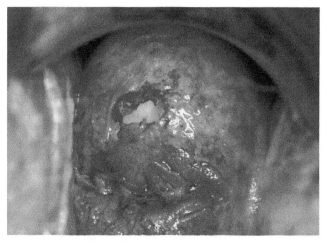

FIGURE 9.74.   An opaque, small CIN 2 on the anterior cervix appearing as an island within a friable transformation zone.

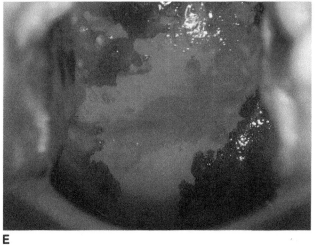

E

FIGURE 9.72.   *(Continued)* **D,E**: In another patient the CIN 2 has an irregular margin (0 points), distinct white color (1 point), and no apparent blood vessels (1 point). The lesion rejects Lugol's iodine (0 points) for a total score of 2, indicating that some histologic CIN 2 will not score high-grade by the Reid Index (≥3 points).

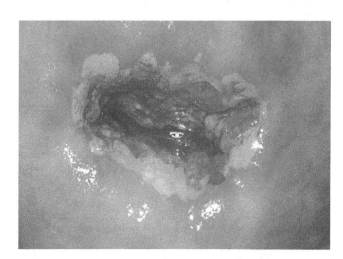

FIGURE 9.75.   A multifocal CIN 2.

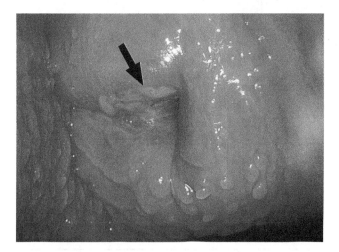

FIGURE 9.73.   A small CIN 2 (*arrow*) on the anterior cervix. The papillary appearance of the cervix is a normal variant, which is rarely seen.

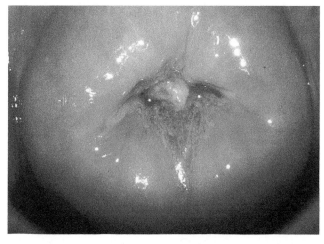

FIGURE 9.76.   A CIN 2 along the SCJ extending from 8 to 12 o'clock into the endocervical canal. Mucous is seen centrally in the canal.

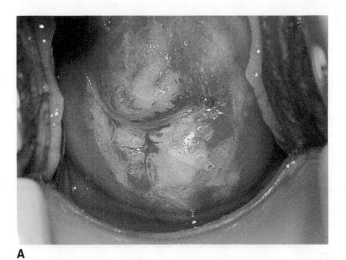

A

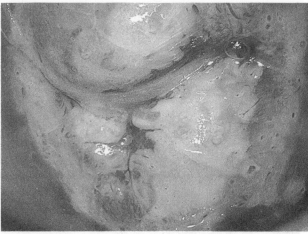

B

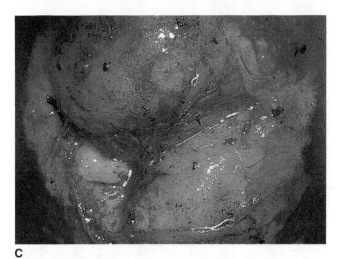

C

FIGURE 9.77. **A:** Fairly opaque acetowhite epithelium is seen in 3 quadrants of the cervix. **B:** Closer inspection discloses no visible vessels and some periglandular cuffing. **C:** The corresponding area is iodine negative. Colposcopically could be either CIN 2 or CIN 3. Biopsy confirmed the severity of this CIN 3. Notice that the areas of densest acetowhite, from 3 -8 o'clock, (**A,B**) correspond to the areas that reject iodine the greatest (**C**). Courtesy of, and reproduced by approval of, the International Cervical Cancer (INCCA) foundation.

9.4.3.3 Margins of CIN 3

The lesion margins of CIN 3 are smooth, gently rounded, or straight, creating a distinct demarcation between normal epithelium and neoplastic epithelium (Figures 9.88A, B and 9.89A–C). These straight margins are the most common presentation for CIN 3 lesions. However, CIN 3 may also have peeling edges or internal margins. "Peeling" margins imply extensive neoplasia within the acetowhite epithelium, and a confident diagnosis of CIN 3 can be made. The only exception would be if nonthickened, normal or minimally abnormal epithelium has been traumatized unintentionally, such as during speculum insertion, and then mistaken for a peeling margin. The thickened epithelium of CIN 3 can be sheared from the underlying stroma because the neoplastic process adversely

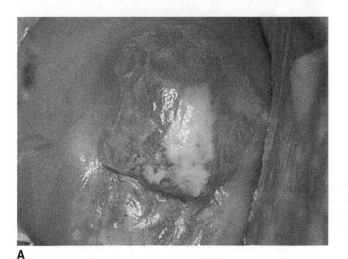

A

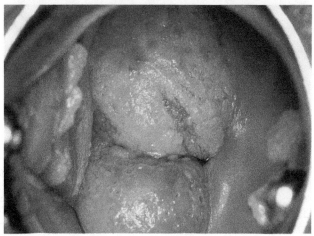

B

FIGURE 9.78. **A–D:** Four different CIN 3 lesions.

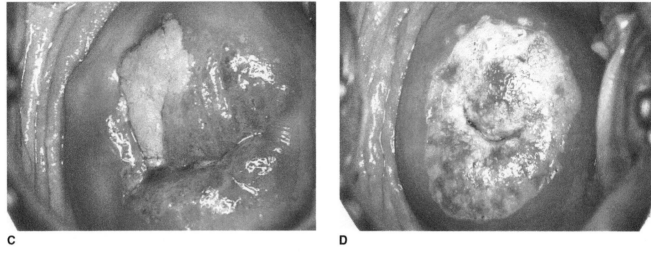

C   **D**

FIGURE 9.78.   *(Continued)*. CIN 3 lesions. Photos A–D courtesy of Dr. Vesna Kesic.

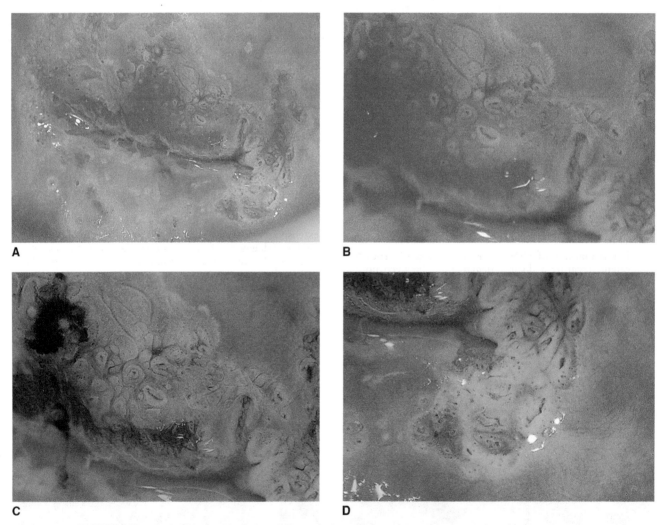

A   **B**

C   **D**

FIGURE 9.79.   **A:** At first glance, a large translucent lesion with irregular margins is noted on the anterior cervix along the SCJ. With closer inspection (**B,C**), we see periglandular cuffing. Yet, fairly opaque acetowhite epithelium with some coarse punctation is seen at 4 o'clock (**D**). This latter area represents CIN 3. Courtesy of, and reproduced by approval of, the International Cervical Cancer (INCCA) foundation.

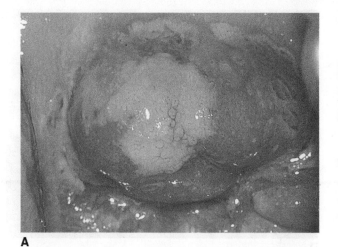

A

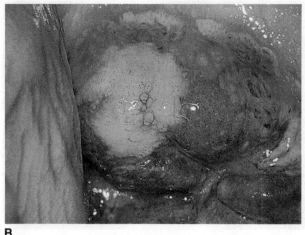

B

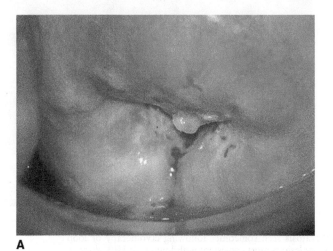

C

FIGURE 9.80.   A prominent opaque, acetowhite lesion is seen along the SCJ on the anterior cervix (**A,B**). The margin is fairly smooth, and a coarse mosaic and punctation is seen in (**C**). Cervical biopsy was diagnosed as CIN 3. Courtesy of, and reproduced by approval of, the International Cervical Cancer (INCCA) foundation.

affects the hemidesmosomes that bind the epithelium to the basement membrane and underlying stroma (Figure 9.90). A small erosion, or ulceration, will usually be seen in the area adjoining the avulsed epithelium. This area must be carefully inspected because cervical ulcerations are also associated with invasive cancer. Biopsy is always indicated in this circumstance.

An internal border or margin that distinctly separates epithelia of differing levels of neoplasia may be noted (Figure 9.91A,B). To form an internal border, a lower-grade lesion encompasses a more centrally located higher-grade lesion along the SCJ (Figure 9.92A,B). Beginning colposcopists tend to overlook internal margins unless taught to recognize this subtle

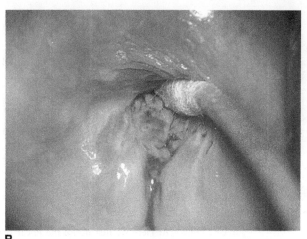

A

B

FIGURE 9.81.   A small opaque acetowhite lesion is seen just at the cervical os, most evident at 7 o'clock (**A**). It appears to extend into the endocervical canal. At this point, the examination is inadequate. A cotton-tipped applicator (**B**) exposes more of the lesion, but its upper margin is still not visible.

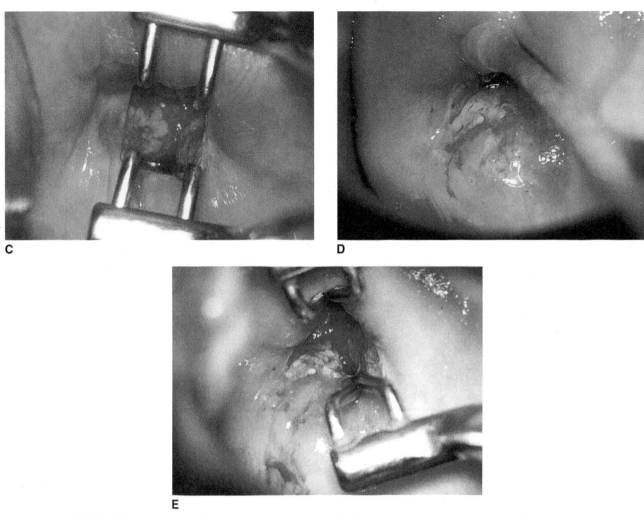

FIGURE 9.81. *(Continued)* Finally, the full extent of the CIN 3 can be seen in the endocervical canal by using the endocervical speculum (**C**). Similarly, another CIN 3 lesion is seen extending into the endocervical canal (**D**). The entire opaque lesion with a coarse mosaic pattern can be seen using the endocervical speculum (**E**).

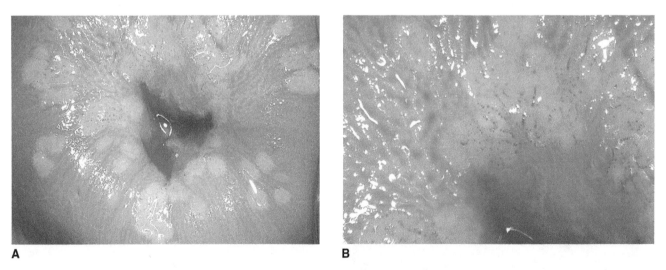

FIGURE 9.82.   A: Here we first notice the linear parakeratosis seen sometimes following cryotherapy or loop excision surgery. There are also diffusely scattered acetowhite lesions most consistent with low-grade HPV disease. However, with closer inspection (**B**), we observe a coarse punctation at 12 to 3 o'clock in this immunocompromised patient. The biopsy was CIN 3.

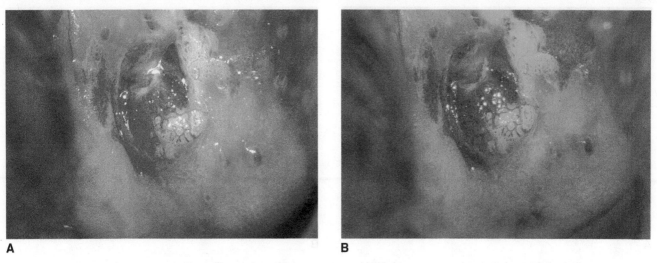

FIGURE 9.83.   A macular CIN 3 is seen at 5 o'clock (**A**). A coarse mosaic vessel pattern is seen using the green filter (**B**).

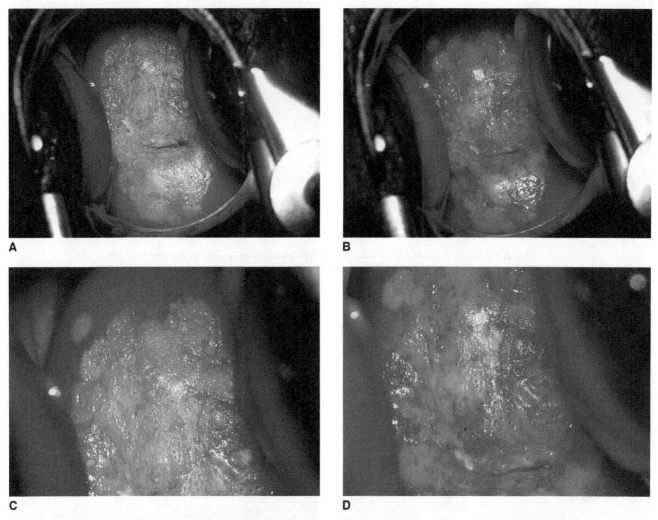

FIGURE 9.84.   A thickened 4-quadrant CIN 3 can be seen in this HIV-positive woman after application of 3% to 5% acetic acid solution and Lugol's iodine solution (**A,B**). No vessels are seen with higher magnification (**C,D**).

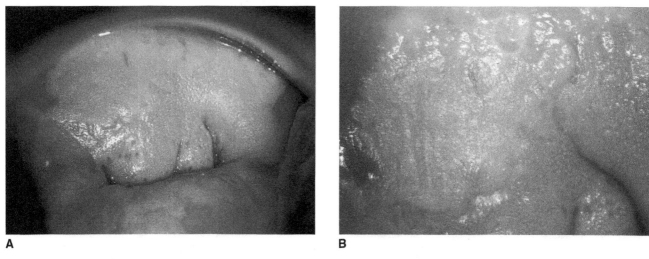

FIGURE 9.85.   **A,B:** Another woman with HIV has a thickened CIN 3 lesion. The epithelium cannot be transilluminated by the white light of the colposcope.

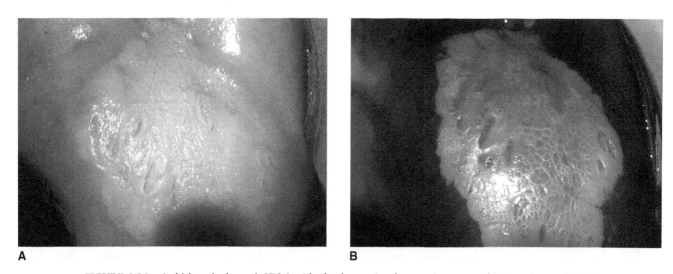

FIGURE 9.86.   A thickened, elevated CIN 3 with gland crypt involvement is seen on the posterior cervix (**A**). Application of Lugol's iodine solution results in an unusual, variegated staining pattern (**B**).

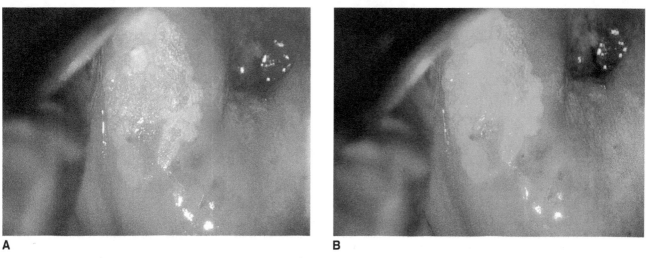

FIGURE 9.87.   **A,B:** An area of leukoplakia covers a CIN 3 at 9 o'clock.

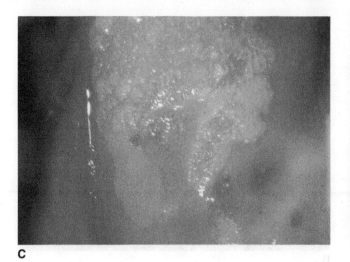

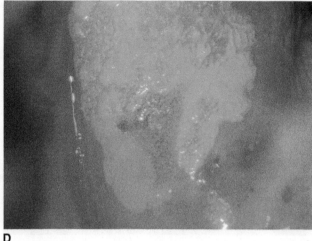

C

D

FIGURE 9.87. *(Continued)* **C,D:** With higher magnification, a coarse punctation can be seen along the posterior margin of the lesion adjacent to the leukoplakia.

change (Figure 9.93A–H). Once the complete circumference of any acetowhite lesion has been outlined, the colposcopist should then look from the margins toward the os. An abrupt change in the appearance of the epithelium, most commonly in color or density, constitutes an internal margin. This may be observed distinctly as one looks from the lateral border across a lesion towards the os, as if following the spokes of a bicycle wheel from the periphery to the central axle. The inner lesion will exhibit more opaque epithelium and a smooth, sometimes slightly elevated, margin can be observed demarcating the central high-grade lesion from the translucent low-grade lesion in the periphery (Figure 9.94). If this inspection process is adopted as routine, colposcopists will rarely fail to identify an internal margin and more centrally positioned CIN 3.

9.4.3.4 Color of CIN 3

Although "dull oyster grey" and "dense white" have been used to describe the color of CIN 3 lesions, it actually may

be better to consider the opacity of the epithelium (Figure 9.95). CIN 3 has a nuclear dense epithelium, with abundant protein and little water.[35] As a result, the epithelium functions like a mirror after acetic acid application, reflecting the intense white light of the colposcope back to the colposcopist's eyes (Figure 9.96). This opaque white color characterizes CIN 3 (Figure 9.97). CIN 3 lesions are typically significantly more acetowhite than CIN 1 lesions and somewhat more acetowhite than CIN 2 (Figure 9.98A–D).[66] CIN 3 lesions resemble a wall that has been painted repeatedly with white latex paint. Both CIN 1 and immature metaplasia more closely resemble a wall that has only received an initial primer coat of white paint or several layers of translucent white watercolor. Moreover, the acetowhite effect persists longer in CIN 3 lesions than in CIN 1 lesions.[66] Therefore, when inspecting a large, complex lesion of the cervix, provided that 3% to 5% acetic acid solution was applied uniformly and at the same time to the cervix, the last area remaining acetowhite will likely be the area of most severe disease.

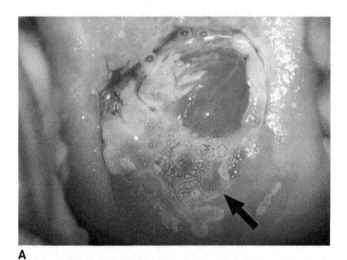

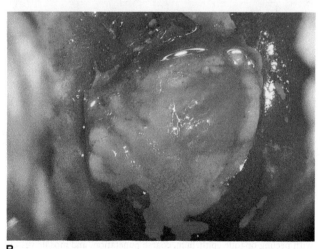

A

B

FIGURE 9.88. A smooth margin is seen in CIN 3 (**A**). This lesion also has an opaque acetowhite color, and a coarse caliber punctation and mosaic (*arrow*). The rounded margin is nicely seen following application of Lugol's iodine solution (**B**).

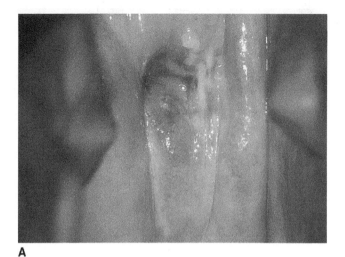

A

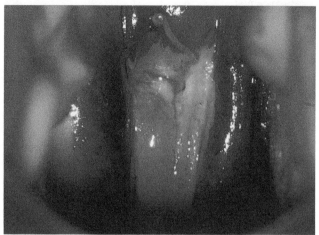

B

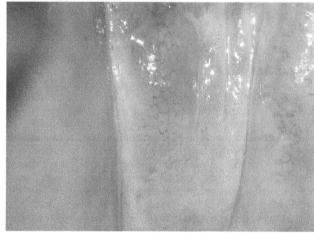

C

FIGURE 9.89.   This CIN 3 on the posterior cervix has a straight, rounded margin (**A,B**). A coarse mosaic vessel pattern is seen using higher magnification (**C**).

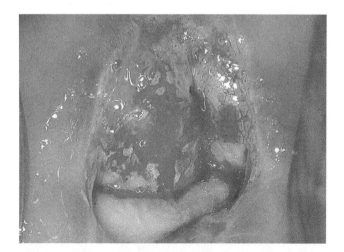

FIGURE 9.90.   An acetowhite lesion is noted on the anterior cervix with peeling opaque epithelium, coarse punctation, and mosaic vessels between 12 o'clock and 3 o'clock. The peeling epithelium on a friable area over the os on the anterior portio is of concern for a microinvasive cancer, but the histology was only CIN 3. Courtesy of, and reproduced by approval of, the International Cervical Cancer (INCCA) foundation.

9.3.3.5 Vessels of CIN 3

Coarsely dilated blood vessels, in either punctation or mosaic patterns, are the classic vascular characteristics of a CIN 3 lesion (Figure 9.99A–D). When coarse mosaic and/or punctation are noted, a diagnosis of CIN 3 must be considered (Figures 9.100A–D, 9.101 A,B, 9.102A–C, and 9.103A–D). Furthermore, the intercapillary distances are greater in CIN 3 than in CIN 1 (Figure 9.104A–L). Vessel patterns and intercapillary distances also tend to be more random, disjointed, and less uniform than in CIN 1 (Figure 9.105A,B). However, it is unusual to see blood vessels in a thick, opaque CIN 3 lesion (Figure 9.106A–C). Physiologically, this can be explained by the fact that expanding blocks of dysplastic epithelium have occluded, or pushed aside, the afferent and efferent capillary loops normally present. A greater pressure is needed to obstruct the arterial side of the vascular system than the venous system. Hence, coarse mosaic and punctation may reflect occlusion of the venous outflow more than the arterial inflow, whereas in very severe CIN 3 lesions, often no vessels are noted (Figure 9.107A–E). Any evidence of atypical vessels suggests cancer, not CIN 3, even though approximately 2% to 6% of histologically confirmed CIN 3 lesions without cancer demonstrate atypical blood vessels.[68,69]

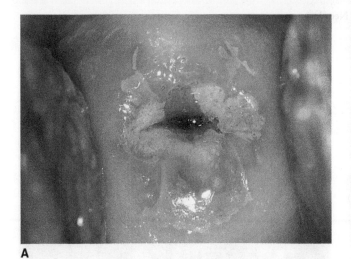 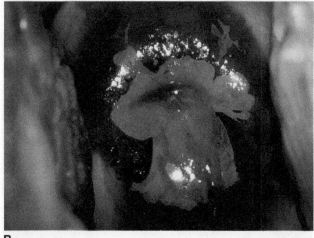

FIGURE 9.91. **A:** A 3-quadrant opaque CIN 3 is seen in A small, translucent CIN 1 can be seen at 6 o'clock. The border between these two lesions is called an internal margin. The demarcation is also seen following application of Lugol's iodine solution (**B**). The low-grade lesion contains glycogen and appears both yellow and brown (variegated). The high-grade lesion does not contain glycogen and as a result appears yellow.

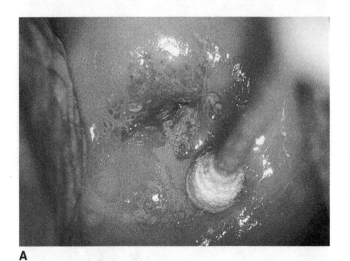 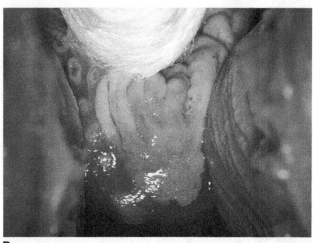

FIGURE 9.92. **A:** An internal margin separates the area of CIN 3 from CIN 1. The CIN 3 has an opaque color and coarse vessels. The CIN 1 is translucent white with a fine punctation and mosaic pattern. In (**B**) an opaque CIN 3 without visible vessels adjoins a more translucent, larger CIN 1 in this pregnant patient.

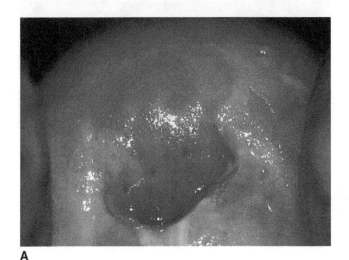 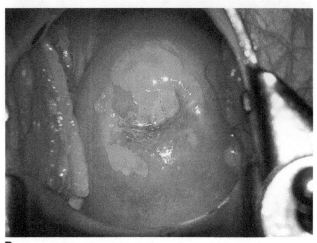

FIGURE 9.93. No lesion is seen on the ectocervix following saline application (**A**). Following application of acetic acid solution, acetowhite lesions are seen on the anterior and posterior cervix (**B**).

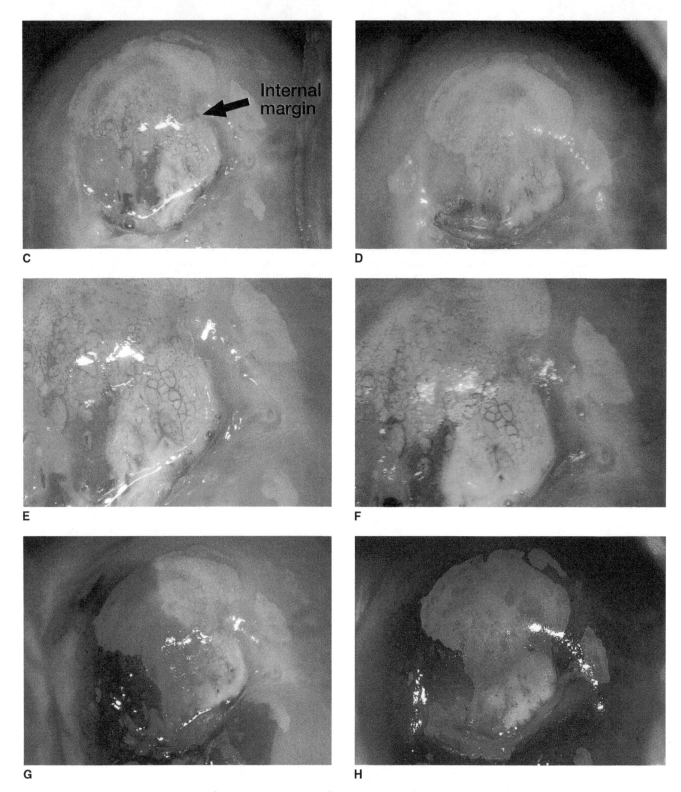

FIGURE 9.93.   *(Continued)* **C,D:** At greater magnification, an internal margin *(arrow)* is seen on the anterior cervix. **E,F:** With even greater magnification, a coarse mosaic and punctation vessel pattern is seen, with several umbilicated mosaic consistent with CIN 3. The translucent and opaque epithelia of CIN 1 and CIN 3 are observed, respectively. **G,H:** The corresponding yellow color following application of Lugol's iodine solution is noted.

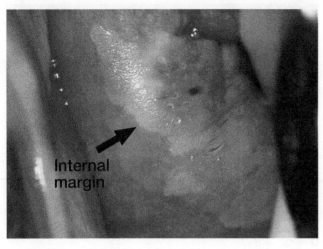

FIGURE 9.94.   An elevated, opaque CIN 3 is demarcated from the surrounding CIN 1 by an internal margin (*arrow*). No blood vessels are seen, but acetowhite rings around crypts are also suggestive of a high-grade lesion.

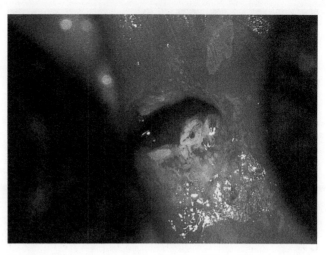

FIGURE 9.95.   A very opaque acetowhite CIN 3 with coarse punctation is seen at the cervical os.

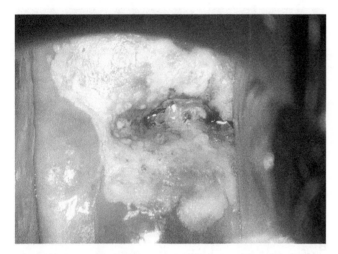

FIGURE 9.96.   A thickened acetowhite CIN 3 involving 3 quadrants of the cervix. This epithelium cannot be transilluminated by the colposcope's white light; hence, most of the white light reflects off the surface.

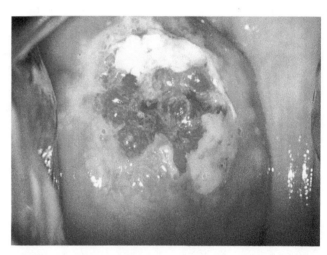

FIGURE 9.97.   An opaque CIN 3 seen at 3–5 o'clock is contrasted with the translucent metaplastic epithelium. The intense white seen at 12 o'clock is mucus.

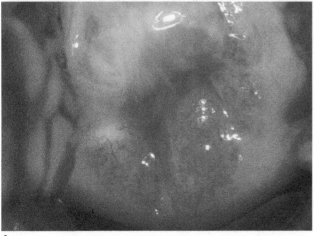

A

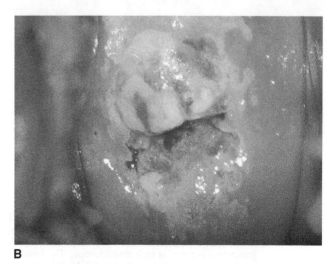

B

FIGURE 9.98.   The cervix is seen in (**A**) following saline application. **B:** An opaque acetowhite lesion is seen on the anterior cervix and at 7 o'clock on the posterior cervix after application of acetic acid solution. An internal margin separates the CIN 3 from a large CIN 1. Less opaque epithelium of CIN 1 is also seen on the posterior cervix.

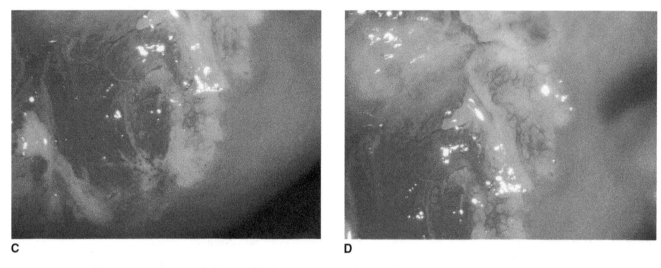

FIGURE 9.98.   *(Continued)* **C,D:** Within the opaque acetowhite epithelium of this CIN 3, coarse caliber mosaic and punctation are observed.

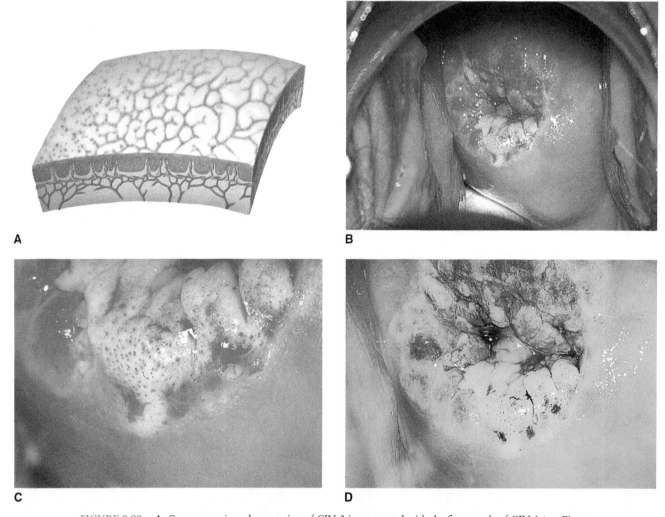

FIGURE 9.99.   **A:** Coarse mosaic and punctation of CIN 3 is contrasted with the fine vessels of CIN 1 (see Figure 9.43b). The intercapillary spacing is wider, the vessels are of greater diameter, and the vessel pattern is more random in CIN 3. **B:** There is an acetowhite lesion at 6 o'clock in this adequate colposcopic examination. **C,D:** A coarse punctation is noted at high magnification. The lesion is very opaque white in color typical of CIN 3. (**A** [illustration]: copyright © 2004, 2011. ASCCP. All rights reserved. **B–D** [Colpophotographs]: courtesy of, and approved for reproduction by, the International Cervical Cancer (INCCA) foundation.)

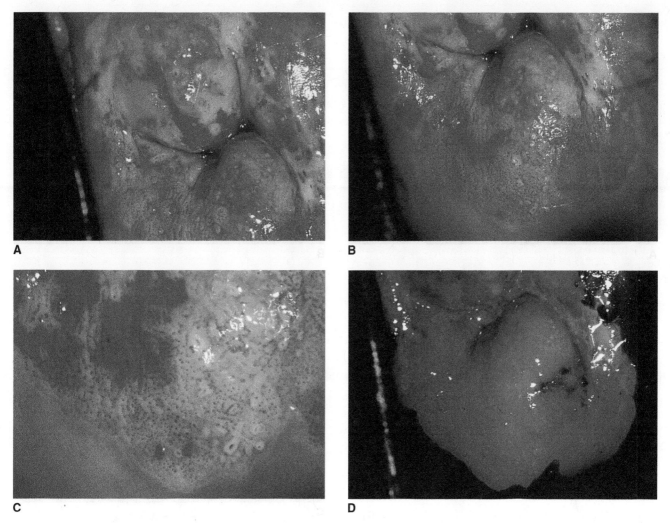

FIGURE 9.100.   **A–C:** A large opaque, peeling acetowhite CIN 3 lesion with a coarse mosaic and punctation pattern. **D:** This lesion contains no glycogen and rejects Lugol's iodine solution, assuming a yellow color. Notice the smooth margin characteristic of CIN 3. Also notice that application of Lugol's solution resulted in losing the fine detail of location of the most abnormal vessels, peeling areas and other signs important for determining best biopsy placement. Hence, it is best to not apply Lugol's solution when important landmarks may be obscured.

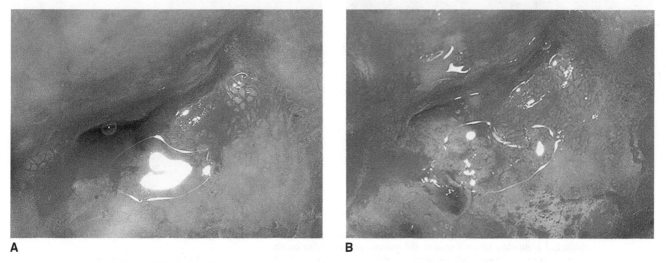

FIGURE 9.101.   **A:** A subtle opaque acetowhite lesion is seen at 4 o'clock near the os. **B:** A coarse mosaic blood vessel pattern is seen in the same area. This small, discrete lesion was diagnosed as CIN 3. Courtesy of, and reproduced by approval of, the International Cervical Cancer (INCCA) foundation.

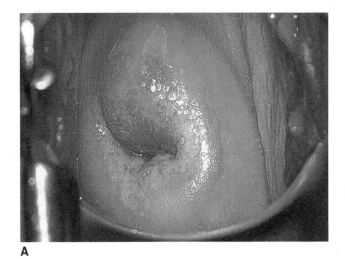

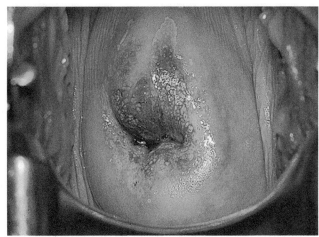

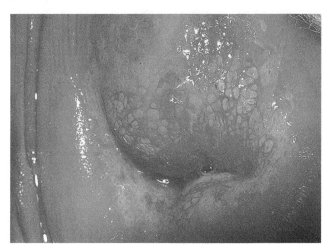

FIGURE 9.102. An acetowhite lesion is seen on both the anterior and posterior cervix (A,B). The high-power image (C) discloses opaque epithelium and a coarse mosaic vessel pattern. Cervical biopsy demonstrated CIN 3. Courtesy of, and reproduced by approval of, the International Cervical Cancer (INCCA) foundation.

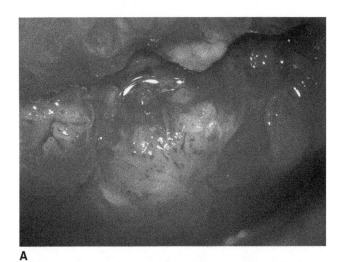

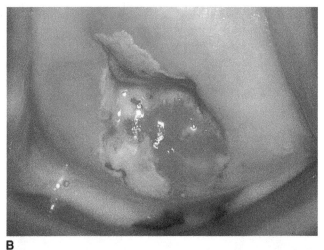

FIGURE 9.103.   A: A coarse punctation pattern can be seen in this small, opaque CIN 3. B: In another patient a thickened acetowhite lesion is seen on the anterior and posterior cervix.

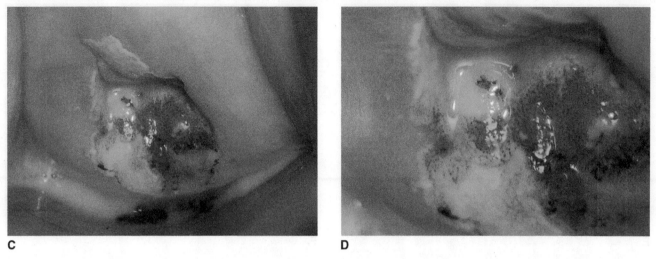

FIGURE 9.103.   *(Continued)* **C,D:** Coarse punctation is seen with the green filter in the cervix in (**B**) on the preceding page.

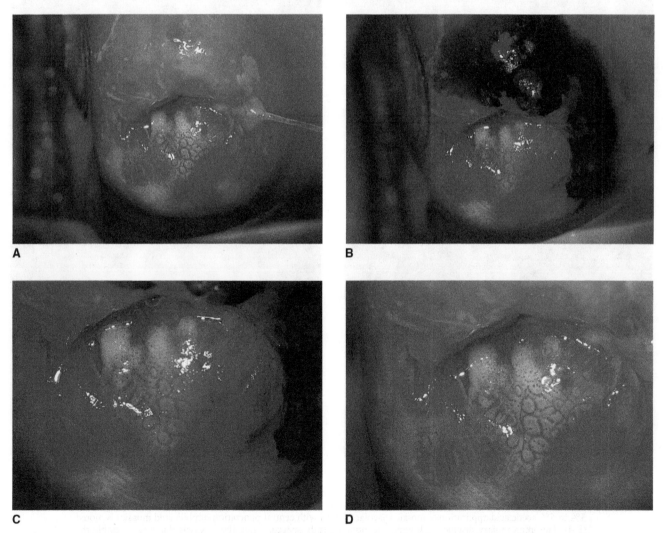

FIGURE 9.104.   **A–D:** A large CIN 3 lesion is seen on the posterior cervix following application of acetic acid (**A**) and Lugol's iodine solution (**B**). With higher magnification (**C,D**), very coarse mosaic and punctation vessel patterns are observed. The intercapillary distance is wide, and the distribution is random.

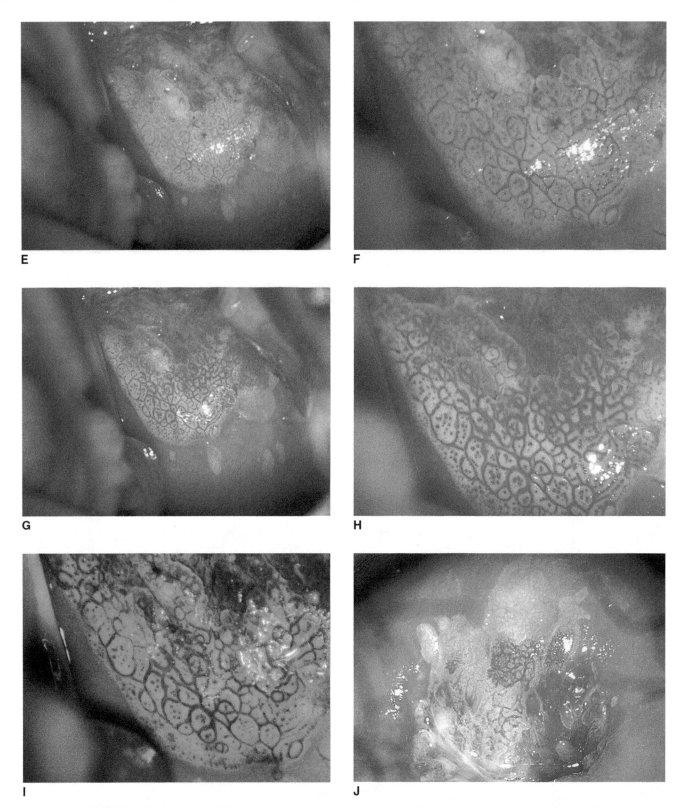

FIGURE 9.104.   *(Continued)* **E–I:** In the second case, an opaque acetowhite lesion with a smooth margin can be seen adjoining the SCJ. Small satellite CIN 1 lesions can be seen in the distant periphery (**E**). Immediately following 3% to 5% acetic acid application, a mosaic vascular pattern with central punctation (umbilicated mosaic) is noted (**E–I**). The intercapillary distances are wide and nonuniformly spaced. Later, these vessels dilate to resemble the coarse-caliber vessels seen with CIN 3 (**G–I**). The green filter examination (**I**) allows clear identification of the mosaic pattern. In the third case (**J–L**), even at low magnification (**J**), a coarse mosaic vessel pattern is seen.

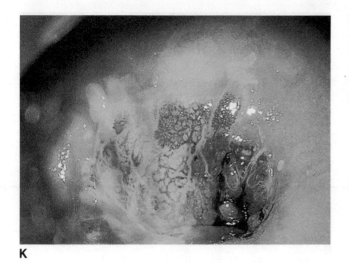

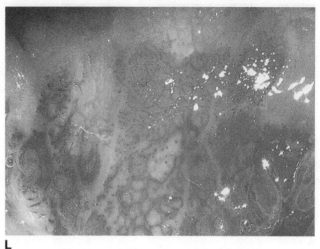

K

L

FIGURE 9.104. *(Continued)* **K:** The green filter highlights the mosaic pattern seen on the previous page in (**J**). Very opaque epithelium is noted closer to the os (**L**). This represents a large CIN 3 within a CIN 1 seen in the periphery. Figure 9.104J–L courtesy of, and reproduced by approval of, the International Cervical Cancer (INCCA) foundation.

9.4.3.6 Iodine Staining of CIN 3

There is no glycogen in CIN 3 lesions. Hence, a yellow, iodine-negative color appears following application of Lugol's iodine solution (Figure 9.108A–J). These iodine-negative areas match the previously detected acetowhite lesions (Figure 9.109A–D). A variegated or speckled pattern is not usually found in CIN 3. Severe CIN 3 lesions may assume a pale, yellowish white, iodine-negative appearance that can be contrasted with the darker yellow, iodine-negative area seen in some CIN 1 lesions.

9.3.3.7 Size and Distribution of CIN 3

CIN 3 lesions tend to be confluent, and longer and wider than CIN 1 or CIN 2 lesions. The mean linear length of CIN 3 is approximately 7.5 mm.[67,70] The maximum linear length of CIN 3 does not usually exceed 15 mm.[70] The mean surface area of CIN 3 measures 63 mm, contrasted with 46 mm for CIN 1,2.[71] Therefore, it is not uncommon to see CIN 3 occupy 2 or 3 quadrants of the cervix (Figure 9.110A–F). Because CIN 3 is more confluent and expansive, many lesions will extend into the external os and beyond colposcopic view (Figure 9.111)

CIN 3 is usually located within the central portion of the cervix, inside the inner curve towards, and often into, the external os (Figure 9.112A,B). In general, CIN 3 is found between 1 mm distal and 21 mm proximal to the most caudal point of the ectocervix.[70] This distribution varies as the SCJ advances within the endocervical canal as a woman ages. The distribution also may differ after cervical surgery, following which the volume and/or normal rounded contour of the cervix may be reduced and the SCJ may be deep within

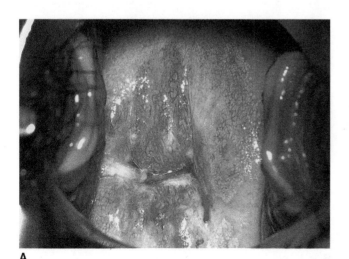

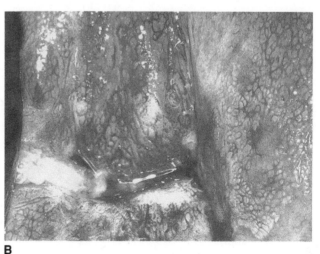

A

B

FIGURE 9.105.   A very large acetowhite lesion with both fine and coarse mosaic is seen (**A**). Opaque epithelium can be seen just above the os (**B**) in this CIN 3. Courtesy of, and reproduced by approval of, the International Cervical Cancer (INCCA) foundation.

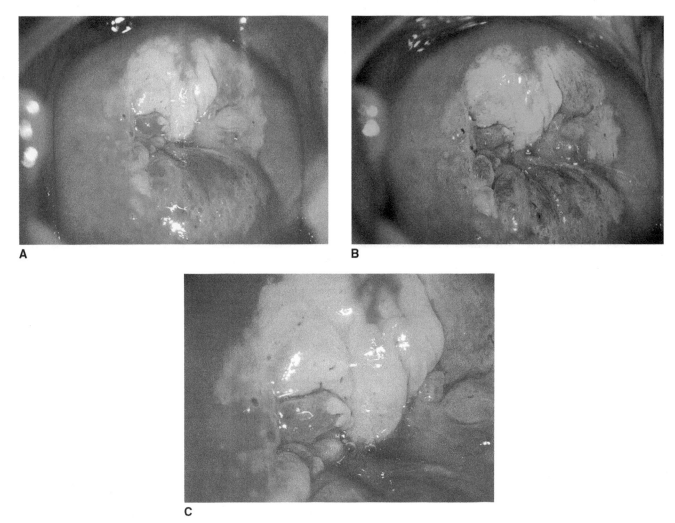

FIGURE 9.106.   **A:** An opaque CIN 3 lesion on the anterior cervix contrasts with the translucent acetowhite immature metaplastic epithelium on the posterior cervix. **B:** No vessels are noted with the green filter. **C:** Most CIN 3 lesions have no visible vessels, as seen at this high magnification.

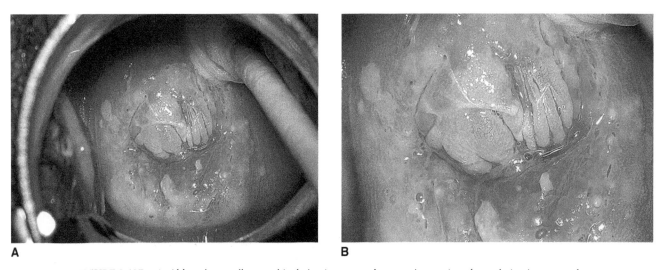

FIGURE 9.107.   **A:** Although a small acetowhite lesion is seen on the posterior cervix, a larger lesion is seen on the anterior cervix. **B:** Immediately after 3% to 5% acetic acid is applied, the lesion appears opaque without visible vessels.

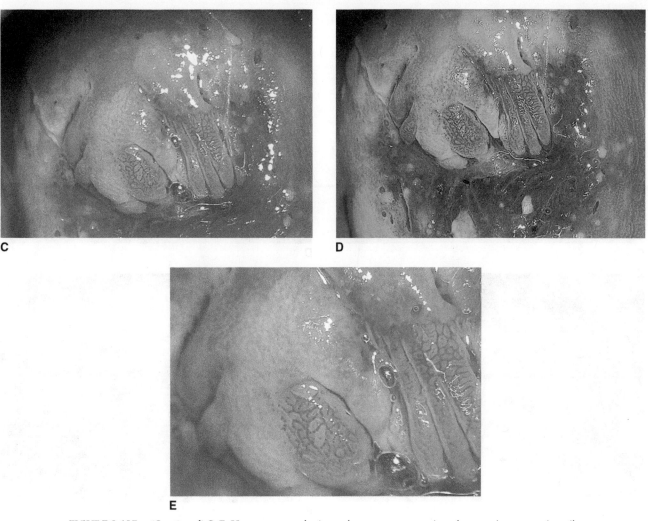

FIGURE 9.107.   *(Continued)* C–E: However, several minutes later, a coarse mosaic and punctation pattern is easily appreciated in this CIN 3.

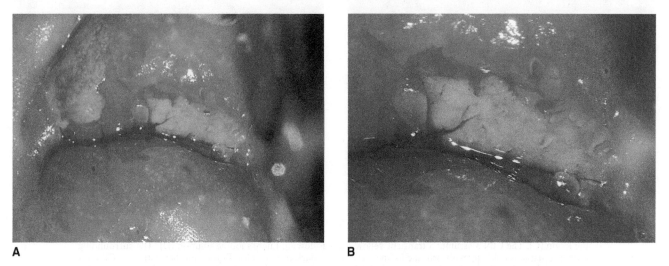

FIGURE 9.108.   A,B: In this first patient, an opaque acetowhite CIN 3 can be seen on the anterior cervix.

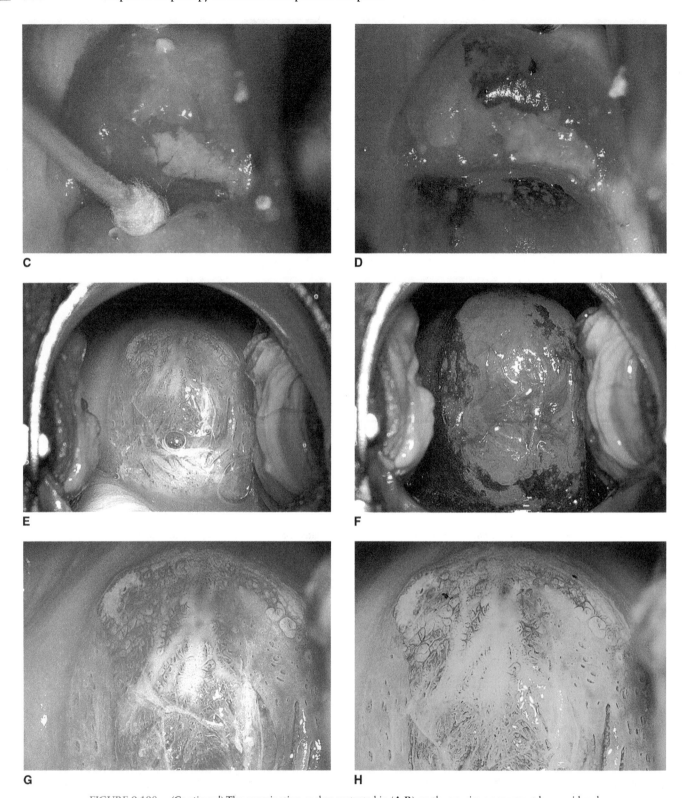

FIGURE 9.108.   *(Continued)* The examination as demonstrated in (**A,B**) on the previous page must be considered inadequate until the assistance provided by a cotton-tipped applicator is able to visualize the proximal extent of the lesion (**C**). The CIN 3 assumes a transient yellow color following Lugol's iodine solution (**D**). The surrounding normal squamous epithelium absorbs the iodine, becoming a dark brown color. **E–J:** In another patient, a CIN 3 is present within a large area of immature metaplasia. **E:** At quick glance, this cervix appears normal. **F:** Since neither stain with Lugol's, iodine staining is not helpful in differentiating between these two areas. **G,H:** With medium magnification, the abnormal blood vessels are more visible.

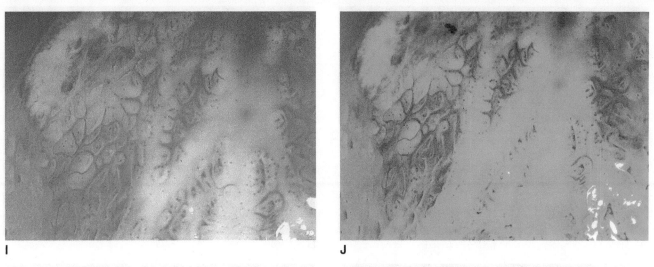

FIGURE 108.   I,J: At higher magnification, we see opaque epithelium with coarsely dilated vessels in this CIN 3 within a field of immature metaplasia. Figure 9.108E–J courtesy of, and reproduced by approval of, the International Cervical Cancer (INCCA) foundation.

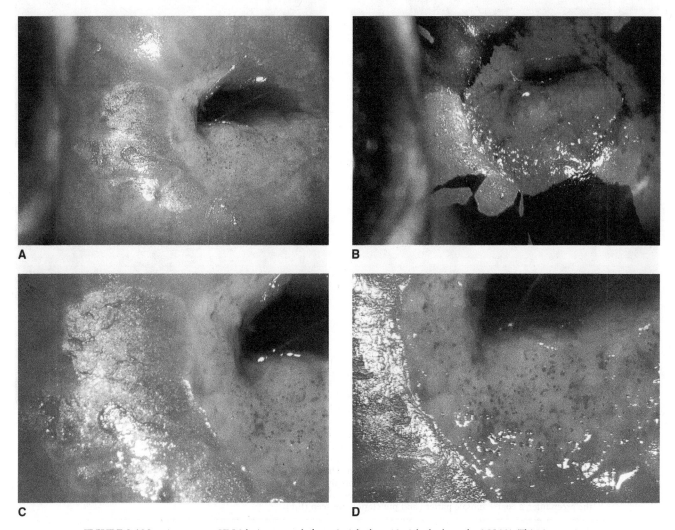

FIGURE 9.109.   An opaque CIN 3 lesion extends from 3 o'clock to 12 o'clock along the SCJ (**A**). This tissue rejects iodine application and appears yellow (**B**). However, a larger yellow area is seen peripheral to the CIN 3. With closer inspection (**C,D**) an area of leukoplakia adjoins the CIN 3 and explains why this area also appears yellow. The CIN 3 has a very coarse, randomly distributed punctation.

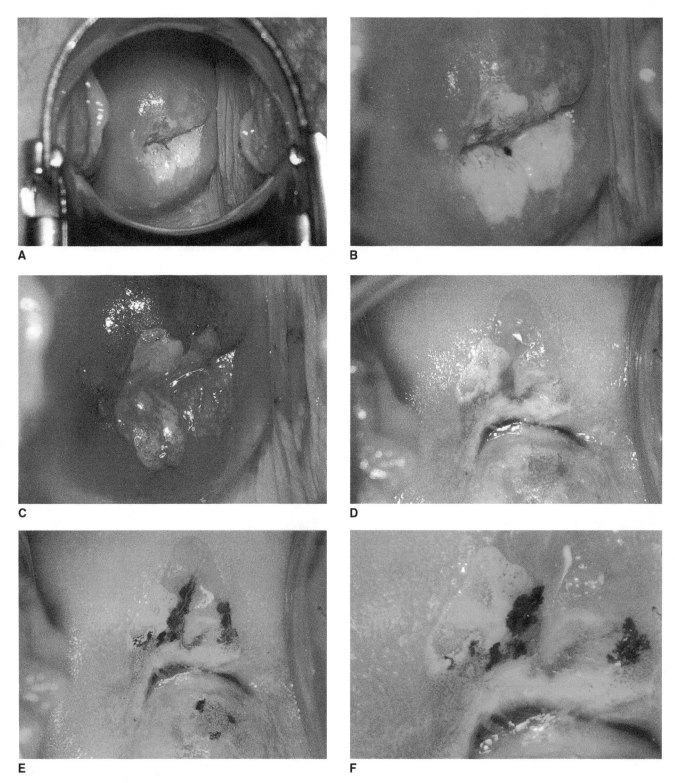

FIGURE 9.110.   A CIN 3 lesion involving 2 or more quadrants of the cervix is not uncommon (A). This CIN 3 is on the anterior and posterior cervix. The margins are smooth, the color is an opaque white, and a coarse mosaic pattern is seen in the anterior lesion. B: No vessels are noted within the posterior cervical lesion, which appears initially to be markedly more acetowhite than the anterior lesion. The Lugol's iodine solution helps to determine the location of the most severe disease (C). The anterior lesion has no glycogen, as evident by its pure yellow color. The lesion at 4 o'clock is variegated. In another patient (D), CIN 3 lesions can be seen on the anterior and posterior cervix. With the green filter, a coarse mosaic pattern and punctation are seen (E,F).

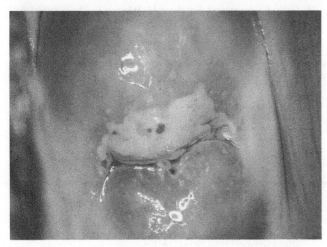

FIGURE 9.111.   This CIN 3 lesion extends within the endocervical canal.

the endocervical canal. It must be remembered that CIN 3 is nearly always found along the SCJ (Figure 9.113).

Except for very thin CIN 3s,[33] occult CIN 3 on the ectocervix is rare. If CIN 3 has penetrated the epithelium surrounding, and within, a gland crypt, then a wide, opaque acetowhite band around a gland opening will be observed. The periglandular acetowhite cuffing can be contrasted with the narrow acetowhite rim of a normal gland opening surrounding a red central area that represents underlying columnar epithelium within the gland crypts (Figure 9.79B,C). Evidence of opaque white, wide, periglandular acetowhite cuffing is almost always pathognomonic of CIN 3. CIN 3 can extend 4.8 mm into gland clefts, but the mean depth is <1.6 mm.[67,70,72] The depth of CIN 3 involvement in gland crypts also appears to correlate, in general, with advancing patient age. Very large CIN 3 lesions may also extend into the vaginal fornices as VaIN 3, or be found to have a separate VaIN 3 lesion (Figure 9.114). When compared with CIN 1, CIN 3 is more likely to be solitary and not multifocal or diffuse in distribution.

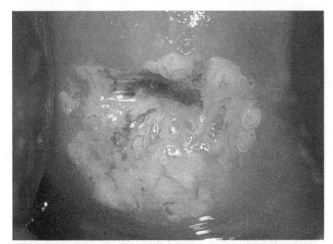

A

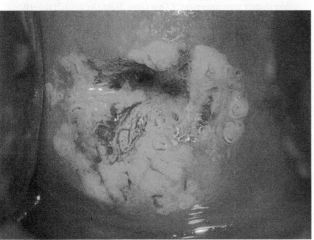

B

FIGURE 9.112.   Most CIN 3 lesions are found in the central portion of the ectocervix (A). This CIN 3 has coarsely dilated blood vessels, including atypical vessels, mosaic, and punctation (B), which are easily visualized using the green filter.

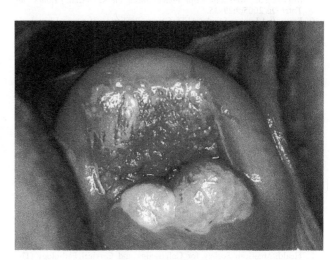

FIGURE 9.113.   This densely acetowhite CIN 3 lesion is located along the SCJ.

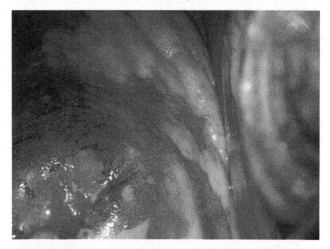

FIGURE 9.114.   This woman with HIV has a VaIN 3 in the left anterior vaginal fornix. The lesion rejects Lugol's iodine solution and has a smooth margin. She also was found to have CIN 3.

References

1. Cox JT. More questions about the accuracy of colposcopy: what does this mean for cervical cancer prevention? *Obstet Gynecol* 2008;111:1266–67.
2. National Cancer Institute Workshop. The 1988 Bethesda System for reporting cervical/vaginal cytologic diagnosis. *JAMA* 1989;262:931–4.
3. Mitchell MF, Schottenfeld D, Tortolero-Luma G, Cantor SB, Richards-Kortum R. Colposcopy for the diagnosis of squamous intraepithelial lesions: a meta-analysis. *Obstet Gynecol* 1998;91:626–31.
4. Hopman EH, Kenemans P, Helmerhorst TJM. Positive predictive rate of colposcopic examination of the cervix uteri: an overview of literature. *Obstet Gynecol Surv* 1998;33:97–106.
5. Benedet JL, Matisic JP, Bertrand MA. An analysis of 84244 patients from the British Columbia cytology-colposcopy program. *Gynecol Oncol* 2004;92(1):127–34.
6. ASCUS LSIL Triage Study (ALTS) Group. Results of a randomized trial on the management of cytology interpretations of atypical squamous cells of undetermined significance. *Am J Obstet Gynecol* 2003;188:1383–92.
7. Massad LS, Collins YC. Strength of correlations between colposcopic impression and biopsy histology. *Gynecol Oncol* 2003;89(3):424–8.
8. Pretorius RG, Zhang WH, Belinson JL, et al. Colposcopically directed biopsy, random cervical biopsy, and endocervical curettage in the diagnosis of cervical intraepithelial neoplasia II or worse. *Am J Obstet Gynecol* 2004;191:430–4.
9. Ferris DG, Litaker M. Interobserver agreement for colposcopy quality control using digitized colposcopic images during the ALTS trial. *J Low Genit Tract Dis* 2005;9:29–35.
10. Ferris and Litaker for the ALTS Group. Prediction of cervical histologic results using an abbreviated Reid Colposcopic Index during ALTS. *Am J Obstet Gynecol* 2006;194:704–10.
11. Pretorius RG, Kim RJ, Belinson JL, Elson P, Qiao YL. Inflation of sensitivity of cervical cancer screening tests secondary to correlated error in colposcopy. *J Low Genit Tract Dis* 2006;10:5–9.
12. Baum ME, Rader JS, Gibb RK, et al. Colposcopic accuracy of obstetrics and gynecology residents. *Gynecol Oncol* 2006;103(3):966–70.
13. Gage JC, Hanson VW, Abbey K, et al. Number of cervical biopsies and sensitivity of colposcopy. *Obstet Gynecol* 2006;108:264–72.
14. Jeronimo J, Massad LS, Castle PE, Wacholder S, Schiffman M; National Institutes of Health (NIH)-American Society for Colposcopy and Cervical Pathology (ASCCP) Research Group. Interobserver agreement in the evaluation of digitized cervical images. *Obstet Gynecol* 2007;110:833–40.
15. Pretorius RG, Bao YP, Belinson JL, Burchette RJ, Smith JS, Qiao YL. Inappropriate gold standard bias in cervical cancer screening studies. *Int J Cancer* 2007;121(10):2218–24.
16. Massad LS, Jeronimo J, Schiffman M; National Institutes of Health/American Society for Colposcopy and Cervical Pathology (NIH/ASCCP) Research Group. Interobserver agreement in the assessment of components of colposcopic grading. *Obstet Gynecol* 2008;111(6):1279–84.
17. Massad LS, Jeronimo J, Katki HA, Schiffman M; National Institutes of Health/American Society for Colposcopy and Cervical Pathology (The NIH/ASCCP) Research Group. The accuracy of colposcopic grading for detection of high-grade cervical intraepithelial neoplasia. *J Low Genit Tract Dis* 2009;13:137–44.
18. Stoler MH, Vichnin MD, Ferenczy A, et al. The accuracy of colposcopic biopsy: analyses from the placebo arm of the Gardasil clinical trials. *Int J Cancer* 2011;128(6):1354–62.
19. Zuchna C, Hager M, Tringler B, et al. Diagnostic accuracy of guided cervical biopsies: a prospective multicenter study comparing the histopathology of simultaneous biopsy and cone specimen. *Am J Obstet Gynecol* 2010;203(4):321, e1–6.
20. Moss EL, Dhar KK, Byrom J, Jones PW, Redman CW. The diagnostic accuracy of colposcopy in previously treated cervical intraepithelial neoplasia. *J Low Genit Tract Dis* 2009;13(1):5–9.
21. Jeronimo J, Schiffman M. Colposcopy at a crossroads. *Am J Obstet Gynecol* 2006;195(2):349–53.
22. Chase DM, Kalouyan M, DiSaia PJ. Colposcopy to evaluate abnormal cervical cytology in 2008. *Am J Obstet Gynecol* 2009;200(5):472–80.
23. Smith HO, Tiffany MF, Qualls CR, Key CR. The rising incidence of adenocarcinoma relative to squamous cell carcinoma of the uterine cervix in the United States—a 24-year population-based study. *Gynecol Oncol* 2000;78:97–105.
24. Kitchener HC, Castle PE, Cox JT. Chapter 7: Achievements and limitations of cervical cytology screening. *Vaccine* 2006;24 (suppl 3):S63–S70.
25. Buxton EJ, Luesley DM, Shafi MI, Rollason M. Colposcopically directed punch biopsy: a potentially misleading investigation. *Br J Obstet Gynaecol* 1991;98(12):1273–6.
26. Etherington IJ, Luesley DM, Shafi MI, Dunn J, Hiller L, Jordan JA. Observer variability among colposcopists from the West Midlands region. *Br J Obstet Gynaecol* 1997;104(12):1380–4.
27. Cox JT, Schiffman M, Solomon D. Prospective follow-up suggests similar risk of subsequent cervical intraepithelial neoplasia grade 2 or 3 among women with cervical intraepithelial neoplasia grade 1 or negative colposcopy and directed biopsy. *Am J Obstet Gynecol* 2003;188:1406–12.

28. Guido RS, Jeronimo J, Schiffman M, Solomon D. The distribution of neoplasia arising on the cervix: results from the ALTS trial. *Am J Obstet Gynecol* 2005;193:1331–7.
29. Ferris DG, Litaker MS. Cervical biopsy sampling variability in ALTS. *J Low Genit Tract Dis* 2011;15(2):163–8.
30. Stoler MH, Schiffman M. Interobserver reproducibility of cervical cytologic and histologic interpretations: realistic estimates from the ASCUS-LSIL Triage Study. *JAMA* 2001;285:1500–5.
31. Cantor SB, Cárdenas-Turanzas M, Cox DD, et al. Accuracy of colposcopy in the diagnostic setting compared with the screening setting. *Obstet Gynecol* 2008;111:7–14.
32. Sherman ME, Wang SS, Tarone R, Rich L, Schiffman M. Histopathologic extent of CIN 3 lesions in ALTS: implications for subject safety and lead-time bias. *Cancer Epidemiol Biomarkers Prev* 2003;12:372–9.
33. Yang B, Pretorius RG, Belinson JL, Zhang X, Burchette R, Qiao YL. False negative colposcopy is associated with thinner cervical intraepithelial neoplasia 2 and 3 lesions. *Gynecol Oncol* 2008;110(1):32–6.
34. Wentzensen N, Zuna RE, Sherman ME, et al. Accuracy of cervical specimens obtained for biomarker studies in women with CIN3. *Gynecol Oncol* 2009;115(3):493–6.
35. Zahm DM, Nindl I, Greinke C, Hoyer H, Schneider A. Colposcopic appearance of cervical intraepithelial neoplasia is age dependent. *Am J Obstet Gynecol* 1998;179(5):1298–304.
36. Jeronimo J, Massad LS, Schiffman M. Visual appearance of the uterine cervix: correlation with human papillomavirus detection and type. *Am J Obstet Gynecol* 2007;197:47–8.
37. Hearp ML, Locante AM, Ben-Rubin M, Dietrich R, David O. Validity of sampling error as a cause of noncorrelation. *Cancer* 2007;111(5):275–9.
38. Elit L, Julian JA, Sellors JW, Levine M. Colposcopists' agreement on cervical biopsy site. *Clin Exp Obstet Gynecol* 2007;34(2):88–90.
39. Sellors J, Qiao Y, Bao Y, et al. False-negative colposcopy: quantifying the problem. In: *Book of abstracts of the 22nd International HPV Conference and Clinical Workshop*. British Columbia, Canada: Vancouver; April 30-May 6, 2005.
40. Solomon D, Stoler M, Jeronimo J, et al. Diagnostic utility of endocervical curettage in women undergoing colposcopy for equivocal or low-grade cytologic abnormalities. *Obstet Gynecol* 2007;10:88–95.
41. Wright TC Jr, Massad LS, Dunton CJ, Spitzer M, Wilkinson EJ, Solomon D; 2006 ASCCP-Sponsored Consensus Conference. 2006 consensus guidelines for the management of women with abnormal cervical screening tests. *J Low Genit Tract Dis* 2007;11(4):201–22.
42. Tidbury P, Singer A, Jenkins D. CIN 3: the role of lesion size in invasion. *Br J Obstet Gynaecol* 1992;99:583–6.
43. Moscicki AB, Ma Y, Wibbelsman C, et al. Rate of and risks for regression of cervical intraepithelial neoplasia 2 in adolescents and young women. *Obstet Gynecol* 2010;116(6):1373–80.
44. Cantor SB, Yamal JM, Guillaud M, et al. Accuracy of optical spectroscopy for the detection of cervical intraepithelial neoplasia: testing a device as an adjunct to colposcopy. *Int J Cancer* 2011;128(5):1151–68.
45. Shaw E, Sellors J, Kaczorowski J. Prospective evaluation of colposcopic features in predicting cervical intraepithelial neoplasia: degree of acetowhite change most important. *J Low Genit Tract Dis* 2003;7(1):6–10.
46. Marana HR, Andrade JM, Duarte G, Matthes AC, Taborda MF, Bighet S. Colposcopic scoring systems for biopsy decisions in different patient groups. *Eur J Gynaecol Oncol* 2000;21:368–70.
47. Stellato G, Paavonen J. A colposcopic scoring system for grading cervical lesions. *Eur J Gynaecol Oncol* 1995;16:296–300.
48. The FUTURE II Study Group. Quadrivalent vaccine against human papillomavirus to prevent high-grade cervical lesions. *N Engl J Med* 2007;356:1915–27.
49. Paavonen J, Naud P, Salmeron J, et al. Efficacy of human papillomavirus (HPV)-16/18 AS04-adjuvanted vaccine against cervical infection and precancer caused by oncogenic HPV types (PATRICIA): final analysis of a double-blind, randomised study in young women. *Lancet* 2009;374:301.
50. Ferris DG, Miller NM. Colposcopic accuracy in a residency training program: defining competency and proficiency. *J Fam Pract* 1993;36:515–20.
51. Benedet JL, Anderson GH, Matisic JP, Miller DM. A quality control program for colposcopic practice. *Obstet Gynecol* 1991;78:873–5.
52. Ferris DG, Cox JT, Burke L, et al. Colposcopy quality control: establishing colposcopy criterion standards for the NCI ALTS trial using cervigrams. *J Lower Genital Tract Dis* 1998;2:195–203.
53. Ferris DG, Litaker MS, ASCUS/LSIL Triage Study (ALTS) Group. Colposcopy quality control by remote review of digitized colposcopic images. *Am J Obstet Gynecol* 2004;191:1934–41.
54. Coppleson M. Colposcopic features of papillomaviral infection and premalignancy in the lower genital tract. *Obstet Gynecol Clin North Am* 1987;14:471–94.
55. Stafl A. Colposcopy. *Clin Obstet Gynecol* 1975;18:195–213.
56. Kolstad P. The development of the vascular bed in tumors as seen in squamous-cell carcinoma of the cervix uteri. *Br J Radiol* 1965;38:216–23.
57. Burke L, Antonioli DA, Ducatman BS. *Colposcopy Text and Atlas*. Norwalk, CT: Appleton and Lange, 1991.

58. Reid R, Scalzi P. Genital warts and cervical cancer. VII An improved colposcopic index for differentiating benign papillomaviral infections from high grade cervical intraepithelial neoplasia. *Am J Obstet Gynecol* 1985;153:611–8.

59. Reid R, Stanhope CR, Herschman BR, Crum CP, Agronow SJ. Genital warts and cervical cancer. IV. A colposcopic index for differentiating subclinical papillomaviral infection from cervical intraepithelial neoplasia. *Am J Obstet Gynecol* 1984;149(8):815–23.

60. Ferris DG, Greenberg MD. Reid's colposcopic index. *J Fam Prac* 1994;39:65–70.

61. Pretorius RG, Belinson JL, Zhang WH, Burchette RJ, Elson P, Qiao YL. The colposcopic impression. Is it influenced by the colposcopist's knowledge of the findings on the referral Papanicolaou smear? *J Reprod Med* 2001;46(8):724–8.

62. Mousavi AS, Fakour F, Gilani MM, Behtash N, Ghaemmaghami F, Karimi Zarchi M. A prospective study to evaluate the correlation between Reid colposcopic index impression and biopsy histology. *J Low Genit Tract Dis* 2007;11(3):147–50.

63. Hong DG, Seong WJ, Kim SY, Lee YS, Cho YL. Prediction of high-grade squamous intraepithelial lesions using the modified Reid index. *Int J Clin Oncol* 2010;15(1):65–9.

64. Strander B, Ellstrom-Andersson A, Franzen S, Milsom I, Radberg T. The performance of a new scoring system for colposcopy in detecting high-grade dysplasia in the uterine cervix. *Acta Obstet Gynecol Scand* 2005;84:1013–17.

65. Bowring J, Strander B, Young M, Evans H, Walker P. The Swede score: evaluation of a scoring system designed to improve the predictive value of colposcopy. *J Low Genit Tract Dis* 2010;14(4):301–5.

66. Sakuma T, Hasegawa T, Tsutsui F, Kurihara S. Quantitative analysis of the whiteness of the atypical cervical transformation zone. *J Reprod Med* 1985;30:773–6.

67. Abdul-Karim FW, Fu YS, Reagan JW, Wentz WB. Morphometric study of intraepithelial neoplasia of the uterine cervix. *Obstet Gynecol* 1982;60:210–4.

68. Sillman F, Boyce J, Fruchter R. The significance of atypical vessels and neovascularization in cervical neoplasia. *Am J Obstet Gynecol* 1981;139:154–9.

69. Sugimori H, Matsuyama T, Kashimura M, Kashimura Y, Tsukamoto N, Taki I. Colposcopic findings in microinvasive carcinoma of the uterine cervix. *Obstet Gynecol Surv* 1979;34:804.

70. Boonstra H, Aalders JG, Koudstaal J, Oosterhuis JW, Janssens J. Minimum extension and appropriate topographic position of tissue destruction for treatment of cervical intraepithelial neoplasia. *Obstet Gynecol* 1990;75:227–31.

71. Rome RM, Urcuyo R, Nelson JH. Observations on the surface area of the abnormal transformation zone associated with intraepithelial and early invasive squamous cell lesions of the cervix. *Am J Obstet Gynecol* 1977;129:565–70.

72. Anderson MC, Hartley RB. Cervical involvement by intraepithelial neoplasia. *Obstet Gynecol* 1980;55:546–50.

Colposcopic, Clinical, and Etiologic Predictors of Invasive Squamous Cell Carcinoma of the Uterine Cervix

10.1 INTRODUCTION
  10.1.1 Etiology
  10.1.2 Incidence and Mortality
  10.1.3 Disparities
  10.1.4 Effect of Screening
10.2 COLPOSCOPIC FINDINGS
  10.2.1 Differentiating Normal from Abnormal
  10.2.2 Adequate versus Inadequate Colposcopic
    Examination

10.2.3 The Correlation Process after a Adequate Colposcopic
    Examination
10.2.4 When Excision Is Required Because of Suspected
    Cancer
10.2.5 Why Cancer Is Missed
10.2.6 Circumstances that Warrant Concern
10.3 COLPOSCOPIC MIMICS OF INVASIVE SQUAMOUS
    CELL CARCINOMA

10.1 INTRODUCTION

10.1.1 Etiology

Human papillomavirus (HPV) is present in 95% to 100% of all squamous cell cancers (SCCs).[1,2] For this reason, the International Agency for Research on Cancer proclaimed in 1999 that cervical cancer may be the first human cancer to have a single necessary cause.[3] The immediate precursor to invasive SCC is cervical intraepithelial neoplasia grade 3/carcinoma *in situ* (CIN 3/CIS), which from hereon will be shortened to CIN 3 because the histology in CIN 3 and CIS are identical. Although persistence of high-risk oncogenic HPV is necessary in the development of CIN 3, the timing from infection to evidence of CIN 3 varies from 1 to 10 years.[4] The peak prevalence of transient infections with carcinogenic types of HPV occurs among women during their teens and early 20s, following the initiation of sexual activity.[5] The peak prevalence of CIN 3 occurs approximately 10 years later in the late 20s and early 30s. That the peak prevalence of invasive cervical cancer (ICC) is at 40 to 50 years of age suggests a long average sojourn time in the precancerous CIN 3 state.[4,5] The median age of cancer moves toward even older ages as the quality of screening decreases,[4] suggesting that when screening is either of poor quality or nonexistent the average invasive cancer is likely to be present for many years before symptoms result in detection. Rapidly invasive, often fatal, cancers among young women are rare but exert a profound influence on prevention strategies in the United States.[4]

10.1.2 Incidence and Mortality

The incidence rate of ICC was 8.9 per 100,000 women during 1998 through 2003.[6] However, the peak ICC incidence varies by age at diagnosis and race.[7] Age at diagnosis peaks for White women between the ages of 35 and 44, whereas incidence peaks for Black and Hispanic women between the ages of 65 and 74.[8] The proportion of cervical cancers that are squamous versus glandular also varies by race, with adenocarcinoma being more common in relation to squamous cell carcinoma (SSC) in Hispanic women compared to other races.[6] In the United States in 2004, there were approximately 12,000 incident cases of ICC and 3850 deaths.[6,9] Incidence and mortality rates have leveled off in the last few years after many decades of continued gains. The American Cancer Society estimates that in 2010, about 12,200 cases of ICC will be diagnosed in the United States and about 4210 women will die from the disease.[10]

The majority of cervical cancers are diagnosed at a localized stage, with regional tumors next most common and distant tumors least common, each peaking at progressively older ages.[11] CIN 3 rates are highest in White women compared with Black women, especially at young ages. Distant stage disease rates are higher in Black women compared with White women, especially at older ages.[11] The 1- and 5-year relative survival rates for women with cervical cancer are 87% and 71%, respectively.[10] The 5-year survival rate for patients diagnosed with localized cervical cancer is 92%, with survival rates decreasing for each increasing stage.

10.1.3 Disparities

Cervical cancer is diagnosed at an early stage more often in Whites (51%) than in African Americans (43%), suggesting that cervical cancer is not being detected and treated as early in this group as in other racial/ethnic groups.[6,10] Women younger than 50 years are also more likely to be diagnosed at an early stage (61%) than in women 50 years and older (36%).[10] Some significant differences in cervical cancer rates persist by race and/or ethnicity but overall some of the disparities have narrowed. Although ICC incidence decreased significantly over the last 10 years, Black or Hispanic US populations continue to have the highest ICC incidence compared to non-Hispanic/Whites.[7] ICC is the 6th most commonly diagnosed cancer in Hispanic and non-Hispanic Black women, whereas it is the 13th most commonly diagnosed cancer in non-Hispanic White women.[12] Higher rates of invasive SCC among Black and Hispanic women may be caused by lower rates of Pap testing or inadequate follow-up.[6,13] In addition, ICC morbidity and mortality rates are higher among women from Black and Hispanic populations compared to non-Hispanic White women, which may be attributed to multiple factors including differences in stage at diagnosis, screening rates, health insurance coverage, poverty, less aggressive therapy following abnormal screening tests, and health beliefs that may affect patient adherence to screening, diagnostic, and treatment protocols.[6,7]

10.1.4 Effect of Screening

In the six decades following the introduction of screening with cervical cytology, cervical cancer incidence fell by 70% to 75%.[2,14] Prior to the introduction of the Papanicolaou smear, cervical cancer was the second most common cancer among women and the second most common cause of cancer death. By 2005, the lifetime risk of a woman dying of cervical cancer had fallen to 1 in 145.[7] Cytology screening is undoubtedly more effective for the detection of SCC than for adenocarcinoma, and this may be one reason that the proportion of cervical cancers that are squamous has fallen in recent decades, as CIN 2,3 has been more successfully detected and treated before invasion than its corresponding high-grade glandular precancer, adenocarcinoma in situ (AIS).[2,11,15] However, screening has had a greater impact on reducing cervical cancer rates in all age groups above the age of 30, than in those younger.[16–18] A 2009 analysis of screening data and cervical cancer rates in the United Kingdom demonstrated that cervical screening in women aged 20 to 24 had little or no impact on rates of ICC up to age 30, although some uncertainty still exists regarding whether it might result in downstaging of tumors detected in women under age 30.[18] In contrast, the same study demonstrated that screening older women leads to a substantial reduction in incidence of and mortality from cervical cancer. The most probable explanation for this discrepancy is that the few cancers that occur in women in their twenties transit through CIN 3 to invasion more rapidly than the typical transit time for women getting cancer in later decades.[16,18] When the progression time from HPV infection through CIN 3 to cancer is much shorter than usual, the opportunities for detecting and treating these lesions prior to invasion are fewer.[18] This is an extreme example of length bias: Most cases of CIN 3 detected will be slow growing and could safely be left for several years, but the rare cases that are progressing rapidly are often missed.[18] Cervical cancer detected in women under the age of 30 is generally at a lower stage at diagnosis, but younger women face an increased risk of dying when controlled for stage compared with older women.[16,19]

10.2 COLPOSCOPIC FINDINGS

Cervical cancer has become so uncommon in well-screened populations that most colposcopists rarely, if ever, see invasive lesions. However, the most fundamental purpose of colposcopy is to determine whether the patient being examined has cancer. This determination is based on information from cervical cytologic screening, the colposcopic impression, and subsequent histologic findings. Each parameter has equal importance, and when either of the first two suggests presence of a squamous cancer that is not confirmed on colposcopically

directed biopsy, excision is required to either confirm the suspicion or rule it out.[20]

Whether microinvasive or frankly invasive, SCC is tissue that has proliferated and transformed, altering cervical surface configuration and causing the formation of exaggerated, contorted, and unusual blood vessels to support tumor growth. Because surface contour and blood vessel patterns are reliable indicators of disease progression, it is essential that all colposcopists learn to recognize the colposcopic signs of microinvasive and more advanced disease. Additionally, it is important to be familiar with the clinical and etiologic predictors such as age, cytology, and location of disease.

10.2.1 Differentiating Normal from Abnormal

Although unusual cervical contour and prominent blood vessels raise concern for cancer, normal women may have these findings. Hence, colposcopists must learn how to differentiate normal cervical findings from cancer and to biopsy when this is not clear. Some women have cervical contour or other irregularities that are congenital in origin (see Chapter 13) (Figure 10.1A–C) or secondary to exposure to diethylstilbestrol (DES) in utero (Figure 10.1D) or to large nabothian or adjacent Gartner's duct cysts (Figure 10.1E–H) or traumatic cervical tears sustained during labor and delivery. Large branching blood vessels in both immature and maturing transformation zones (Figure 10.2A–F) are very common but are occasionally so prominent as to be alarming. Hence, in order to be able to determine whether findings are significant or insignificant, the colposcopist must be able to recognize the normal presentations of native, metaplastic, and neoplastic squamous epithelium (see Chapters 8 and 9). This includes familiarity with normal blood vessel patterns in an original cervix and in a developing and matured transformation zone.

The colposcopic study of vascular patterns and intercapillary distance should begin before the colposcopist applies acetic acid. Following the application of acetic acid, surface contours become more evaluable, as does color, tone, and the lines of demarcation between normal and abnormal areas, with or without iodine solution (the standard colposcopic criteria of Kolstad and Stafl).[21] Insignificant findings include benign polyps, inflammation, and large nabothian cysts (see Chapter 13). Significant findings include an abnormal transformation zone, and colposcopic mimics of cancer that are insignificant with regard to cancer including postradiation changes, condylomata, traumatic ulcers, and microglandular hyperplasia.

Following the application of acetic acid, important squamous lesions become densely acetowhite with sharp borders and exhibit punctation of coarse or unequal caliber. These lesions also may develop coiled or bizarrely branching vessels that vary in intercapillary distances and have irregular surfaces. Excessively abnormal vessels or irregular surfaces observed colposcopically are early indications of an imminent microinvasive or invasive SCC.[21,22]

10.2.2 Adequate versus Inadequate Colposcopic Examination

The second most important consideration is whether cancer can be reliably excluded when no suspicious lesion is seen. One of the issues that increase concern for cancer is an inadequate colposcopic exam, where the examiner

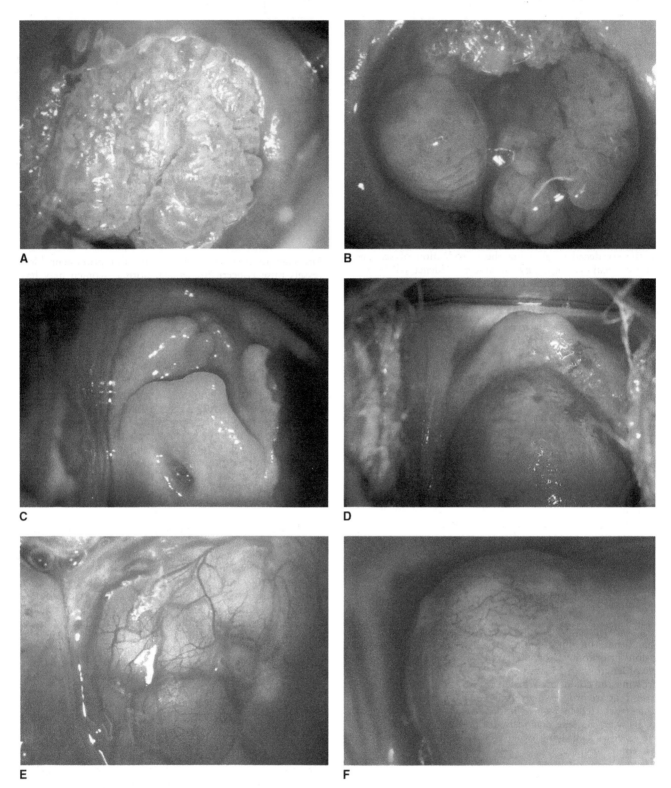

FIGURE 10.1.   **A:** Glazing and fusion of metaplasia producing a markedly irregular surface contour as it appears after acetic acid application. **B:** Prolapsing polypoid masses of normal endocervical epithelium with immature metaplasia producing a grossly irregular ectocervical surface. **C:** Shortened, irregular cervix with a "cockscomb-like" formation of a DES-exposed cervix. Unusual, but normal, cervical contours such as this can also be seen in women with no history of DES exposure. **D:** Cervical hood formation of a DES-exposed cervix. Note large ectopy demonstrating immature metaplasia below the hood. **E:** Retention cyst (nabothian cyst) occupying the left lower quadrant of the cervix extending from the external OS to the periphery of the cervix. Note the numerous, normal, long branching blood vessels coursing over its surface. Some of the vessels appear to be congested. Note the classic yellow hue of the content of the retention cyst as it appears through the cervical epithelium. **F:** Large nabothian cysts and mesonephric duct (Gartner's) cysts near the cervicovaginal border can also distort cervical contour, as this nabothian cyst does on the right superior portio of the cervix.

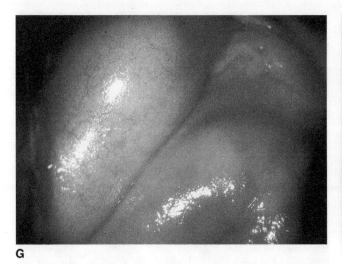

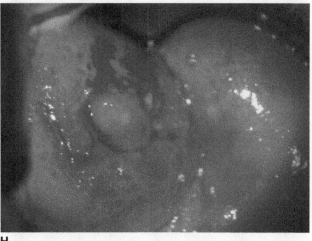

G   **H**

FIGURE 10.1.   *(Continued)* **G:** Large mesonephric duct (Gartner's duct) cyst of the anterior right vaginal apex in a pregnant woman. Note the compression against the cervix. **H:** Large mesonephric duct (Gartner's duct) cyst of the anterior left upper vagina also noted in pregnancy. Note that it is in contact with the outer rim of the cervix partly obscuring it. (Parts [A], [B], [D], [G], and [H] reproduced with permission from Wright VC. *Principles of Cervical Colposcopy*. Houston, TX: Biomedical Communications, 2004. Parts [C] and [E] reproduced with permission from Wright VC. *Color Atlas of Colposcopy—Cervix, Vagina and Vulva*. Houston, TX: Biomedical Communications, 2003. Part [F], Colpophoto thanks to J. Thomas Cox, MD.)

cannot see the transformation zone or cannot see the entire lesion or cannot achieve exposure to evaluate the cervix. An abnormal discharge or exudate may also obscure cervical evaluation.

10.2.3 The Correlation Process after a Adequate Colposcopic Examination

Once the colposcopic examination has been determined to be adequate and the biopsy report has been received, the practitioner can carry out the correlation process. This process determines whether the patient can be managed by observation in the absence of a high-grade lesion, by an ablative or cytodestructive treatment such as cryosurgery or CO_2 laser

ablation, or by excision to determine whether the patient has a malignancy. Excision is required when (1) any lesion extends into the endocervical canal; (2) the endocervical curettage (ECC) specimen is read as showing high-grade or unclassified CIN, AIS, or cancer; (3) microinvasive or invasive disease is suspected colposcopically or cytologically but not proven histologically; (4) microinvasive squamous disease is detected by biopsy; (5) there is a failure to correlate within one CIN grade between cytology, colposcopy and histology, unless histology is two or more grades more severe than cytology or colposcopy (e.g., if biopsy is CIN 2 but impression is metaplasia and Pap test is ASC, excision is not required for diagnosis); (6) AIS is reported on biopsy; or (7) there are colposcopic indications of glandular disease that is not proven histologically.

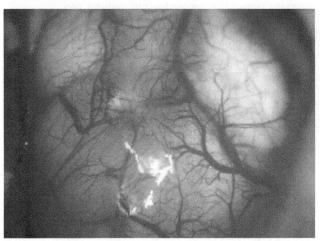

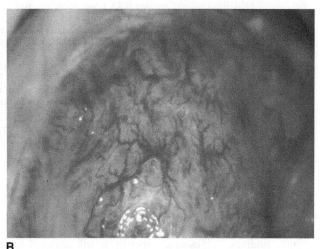

A   **B**

FIGURE 10.2.   **A:** Large normal tapering and branching blood vessels coursing over a large nabothian cyst. **B:** Matured transformation zone with blood vessels that taper off in a uniform manner and anastomose with similar blood vessels.

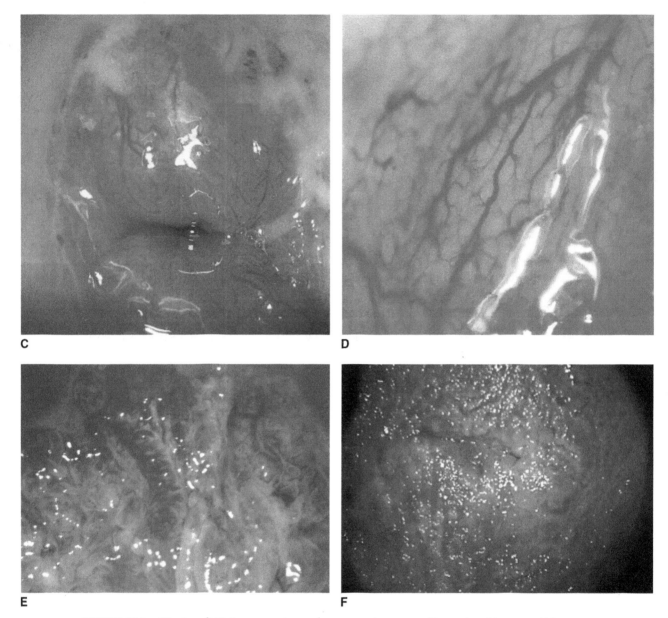

FIGURE 10.2. *(Continued)* C: Long, tapering, and anastomosing taproot-like angioarchitecture within a normal developing transformation zone. D: High magnification view of tapering, taproot-like vessels in a matured transformation zone. E: Lateral branching vessels off a main vertical trunk as seen in this immature metaplasia. F: Vascularity of columnar epithelium that has become congested as a result of continuous hormone stimulation. This condition can occur in pregnancy and because of use of contraceptive hormones, in this case medroxyprogesterone. (Parts [A,B] reproduced with permission from Wright VC. *Color Atlas of Colposcopy—Cervix, Vagina and Vulva.* Houston, TX: Biomedical Communications, 2003. Parts [C–E] reproduced with permission from Wright VC. *Principles of Cervical Colposcopy.* Houston, TX: Biomedical Communications, 2004. Part [F] reproduced with permission from Wright VC. *Comprehensive Colposcopy Review: Cervix, Vagina, Vulva and Adjacent Sites CD-ROM.* Houston, TX: Biomedical Communications, 2008.)

10.2.4 When Excision Is Required Because of Suspected Cancer

Although monopolar electrosurgical loop excision is available and frequently used, especially in the presence of high-grade cytologic findings, colposcopic expertise is still required to identify the location and extent of abnormal squamous disease. Colposcopy is also used to plan the surgical configuration of the specimen. In the presence of suspected or confirmed microinvasive squamous disease or a glandular lesion, excision by cold knife cone (CKC) is often preferable to the "loop" electrosurgical excision procedure (LEEP) because electric current follows the path of least resistance, which is offered by mucus in the endocervical crypts. This can result in excessive thermal burns with or without pseudostratification of glandular epithelium, or fragmentation and denudation that make margins pathologically uninterpretable. These artifacts make it difficult or impossible to differentiate between microinvasive and invasive SCC or between AIS and adenocarcinoma.[23–26] Additionally, artifacts in the intact cervix may interfere with follow-up assessment. For these reasons, the author prefers to not use electrosurgical excision when AIS or microinvasive cancer is found on biopsy or is suspected on cytology or colposcopy. The 2006 American Society for Colposcopy and Cervical Pathology (ASCCP) Guidelines changed an earlier recommendation to use only CKC for management of a suspected glandular lesion to "a diagnostic excisional procedure that provides an intact specimen with interpretable margins" in recognition of declining expertise in the CKC procedure and the lack of evidence that CKC is superior in most situations.[20] The ASCCP Guidelines do not identify a specific procedure for suspected or confirmed microinvasive squamous disease.

10.2.5 Why Cancer Is Missed

Missing a cervical cancer has serious ramifications, for both the patient and the clinician. It happens because of any of several potential inadequacies: (1) an inadequate case load (i.e., not enough patients to develop an adequate level of expertise); (2) a poor understanding of the disease processes; (3) deviation from or deficiencies in a diagnostic protocol; (4) insufficient biopsies (i.e., too small, no stroma, inadequate number) or samples from the wrong sites; (5) failure to perform an ECC when indicated; (6) failure to excise when ECC is positive; (7) cervical ablation without prior biopsy; (8) failure to correlate cytologic, colposcopic, and histologic findings; (9) failure to appreciate the indications for excision; (10) failure to refer in difficult cases, such as in the presence of exaggerated patterns of pregnancy; and (11) miscommunication with the pathologist. Being aware of and avoiding these pitfalls will reduce the likelihood of missed cancers.[27]

10.2.6 Circumstances That Warrant Concern

10.2.6.1 Patient Age

Cancer of the cervix is very rare in patients younger than 25 years. Between 1998 and 2006, an average of 14 cervical cancers were reported annually in the United States in girls aged 15 to 19 and only 123 cases annually in the 20- to 24-year-old age group, for an incidence of 0.1/100,000 and 1.1/100,000, respectively.[6] Cervical cancer continues to be uncommon under the age of 30, with only 680 cases reported annually in the United States for all women under this age,

whereas the median age of screen-detected CIN 3 is between 27 and 30 years.[4,28] However, the incidence of microinvasive and occult invasive cancers increases as women grow older. The incidence begins to gradually rise in the late 20s, reaching a plateau in the 40s and peaking in the late 50s (Table 10.1).[6] From 2002 to 2006 the median age at diagnosis and death from cervical cancer was 48 and 57, respectively.[29] While increasing age increases the risk for invasive cancer, the risk for the colposcopist in missing cancer may be greatest for young women with cancer because of its extreme rarity.

10.2.6.2 Cytology

Although cancer can be found with any grade of cytologic finding, more severe cytologic abnormalities correlate with a greater likelihood of cancer. Cytologic findings demonstrating SCC will almost invariably be associated with a significant cervical or vaginal neoplasm, with only rare reports of cells shed from an intraepithelial lesion that are so abnormal in appearance to be interpreted as malignant. Patients with malignant cells on cytologic testing require immediate colposcopic assessment with biopsy, ECC, and excision if biopsy does not confirm cancer. Glandular and squamous lesions may be present together even though the cytology result may demonstrate only abnormal squamous cells. Two to three percent of CIN 3 lesions will have a coexistent glandular component,[30,31] but cytologic testing often will not demonstrate abnormal glandular cells.[32,33] To some degree, cytologic severity should be considered in connection with the patient's age although markedly abnormal cells at any age should raise concern. Markedly abnormal cells in a patient 40 years or older should suggest a high risk of cancer to the colposcopist.

10.2.6.3 Linear Length, Surface Area of Lesions, and Cervical Diameter

The linear length of a lesion is defined as the distance over the tissue surface between the caudal and cephalad edges of the lesion (Figure 10.3A,B). During the first four decades after screening was introduced, the linear length of CIN 3 lesions was generally greater than that reported in the last two decades. In the ASCUS LSIL Triage Study, the median length of CIN 3 was only 6.5 mm and lesions in one-third were so small that colposcopic biopsy did not leave any residual CIN 3 to be detected in the LEEP specimen.[34] In the HPV

TABLE 10.1	ANNUAL COUNTS, AGE-ADJUSTED INCIDENCE RATES, AND MEDIAN AGE AT DIAGNOSIS OF INVASIVE CERVICAL CARCINOMA AGE: UNITED STATES, 1998–2003*			
■ AGE, Y	■ AVERAGE ANNUAL	■ INCIDENCE (95% CI)	■ % INCIDENCE RATE	■ MEDIAN AGE
All ages	10,846	8.9 (8.8–9)	100	47
0–14	0	0.0		
15–19	14	0.2 (0.1–0.2)	0.1	
20–24	123	1.6 (1.5–1.7)	1.1	
25–29	543	6.9 (6.7–7.2)	5.0	
30–34	1045	12.3 (12–12.6)	9.6	
35–39	1350	14.6 (14.3–14.9)	12.5	
40–44	1534	16.3 (15.9–16.6)	14.1	
45–49	1323	15.4 (15–15.7)	12.2	
50–59	1958	14.5 (14.2–14.7)	18.0	
60–69	1352	14.8 (14.5–15.1)	12.5	
70–79	1008	12.9 (12.6–13.3)	9.3	
≥80	595	11.2 (10.9–11.6)	5.5	

*From Watson M, Saraiya M, Benard V, et al. Burden of cervical cancer in the United States, 1998–2003. *Cancer* 2008;113(10 suppl):2855–64.

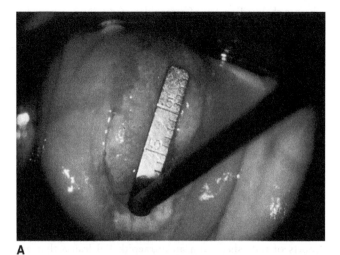

A

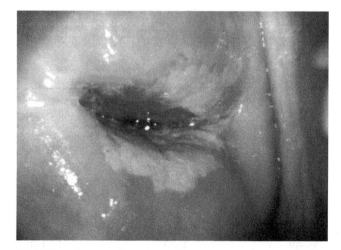

B

FIGURE 10.3. **A:** Measuring the linear length (>20 mm) of the high-grade epithelial lesion on the ectocervical portion. The lesion however extends into the endocervical canal where most cancers are located. **B:** Linear measurements and surface area of intraepithelial lesions are exaggerated in pregnancy. This CIN 3 lesion measures over 20 mm due to the increased size of the cervix in pregnancy. (Part [A] reproduced with permission from Wright VC. *Color Atlas of Colposcopy—Cervix, Vagina and Vulva.* Houston, TX: Biomedical Communications, 2003. Part [B] reproduced with permission from Wright VC. *Principles of Cervical Colposcopy.* Houston, TX: Biomedical Communications, 2004.)

vaccine trials, CIN 3 detected within 30 months of incident oncogenic HPV infection was often so small as to not be colposcopically identifiable. In contrast, the median length of CIN 3 lesions reported in the literature from 1953 to 1990 was 6 to 10 mm, with a range of <2 mm up to 22 mm.[35–38] Hence, screen-detected CIN 3 is generally larger for populations with recently introduced screening, than for populations well-screened over a period of decades. The size of a CIN 3 lesion with associated invasion is, on average, seven times larger than that without invasion.[39] Therefore, long linear lesions—those >10 mm, particularly when there is endocervical involvement—are always suspicious for cancer (Figure 10.3A,B). As the surface area of lesions increases to more than 40 mm², so should the suspicion for cancer. Since the size of the cervix itself increases due to tumor infiltration and proliferation in invasive cancer, an unusually large cervix may also be indicative of cancer.

10.2.6.4 High-grade Lesions with Complete or Partial Canal Involvement

Squamous disease develops and worsens within oncogenic HPV-infected metaplastic cells. As women age, if this process is persistent and progressive, the normal advancement of the metaplastic transformation zone toward, into, and up the endocervical canal typically results in the most abnormal area being most central. Thus, disease on the periphery of the cervix can be of lesser severity than that located more centrally (Figure 10.4). Low-grade disease is not infrequently peripheral to coexisting high-grade disease, which is peripheral to any coexisting cancer.[40–42] Biopsies, therefore, should be taken from the leading edge of the lesion where the most severe histologic results will likely be found. CIN 3 lesions often involve the endocervical canal (Figure 10.4).[35] The worst disease will always be located centrally, with invasive cancer found at the inner/upper lesion border.[36,37,40–43] When lesions are located high in the canal, the upper margin must be sampled, most often requiring a cylindrical excision (Figure 10.5). Missing cancer—the most serious error made in colposcopy—usually can be attributed to inadequate evaluation of the endocervical canal. When squamous cancer is found more peripherally on the cervix, it is more likely to be highly differentiated and have

FIGURE 10.4. A high-grade squamous intraepithelial lesion, specifically CIN 3, extending into the endocervical canal. Potentially, the worst disease is located cephalad, which, in this case, is in the endocervical canal. Excision is required to exclude malignancy if not proven on biopsy. (Reproduced with permission from Wright VC. *Color Atlas of Colposcopy—Cervix, Vagina and Vulva.* Houston, TX: Biomedical Communications, 2003.)

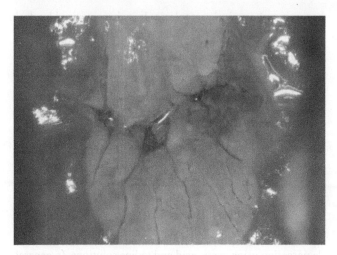

FIGURE 10.5.   A large area of high-grade squamous intraepithelial lesion covers the ectocervix with canal extension. Some method of excision in the endocervical canal is necessary to exclude malignancy if not already proven on biopsy. (Reproduced with permission from Wright VC. *Color Atlas of Colposcopy—Cervix, Vagina and Vulva*. Houston, TX: Biomedical Communications, 2003.)

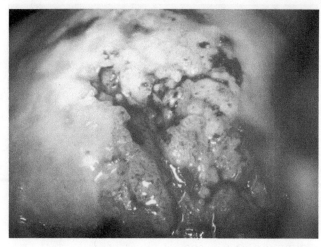

FIGURE 10.7.   A large SCC with surface irregularities and ulceration. Irregular punctation is seen and, in some areas, elongated irregular vessels are forming. (Reproduced with permission from Wright VC. *Color Atlas of Colposcopy—Cervix, Vagina and Vulva*. Houston, TX: Biomedical Communications, 2003.)

a better prognosis.[37] Cancers found within the canal can be of any degree of severity.

10.2.6.5 Surface Contour

Microinvasive and occult cancers can produce irregular surfaces, erosions, granular appearances, or in more advanced disease, necrosis (Figures 10.6 and 10.7).

10.2.6.6 Color

A dense acetowhite color after the application of acetic acid is a distinct colposcopic feature of most concern for a high-grade squamous intraepithelial neoplasia. In contrast, if the lesion is already white prior to the application of acetic acid, even to the naked eye, the color is secondary to the presence

of keratin. Keratin is expressed in both benign and malignant conditions. Benign conditions displaying keratin include condyloma, chronic trauma (such as from a pessary), and posttreatment states. The degree of acetowhiteness in neoplasia is a reflection of the amount of nuclear activity (Figure 10.8).[21,22] Visualization using a blue or green filter often reveals punctation or mosaicism and white epithelium after the application of acetic acid. High-grade squamous lesions are usually dense white from border to border, whereas glandular lesions often exhibit a variegated red and white coloration. Squamous cancers can be yellowish, a characteristic associated with necrosis (Figure 10.9). A red color reflects marked vascularity (Figure 10.10A). Invasive lesions with marked vascularity are often symptomatic, with vaginal bleeding, most commonly postcoital, and/or a watery discharge (Figure 10.10B).

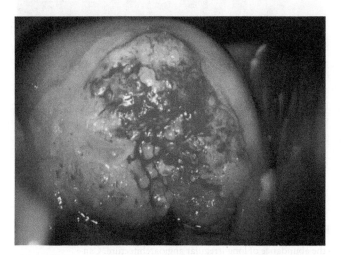

FIGURE 10.6.   A large SCC of the anterior cervical lip with an irregular ulcerative surface. A high-grade squamous intraepithelial lesion is noted peripherally from 7 to 12 o'clock. (Reproduced with permission from Wright VC. *Color Atlas of Colposcopy—Cervix, Vagina and Vulva*. Houston, TX: Biomedical Communications, 2003.)

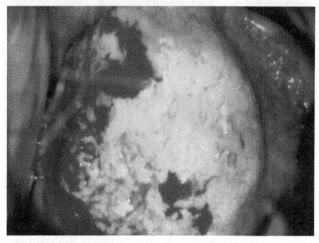

FIGURE 10.8.   A large SCC producing an enlarged cervix. It is dense white due to keratin and increased nuclear activity. (Reproduced with permission from Wright VC. *Color Atlas of Colposcopy—Cervix, Vagina and Vulva*. Houston, TX: Biomedical Communications, 2003.)

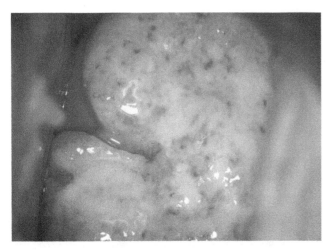

FIGURE 10.9.   A large SCC with necrosis, demonstrating a yellow hue. (Reprinted with permission from Wright VC. *Principles of Cervical Colposcopy*. Houston, TX: Biomedical Communications, 2004.)

10.2.6.7 Atypical Vessels

Abnormality of angioarchitecture is an expression of stage of disease. Mosaicism and punctation, whether regular, irregular, fine, or coarse, are usually indicative of some grade of intraepithelial neoplasia. In microinvasive cancer, the punctate and mosaic patterns become degraded and disorganized as if the vessels are breaking out of the typical arrangements and transmuting into more atypical vessels (Figures 10.11–10.14A).[21,22] Such atypical vascular formations should not be confused with the pseudomosaic (reverse mosaic) angioarchitecture that is seen in immature metaplasia and in the

beginning of atypical metaplasia. It is characterized by dark dilated vessels centrally surrounded by acetowhite-appearing immature metaplastic squamous epithelium (Figure 10.14B,C). True atypical vessels are commonly referred to as corkscrew, spaghetti, irregular coarse, irregular parallel, comma, tendril, and waste-thread depending on what they resemble (Figures 10.10 and 10.15–10.19). Other atypical forms have nonbranching vessels that bulge and constrict, exhibiting variable calibers (Figure 10.18). The vessels sometimes appear within an area of uneven surface contour because these vessels are supporting active, proliferating tumors (Figure 10.19).

10.2.6.8 Colposcopic Grading Systems

Various colposcopic grading systems have been described (see Chapter 9).[22,44,45] They address the angioarchitecture of squamous lesions, their surface contour, acetowhiteness, and demarcation using acetic acid and iodine solutions. In general, a greater severity of disease correlates with more pronounced findings, and any area with atypical vessels is suspicious for malignancy. None of the grading schemes is applicable to glandular lesions and grading systems are not applicable to cancer staging.

10.2.6.9 Persistence or Recurrence of High-grade Lesions after Treatment

When high-grade squamous disease persists or returns after treatment (Figures 10.20 and 10.21), colposcopy is frequently inadequate because the remaining lesion may be buried under normal epithelium or lies within the endocervical canal.[18] Since this is where most cancers occurring posttreatment are located, there is a higher likelihood of cancer, warranting some method of excision for diagnosis.

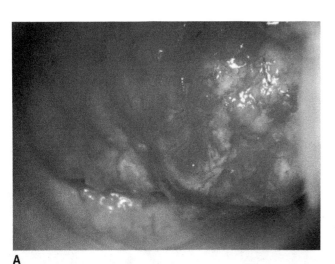

A

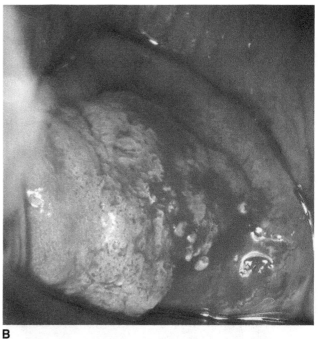

B

FIGURE 10.10.   **A:** This very large SCC appears red due to the abundance of long irregular angioarchitecture. Cancer bleeds easily with physical trauma. **B:** Marked abnormal angiogenesis in a clinical stage 1b SCC. This is because the vasculature proliferates to try to support the rapid tumor growth. (Parts [A] and [B] reprinted with permission from Wright VC. *Principles of Cervical Colposcopy*. Houston, TX: Biomedical Communications, 2004.)

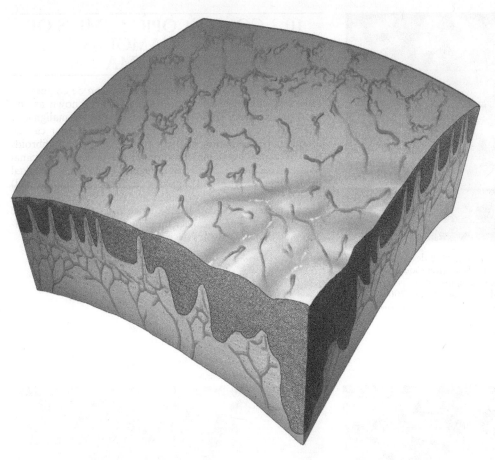

FIGURE 10.11.   Schematics of the mosaic pattern breaking up, as seen in the beginning stages of squamous cell invasion.

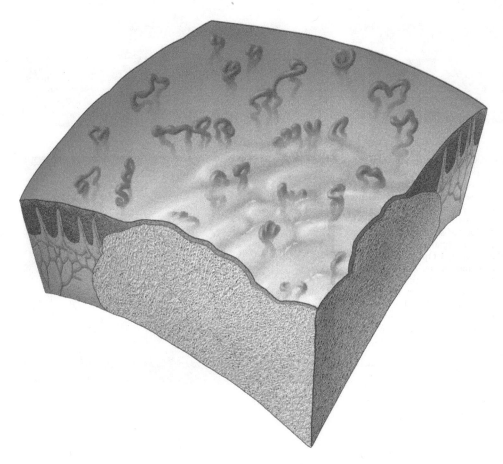

FIGURE 10.12.   Schematics of irregular blood vessels of an invasive SCC demonstrating corkscrew-like formations.

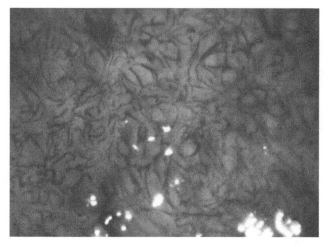

FIGURE 10.13. The mosaic pattern is becoming degraded and disorganized, a finding seen in early invasive SCC. (Reproduced with permission from Wright VC. *Color Atlas of Colposcopy—Cervix, Vagina and Vulva*. Houston, TX: Biomedical Communications, 2003.)

10.3 COLPOSCOPIC MIMICS OF INVASIVE SQUAMOUS CELL CARCINOMA

A number of histologically benign entities can be colposcopically suspicious for cancer and are therefore known as colposcopic mimics. These colposcopic mimics of malignancy relate to surface contours and atypical vessels that can be found in postradiation changes (Figure 10.22A,B), fibroids that have prolapsed into or through the endocervical canal (Figure 10.23A,B), condyloma (Figure 10.24A–C), decidual tissue (Figure 10.25A,B), polyps (cervical or endometrial) (Figure 10.26A,B), and granulation tissue postcervical treatment (Figures 10.27 and 10.28). Since all of these entities are only proven to *not be* cancer upon histologic evaluation, colposcopic biopsy is always necessary.

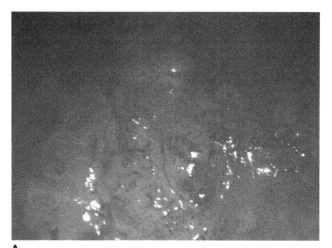

A

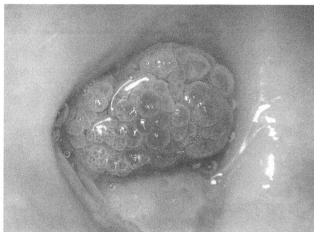

B

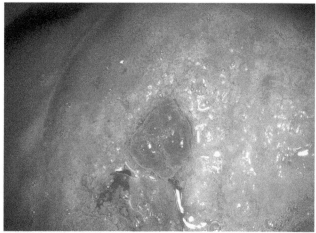

C

FIGURE 10.14. **A:** A microinvasive SCC in which the punctate pattern is becoming disorderly and irregular elongated vessels are seen. **B:** A protruding endocervical polypoid mass with immature metaplastic changes. Note the pseudomosaic/reverse mosaic angioarchitecture with dilated vascular centers surrounded by acetowhiteness. It is frequently confused with malignancy and tissue sampling is required. Posterior acetowhiteness is mature transformed squamous epithelium (from columnar), and peripheral to that is original squamous epithelium. **C:** A low magnification view of immature metaplastic epithelium demonstrating pseudomosaicism/reverse mosaicism. Centrally is a mound (bouquet) of immature metaplastic epithelium that also shows this pattern. (Part [A] reproduced with permission from Wright VC. *Color Atlas of Colposcopy—Cervix, Vagina and Vulva*. Houston, TX: Biomedical Communications, 2003. Parts [B] and [C] reprinted with permission from Wright VC. *Comprehensive Colposcopy Review: Cervix, Vagina, Vulva and Adjacent Sites CD-ROM*. Houston, TX: Biomedical Communications, 2008.)

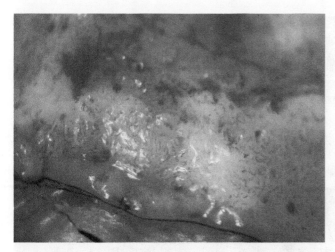

FIGURE 10.15. Irregular blood vessel formations over the surface of an invasive SCC. (Reproduced with permission from Wright VC. *Color Atlas of Colposcopy—Cervix, Vagina and Vulva—Cervix, Vagina and Vulva.* Houston, TX: Biomedical Communications, 2003.)

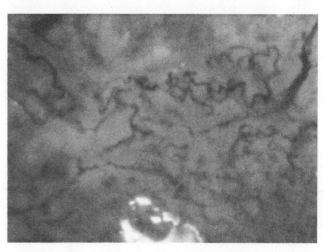

FIGURE 10.18. A high-power colposcopic view of irregular angioarchitecture seen in squamous cancer. (Reproduced with permission from Wright VC. *Color Atlas of Colposcopy—Cervix, Vagina and Vulva.* Houston, TX: Biomedical Communications, 2003.)

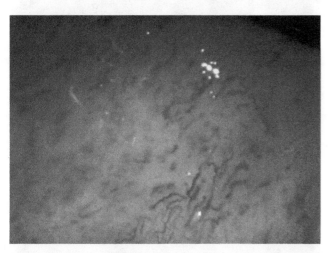

FIGURE 10.16. Irregular dilated (corkscrew) blood vessels of a SCC. (Reproduced with permission from Wright VC. *Color Atlas of Colposcopy—Cervix, Vagina and Vulva.* Houston, TX: Biomedical Communications, 2003.)

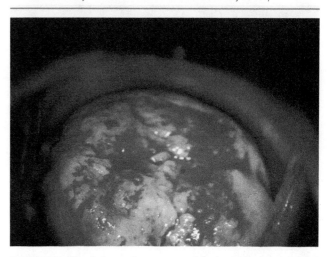

FIGURE 10.19. Advanced tumor growth and proliferation of blood vessels with bleeding associated with trauma. (Reproduced with permission from Wright VC. *Color Atlas of Colposcopy—Cervix, Vagina and Vulva.* Houston, TX: Biomedical Communications, 2003.)

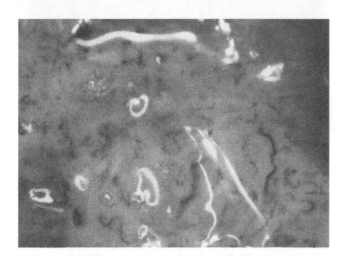

FIGURE 10.17. Numerous different blood vessel formations seen in SCC. (Reproduced with permission from Wright VC. *Color Atlas of Colposcopy—Cervix, Vagina and Vulva.* Houston, TX: Biomedical Communications, 2003.)

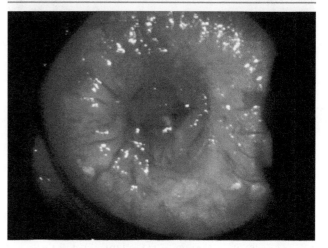

FIGURE 10.20. Recurrent/persistent disease after laser ablation for high-grade squamous intraepithelial lesion. This distribution is characteristic and resembles a white-walled tire. It is most likely related to activation of latent HPV during the healing phase. (Reproduced with permission from Wright VC. *Color Atlas of Colposcopy—Cervix, Vagina and Vulva.* Houston, TX: Biomedical Communications, 2003.)

FIGURE 10.21.   Irregular vascularity is seen after electrosurgery for a high-grade squamous intraepithelial lesion. Such a formation requires excision to exclude malignancy. (Reproduced with permission from Wright VC. *Color Atlas of Colposcopy—Cervix, Vagina and Vulva*. Houston, TX: Biomedical Communications, 2003.)

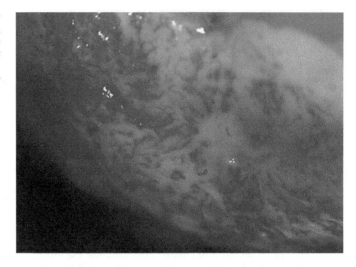

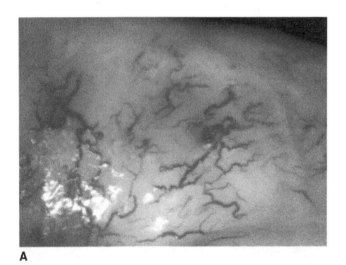

A

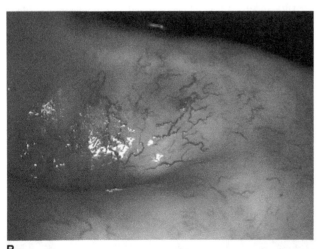

B

FIGURE 10.22.   **A:** The angioarchitecture seen in normal cervical squamous epithelium after radiation for cancer of the cervix. The spatial distribution and corkscrew-like formations are characteristic. **B:** Lower magnification of (**A**). (Parts [**A**] and [**B**] reproduced with permission from Wright VC. *Color Atlas of Colposcopy—Cervix, Vagina and Vulva*. Houston, TX: Biomedical Communications, 2003.)

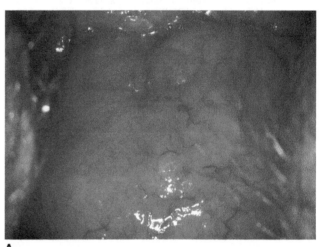

A

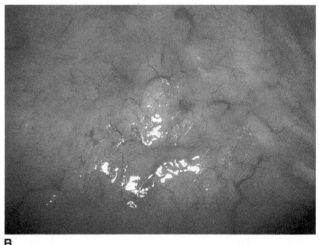

B

FIGURE 10.23.   **A:** A prolapsed endocervical fibroid. **B:** Higher magnification of (**A**) showing the characteristic distribution of normal blood vessels. (Part [**A**] reproduced with permission from Wright VC. *Color Atlas of Colposcopy—Cervix, Vagina and Vulva*. Houston, TX: Biomedical Communications, 2003. Part [**B**] reprinted with permission from Wright VC. *Principles of Cervical Colposcopy—A Text and Atlas*. Houston, TX: Biomedical Communications, 2004.)

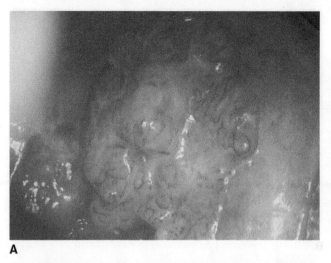

A

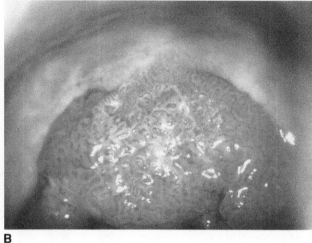

B

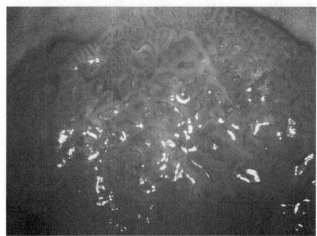

C

FIGURE 10.24.   **A:** The irregular vascularity of a cervical condyloma resembling the angioarchitecture of malignancy. **B:** Cervical condyloma before acetic acid demonstrating a variety of abnormal blood vessels. These include tendril-like, waste thread-like, and single and multiple dot-like forms. Similar vessel patterns are seen in SCCs. **C:** Higher magnification view of previous lesion. (Parts [A] and [B] reproduced with permission from Wright VC. *Color Atlas of Colposcopy— Cervix, Vagina and Vulva.* Houston, TX: Biomedical Communications, 2003. Part [C] reprinted with permission from Wright VC. *Principles of Cervical Colposcopy.* Houston, TX: Biomedical Communications, 2004.)

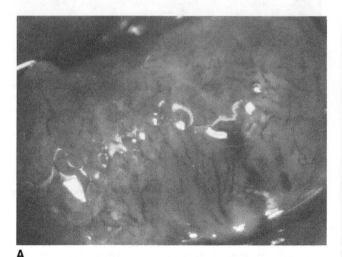

A

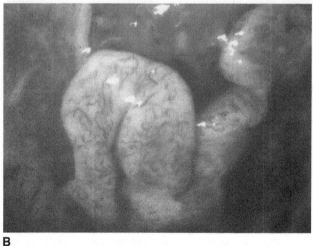

B

FIGURE 10.25.   **A:** The characteristic distribution of blood vessels coursing over the surface of a large mass of decidual tissue, as seen in pregnancy. **B:** Mounds of decidual tissue on the posterior cervical lip with atypical-appearing vascularity that is characteristic of this entity. It mimics a SCC; hence, biopsy is recommended for the inexperienced colposcopist. (Parts [A] and [B] reprinted with permission from Wright VC. *Color Atlas of Colposcopy—Cervix, Vagina and Vulva.* Houston, TX: Biomedical Communications, 2003.)

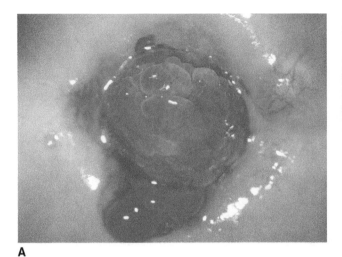
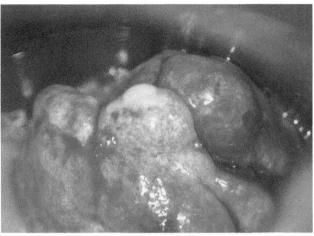

A   **B**

FIGURE 10.26.   **A:** A large endocervical polypoid mass. Removal is necessary to exclude malignancy. In this case, the lesion was benign polyp. **B:** A large, uterine, atypical polypoid adenomyofibroma prolapsing through the endocervical canal mimicking a cervical malignancy. To find such an entity intact is a rarity because most are fragmented by dilation and curettage for investigating abnormal vaginal/uterine bleeding. (Part [A] reproduced with permission from Wright VC. *Color Atlas of Colposcopy—Cervix, Vagina and Vulva.* Houston, TX: Biomedical Communications, 2003. Part [B] Reprinted with permission from Wright VC. *Principles of Cervical Colposcopy.* Houston, TX: Biomedical Communications, 2004.)

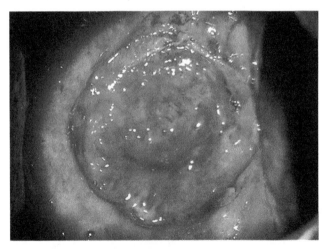
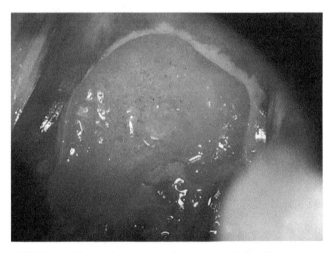

FIGURE 10.27.   Cervix at 8 days after a laser cylindrical excisional procedure. To the colposcopist without a patient history, this could be mistaken for a cancer. (Reprinted with permission from Wright VC. *Carbon Dioxide Laser Surgery for Lower Genital Tract Disease CD-ROM.* Houston, TX: Biomedical Communications, 2006.)

FIGURE 10.28.   A large, somewhat symmetrical iodine-negative mass seen colposcopically 6 weeks after electrosurgical desiccation of cervical condyloma. It mimics a SCC. Biopsy confirmed granulation tissue. (Courtesy of V. C. Wright.)

References

1. Walboomers JMM, Jacobs MV, Manos MM, et al. Human papillomavirus is a necessary cause of invasive cancer worldwide. *J Pathol* 1999;189:12–9.
2. Tjalma WA, Van Waes TR, Van den Eeden LE, Bogers JJ. Role of human papillomavirus in the carcinogenesis of squamous cell carcinoma and adenocarcinoma of the cervix. *Best Pract Res Clin Obstet Gynaecol* 2005;19:469–83.
3. Bosch FX, Munoz N. The viral etiology of cervical cancer. *Virus Res* 2002;89:183–90.
4. Moscicki AB, Schiffman M, Kjaer S, Villa LL. Chapter 5: Updating the natural history of HPV and anogenital cancer. *Vaccine* 2006;24S3:S3/42–51.
5. Schiffman M, Castle PE. The promise of global cervical-cancer prevention. *N Engl J Med* 2005;353:2101–4.
6. Watson M, Saraiya M, Benard V, et al. Burden of cervical cancer in the United States, 1998–2003. *Cancer* 2008;113(10 suppl):2855–64.
7. Barnholtz-Sloan J, Patel N, Rollison D, et al. Incidence trends of invasive cervical cancer in the United States by combined race and ethnicity. *Cancer Causes Control* 2009;20(7):1129–38. doi:10.1007/s10552-009-9317-z.
8. Saraiya M, Ahmed F, Krishnan S, et al. Cervical cancer incidence in a prevaccine era in the United States, 1998–2002. *Obstet Gynecol* 2007;109:360–70.
9. US Cancer Statistics Working Group. *United States Cancer Statistics: 2004 Incidence and Mortality.* Atlanta, GA: Department of Health and Human Services, Centers for Disease Control and Prevention and National Cancer Institute, 2007.
10. American Cancer Society. Cancer Facts & Figures 2010. http://www.cancer.org/acs/groups/content/@nho/documents/document/acspc-024113.pdf. Accessed May 08, 2010.

11. Wang SS, Sherman ME, Hildesheim A, Lacey JV Jr, Devesa S. Cervical adenocarcinoma and squamous cell carcinoma incidence trends among white women and black women in the United States for 1976–2000. *Cancer* 2004;100:1035–44.
12. Howe HL, Wu X, Ries LA, et al. Annual report to the nation on the status of cancer, 1975–2003, featuring cancer among U.S. Hispanic/Latino populations. *Cancer* 2006;107:1711–42.
13. Farley J, Risinger JI, Rose GS, Maxwell GL. Racial disparities in blacks with gynecologic cancers. *Cancer* 2007;110:234–43.
14. Solomon D, Breen N, McNeel T. Cervical cancer screening rates in the United States and the potential impact of implementation of screening guidelines. *CA Cancer J Clin* 2007;57:105–11.
15. Castellsagué X, Díaz M, de Sanjosé S, et al. International Agency for Research on Cancer Multicenter Cervical Cancer Study Group. Worldwide human papillomavirus etiology of cervical adenocarcinoma and its cofactors: implications for screening and prevention. *J Natl Cancer Inst* 2006;98:303–15.
16. Gustafsson L, Ponten J, Zack M, Adami HO. International incidence rates of invasive cervical cancer after introduction of cytological screening. *Cancer Causes Control* 1997;8:755–63.
17. Chan PG, Sung HY, Sawaya GF. Changes in cervical cancer incidence after three decades of screening US women less than 30 years old. *Obstet Gynecol* 2003;102:765–73.
18. Sasieni P, Castanon A, Cuzick J. Effectiveness of cervical screening with age: population-based case-control study of prospectively recorded data. *BMJ* 2009;339:b2968.
19. Sparén P, Gustafsson L, Friberg LG, Pontén J, Bergström R, Adami HO. Improved control of invasive cervical cancer in Sweden over six decades by earlier clinical detection and better treatment. *J Clin Oncol* 1995;13:715–25.
20. Wright TC Jr, Massad LS, Dunton CJ, Spitzer M, Wilkinson EJ. 2006 consensus guidelines for the management of women with cervical intraepithelial neoplasia or adenocarcinoma in situ. *J Low Genit Tract Dis* 2007;11:223–39.
21. Kolstad P, Stafl A. Terminology and definition. In: Kolstad P, Stafl A, eds. *Atlas of Colposcopy* (1st ed.). Oslo, Norway: Universitetsforlaget, 1972:21–5.
22. Coppleson M, Pixley EC, Reid BL. *Colposcopy: A Scientific and Practical Approach to the Cervix, Vagina and Vulva in Health and Disease* (3rd ed.). Springfield, IL: Charles C. Thomas, 1986.
23. Dalrymple C, Russell P. Thermal artifact after diathermy loop excision cone biopsy. *Int J Gynecol Can* 1999;9:238–42.
24. Ioffe OB, Brooks SE, DeRezende RB, Silverberg SG. Artifact in cervical LLETZ specimens: correlation with follow-up. *Int J Gynecol Pathol* 1999;18:115–21.
25. Missing MJ, Otken L, King LA, Gallup DG. Large loop excision of the transformation zone (LLETZ): a pathologic evaluation. *Gynecol Oncol* 1994;52:207–11.
26. Montz FJ, Holschneider CH, Thompson LD. Large loop excision of the transformation zone: effect on the pathologic interpretation of resection margins. *Obstet Gynecol* 1993;81:976–82.
27. Powell JL. Pitfalls in cervical colposcopy. In: Wright VC, ed. *Contemporary Colposcopy. Obstet Gynecol Clin* NA 1993;20:177–88.
28. Bosch FX, de Sanjose S. Chapter 1: Human papillomavirus and cervical cancer-burden and assessment of causality. *J Natl Cancer Inst Monogr* 2003;31:3–13.
29. Horner MJ, Ries LAG, Krapcho M, et al., eds. *SEER Cancer Statistics Review, 1975–2006*. Bethesda, MD: National Cancer Institute. http://seer.cancer.gov/csr/1975_2006/, based on November 2008 SEER data submission, posted to the SEER web site, 2009.
30. Christopherson WM, Nealson N, Gray LA. Noninvasive precursor lesions of adenocarcinoma and mixed adenosquamous carcinoma of the cervix uteri. *Cancer* 1979;44:975–83.
31. Boon ME, Baak JPA, Kurver PGH, et al. Adenocarcinoma in situ of the cervix. An underdiagnosed lesion. *Cancer* 1981;48:768–73.
32. Nguyen G-K, Jeannot AB. Exfoliative cytology of in situ and microadenocarcinoma of the uterine cervix. *Acta Cytol* 1984;28:461–7.
33. Östör AG, Duncan A, Quinn M, et al. Adenocarcinoma in situ of the uterine cervix: an experience with 100 cases. *Gynecol Oncol* 2000;79:207–10.
34. Sherman ME, Wang SS, Tarone R, Rich L, Schiffman M. Histopathologic extent of CIN 3 lesions in ALTS: implications for subject safety and lead-time bias. *Cancer Epidemiol Biomarkers Prev* 2003;12:372–9.
35. Przybora LA, Plutowa A. Histological topography of carcinoma in situ of the cervix uteri. *Cancer* 1959;12:268–73.
36. Abdul-Karim FW, Yao SF, Reagan JW, et al. Morphometric study of intraepithelial neoplasia of the uterine cervix. *Obstet Gynecol* 1982;60:210–4.
37. Boonstra H, Aalders JG, Koudstaal J, et al. Minimum extension and appropriate topographic and position of tissue destruction for treatment of cervical intraepithelial neoplasia. *Obstet Gynecol* 1990;75:227–31.
38. Reagan JW, Hicks DJ. A study of in situ and squamous-cell cancer of the uterine cervix. *Cancer* 1953;6:1200–14.
39. Tidbury P, Singer A, Jenkins D. CIN 3: the role of lesion size in invasion. *Br J Obstet Gynaecol* 1992;99:583–6.
40. Holzner JH. Dysplasia of cervical epithelium—an intermediate or final stage in the development of epithelial atypia. In: Burghardt E, Holzer E, Jordan JA, eds. *Cervical Pathology and Colposcopy*. Stuttgart, Germany: George Thieme Publishers, 1978:46–57.
41. Reagan JW, Patten F Jr. Dysplasia: a basic reaction to injury in the uterine cervix. *Ann NY Acad Sci* 1962;97:662–7.
42. Holzer E. Localization of dysplasic epithelium. In: Burghart E, Holzer E, Jordan JA, eds. *Cervical Pathology and Colposcopy*. Stuttgart, Germany: George Thieme Publishers, 1978:49–57.
43. Roman LD, Felix JC, Muderspach LI, et al. Risk of residual invasive disease in women with microinvasive squamous cancer in a conization specimen. *Obstet Gynecol* 1997;90:759–64.
44. Stafl A, Mattingly RF. Colposcopic diagnosis of cervical neoplasia. *Obstet Gynecol* 1973;41:168–72.
45. Reid R, Stanhope CR, Herschman BR, et al. Genital warts and cervical cancer IV. A colposcopic index for differentiating subclinical papillomaviral infection from cervical intraepithelial neoplasia. *Am J Obstet Gynecol* 1984;149:815–9.

Colposcopy of Adenocarcinoma *In Situ* and Adenocarcinoma of the Uterine Cervix

11.1 INTRODUCTION
11.2 THE COLUMNAR EPITHELIUM
11.3 THE FATE OF COLUMNAR EPITHELIUM
11.4 NEOPLASTIC TRANSFORMATION OF COLUMNAR EPITHELIUM
11.5 STIMULUS OF DISEASE DEVELOPMENT
11.6 MORPHOLOGIC SPECTRUM OF GLANDULAR INTRAEPITHELIAL LESIONS
11.7 PROBLEMS DETECTING ADENOCARCINOMA *IN SITU* AND ADENOCARCINOMA
    11.7.1 Reduced Sensitivity of Cytologic Screening
    11.7.2 Colposcopic Inexperience and Subtle Findings
    11.7.3 Lesion Size and Location

11.7.4 Skip (Multifocal) Lesions
11.7.5 Buried Disease
11.7.6 Mixed Disease
11.8 THREE COLPOSCOPIC PRESENTATIONS OF AIS AND ADENOCARCINOMA
11.9 DIFFERENTIATING GLANDULAR DISEASE FROM OTHER ENTITIES
    11.9.1 Surface Patterns in Glandular Disease
    11.9.2 Atypical Blood Vessels
11.10 CONFIRMING THE DIAGNOSIS
    11.10.1 Management of the Patient Desiring to Maintain Fertility
    11.10.2 2006 ASCCP Guidelines for Postcone AIS Management

11.1 INTRODUCTION

Cervical adenocarcinoma (AC) is much less common than cervical squamous cell carcinoma (SCC), comprising about 20% of all cervical cancers.[1] The mean annual incidence for cervical adenocarcinoma is 1.2 per 100,000 women, compared to 6.6 for SCC and 0.06 for extremely rare small cell carcinoma.[2] The immediate precursor to adenocarcinoma of the cervix, adenocarcinoma *in situ* (AIS), is also relatively rare. The ratio of AIS to CIN 3 (cervical intraepithelial neoplasia Grade 3) has varied from 1:26 to 1:239, an average of approximately 50 cases of CIN 3 for each case of AIS.[3–5] Perhaps the relative infrequency of AIS and adenocarcinoma is one reason why the descriptive terminology of colposcopy has focused almost entirely on findings related to squamous lesions. Additionally, colposcopic findings of AIS are much more subtle than those found in CIN 3/carcinoma *in situ* (CIS) and typically cannot definitively be differentiated from metaplasia except on histology. Hence, historically, colposcopy was primarily directed to the identification of squamous lesions. However, over the past 20 years, the colposcopic findings of AIS and cervical adenocarcinoma have been intensively studied and described through the work of Cecil Wright, Gordon Lickrish, RM Shier, and others.[3,6–9] Their work enables us to appreciate that there are valid and reliable colposcopic findings when a glandular lesion is present on the cervix. These lesions can develop solely in the glandular epithelium or with a coexistent squamous abnormality. Colposcopists can learn when to suspect that an AIS or adenocarcinoma may be present, but confirmation always requires histology.

In this chapter, the author describes the origin of glandular neoplasia as it is presently understood, the colposcopic findings of AIS and cervical adenocarcinoma, and the treatment and posttreatment follow-up of AIS. Further discussion of treatment of AIS can be found in Chapter 20.

11.2 THE COLUMNAR EPITHELIUM

The cervical columnar epithelium extends from its junction with the endometrium at the internal cervical os down the canal to either metaplastic or to native squamous epithelium.[10–12] In young women, in particular, the columnar epithelium often extends out the external os to various degrees on the cervical portio and rarely to the adjacent cervical-vaginal margin. The columnar epithelium that lines the endocervical canal consists mostly of tall, cylindrical, single-layer, secretory cells with basally situated nuclei (Figure 11.1). The majority of endocervical cells secrete mucus, but approximately 4% to 6% are ciliary cells that may facilitate sperm transport (see Chapter 2). Reserve cells lie immediately beneath the basal zone of the epithelium. The columnar cells lie over stroma in the form of ridges and clefts. Columnar epithelium on the ectocervix colposcopically presents as villous structures measuring 1.0 mm × 0.2 mm. (Figure 11.2). Histologically, these villi demonstrate a central core covered by a similar single layer of columnar cells (Figure 11.1).

11.3 THE FATE OF COLUMNAR EPITHELIUM

Glandular epithelium can present in many different ways. It can remain in its original form, be transformed to normal squamous epithelium through the process of metaplasia, or undergo an atypical metaplastic process producing squamous neoplasia. Least common is transformation into glandular neoplasia. Furthermore, more than one process may occur at any one time. So, a field of AIS may coexist with normal metaplasia, or a glandular lesion may coexist with squamous disease. The latter is termed "mixed disease" and

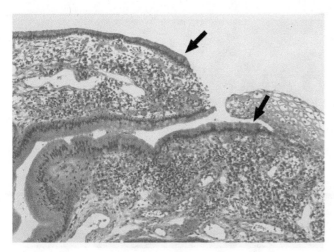

FIGURE 11.1.   Histology of the villous structures of an ectopy demonstrating tall columnar epithelium with basally situated nuclei (see *arrows*). (Note that one *arrow* shows the SCJ) Hematoxylin and eosin stain, medium-power magnification. (Reprinted from Wright VC. *Color Atlas of Colposcopy—Cervix, Vagina and Vulva.* Houston, TX: Biomedical Communications, 2003, with permission.)

is found in 46% to 72% of AIS cases, with CIN 3 being the most common squamous lesion.[3] Also, about 2% of CIN 2,3 lesions are found to have a coexisting glandular lesion.[3,7,13]

11.4 NEOPLASTIC TRANSFORMATION OF COLUMNAR EPITHELIUM

The exact nature of the cytologic and histologic transformation from normal glandular cells to neoplastic cells is poorly understood. Although controversy exists about whether the process that leads to glandular neoplasia is initiated in reserve cell hyperplasia, as in squamous disease, it is clear that the undifferentiated bipotential reserve cell can

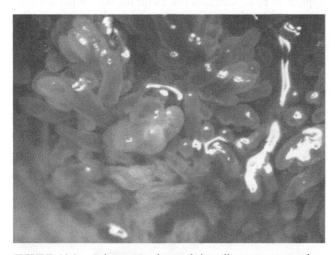

FIGURE 11.2.   Colposcopic photo of the villous structures of an ectopy. They remain transparent after acetic acid is applied, and blood vessels are not well defined. (Reprinted from Wright VC, Shier RM. *Colposcopy of Adenocarcinoma In Situ and Adenocarcinoma of the Cervix—Differentiation from other Cervical Lesions.* Houston, TX: Biomedical Communications, 2000, with permission.)

differentiate into either a squamous or a glandular cell. As discussed previously, most cases of AIS occur in the company of squamous disease.[6,8] However, squamous metaplasia itself, either normal or abnormal, does not produce glandular disease. Two types of glandular metaplasia have been identified: tubal (ciliated cell) and intestinal (goblet cell). Although 48% of cervical glandular and squamous neoplasias contain glandular metaplasia, there is no clear evidence that the changes are precursors to AIS and adenocarcinoma.[14] Once abnormal cells develop, they can exist in single or multiple layers and can be stratified or pseudostratified. The underlying villous structures in disease can remain as single structures (Figure 11.3) or colposcopically appear as coalescing or clumping masses (Figure 11.4). The result produces colposcopic findings that are different from those of squamous disease.

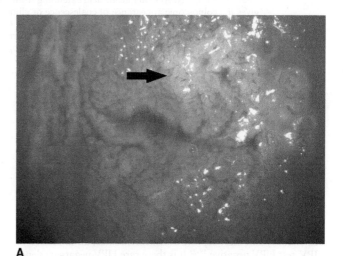

A

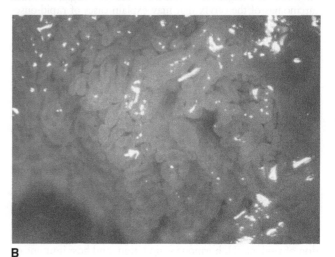

B

FIGURE 11.3.   **A:** AIS of the anterior cervical lip demonstrating simple villous structures that stain faintly acetowhite (see *arrow*). The area is surrounded by typical normal villi. (Reprinted from Wright VC, Shier RM. *Colposcopy of Adenocarcinoma In Situ and Adenocarcinoma of the Cervix—Differentiation from other Cervical Lesions.* Houston, TX: Biomedical Communications, 2000, with permission.) **B:** Higher magnification of previous lesion. (Reprinted from Wright VC. *Comprehensive Colposcopy Review—Cervix, Vagina, Vulva and Adjacent Sites CD-ROM.* Houston, TX: Biomedical Communications, 2008, with permission.)

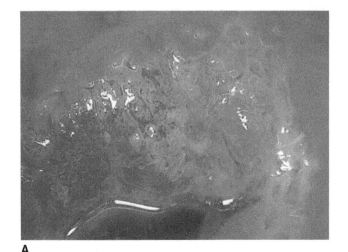

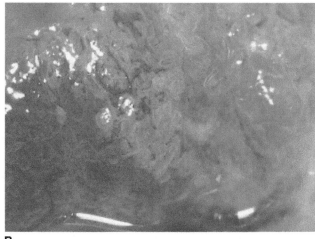

A

B

FIGURE 11.4. **A:** AIS after acetic acid extending from 12 o'clock to 4 o'clock. The glandular proliferative process gives the colposcopic appearance of coalescence or clumping. (Reprinted from Wright VC, Shier RM. *Colposcopy of Adenocarcinoma In Situ and Adenocarcinoma of the Cervix—Differentiation from other Cervical Lesions.* Houston, TX: Biomedical Communications, 2000, with permission.) **B:** Higher magnification view of previous lesion. (Reprinted from Wright VC. *Color Atlas of Colposcopy—Cervix, Vagina and Vulva.* Houston, TX: Biomedical Communications, 2003, with permission.)

11.5 STIMULUS OF DISEASE DEVELOPMENT

The process that leads from normal columnar epithelium to cervical adenocarcinoma requires human papillomavirus (HPV), just as the oncogenic process leading to SCC requires HPV.[15–18] Using PCR-based tests, 99.7% of cervical squamous cell cancers and 93% of adenocarcinomas test positive for HPV.[15,18] Only misclassified true endometrial carcinomas of the cervix and rare clear cell, serous, and mesonephric adenocarcinomas, all unrelated to HPV, test HPV negative.[18–23] It is these rare HPV-negative adenocarcinomas of the cervix that may explain cases of rapid-onset cervical cancer in virgins and, in some cases, in nonvirgin young women.[19] A number of studies have demonstrated that the frequency of HPV-negative cervical adenocarcinomas increases with age, adding further support to molecular and histologic evidence of misclassification of endometrial carcinomas as cervical.[20–23]

Over 80% of cervical adenocarcinomas are found to have one of two high-risk HPV types, either HPV 16 or HPV 18.[18] Some of the remainder have HPV 45, which is closely related to phylogenetically to HPV 18.[17,18] This predominance of two HPV types is more dramatic than for SCC, in which HPV 16 and 18 account for 70% compared to 86% in adenocarcinoma.[18] While HPV 18 is more common in adenocarcinoma than it is in SCC, HPV 16 is still the most prevalent type in glandular cervical cancer in all areas of the world other than Southeast Asia.[18] HPV 16 is also the most common HPV type found in AIS. This indicates that certain HPV types in association with potential cofactors (trauma to columnar cells, alteration of vaginal pH, hormone stimulation, and host immune or other external cofactors) produce two types of abnormal histological findings by reserve cell stimulation occurring either independently or simultaneously.[7,13] This is further supported by the presence of AIS within superficial and deep endocervical crypts whose surface epithelium has been replaced by benign metaplastic or dysplastic epithelium (Figure 11.5).[3,6,18]

A number of studies demonstrate an increased risk for cervical cancer that may reflect hormonal influence on the cervix. Included risk factors are high parity, early age at first full-term pregnancy, and long-term OC use.[24–29] Moreover, it has been suggested that long-term use of OCs, particularly among young women, increases the risk of adenocarcinoma of the cervix.[24,26] A pooled analysis of IARC HPV prevalence surveys confirmed that the probable cofactors noted above are not associated with HPV prevalence but are more likely involved in the transition from HPV infection to neoplastic cervical lesions through direct influence of increased levels of estrogen on HPV promoter regions.[17] Overall cervical cancer risk appears to double with 5 or more years of OC use but returns to that of "never users" 10 years following cessation of use.[29] A 2004 evaluation of US SEER data demonstrated an increased risk for AIS with duration of OC use, with the highest risk for 12 or more years of use (odds ratio, 5.5).[26] Progestin-only contraceptives appear to increase the risk of cervical cancer only slightly.[17] Obesity appears to be a risk factor for adenocarcinoma but not squamous cell cancer, also suggesting that estrogen may be a cofactor in glandular oncogenesis. Although current smoking appears to be an increased risk factor for SCC, it has not been shown to have the same association with adenocarcinoma.[28]

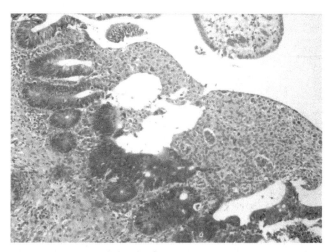

FIGURE 11.5. Histology of buried disease beneath dysplastic epithelium. It is obviously not visible colposcopically. Hematoxylin and eosin stain, medium-power magnification. (Photo courtesy of Dr. V. Cecil Wright.).

11.6 MORPHOLOGIC SPECTRUM OF GLANDULAR INTRAEPITHELIAL LESIONS

In 1953, Friedell and McKay[30] were the first to describe AIS. Intraepithelial glandular lesions of the cervix likely have a morphologic spectrum (like squamous) from mild to severe, but changes less than AIS have been much more difficult to reliably categorize than grades of CIN. This is because the grading of squamous intraepithelial lesions is based primarily on the percent of the epithelial thickness involved with dysplastic cells, whereas all grades of glandular intraepithelial neoplasia (GIN) less than AIS have the same changes as AIS but are just less severe. Hence, severe glandular atypia, also known as GIN Grade 2, has fewer mitotic figures, more preservation of polarity, less stratification, and more mucin than AIS, also known as GIN Grade 3. Mild glandular atypia, or GIN Grade 1, has even less prominent findings. Because classification of glandular abnormalities based on these findings is even more arbitrary than classification of squamous lesions, the GIN grading system is not used widely in the United States.[31]

11.7 PROBLEMS DETECTING ADENOCARCINOMA *IN SITU* AND ADENOCARCINOMA

The incidence of both squamous cell CIS and AIS has increased over the past 40 years, but screening, detection, and treatment of precancer appear to have only impacted the incidence of SCC, which has decreased by at least 75%, while the incidence of cervical adenocarcinoma has remained relatively stable or increased.[32-34] Compared to SCC, adenocarcinomas comprise a disproportionate percentage of tumors occurring among women screened within the past 5 years,[35] and a negative cytology report affords less protection against adenocarcinoma than SCC,[36] suggesting that some AIS lesions may progress rapidly to invasion or fail to be detected by cytologic screening.[33] Additionally, data suggest that cytologic screening may be less sensitive in detecting lesions caused by HPV 18, found more commonly in adenocarcinoma than in SCC.[37] This strong association of HPV 18 with adenocarcinoma may be secondary to a predilection of this HPV type for the endocervical canal, where persistence would be more occult and less likely to produce the early cytologic findings of koilocytotic atypia/LSIL so clearly demonstrated on screening for squamous cell precursor lesions.[33]

Hence, the prevention of invasive cervical adenocarcinoma presents specific challenges: (1) The morphology of precursors to AIS has not been well defined, (2) AIS typically involves the endocervical canal, making sampling more difficult, (3) invasive adenocarcinoma may develop from small foci of AIS, and (4) historically the diverse and sometimes subtle cytologic and colposcopic features of AIS have not been widely appreciated.[33,38,39]

Problems impacting the detection and management of cervical glandular precancer and cancer include reduced sensitivity of screening with cervical cytology, colposcopic inexperience and subtle colposcopic findings, lesion size and location, skip lesions, buried disease, and mixed lesions.

11.7.1 Reduced Sensitivity of Cytologic Screening

The prognostic value of cytology has been shown to be less in both magnitude and duration for adenocarcinoma than for squamous carcinoma, whereas the impact of screening on adenosquamous carcinoma is similar to its impact on squamous carcinoma.[40] Pap tests may not contain cells suggestive of glandular disease. Atypical glandular cells are noted on cytology reports in only 41% to 70% of cases of AIS.[38-46] Cytology is more likely to detect a coexisting squamous abnormality because these are more likely to be ectocervical, and if in the canal, more likely to be proximal to a glandular lesion and therefore sampled. In contrast, glandular lesions, in the absence of a squamous abnormality, or if buried beneath one, are less likely to be sampled.

Cullimore et al. noted that women found to have only AIS were 4.8 years older than women having both CIN and AIS.[41] This finding suggests that cytology is more sensitive in identifying squamous neoplasia than glandular neoplasia. It also suggests that earlier diagnosis of mixed disease may be possible when colposcopists are motivated to search for, and find, coexistent glandular and squamous lesions.[41] In addition to the reduced protection of cervical screening for adenocarcinoma, protection from developing any cervical carcinoma has been shown to be shorter in younger women (<40 years) than in older (>40 years),[46] confirming results of a prior large study carried out in UK.[47] Endocervical sampling, using an endocervical brush, may improve the detection of AIS. However, cells demonstrating AIS, even if present on the smear, may not be noticed.[45]

The Bethesda System 2001 removed the term "of undetermined significance" from the prior glandular cell category of AGUS, creating the category of atypical glandular cells (AGC) (see Chapter 2).[48] Importantly, endocervical AIS now has its own category. Although a cytologic interpretation of AIS is highly correlated with risk for a similar high-grade glandular histologic finding, AGC Pap results are not often found to be highly associated with a glandular lesion at colposcopy, nor is it possible to differentiate between AIS and adenocarcinoma.[49-53] A recent review of seven large studies of AGC found significant cervical neoplasia (CIN 2,3 or AIS) in 23.3%,[54] and numerous other studies have reported CIN 2,3, AIS, or cancer in 9% to 38%, and invasive cervical cancer in 3% to 17%.[50-53] The rate and type of high-grade squamous and glandular abnormalities in women with AGC varies with age; women under 35 rarely have gynecologic malignancy but have CIN more commonly than older women.[52,53] Cumulative studies of cases presenting with AGC cytologic findings qualified as "favor neoplastic" indicate that a significant pathologic component will be found in 46% to 72% of cases, whereas for AGC "not otherwise specified" the rate of significant abnormalities is much lower (11% to 33%).[55-57] One large retrospective study found some grade of CIN in 28.3%, AIS in 3.5%, endometrial hyperplasia in 4.7%, and cancer in 5.5%, but these rates vary widely between studies.[49] Wide ranges reported between studies reflect interobserver and interlaboratory variation in the cytologic interpretation of AGC, as well as differences in the median age of the population evaluated. Risk for CIN 2,3 is significantly increased for HPV-positive women with AGC in comparison with those testing HPV negative (odds ratio 39.6), whereas the rate of HPV–non-associated cancers is significantly higher in patients HPV negative versus those HPV positive (4% vs. 0.4%).[54] In 98% of cases, an AIS cytology result indicates that a glandular lesion will be found.[41]

All atypical glandular cell interpretations, including AIS, must be differentiated from the following benign changes: (1) reactive and regenerative changes in the columnar and squamous epithelium; (2) Arias-Stella changes in the cervix (a rare pregnancy change of endocervical crypts characterized by enlarged hyperchromatic nuclei of irregular shape with abundant cytoplasm +/− increased secretory activity—however, mitotic changes are not seen); (3) cervical polyp; (4) mesonephric duct hyperplasia; (5) tubal or serous metaplasia; (6) cervical endometriosis; (7) microglandular hyperplasia; (8) endocervical changes associated with an intrauterine device; (9) squamous dysplasia involving glandular epithelium; (10) cervical adenocarcinoma; and (11) invasive endometrial carcinoma.[8,58]

11.7.2 Colposcopic Inexperience and Subtle Findings

Most colposcopists have found colposcopy to be of little value in recognizing AIS. The barriers to colposcopic detection of AIS include a number of issues already discussed: inexperience of the colposcopist in recognizing glandular lesions, more frequent location of lesions within the endocervical canal, subjective colposcopic findings that often look similar to a normal ectopy, and the frequent finding of more dramatic colposcopic changes in adjacent CIN and the occasional buried glandular disease under squamous abnormality.[33] Additionally, a cytologic report of a squamous abnormality most often motivates the colposcopist to search for a squamous lesion and be satisfied if it is found, rather than suspecting the presence of a glandular lesion as well. The lack of firm criteria to base a suspicion of glandular disease is due in part to the rarity of these cases and, hence, the inexperience of even the most "experienced" colposcopists. Thus, AIS is less commonly diagnosed than its malignant counterpart, indicating that colposcopists are often missing AIS and probably unknowingly destroying AIS when ablating squamous lesions. This is also why AIS comes as a surprise finding on biopsy reports and loop specimens. Missing AIS is of increasing concern due to the rising incidence of both AIS and adenocarcinoma.[5,33,59] Concerted efforts must be made through increased education of colposcopists in the detection of glandular lesions and heightened vigilance towards finding AIS and adenocarcinoma.

11.7.3 Lesion Size and Location

Studies indicate that most glandular lesions are located within the transformation zone.[4,7,60,61] Specifically, Muntz et al. found AIS lesions to involve the ectocervical transformation zone exclusively in 53% of cases and the endocervical canal exclusively in only 5%.[60] Contiguous involvement was noted in 38%, indicating that 95% of cases were available for partial or complete visualization through the colposcope. Many of the lesions are small, with 48% of AIS lesions involving only one cervical quadrant versus only 10% occupying four quadrants.[13,41,62] The linear length of AIS disease (the distance over the tissue surface between caudal and cephalad edges) usually does not exceed 15 mm.[13,41,62] Women younger than 36 years of age have a significantly lower disease volume than do women over this age, suggesting that the precursor lesion increases in extent and depth prior to becoming invasive.[63] The largest lesions with the greatest linear length and underlying crypt involvement are found in older patients.[63] The most abnormal histologic findings occur centrally, meaning that adenocarcinoma is more likely to be located toward or within the canal than widely out on the ectocervix, especially in older women.

Bertrand et al. studied the highest focus of cervical involvement of AIS measured from the maximal convexity of the cervix in hysterectomy specimens and from the resection margin in excisional specimens.[6] Using these measurement parameters, the highest focus did not exceed 19.9 mm in 78.9% of cases. Among the 21.1% extending beyond 19.9 mm, none exceeded 29.9 mm. Such measurements do not reflect the true linear length of disease but provide guidelines for designing the cylindrical excision to maximize encompassing and removing the disease.

11.7.4 Skip (Multifocal) Lesions

Unlike high-grade cervical squamous lesions, which present as "skip lesions" only in posttreatment failures, glandular lesions can present *de novo* as skip lesions (i.e., lesions which are not

contiguous).[64] Skip glandular lesions are foci involving different portions of the endocervical mucosa separated by normal epithelium. Multifocal AIS by definition is a complete normal radial histologic section separating two or more areas of AIS. The finding of normal and involved glands within the same slide is not accepted as multifocal as this may merely represent fingers of contiguous abnormality extending into normal mucosa.[6,62] Skip lesions occur in 6.5% to 15% of AIS lesions.[6,62] Skip lesions are uncommon, but when they do exist and are not far apart, they rarely interfere with colposcopic assessment. However, because skip lesions do occur and most often are not identified at colposcopy, negative margins on a diagnostic excisional specimen demonstrating AIS do not necessarily mean that the lesion has been completely excised.[64] Therefore, the primary importance of skip lesions with AIS is diminished predictive value of negative margins for absence of residual disease.

11.7.5 Buried Disease

Glandular disease can involve the superficial and deep crypts that are covered by benign metaplastic or dysplastic squamous epithelium (Figure 11.5).[6,7,65] Although the crypts usually open through such tissue, the glandular component may not be colposcopically visible. Such buried disease occurs in 60% of cases of AIS.[63,65]

11.7.6 Mixed Disease

A squamous lesion coexists with AIS in more than one half of AIS cases.[3,7,9] More than 80% of the squamous lesions will be CIN 3. Less than 3% to 4% of squamous disease cases are invasive, but when they are, they are usually microinvasive. The squamous component is usually colposcopically visible. The glandular area can be adjacent to the squamous lesion (Figure 11.6), be sandwiched between two squamous lesions (Figure 11.7), or be cephalad to the squamous lesion (the most common location) (Figure 11.8). Studying the vascular patterns, intercapillary distance, surface contour, color tone and opacity, and clarity of demarcation (both before and after the application of acetic acid) can enable the colposcopist to grade the squamous lesion(s).[66] The glandular component, when seen, often can be differentiated from other cervical lesions using the criteria described below.[67]

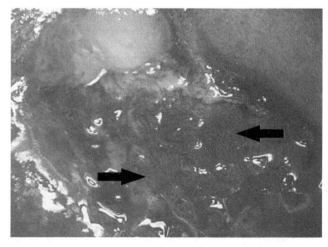

FIGURE 11.6. AIS appearing like the villous structures of an ectopy on the posterior cervical lip. A well-defined afferent and efferent vessel can be seen (see *arrows*). Abutting it anteriorly is a well-defined densely acetowhite CIN 3 lesion. (Photo courtesy of Dr. V. Cecil Wright.)

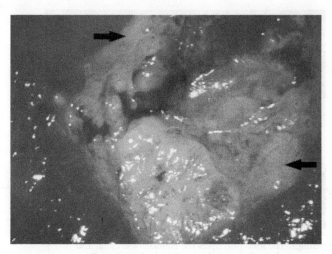

FIGURE 11.7. A well-defined AIS lesion from the 5 o'clock to 10 o'clock positions separates two high-grade squamous lesions (see *arrows*). (Reprinted from Wright VC, Shier RM. *Colposcopy of Adenocarcinoma In Situ and Adenocarcinoma of the Cervix—Differentiation from other Cervical Lesions.* Houston, TX: Biomedical Communications, 2000, with permission.)

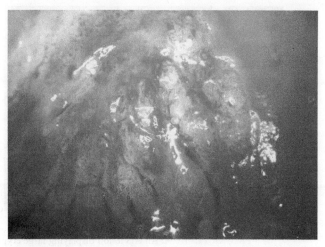

FIGURE 11.9. An AIS lesion after acetic acid application demonstrating discrete patches of budding, proliferating villi of different sizes. Single and multiple dots created by vessel loops within the growing projections are visible. The areas resemble the fused villous processes of early normal metaplasia. (Reprinted from Wright VC, Shier RM. *Colposcopy of Adenocarcinoma In Situ and Adenocarcinoma of the Cervix—Differentiation from other Cervical Lesions.* Houston, TX: Biomedical Communications, 2000, with permission.)

11.8 THREE COLPOSCOPIC PRESENTATIONS OF AIS AND ADENOCARCINOMA

Three colposcopic appearances of glandular disease have been described.[67] The most common form is a papillary expression resembling an immature transformation zone. After acetic acid is applied, discrete patches of somewhat acetowhite, proliferating villi, varying in size, can be identified. They look like the fused villous processes of early, normal metaplasia (Figures 11.9 and 11.10), which is why these lesions are often dismissed without sampling.[3,9,67,68] The second most common form is that of a flat, variegated red and white area resembling an immature transformation zone (Figure 11.11).[3,9,67] The least common presentation consists of one or more individual, isolated, elevated, densely acetowhite lesion(s) overlying columnar epithelium (Figure 11.12).[3,9,67] The degree of acetowhiteness exhibited by glandular disease reflects the degree of the villous proliferative process, multiplication of the central villous core (the more, the whiter), and the histologic pseudostratification of columnar cells with their enlarged hyperchromatic nuclei (Figsure 11.13–11.16).[3,9,67] In most cases, when glandular and squamous diseases coexist, the squamous component is more likely to be noted because it is more likely to be visible and distinct (Figure 11.6).

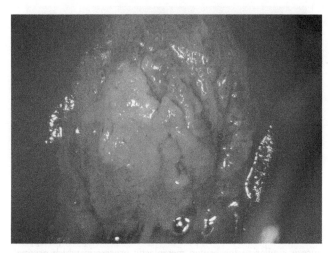

FIGURE 11.8. A densely acetowhite papillary AIS lesion lies centrally. Peripherally, it is surrounded by a high-grade squamous lesion. (Reprinted from Wright VC, Shier RM. *Colposcopy of Adenocarcinoma In Situ and Adenocarcinoma of the Cervix—Differentiation from other Cervical Lesions.* Houston, TX: Biomedical Communications, 2000, with permission.)

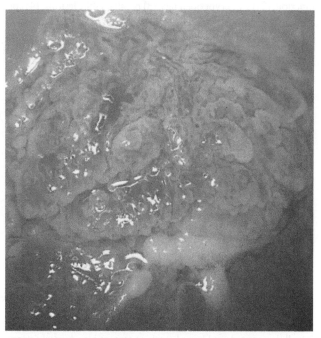

FIGURE 11.10. Benign metaplasia with formation of discrete patches of fused villi after the application of acetic acid. It easily could be confused with an AIS lesion (compare with Figure 11.9). (Reprinted from Wright VC. *Color Atlas of Colposcopy—Cervix, Vagina and Vulva.* Houston, TX: Biomedical Communications, 2003, with permission.)

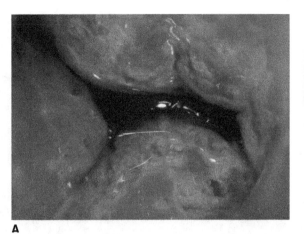

A

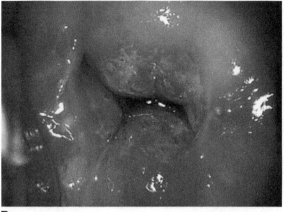

B

FIGURE 11.11. **A:** An AIS lesion displaying large crypt openings. The lesion occupies the endocervical canal and exhibits a patchy red and white color after acetic acid has been applied. (Reprinted from Wright VC, Shier RM: *Colposcopy of Adenocarcinoma In Situ and Adenocarcinoma of the Cervix—Differentiation from other Cervical Lesions.* Houston, TX: Biomedical Communications, 2000, with permission.) **B:** Lower magnification of previous lesion. (Reprinted from Wright VC. *Comprehensive Colposcopy Review—Cervix, Vagina, Vulva and Adjacent Sites CD-ROM.* Houston, TX: Biomedical Communications, 2008, with permission.)

11.9 DIFFERENTIATING GLANDULAR DISEASE FROM OTHER ENTITIES

There is no single colposcopic appearance that characterizes glandular dysplasia, AIS, or adenocarcinoma. To complicate matters, colposcopic appearances of these entities often mimic other conditions. The generally accepted colposcopic criteria for grading squamous lesions do not apply to glandular lesions.[3,9,66,67,69,70]

Glandular lesions are to be suspected when any of the following colposcopic findings are observed: (1) a lesion overlying columnar epithelium not contiguous with the squamocolumnar junction, (2) large crypt openings, (3) papillary-like lesions, (4) epithelial budding, (5) variegated red and white lesions, (6) waste-thread-like vessels, (7) tendril-like vessels, (8) root-like vessels, (9) character-writing-like vessels, and (10) single- or multiple-dot formations as seen in the tips of the papillary excrescences.[67,71,72]

11.9.1 Surface Patterns in Glandular Disease

11.9.1.1 Elevated Lesions

When elevated lesions, particularly those exhibiting irregular surfaces, are lying over columnar epithelium, the differential diagnosis includes metaplasia (Figure 11.17), condylomata, AIS (Figures 11.3, 11.4, 11.9, and 11.12), adenocarcinoma, and microglandular hyperplasia. In glandular disease, after the application of acetic acid, proliferating villi appear in discrete patches that vary in size resembling immature metaplasia. This is the most common colposcopic presentation of AIS.[68,69,72] Less commonly, a single, densely acetowhite lesion overlies columnar epithelium with no contact with the squamous border (Figure 11.12). Metaplastic-looking areas, particularly in the presence of a glandular cytology result, should be biopsied since this may actually be a glandular lesion.

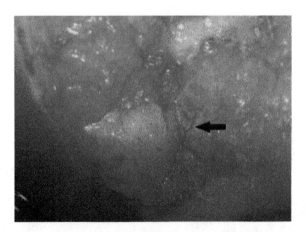

FIGURE 11.12. A well-defined AIS lesion overlying columnar epithelium and not in contact with the squamous border. It is elevated, is well demarcated, and has a branching taproot blood vessel (*arrow*) coursing over its surface. (Reprinted from Wright VC, Shier RM. *Colposcopy of Adenocarcinoma In Situ and Adenocarcinoma of the Cervix—Differentiation from other Cervical Lesions.* Houston, TX: Biomedical Communications, 2000, with permission.)

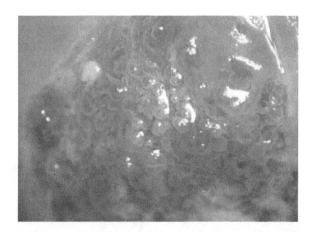

FIGURE 11.13. An AIS lesion after acetic acid exhibiting original, individual villi as well as proliferating villi. The colposcopic appearance is similar to the benign metaplastic process in which original, individual villi fuse together, creating clumps or tongues in their transformation into squamous epithelium. (Reprinted from Wright VC, Shier RM. *Colposcopy of Adenocarcinoma In Situ and Adenocarcinoma of the Cervix—Differentiation from other Cervical Lesions.* Houston, TX: Biomedical Communications, 2000, with permission.)

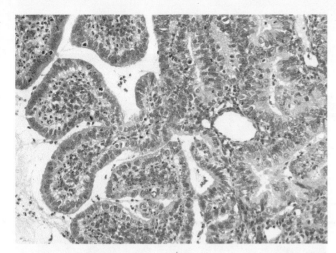

FIGURE 11.14. The histology of the AIS lesion in Figure 11.13 showing multiplication of the central villous core. The colposcopic impression is very similar to that caused by the fusing of villous structures that occurs in active metaplasia. Hematoxylin and eosin stain, medium-power magnification. (Reprinted from Wright VC, Shier RM. *Colposcopy of Adenocarcinoma In Situ and Adenocarcinoma of the Cervix—Differentiation from Other Cervical Lesions.* Houston, TX: Biomedical Communications, 2000, with permission.)

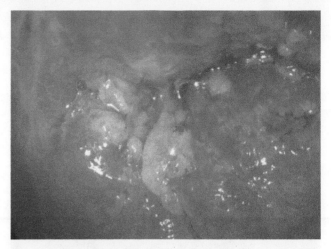

FIGURE 11.17. Metaplasia after acetic acid has been applied. Elevated, well-defined acetowhite areas lie over columnar epithelium. Biopsy is recommended to exclude glandular disease. (Reprinted from Wright VC. *Color Atlas of Colposcopy—Cervix, Vagina and Vulva.* Houston, TX: Biomedical Communications, 2003, with permission.)

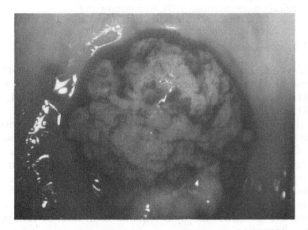

FIGURE 11.15. An invasive cervical adenocarcinoma after acetic acid application. It is papillary and more densely acetowhite than is the AIS lesion shown in Figure 11.13. Numerous atypical blood vessels are evident. (Reprinted from Wright VC, Shier RM. *Colposcopy of Adenocarcinoma In Situ and Adenocarcinoma of the Cervix—Differentiation from Other Cervical Lesions.* Houston, TX: Biomedical Communications, 2000, with permission.)

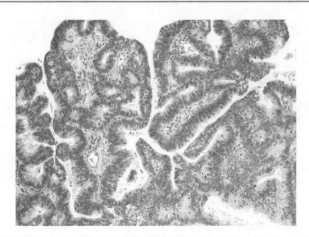

FIGURE 11.16. The histology of the lesion in Figure 11.15 revealing the proliferative process and multiplication of the central villous core that is responsible for the dense acetowhiteness. Hematoxylin and eosin stain, medium-power magnification.

11.9.1.2 Lesions with Large Crypt Openings

Some AIS demonstrate a patchy red and white surface rather than the uniform dense acetowhiteness as seen in high-grade squamous intraepithelial neoplasia (Figures 11.11, 11.18, and 11.19).[3,9] Frequently, very large crypt openings are seen (Figure 11.11).

11.9.1.3 Papillary Lesions

Papillary excrescences must be differentiated from normal papillary glandular mucosa (the villous structures of columnar epithelium constituting the ectopy) (Figure 11.2) and also from metaplasia (Figure 11.10), condylomata (Figure 11.20), AIS (Figures 11.3, 11.4, 11.9, and 11.21–11.23), adenocarcinoma (Figures 11.15 and 11.24–11.27), SCC, and microglandular hyperplasia (Figures 11.28 and 11.29). MGH represents a florid example of reserve cell hyperplasia with glandular differentiation in response to hormone stimulation. Colposcopically it appears yellow (similar to the color of chicken fat).[62,72,73] In AIS, the papillary processes may appear colposcopically as single villi (Figures 11.3 and 11.6) or as proliferative villi, appearing clumped in a manner similar to that of a developing metaplastic transformation zone (Figures 11.4, 11.9, 11.10, 11.13, 11.15, 11.21, and 11.22).[3,9,73] Differentiating colposcopically between these entities may be impossible, hence the need for biopsies.

11.9.1.4 Epithelial Budding

AIS can cause villi to proliferate in a "budding" fashion (Figure 11.30). The proliferations have broad bases and many have serrated outer edges. In the case of budding, differentiation should be made between the budding of immature metaplastic epithelium (Figure 11.31), budding of immature condylomata (Figure 11.32), and that of AIS (Figure 11.30).[3,9,73,74] Colposcopically directed biopsy is always necessary to differentiate.

11.9.1.5 Lesions with a Patchy (Variegated) Red and White Surface

This is the second most common expression of glandular disease.[3,9,75] The surface may be slightly uneven or rough (Figures 11.11, 11.18, 11.33, and 11.34), or it can simply resemble an immature transformation zone. When a variegated coloration

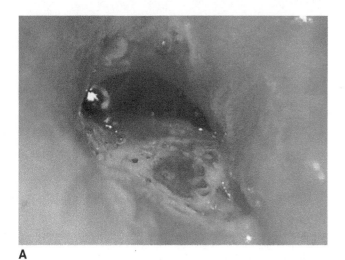

A

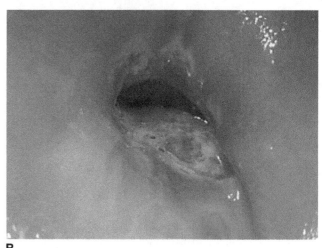

B

FIGURE 11.18.   **A:** An AIS lesion occupies the endocervical canal. It is patchy red and white (variegated) after acetic acid. A large "gland"/crypt opening can be seen at the 11 o'clock position with glandular proliferation surrounding it. (Reprinted from Wright VC, Shier RM. *Colposcopy of Adenocarcinoma In Situ and Adenocarcinoma of the Cervix—Differentiation from Other Cervical Lesions*. Houston, TX: Biomedical Communications, 2000, with permission.) **B:** Lower magnification of previous cervix. (Reprinted from *Wright VC: Comprehensive Colposcopy Review—Cervix, Vagina, Vulva and Adjacent Sites CD-ROM*. Houston, TX: Biomedical Communications, 2008, with permission.)

is seen after acetic acid application, the colposcopist should differentiate between a developing normal transformation zone (Figure 11.35), AIS (Figures 11.11, 11.18, 11.33, and 11.34), and adenocarcinoma (Figure 11.36), only possible through biopsy.

11.9.2 Atypical Blood Vessels

Glandular disease causes a variety of atypical blood vessels to form (Figures 11.37–11.39). The most common are the single and multiple dots that can be seen in the tips of single or proliferating excrescences (Figures 11.40 and 11.41).[3,9,74]

Less common are waste-thread, tendril (Figures 11.15, 11.42, and 11.43), tap and tuberous root shaped (Figures 11.44 and 11.45), and character-writing blood vessels (Figures 11.46–11.49).[3,9,75] Some of these configurations are also found in other cervical entities such as metaplasia (Figure 11.50), condylomata (Figures 11.20, 11.32, and 11.51), and squamous cell cancer (Figure 11.52). Punctation, mosaicism, and corkscrew vessels, although common in squamous disease, do not appear in glandular disease (see Chapter 10). While all these findings have been associated with AIS, the sensitivity, specificity, and positive and negative predictive values of these findings are unknown. Biopsy is required in all cases to confirm the diagnosis.

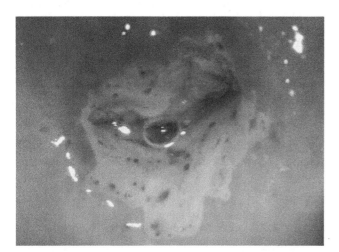

FIGURE 11.19.   A high-grade cervical intraepithelial squamous neoplastic lesion (CIN 3) occupies the endocervical canal. After acetic acid, the lesion has become densely acetowhite from border to border and does not exhibit the red and white coloration seen with glandular lesions. (Reprinted from Wright VC. *Color Atlas of Colposcopy—Cervix, Vagina and Vulva*. Houston, TX: Biomedical Communications, 2003, with permission.)

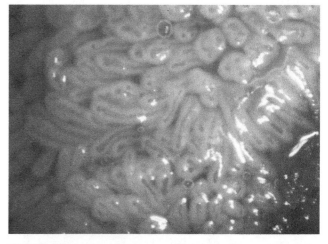

FIGURE 11.20.   The papillary proliferations of a cervical condyloma. It is villous appearing, and each excrescence has a very well-defined afferent and efferent blood vessel. This angioarchitecture produces single or multiple dots in their tips. (Reprinted from Wright VC, Shier RM. *Colposcopy of Adenocarcinoma In Situ and Adenocarcinoma of the Cervix—Differentiation from Other Cervical Lesions*. Houston, TX: Biomedical Communications, 2000, with permission.)

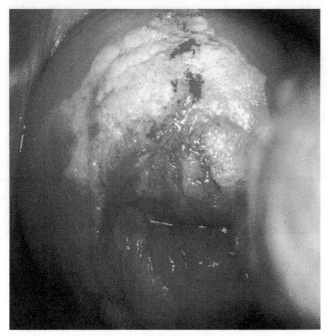

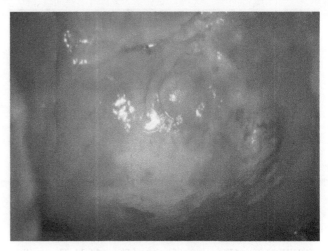

FIGURE 11.23. An AIS lesion appearing densely acetowhite and elevated is visible on the patient's left posterior cervical quadrant. Biopsy and excision proved AIS disease. (Reprinted from Wright VC. *Principles of Cervical Colposcopy*. Houston, TX: Biomedical Communications, 2004, with permission.)

FIGURE 11.21. Extensive AIS of the cervix looking much like the fused, acetowhite excrescences of metaplasia. Small dots are created by internal vessel loops. (Reprinted from Wright VC, Shier RM. *Colposcopy of Adenocarcinoma In Situ and Adenocarcinoma of the Cervix—Differentiation from Other Cervical Lesions*. Houston, TX: Biomedical Communications, 2000, with permission.)

11.10 CONFIRMING THE DIAGNOSIS

When AIS is obtained on biopsy or is suspected cytologically or colposcopically, an excisional procedure producing negative margins is required to be sure no invasive disease is present. Some consideration should be given to the size and configuration (height and radius) of the specimen. Basically, it should be cylindrical and deep enough to account for the depth of

crypt involvement and long enough to encompass the length of disease.[6,76] Both of these measurements are influenced by age as well as disease extent and location. The excision should be carried out under colposcopic guidance.[67,71] If the colposcopic biopsy or biopsies confirm AIS, and the lesion was not predicted by colposcopy, the practitioner should reexamine the cervix with the colposcope, noting the lower border and, if possible, the upper margin (i.e., the entire linear extent of the lesion). These measurements serve as a guide for determining the dimensions of the specimen to be produced by the excisional procedure.[71]

In the hands of a surgeon skilled in the use of a high-energy carbon dioxide (CO_2) laser under colposcopic visualization,

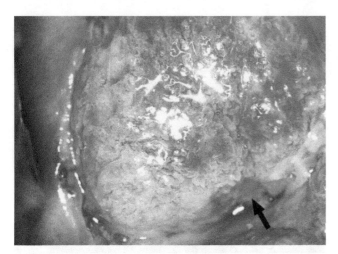

FIGURE 11.22. After acetic acid is applied, normal metaplastic epithelium can be identified between the 12 o'clock and 5 o'clock positions. In contrast, AIS exists between the 5 o'clock and 12 o'clock positions. Note that the two lesions look almost identical except that the AIS is slightly more papillary. The *arrow* depicts the external os. (Reprinted from Wright VC, Shier RM. *Colposcopy of Adenocarcinoma In Situ and Adenocarcinoma of the Cervix—Differentiation from Other Cervical Lesions*. Houston, TX: Biomedical Communications, 2000, with permission.)

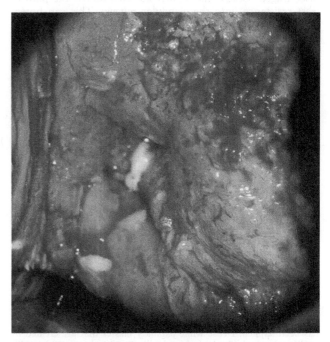

FIGURE 11.24. Papillary villous-like excrescences of an adenocarcinoma. (Reprinted from Wright VC, Shier RM. *Colposcopy of Adenocarcinoma In Situ and Adenocarcinoma of the Cervix—Differentiation from Other Cervical Lesions*. Houston, TX: Biomedical Communications, 2000, with permission.)

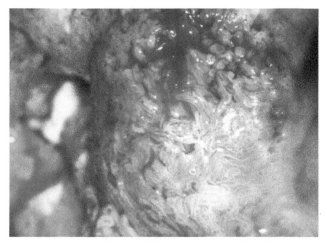

FIGURE 11.25. Higher magnification of Figure 11.24. The papillary structures resemble the villous structures of an ectopy. In some of the projections, afferent and efferent vessels can be identified. (Reprinted from Wright VC, Shier RM. *Colposcopy of Adenocarcinoma In Situ and Adenocarcinoma of the Cervix—Differentiation from Other Cervical Lesions.* Houston, TX: Biomedical Communications, 2000, with permission.)

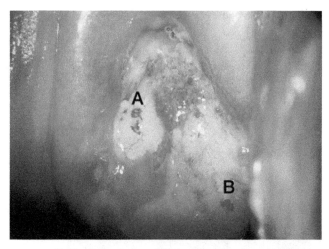

FIGURE 11.27. The smaller, densely acetowhite lesion is AIS (*Site A*). It is separated by normal tissue from a large acetowhite microinvasive squamous cell cancer (*Site B*). (Reprinted from Wright VC, Shier RM. *Colposcopy of Adenocarcinoma In Situ and Adenocarcinoma of the Cervix—Differentiation from Other Cervical Lesions.* Houston, TX: Biomedical Communications, 2000, with permission.)

cylindrical laser excision with scalpel excision of the apex can provide a superb specimen. However, cold knife conization with a scalpel alone, or loop electrosurgical excision procedure (LEEP) with a second (top hat) excision up the canal are the procedures more commonly performed because of the lack of availability of CO_2 lasers and of surgeons skilled in this procedure. However, LEEP excision is not ideal because the requirement of obtaining nearly 2.5 cm of endocervical canal in the cone requires a "top-hat" excision that by necessity has a burn margin through the center of the excised specimen. Excision using a monopolar electrosurgical (loop) excision is discouraged because monopolar currents follow the path of least resistance (into the glandular mucus). This can potentially distort benign as well as diseased glandular epithelium, making histologic interpretation difficult, if not impossible.[69]

11.10.1 Management of the Patient Desiring to Maintain Fertility

The safety of conservative management of the patient with AIS desiring to maintain fertility depends on the status and interpretability of the surgical margin of the cone specimen.[77] For optimal safety in the absence of hysterectomy, the adequacy and accuracy of follow-up by cytology alone are inadequate to rule out persistence, recurrence, or invasive disease beyond the cone margins.[36,42,78,79] Hence, patients who choose conservative management for AIS must be counselled regarding the importance of compliance with long-term follow-up and the potential risks of undetected persistent and recurrent glandular disease, including adenocarcinoma, despite negative screening results.[77–80]

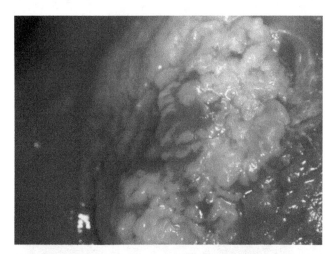

FIGURE 11.26. A large cervical adenocarcinoma after acetic acid has been applied. Dense white papillary masses that are created by proliferation look like agglutinated villi. (Reprinted from Wright VC, Shier RM. *Colposcopy of Adenocarcinoma In Situ and Adenocarcinoma of the Cervix—Differentiation from Other Cervical Lesions.* Houston, TX: Biomedical Communications, 2000, with permission.)

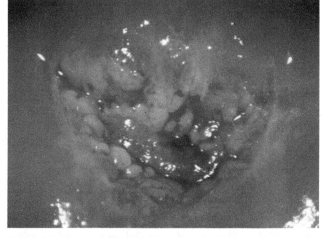

FIGURE 11.28. Microglandular hyperplasia. Large, yellow globular masses (with the color of chicken fat) lie over columnar epithelium. (Reprinted from Wright VC, Shier RM. *Colposcopy of Adenocarcinoma In Situ and Adenocarcinoma of the Cervix—Differentiation from Other Cervical Lesions.* Houston, TX: Biomedical Communications, 2000, with permission.)

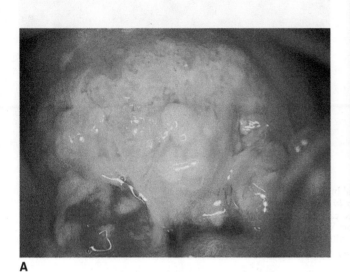
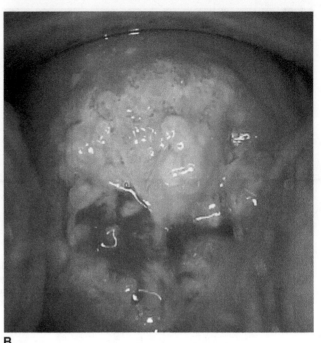

A   **B**

FIGURE 11.29. **A:** Extensive microglandular hyperplasia in a patient who is 6 weeks postpartum. Large papillary, globular masses having a whitish-yellow texture are noted. This mimics an adenocarcinoma (see Figure 11.26). (Reprinted from Wright VC, Shier RM. *Colposcopy of Adenocarcinoma In Situ and Adenocarcinoma of the Cervix—Differentiation from Other Cervical Lesions.* Houston, TX: Biomedical Communications, 2000, with permission.) **B:** Lower magnification of previous lesion. (Reprinted from Wright VC. *Comprehensive Colposcopy Review—Cervix, Vagina, Vulva and Adjacent Sites CD-ROM.* Houston, TX: Biomedical Communications, 2008, with permission.)

11.10.2 2006 ASCCP Guidelines for Postcone AIS Management

Hysterectomy is the *preferred* management postcone for AIS when no further childbearing is contemplated.[64] An excisional cone must always precede a hysterectomy to avoid the

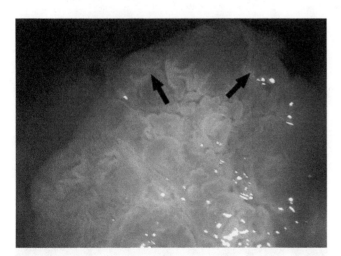

FIGURE 11.30. An AIS lesion demonstrating papillary features and scalloped-edged epithelial budding. Blood vessel patterns resembling character writing are noted in several peripheral locations (see *arrows*). (Reprinted from Wright VC, Shier RM. *Colposcopy of Adenocarcinoma In Situ and Adenocarcinoma of the Cervix—Differentiation from Other Cervical Lesions.* Houston, TX: Biomedical Communications, 2000, with permission.)

possibility that an occult invasive adenocarcinoma exists that would require a more radical surgical approach.[64] For women desiring continued fertility, postcone management depends on whether the margins of the excised cone specimen are negative or positive.

11.10.2.1 Significance of Negative Margins in the Excised Specimen

Most studies indicate that if the excised specimen's margins are negative, conservative management is permissible in women desiring future childbearing.[13,41,60,64,78,79,81–84] Because of skip lesions, negative margins are associated with persistent AIS in the extirpated uterus in up to 9% of cases.[64,79,81–84] On occasion, studies identified adenocarcinoma even when specimens had negative margins.[77,85,86]

If the patient elects to be managed conservatively, reevaluation at 6 months using a combination of cervical cytology, HPV DNA testing, and colposcopy with endocervical sampling is acceptable. Long-term follow-up is recommended for women who do not undergo hysterectomy.[64]

11.10.2.2 Significance of Positive Margins in the Excised Specimen

Cumulative studies indicate that positive margins in the excised specimen are of great clinical importance because of the high risk of remaining AIS (46% of cases) and invasive adenocarcinoma (16.7% of cases).[41,60,62,77,86–88] Repeat excision is therefore *preferred* to obtain negative margins for the conservatively managed patient with either a positive margin or a positive endocervical sampling obtained immediately after excision.[65] This is recommended both for women desiring further childbearing and for women choosing to have a simple hysterectomy. Failure to do so in the latter circumstance may

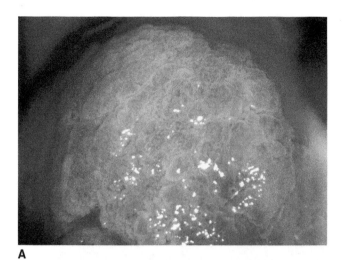

A

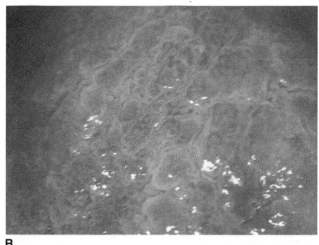

B

FIGURE 11.31.   **A:** Metaplasia demonstrating epithelial budding similar to that in Figure 11.30. (Reprinted from Wright VC, Shier RM. *Colposcopy of Adenocarcinoma In Situ and Adenocarcinoma of the Cervix—Differentiation from Other Cervical Lesions.* Houston, TX: Biomedical Communications, 2000, with permission.) **B:** Higher magnification view of the previous cervix. (Reprinted from Wright VC. *Color Atlas of Colposcopy—Cervix, Vagina and Vulva.* Houston, TX. Biomedical Communications, 2003, with permission.)

result in inadequate surgery (simple hysterectomy instead of radical hysterectomy) should invasive adenocarcinoma be found in the extirpated uterine cervix. When it is elected to manage women with positive margins conservatively, rather than by first repeating the conization, follow-up should be with a combination of cervical cytology, HPV DNA testing, and colposcopy with endocervical sampling as discussed for women with negative margins on the initial cone. Long-term follow-up is recommended for women who do not undergo hysterectomy, but is not further defined by the 2006 ASCCP

guidelines. Considering the potential for persistence and recurrence, it would seem to be prudent to repeat all four modalities every 6 months until at least four completely negative screens on all modalities have been obtained. Once this goal had been achieved, strict annual screening for at least 20 years, as recommended for the follow-up of women treated for CIN 2,3 would seem advisable.[64] Once reproduction is complete, hysterectomy has been advocated. It is not known whether this is necessary in the highly compliant patient without evidence of persistent disease.

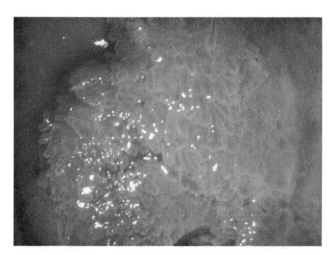

FIGURE 11.32.   Epithelial budding structures in a cervical condyloma. Many of the structures contain proliferating angioarchitecture resembling character writing. (Reprinted from Wright VC. *Color Atlas of Colposcopy—Cervix, Vagina and Vulva.* Houston, TX: Biomedical Communications, 2003, with permission.)

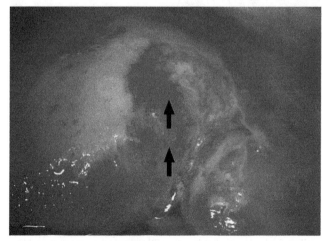

FIGURE 11.33.   A variegated red and white AIS lesion (*see arrows*) splits two acetowhite epithelial lesions. The indication that there is a glandular lesion is that squamous intraepithelial lesions are densely acetowhite from border to border. (Photo courtesy of Dr. V. Cecil Wright.)

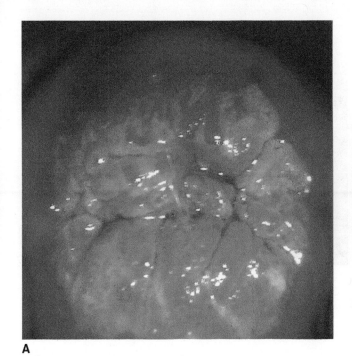

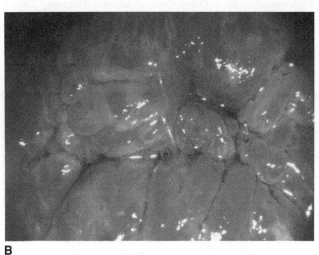

A

B

FIGURE 11.34. **A:** An extensive AIS lesion involving all cervical quadrants. It is patchy red and white after acetic acid. (Reprinted from Wright VC, Shier RM. *Colposcopy of Adenocarcinoma In Situ and Adenocarcinoma of the Cervix—Differentiation from Other Cervical Lesions.* Houston, TX: Biomedical Communications, 2000, with permission.) **B:** Higher magnification of previous cervix. (Reprinted from Wright VC. *Comprehensive Colposcopy Review—Cervix, Vagina, Vulva and Adjacent Sites CD-ROM.* Houston, TX: Biomedical Communications, 2008, with permission.)

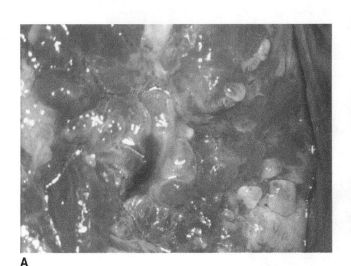

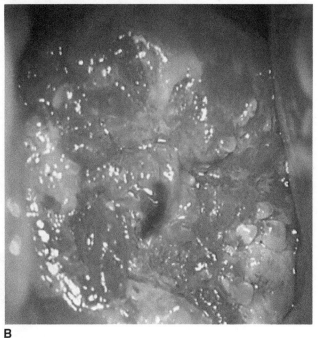

A

B

FIGURE 11.35. **A:** The variegated red and white acetowhite appearance of metaplasia. Metaplasia is forming glazed villi and bouquets of well-demarcated acetowhite epithelium overlying columnar epithelium. It mimics glandular disease. (Reprinted from Wright VC, Shier RM. *Colposcopy of Adenocarcinoma In Situ and Adenocarcinoma of the Cervix—Differentiation from Other Cervical Lesions.* Houston, TX: Biomedical Communications, 2000, with permission.) **B:** Lower magnification of previous lesion. (Reprinted from Wright VC. *Comprehensive Colposcopy Review—Cervix, Vagina, Vulva and Adjacent Sites CD-ROM.* Houston, TX: Biomedical Communications, 2008, with permission.)

FIGURE 11.36. The densely acetowhite high-grade squamous intraepithelial lesion is easily identified peripherally. Beneath it and extending into the endocervical canal is a variegated red and white lesion with dilated blood vessels representing an adenocarcinoma. (Reprinted from Wright VC, Shier RM. *Colposcopy of Adenocarcinoma In Situ and Adenocarcinoma of the Cervix— Differentiation from Other Cervical Lesions.* Houston, TX: Biomedical Communications, 2000, with permission.)

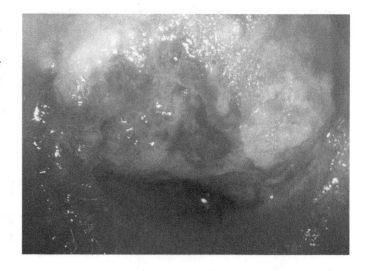

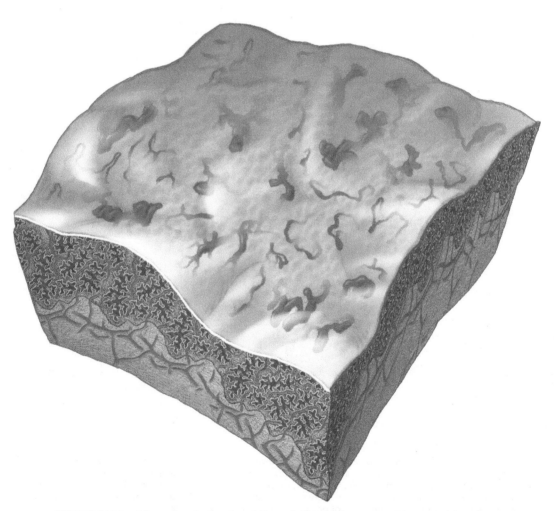

FIGURE 11.37.   Schematics of waste-thread-like and dilated tuberous-root-like angioarchitecture.

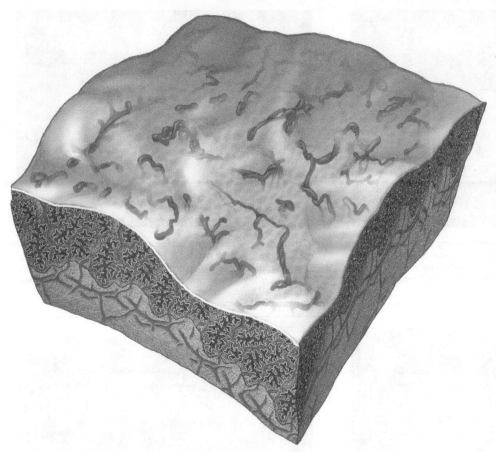

FIGURE 11.38. Schematics of character-writing-like and waste-thread-like blood vessel formations.

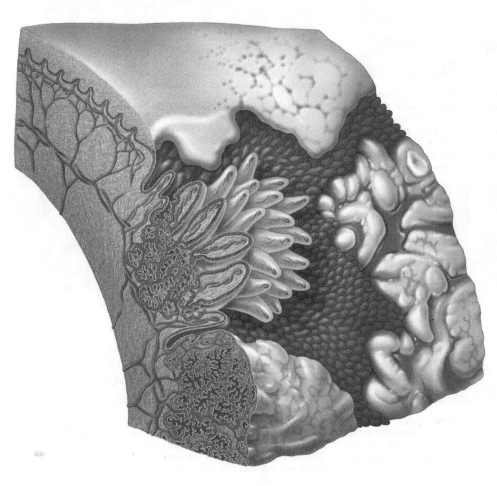

FIGURE 11.39. Schematics of character-writing-like blood vessels coursing over the surface of glandular disease. Dot-like angioarchitecture is seen in the tips of the villous processes. In contrast, anteriorly are punctate and mosaic patterns of a high-grade intraepithelial squamous lesion. These latter two blood vessel patterns are not seen in areas of glandular disease.

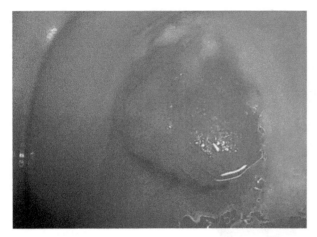

FIGURE 11.40.   An AIS lesion demonstrating patches of multiple dots on the anterior cervical lip lies over columnar epithelium prior to the application of acetic acid. (Reprinted from Wright VC. *Principles of Cervical Colposcopy*. Houston, TX: Biomedical Communications, 2004, with permission.)

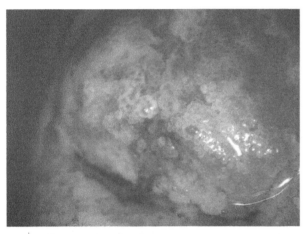

FIGURE 11.41.   The lesion in Figure 11.40 after application of acetic acid. The AIS lesion contains proliferating excrescences that look like the fusing villi of metaplasia. Dots are seen in the tips. (Reprinted from Wright VC, Shier RM. *Colposcopy of Adenocarcinoma In Situ and Adenocarcinoma of the Cervix—Differentiation from Other Cervical Lesions*. Houston, TX: Biomedical Communications, 2000, with permission.)

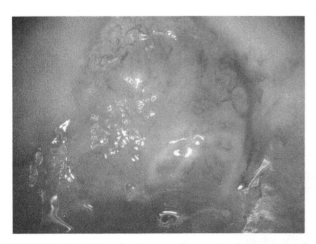

FIGURE 11.42.   This colpophotograph was taken before the application of acetic acid. Note the papillary excrescences, irregular waste thread, and other looped and tendril vessels. (Reprinted from Wright VC. *Principles of Cervical Colposcopy*. Houston, TX: Biomedical Communications, 2004, with permission.)

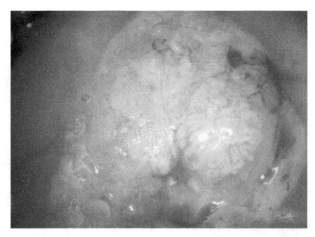

FIGURE 11.43.   The lesion in Figure 11.42 after acetic acid. The vessels are obscured by the dense acetowhiteness. An irregular, papillary proliferative process is evident. (Reprinted from Wright VC, Shier RM. *Colposcopy of Adenocarcinoma In Situ and Adenocarcinoma of the Cervix—Differentiation from Other Cervical Lesions*. Houston, TX: Biomedical Communications, 2000, with permission.)

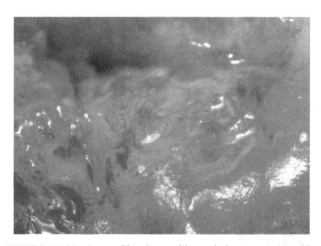

FIGURE 11.44.   Large dilated, root-like and character-writing-like blood vessels in a cervical adenocarcinoma. (Reprinted from Wright VC, Shier RM. *Colposcopy of Adenocarcinoma In Situ and Adenocarcinoma of the Cervix—Differentiation from Other Cervical Lesions*. Houston, TX: Biomedical Communications, 2000, with permission.)

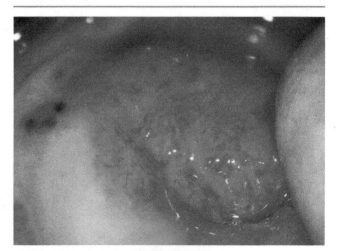

FIGURE 11.45.   Large, dilated, tuberous root-like blood vessels in an adenocarcinoma. (Reprinted from Wright VC, Shier RM. *Colposcopy of Adenocarcinoma In Situ and Adenocarcinoma of the Cervix—Differentiation from Other Cervical Lesions*. Houston, TX: Biomedical Communications, 2000, with permission.)

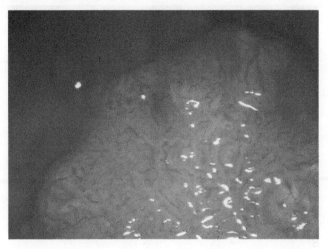

FIGURE 11.46. A variety of blood vessel patterns are contained in this AIS lesion. They are character-writing, taproot-like and tendril-like. (Reprinted from Wright VC, Shier RM. *Colposcopy of Adenocarcinoma In Situ and Adenocarcinoma of the Cervix—Differentiation from Other Cervical Lesions*. Houston, TX: Biomedical Communications, 2000, with permission.)

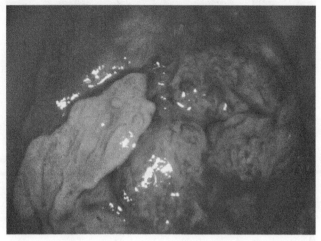

FIGURE 11.48. A mixed lesion. The very densely acetowhite, well-demarcated, high-grade squamous intraepithelial lesion is easily identified extending from the 7 o'clock to 10 o'clock positions. Centrally and also involving the endocervical canal is the AIS component exhibiting numerous root-like and character-writing-like patterns. (Reprinted from Wright VC, Shier RM. *Colposcopy of Adenocarcinoma In Situ and Adenocarcinoma of the Cervix—Differentiation from other Cervical Lesions*. Houston, TX: Biomedical Communications, 2000, with permission.)

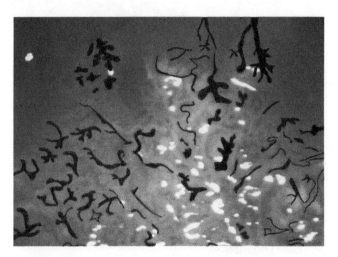

FIGURE 11.47. Vessels in the above lesion that have been "inked in" for easier identification. (Reprinted from Wright VC, Shier RM. *Colposcopy of Adenocarcinoma In Situ and Adenocarcinoma of the Cervix—Differentiation from other Cervical Lesions*. Houston, TX: Biomedical Communications, 2000, with permission.)

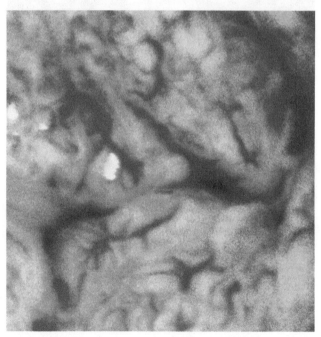

FIGURE 11.49. A higher magnification of the vessels in the lesion illustrated in Figure 11.48. (Reprinted from Wright VC, Shier RM. *Colposcopy of Adenocarcinoma In Situ and Adenocarcinoma of the Cervix—Differentiation from other Cervical Lesions*. Houston, TX: Biomedical Communications, 2000, with permission.)

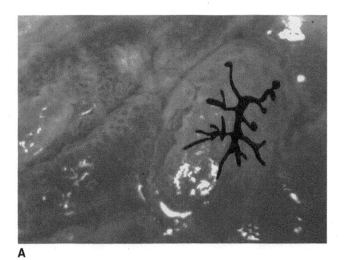

A

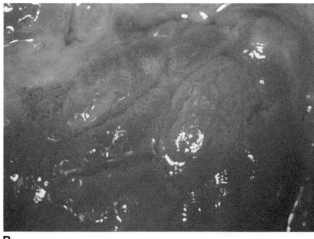

B

FIGURE 11.50. **A:** "Inked-in" character-writing vessels as seen in benign metaplasia similar to that seen in AIS. Differentiation cannot be made from AIS without a punch biopsy. (Reprinted from Wright VC, Shier RM. *Colposcopy of Adenocarcinoma In Situ and Adenocarcinoma of the Cervix—Differentiation from other Cervical Lesions.* Houston, TX: Biomedical Communications, 2000, with permission.) **B:** Another view of the character-writing vasculature without the ink. (Reprinted from Wright VC. *Comprehensive Colposcopy Review—Cervix, Vagina, Vulva and Adjacent Sites CD-ROM.* Houston, TX: Biomedical Communications, 2008, with permission.)

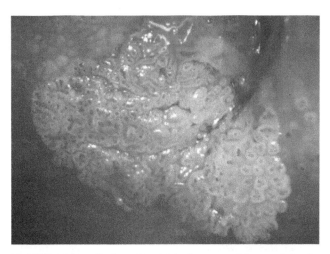

FIGURE 11.51. Single and multiple dots created by vessels in the tips of the proliferations of a cervical condyloma. (Reprinted from Wright VC. *Color Atlas of Colposcopy—Cervix, Vagina and Vulva.* Houston, TX: Biomedical Communications, 2003, with permission.)

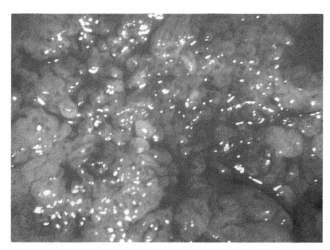

FIGURE 11.52. Single and multiple dots in a papillary squamous cell cancer. (Reprinted from Wright VC, Shier RM. *Colposcopy of Adenocarcinoma In Situ and Adenocarcinoma of the Cervix—Differentiation from other Cervical Lesions.* Houston, TX: Biomedical Communications, 2000, with permission.)

References

1. Reimers LL, Anderson WF, Rosenberg PS, Henson DE, Castle PE. Etiologic heterogeneity for cervical carcinoma by histopathologic type, using comparative age-period-cohort models. *Cancer Epidemiol Biomarkers Prev* 2009;18:792–800.
2. Chen J, Macdonald OK, Gaffney DK. Incidence, mortality, and prognostic factors of small cell carcinoma of the cervix. *Obstet Gynecol* 2008;111:1394–402.
3. Wright VC. Cervical squamous and glandular intraepithelial neoplasia: identification and current management approaches. *Salud Publica Mex* 2003;45(suppl 3):S417–29.
4. Farnsworth A, Laverty C, Stoler MH. Human papilloma virus messenger RNA expression in adenocarcinoma in situ of the uterine cervix. *Int J Gynecol Pathol* 1989;8:321–30.
5. Watson M, Saraiya M, Benard V, et al. Burden of cervical cancer in the United States, 1998–2003. *Cancer* 2008;113(10 suppl):2855–64.
6. Bertrand M, Lickrish GM, Colgan TJ. The anatomical distribution of cervical adenocarcinoma *in situ. Am J Obstet Gynecol* 1987;1:21–6.
7. Colgan TJ, Lickrish GM. The topography and invasive potential of cervical adenocarcinoma *in situ*, with or without associated dysplasia. *Gynecol Oncol* 1990;36:246–9.
8. Lickrish GM, Colgan TJ, Wright VC. Colposcopy of adenocarcinoma in situ and invasive adenocarcinoma of the cervix. *Obstet Gynecol Clin North Am* 1993;20:111–22.
9. Wright VC. Colposcopic features of cervical adenocarcinoma *in situ* and adenocarcinoma and management of preinvasive disease. In: Apgar B, Bronztman GL, Spitzer M, eds. *Colposcopy—Principles and Practice.* Philadelphia, PA: WB Saunders, 2001:301–20.
10. Hafez ESE. Structural and ultrastructural parameters of the uterine cervix. *Obstet Gynecol Surv* 1982;37:507–16.
11. Philipp E. Normal endocervical epithelium. *J Reprod Med* 1975;14:188–191.
12. Fluhmann CF, Dickman Z. The basic pattern of glandular structures of the cervix uteri. *Obstet Gynecol* 1958;11:543–55.
13. Anderson ES, Arfmann E. Adenocarcinoma in situ of the uterine cervix: a clinico-pathologic study of 36 cases. *Gynecol Oncol* 1989;35:1–7.
14. Dlott JS, Dlott TR, Matthews TH, et al. Endocervical metaplasias and their association with squamous abnormalities. *J Low Genit Tract Dis* 1999;3:77–82.

15. Walboomers JMM, Jacobs MV, Manos MM, et al. Human papillomavirus is a necessary cause of invasive cancer worldwide. *J Pathol* 1999;189:12–9.

16. Bosch FX, Lorincz A, Munoz N, Meijer CJ, Shah KV. The causal relation between human papillomavirus and cervical cancer. *J Clin Pathol* 2002;55:244–65.

17. Munoz N, Bosch FX, de Sanjose S, et al. International agency for research on cancer multicenter cervical cancer study group. Epidemiologic classification of human papillomavirus types associated with cervical cancer. *N Engl J Med* 2003;348: 518–27.

18. Castellsagué X, Díaz M, de Sanjosé S, et al.; International Agency for Research on Cancer Multicenter Cervical Cancer Study Group. Worldwide human papillomavirus etiology of cervical adenocarcinoma and its cofactors: implications for screening and prevention. *J Natl Cancer Inst* 2006;98:303–15.

19. Liebrich C, Brummer O, Von Wasielewski R, et al. Primary cervical cancer truly negative for high-risk human papillomavirus is a rare but distinct entity that can affect virgins and young adolescents. *Eur J Gynaecol Oncol* 2009;30:45–8.

20. Tjalma WA, Van Waes TR, Van den Eeden LE, Bogers JJ. Role of human papillomavirus in the carcinogenesis of squamous cell carcinoma and adenocarcinoma of the cervix. *Best Pract Res Clin Obstet Gynaecol* 2005;19:469–83.

21. Zielinski GD, Snijders PJ, Rozendaal L, et al. The presence of high-risk HPV combined with specific cp53 and p16INK4a expression patterns points to high-risk HPV as the main causative agent for adenocarcinoma in situ and adenocarcinoma of the cervix. *J Pathol* 2003;201:535–43.

22. Andersson S, Rylander E, Larson B, et al. Types of human papillomavirus revealed in cervical adenocarcinomas after DNA sequencing. *Oncol Rep* 2003;10:175–9.

23. Pirog EC, Kleter B, Olgac S, et al. Prevalence of human papillomavirus DNA in different histological subtypes of cervical adenocarcinoma. *Am J Pathol* 2000;157:1055–62.

24. Jones MW, Silverberg SG. Cervical adenocarcinoma in young women: possible relationship to microglandular hyperplasia and use of oral contraceptives. *Obstet Gynecol* 1989;73:984–8.

25. Brinton LA, Reeves WC, Herrero R, et al. Oral contraceptive use and risk of invasive cervical cancer. *Int J Epidemiol* 1990;19:4–11.

26. Madeleine MM, Daling JR, Schwartz SM, et al. Human papillomavirus and long-term oral contraceptive use increase the risk of adenocarcinoma *in situ* of the cervix. *Cancer Epidemiol Biomarkers Prev* 2001;10:171–7.

27. Vaccarella S, Herrero R, Dai M, et al.; IARC HPV Prevalence Surveys Study Group. Reproductive factors, oral contraceptive use, and human papillomavirus infection: pooled analysis of the IARC HPV prevalence surveys. *Cancer Epidemiol Biomarkers Prev* 2006;15:2148–53.

28. Berrington de González A, Sweetland S, Green J. Comparison of risk factors for squamous cell and adenocarcinomas of the cervix: a meta-analysis. *Br J Cancer* 2004;90:1787–91.

29. International Collaboration of Epidemiological Studies of Cervical Cancer (IARC). Cervical cancer and hormonal contraceptives: collaborative reanalysis of individual data for 16,573 women with cervical cancer and 35,509 women without cervical cancer from 24 epidemiological studies. *Lancet* 2007;370:1609–21.

30. Friedell GH, McKay DG. Adenocarcinoma in situ of the endocervix. *Cancer* 1953;6:887–97.

31. El-Ghobashy AA, Shaaban AM, Herod J, Herrington CS. The pathology and management of endocervical glandular neoplasia. *Int J Gynecol Cancer* 2005;15:583–92.

32. Wang SS, Sherman ME, Hildesheim A, Lacey JV Jr, Devesa S. Cervical adenocarcinoma and squamous cell carcinoma incidence trends among white women and black women in the United States for 1976–2000. *Cancer* 2004;100:1035–44.

33. Sherman ME, Wang SS, Carreon J, Devesa SS. Mortality trends for cervical squamous and adenocarcinoma in the United States: relation to incidence and survival. *Cancer* 2005;103:1258–64.

34. Chan PG, Sung HY, Sawaya GF. Changes in cervical cancer incidence after three decades of screening US women less than 30 years old. *Obstet Gynecol* 2003;102:765–73.

35. Hildesheim A, Hadjimichael O, Schwartz PE, et al. Risk factors for rapid-onset cervical cancer. *Am J Obstet Gynecol* 1999;180:571–7.

36. Mitchell H, Medley G, Gordon I, Giles G. Cervical cytology reported as negative and risk of adenocarcinoma of the cervix: no strong evidence of benefit. *Br J Cancer* 1995;71:894–7.

37. Woodman CB, Collins S, Rollason TP, et al. Human papillomavirus type 18 and rapidly progressing cervical intraepithelial neoplasia. *Lancet* 2003;361:40–3.

38. Ruba S, Schoolland M, Allpress S, Sterrett G. Adenocarcinoma in situ of the uterine cervix: screening and diagnostic errors in Papanicolaou smears. *Cancer* 2004;102:280–7.

39. Schoolland M, Segal A, Allpress S, Miranda A, Frost FA, Sterrett GF. Adenocarcinoma in situ of the cervix. Sensitivity of detection by cervical smear. *Cancer (Cancer Cytopathol)* 2003;96:330–7.

40. Sasieni P, Castanon A, Cuzick J. Screening and adenocarcinoma of the cervix. *Int J Cancer* 2009;125:525–9.

41. Cullimore JE, Luesley DM, Rollason TP, et al. A prospective study of conization of the cervix in the management of cervical intraepithelial

42. Laverty CR, Farnsworth A, Thurloe T, et al. The reliability of a cytological prediction of cervical adenocarcinoma in situ. *Aust NZ J Obstet Gynecol* 1998;28:307–12.

43. Roberts JM, Thurloe JK, Bowditch RC, Humcevic J, Laverty CR. Comparison of ThinPrep and Pap smear in relation to prediction of adenocarcinoma in situ. *Acta Cytol* 1999;43:74–80.

44. Ashfaq R, Gibbons D, Vela C, Saboorian MH, Iliya F. ThinPrep Pap test. Accuracy for glandular disease. *Acta Cytol* 1999;43:81–5.

45. van Aspert-van Erp AJM, Smedts FMM, Vooijs JP. Severe cervical glandular cell lesions and severe cervical combined lesions: predictive value of the Papanicolaou smear. *Cancer Cytopathol* 2004;102:210–7.

46. Zappa M, Visioli CB, Ciatto S, Iossa A, Paci E, Sasieni P. Lower protection of cytological screening for adenocarcinoma and shorter protection for younger women: the results of a case-control study in Florence. *Br J Cancer* 2004;90:1784–6.

47. Sasieni P, Adams J, Cuzick J. Benefit of cervical screening at different ages: evidence from the UK audit of screening histories. *Br J Cancer* 2003;89:89–93.

48. Solomon D, Davey D, Kurman R, et al. The 2001 Bethesda System: terminology for reporting results of cervical cytology. *JAMA* 2002;287:2114–9.

49. Veljovich DS, Stoler MH, Andersen WA, et al. Atypical glandular cells of undetermined significance. A five-year retrospective histopathologic study. *Am J Obstet Gynecol* 1998;179:382–90.

50. Nasu I, Meurer W, Fu YS. Cytological features alone do not allow accurate distinction between in situ and invasive adenocarcinoma. *Int J Gynecol Pathol* 1993;12:208–18.

51. Sharpless KE, Schnatz PF, Mandavilli S, Greene JF, Sorosky JI. Dysplasia associated with atypical glandular cells on cervical cytology. *Obstet Gynecol* 2005;105:494–500.

52. DeSimone CP, Day ME, Tovar MM, Dietrich CS III, Eastham ML, Modesitt SC. Rate of pathology from atypical glandular cell Pap tests classified by the Bethesda 2001 nomenclature. *Obstet Gynecol* 2006;107:1285–91.

53. Wright TC Jr, Massad LS, Dunton CJ, Spitzer M, Wilkinson EJ, Solomon D; 2006 American Society for Colposcopy and Cervical Pathology-sponsored Consensus Conference. 2006 consensus guidelines for the management of women with cervical intraepithelial neoplasia or adenocarcinoma in situ. *Am J Obstet Gynecol* 2007;197:346–55.

54. Sharpless KE, O'Sullivan DM, Schnatz PF. The utility of human papillomavirus testing in the management of atypical glandular cells on cytology. *J Low Genit Tract Dis* 2009;13:72–8.

55. Lai CR, Hsu CY, Tsay SH, Li AF. Clinical significance of atypical glandular cells by the 2001 Bethesda System in cytohistologic correlation. *Acta Cytol* 2008;52:563–7.

56. Haidopoulos DA, Stefanidis K, Rodolakis A, Pilalis A, Symiakaki I, Diakomanolis E. Histologic implications of Pap smears classified as atypical glandular cells. *J Reprod Med* 2005;50:539–42.

57. Zhao C, Austin RM, Pan J, et al. Clinical significance of atypical glandular cells in conventional Pap smears in a large, high-risk U.S. west coast minority population. *Acta Cytol* 2009;53:153–9.

58. Lickrish GM, Colgan T. Management of adenocarcinoma in situ of the uterine cervix. In: Wright VC, Lickrish GM, Shier RM, eds. *Basic and Advanced Colposcopy—A Practical Handbook for Treatment* (2nd ed.). Houston, TX: Biomedical Communications, 1995;30-1–8.

59. Plaxe SC, Saltzstein SL. Estimation of the duration of the preclinical phase of cervical adenocarcinoma suggests there is ample opportunity for screening. *Gynecol Oncol* 1999;75:55–61.

60. Muntz HG, Bell DA, Lage JM, et al. Adenocarcinoma in situ of the uterine cervix. *Obstet Gynecol* 1992;80:935–9.

61. Jaworski RC, Pacey NF, Greenberg ML. The histologic diagnosis of adenocarcinoma in situ and related lesions of the cervix uteri. *Cancer* 1988;61:1171–81.

62. Östör AG, Paganor, Davoran AM, et al. Adenocarcinoma in situ of the cervix. *Int J Obstet Gynecol Pathol* 1984;3:179–90.

63. Nicklin JL, Wright RG, Bell JR, et al. A clinicopathological study of adenocarcinoma in situ of the cervix. The influence of HPV infection and other factors, and the role of conservative surgery. *Aust NZ Obstet Gynecol* 1991;31:179–83.

64. Wright TC Jr, Massad LS, Dunton CJ, Spitzer M, Wilkinson EJ, Solomon D; 2006 American Society for Colposcopy and Cervical Pathology-sponsored Consensus Conference. 2006 consensus guidelines for the management of women with cervical intraepithelial neoplasia or adenocarcinoma in situ. *Am J Obstet Gynecol* 2007;197:340–5.

65. Christopherson WM, Nealson N, Gray L Sr. Noninvasive precursor lesions of adenocarcinoma and mixed adenosquamous carcinoma of the cervix uteri. *Cancer* 1979;44:975–83.

66. Kolstad P, Stafl A. Terminology and definition. In: Kolstad P, Stafl A, eds. *Atlas of Colposcopy* (1st ed.). Oslo, Norway: Universitetsforlaget, 1972;21–5.

67. Wright VC. Colposcopy of adenocarcinoma in situ and adenocarcinoma of the uterine cervix: differentiation from other cervical lesions. *J Low Genit Tract Dis* 1999;2:83–97.

68. Coppleson M, Atkinson KH, Dalrymple JC. Cervical squamous and glandular neoplasia: clinical features and review of management. In: Coppleson M, ed. Gynecologic Oncology Edinburgh: Churchill Livingston, 1992;571–607.

glandular neoplasia (CIGN)—a preliminary report. *Br J Obstet Gynecol* 1992;99:314–8.

69. Coppleson M, Pixley EC, Reid BL. *Colposcopy: A Scientific and Practical Approach to the Cervix, Vagina and Vulva in Health and Disease* (3rd ed.). Springfield, IL: Charles C Thomas, 1986.
70. Reid R, Stanhope CR, Herschman BR, et al. Genital warts and cervical cancer IV. A colposcopic index for differentiating subclinical papillomaviral infection from cervical intraepithelial neoplasia. *Am J Obstet Gynecol* 1984;149:815–9.
71. Wright VC, Dubue-Lissoir J, Ehlen T, et al. Guidelines on adenocarcinoma in situ of the cervix: clinical features and review of management. *J Soc Obstet Gynaecol Can* 1999;21:699–706.
72. Wright VC, Shier RM. Differentiating adenocarcinoma in situ and invasive adenocarcinoma from other cervical lesions. In: Wright VC, Shier RM, eds. *Colposcopic Features of Adenocarcinoma In Situ and Invasive Adenocarcinoma of the Cervix.* Houston, TX: Biomedical Communications, 2000.
73. Wright VC. Home study course: summer 2001. *J Low Genit Tract Dis* 2001;5:189–92.
74. Wright VC. Home study course: winter 2002. *J Low Genit Tract Dis* 2002;6:53–56.
75. Wright VC. Home study course: autumn 2001. *J Low Genit Tract Dis* 2001;5:226–9.
76. Wright VC, Davies E, Riopelle MA. Laser cylindrical conization to replace conization. *Am J Obstet Gynecol* 1983;145:181–5.
77. Poynor EA, Barakat RR, Hoskins WJ. Management and follow-up of patients with adenocarcinoma in situ of the uterine cervix. *Gynecol Oncol* 1995;57:158–64.
78. Wolf J, Levenback C, Malpica A, et al. Adenocarcinoma in situ of the cervix: significance of cone biopsy margins. *Obstet Gynecol* 1996;88:82–6.
79. Soutter WP, Haidopoulos D, Gornall RJ, et al. Is conservative treatment for adenocarcinoma in situ of the cervix safe? *BJOG* 2001;108:1184–9.
80. Hwang DM, Lickrish GM, Chapman W. Long-term surveillance is required for all women treated for adenocarcinoma in situ. *J Low Genit Tract Dis* 2004;8:125–31.
81. Azodi M, Chambers SK, Rutherford TJ, Kohorn EI, Schwartz PE, Chambers JT. Adenocarcinoma in situ of the cervix: management and outcome. *Gynecol Oncol* 1999;73:348–53.
82. Andersen ES, Nielsen K. Adenocarcinoma in situ of the cervix: a prospective study of conization as definitive treatment. *Gynecol Oncol* 2002;86:365–9.
83. Kennedy AW, Biscotti CV. Further study of the management of cervical adenocarcinoma in situ. *Gynecol Oncol* 2002;86:361–4.
84. Krivak TC, Rose GS, McBroom JW, Carlson JW, Winter WE III, Kost ER. Cervical adenocarcinoma in situ: a systematic review of therapeutic options and predictors of persistent or recurrent disease. *Obstet Gynecol Surv* 2001;56:567–75.
85. Widrich T, Kennedy AW, Myers TM, et al. Adenocarcinoma in situ of the uterine cervix: management and outcome. *Gynecol Oncol* 1996;61:304–8.
86. Kennedy AW, Tabbakh GH, Biscotti CV, et al. Invasive adenocarcinoma of the cervix following LLETZ (large loop excision of the transformation zone) for adenocarcinoma in situ. *Gynecol Oncol* 1995;58:274–7.
87. Im DI, Duska LR, Recension NB. Adequacy of conization margins of adenocarcinoma in situ of the cervix as a predictor of residual disease. *Gynecol Oncol* 1995;59:179–82.
88. Hopkins M, Roberts JA, Schmidt RW. Cervical adenocarcinoma in situ. *Obstet Gynecol* 1988;7:842–4.

CHAPTER 12

DARON G. FERRIS
J. THOMAS COX
EDWARD J. MAYEAUX, JR.

Colposcopy and Pregnancy

12.1 INTRODUCTION
12.2 HUMAN PAPILLOMAVIRUS AND PREGNANCY
  12.2.1 Epidemiology of Human Papillomavirus in Pregnancy
  12.2.2 Natural History of HPV during Pregnancy
  12.2.3 Potential Complications from HPV Infections during Pregnancy
12.3 CERVICAL INTRAEPITHELIAL NEOPLASIA AND PREGNANCY
  12.3.1 Epidemiology of CIN during Pregnancy
  12.3.2 Natural History of CIN during Pregnancy
  12.3.3 Complications of CIN during Pregnancy
12.4 CERVICAL CANCER AND PREGNANCY
  12.4.1 Epidemiology of Cervical Cancer during Pregnancy
  12.4.2 Natural History of Cervical Cancer during Pregnancy
  12.4.3 Potential Complications from Cervical Cancer Diagnosed during Pregnancy
12.5 LOWER GENITAL TRACT MODIFICATIONS OF PREGNANCY
  12.5.1 Physiology
  12.5.2 Cytology
  12.5.3 Histology
12.6 COLPOSCOPY OF PREGNANT WOMEN
  12.6.1 Indications for Colposcopy during Pregnancy
  12.6.2 Objectives of Colposcopy during Pregnancy
  12.6.3 Colposcopic Examination of Pregnant Women
12.7 COLPOSCOPIC FINDINGS OF CERVICAL NEOPLASIA IN PREGNANCY

12.7.1 Colposcopy of Low-Grade Cervical and Vaginal Lesions in Pregnancy
12.7.2 Colposcopy of High-Grade Cervical Lesions (CIN 2,3) in Pregnancy
12.7.3 Colposcopy of Carcinoma of the Cervix in Pregnancy
12.8 ANTEPARTUM MANAGEMENT OF PREGNANT WOMEN WITH ABNORMAL CERVICAL CYTOLOGY
  12.8.1 Management of Pregnant Women with ASC and LSIL Pap Results
  12.8.2 Management of Pregnant Women with ASC-H, AGC, and HSIL Pap Results
  12.8.3 Management of Pregnant Women with a Pap Test Report Suspect for Cancer
12.9 MANAGEMENT OF CERVICAL NEOPLASIA IN PREGNANCY
  12.9.1 Management of Pregnant Women with CIN 1
  12.9.2 Management of Pregnant Women with CIN 2,3
  12.9.3 Management of Invasive Cervical Cancer in Pregnancy
12.10 COMPLICATIONS REPORTED IN THE MANAGEMENT OF PREGNANT WOMEN WITH CERVICAL NEOPLASIA
  12.10.1 Abortion
  12.10.2 Hemorrhage
  12.10.3 Other Conization-Related Complications
12.11 POSTPARTUM MANAGEMENT OF WOMEN WITH CERVICAL NEOPLASIA

12.1 INTRODUCTION

The management of abnormal cervical screening tests and cervical neoplasia in pregnancy presents challenges not found in the management of nonpregnant women due to the necessity to balance maternal and fetal risks in avoiding compromise to either. The close proximity of the uterine cervix to the fetus and the importance of maintaining cervical integrity require modified management strategies that maintain fetal viability and maturation to the maximum extent possible without jeopardizing the life and welfare of the mother. Although evaluation of minor cytologic abnormalities detected during pregnancy may be deferred until postpartum, when evaluation is indicated, colposcopy remains the assessment method of choice.[1] Many of the basic principles of colposcopy discussed previously also apply to this special population. However, hampered visualization, altered vascularity, challenging assessment secondary to cervical decidual changes, and a need for cautious, conservative sampling require a unique approach to colposcopic evaluation during pregnancy. When a colposcopist has limited prior experience with colposcopy during pregnancy, consultation with a colposcopist with expertise in this area is ideal when available. This chapter discusses the basic principles and findings of colposcopy during pregnancy.

The management of pregnant women with abnormal cervical cytology is discussed further in Chapter 19, and additional discussion on the management of cervical intraepithelial neoplasia (CIN) found during pregnancy is discussed in Chapter 20.

12.2 HUMAN PAPILLOMAVIRUS AND PREGNANCY

12.2.1 Epidemiology of Human Papillomavirus in Pregnancy

The natural history of human papillomavirus (HPV) infection and associated cervical neoplasia is modified by naturally occurring changes in host immunity and hormone levels during pregnancy.[2-4] Pregnancy typically induces a temporary impaired cell-mediated immunity that often facilitates clinical expression of both recently acquired and long-term latent

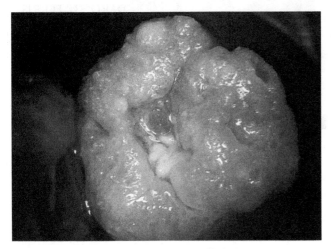

FIGURE 12.1.   Condylomas on the cervix of a woman at 16 weeks' gestation.

HPV infection.[3] The result for both new lesions and lesions already present can be the acceleration of rapid growth of HPV lesions (Figure 12.1).[3,4] This suggests that both cervical cytologic changes and HPV lesions should be more common in pregnancy. Some case–control studies of pregnant and nonpregnant women support these hypotheses. The incidence of HPV in pregnant women when compared to matched nonpregnant controls has been shown to be from 48% to 72% higher in the pregnant cohort.[5] Likewise, the incidence of high-risk (oncogenic) HPV has been from 52% to >100% higher for the pregnant cohort than for the nonpregnant cohort.[5,6] In these studies, this increased HPV detection in the first trimester persists through the third trimester without significant change but drops by about a third within 4 to 12 weeks from delivery.[7] These observations are most consistent with transient activation of the virus by the physiologic changes of pregnancy and/or reduced host immunity.[6] These data are consistent with the long-standing impression by obstetricians that sudden appearance, or increased proliferation, of genital warts and other HPV-induced changes is more common in pregnancy.

However, the picture is not entirely clear. The incidence and prevalence of HPV may vary because of the specific population sampled and the type and sensitivity of the particular HPV DNA test used to detect infection. While some studies have not demonstrated higher HPV DNA or serologic detection rates in pregnancy,[8–10] many have, and in general, the question of whether pregnancy increases HPV detection remains controversial. Hildesheim et al.[11] found a positive association between current pregnancy and HPV prevalence in a study of inner city low-income women. Fife et al.[2] compared the rate of HPV detection in a pregnant cohort compared with nonpregnant women attending either a sexually transmitted disease clinic or a general gynecology clinic, demonstrating that pregnancy was an independent predictor for the presence of carcinogenic HPV (odds ratio [OR] 1.79). On the other hand, Chan et al. did not detect a difference in HPV prevalence between pregnant women (10.1%) and nonpregnant women (11.4%), consistent with the findings of several other studies.[8,10,12–14]

The absence of an increase in HPV-related cytologic findings on Pap screening in pregnant women compared with that found in nonpregnant women[15] supports similar HPV prevalence in each group. The median prevalence rate for HPV infection detected during pregnancy is approximately 25%, with a range of 6.5% to over 50%.[8,10,12,13,16–20] Despite increased HPV detection during pregnancy, the majority of pregnant women testing positive for HPV have no obvious HPV lesions, nor have there been reports of an increase in HPV-associated abnormal cytologic changes.[21] Those that do have HPV expression may have only subclinical changes not visible without colposcopic examination or may have clinically detectable genital warts or cervical neoplasia.

The presence of HPV during specific intervals of pregnancy has also been evaluated. Findings vary in respect to fluctuations in HPV positivity during the course of pregnancy.[12,22] Several studies have shown increased HPV detection in the first and second trimesters followed by decreased HPV beginning either in the third trimester[22] or in the postpartum.[7,23] Multiple HPV types have also been reported to be more frequent in the first trimester.[23] Whether these findings are related more to sexual activity differences by trimester or to immunologic factors is not clear. In contrast, a number of studies have not found a significant variation in detection of HPV during pregnancy.[10,12] Additional prospective studies are needed to better understand the epidemiology of HPV infection during pregnancy.

12.2.2 Natural History of HPV during Pregnancy

Few data are available concerning the natural history of HPV infections in pregnant women. Epidemiologic studies have not clearly substantiated whether pregnant women are more susceptible to acquiring or reactivating HPV. However, although a fetus is inherently antigenic to its mother, it is not rejected at least in part because the T regulatory subset of CD4+ T cells can limit the maternal immune response. While this mechanism has been implicated in the maternal tolerance of the fetus, it is not clear whether such immune suppression extends to tolerance of HPV. Pregnant women are known to have fewer T lymphocytes, particularly a reduced level of CD4+ T lymphocytes, especially during the third trimester.[24] While alterations to the immune system from changes associated with pregnancy may influence susceptibility to HPV, additional negative effects on the immune system, such as are posed by diabetes mellitus, were not found to compound risk for harboring HPV during pregnancy.[25]

As in the general nonpregnant population, subclinical HPV expression is more common during pregnancy than is actual clinical expression such as genital warts.[12] The concept that HPV infections are more prominent in pregnancy has been accepted by many clinicians on the basis of clinical experience, particularly the anecdotal impression that external genital warts occur more commonly in pregnancy, grow more dramatically, and become friable.[10,26] Occasionally, they may become very large, bulky lesions, though only rarely do they enlarge to a size that might obstruct vaginal delivery (Figure 12.2). Just as in nonpregnant women, condylomas may be distributed throughout the epithelium of the lower genital tract, affecting the cervix, vagina, vulva, and perianal regions.

Personal experience of the authors suggests that genital warts present during pregnancy are more recalcitrant to treatment. However, solid data documenting success rates for treatment of genital warts in pregnant versus nonpregnant women do not exist. Many subclinical and clinically evident HPV lesions will regress spontaneously in the postpartum period as immunity recovers, and some will persist. Some effective therapies are contraindicated in pregnancy, further complicating comparisons.

12.2.3 Potential Complications from HPV Infections during Pregnancy

In most pregnant women, HPV infections are unnoticed: either latent (nonexpressed) or expressed but detected neither by the patient nor by her clinician (subclinical disease). However, in some patients, HPV has the potential to impair the birth process or afflict the baby. Pap test sampling performed during pregnancy

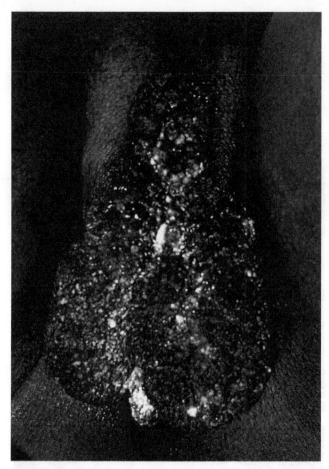

FIGURE 12.2.   Extensive, bulky condylomas involving the vulva and also the vagina. This woman's baby was delivered by cesarean section because of severe outlet obstruction.

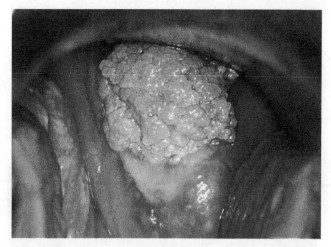

FIGURE 12.3.   Large condyloma on the anterior cervix in a pregnant women. (Photo courtesy of Dr. Vesna Kesic.)

may detect cytologic evidence of HPV but should only be done if the appropriate interval since the last Pap test has elapsed. As with nonpregnant women, pregnant women most at risk for the consequences of HPV infection are those with a history of multiple sexual partners or whose partner(s) have had multiple partners. Previous HPV exposure without evidence of present HPV expression, as demonstrated by HPV 16–seropositive but HPV 16 DNA–negative results, was not shown to increase the risk of an adverse obstetric outcome.[9] Likewise, subclinical and most clinical expressions of HPV pose no serious hazard to pregnant patients (Figure 12.3). Small condylomas of the cervix, vagina, vulva, or perianal regions are usually more of a nuisance than a threat. Even high-grade HPV-associated intraepithelial neoplasia of the cervix, vagina, or vulva rarely influences pregnancy outcomes. Only HPV-induced lower genital tract malignancies pose a serious risk for the pregnant patient.

Several complications may ensue when condylomas, large or small, occupy space within the birth canal. Shearing forces generated during delivery may tear condylomas and cause bleeding, particularly if large. Warts on the perineum or in the midline may be problematic if an episiotomy is indicated or a significant tear occurs. Proper wound closure may be challenging because of relatively friable tissue and uneven, irregular epithelial surfaces, and wound dehiscence may be more likely. More importantly, if large condylomas are present within the vagina, or at the introitus, dystocia may occur. Consequently, when very large condylomas are encountered in pregnant women, aggressive treatment should be initiated early to minimize the chance of mechanical outlet obstruction. However, although lesions are rarely large enough to prevent a normal vaginal delivery, the risk

of obstruction or excessive bleeding from massive condylomas occasionally necessitates cesarean delivery (Figure 12.2).[26] In the absence of obstruction, the mere presence of lower genital tract condylomas is not an indication for cesarean section.

The one definite risk to the neonate is the rare, but potentially devastating, development of condylomas in the upper respiratory tract of infants or young children born to mothers with HPV 6 or 11 lower genital tract HPV expression. Known as juvenile-onset recurrent respiratory papillomatosis (JORRP), this condition challenges otolaryngologists, frustrates parents, and may severely impact the affected child (Figure 12.4).[27,28] Even though the consequences of JORRP are serious, it must be emphasized that most infants born to mothers with lower genital tract condylomas do not develop JORRP. Based on evidence from several studies,[28–31] vertical transmission of both low- and high-risk HPV types from mother to offspring occurs, but only transmission of these low-risk types has been shown to cause definite disease. A number of studies have demonstrated a median 39% (0.2% to 73%) concordance between cervical HPV detected in the mother and HPV detected soon after birth on the infant.[28] At one time, JORRP was thought to be acquired only by direct contact or aspiration during vaginal delivery in women with lower genital tract HPV. However, infants born by cesarean section have been shown to harbor the same HPV type detected in the mother's lower genital tract.[31] The retrieval of HPV DNA in amniotic fluid aspirates of women with cervical HPV lesions appears

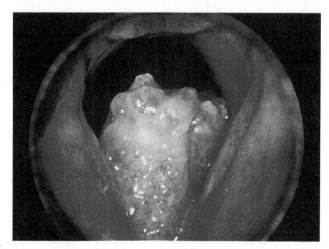

FIGURE 12.4.   Recurrent respiratory papillomatosis of the larynx.

to support theoretical transmission across the amnion.[32] HPV DNA has also been found in placental tissue obtained by transabdominal chorionic villus sampling,[33] umbilical cord, fetal membranes, and amniotic fluid.[34–37] Thus, some oral and airway infections are probably established in utero.[28,38]

The primary symptom of JORRP is hoarseness. Because the larynx and trachea are narrow, airway compromise of variable severity may develop and may rarely lead to suffocation if rapid proliferation of therapy-resistant warts should ensue. The majority of cases of JORRP are diagnosed prior to 5 years of age. The course of the disease is variable. Laryngeal HPV disease is currently best managed by laser excision and ablation or microdebrider. Adjuvant medical therapies include cidofovir, interferon, indole-3-carbinol, and heat shock protein.[39] Some children may require repeated surgical procedures. The mortality rate is <5%, and the disease usually resolves spontaneously by adulthood.[39] While more than 50% of mothers whose offspring develop JORRP had genital tract condylomas diagnosed at the time of birth, a substantial number have only subclinical genital HPV infections (Figure 12.5A–E).

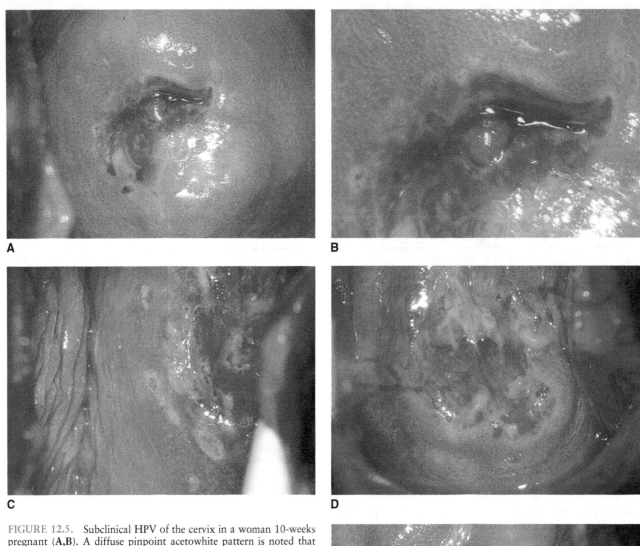

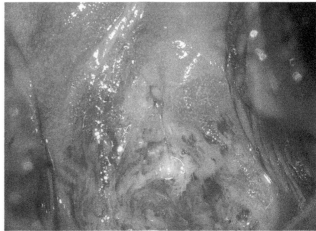

FIGURE 12.5. Subclinical HPV of the cervix in a woman 10-weeks pregnant (A,B). A diffuse pinpoint acetowhite pattern is noted that represents micropapillary surface projections. These are also appreciated at higher magnification in another woman with subclinical HPV changes (C). Similar viral changes are also seen in (D) and (E).

Therefore, the absence of clinically obvious lower genital tract condylomas in the mother does not eliminate the risk of JORRP in the infant.[28] The corollary, however, is that most children born to mothers with known condylomata at delivery do not get JORRP, as only 7 of every 1000 births with a maternal history of genital warts during pregnancy are subsequently found to result in the development of JORRP in the child.[28] With this low risk, cesarean section as prophylaxis against JORRP is not indicated for pregnant women with lower genital tract HPV even when condyloma are present.[26] For more discussion on JORRP, refer to the section on Vertical Transmission in Chapter 5 (see Section 5.3.1.3).

12.3 CERVICAL INTRAEPITHELIAL NEOPLASIA AND PREGNANCY

12.3.1 Epidemiology of CIN during Pregnancy

For some women, contact with medical care for pregnancy may be an important opportunity to receive delayed cervical screening or even to initiate screening. For these women, receiving a Pap test at the first prenatal visit is standard and very important. Although cervical cytologic sampling during the first trimester of pregnancy was long considered routine care, recent guidelines have clarified that cervical screening, even in pregnancy, is only indicated if the woman is otherwise due for her next cervical screen.[40,41] In other words, cytology screening is no longer part of the routine new obstetrical panel.

Approximately 4 million pregnancies occur in the United States annually, and if all had cervical cancer screening, between 80,000 and 320,000 would have an abnormal Pap test result.[42] Overall, the prevalence of abnormal cervical cytology in pregnancy is similar to that of age-matched, nonpregnant women.[41] The incidence of CIN in pregnancy varies among different patient populations, as it does in nonpregnant women, but when age-matched, risk is not higher than that among women who are not pregnant, ranging from 3.4% to as high as 10%.[43,44] Generally, the majority of pregnant women with CIN have CIN 1 or other evidence of HPV infection. CIN 3 is much less common, occurring at rates consistent with that found in the nonpregnant population and depending on age and history of prior screening (0.1% to 1.8%) (Figure 12.6).[44,45]

12.3.2 Natural History of CIN during Pregnancy

Only recently has there been improved documentation of the natural history of CIN during pregnancy. In the largest retrospective review of pregnant patients with abnormal cervical cytology and antepartum colposcopic assessment, progression of biopsy-proven CIN in the intrapartum and postpartum periods was uncommon, and spontaneous resolution was frequent.[43] Sixty-one percent of the women having follow-up postpartum reverted to normal and no progression to cancer occurred during pregnancy, consistent with other reports that CIN 3 is unlikely to progress to frankly invasive cancer during pregnancy.[43,46] In fact, there is a surprisingly high rate of regression from high-grade intraepithelial neoplasia to low grade and from low-grade lesions to normal histology, during pregnancy and in the postpartum.[42] Even among patients referred initially with a high-grade squamous intraepithelial lesion (HSIL) Pap result, 53% regressed to normal, 16% regressed to a lower-grade lesion, only 31% had persistent high-grade dysplasia, and none developed cancer.[43]

This supports previous findings that CIN does not progress to high-grade disease or cancer more rapidly during this 9-month time frame than comparably severe levels of CIN do in nonpregnant women. Smoking during pregnancy does adversely affect spontaneous resolution. Other studies have shown similar results. Patsner,[47] in a much more limited sample size, demonstrated that 45% of pregnant women with cytologic and histologic evidence of CIN 1 had disease regression at a postpartum evaluation, the remainder (55%) had persistence of CIN 1, and none progressed. It is likely that longer follow-up would demonstrate significantly higher spontaneous remission rates consistent with the 70% to 90% remission noted in large prospective studies of nonpregnant women with CIN 1.[48] Palle[49] found that 25% of all CIN grades regressed from pregnancy to the postpartum, 47% persisted, and 28% progressed. Of the women who progressed (or disease was missed on colposcopy), fewer than 1% had microinvasive cancer. Others have shown that CIN either regresses or persists at the same severity level for approximately 98% of pregnant women, and thus, rarely advances in severity.[43,50] We conclude, therefore, that CIN during pregnancy generally regresses or remains stable (Figure 12.7). Only a minority appears to have progressed at the postpartum examination, and because histologic sampling is generally minimized in pregnancy, predicting

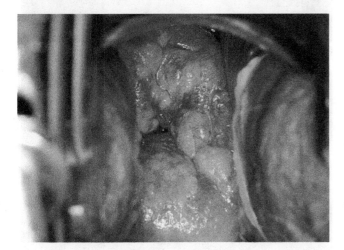

FIGURE 12.6.   A large four-quadrant CIN 3 lesion in a pregnant woman with an estimated gestational age of 7 months. A dense acetowhite epithelium with a coarse mosaic vascular pattern is seen.

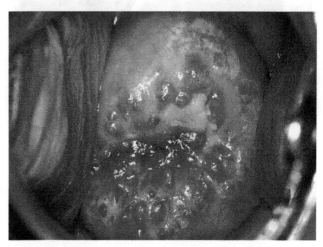

FIGURE 12.7.   A large CIN 3 seen postpartum that did not progress during pregnancy. (Photo courtesy of Dr. Vesna Kesic.)

whether a lesion has progressed or merely was not sampled previously is almost impossible. These findings further support the consensus that biopsy-proven CIN in pregnancy does not warrant interruption of the gestation, as CIN 1, 2, and 3 have all been associated with acceptably low rates of progression during pregnancy.[42,51,52]

12.3.3 Complications of CIN during Pregnancy

In the absence of treatment, CIN does not cause complications during pregnancy (Figure 12.8A–C). Yet, the diagnosis of CIN may result in psychological distress. Clinicians caring for pregnant women must be able to appropriately reassure women with most abnormal Pap test results that the risk of having a significant abnormality is extremely low and the risk to the fetus nil. It is important to explain the guidelines and reasoning appropriate for the Pap result. In this context, the importance of adherence to follow-up recommendations can be made without creating undue anxiety. The noninvasive nature of CIN should be emphasized, while conveying the importance of follow-up according to recommendations, including postpartum evaluation.

The morbidity associated with the evaluation of CIN during pregnancy was drastically reduced when colposcopy and targeted biopsy supplanted cold-knife conization (CKC).[15] Severe hemorrhage, postoperative infection, premature labor, and even fetal and maternal death reported with CKC during pregnancy are now practically nonexistent as a consequence of the more conservative colposcopic evaluation and management of neoplasia during pregnancy. Use of smaller biopsy forceps such as the mini-Tischler has also reduced bleeding. The only reason for performing a surgical excision procedure during pregnancy is if invasive cervical cancer is suspect. In this situation, the risks and benefits to the fetus and mother must be carefully assessed and discussed with the patient. In some cases of CIN 3 during pregnancy, the colposcopic appearance can be of more severe disease than truly exists, prompting more aggressive evaluation. Large CIN 3 lesions may also contain small, focal areas of microinvasion that are not readily detected. The presence of CIN is not an indication for a cesarean delivery.[51,52]

12.4 CERVICAL CANCER AND PREGNANCY

12.4.1 Epidemiology of Cervical Cancer during Pregnancy

Few clinicians will ever diagnose cervical cancer in a pregnant woman (Figure 12.9). Approximately 30% of women diagnosed with cervical cancer are in their reproductive years, and 3% of cervical cancer cases are diagnosed during pregnancy.[15,53,54] Although cervical cancer is the most common cancer in pregnancy, it is still rare, occurring in only 1/1200 to 1/10,000 pregnancies.[53] As in the nonpregnant population, squamous cell carcinoma constitutes about 80% of the cancers and adenocarcinoma the remainder.[54–57] Because the majority

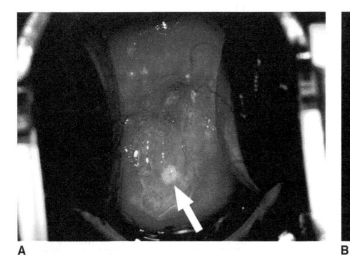

A

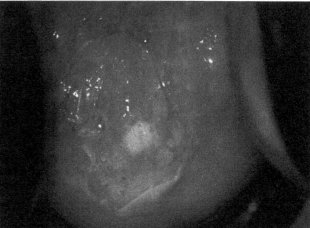

B

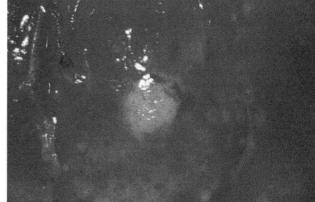

C

FIGURE 12.8.   **A–C:** A small CIN 3 (*arrow*) within metaplastic epithelium in this pregnant patient.

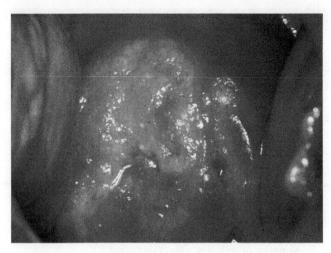

FIGURE 12.9.   Cervical cancer in pregnant woman. (Photo courtesy of Dr. Vesna Kesic.)

of pregnancies occur in women between the ages of 18 and 35, pregnant women with cervical cancer are often younger than the general population of women with cervical cancer, with a mean age of cervical cancer in pregnant women of 33.8 years, with a range of 17 to 47 years.[53] This is approximately 15 years younger than the mean age of cervical cancer in nonpregnant women. Even though cervical cancer is uncommon in pregnancy, the goal of colposcopy in the evaluation of abnormal cervical cytology in pregnancy is to identify microinvasive or invasive disease.[1,58,59] It is unlikely that the diagnosis of cervical neoplasia will affect the clinical outcome of a pregnant patient, even when the diagnosis is a small stage 1 invasive cervical cancer, for tumor characteristics and maternal survival have not been shown to be adversely affected by pregnancy.[52] Obviously, any pregnant patient with either microinvasive or frankly invasive cervical cancer should be managed by a specialist in gynecologic cancer. Current American Society for Colposcopy and Cervical Pathology (ASCCP) and American College of Obstetricians and Gynecologists (ACOG) Guidelines recommend that women diagnosed with CIN 2,3 should be managed without treatment until postpartum because progression to invasive disease is unlikely.[1,51,52,59,60]

The most common presenting symptom of cervical cancer in pregnancy is painless vaginal bleeding occurring in 41% to 63%.[15,51,52,55–57,61] Bleeding may be minor spotting, postcoital bleeding, or massive hemorrhage. Clinicians must remember that vaginal bleeding in pregnant women may result from cancer, but cancer is an extremely uncommon cause of antepartum bleeding when compared to pregnancy-related causes such as placenta previa, abruptio placentae, ectopic pregnancy, other early pregnancy loss, or trophoblastic disease. Nevertheless, it is important to evaluate for lower genital tract malignancy by cytology and colposcopy and, when indicated, by biopsy, when the bleeding cannot be explained by pregnancy-related causes. Other, less common presenting symptoms of cervical cancer during pregnancy are vaginal discharge, lower extremity edema, and pelvic pain. These symptoms are also very common in pregnant women without cervical cancer. Overall, 18% to 59% of pregnant women with cervical cancer will have no symptoms, usually reflecting earlier disease.[44,55–57] Almost all pregnant women with microinvasive cervical cancer are asymptomatic.

Except where screening is organized and population coverage is almost universal, cervical cancer stage at diagnosis is generally earlier for pregnant women than stage at diagnosis among nonpregnant women. This is likely because of the increased opportunity for screening pregnant women attending medical care and that pregnant women are younger than

the general population of women screened. In a recent review, the majority of women with cervical cancer in pregnancy have stage IB (76%) or stage II disease (11% to 20%), with only 3% to 8% reported to have stage III and 0% to 3% stage IV.[15,54,62,63] This is in comparison to 23% of nonpregnant women with cervical cancer diagnosed at stage III or greater (21% stage III and 2% stage IV).

12.4.2 Natural History of Cervical Cancer during Pregnancy

Once reports confirmed that pregnancy down-regulates the immune system, many oncologists presumed that pregnancy would accelerate disease in women diagnosed with invasive cervical cancer. This premise resulted in interventions that caused many cases of fetal demise while attempting to optimize maternal outcomes. However, careful studies have shown that the course of cervical cancer is not accelerated in pregnancy.[15] In fact, the 5-year and 30-year survival data for women with early cervical cancer demonstrate no difference in survival among women whether pregnant or nonpregnant at the time of cervical cancer diagnosis.[15,57,64,65] Although systematic studies of cervical cancer in pregnancy are somewhat limited, it does appear that the survival profile of pregnant women with cervical cancer closely approximates that of the nonpregnant population, despite the common delay in treating early-stage cervical cancer during pregnancy in order to achieve fetal maturation.[57,61,65] This knowledge is helpful in planning appropriate management.

The maternal prognosis has not been shown to be adversely affected in patients with a diagnosis made after 16 weeks of pregnancy with postponement of treatment in order to wait for fetal pulmonary maturity.[15,66–68] The rate of recurrence in these cases is similar to that observed among nonpregnant women. The fetal prognosis is influenced by the type of treatment and by the choice of time when the treatment should be performed, since neonatal morbidity and mortality are related to prematurity.

Infants born to mothers with cervical carcinoma have lower birth weight and higher risk of death on delivery, but even a brief increase in the length of the gestation can have a profound effect on infant survival.[15,61] Fetal prognosis also depends on intrauterine exposure to chemotherapeutic drugs and radiation.[61] Once a diagnosis of invasive cervical cancer has been established in a pregnant patient, a multidisciplinary meeting between representatives from gynecologic oncology, maternal–fetal medicine, neonatology, social work, and radiation oncology is ideal and should be arranged if at all possible.[61] The decision to delay or initiate treatment has religious, ethical, moral, and cultural implications that need to be carefully addressed.[61] Once cancer is identified and a decision made to observe until improved fetal viability, ongoing monitoring is required. Again, referral to a gynecologic oncologist is indicated.

12.4.3 Potential Complications from Cervical Cancer Diagnosed during Pregnancy

Having cervical cancer diagnosed during pregnancy obviously complicates care plans. Other than an increased rate of cesarean section, maternal medical complications are similar to those expected for nonpregnant women. Because most cancers in pregnancy are early-stage disease, maternal deaths during pregnancy, independent of intervention, are extremely uncommon.[15] When adverse events occur, they usually result from diagnostic and therapeutic intervention. Colposcopic visualization, assessment, and cervical biopsy may be complicated

TABLE 12.1	PHYSIOLOGIC CHANGES OF PREGNANCY AND COLPOSCOPIC CONSEQUENCES
■ **PHYSIOLOGIC CHANGES**	■ **COLPOSCOPIC CONSEQUENCES**
Abundant cervical mucus Vaginal wall prolapse Stromal hypertrophy	Visualization hindered
Cervical eversion External os and endocervical canal dilation	Visualization enhanced
Presence of decidual tissue Increased blood volume and cardiac output, dilated blood vessels Active immature squamous metaplasia Epithelial cyanosis Edema and glandular hyperplasia	Assessment challenge
Increased vascularity Intrauterine pregnancy Decidua, immature metaplasia and glandular neoplasia	Sampling complication from bleeding Sampling of endocervix contraindicated Correlation challenge

by bleeding since the tissue may be friable and necrotic. Cone biopsy during pregnancy poses increased risks for the patient, being a greater risk for hemorrhage that frequently requires transfusion. Fetal complications also result from conization, including spontaneous abortion, preterm labor, premature delivery, infection, and stillbirth.[64] Fetal demise is an inevitable complication of immediate cervical cancer therapy in the first two trimesters. Fetal complications resulting from preterm birth during the early third trimester may create additional hazards. Because of the potential for these rather common serious complications, a gynecologic oncologist should be consulted as soon as a pregnant woman is diagnosed with cervical cancer.

12.5 LOWER GENITAL TRACT MODIFICATIONS OF PREGNANCY

12.5.1 Physiology

The cervix serves many functions during a woman's lifetime and undergoes alterations accordingly. The greatest modifications of the cervix occur during pregnancy. Shortly following fertilization, the cervix induces changes to preserve the pregnancy until shortly before delivery when very different characteristics are demanded of the tissue to facilitate birth. The vagina also prepares to permit delivery without associated trauma or obstruction. The degree of physiologic change varies depending on parity.[69]

Uterine blood flow increases during pregnancy to support fetal growth. The more rapid blood flow, a result of increased cardiac output and reduced vascular resistance, causes increased cervical vascularity and a bluish cervical hue (Chadwick sign, or epithelial cyanosis) (Table 12.1). Moreover, the vaginal portion of the cervix softens gradually throughout pregnancy (Goodell sign) until the initiation of cervical effacement. Endocervical epithelium proliferates, and an abundance of thick mucus congeals to produce the mucus plug that seals the cervix from unwanted pathogens or other intrusion (Figure 12.10A,B). The voluminous production of tenacious mucus may make colposcopic visualization challenging.

The most noteworthy changes are a result of the high estrogen levels during pregnancy, because cervical epithelium is highly sensitive to alterations in estrogen levels. Higher estrogen levels in early pregnancy increase cervical volume through hypertrophy of the fibromuscular stroma. As the diameter of the cervix increases, the endocervical epithelium everts onto the ectocervix (Figure 12.11A,B).[70] Additionally, the external os dilates slightly.[69,70] These events differ in extent depending on parity.

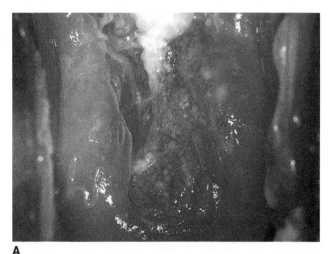
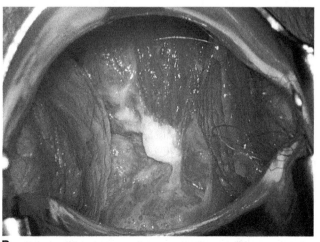

A   **B**

FIGURE 12.10.   **A,B:** Proliferation of the columnar epithelium with mucus production during pregnancy in two women.

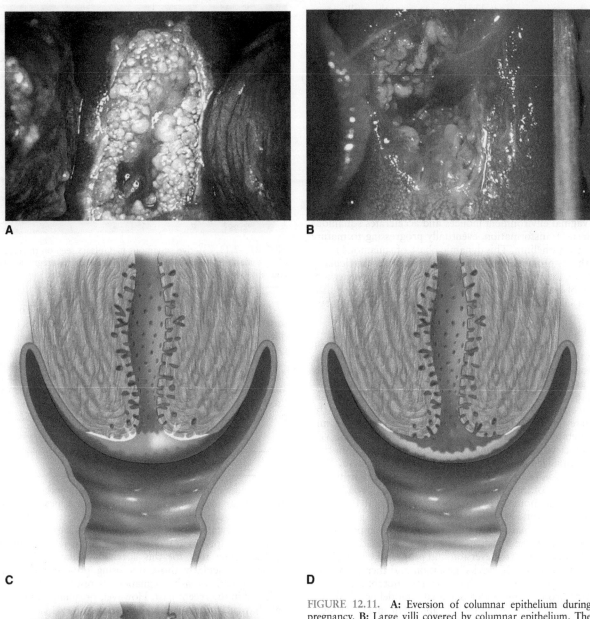

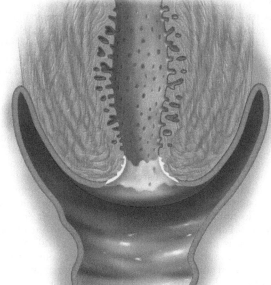

FIGURE 12.11. **A:** Eversion of columnar epithelium during pregnancy. **B:** Large villi covered by columnar epithelium. The cervix in early pregnancy (**C**) resembles the nonpregnant cervix. In the nulliparous women, an active transformation zone with abundant immature metaplasia and eversion is noted in (**D**). Note the os remains in constant diameter and narrow. In contrast, the multiparous woman (**E**) has more gaping of the os along with active transformation. (Photos courtesy of Dr. Vesna Kesic.)

Cervical eversion is more likely to occur in the nulliparous patient, while mild canal dilation, or gaping, is more typical in the parous woman (Figure 12.11C–E).[69] Eversion begins during the early weeks of pregnancy and usually will be apparent in the early second trimester. When an inadequate colposcopic examination results from the inability to observe the entire squamo-columnar junction (SCJ) during early pregnancy, eversion and mild canal dilation facilitate colposcopy later in pregnancy. By reexamining the patient at approximately 20 weeks' gestation, when eversion and gaping are normally pronounced, a previously inadequate colposcopic examination will often become adequate as the SCJ everts onto the exocervix where it may readily be seen in its entirety (Figure 12.12).

By the physiologic processes of eversion and dilation, columnar epithelium becomes exposed to the acidic vaginal environment mediated by *Lactobacillus acidophilus*. The acidic vaginal environment induces and accelerates squamous metaplastic transformation, eventually progressing to mature squamous epithelium. This dynamic phase of squamous metaplasia that is progressive throughout pregnancy is particularly striking in the primipara (Figure 12.13). In the puerperium, the area of metaplasia is returned, partly or completely, to the canal. In subsequent pregnancies, the preexistent area of metaplasia may again evert. However, more commonly, a gaping or widening of the endocervical canal predominates over eversion and is progressive throughout pregnancy, typically peaking during the third trimester. As a result, in parous women, the squamous metaplastic process tends to occur predominantly in late pregnancy, but there is variability among women.

These changes result in colposcopic findings that are determined largely by gestational age. Toward the end of the first trimester, eversion of columnar epithelium and dynamic phase metaplasia produce areas of fusion of columnar villi and distinct islands of immature metaplastic epithelium that can be visualized after the application of acetic acid. This process is rapidly progressive through the second trimester. As the islands of immature metaplasia coalesce, broad areas of smooth squamous metaplasia become apparent following application of acetic acid (Figure 12.14A–D). The acetic acid reaction of the immature metaplastic epithelium in pregnancy is exaggerated by the bluish hue caused by increased vascularity. In the third trimester, eversion and progressive metaplasia continue until about 36 weeks' gestation and then slow. The dimensions of the cervix at this time have notably increased in varying proportions, with associated remodeling of surface contours. Increased vascularity and abundant mucus production are clearly evident.

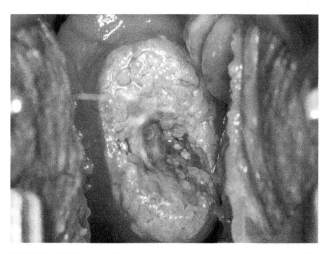

FIGURE 12.12.   Maximum eversion of columnar epithelium at 20 weeks' estimated gestational age.

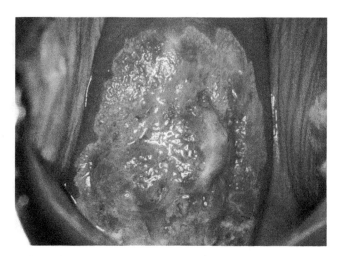

FIGURE 12.13.   Active squamous metaplasia seen on the ectocervix of a woman at 14 weeks' gestation during her first pregnancy. (Photo courtesy of Dr. Vesna Kesic.)

Physiologic changes are not limited to the cervix. The vaginal squamous mucosa thickens, and the vagina increases in length during pregnancy. As is true for the cervix, an increase in vascularity gives the vaginal epithelium a blue hue. A softening of the vaginal and cervical connective tissue is essential to accommodate birth. Therefore, the vaginal sidewalls develop some laxity and become redundant, prolapsing into the middle of the vagina. Prolapsing of the vaginal walls may significantly hinder the colposcopic examination in late pregnancy (Figure 12.15A–C).

12.5.2 Cytology

Even though impressive physiologic changes in the cervix occur during pregnancy, these alterations do not appear to affect the diagnostic accuracy of cervical cytologic examinations.[42,71] Because cervical neoplasia prevalence rates are similar for pregnant and nonpregnant women, the Pap test remains an important screening tool for this special population.[71] For many women, particularly those not using prescription-dependent contraceptives, an early pregnancy Pap test may be the only one collected in the recent past. However, pregnant women should only have a Pap test if the appropriate interval since their last test has elapsed, as determined by recent screening guidelines. Pregnancy is not an indication for early screening.[40,41]

For many years, Pap tests were collected from pregnant women using an Ayre spatula and a moistened cotton-tipped applicator. However, studies found that cotton fibers trap cervical cells, appreciably hindering cellular transfer to the glass slide.[72] Additionally, most Pap tests done today are liquid based and cannot be done with a cotton-tipped applicator. Although some concerns were initially raised about their safe use during pregnancy, several studies have now documented the safety of the endocervical brush (Cytobrush) and broom devices (Cervex-Brush) during pregnancy, even though the former device does not carry a product indication for use in pregnancy.[73–75] Moreover, these endocervical sampling devices yield significantly more endocervical cells in pregnant women than do cotton or Dacron swabs.[73–76] As a result, fewer unsatisfactory Pap tests will be reported.[77] Because of cervical eversion during pregnancy, a sufficient endocervical cellular yield is expected. Satisfactory Pap tests are more common for pregnant women compared with those for nonpregnant women.[78]

In general, interpretation of Pap tests collected from pregnant women does not differ from Pap tests collected from nonpregnant women. Because large areas of squamous metaplasia

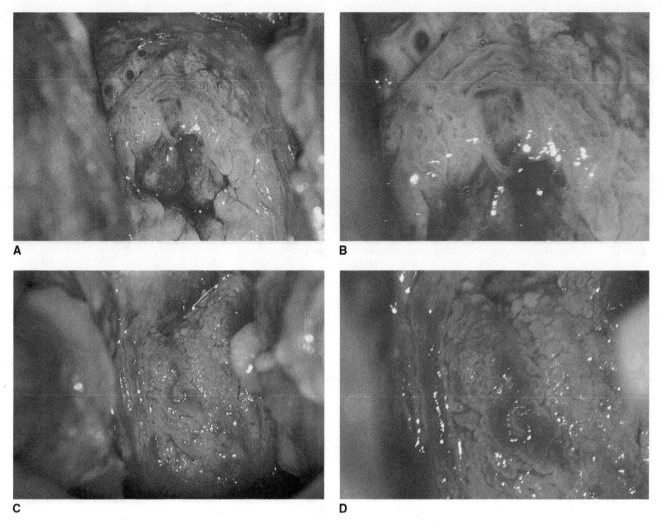

A   **B**

C   **D**

FIGURES 12.14.   Immature metaplasia on the anterior and posterior lip of the cervix during the second trimester of pregnancy (**A,B**). Active metaplasia in a woman 7½ months pregnant (**C,D**). Tongue-like projections of translucent acetowhite epithelium are seen along with focal changes on the tips of columnar villi.

may be sampled, a shift in proportion of types of cervical cells may be observed. Inflammatory cells are commonly noted in association with immature metaplasia. Navicular and decidual cells (Figure 12.16) may be seen. Decidual cells, or Arias-Stella reaction, are large, hypervacuolated cells with variably staining cytoplasm and a large nucleus.[42] Hence, they may be confused with neoplasia or reparative change. This potential may be minimized by providing the cytologist with a detailed patient history, including that the patient is pregnant.

12.5.3 Histology

With few exceptions, the evaluation of lower genital tract histology is similar for pregnant and nonpregnant women. However, just as colposcopic findings change during pregnancy, so does histology. Basal cell and columnar cell hyperplasia may be noted, and a greater percentage of mitotic figures may be detected in the basal layers. Evidence of immature metaplasia associated with a submucosal inflammatory process is commonly seen. Stromal edema and an increased vascularity are also observed. None of these findings are pathognomonic for pregnancy, since they can be noted with other entities. However, the presence of decidual cells in a histologic specimen suggests pregnancy (Figure 12.17). Decidual cells may

exhibit cytoplasmic vacuolization and nuclear enlargement that mimic neoplasia. Occasionally, these specialized cells, which are thought to help maintain pregnancy and initiate labor, will be found on the ectocervix because of cervical eversion and dilation of the external os. Stromal decidualization occurs in the second and third trimesters in about 30% of pregnant women. Decidual tissue can also mimic neoplasia colposcopically as an irregular exophytic projection from the surface of the cervix (Figure 12.18). Prominent atypical blood vessels may also be seen with decidua. However, decidual changes are benign and do not require intervention.

12.6 COLPOSCOPY OF PREGNANT WOMEN

12.6.1 Indications for Colposcopy during Pregnancy

The 2012 ASCCP and 2008 ACOG Guidelines clearly state that the only indication for therapy of cervical neoplasia in pregnant women is invasive cancer, although diagnostic excision may be indicated when cancer is suspected based on cytology, colposcopy, or biopsy findings.[1,52] Therefore, it is

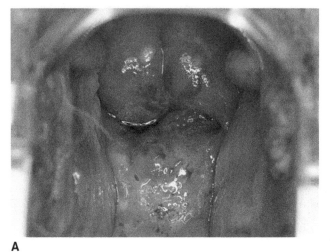

A

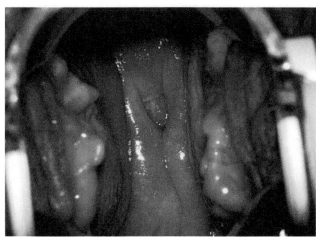

B

FIGURES 12.15.   **A–C:** Prolapsing vaginal sidewalls noted during pregnancy. In these cases, the prolapse is mild to moderate.

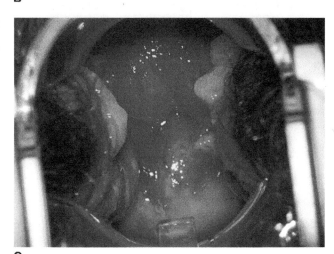

C

reasonable to defer colposcopy in pregnant women with Pap test results that convey a low risk for having cancer. This is particularly true for atypical squamous cells of undetermined significance (ASC-US) because the risk of cancer is relatively low in women with this cytologic abnormality, and some studies have shown that antepartum colposcopic evaluation does not add to management.[1,52] However, despite relatively low risk for cancer for pregnant women with either ASC-US or low-grade squamous intraepithelial lesion (LSIL), colposcopy is still the preferred initial management for all pregnant women ≥25 years with LSIL, with the caveat that it is acceptable to delay colposcopic evaluation until at least 6 weeks postpartum for pregnant women of any age with ASC-US or LSIL.[1] When ASC-US or LSIL are found in pregnant women aged 21 to 24 years, repeat cytology in 1 year rather than colposcopy is indicated. Pregnant women with any of the other abnormal

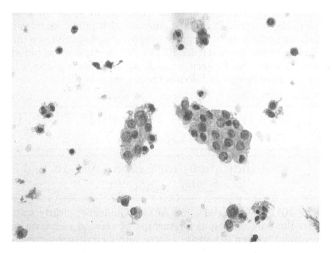

FIGURE 12.16.   Decidual cells seen on the Pap test from a pregnant woman. (Papanicolaou stain; high-power magnification.)

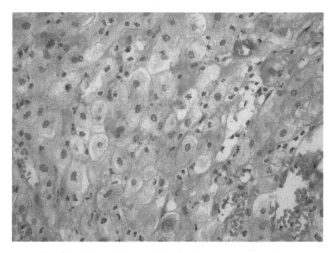

FIGURE 12.17.   Histologic specimen demonstrating decidua. (Hematoxylin-eosin stain; high-power magnification.)

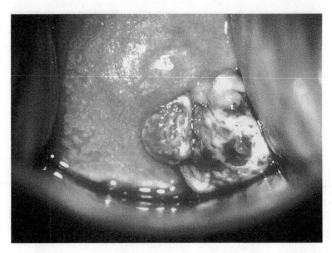

FIGURE 12.18. Decidua of the cervix that mimics an invasive cancer. (Photo courtesy of Dr. Burton Krumholz.)

Pap results should have colposcopy during pregnancy.[1,52,58] The other indications for colposcopy are essentially the same for pregnant and nonpregnant women. These include (1) a cervical mass or clinically apparent abnormality observed or palpated during a pelvic exam, (2) clinical or histologic evidence of neoplasia, or (3) any history of unexplained, nonobstetric vaginal bleeding or postcoital spotting. The latter indication may more frequently represent specific complications of pregnancy, such as early pregnancy loss, placenta previa, and placental abruption, which should be excluded prior to colposcopy. Despite its infrequency, it is important to consider the risk of cervical carcinoma when evaluating pregnancy-related bleeding problems.

When colposcopy is indicated, pregnant women should be scheduled for the examination as soon as possible. In early pregnancy, the cervix and lower genital tract retain features similar to the nonpregnant anatomy. Therefore, an examination in the early weeks of pregnancy will avoid late pregnancy changes that hinder the colposcopic exam. A thorough discussion of the procedures, risks, and alternatives to colposcopy and a discussion about the frequency of spontaneous abortion in routine pregnancies in the absence of colposcopy are important. Colposcopy with biopsy has not been associated with subsequent miscarriage. Such discussion should facilitate the assurance of the patient and family about the safety and importance of the colposcopic procedures in this setting and reduce the possibility of misinterpretation of the cause of a subsequent spontaneous miscarriage were this to occur. Immediate intervention also helps allay the psychological concerns of the pregnant woman regarding the potential for cervical disease interfering with a positive obstetrical outcome. Although colposcopic examinations can be performed throughout pregnancy, inspection during the first two trimesters is optimal. Women with previously detected cervical lesions can also be monitored by colposcopic and cytologic examinations during the course of the pregnancy and postpartum period as indicated.

12.6.2 Objectives of Colposcopy during Pregnancy

The main objective of colposcopy for nonpregnant women is to identify the presence, severity, and extent of neoplasia involving the lower genital tract so precancerous lesions can be destroyed. In contrast, the objective of colposcopy in pregnancy is to find or exclude cancer. Compared with the examination of the cervix in the nonpregnant patient, examination of colposcopic changes of the cervix during pregnancy demands

more experienced pattern-recognition skills by the colposcopist. When experience with the colposcopic evaluation of pregnant women is limited and a colposcopist with greater expertise in this area is available, consultation is appropriate. Of course, managing pregnant women with abnormal cervical cytology must take into account the welfare of both the mother and the fetus. Consequently, endocervical curettage (ECC) is contraindicated during pregnancy because it could accidentally rupture the amnion or lacerate the soft endocervix. Hypotension from inferior vena cava compression during a colposcopic examination in late pregnancy can be prevented by selective patient positioning and expedited inspection. Biopsy of areas with high-grade colposcopic appearance is recommended, while biopsy of lesser lesions may be elected. Biopsy sampling should be representative, but conservative and limited in number, and limited in size. Cervical conization, including loop electrosurgical excision procedure (LEEP), should be considered only when invasive cancer is suspected.

In summary, colposcopy of pregnant women is undertaken to rule out cancer. CIN detected should not be treated until the postpartum visit. At that time, women with CIN should be reevaluated by colposcopy and cytologic testing, since even CIN 3 has been shown to regress during and after pregnancy. Determining the adequacy of the colposcopic examination may be more challenging late in pregnancy when a larger cervix, thick mucus, and prolapsing vaginal sidewalls complicate colposcopic inspection. As with nongravid women, the correlation of cytologic, histologic, and colposcopic impressions should guide management strategy for pregnant women.

12.6.3 Colposcopic Examination of Pregnant Women

Colposcopic technique is identical for pregnant and nonpregnant women. The steps of visualization, assessment, sampling, and correlation must be followed as usual.

12.6.3.1 Visualization

Even though colposcopic visualization of the lower genital tract during pregnancy may be difficult, unobstructed visualization of the cervix is mandatory. As pregnancy progresses, there is increased laxity of the vaginal walls allowing the lateral walls to prolapse through the vaginal speculum blades, impairing visualization (Figure 12.19). As

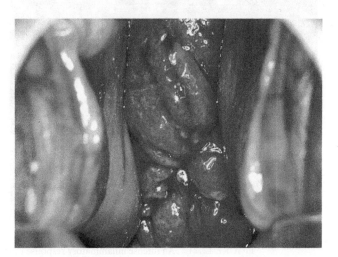

FIGURE 12.19. Prolapsing vaginal sidewalls hinder colposcopy during pregnancy. Decidual changes can be seen on the ectocervix.

the cervix enlarges during pregnancy, the vaginal wall pro-lapse increases, progressively reducing the proportion of the ectocervix that can be easily visualized. A large speculum is frequently necessary, and the use of a lateral vaginal side-wall retractor will often permit improved access to the cervix. Use of condoms or a cut latex glove finger with the tip removed and rolled onto the speculum blades is an inexpensive way to achieve a similar level of visualization in patients not allergic to latex. The latex barriers also minimize the risk for painful pinching by speculum blades that may be encountered with use of the lateral sidewall retractor. Otherwise, colposcopists can examine the entire ectocervix by inspecting smaller, visible portions of the ectocervix separately, using a large swab for manipulation. This restricted examination requires repositioning the cervix so that all sections have been colposcopically inspected by the completion of the examination.

Tenacious endocervical mucus encountered in pregnancy may also hamper adequate visualization (Figure 12.10A,B), although a deeply positioned mucus plug rarely interferes. Application of 3% to 5% acetic acid as a mucolytic will aid in mucus removal. Sponge-holding forceps or small tissue forceps may be used to carefully remove viscous mucus from the ectocervix or endocervical canal. If the mucus cannot be satisfactorily removed, it can be manipulated gently using moistened cotton-tipped applicators, allowing for a systematic examination of the cervix in quadrants. Finally, gently pushing the mucus a short distance back up, the endocervical canal with a small cotton-tipped applicator will sometimes facilitate proper inspection.

Visualization may be impaired further by bleeding if the vascular cervical epithelium is traumatized (Figure 12.20). This is particularly true in late pregnancy, when vascularity is most pronounced. Any associated inflammation further accentuates tissue friability (Figure 12.21A,B). Bleeding can be easily controlled with gentle pressure exerted by a large swab. Bleeding observed from the external os should be evaluated for more typical pregnancy-associated causes.

Regardless of these pregnancy-induced changes, the vast majority of pregnant women actually have adequate colposcopic examinations (Figure 12.22A,B).[79] Moreover, the cervical tissue gradually becomes softer and more amenable to gentle manipulation as the pregnancy progresses, so reinspection 6 to 12 weeks after an initial inadequate colposcopic examination early in pregnancy may be helpful in fully assessing the transformation zone.

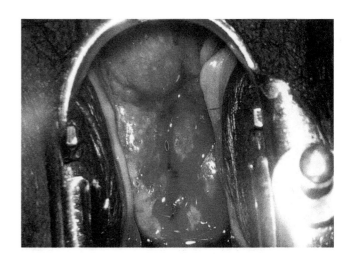

FIGURE 12.20. Bleeding during the third trimester of pregnancy obscures a CIN 3.

12.6.3.2 Assessment

Although colposcopic assessment of pregnant women may be difficult, particularly for the novice, most cervical lesions seen during pregnancy appear remarkably similar to those seen in nonpregnant women. As in the evaluation of nonpregnant women, colposcopists should consider the margin, color, vessels, and contour. Occasionally, iodine staining may also be helpful. Critical appraisal of these colposcopic findings enables reaching a meaningful colposcopic impression.

Many of the colposcopic features found in pregnancy are secondary to the normal pregnancy-induced physiologic changes discussed previously. Acetowhite areas of immature metaplastic epithelium are clearly visualized, becoming increasingly prominent as pregnancy proceeds. However, the acetowhite color of immature metaplasia is typically somewhat translucent and fades more quickly following the application of 3% to 5% acetic acid than does acetowhitening secondary to CIN. A fine punctation and mosaic vessel pattern may be noted within acetowhite areas of physiologic immature metaplasia (Figure 12.23A–C). These small-caliber vessels are closely and uniformly spaced. An associated cyanosis of pregnancy may alter the contrast between acetowhite epithelium and the normal epithelial background color. The prominent

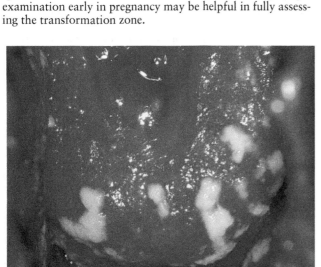

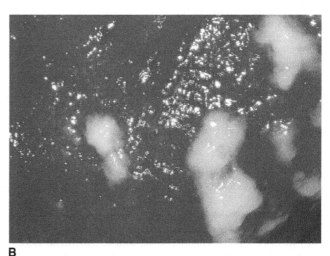

A   **B**

FIGURE 12.21.   An intense inflammatory response to vulvovaginal candidiasis of the cervix during pregnancy (**A**). At higher magnification, dilated loop capillaries can be seen (**B**).

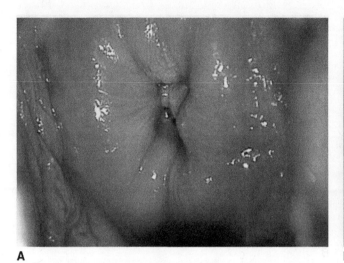

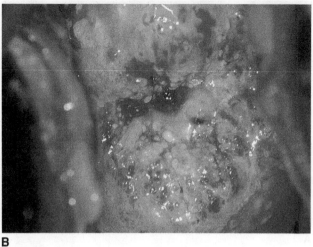

A   **B**

FIGURE 12.22.   An inadequate colposcopic examination (**A**) of this pregnant woman at 12 weeks' gestation. Her examination showed parakeratosis secondary to prior loop conization. It is doubtful that her examination will be adequate at 20 weeks because of her postsurgical changes. An adequate colposcopic examination is seen in a pregnant woman with CIN 1 (**B**).

increased vascularity of the cervix during pregnancy may be exaggerated against acetowhite epithelium. Consequently, a confusing angioarchitecture may be observed. This appearance may lead to normal physiologic changes being misinterpreted as neoplasia, particularly as low-grade lesions.

Excluding low- and moderate-grade CIN in extensive areas of immature metaplasia may be difficult since the appearances are similar in pregnancy (Figure 12.24A–D). However, precise discrimination is not critical since CIN 1 and CIN 2 do not require further observation through pregnancy; only

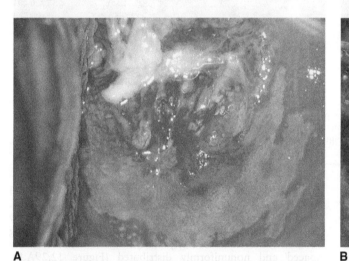

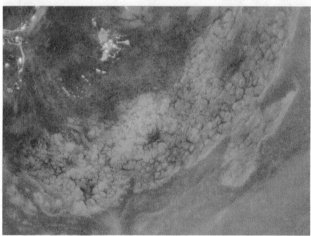

A   **B**

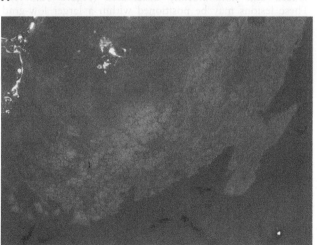

FIGURE 12.23.   An area of faint acetowhite epithelium with irregular margins is noted in this pregnant woman with immature metaplasia (**A**). A fine-caliber, lacy mosaic pattern is seen with the green filter (**B**). This same fine mosaic is also seen in iodine-negative epithelium of immature metaplasia following the application of half-strength Lugol iodine solution (**C**).

C

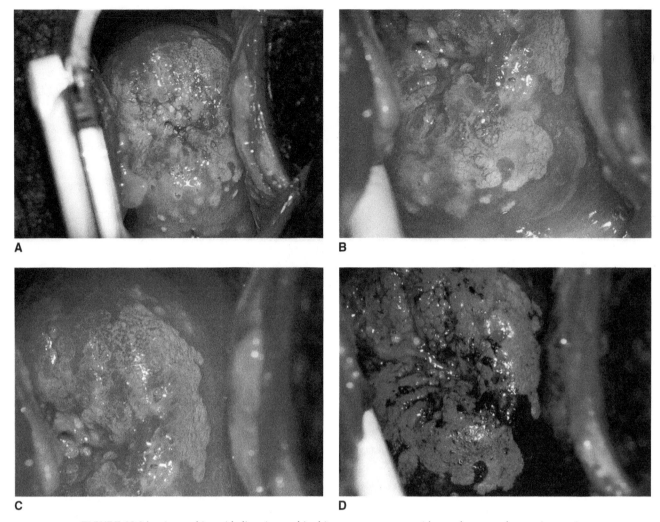

FIGURE 12.24. Acetowhite epithelium is noted in this pregnant woman with an adequate colposcopic examination (**A**). At higher magnification, a fine mosaic and punctation vascular pattern can be seen (**B,C**). Iodine-negative staining (**D**) confirms the colposcopic findings seen in Figure 12.24C. It is difficult to discriminate immature metaplasia from CIN 1 as seen.

reassessment in the puerperium. During the second and third trimesters, normally fine-caliber vessels change appearance secondary to increased blood volume, cardiac output, and vascular dilation.[80] Low-grade lesions may be colposcopically overinterpreted as high-grade lesions because of the physiologic dilation. However, if the colposcopist also considers other colposcopic signs, such as color, contour, and lesion margin (Figure 12.25A–D), proper discrimination is still possible.

In pregnancy, as in nonpregnancy, condylomas appear as exophytic growths, with a shiny acetowhite color and fine-caliber loop capillaries. They may be isolated on the cervix or distributed throughout the lower genital tract. Low-risk HPV types induce lesions that may vary in morphology, including flat, raised, papillary, cerebriform, inverted, or micropapillary (Figure 12.26A,B). Noncervical lesions caused by high-risk HPV types are more commonly papular in morphology. All HPV-induced lesions may proliferate rapidly during pregnancy.

CIN 1 lesions are flat, with irregular or geographic margins, mildly and transiently acetowhite epithelium, iodine-negative or iodine-positive (tortoise-shell) staining, and fine, closely spaced but evenly distributed blood vessels (Figures 12.24 and 12.27A,B). These lesions can be small or may occupy all four quadrants. They are usually located on the ectocervix, particularly in younger women.

The colposcopic features of CIN 2,3 during pregnancy may be obvious, but again must be discriminated from immature metaplasia, CIN 1, and cancer (Figure 12.28A–C). CIN 2,3 lesions are more likely to display smooth, straight margins, opaque acetowhite epithelium that may be easily dislodged by cervical sampling or manipulation, iodine-negative staining (if done), and rather coarsely dilated vessels that are widely spaced and nonuniformly distributed (Figure 12.29A,B). These lesions may be positioned within a larger low-grade lesion, and an abrupt interface or internal margin may be delineated between the two types of lesions (Figure 12.30A,B). Some high-grade lesions are opaque acetowhite with no blood vessels observed on the surface. The acetowhite reaction will also persist longer in high-grade lesions, helping to isolate the area of most severe colposcopic atypia.

Cervical cancer, particularly of advanced stage, should be readily identifiable during pregnancy (Figure 12.9). Large exophytic tumors may demonstrate leukoplakia, yellow necrotic epithelium, or a dense acetowhite color. The margins are usually well defined, especially when adjoining normal epithelium. Atypical blood vessels may be particularly prominent, coarsely dilated, and nonbranching. Superficial erosions or ulcerations and tissue friability with necrosis may be seen when the rapidly expanding cancer exceeds its vascular supply.

Knowledge of the warning signs of early invasive cancer is critical in colposcopic assessment of the cervix in pregnancy. The presence of any finding suspicious for invasive disease requires biopsy at a minimum and the most conscientious

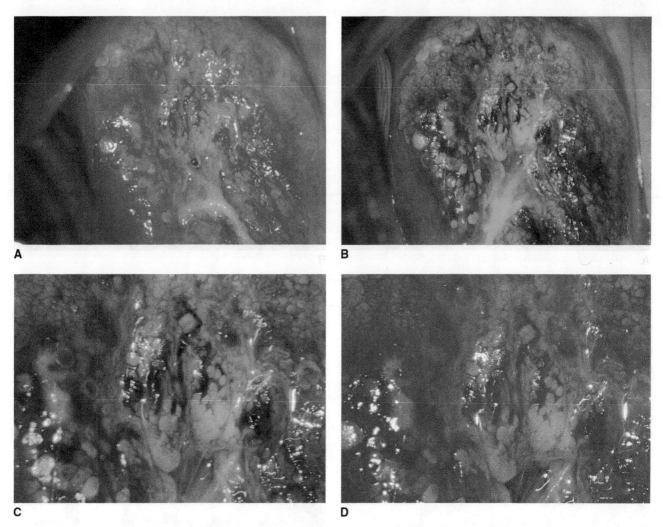

FIGURE 12.25.   A large CIN 3 lesion is seen in the pregnant woman (**A,B**). With closer inspection (**C,D**), a very coarsely dilated mosaic pattern is seen. These vessels mimic those associated with cancer.

colposcopic, histologic, and cytologic review. The surface contour changes associated with mucus-filled glands and decidual reaction may create diagnostic problems. Decidua frequently has a polypoid or exophytic appearance that can be confused with condylomas or cancer (Figure 12.31A–F). When

prominent vascular changes accompany decidual reaction, the appearance may mimic an invasive cancer.

The ability of experienced colposcopists to formulate colposcopic impressions reliably in pregnant women supports the use of this procedure for the diagnosis of cervical neoplasia in

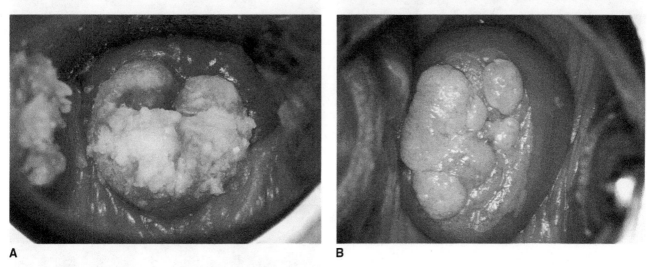

FIGURE 12.26.   **A,B:** Large condylomatous lesions of the ectocervix. These large lesions could be confused with an exophytic invasive cancer. (Photo courtesy of Dr. Vesna Kesic.)

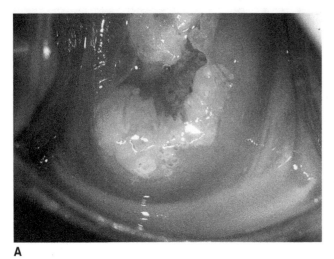
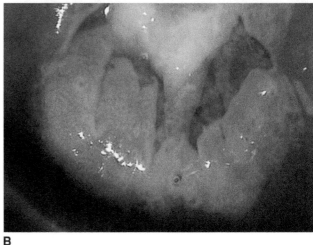

A   **B**

FIGURE 12.27.   A CIN 1 on the posterior lip of the cervix (**A**). No vessels are seen at higher magnification in this pregnant woman (**B**).

pregnancy. In one study, the antepartum colposcopic interpretation correlated within one degree with patients' postpartum histologic diagnoses in 87%, with 11% found to have a colposcopic impression more severe than the histologic impression, and colposcopic under interpretation noted for only 2% of women with more severe lesions found by histology.[81] In a study of over 1000 pregnant patients having colposcopy for abnormal cervical cytology, of patients who had biopsy, results correlated with or were less severe than the colposcopic

impression in 83% with CIN 1 and 56% with CIN 2,3.[43] The authors concluded that colposcopic impression in pregnancy correlated with cervical biopsy results and postpartum colposcopic findings when performed by expert colposcopists. They also noted that 61% of CIN regressed postpartum. Another large retrospective study of 811 women referred with abnormal cervical cytology in pregnancy also supported the safety and accuracy of managing dysplasia in pregnancy with colposcopy, directed punch biopsy as needed, and deferral of

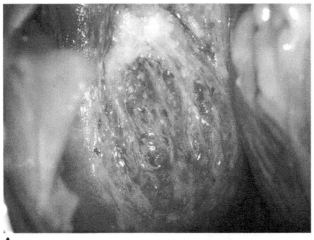
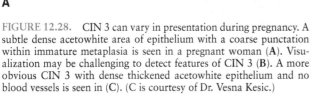

A

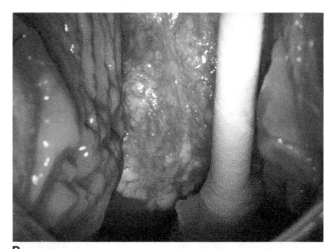

B

FIGURE 12.28.   CIN 3 can vary in presentation during pregnancy. A subtle dense acetowhite area of epithelium with a coarse punctation within immature metaplasia is seen in a pregnant woman (**A**). Visualization may be challenging to detect features of CIN 3 (**B**). A more obvious CIN 3 with dense thickened acetowhite epithelium and no blood vessels is seen in (**C**). (C is courtesy of Dr. Vesna Kesic.)

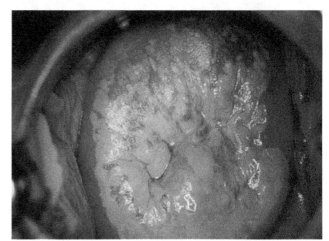

C

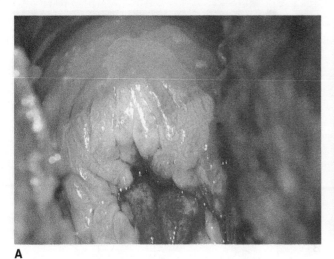
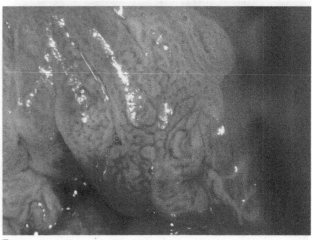

FIGURE 12.29. A high-grade lesion of the cervix in a pregnant woman (**A**). An internal margin, dense acetowhite epithelium and a coarse mosaic pattern with punctation can be seen (**B**).

treatment until the postpartum period.[82] Histologic progression during pregnancy to a higher grade of CIN in the postpartum period was only 7%. None of the women developed microinvasive or invasive cancer between antenatal assessment and postpartum review. Siddiq et al.[83] also demonstrated a significant decrease in colposcopically detected CIN 2,3 between the antenatal and postpartum period. As noted earlier, there is a small propensity to overinterpret cervical neoplasia colposcopically during pregnancy.[79,84–86] However, underdiagnoses of 54% of women with CIN 1 or 2 as normal was reported in a larger retrospective study of pregnant women evaluated during the period from 1975 to 1992.[85] Of greater importance was the finding of CIN 3 in 14% of women with a colposcopic impression of CIN 1. Hence, if uncertain whether high-grade disease is present colposcopically, one or more biopsies are indicated.

12.6.3.3 Sampling

Histologic sampling can be done safely during pregnancy but must be performed carefully (Figure 12.32A,B).[79] Selective biopsy of the most severe areas of colposcopic atypia minimizes potential complications from noncritically assessed sampling. Because of a potential for excessive bleeding following cervical biopsy

during pregnancy, the 2012 ASCCP Guidelines recommend that biopsy of cervical lesions suspicious for CIN 2,3 or cancer is preferred but that biopsy of other lesions is acceptable.[1] Although multiple biopsies of all colposcopically abnormal areas are advised in nonpregnant women to maximize detection of CIN 2,3, bleeding may not allow this during pregnancy.

Bleeding is the main concern when obtaining biopsies in pregnancy. Marked edema and vascularity of the cervix contribute to potentially significant bleeding after biopsy. Bleeding is brisker in late pregnancy than during the earlier weeks of pregnancy. However, serious bleeding complications from biopsy are actually rare in pregnancy,[42,86] and hemostasis is usually readily secured. The risks of severe hemorrhage associated with biopsy are notably less than those associated with conization or missed diagnosis of early invasive cancer.

Biopsy techniques for pregnant and nonpregnant women are the same. However, biopsy forceps that take smaller bites are more likely to reduce the risk of heavy bleeding than those that take a large amount of tissue and should be available to clinicians who elect to do colposcopy in pregnant women. Colposcopists must ascertain whether an adequate specimen has been obtained once the jaws are removed from the cervix and should be prepared to rapidly administer a hemostatic agent. Silver

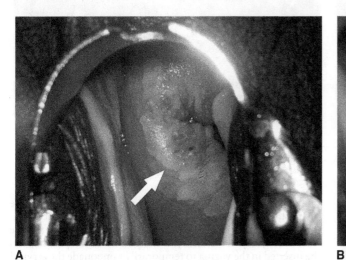
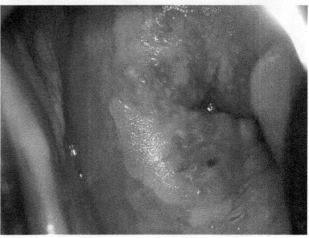

FIGURE 12.30. A high-grade lesion is positioned within a low-grade lesion seen in this pregnant patient (**A**). Some leukoplakia precluded visualization of blood vessels (**B**). An internal margin can be seen demarcating the low- from high-grade lesion (*arrow*).

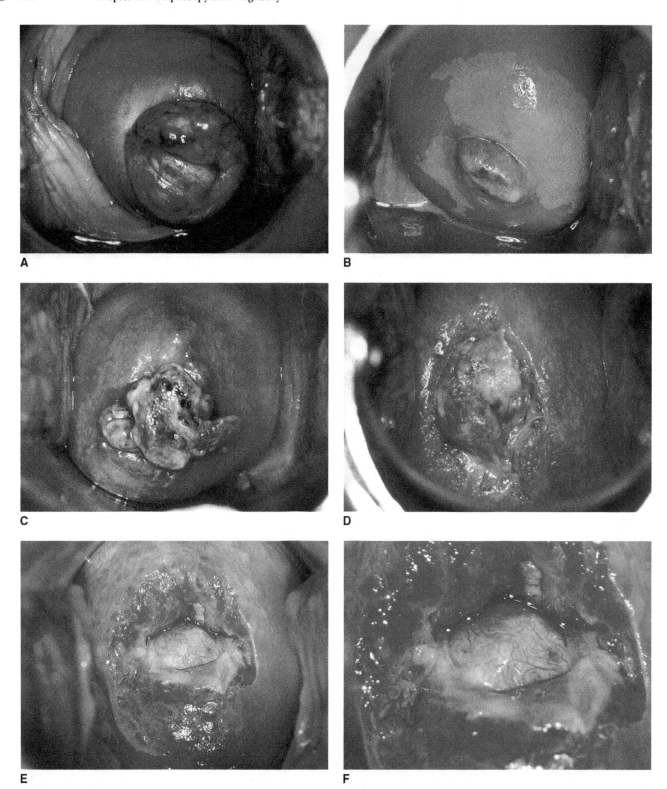

FIGURE 12.31.   A–F: No two decidual polyps of the cervix are alike. Many mimic invasive cancer. Note the prominent blood vessels in (**F**). (Photos **A–D** courtesy of Dr. Vesna Kesic.)

nitrate sticks or cotton-tipped applicators soaked in Monsel paste should be readily available during biopsy for immediate placement at the biopsy site as needed. Once the biopsy is taken with one hand, the Monsel-soaked cotton-tipped applicator or silver nitrate stick is pressed firmly onto the bleeding site with the other hand without delay. The applicator should be held in place, covering the base of the wound and wound edges until hemostasis is achieved. Additional Monsel or silver nitrate

may need to be applied. Sutures are rarely necessary to secure hemostasis when cautery methods fail, but an experienced colposcopist will have the required equipment available for the rare emergency. If necessary, a tampon or gauze packing can be inserted in the vagina to temporarily tamponade the cervical biopsy site(s), and the patient should rest in the office/clinic for 15 to 30 minutes. If bleeding was heavy or difficult to stop, she should be counseled to avoid vigorous activity for 48 hours

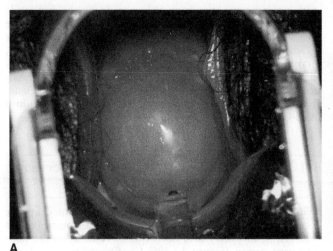
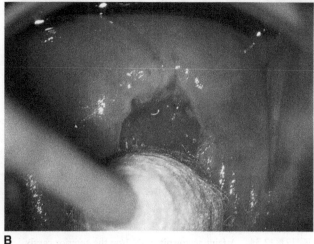

A   B

FIGURE 12.32.   Histologic sampling of this pregnant woman (24 weeks) with an LSIL Pap test was delayed upon visual detection of amniotic membranes (**A**). Her postpartum colposcopic examination was normal (**B**).

afterward and intercourse for up to 5 to 7 days; otherwise a shorter period of these restrictions can be advised. Also advise that some bright red spotting and serous vaginal discharge is normal and may continue for several days, but caution that heavy bleeding requires medical attention.

Occasionally, high-grade disease may extend deep into the endocervical canal, rendering the assessment of the upper extent of the lesion very difficult. A carefully placed endocervical speculum can improve assessment of the distal endocervical canal in some pregnant patients. If this approach fails to improve visualization, reevaluation at around 20 weeks' gestation may permit an unencumbered view of the entire lesion and SCJ. The delay may be appropriate if invasive disease is not suspected. Remember that ECC is contraindicated in pregnancy.[1,42,52] Although cervical biopsy is a relatively benign procedure, patients may be particularly frightened. Auscultation of fetal heart tones following histologic sampling may reassure the patient that the procedure has not harmed the fetus.

12.6.3.4 Correlation

Finally, the correlation of cytologic, histologic, and colposcopic impressions determines proper management of pregnant women with cervical neoplasia. Agreement within one degree of severity should be expected just as for nonpregnant women.[79,84–86] Discordance may prompt further diagnostic evaluation.[83] Diagnostic excision is unacceptable unless invasive cancer is suspected based on the referral cytology, colposcopic appearance, or cervical biopsy.[1,52] Provided cancer has been excluded, minor discordance will generally require only serial cytologic and colposcopic monitoring.

12.7 COLPOSCOPIC FINDINGS OF CERVICAL NEOPLASIA IN PREGNANCY

12.7.1 Colposcopy of Low-Grade Cervical and Vaginal Lesions in Pregnancy

In general, CIN 1 lesions appear the same in pregnant and non-pregnant women (Figures 12.33A,B, 12.34, and 12.35A–C). Low-grade lesions noted during pregnancy may be exophytic or papular condylomas, or acetowhite macular lesions with irregular margins. Condylomas may be snowy white after acetic acid application or opaque white prior to acetic acid

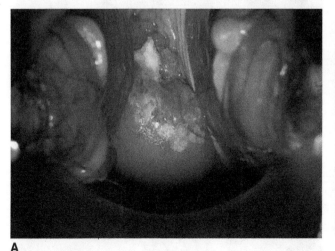
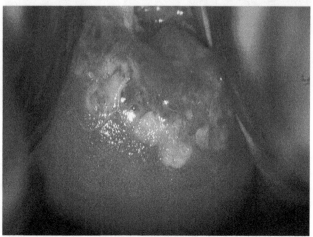

A   B

FIGURE 12.33.   **A,B:** A CIN 1 on the posterior cervix in this pregnant woman.

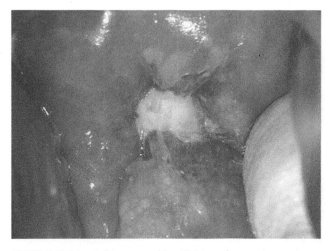

FIGURE 12.34.   A faint acetowhite CIN 1 on the anterior cervix.

application, denoting the presence of HPV-related leukoplakia (Figure 12.26A,B). Raised, exophytic condylomas of the cervix may be luxuriant in pregnancy and should be biopsied to rule out cancer. Macular lesions have a transient, faint acetowhite color. The blood vessels are of fine caliber, closely spaced, and arranged in a uniform pattern. Later in pregnancy, these vessels may dilate as cardiac output and blood volume increase. However, intercapillary distances remain constant. If Lugol iodine staining is used, the lesion may appear iodine positive or negative, depending on the amount of glycogen in the tissue (Figure 12.24D). Lesions

with a colposcopic impression of low grade may be seen inside or outside the transformation zone but, if positioned along the SCJ, are potentially of greater risk for underdiagnosing CIN 2 or 3. Small, diffuse micropapillary projections, known as asperities, may be noted on the cervix or in the proximal vagina. These subclinical HPV changes may appear with distinct unifocal or multifocal low-grade lesion(s), or they may exist independently (Figure 12.36A–C). Such findings are not uncommon with HPV-positive ASC-US and LSIL cytology (Figures 12.37 and 12.38A,B).

12.7.2 Colposcopy of High-Grade Cervical Lesions (CIN 2,3) in Pregnancy

While many high-grade lesions during pregnancy appear similar to the same lesions seen in nongravid women (Figure 12.39A,B), they may also not be as obvious as in the nonpregnant cervix (Figure 12.39C–G). Others may be large, involving multiple quadrants of the cervix. As in the nonpregnant cervix, CIN 2,3 lesions typically have margins that are smooth, peeling, or may exhibit an internal border separating the high-grade lesion from a larger surrounding low-grade lesion (Figure 12.40). Epithelial thickening may be observed as an opaque dull acetowhite color that persists for a prolonged time following 3% to 5% acetic acid application (Figure 12.41A–D). Prominent coarsely dilated blood vessels with an irregular, nonuniform, and widely spaced capillary pattern (Figure 12.42) may be seen and are often exaggerated later in pregnancy. However, many high-grade lesions contain no colposcopically observable blood vessels.

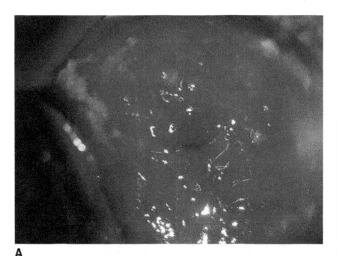

A

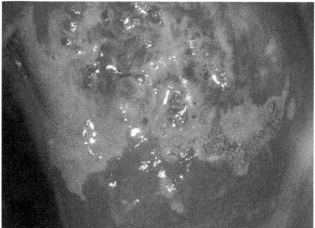

B

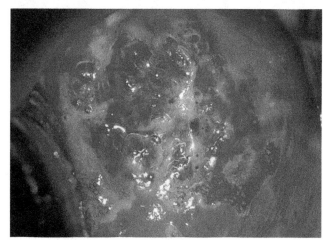

C

FIGURE 12.35.   Nabothian follicles are seen on this pregnant woman's cervix prior to the application of acetic acid (**A**). After acetic acid has been applied, a geographic acetowhite lesion can be seen (**B**). The lesion is still apparent as the effects of the 3% to 5% acetic acid diminish (**C**).

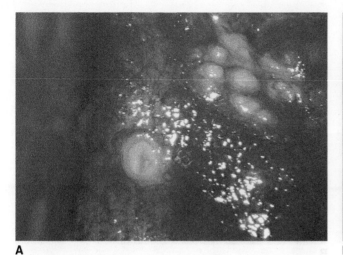

A

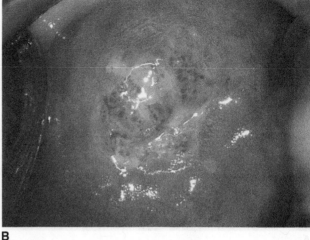

B

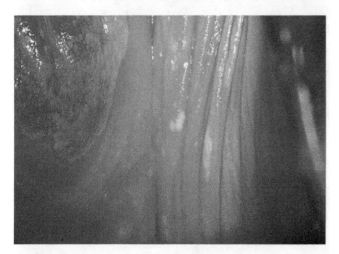

C

FIGURE 12.36.   CIN 1 noted in a pregnant women with an LSIL Pap test report (**A**). Involvement of a gland cleft can also be appreciated by the wide acetowhite band of CIN 1 encompassing the gland opening. A small low-grade lesion is seen at the 10 o'clock position in the next pregnant patient (**B**). With closer inspection (**C**), a faint acetowhite lesion is seen along the SCJ. In the periphery small, diffuse micropapillary projections, known as asperities, can be seen. A small area of fine mosaic appears to be developing.

12.7.3 Colposcopy of Carcinoma of the Cervix in Pregnancy

12.7.3.1 Colposcopy of Microinvasive Cancer

Large high-grade lesions may harbor an area of microinvasive cancer. Colposcopists may not notice a focal contour

FIGURE 12.37.   A vaginal flat condyloma is seen in this pregnant woman with CIN 3.

change or early atypical vessel that may accompany an evolving microinvasion. The microinvasion may present as a small opaque, acetowhite lesion with short atypical vessels (Figure 12.43). Prominent, dilated vasculature noted during late pregnancy may make a severe high-grade lesion appear as a potential microinvasive lesion. Therefore, microinvasion can either be easily overlooked colposcopically or overdiagnosed. Furthermore, a simple cervical biopsy may miss a small microinvasive lesion, particularly if the area of microinvasion is focal in nature, as it frequently is, or the biopsy may not obtain sufficient depth to allow a diagnosis of microinvasion. Thus, if the colposcopic impression and cytology continue to be of concern for cancer despite the absence of microinvasion or invasion on biopsy, a large wedge biopsy, cone biopsy, or electrosurgical loop excision (LEEP) may be required for confirmation. Prior to electing an excisional procedure, consultation with a gynecologic oncologist for diagnostic and therapeutic assistance should be obtained. If conization is elected, it is best performed in midpregnancy or following fetal maturity. The goal of conization is to identify suspected cancer, not treatment of all disease on the transformation zone; for this reason, the size of the excision may be restricted. However, conization may not be required even if microinvasion is diagnosed on biopsy, as the pregnancy may be allowed to continue even if frank invasion is present, for delaying treatment of an occult malignancy may have no impact on survival, especially when diagnosed near fetal maturity.[62] These decisions should be made in consultation with a gynecologic oncologist.

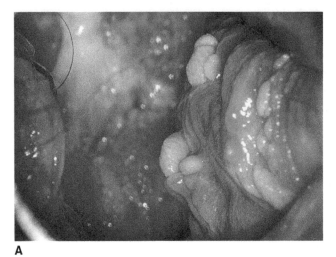
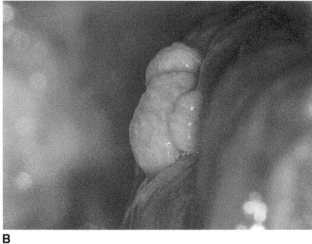

A   **B**

FIGURE 12.38.   **A,B:** Condylomas are seen in this pregnant woman's vagina.

12.7.3.2 Colposcopy of Invasive Carcinoma

Because cervical cancer is so uncommon, it can be missed unless a very high index of suspicion is maintained for symptoms and signs of cervical cancer in pregnant women. If there is no apparent pregnancy-related cause for bleeding, a colposcopic examination should be performed to exclude a rare occult invasive cancer. Also, if the cervix feels abnormally firm and indurated or demonstrates an unusual surface contour during pelvic examination in pregnancy, colposcopy is indicated to exclude cervical cancer. The same colposcopic warning signs for cervical cancer in nonpregnant women also apply for pregnant women (see Chapter 10). Atypical blood vessels are the hallmark of cervical cancer. During pregnancy, these large caliber vessels may be particularly engorged. Exophytic

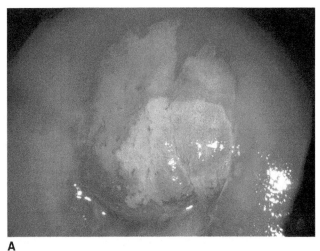
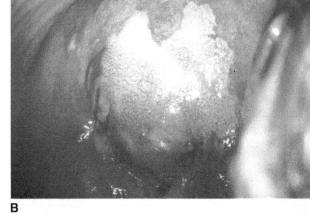

A   **B**

FIGURE 12.39.   CIN 2 (**A**) and CIN 3 (**B**) seen in pregnant women. The CIN 2 is seen demarcated from immature metaplasia by an internal margin. The CIN 3 has an opaque acetowhite color with a coarse punctation and mosaic vascular pattern. (Reprinted with permission from Wright VC. Color Atlas of colposcopy: cervix, vagina, and vulva. Houston: Biomedical Communications, 2000*). A less obvious CIN 3 is seen in (**C**).

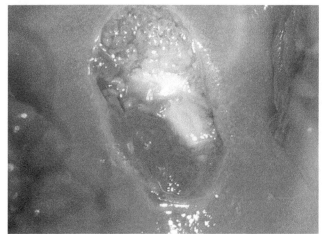

C

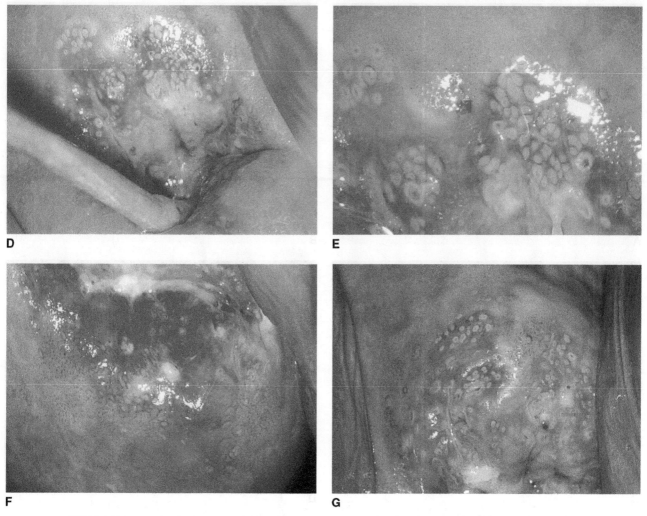

FIGURE 12.39. (*continued*) There is a red, non acetowhite lesion from the 6 o'clock to the 8 o'clock position along the SCJ; a faintly acetowhite lesion is seen in (**D**) and (**E**). The wide opaque periglandular cuffing suggests a high-grade lesion. The other lesion in (**F**) and (**G**) is also similar, faintly acetowhite but with opaque periglandular cuffing.

cancers may be readily detected by an irregular contour change of the ectocervix (Figure 12.44). Decidual tissue of pregnancy may be confused easily with small exophytic tumors (Figure 12.45). Uncertainty of etiology always demands appropriate

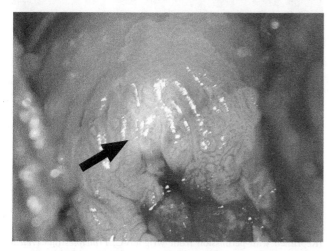

FIGURE 12.40. A high-grade lesion (*arrow*) is demarcated from a low-grade lesion by an internal margin in this pregnant woman.

histologic sampling. Since cervical volume enlarges in both pregnancy and invasive cancer, endophytic cancers may not be as easily noted. Ulcerations may indicate cancer in a necrotic area surrounded by yellow, friable epithelium. Large four-quadrant, opaque acetowhite lesions are more likely to harbor cancer, as are the same lesions that extend deeply within the endocervical canal.

A colposcopic impression of cervical cancer in pregnancy requires an appropriate biopsy for confirmation. If the histologic diagnosis of invasive cancer is in doubt, an additional pathologist's opinion should be obtained. If the tumor is clinically obvious, colposcopy is redundant and a directed biopsy may be adequate to establish the diagnosis. As noted for microinvasive disease, in some cases, however, a larger tissue sample, either a wedge or cone biopsy, may be required to determine depth of invasion. Colposcopists must be prepared for the extensive bleeding that may be experienced after pregnant woman are biopsied or excisional procedures are performed. Therefore, histologic sampling of pregnant patients with lesions suggestive of cancer should be performed by colposcopists experienced in the evaluation and management of pregnant women with abnormal cervical cytology or by gynecologic oncologists. Performing the procedure under sedation or general anesthesia in an operating theater with intravenous access and ready access to suture supplies is often advisable.

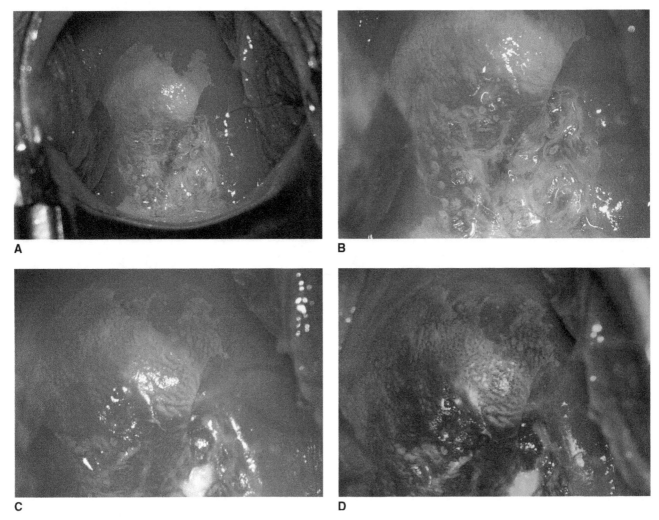

FIGURE 12.41.   **A–D:** A high-grade lesion with opaque acetowhite epithelium and a coarse mosaic in this pregnant woman.

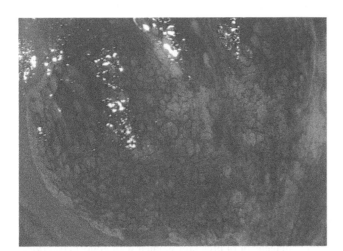

FIGURE 12.42.   A CIN 3 with a smooth margin and a coarse, widely spaced mosaic vessel pattern in this pregnant woman.

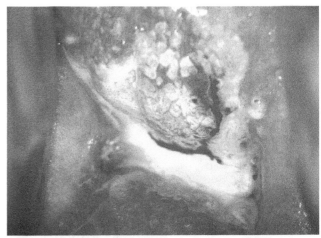

FIGURE 12.43.   Microinvasive cervical cancer in a pregnant woman. (Reprinted with permission from Wright VC. *Principles of Cervical Colposcopy*. Houston: Biomedical Communications, 2004.)

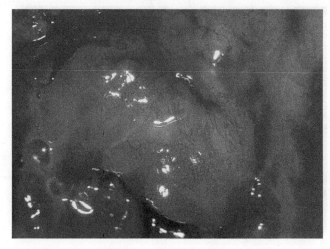

FIGURE 12.44. Cervical cancer in a pregnant woman. A *yellow* color and atypical blood vessels are seen. (Reprinted with permission from Wright VC. *Color Atlas of Colposcopy—Cervix, Vagina and Vulva.* Houston: Biomedical Communications, 2003.)

12.8 ANTEPARTUM MANAGEMENT OF PREGNANT WOMEN WITH ABNORMAL CERVICAL CYTOLOGY

The management of pregnant women with abnormal cytology depends on the degree of cytologic abnormality, the outcome of colposcopy, and, when necessary, directed biopsy. Because the only diagnosis that may alter management in pregnancy is invasive cancer, the management of pregnant women with abnormal cervical cytology or biopsy-proven CIN is generally more conservative than management of similar cytology and histology in nonpregnant women. Colposcopic examination during pregnancy should have as its primary goal the exclusion of invasive cancer.[1,52] (see Chapter 19 for full discussion of the management guidelines for abnormal cervical cytology in pregnancy.)

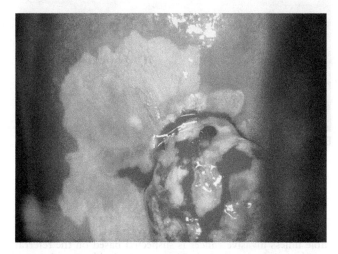

FIGURE 12.45. A macular acetowhite high-grade lesion can be seen alongside decidual tissue that mimics invasive cancer. Biopsy of both lesions is mandatory, given this women's HSIL Pap test report. (Photo courtesy of Dr. Burton Krumholz.)

12.8.1 Management of Pregnant Women with ASC and LSIL Pap Results

A number of studies have supported a conservative approach to the management of CIN during pregnancy. In patients with ASC-US or LSIL cytology, CIN 2,3 warranting biopsy is not commonly found with these minor cytologic findings, regression to normal in the postpartum is frequent, and invasive cancer is very rare (Figure 12.46A–E).[42,43,60,61,87] Therefore, the 2012 ASCCP management options for pregnant women ≥21 years of age with ASC-US are identical to those described for nonpregnant women, with the exception that it is acceptable to defer colposcopy until at least 6 weeks postpartum.[1] Additionally, ECC is unacceptable in pregnant women. If colposcopy is performed during pregnancy for ASC-US, women with no histologic or colposcopically suspected CIN 2+ at the initial colposcopy should have follow-up postpartum (see Chapter 19, Section 19.3.2.2.2.2 Management of Pregnant Women with ASC-US, Table 19.18).[1]

The guidelines for managing pregnant women ≥25 years with LSIL cytology are also in Chapter 19, Section 19.3.4.3.3. Colposcopy is preferred for pregnant women with LSIL cytology just as it is for nonpregnant women, although deferring colposcopy until postpartum is also acceptable because of the low risk for cancer[1] (Figure 12.47). ECC is *unacceptable* in pregnant women. Postpartum follow-up is recommended for pregnant women without cytologic, histologic, or colposcopically suspected CIN 2,3 or cancer at the initial colposcopy. Additional colposcopic and cytologic examinations during pregnancy are unacceptable.[1]

Management of pregnant women aged 21 to 24 years with LSIL cytology should be the same as for management of non-pregnant women in this age group with LSIL, namely repeat cytology in 1 year without colposcopy.

12.8.2 Management of Pregnant Women with ASC-H, AGC, and HSIL Pap Results

All other cytologic interpretations, that is, ASC-H, atypical glandular cells (AGC), and HSIL, should all have colposcopy as soon as possible after the laboratory report is received.[1,52] Immediate excision of the transformation zone for women referred for the evaluation of any abnormal cytology, including HSIL ("see and treat,") is not acceptable in pregnancy. It is preferred that the colposcopic evaluation of pregnant women with HSIL be conducted by a clinician experienced in the evaluation of colposcopic changes induced by pregnancy.[1,52] These include cervical hyperemia, the development of prominent normal epithelial changes that colposcopically mimic preinvasive disease, obscuring mucus, contact bleeding, prolapsing vaginal walls, and bleeding after biopsy. This caution could be prudently extended to the evaluation of pregnant women with ASC-H and AGC cytology. Occasionally, the interpretation of HSIL reflects misclassified pregnancy-induced cytologic changes, including immature squamous metaplasia, decidual changes, and inflammation. However, the majority of pregnant women with HSIL cytology will have CIN 2,3 detected during colposcopic examination (Figure 12.48A–D). ECC is contraindicated in pregnancy regardless of the cytology result because an ECC can result in laceration of the soft cervix with consequent hemorrhage, and it also may rupture the amniotic membranes.[1,52] Biopsy is important if the colposcopy impression is high grade, especially in older pregnant women at higher risk of occult invasive cancer, for the primary goal is excluding the presence of invasive cervical cancer (Figure 12.9).[1,80]

Once cancer has been excluded, cervical therapy can be deferred until postpartum.[1] CIN may regress during the interval between antenatal cytology and a postpartum examination

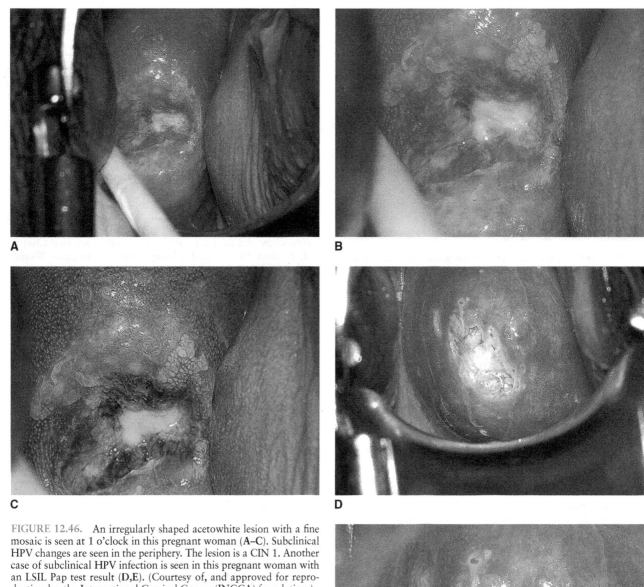

FIGURE 12.46.   An irregularly shaped acetowhite lesion with a fine mosaic is seen at 1 o'clock in this pregnant woman (A–C). Subclinical HPV changes are seen in the periphery. The lesion is a CIN 1. Another case of subclinical HPV infection is seen in this pregnant woman with an LSIL Pap test result (D,E). (Courtesy of, and approved for reproduction by, the International Cervical Cancer (INCCA) foundation.)

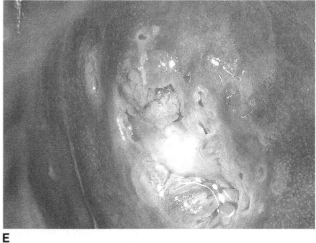

and progression to invasion during pregnancy is unlikely. Additionally, colposcopy becomes increasingly difficult as pregnancy proceeds. Therefore, once invasion has been ruled out, repeat colposcopy is not usually helpful until postpartum. Reassessment with cytology and colposcopy no sooner than 6 weeks after delivery is important in tailoring therapy (see 19.3.6.3.2 Management of HSIL in pregnancy and Table 19.22).[1]

If the colposcopic examination is inadequate, reappraisal with Pap test and colposcopic evaluation at approximately 20 weeks' gestational age, or 12 weeks from the initial colposcopy, may be beneficial as more of the cervix is everted. When CIN 2,3 is not found in the evaluation of a pregnant women with HSIL cytology, a diagnostic excision is unacceptable unless invasive cancer is suspected based on the referral cytology, colposcopic appearance, or cervical biopsy.[1] Instead, if the colposcopy is adequate, reevaluation with cytology and colposcopy is recommended no sooner than 6 weeks postpartum for pregnant women with HSIL in whom CIN 2,3 is not diagnosed.[1] If the colposcopic impression is of early invasion

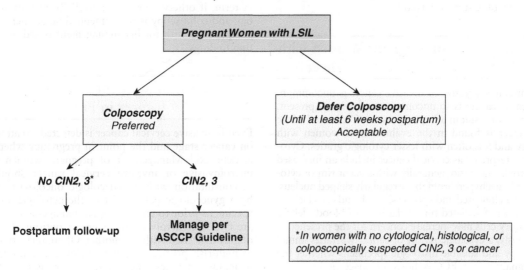

Management of Pregnant Women with Low-grade Squamous Intraepithelial Lesion (LSIL) Cytology
Except women 21–24

Pregnant Women with LSIL

Colposcopy
Preferred

Defer Colposcopy
(Until at least 6 weeks postpartum)
Acceptable

No CIN2, 3*

CIN2, 3

Postpartum follow-up

Manage per ASCCP Guideline

**In women with no cytological, histological, or colposcopically suspected CIN2, 3 or cancer*

FIGURE 12.47.   Algorithm for management of pregnant women with an abnormal ASC-US or LSIL Pap test report. Colposcopy is preferred for adult women. However, it is acceptable to defer colposcopy until at least 6 weeks postpartum.

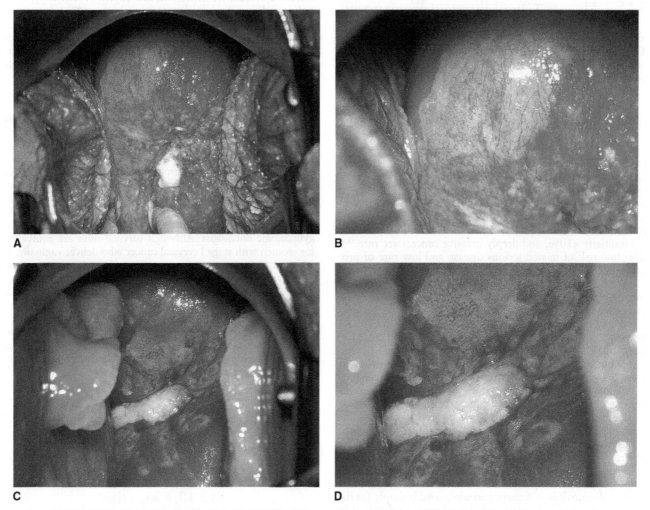

A

B

C

D

FIGURE 12.48.   A large opaque CIN 2 with coarse punctation and mosaic is seen on the anterior cervix (**A,B**). The next pregnant woman with an HSIL Pap test had this CIN 2 with coarse punctation at 10 o'clock (**C,D**). (Courtesy of, and approved for reproduction by, the International Cervical Cancer (INCCA) Foundation.)

and biopsy does not confirm the impression, referral to an expert in the colposcopic evaluation of pregnant women or to a gynecologic oncologist is preferred.[1]

12.8.3 Management of Pregnant Women with a Pap Test Report Suspect for Cancer

A cytologic finding suggestive of invasive cancer is uncommon, primarily because cancer is so uncommon and, even if present, sometimes does not result in a Pap test result of "cancer." More frequently, cancer is found in the evaluation of women with HSIL cytology and less often with lesser cytologic grades. Cytologic changes interpreted as cervical cancer include an increased nuclear-to-cytoplasmic ratio, generally with a scant rim of cytoplasm surrounding a hyperchromatic, irregularly shaped nucleus, cells that may be elongated and spindle shaped, and cells lacking uniform shape. An associated tumor diathesis of blood, debris, and inflammatory cells may increase concern for the presence of cancer. Obviously, a cytologic report of cancer warrants immediate colposcopy and suitable histologic specimens whether the patient is pregnant or not. ECC is, however, unacceptable.

12.9 MANAGEMENT OF CERVICAL NEOPLASIA IN PREGNANCY

12.9.1 Management of Pregnant Women with CIN 1

The management of pregnant women with a histology diagnosis of CIN 1 is follow-up without treatment. Treatment of pregnant women for CIN 1 is unacceptable.[1,52]

12.9.2 Management of Pregnant Women with CIN 2,3

Once cancer has been excluded, cervical therapy of high-grade CIN can be deferred until the postpartum period, as a cervical excision procedure during pregnancy should only be done if invasion is suspected[1,52] (see Section 20.2.3.2.3). The risk of missed microinvasive cancer in a pregnant woman with histologic CIN 2 is negligible, whereas the risk after CIN 3 is substantially <10%, and deeply invasive cancers are rare.[88,89] This low risk of missed serious disease and low rate of progression prompted guidelines recommending that high-grade CIN not be treated in pregnancy because of the risk of serious complications, including abortion, hemorrhage, cervical incompetence, cervical stenosis, infection, stillbirth, preterm labor, and maternal death.[51,52] Pregnant women with CIN 2,3 may be reevaluated during pregnancy at intervals no more frequent than every 12 weeks by repeat colposcopy and cytology,[51] but it is acceptable to defer their reevaluation until at least 6 weeks postpartum. Repeat biopsy during pregnancy is recommended only if the appearance of the lesion worsens or if cytology suggests invasive cancer. Unless invasive cancer is identified, or concern remains that invasive cancer has not been ruled out, treatment is unacceptable because documented progression of a high-grade lesion to cancer during pregnancy is rare.[1,42,55,81] Most commonly, a cervical excision procedure is reserved for those situations at high concern for cancer when colposcopy and biopsy do not confirm. Hence, its use for antepartum diagnosis is infrequent and when used is simply for the purpose of ruling out cancer and should never be designed to be therapeutic.[86] In other words, in order to conserve as much cervical structure as possible, excision of the full transformation zone is not required, and reexcision is not indicated when

margins are positive for CIN but not cancer. Pregnant women with high-grade CIN should be permitted to deliver vaginally at term, if otherwise appropriate.[42] Reevaluation with cytology and colposcopy is recommended no sooner than 6 weeks postpartum, with further management based on the postpartum findings.

12.9.3 Management of Invasive Cervical Cancer in Pregnancy

Even if invasive cervical cancer is detected, treatment depends on cancer stage and the point in pregnancy when the cancer is detected.[1] Management of pregnant women with either microinvasive or invasive cervical cancer should be done in consultation with a gynecologic oncologist, with review by a gynecologic pathologist of the cytologic and histologic specimens prior to embarking on management. Because there are two lives involved, management options should be thoroughly discussed with the mother. Often, input from an expert in high-risk pregnancy can be helpful in outlining potential neonatal outcomes when early delivery is considered. Management options should be individualized and influenced by gestational length, cell type, tumor size, lymphovascular space involvement, cone margin status, disease stage, and patient preference.[62,90] As in nonpregnant women, management is based on clinical staging, along with ancillary studies that may include cystoscopy, intravenous urography, proctoscopy, chest radiography, and magnetic resonance imaging.[90]

If the pregnancy is not desired or the fetus is not viable, immediate treatment may be undertaken. If the diagnosis is made late in pregnancy, some delay in definitive management to permit fetal viability usually should not negatively affect treatment outcome, particularly for stage I lesions.[57,62,65] Women diagnosed with small stage IA2 or IB1 invasive cancers and more than 20 weeks' gestation are most often managed at fetal viability by cesarean delivery and radical hysterectomy with pelvic lymphadenectomy.[62] Management of cervical cancer during pregnancy should be deferred to gynecologic oncologists and associated cancer specialists.

Survival is primarily determined by the FIGO stage of disease at the time of treatment.[62] Pregnancy does not appear to modify the prognosis when controlling for age and disease stage as compared with the nonpregnant state.[62,65] The method of delivery should also be carefully planned in consultation with the gynecologic oncologist. Although survival rates are equivalent for women with stage I cervical cancer who deliver vaginally, as opposed to cesarean section, concerns about intrapartum and postpartum hemorrhage from the cervical cancer, and reports of recurrence of cervical cancer in the episiotomy, favor abdominal delivery.[62,91,92] This approach may also decrease the risk of pulmonary embolism.[62] When counting all stages, vaginal delivery is a significant predictor of recurrence (OR = 6.9), as is increasing stage of disease (OR = 4.7).[93] Additionally, patients in whom radical hysterectomy is the treatment of choice should be delivered by cesarean section concomitant with their cancer surgery.[62]

12.10 COMPLICATIONS REPORTED IN THE MANAGEMENT OF PREGNANT WOMEN WITH CERVICAL NEOPLASIA

12.10.1 Abortion

Certain complications unique to pregnant women may be encountered during the management of their cervical neoplasia. One risk is iatrogenic abortion or preterm delivery (when the intervention is after 20 weeks' gestation). CIN, per se, does not increase the risk for spontaneous abortion, but pregnancy loss in a woman with cervical neoplasia may be erroneously blamed on the disease process or on the procedures to evaluate it. However, inadvertent trauma from procedures required for proper evaluation may result in an accidental iatrogenic abortion, although this should be a rare event with the precautions outlined in the guidelines. In the era when CKC was the only surgical excision procedure, up to 27% of pregnant women experienced abortion following first-trimester diagnostic conization.[94] In comparison, a mean spontaneous abortion rate of 18% during the first trimester can normally be expected,[95] although the rate is likely significantly higher when pregnancy loss occurring before definitive confirmation of pregnancy is counted. Abortion rates following CKC in the second trimester have been reported to be as high as 19%.[94] ECC in the early first trimester before either the patient or the clinician recognizes the pregnancy could occasionally contribute to pregnancy loss. Additionally, induced abortion resulting from radiation therapy or surgical treatment of women with invasive cervical cancer is an unfortunate but predictable outcome. Preterm labor and premature delivery also may result as consequences of necessary diagnostic or therapeutic interventions.

12.10.2 Hemorrhage

Hemorrhage during pregnancy is most commonly a result of pregnancy-related complications, such as placenta previa or abruptio placentae, particularly in the third trimester. Abnormal bleeding from diagnostic procedures during pregnancy has been reported in as many as 12% of patients,[95] with 6% to 9% requiring transfusion following conization.[42,94,95,96] Clinicians should be cognizant of this potential serious complication (Table 12.2). Measures should be taken to minimize bleeding when diagnostic interventions such as wedge biopsy or conization are required. Hemostatic sutures, vasoconstrictive drugs, and minimal, but sufficient excision of tissue should limit operative and postoperative hemorrhage. Operative bleeding complications are experienced most frequently during the third trimester.[42,94,97,98] Therefore, it is preferable to do conizations during the late first or early second trimester. Because the complications of CKC in pregnancy are higher than with limited loop excision of the transformation zone (limited LEEP), the latter is advisable when an excisional procedure is necessary.[42]

12.10.3 Other Conization-Related Complications

Postcone cervical stenosis and cervical incompetence are always potential complications that should be recognized and discussed preoperatively with the patient before proceeding with a cervical excision procedure. These problems are also of increased risk when performing CKC in comparison with LEEP excision. Cervical lacerations requiring repair at the time of spontaneous vaginal delivery may occur in as many as 18% of pregnant women who had a prior conization during pregnancy. It is important to note that cervical conization performed during pregnancy is rarely therapeutic and should not aim to be. This may be partly due to the need to make cervical excision in pregnancy smaller and shallower to minimize complications for the patient and fetus. Approximately 50% of patients will have recurrent CIN following an antepartum conization, presumably at least partly secondary to smaller-than-usual excisions that deliberately leave portions of at-risk transformation zone intact.[42,55,95] The majority of residual disease is located deep within the endocervical glands. Larger or repeat excisions are not needed during pregnancy to minimize this risk of persistence. Rather, women who receive diagnostic conization during pregnancy but do not undergo hysterectomy should be reevaluated postpartum with cytologic, colposcopic, and histologic sampling, as appropriate. Residual disease may require retreatment.

12.11 POSTPARTUM MANAGEMENT OF WOMEN WITH CERVICAL NEOPLASIA

Provided cancer has been excluded during pregnancy, further evaluation and treatment of cervical neoplasia are postponed until postpartum. Treatment for preinvasive disease identified on biopsy antepartum is not initiated postpartum based on antepartum findings because of the substantial potential for regression and the small but real possibility of progression to cancer since the antepartum assessment. Instead, women with preinvasive disease identified antepartum should be reevaluated postpartum with cervical cytology, colposcopy, and histologic sampling, when indicated, and management should be determined based on the postpartum results. Women are generally examined around 6 weeks postpartum to allow time for the cervix to complete involution. In some cases, no disease is detected in women who had a CIN documented during pregnancy. This is particularly true for women with CIN 1 or condylomas, which are apt to regress or resolve spontaneously. However, CIN 2 and even CIN 3 may also vanish without surgical intervention. Clinicians should obtain a Pap test at the time of the colposcopic examination, even if not otherwise indicated. The increased sensitivity of a cotest (Pap plus HPV test) may justify its use in this setting. Visible acetowhite lesions should be biopsied and ECC performed as indicated. Clinicians should follow the management guidelines outlined in Chapter 20. It is important to reemphasize that women with antepartum preinvasive disease are usually managed based on postpartum findings.

Women having conization during pregnancy for CIN 2,3 should undergo similar postpartum reevaluation because the rate of residual disease often exceeds 50%.[42,45,95] A small but definite risk exists that new disease may evolve or small foci of existing disease may become apparent later within the transformation zone. In addition, if previously adequate colposcopy has become inadequate, ablative therapies and observation without treatment will be contraindicated. Therefore, it is critical that a patient with postpartum regression of histologically proven antepartum CIN 2,3 adhere to recommended follow-up. There are no specific guidelines for the follow-up of women with spontaneous remission of CIN 2,3 postpartum, but follow-up similar to that recommended posttreatment for CIN 2,3 seems reasonable. As discussed in Chapter 20, follow-up post treatment should be with cotesting performed at 12 and 24 months.[1] If both cotests are negative/negative, an additional co-test should be performed 3 years later. If this cotest is also negative, the woman can return to routine age-appropriate screening for at least 20 years. Alternatively, if any of the cotests

▪ STUDY	▪ IMMEDIATE HEMORRHAGE	▪ DELAYED HEMORRHAGE
TABLE 12.2 CONIZATION-INDUCED MATERNAL BLOOD LOSS IN PREGNANT WOMEN		
Hannigan et al.[95]	12.4%	3.7%
Daskal and Pitkin.[98]	5.2%	5.2%
Averette et al.[94]	7.2%	4.4%

during the first three follow-ups are positive, the patient should be assessed with colposcopy and endocervical sampling.[1]

Although the option of following a woman with apparent postpartum spontaneous regression of CIN 2,3 without treatment is reasonable, an argument can also be made for empiric transformation zone treatment to reduce the risk of recurrence of undetected disease, particularly if the antepartum histology was CIN 3. If CIN 2,3 is histologically documented at the postpartum follow-up evaluation, treatment should proceed by either ablative or excisional modalities according to the 2012 guidelines (see Chapter 20). Cytologic, histologic, or colposcopic findings of cancer may require further diagnostic evaluation prior to definitive treatment.

References

1. Massad LS, Einstein MH, Huh WK, et al.; 2012 ASCCP Consensus Guidelines Conference. 2012 updated consensus guidelines for the management of abnormal cervical cancer screening tests and cancer precursors. *Obstet Gynecol* 2013;121(4):829–46.
2. Fife KH, Katz BP, Roush J, Handy VD, Brown DR, Hansell R. Cancer associated human papillomavirus types are selectively increased in the cervix of women in the first trimester of pregnancy. *Am J Obstet Gynecol* 1996;174:1487–93.
3. Szekeres-Bartho J. Immunological relationship between the mother and the fetus. *Int Rev Immunol* 2002;21(6):471–95.
4. Vaccarella S, Herrero R, Dai M, et al. Reproductive factors, oral contraceptive use, and human papillomavirus infection: pooled analysis of the IARC HPV prevalence surveys. *Cancer Epidemiol Biomarkers Prev* 2006;15(11):2148–53.
5. Aydin Y, Atis A, Tutuman T, Goker N. Prevalence of human papilloma virus infection in pregnant Turkish women compared with non-pregnant women. *Eur J Gynaecol Oncol* 2010;31(1):72–4.
6. Fife KH, Rogers RE, Zwickl BW. Symptomatic and asymptomatic cervical infections with human papillomavirus during pregnancy. *J Inf Dis* 1987;156:904–11.
7. Fife KH, Katz BP, Brizendine EJ, Brown DR. Cervical human papillomavirus deoxyribonucleic acid persists throughout pregnancy and decreases in the postpartum period. *Am J Obstet Gynecol* 1999;180:1110–4.
8. deRoda Husman AM, Walboomers JM, Hopman E, et al. HPV prevalence in cytomorphologically normal cervical scrapes of pregnant women as determined by PCR: the age related pattern. *J Med Virol* 1995;46:97–102.
9. Hagensee ME, Slavinsky J III, Gaffga CM, Suros J, Kissinger P, Marti DH. Seroprevalence of human papillomavirus type 16 in pregnant women. *Obstet Gynecol* 1999;94:653–8.
10. Chan PK, Chang AR, Tam WH, Cheung JL, Cheng AF. Prevalence and genotype distribution of cervical human papillomavirus infection: comparison between pregnant women and non-pregnant controls. *J Med Virol* 2002;67:583–8.
11. Hildesheim A, Gravitt P, Schiffman MH, et al. Determinants of genital human papillomavirus infection in low income women in Washington, D.C. *Sex Trans Dis* 1993;20:279–85.
12. Kemp EA, Hakenewerth AM, Laurent SL, Gravitt PE, Stoerker J. Human papillomavirus prevalence in pregnancy. *Obstet Gynecol* 1992;79:649–56.
13. Tenti P, Zappatore R, Migliora P, et al. Latent human papillomavirus infection in pregnant women at term: a case–control study. *J Inf Dis* 1997;176:277–80.
14. Chang-Claude J, Schneider A, Smith E, Blettner M, Wahrendorf J, Turek L. Longitudinal study of the effects of pregnancy and other factors on detection of HPV. *Gynecol Oncol* 1996;60:355–62.
15. Gonçalves CV, Duarte G, Costa JS, et al. Diagnosis and treatment of cervical cancer during pregnancy. *Sao Paulo Med J* 2009;127(6):359–65.
16. Peng TC, Searle CP, Shah KV, Repke JT, Johnson TR. Prevalence of human papillomavirus infections in term pregnancy. *Am J Perinatol* 1990;7:189–92.
17. Castellsagué X, Drudis T, Cañadas MP, et al. Human papillomavirus (HPV) infection in pregnant women and mother-to-child transmission of genital HPV genotypes: a prospective study in Spain. *BMC Infect Dis* 2009;9:74.
18. Hernandez-Giron C, Smith JS, Lorincz A, et al. The prevalence of high-risk HPV infection in pregnant women from Morelos, Mexico. *Salud Publica Mex* 2005;47:423–9.
19. Gajewska M, Wielgos M, Kaminski P, et al. The occurrence of genital types of human papillomavirus in normal pregnancy and in pregnant renal transplant recipients. *Neuro Endocrinol Lett* 2006;27:529–34.
20. Nobbenhuis MAE, Helmerhorst TJM, van den Brule ACJ, et al. High-risk human papillomavirus clearance in pregnant women: trends for lower clearance during pregnancy with a catch-up postpartum. *Br J Cancer* 2002;87:75–80.
21. McIntyre-Seltman K, Lesnock JL. Cervical cancer screening in pregnancy. *Obstet Gynecol Clin North Am* 2008;35(4):645–58.
22. Rando RF, Lindheim S, Hasty L, Sedlacek TV, Woodland M, Eder C. Increased frequency of detection of human papillomavirus DNA in exfoliated cervical cells during pregnancy. *Am J Obstet Gynecol* 1989;161:50–5.
23. Yamasaki K, Miura K, Shimada T, et al. Epidemiology of human papillomavirus genotypes in pregnant Japanese women. *J Hum Genet* 2011;56(4):313–5.
24. Sridama V, Pacini F, Yang SL, Moawad A, Reilly M, Degroot LJ. Decreased levels of helper T cells: a possible cause of immunodeficiency in pregnancy. *N Engl J Med* 1982;307:352–6.
25. Hietanen S, Ekblad A, Pellinieng TT, Syrjanen K, Helenius H, Syrjanen S. Type I diabetic pregnancy and subclinical human papillomavirus infection. *Clin Inf Dis* 1997;24:153–6.
26. Workowski KA, Berman S; Centers for Disease Control and Prevention (CDC). Sexually transmitted diseases treatment guidelines, 2010. *MMWR Recomm Rep* 2010;59(RR-12):1–110.
27. Kashima HK, Shah K. Recurrent respiratory papillomatosis. *Obstet Gynecol Clin N Am* 1987;14:581–8.
28. Syrjanen S. Current concepts on human papillomavirus infections in children. *APMIS* 2010;118(6–7):494–509.
29. Rintala MA, Grénman SE, Puranen MH, et al. Transmission of high-risk human papillomavirus (HPV) between parents and infant: a prospective study of HPV in families in Finland. *J Clin Microbiol* 2005;43(1):376–81.
30. Puranen M, Yliskoski M, Saarikoski S, Sydanen K, Syjanen S. Vertical transmission of human papillomavirus from infected mothers to their newborn babies and persistence of the virus in childhood. *Am J Obstet Gynecol* 1996;174:694–9.
31. Puranen MH, Yliskoski MIR, Saarikoski SV, Sydanen KJ, Syrjanen SM. Exposure of an infant to cervical human papillomavirus infection of the mother is common. *Am J Obstet Gynecol* 1997;176:1039–45.
32. Armbruster-Moraes E, Ioshimoto LM, Leao E, Zugaib M. Presence of human papillomavirus DNA in amniotic fluids of pregnant women with cervical lesions. *Gynecol Oncol* 1994;54:152–8.
33. Weyn C, Thomas D, Jani J, et al. Evidence of human papillomavirus in the placenta. *J Infect Dis* 2011;203(3):341–3.
34. Wang X, Zhu Q, Rao H. Maternal-fetal transmission of human papillomavirus. *Chin Med J* 1998;111:726–7.
35. Gomez LM, Ma Y, Ho C, McGrath CM, Nelson DB, Parry S. Placental infection with human papillomavirus is associated with spontaneous preterm delivery. *Hum Reprod* 2008;23:709–815.
36. Sarkola ME, Grénman SE, Rintala MA, Syrjanen KJ, Syrjanen SM. Human papillomavirus in the placenta and umbilical cord blood. *Acta Obstet Gynecol Scand* 2008;87:1181–8.
37. Sedlacek TV, Lindheim S, Eder C, et al. Mechanism for human papillomavirus transmission at birth. *Am J Obstet Gynecol* 1989;161:55–9.
38. Chow LT, Broker TR, Steinberg BM. The natural history of human papillomavirus infections of the mucosal epithelia. *APMIS* 2010;118(6–7):422–49.
39. Schraff S, Derkay CS, Burke B, Lawson L. American Society of Pediatric Otolaryngology members' experience with recurrent respiratory papillomatosis and the use of adjuvant therapy. *Arch Otolaryngol Head Neck Surg* 2004;130(9):1039–42.
40. American College of Obstetricians and Gynecologists. Screening for cervical cancer. American College of Obstetricians and Gynecologists (ACOG) Practice Bulletin No. 131, November 2012.
41. Saslow D, Solomon D, Lawson HW, et al.; for the American Cancer Society; American Society for Colposcopy and Cervical Pathology; American Society for Clinical Pathology. American Cancer Society, American Society for Colposcopy and Cervical Pathology, and American Society for Clinical Pathology screening guidelines for the prevention and early detection of cervical cancer. *Am J Clin Pathol* 2012;137(4):516–42.
42. Hunter MI, Monk BJ, Tewari KS. Cervical neoplasia in pregnancy. Part 1: screening and management of preinvasive disease. *Am J Obstet Gynecol* 2008;199(1):3–9.
43. Fader AN, Alward EK, Niederhauser A, et al. Cervical dysplasia in pregnancy: a multi-institutional evaluation. *Am J Obstet Gynecol* 2010;203(2):113.e1–e6.
44. Hannigan EV. Cervical cancer in pregnancy. *Clin Obstet Gynecol* 1990;33:837–45.
45. Dudan RC, Yon JL, Ford JH, Averette HE. Carcinoma of the cervix and pregnancy. *Gynecol Oncol* 1973;1:283–9.
46. Yost NP, Santoso JT, McIntire DD, Iliya FA. Postpartum regression rates of antepartum cervical intraepithelial neoplasia II and III lesions. *Obstet Gynecol* 1999;93:359–62.
47. Patsner B. Management of low-grade cervical dysplasia during pregnancy. *South Med J* 1990;83:1405–6.
48. Moscicki AB, Ma Y, Wibbelsman C, et al. Rate of and risks for regression of cervical intraepithelial neoplasia 2 in adolescents and young women. *Obstet Gynecol* 2010;116(6):1373–80.
49. Palle C, Bangsboll S, Andreasson B. Cervical intraepithelial neoplasia in pregnancy. *Acta Obstet Gynecol Scand* 2000;79:306–10.
50. Ueda Y, Enomoto T, Miyatake T, et al. Postpartum outcome of cervical intraepithelial neoplasia in pregnant women determined by route of delivery. *Reprod Sci* 2009;16(11):1034–9.

51. Wright TC Jr, Massad S, Dunton CJ, Spitzer M, Wilkinson EJ, Solomon D. 2006 consensus guidelines for the management of women with cervical intraepithelial neoplasia or adenocarcinoma in situ. *Am J Obstet Gynecol* 2007;197:340–5.

52. ACOG Practice Bulletin No. 99: Management of abnormal cervical cytology and histology. *Obstet Gynecol* 2008;112:1419–44.

53. Nguyen C, Montz FJ, Bristow RE. Management of stage I cervical cancer in pregnancy. *Obstet Gynecol Surv* 2000;55:633–43.

54. Frega A, Scirpa P, Corosu R, et al. Clinical management and follow-up of squamous intraepithelial cervical lesions during pregnancy and postpartum. *Anticancer Res* 2007;27(4C):2743–6.

55. Hacker NF, Berek JS, Lagasse LD, Charles EH, Savage EW, Moore JG. Carcinoma of the cervix associated with pregnancy. *Obstet Gynecol* 1982;59:735–46.

56. Norstrom A, Jansson I, Andreasson H. Carcinoma of the uterine cervix in pregnancy. A study of the incidence and treatment in the western region of Sweden 1973 to 1992. *Acta Obstet Gynecol Scand* 1997;76:583–9.

57. Duggan B, Maderspach LL, Roman LD, Curtin JP, d'Ablaing G, Morrow CP. Cervical cancer in pregnancy: reporting on planned delay in therapy. *Obstet Gynecol* 1993;82:598–602.

58. Dunn TS, Bajaj JE, Stamm CA, Beaty B. Management of the minimally abnormal Papanicolaou smear in pregnancy. *J Low Genit Tract Dis* 2001;5:133–7.

59. Wetta LA, Matthews KS, Kemper ML, et al. The management of cervical intraepithelial neoplasia during pregnancy: is colposcopy necessary. *J Low Genit Tract Dis* 2009;13(3):182–5.

60. Vlahos G, Rodolakis A, Diakomanolis E, et al. Conservative management of cervical intraepithelial neoplasia (CIN 2,3) in pregnant women. *Gynecol Obstet Invest* 2002;54:78–81.

61. Hunter MI, Tewari K, Monk BJ. Cervical neoplasia in pregnancy. Part 2: current treatment of invasive disease. *Am J Obstet Gynecol* 2008;199(1):10–8.

62. Lishner M. Cancer in pregnancy. *Ann Oncol* 2003;14(suppl 3):iii31–6.

63. Pavlidis NA. Coexistence of pregnancy and malignancy. *Oncologist* 2002;7(4):279–87.

64. Zemlickis D, Lishner M, Degendorfer P, Panzarella T, Sutcliffe SB, Koren G. Maternal and fetal outcome after invasive cervical cancer in pregnancy. *J Clin Oncol* 1991;9:1956–61.

65. Hopkins NW, Morley GW. The prognosis and management of cervical cancer associated with pregnancy. *Obstet Gynecol* 1992;80:9–13.

66. Van Calsteren K, Vergote I, Amant F. Cervical neoplasia during pregnancy: diagnosis, management and prognosis. *Best Pract Res Clin Obstet Gynaecol* 2005;19(4):611–30.

67. Simcock B, Shafi M. Invasive cancer of the cervix. *Obstet Gynaecol Reprod Med* 2007;17(6):181–7.

68. Jacobs IA, Chang CK, Salti GI. Coexistence of pregnancy and cancer. *Am Surg* 2004;70(11):1025–9.

69. Singer A. The cervical epithelium during pregnancy and the puerperium. In: Jordan JA, Singer A, eds. *The Cervix*. London, UK: WB Saunders Co., 1976.

70. Coppleson M, Reid B. A colposcopic study of the cervix during pregnancy and the puerperium. *J Obstet Gynecol Br Commonwealth* 1966;73:575–85.

71. Ueki M, Ueda M, Kumagai K, Okamoto Y, Noda S, Matsuoka M. Cervical cytology and conservative management of cervical neoplasia. *Int J Gynecol Pathol* 1995;14:63–9.

72. Ruffin MT IV, Van Noord GR. Improving the yield of endocervical elements in a Pap smear with the use of the cytology brush. *Fam Med* 1991;23(5):365–9.

73. Rivlin ME, Woodliff JM, Bowlin RB, et al. Comparison of cytobrush and cotton swab for Papanicolaou smears in pregnancy. *J Reprod Med* 1993;38:147–50.

74. Orr JW, Barrett JM, Orr PF, Holloway RW, Holimon JL. The efficacy and safety of the cytobrush during pregnancy. *Gynecol Oncol* 1992;44:260–2.

75. Paraiso NTR, Brady K, Helmchen R, Roat TW. Evaluation of the endocervical cytobrush and Cervex-Brush in pregnant women. *Obstet Gynecol* 1994;84:539–43.

76. Stillson T, Knight AL, Elswick RK Jr. The effectiveness and safety of two cervical cytologic techniques during pregnancy. *J Fam Pract* 1997;45:159–63.

77. Davey D, Cox JT, Austin M, et al. Cervical cytology specimen adequacy: patient management guidelines and optimizing specimen collection. *J Low Gen Tract Dis* 2008;12(2):71–81.

78. Ferris DG, Berrey MM, Ellis KE, Petry LJ, Voxnaes J, et al. The optimal technique for obtaining a Papanicolaou smear with the Cervex-Brush. *J Fam Pract* 1992;34:276–80.

79. Kohan S, Beckman EM, Bigelow B, Klein SA, Douglas GW. The role of colposcopy in the management of cervical intraepithelial neoplasia during pregnancy and postpartum. *J Reprod Med* 1980;25:279–84.

80. Benedet JL, Boyes DA, Nichols TM, Nfillner A. Colposcopic evaluation of pregnant patients with abnormal cervical smears. *Br J Obstet Gynecol* 1977;84:517–21.

81. Benedet JL, Selke PA, Nickerson KG. Colposcopic evaluation of abnormal Papanicolaou smears in pregnancy. *Am J Obstet Gynecol* 1987;157:932–7.

82. Woodrow N, Permezel M, Butterfield L, Rome R, Tan J, Quinn M. Abnormal cervical cytology in pregnancy: experience of 811 cases. *Aust NZ J Obstet Gynaecol* 1998;38(2):161–5.

83. Siddiq TS, Twigg JP, Hammond RH. Assessing the accuracy of colposcopy at predicting the outcome of abnormal cytology in pregnancy. *Eur J Obstet Gynecol Reprod Biol* 2006;124:93–7.

84. Ostergard DR, Nieberg RK. Evaluation of abnormal cervical cytology during pregnancy with colposcopy. *Am J Obstet Gynecol* 1979;134:756–8.

85. Economos K, Veridiano NP, Delke I, Collado ML, Tancer ML. Abnormal cervical cytology in pregnancy: a 17-year experience. *Obstet Gynecol* 1993;81:915–8.

86. Baldauf JJ, Dreyfus M, Ritter J, Phillippe E. Colposcopy and directed biopsy reliability during pregnancy: a cohort study. *Eur J Obstet Gynecol Reprod Biol* 1995;62:31–6.

87. Murta EF, de Andrade FC, Adad SJ, de Souza H. Low-grade cervical squamous intraepithelial lesion during pregnancy: conservative antepartum management. *Eur J Gynaecol Oncol* 2004;25:600–2.

88. Roberts CH, Dinh TV, Hannigan EV, Yandell RB, Schnadig VJ. Management of cervical intraepithelial neoplasia during pregnancy: a simplified and cost-effective approach. *J Low Genit Tract Dis* 1998;2:67–70.

89. Boardman LA, Goldman DL, Cooper AS, Heber WW, Weitzen S. CIN in pregnancy: antepartum and postpartum cytology and histology. *J Reprod Med* 2005;50:13–8.

90. Zanotti KM, Belinson JL, Kennedy AW. Treatment of gynecologic cancers in pregnancy. *Semin Oncol* 2000;6:686–98.

91. Gordon AN, Jensen R, Jones HW. Squamous carcinoma of the cervix complicating pregnancy: recurrence in episiotomy after vaginal delivery. *Obstet Gynecol* 1989;73:850–2.

92. Cliby WA, Dodson NM, Podratz KC. Cervical cancer complicated by pregnancy: episiotomy site recurrences following vaginal delivery. *Obstet Gynecol* 1994;84:179–82.

93. Sood AK, Sorosky JI, Mayr N, Anderson B, Buller RE, Niebyl J. Cervical cancer diagnosed shortly after pregnancy: prognostic variables and delivery routes. *Obstet Gynecol* 2000;95:832–8.

94. Averette BE, Nasser N, Yankow SL, Little WA. Cervical conization in pregnancy. *Am J Obstet Gynecol* 1970;106:543–9.

95. Hannigan EV, Whitehouse HH, Atkinson WD, Becker SN. Cone biopsy during pregnancy. *Obstet Gynecol* 1982;60:450–5.

96. Carter PM, Coburn TC, Luszczakm. Cost-effectiveness of cervical cytologic examination during pregnancy. *J Am Board Fam Pract* 1993;6:537–45.

97. Robinson WR, Webb S, Tirpack J, Degefu S, O'Quinn AG. Management of cervical intraepithelial neoplasia during pregnancy with LOOP excision. *Gynecol Oncol* 1997;64:153–5.

98. Daskal JL, Pitkin RM. Cone biopsy of the cervix during pregnancy. *Am J Obstet Gynecol* 1968;32:1–5.

CHAPTER 13

J. THOMAS COX
EDWARD J. MAYEAUX, JR.

Colposcopy in Special Situations

13.1 INTRODUCTION
13.2 HORMONALLY INDUCED CHANGES
    13.2.1 Changes Due to Estrogen-Progestin–Releasing Contraceptives
    13.2.2 Changes Due to Progestin-Only Contraceptives
    13.2.3 Microglandular Hyperplasia
    13.2.4 Vaginal Adenosis and In Utero Diethylstilbestrol Exposure
    13.2.5 Estrogen Deficiency
13.3 RADIATION-INDUCED CHANGES
13.4 CERVICAL POLYPS
13.5 POSTTREATMENT FINDINGS

13.5.1 Mimics of Cervical Neoplasia
13.5.2 Other Posttreatment Findings
13.6 DEVELOPMENTAL MALFORMATIONS
    13.6.1 Transverse Vaginal Septum
    13.6.2 Vaginal and Cervical Duplication
    13.6.3 Cervical Anomalies
13.7 COLPOSCOPY OF SEXUAL ASSAULT VICTIMS
    13.7.1 The Use of Colposcopy in the Sexual Assault Examination
    13.7.2 Findings in Consensual Intercourse and Nonintercourse-Related Trauma
    13.7.3 Findings in Sexual Assault

13.1 INTRODUCTION

The single most consistent characteristic of all life is that it is a dynamic system. This is certainly true for the human body. Age, hormones, intravaginal products, contraceptive agents and devices, and trauma from both consensual and nonconsensual sexual relations influence the colposcopic appearance of the lower genital tract. Colposcopists must be able to recognize and separate the normal and abnormal modifications that are the result of external, natural, or developmental influences. For example, hormonal changes induced by oral contraceptive pills and other factors can cause benign pseudoneoplastic glandular lesions of the uterine cervix that may mimic normal benign changes of pregnancy or glandular neoplasia.[1] Exposure to diethylstilbestrol (DES) in utero later resulted in some women developing columnar epithelium in the vaginal mucosa (adenosis), having an increased risk of clear cell adenocarcinoma of the vagina, and developing structural changes in the cervix and other areas of the genital tract.[2–8] Loss of estrogen in menopausal and postmenopausal women results in structural changes to the cervical stroma, as well as alterations in epithelial thickness and glycogen content.

In addition to the myriad of changes that may be caused by hormones, the effects of foreign objects on the vaginal and cervical epithelium may result in confusing colposcopic findings. Tampons, vaginal spermicides, lubricants, diaphragms, cervical caps, and a host of sexually introduced objects may irritate or traumatize the epithelium. Consequently, erosions, tears, abrasions, and epithelial regeneration patterns may hamper the colposcopist's ability to identify and diagnose epithelial abnormalities. Colposcopists must recognize these effects if underdiagnosis and overdiagnosis are to be avoided.

As society has moved toward greater protection of individuals from unwanted sexual contact, a new colposcopic subspecialty, the colposcopy of sexual assault victims, has become very important.[9,10] Well-trained sexual assault response teams (SARTs) have been established in many communities. Members of these teams are trained in the use of the colposcope, particularly for identification of normal anatomic and mucosal findings seen with consensual sexual relations and abnormal changes seen in victims of sexual assault. While it is not within the scope of Modern Colposcopy to provide a complete review of the forensics and major colposcopic findings associated with unwanted sexual advances, some familiarity with these issues is an important part of every colposcopist's training.

13.2 HORMONALLY INDUCED CHANGES

13.2.1 Changes Due to Estrogen-Progestin–Releasing Contraceptives

Combination estrogen-progestin oral contraceptive pills (OCPs) and other estrogen-progestin–containing contraceptives can induce both stromal and epithelial changes (Table 13.1). Hypertrophy of the stroma causes enlargement of the cervix that often causes the columnar epithelium to evert and increases vascularity.[11] Increasing duration of oral contraceptive use appears to have some influence on the size of the ectopy.[12] Prominent vascularity may be noted colposcopically as hyperemia of the exposed columnar epithelium.[12] Abundant mucus may be observed, and the fusing of enlarged columnar villi may produce globular, hyperemic, polypoid shapes. Prior to the application of a 5% acetic acid solution, this hyperemic ectopy may appear to be eroded, hence the misnomer "cervical erosion."[12] However, a typical, faint, and transient acetowhitening of these polypoid villi clearly delineates the tissue as normal, frond-like columnar villi (Figure 13.1A,B). Particularly large, irregular villi may appear similar in shape to small condylomata, and their prominence can be confusing. Similar findings may also be seen in patients using other estrogen-progestin–releasing contraceptives such as the

TABLE 13.1	EFFECTS OF COMBINATION ESTROGEN-PROGESTIN–CONTAINING CONTRACEPTIVES ON THE UTERINE CERVIX	
■ EFFECT	■ OBSERVED CHANGE	
Hypertrophy of the stroma	Enlargement of the cervix	
	Eversion of columnar epithelium	
	Cervix feels softer than expected	
Increased vascularity	Cervical hyperemia	
Abundant mucus	May obscure cervical os	
Fusing of enlarged columnar villi	Globular polypoid shapes	
	May be confused with small condylomata	

etonogestrel/ethinyl estradiol vaginal ring (NuvaRing) and ethinyl estradiol/norelgestromin transdermal patch. In addition, the close proximity of the hormone-infused vaginal ring (NuvaRing) to the cervix occasionally produces decidual-like changes in the columnar ectopy.

13.2.2 Changes Due to Progestin-Only Contraceptives

Progestin-only contraceptives, such as progestin-only contraceptive pills (minipills), depo-medroxyprogesterone (Depo-Provera), and etonogestrel implant (Implanon), can also induce epithelial and stromal changes that may become apparent during colposcopy. Increased vascularity and vascular congestion may produce a blue tint to the cervical epithelium similar to that found in early pregnancy. Abundant, thick cervical mucus may also be found, further confusing the appearance of the cervix with that seen in pregnancy. Rarely, glandular hypertrophy may be found.

13.2.3 Microglandular Hyperplasia

An exaggeration of tissue response to hormonal contraceptives, called microglandular hyperplasia (MGH), is another example of lower genital tract epithelial alterations caused by hormones. MGH was first described in 1967 by Taylor et al.

and was felt to be a consequence of oral contraceptives.[13,14] However, it is now known that progestins are the inciting hormone in MGH.[15] Hence, MGH is found not only with combined oral contraceptives but also in women on progestin-only contraceptives, and in pregnancy due to the increased progesterone levels. The columnar cellular changes that result are often difficult to reliably discriminate colposcopically from glandular neoplasia.[12] Similar changes have also been noted in menopausal women.[14] These hormonal changes can induce cellular proliferation and budding of the endocervical crypts.[16] Proliferation of these crypts expands the columnar villi, producing polypoid excrescences (Figure 13.2A,B). Individual villi typically swell, and may be hyperemic. Clumping of these structures produces irregular masses that may appear quite abnormal. A yellow hue in areas of MGH should raise concern about the presence of occult cancer, even when the vascular pattern is normal (Figure 13.2C).

Histologically, numerous gland crypts lined by cuboidal cells with regular nuclei are noted.[16] Mitotic figures can be found, but they are not abnormal. Budding of these endocervical crypts produces a microglandular pattern against a background of reserve cell hyperplasia.[17] Maturing metaplasia within gland crypts that appears to be separate from the surface epithelium occasionally has been confused with carcinoma, and the atypical glandular cells sometimes seen in cytology of cells from women with MGH can be confused with adenocarcinoma in situ.[17] However, the normal appearance of the nuclei and the normal appearance and minimal

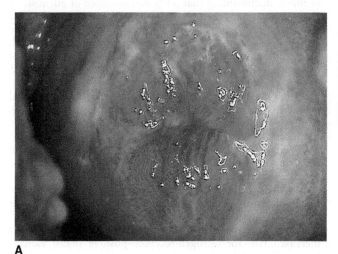

A

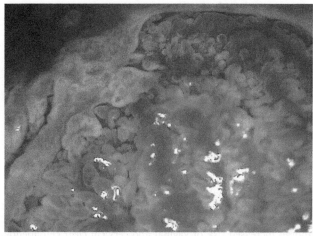

B

FIGURE 13.1. **A:** Hyperemic ectopy accentuated by oral contraceptive use appears "eroded" because of the increased vascular congestion. **B:** After the application of acetic acid, acetowhitening of these polypoid villi clearly delineates the area as normal, fused columnar villi.

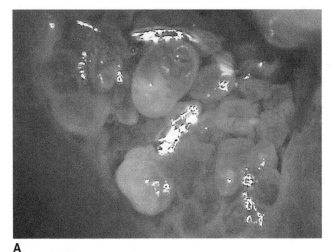

A

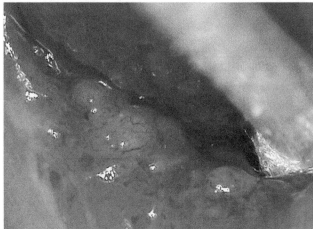

B

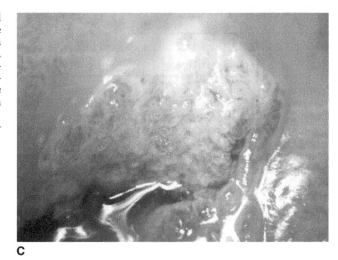

C

FIGURE 13.2.   Colposcopy of MGH. **A:** Individually, the polypoid structures of MGH may resemble small polyps. **B:** Clumping of these polypoid structures produces irregular polypoid masses that are often cream to yellow in color. **C:** Fused papillary excrescences of MGH. These areas have a yellow hue similar to chicken fat. Angioarchitectural formations are not a prominent feature in MGH. (Reproduced from Wright VC. *Color Atlas of Colposcopy—Cervix, Vagina and Vulva.* Houston, TX: Biomedical Communications, 2003, with permission.)

number of mitotic figures should reassure the colposcopist that the lesion is benign.

13.2.4 Vaginal Adenosis and *In Utero* Diethylstilbestrol Exposure

Vaginal adenosis is simply the presence of glandular cells in the vaginal epithelium, thought to be derived from persistent paramesonephric epithelial islets in postembryonic life.[18,19] Columnar epithelial cells have been detected in vaginal histologic specimens in approximately 10% to 15% of female infants under the age of 1 month and in a similar percent of women between the onset of puberty and 25 years of age.[18] Vaginal adenosis has also been described in patients after Stevens-Johnson syndrome,[20] following vaginal CO_2 laser ablation,[21] and following treatment of vaginal condylomata with 5-flurouracil,[22–24] prompting increased vigilance when evaluating these women.[20–24]

Although vaginal adenosis was originally considered an entirely benign process, Herbst et al. described in 1971 an association between *in utero* exposure to DES, vaginal adenosis, and an increased risk of vaginal and cervical clear cell adenocarcinoma (CCAC).[4] Although long-term follow-up of women with vaginal adenosis has not documented a definitive case of transformation of CCAC directly from an area of benign adenosis,[25–28] the relationship of DES with both vaginal adenosis and with clear cell adenocarcinoma is clearly established.[4]

For several decades prior to 1971, the synthetic estrogen DES was given to millions of pregnant women, as it was thought to reduce the risk of miscarriage. The National Diethylstilbestrol Screening Project evaluated 1275 women exposed to DES *in utero*, documenting that 34% had evidence of adenosis or areas of squamous metaplasia in the vagina or byproducts of this activity, such as gland openings and nabothian cysts.[8] The frequency of the presence of these findings was associated with the gestational age at which DES exposure began, the length of exposure, and the dose.[27,28] Prenatal exposure of males to DES has also been shown to increase the rate of male urogenital abnormalities including cryptorchidism (RR 1.9), epididymal cyst (RR 2.5), and testicular inflammation/infection (RR 2.4), with even higher risk for DES exposure that began before the 11th week of pregnancy.[29]

The risk of developing clear cell adenocarcinoma from birth through the fourth decade of life for individuals exposed to DES has been estimated to be approximately 1 in 1000, for a standardized incidence ratio of over 24.[27,28,30] The concern that DES exposure might place women at increased risk for developing other cancers so far has not been realized.[25–28,30,31] However, concern that DES-exposed women may have an increased risk for estrogen-receptor–positive breast cancers later in life remains.[30,31]

The mechanism for DES induction of vaginal adenosis appears to be transient disruption of developmental signals by DES that permanently changed expression of p63, thereby altering the developmental fate of müllerian duct epithelium.[32]

p63 is critical for the development of stratified squamous epithelial tissues, and has high homology with p53, one of our two most important antioncogenes.[33] For most DES-exposed women, the vaginal adenosis is replaced by benign squamous metaplasia that eventually transforms into mature squamous epithelium, which has no increased risk of developing into vaginal neoplasia, but for some, cervicovaginal epithelial cells fail to express p63, remain columnar, and persist into adulthood as adenosis.[32] Vaginal adenosis occurring following CO_2 laser treatment of vaginal condyloma or after Stevens-Johnson syndrome or other inflammatory conditions affecting the vagina appears to be secondary to the "unmasking" (denuding) of an occult (submucosal) vaginal adenosis by destruction of the overlying stratified vaginal epithelium.[20]

Benign structural changes within the lower genital tract have also been reported more frequently in women exposed to DES *in utero*.[8,19] These changes include cervical pseudopolyps,

grossly irregular cervix, rough or smooth anterior cervical protuberance ("cockscomb"), columnar ectopy completely covering the portio or beyond the cervical-vaginal margins, hypertrophy of tissue surrounding the cervical ectopy (cervical collar), and circular or irregular sulci on the portio (Figure 13.3A–G). While more commonly seen in DES-exposed women, each of these structural changes can also be found in women who have not been exposed to DES.

Women with vaginal adenosis are usually asymptomatic, although some may experience a greater-than-usual volume of mucoid vaginal discharge or have postcoital bleeding. Gross inspection of the vagina may reveal erythematous areas similar in color and texture to cervical ectopy.[19] Rarely, eroded or ulcerated areas may be present, and these may be associated with dyspareunia. Colposcopic evaluation using high magnification will better demonstrate well-circumscribed erythematous vaginal lesions surrounded by the homogeneous

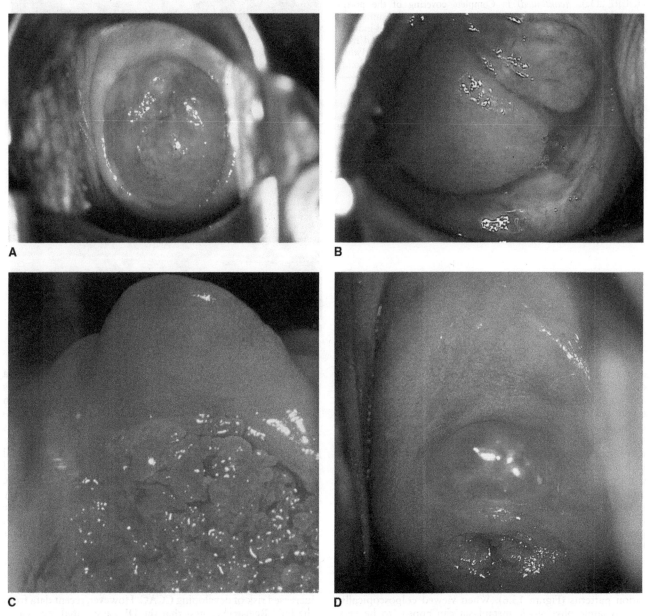

A **B** **C** **D**

FIGURE 13.3. Benign structural changes noted in women who were exposed to DES *in utero*. **A:** Cervical pseudopolyp. **B:** Grossly irregular cervix in a non–DES-exposed woman, raising the question of DES exposure. **C,D:** "Cockscomb."

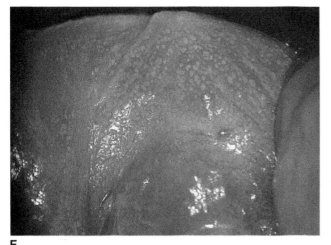

E

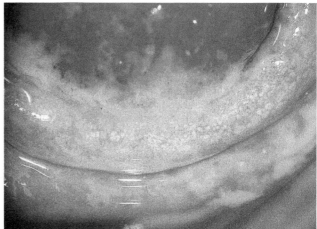

F

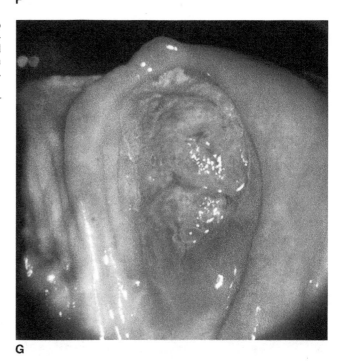

G

FIGURE 13.3. *(continued)* **E:** Complete covering of the portio beyond the cervical-vaginal margin with columnar epithelium undergoing metaplasia. **F:** Cervical collar. **G:** A diethylstilbestrol-induced shortened cervix with a complete cervical collar. (Reproduced from Wright VC. *Color Atlas of Colposcopy-Cervix, Vagina and Vulva.* Houston, TX: Biomedical Communications, 2003, with permission.)

appearance of normal, pink squamous epithelium. However, only after application of acetic acid will the colposcopist be able to conclusively demonstrate the typical "grapelike" clusters of columnar epithelium that confirm the glandular nature of the lesion.[19,34] When vaginal adenosis is precipitated by *in utero* exposure to DES, the benign nature of similar findings that indicate an increased glandular presence on the ectocervix, including irregularity, pseudopolyps, and sulci, can be confirmed colposcopically by the absence of atypical vessels and other warning signs of cancer. Adenosis is most commonly associated with large cervical ectopy that extendss onto the vaginal walls (Figure 13.4). However, diffuse small patches of adenosis may be noted throughout the vagina, and larger isolated patches may be found within the vaginal fornices (Figure 13.5A,B). Extensive immature metaplasia within the transforming adenosis often produces readily apparent acetowhite areas with striking fine-caliber mosaic and punctation patterns (Figure 13.6). When viewed colposcopically, this dynamic physiologic metaplasia can appear to be very similar to intraepithelial neoplasia (Figure 13.7A,B). Detection of other suspicious-looking benign entities can be equally worrisome (Figure 13.8A,B). High-grade CIN can develop

within large areas of ectopy and immature metaplasia (Figure 13.9A,B), which can complicate the diagnosis, just as it can when present within a large congenital transformation zone (Figure 13.10). Patches of adenosis can bleed on contact, heightening the colposcopist's concern that neoplasia is present, as can an irregular surface contour. Hormonal contraceptives can stimulate hyperplasia within areas of vaginal adenosis, in much the same way they affect areas of normal cervical columnar epithelium. The resulting MGH can mimic adenocarcinoma. Additionally, palpation of the vagina may detect large nabothian cysts in areas of adenosis that may be confused with tumors.[19] Puncturing these palpable cysts with a small needle will produce clear mucus as evidence of their benign nature.

Previously, it was thought that by the year 2011 (40 years from the date DES was last administered to a woman during pregnancy), DES-exposed women would no longer be at increased risk of developing CCAC. However, recent data from the DES Registry suggest that the DES-associated increase in the incidence of CCA remains elevated through the reproductive years.[35] The data do not demonstrate any consistent evidence of risk excesses for cancers other than CCA, and breast

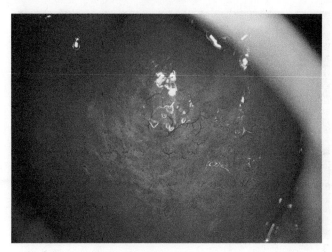

FIGURE 13.4.   Large portio ectopy extending to the vaginal wall entirely around the circumference of the cervix is seen in this DES-exposed woman.

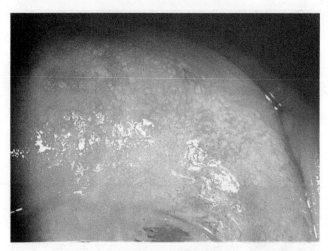

FIGURE 13.6.   Fine mosaic is present in this area of adenosis that is undergoing metaplasia. Biopsy confirmed that this was normal immature metaplasia.

cancer in older women. The DES Registry now has identified at least six cases in which CCAC has been detected in DES-exposed women over the age of 40 years, and one CCAC has been reported in a DES-exposed woman aged 54.[36] Furthermore, a bimodal curve noted for CCAC for both women exposed to DES and for unexposed women raises concern that new cases could occur in the postmenopausal years.[36] Because clinicians had become less concerned about detecting clear cell adenocarcinoma in DES-exposed women, the DESAD Project has begun a national education campaign to alert clinicians that DES-exposed women continue to be at some risk. One sign of hope that risk may be declining is a marked drop in the incidence of CCAC of the vagina and cervix in the Netherlands in the first decade of the 21st century compared to the two decades prior.[37]

The original DESAD protocol called for obtaining two separate Papanicolaou (Pap) smears, with one smear taken from the cervix and the other from the vaginal fornices; conducting a full colposcopic evaluation following application of acetic acid to the cervix and entire vagina and repeat of the entire procedure following similar application of aqueous iodine and palpating the entire vagina and cervix after the speculum was removed.[2,6,16] Others have argued that adequate evaluation can be accomplished by conducting a gross inspection before and after applying Lugol's solution, and that conducting a full colposcopic examination is not necessary unless inspection and palpation of the vaginal wall raises concerns. Any patient in whom an abnormality is detected could then be referred for a more comprehensive colposcopic evaluation.

13.2.5 Estrogen Deficiency

Up to 40% of postmenopausal women have symptoms of atrophic vaginitis, as do some premenopausal women taking antiestrogenic medications and some women on progestin-only contraception.[38,39] Vaginal epithelial integrity is highly dependent upon adequate estrogen. In its absence, the epithelium becomes thin and atrophic and capillary fragility may result in punctate hemorrhages into the mucosa and hemosiderin deposits. Cytologic smears can become quite difficult to interpret, as parabasal cells with an increased nuclear:cytoplasmic

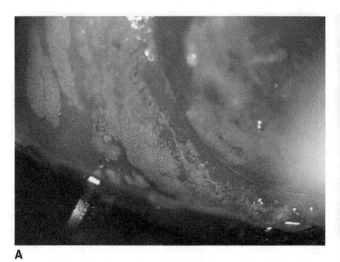

A

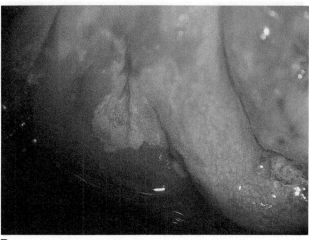

B

FIGURE 13.5.   A: A large area of adenosis extends to the right posterior vaginal fornix in this DES-exposed woman. B: Vaginal adenosis undergoing metaplasia extending beyond a cervical collar.

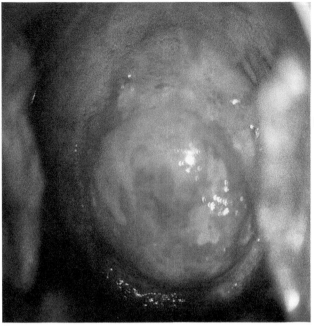

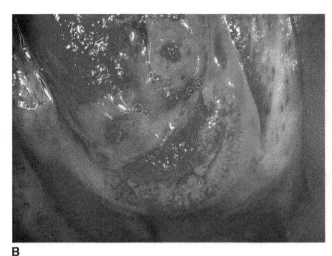

FIGURE 13.7.   **A,B:** DES adenosis with extensive metaplasia extends to the vagina.

ratio predominate.[40,41] As a result, estrogen-deficient women are commonly referred for colposcopic evaluation for such "atypical" smears. Colposcopically, the vaginal epithelium appears thin, with enhancement of the underlying vasculature (Figure 13.11).[42] The epithelium is friable, often bleeding upon contact with the vaginal speculum or a cotton swab. Ulcerations, erosions, or epithelial tears may result from minor trauma precipitated by intercourse, pessaries, or the introduction of the vaginal speculum. Loss of the protective effect of full epithelial thickness often results in inflammation of the vaginal mucosa that produces a thin discharge with profuse numbers of WBCs noted on wet mount examination.[19,38,39] Lugol's uptake is minimal due to the lack of estrogen-induced glycogen in the epithelium. Consequently, ina diffusely light brown-to-yellow color results from the application of Lugol's iodine.

Women with atrophic vaginitis commonly have symptoms that warrant treatment. Although vaginal atrophy occurs in the majority of postmenopausal women, not all women will be symptomatic.[38,43] Typical symptoms are vaginal dryness in 27% to 55%; introital itching, irritation, and introital dyspareunia in 37% to 41%; and recurrent urinary tract infections in 4% to 15%.[43,44] The most effective therapy has been the application of vaginal estrogen cream, but for women wishing to avoid the use of hormones, the application of vaginal moisturizers applied on a regular basis have an efficacy equivalent to local hormone replacement for the treatment of local urogenital symptoms.[44] However, when estrogen is not contraindicated, the following intravaginal estrogen therapies have been recommended by the Society of Obstetricians and Gynecologists of Canada (SOGC): conjugated equine estrogen

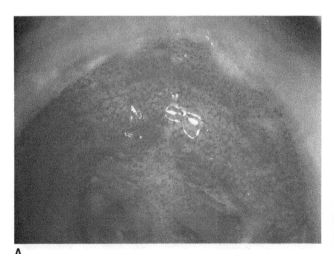

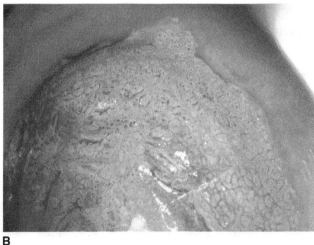

FIGURE 13.8.   **A,B:** DES-exposed woman with a minor cervical collar and a protuberant large area of columnar epithelium (**A**) preacetic acid and (**B**) postacetic acid.

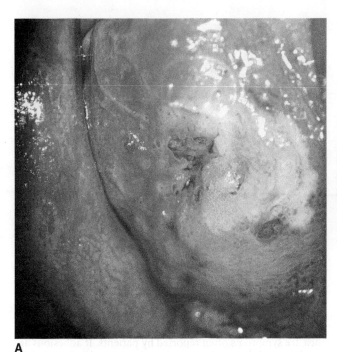

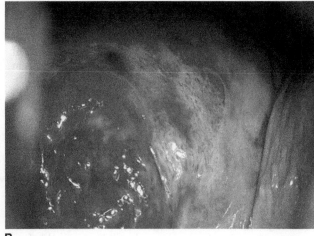

B

A

FIGURE 13.9.   **A:** CIN 2,3 within a pseudopolyp surrounded by a prominent cervical collar. **B:** Same patient postlaser.

cream (I-A), a sustained-release intravaginal estradiol ring (I-A), or a low-dose estradiol tablet (I-A).[44] Although systematic absorption of estrogen can occur with local preparations, the 2004 SOGC guidelines stated that there were insufficient data to recommend annual endometrial surveillance in asymptomatic women using local estrogens (III-C).

For the asymptomatic patient with vaginal atrophy requiring colposcopy, any of these treatments applied for only 3 weeks may be used to significantly improve the adequacy of the colposcopic evaluation for the presence of a vaginal or cervical lesion.[42] Ideally, the colposcopy should be performed several days to a week following discontinuation of the medication. Following estrogen replacement, parabasal cells will quickly mature into intermediate and superficial squamous cells that convey a typical colposcopic appearance. If a lesion is present, it is often not possible to detect it until this step is taken. It must also be remembered that occasionally a woman may be on adequate exogenous oral estrogen replacement for hot flashes, and yet have atrophic vaginal epithelium.[19] Additionally, premenopausal women on Depo-Provera or Lupron may have similar atrophic findings from suppression of the production of endogenous estrogen.[39]

New therapies for vaginal atrophy are being investigated.[40,43] Lower doses of existing vaginal estrogen formulations have

FIGURE 13.10.   Large symmetrical acetowhite with fine mosaic in a young DES-exposed woman resembles the congenital transformation zone seen in 3% of non-DES exposed women.

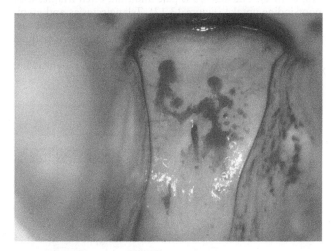

FIGURE 13.11.   The classic thin, friable epithelium of the atrophic vagina and cervix. Note the subepithelial hemorrhagic appearance.

proven to be efficacious, and certain selective estrogen receptor modulators (SERMs) and intravaginal dehydroepiandrosterone (DHEA) have both been shown to positively affect vaginal atrophy and symptoms without inducing endometrial proliferation.[43,45,46] The ability of SERMs to act as estrogens in certain tissues while remaining inert or acting as an antiestrogen in other tissues stimulated interest in their possible use in treating vaginal atrophy. However, the two investigated thus far that have shown to be effective against postmenopausal vaginal atrophy (ospemifene and lasofoxifene) have, in a few cases, appeared to be associated with hot flushes and muscle cramps.[46] A 2010 randomized control trial of 0.5% DHEA daily intravaginal dose reported a highly significant improvement in all parameters of vaginal atrophy including sexual function, without causing any, or at most minimal, changes in serum sex steroid levels, which all remained within the normal postmenopausal range.[45] Although these potential new treatments are promising, further research will be required before they will be ready to be used outside the research setting.[43]

13.3 RADIATION-INDUCED CHANGES

Radiation of cervical, vaginal, endometrial, sigmoid colon, or rectal cancer may result in thinned, friable epithelium and atypical blood vessels in the lower genital tract.[47] These radiation-induced changes may be extremely worrisome and difficult to interpret colposcopically. The majority of these women are also estrogen deficient because they are postmenopausal, either having gone through menopause prior to radiation treatment or having had radiation-reduced menopause through ablation of ovarian function. In either case, atrophic vaginitis further complicates the colposcopic interpretation. Long-term changes to the cervical and vaginal epithelium caused by radiation are often seen cytologically.[48] Benign postradiation cytologic changes can range from mild to severe and may consist of cytoplasmic vacuolization, nuclear wrinkling and enlargement, and multinucleation (see Chapter 2). These cytologic findings may be confused with dysplastic changes. The presence of large, bizarre, hyperchromatic nuclei should increase the colposcopist's concern and dictates the need for vigilance, especially when the patient has a history of genital tract cancer that may recur in the vagina.

Radiation-induced colposcopic findings may be difficult to discriminate from similar findings associated with cancer (Table 13.2). The mucosa is pale and thin, often friable, with poor iodine uptake (Figure 13.12). Telangiectasias and atypical blood vessels are usually present (Figure 13.13).[19] Neovascularization resulting from the effects of radiation can be quite bizarre. Dilated, tortuous, or elongated nonbranching vessels may be seen. The thin epithelium is susceptible to trauma;

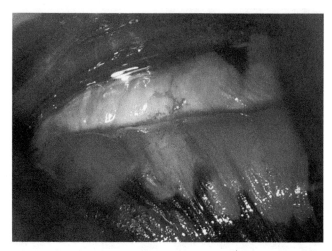

FIGURE 13.12. A sharply demarcated iodine-negative area is seen in this vaginal cuff postradiation.

hence, postcoital bleeding, petechiae or purpura, and leukorrhea are symptoms often reported by patients. If adhesions are not disrupted during the several weeks or months required for healing following radiation treatment, the vagina will become foreshortened and areas of the lower genital tract that are at risk for recurrent disease will become inaccessible to colposcopic evaluation. Atrophy secondary to estrogen deficiency further complicates the evaluation. When estrogen deficiency is likely, the application of 1 g of vaginal estrogen cream daily for 3 to 4 weeks prior to the colposcopic examination will increase the thickness of the vaginal epithelium, resulting in less patient discomfort and minimizing the confusion caused by atrophic changes.[19,49] Frequent follow-up examinations and biopsy of suspicious areas are mandatory to ensure positive outcomes in these patients. Palpation of the vaginal wall prior to inserting a speculum also can be helpful, since areas of

TABLE 13.2	EFFECTS OF RADIATION ON THE LOWER GENITAL TRACT EPITHELIUM
▪ EFFECT	▪ OBSERVED CHANGE
Thinned, friable epithelium	Pale thin mucosa
	Friable mucosa
	Poor iodine uptake
Neovascularization	Telangiectasias
	Atypical blood vessels
	Increased susceptibility to trauma
Narrowed vagina	Inaccessibility to colposcopic evaluation

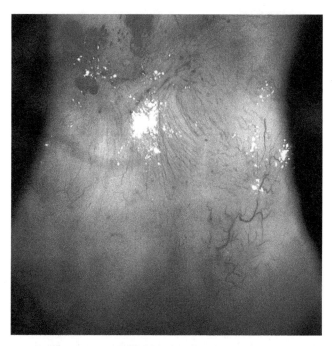

FIGURE 13.13. Friable thinned epithelium with atypical vessels can be seen in this woman treated previously by radiation for a vaginal sarcoma. Such findings are extremely difficult to interpret.

localized thickened epithelium found will need to be inspected visually during the subsequent colposcopic examination.

13.4 CERVICAL POLYPS

Polyps that develop on the cervical os are almost always benign extensions of endocervical or endometrial epithelium. They are most commonly asymptomatic findings noted during routine examination. Although women with polyps typically are asymptomatic, occasionally they may present with complaints of postcoital bleeding, or, if the polyps are necrotic, with a foul-smelling yellow discharge. Virtually all cervical polyps arise from the columnar epithelium of the endocervix. Most evolve from a single enlarged endocervical villus.[16] Extension of the tip of the polyp into the acidic vaginal environment beyond the cervical os will initiate the metaplastic process. Single and multiple polyps may contain both immature and mature metaplasia, while columnar epithelium may cover the stalk (Figure 13.14A–E). This combination of immature metaplasia and inflammation may produce an acetowhite area with a fine mosaic vascular pattern that may be confused with neoplasia. Women with endocervical polyps may have abnormal Pap smear results that indicate the presence of inflammatory or atypical glandular cells.[50] The differential diagnosis for polyps presenting at the cervical os includes pseudopolyps, rare prolapsing submucosal fibroids, nabothian cysts, and polypoid endocervical or endometrial adenocarcinoma (Figure 13.15A,B). Rarely, premalignant squamous neoplasia and adenocarcinoma may present exclusively on the tips of cervical polyps (Figure 13.16).

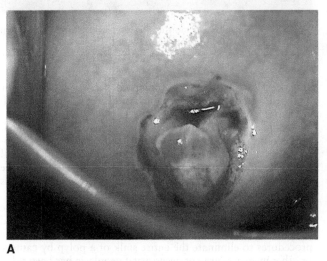

A

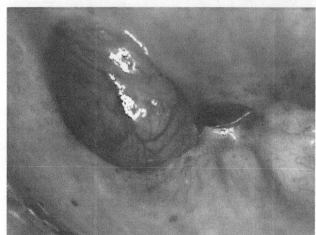

B

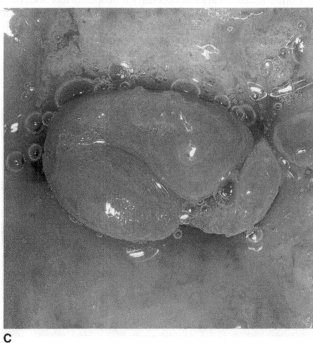

C

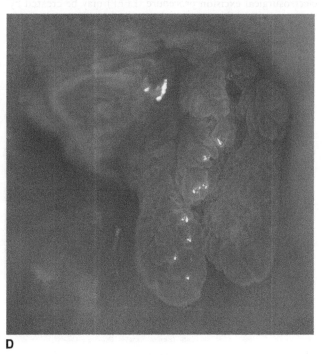

D

FIGURE 13.14.   **A:** Cervical polyps often demonstrate metaplasia in various stages of maturity on the tip of the polyp and columnar epithelium on the more protected stalk. **B:** Polyp with prominent branching blood vessels. (Colpophoto courtesy of J. Thomas Cox, MD.) **C:** Multiple endocervical polyps with immature metaplasia. (Reproduced from Wright VC. *Principles of Cervical Colposcopy—A Text and Atlas*. Houston, TX: Biomedical Communications, 2004, with permission.) **D:** A large endocervical polyp demonstrating immature metaplastic changes. (Reproduced from Wright VC. *Principles of Cervical Colposcopy—A Text and Atlas*. Houston, TX: Biomedical Communications, 2004, with permission.)

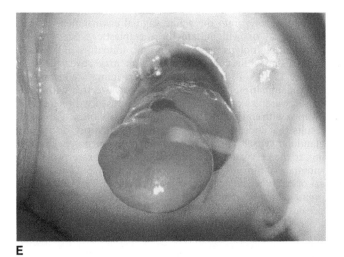

E

FIGURE 13.14.   *(continued)* **E:** A benign, cylindrical, fibroepithelial endocervical polyp. (Reproduced from Wright VC. *Color Atlas of Colposcopy—Cervix, Vagina and Vulva.* Houston, TX: Biomedical Communications, 2000, with permission.)

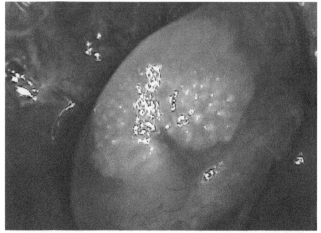

FIGURE 13.16.   CIN 1 demonstrating a typical acetowhite lesion on the tip of a polyp. (Colpophoto courtesy of J. Thomas Cox, MD.)

A pseudopolyp is an accentuated outfolding of the endocervical canal that appears to be a polyp, but on close inspection the colposcopist will see that it does not have a stalk. Rather, the apparent polypoid surface has a broad base (Figure 13.17A,B). Differentiating pseudopolyps from true polyps is important because attempted removal may cause excessive bleeding. Pseudopolyps are not an abnormality. Colposcopic identification of the broad base and healthy surface epithelium should reassure the colposcopist that this finding is normal. Iatrogenic pseudopolyps that develop following loop electrosurgical excision procedure (LEEP) may be created by the button-like appearance of the cervical portio seen in many women who have undergone LEEP.

Submucosal fibroids can extrude through the external cervical os. Compromise of the vascular supply can cause necrosis that may colposcopically and histologically mimic carcinoma (see Chapter 10). Endocervical adenocarcinoma may occasionally present as a polypoid, necrotic lesion similar in appearance to necrotic submucosal fibroids, however; both are extremely uncommon.

Single large or multiple small grouped nabothian cysts that are near the os may protrude over the os and appear more polypoid, especially to the naked eye. Under magnification, the typical yellow color and superficial arborizing vessels may usually be observed. When in doubt, a biopsy usually releases the mucus contained in the cyst or cysts, and the diagnosis is obvious.

Endocervical polyps will frequently recur if the stalks are not completely eliminated. However, polyps are common and pose little risk of becoming malignant. Therefore, extensive procedures to eliminate the entire stalk of a polyp by cautery or other measures are not necessary if neoplasia has been ruled out. Grasping the polyp with a ring forceps and repeatedly rotating the forceps 360° until the polyp "twists" off at the base is an easy way of removing most polyps with thin stalks. Polyps on thick stalks also can be removed either by using biopsy forceps to sever the stalk at the base or, if the polyp is small, simply by biopsying the entire polyp. Wire loop snares

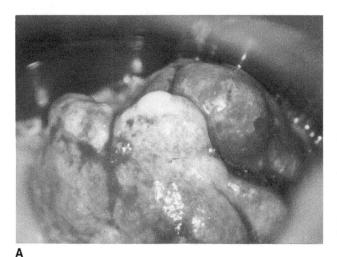

A

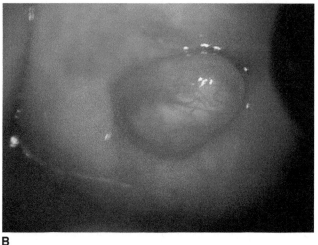

B

FIGURE 13.15.   **A:** A large, uterine, atypical polypoid adenomyofibroma prolapsing through the endocervical canal. (Reproduced from Wright VC. *Color Atlas of Colposcopy—Cervix, Vagina and Vulva.* Houston, TX: Biomedical Communications, 2003, with permission.) **B:** Large nabothian cyst located at the edge of the cervical os that appeared to the naked eye to be a cervical polyp, Note the typical yellow color and superficial arborizing vessels typical of nabothian cysts. When punctured, the cyst completely disappeared. (Colpophotograph courtesy of EJ Mayeaux, MD.)

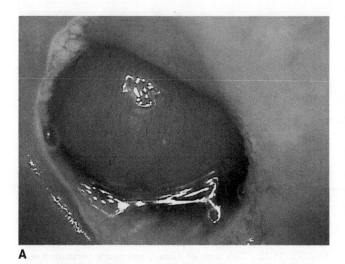

A

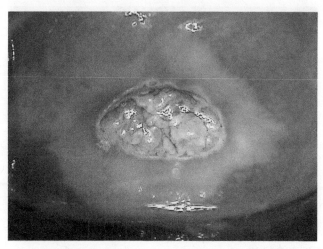

FIGURE 13.18. Four weeks after loop excision was performed, this cervix appears to be almost back to normal. (Colpophoto courtesy of J. Thomas Cox, MD.)

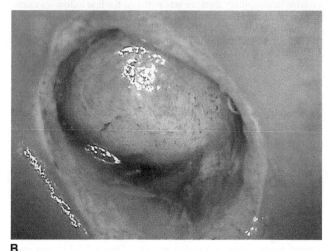

B

FIGURE 13.17. **A:** Pseudopolyp. An apparent cervical polyp is found to have a broad base, which is consistent with an outfolding of the stroma and columnar epithelium of the endocervical canal. This patient was not exposed to DES. (Colpophoto courtesy of J. Thomas Cox, MD.) **B:** After the application of acetic acid, the villi of normal columnar epithelium covering the surface of this cervical pseudopolyp seen in (**A**) can be easily delineated. (Colpophoto courtesy of J. Thomas Cox, MD.)

colposcopic, and histologic findings that may mimic residual intraepithelial neoplasia. The cervix generally heals more rapidly after excision than after ablation. This is because ablation leaves nonviable tissue that must first undergo necrosis and sloughing before repair and reepithelialization can occur. Therefore, cervical tissue treated by electrosurgical loop excision, laser, or cold-knife conization often appears colposcopically to have healed completely within 3 to 4 weeks (Figure 13.18). However, cytology will usually continue to show reparative changes for many more weeks, which may appear to be quite atypical even when the lesion has been successfully treated. In contrast, a cervix that has undergone cryotherapy may continue to slough residual necrotic eschar for 4 to 6 weeks and may have colposcopically identifiable areas still undergoing regeneration for up to 6 months (Figure 13.19). Therefore, the ASCCP Guidelines recommend that the first posttreatment examination be delayed until 4 to 6 months after either ablation or excision.[51]

may also be used. Bleeding from polyps removed by these techniques is usually minimal.

Although most endocervical polyps are benign, removed polyps should always be sent for histologic evaluation. In most cases, histology will reveal normal, endocervical epithelium covering normal lamina propria. The presence of metaplasia of varying degrees of maturity and an inflammatory stromal infiltrate of predominantly plasma cells is typical. Necrosis results in loss of surface epithelium and granulation. Dilated endocervical crypts are also common. In rare cases, involvement of the surface epithelium with HPV-induced intraepithelial neoplasia or cancer can occur, sometimes without evidence of other cervical involvement.

13.5 POSTTREATMENT FINDINGS

13.5.1 Mimics of Cervical Neoplasia

Cellular and tissue regeneration and repair within the cervix following treatment often creates confusing cytologic,

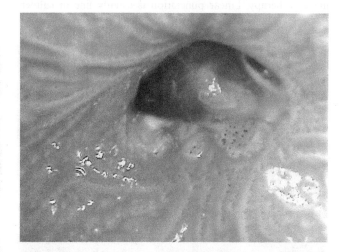

FIGURE 13.19. Four months after this patient underwent cryotherapy, a small dense acetowhite area with sharp margins and punctation is seen at the SCJ, a finding usually suspect for persistent CIN. However, a biopsy was performed and the histology interpreted as only metaplasia and inflammation. Leukoplakic ridges with fine punctation radiate out from the os, a common benign finding postcryotherapy. (Colpophoto courtesy of J. Thomas Cox, MD.)

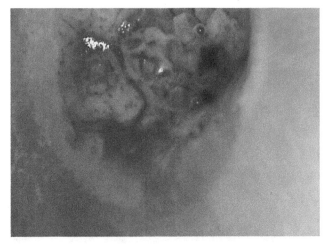

FIGURE 13.20.   A regenerating area at the squamocolumnar junction and over the tips of villi is transiently acetowhite and appears more translucent than is usually seen with persistent CIN. Punctation and mosaic are also seen but the translucent and transient nature of the acetowhitening are more consistent with a diagnosis of normal regenerating immature metaplasia. (Colpophoto courtesy of J. Thomas Cox, MD.)

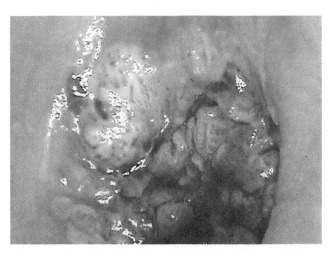

FIGURE 13.22.   This area of dilated, worrisome punctation with variable intercapillary distance was noted on the first follow-up examination of a patient who had undergone cryotherapy. The colposcopic impression of high-grade CIN (CIN 2). However, the results of both the Pap smear and the biopsy were normal. (Colpophoto courtesy of J. Thomas Cox, MD.)

The most common colposcopic finding during the first posttreatment examination is an acetowhite reaction within the regenerating epithelium that follows the application of an acetic acid solution. When the acetowhite effect is quite transient and the whitening appears more translucent than opaque, the area may be readily identified as normal immature metaplasia (Figure 13.20). However, areas in which the acetowhite effect persists and appears more opaque can be seen during epithelial regeneration within a cervix that is free of HPV-induced changes and residual intraepithelial neoplasia. Often the colposcopic picture is further complicated by the presence of punctation. When this punctation assumes a linear pattern radiating out from the os, it usually indicates that the area is undergoing healing and repair (Figure 13.21A,B). Linear punctation may be found following cervical laser, loop excision, or conization, but occurs more commonly following cryotherapy. Linear punctation is usually fine in caliber and evenly spaced. The punctation may protrude slightly above the surface plane of the epithelium, commonly within a ridge of parakeratosis. Benign linear punctation can usually be discriminated from neoplasia-associated punctation by the absence of surrounding dense acetowhite epithelium as well as by the linear pattern. However, dilated punctation with variable intercapillary distances is occasionally present in areas histologically confirmed to be normal (Figure 13.22).

Hyperkeratotic epithelium may also be present as part of normal repair. Most commonly, these leukoplakic excrescences extend from the os in a radial pattern (Figure 13.23), but they also can have a random distribution. Since they are either hyperkeratotic or parakeratotic, they do not absorb iodine and appear as tiny yellow dots against a brown background when Lugol's solution is applied. Their appearance may be strikingly similar to that of HPV-induced colpitis, except that the HPV-induced changes are in a more random pattern. Many

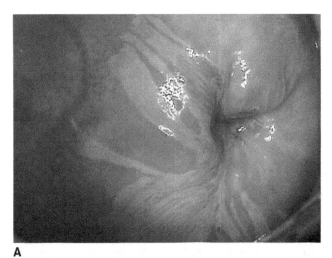

A

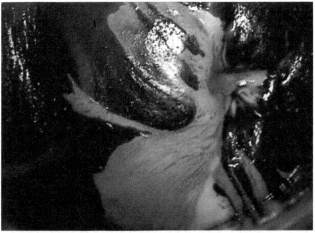

B

FIGURE 13.21.   **A:** Almost 4 months after cryotherapy was performed, an acetowhite geographic area is noted following acetic acid application. (Colpophoto courtesy of J. Thomas Cox, MD.) **B:** Same cervix postapplication of Lugol's iodine stain. Biopsy read as metaplasia with mild atypia. (Colpophoto courtesy of J. Thomas Cox, MD.)

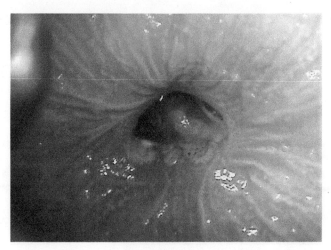

FIGURE 13.23. Radially distributed leukoplakic excrescences extending out as far as the tissue destruction of the cryoprobe are noted 4 months after cryotherapy. The radial distribution of these hyperkeratotic ridges can also be highlighted by the absence of iodine staining. (Colpophotos courtesy of J. Thomas Cox, MD.)

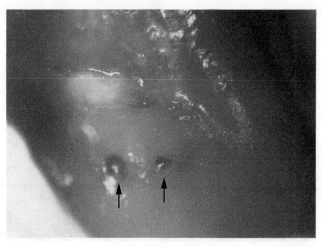

FIGURE 13.25. This colposcopic examination was performed 1 year after LEEP excision. The cervical os is bisected by a "T" shaped band that gives the appearance of three separate openings (2 smaller openings shown by *arrows*). The patient was asymptomatic from the condition with normal menstrual periods. (Colpophoto courtesy of EJ Mayeaux, MD.)

of these colposcopically identified minor changes will resolve spontaneously within 6 to 12 months after treatment. Major acetowhite lesions with or without punctation (Figure 13.24) should always be biopsied.

13.5.2 Other Posttreatment Findings

Other cervical findings include a "flush" cervix, coaptation of the external os following formation of occluding bands of tissue (Figure 13.25), or even complete stenosis and a completely distorted (knobby) cervix. Many posttreatment findings are fairly specific for the type of treatment that the patient received. For instance, a "puckered" appearance to the cervix is a typical effect of cryotherapy (Figure 13.26). A pronounced endocervical "button" may develop following laser or loop excision (Figure 13.27A,B). Marked accentuation of a "button" may occur when a "groove" is sculpted into the cervical portio at the ectocervical margin of the ablated or excised area.

The healing endocervical epithelium essentially everts onto the cervical portio, producing a red mushroom-like mass surrounding the endocervical os. The resulting "button" may look like a protruding endocervical polyp when present on only one side of the os (Figure 13.28). Such "pseudopolyps" can be differentiated from true polyps by gentle exploration of the broad base of the protruding columnar epithelium. Any excisional or ablative treatment may narrow the cervical os and endocervical canal. The new squamocolumnar junction may assume an endocervical position beyond the field of colposcopic view. When this occurs, cytologic testing and colposcopy become less reliable follow-up procedures. Inadequate sampling and poor visualization are less common problems in patients who undergo loop excision, laser ablation or excision, or cryotherapy in which a flat or very shallow cone probe is used. Any surgical procedure performed within the lower genital tract can cause cervical stenosis, but it occurs most frequently (in 1% to 4% of cases) following laser or cold-knife conization (Figure 13.29).[52–56] Cervical stenosis can also occur

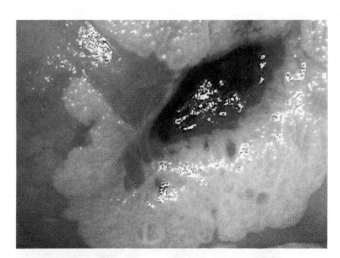

FIGURE 13.24. Extensive recurrence of CIN 1 4 months postcryotherapy. The rectangular cleared area at 11 o'clock is the healed biopsy site. This patient went on to spontaneously clear the recurrent low-grade lesion. (Colpophoto courtesy of J. Thomas Cox, MD.)

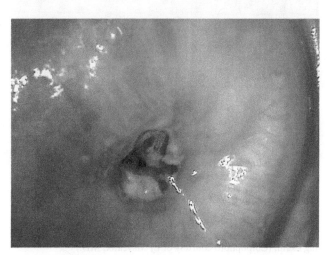

FIGURE 13.26. This "puckered" appearance is a typical finding in women who have undergone cryotherapy. Minor degrees of puckering can be seen after any ablative or excisional procedure. An area of recurrent CIN 2 is present at the new SCJ at 7 o'clock. (Colpophoto courtesy of J. Thomas Cox, MD.)

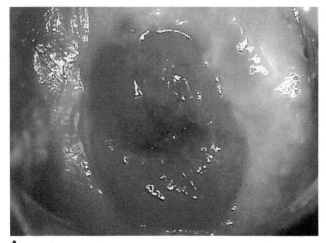

A

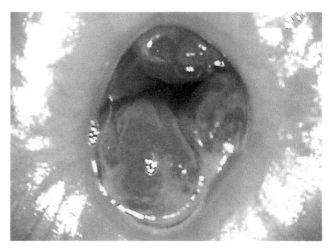

FIGURE 13.28.   A groove at the edge of the treatment area during laser ablation of a high-grade lesion resulted in the appearance of several small polyps. These iatrogenically created pseudopolyps were recognized as not being true polyps because none were on a stalk. (Colpophoto courtesy of J. Thomas Cox, MD.)

when flat or minimally sculpted cryoprobes are used. Cervical stenosis resulting from a cervical procedure is more common in older women because of their lower estrogen levels and the increased incidence of disease within the endocervical canal requiring deeper excisional procedures.

Posttreatment administration of a gram of vaginal estrogen daily for 4 to 8 weeks during the healing phase may decrease the risk of stenosis in these women. Similarly, posttreatment stenosis may be more common in women who use contraceptives containing only progestin. Women who were exposed to DES *in utero* have been reported to have an increased risk for developing cervical stenosis of up to 75% following cervical treatment.[55,56] Cervical stenosis may be either complete, in which the os is closed, or incomplete, in which the cervix is narrowed, but still open. Usually therapeutic intervention is necessary only when a significant change in the menstrual history is reported. In a premenopausal woman, complete stenosis will result in entrapment of menstrual blood (hematometra), amenorrhea, severe cyclic dysmenorrhea, and infertility.

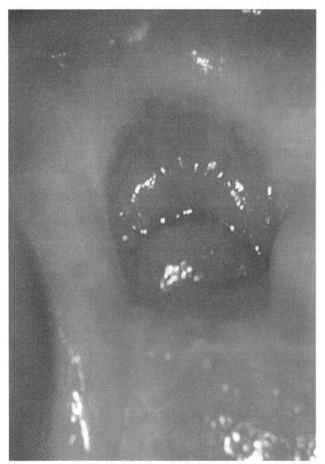

B

FIGURE 13.27.   **A:** This pronounced endocervical "button" is typically seen following laser treatment and occurs when a "groove" is sculpted into the ectocervix to deliberately evert endocervical mucosa onto the portio. It may also occasionally be noted following LEEP. (Colpophoto courtesy of J. Thomas Cox, MD.) **B:** LEEP button. Colposcopy of a 6 month post-LEEP cervix demonstrating a red mass surrounding the endocervical os, commonly referred to as a "button." This lesion completely disappeared at her 1-year posttreatment screening exam. (Colpophoto courtesy of EJ Mayeaux, MD.)

after any ablative procedure, including laser ablation, diathermy, and cryotherapy when performed with a cryoprobe tip that extends more than 5 mm into the endocervical canal. The development of cervical stenosis following cryotherapy is rare

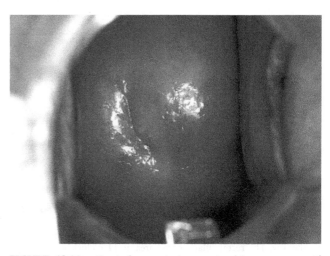

FIGURE 13.29.   Cervical stenosis is seen in this premenopausal woman who began experiencing cyclic pain and amenorrhea after undergoing laser treatment for CIN.

Significant narrowing of the os may lead to diminished menstrual flow and increased dysmenorrhea. For the purpose of conducting a cervical examination in a patient with cervical stenosis, local anesthesia should be administered to the cervix, followed by dilation of the cervical canal with a series of increasingly larger cervical dilators. The most effective treatments for complete cervical stenosis are carbon dioxide laser vaporization of a few millimeters of tissue at the proximal end of the stenosed os,[57] or loop excision of the occluding tissue using a small (10 mm) loop electrode. Following either procedure, the patient should be rechecked weekly for the first several weeks to ensure that the os remains open. If the os begins to close, it should be gently reopened with a cervical dilator. Vaginal estrogen cream applied nightly for several weeks may decrease the risk of recurrent stenosis, as estrogen deficiency has been reported to increase the incidence of this problem after laser ablation.[57]

13.6 DEVELOPMENTAL MALFORMATIONS

Several developmental anomalies of the cervix and vagina may contribute to difficulties in obtaining an adequate cytologic sample or to colposcopic evaluation of the cervix following an abnormal Pap smear. Congenital malformations of the female genital tract result from abnormal development of the müllerian or paramesonephric ducts during fetal life.[58] Failure of one or more müllerian ducts to develop results in aplasia in parts of the system, such as a unicornuate uterus without rudimentary horn. Failure to canalize is best demonstrated by the unicornuate uterus with a rudimentary horn but without a proper cavity.[59,60] Abnormal fusion of the ducts, or a lack of duct fusion, results in uterus didelphys or a bicornuate uterus. Failure to absorb the septum, either totally or partially, results in a septate or arcuate uterus or an obstructing or nonobstructing cervical or vaginal septum.[58–67]

The primary colposcopic challenges resulting from congenital malformations of the female lower genital tract are primarily cervical and vaginal. Hence, although uterine and the frequently associated renal malformations are extremely important, for the purposes of Modern Colposcopy, this section will be limited to discussion of malformations of the cervix and vagina. Vaginal malformations include transverse vaginal septa, complete and partial vaginal duplication, and Gartner's duct cysts derived from wolffian duct remnants (discussed in Chapter 14). Vaginal agenesis and imperforate hymen are not discussed here since these conditions prohibit cervical screening and are therefore irrelevant to the colposcopist. Cervical malformations include a double cervical os and complete duplication of the cervix.

13.6.1 Transverse Vaginal Septum

Recanalization of the vaginal plate by the 20th week of gestation usually produces a completely patent vaginal canal.[19] However, in rare cases, failure to completely canalize the plate results in the formation of a transverse vaginal septum that can be located anywhere in the vagina.[61] Most commonly, the septa can be found in the cephalad or middle third of the vagina.[19] If the septum is completely imperforate, cyclic pain similar to that caused by an imperforate hymen will be felt at menarche, prompting the patient to seek medical help.[62–64] Often the presenting complaint will be mucocolpos or hematocolpos,[63,64] usually identifiable by ultrasound.[65,66] Degeneration of cells within the septum during vaginal recanalization will result in a perforated septum that often is not detected until the first attempt at sexual intercourse or vaginal speculum insertion. Increased canalization may leave only vaginal

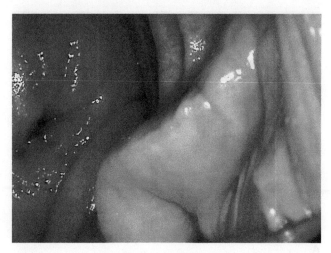

FIGURE 13.30.   Large partial vaginal septum extends from near the hymen to the posterior cul de sac. (Colpophoto courtesy of J. Thomas Cox, MD.)

bands, rather than septa (Figure 13.30). Small openings in the septa may permit cervical evaluation. The most common complaint reported by patients who have incomplete transverse vaginal septa is dyspareunia. Significant vaginal discomfort may warrant surgical extirpation of the septum. When only vaginal bands are present, simple division of the bands using a surgical knife (a procedure that is easily accomplished in the office) usually suffices. Several incisions (such as at the 10 o'clock, 2 o'clock and 4 o'clock positions) may be necessary to open more extensive septa.[19] Excision also may be necessary if the septum is fibrotic.

13.6.2 Vaginal and Cervical Duplication

When the paramesonephric ducts fail to fuse at their caudal end, duplication of the vagina, cervix, and uterus may occur.[19] Partial fusion at the extreme distal end of the paramesonephric ducts produces partial vaginal duplication. Partial or complete vaginal duplication is not extremely uncommon; therefore, colposcopists are likely to encounter this situation a number of times. The colposcopist is sometimes first alerted to the problem when colposcopy results do not correlate with cytologic results. This occurs when the Pap test is taken from one cervix and the colposcopic evaluation is performed on the other cervix. A diligent search for the cause of a noncorrelating colposcopy examination should lead to detection of the second vagina and cervix. When duplication is complete, the presence of an anterior-posterior septum and left and right vaginas adjacent to the hymenal ring usually are easily identifiable. However, it is not uncommon to see a woman with either complete or partial vaginal duplication who has been sexually active for years and has had several gynecologic exams without identification of the duplication. When vaginal duplication is only partial, the introduction of the speculum commonly displaces the septum laterally where it may become indistinguishable from the lateral vaginal wall. In this situation, the only finding on colposcopic examination will be a crease in the vaginal wall. Whether the septum is full or only partial, exploration with a cotton-tipped applicator will facilitate demonstration of the duplicated canal and septum (Figure 13.31A–D). The speculum can then be repositioned to evaluate the duplicated canal and cervix or, in the case of partial duplication, a blind "pouch."

Alternatively, a longitudinal vaginal septum may be detected accidentally during bimanual examination of the cervix if one finger of the examiner's hand is inserted into one compartment

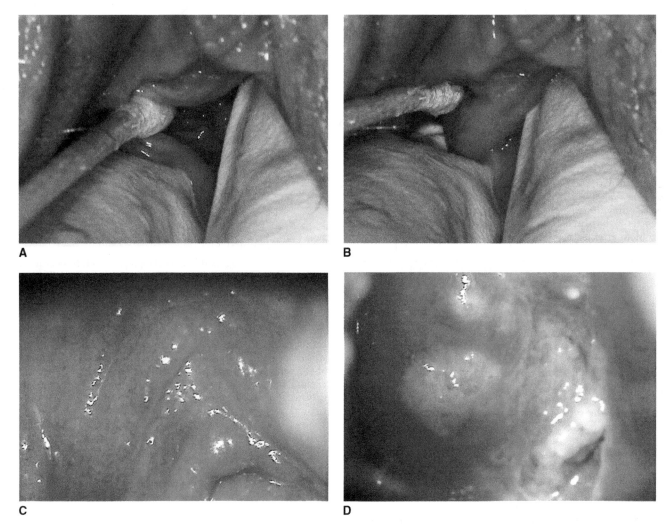

A   **B**

C   **D**

FIGURE 13.31.   **A:** Insertion of a cotton-tipped applicator into the left side of a midline anterior-posterior apparent septum helps verify that the space beyond is the entrance to a vaginal tube. (Colpophoto courtesy of J. Thomas Cox, MD.) **B:** Insertion of a cotton-tipped applicator into the right side of the same midline anterior-posterior septum helps verify that the space beyond is also the entrance to a vaginal tube. Insertion of a speculum into the right, and then the left, side of the septum confirmed that there was no communication between the left and right vaginal tube. (Colpophoto courtesy of J. Thomas Cox, MD.) **C,D:** However, until the cervix was visualized in the left vaginal tube and compared with the cervix visualized in the right vaginal tube, it was not yet clear whether this was a complete duplication of the müllerian system. The cervix in the left vaginal tube was somewhat hypoplastic and completely different in colposcopic appearance from the cervix in the right vaginal tube. (Colpophotos courtesy of J. Thomas Cox, MD.)

and the other finger into the other compartment. In rare cases, duplication of the vagina causes dyspareunia; otherwise, most women with this condition are completely asymptomatic. Soft tissue damage may be noted during childbirth; however, the septum is usually able to stretch to accommodate the neonate. The finding of a duplicated vagina or cervix should instigate a thorough evaluation of the upper genital and urinary tracts to determine whether other areas of duplication exist. Complete duplication of the vagina is often associated with other anomalies within the genitourinary tract, such as duplication of the ureters and kidneys, whereas partial duplication is not.[19,56,57] If the patient is symptomatic, surgically separating the septum will eliminate dyspareunia.

13.6.3 Cervical Anomalies

The most common cervical anomalies seen are the distorted shapes related to DES exposure *in utero*. These findings are

discussed under "Vaginal Adenosis," in Section 13.2.4 of this chapter. Duplication of the cervix is usually accompanied by a uterus didelphys and a complete or partial duplication of the vagina. However, occasionally a double os or a complete double cervix will be present without a vaginal septum (Figure 13.32). A false double os endocervical canal occurs when canalization of the cervical canal leaves a band of cervical tissue through the center of the cervical os. Exploration of each os with a small dilator or other probe will reveal a common endocervical canal.

13.7 COLPOSCOPY OF SEXUAL ASSAULT VICTIMS

Although most urban areas now have specially trained SARTs, every colposcopist should develop basic skills in evaluation of the injuries associated with sexual assault in order to identify

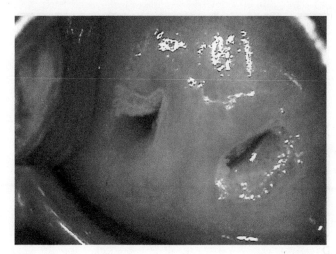

FIGURE 13.32.   Double os cervix. In this case, each os appeared to have its own endocervical canal. (Colpophoto courtesy of J. Thomas Cox, MD.)

women who may have been assaulted but are reluctant to initiate the conversation, and to be proficient when a SART is not available or the patient declines transport to a SART facility. Approximately 6.8 million women are sexually or physically (without sex) assaulted in the United States every year, resulting in physical injury for 2.6 million, with 800,000 receiving health care.[68–71] Emergency management of sexual assault survivors has two primary components: (1) assessment/treatment of injuries and (2) evidence collection important for the outcome of criminal justice proceedings that may result.[71,72]

13.7.1 The Use of Colposcopy in the Sexual Assault Examination

Colposcopy is a critical procedure in the evaluation of genital injuries from sexual assault, as only 5% of women sexually assaulted will be found to have genital injuries on direct visualization compared to 87% with colposcopic evaluation.[69] The sexual assault forensic examination may include direct visualization, colposcopy, and the application of a contrast medium such as toluidine blue, gentian violet, Lugol's solution, and fluorescein to enhance difficult-to-visualize injuries. In the setting of a forensic examination following sexual assault, colposcopy allows practitioners to identify the location and extent of injury and potentially photograph genital injury not readily visible to the unaided eye. This provides strong evidence for court proceedings. Of the 231 responding programs in a 2007 survey of the 549 active sexual assault nurse examiner programs in the United States, 64% always used a colposcope and 32% always used toluidine-blue contrast during assault examinations.[73]

The prevalence of genital injury found on forensic examination varies by the method used for the examination, with genital injuries reported in 5% to 57% of sexual assault survivors examined by direct visualization, in 40% to 58% who were examined using toluidine blue as a contrast agent, and in up to 87% who had a forensic examination using colposcopy.[74] Injury documentation is important in the forensic examination of sexual assault victims. Over the last two decades in the United States, the use of photocolposcopy to document anogenital injury in the sexually assaulted child or adult has become standard practice. However, photodocumentation in adult rape is still not widely accepted in Europe and is actively discouraged in most jurisdictions in Australia, at least partially due to concerns about privacy issues for the victim.[75] Trained forensic examiners may also provide expert testimony regarding the physical findings discovered during the sexual assault examination.[76]

While genital injury may not always occur during sexual assault, the majority (87%) of female rape victims will sustain one or more of the following injuries (Figures 13.33A–D): (1) swelling, abrasions, and/or tears in the labia minora, posterior fourchette, fossa navicularis, and/or hymen; (2) abrasions, ecchymoses, and lacerations in the vagina; and (3) ecchymoses and erosions on the cervix. These injuries have been given the acronym TEARS, which stands for tears (T), ecchymoses (E), abrasions (A), redness (R), and swelling (S).[9,76] All of these injuries are more likely to occur during nonconsensual

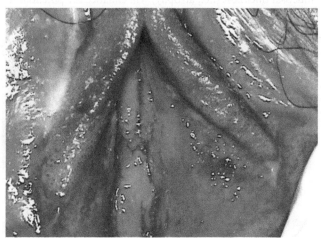

A

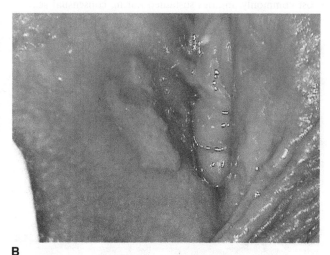

B

FIGURE 13.33.   **A:** Swelling and abrasions can be identified in the labia minora and introitus of this young assault victim. **B:** Abrasions 6 days postrape reveal a yellow granulation to the base noted when the abrasion is several days old.

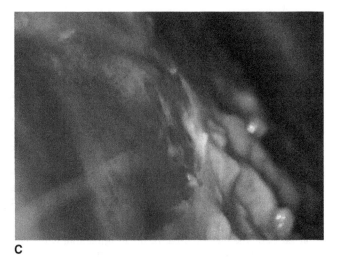

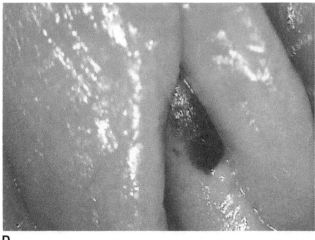

C

D

FIGURE 13.33. *(continued)* **C:** A vaginal abrasion was sustained when this woman was assaulted with a blunt object. **D:** An ecchymotic area next to the clitoris is present postassault.

penetration rather than during consensual intercourse. In cases of sexual assault, the victim's vagina is not lubricated, physical constraints may place the pelvis in an awkward position, and insertion of the penis or other object into the vagina is usually by excessive force.[9,77] The anus is even more vulnerable to laceration during sexual assault because of the greater sphincter tone surrounding this orifice. Hence, forced anal copulation almost always causes perianal tears (Figure 13.34).[9]

13.7.2 Findings in Consensual Intercourse and Nonintercourse-Related Trauma

Although the introital mucosa is quite elastic, even consensual sexual relations may produce traumatic microtears, superficial abrasions, and ecchymoses. The number and severity of injuries are usually less in women injured while having consensual relations, but the sites where injuries occur are the same for women in both groups.[9,77,78] This is because the sites of tissue stress and the position of the male are usually the same. Most commonly, injuries sustained during consensual sexual

relations occur because the female is not aroused adequately; thus, the introital mucosa is dry and not receptive to penetration except by force.[77-80] Since these characteristics differ from those of a woman being sexually assaulted only by the degree of force used during entry, it is not surprising that the locations of injuries in these two groups of patients are similar.[9,81]

Of women who sustained injuries while having consensual intercourse, 4% to 10% will have fissures in the posterior fourchette that can be identified without magnification (Figure 13.35).[9,77] Erythema in the mucosa of the hymen, introitus, and vagina secondary to vascular engorgement may also be seen in both women injured during consensual intercourse and those injured during sexual assault (Figure 13.36). When the trauma is minimal, the engorgement will be transitory, usually disappearing within minutes to hours after the sexual encounter occurs. However, with increasing friction and force against the dry mucosa, capillary walls rupture and ecchymoses appear. Prolonged, dry intercourse can occasionally cause abrasions at the introitus that can be quite painful, particularly during urination (Figure 13.37). Any decrease in normal mucosal thickness (i.e., atrophy) will enhance the potential for

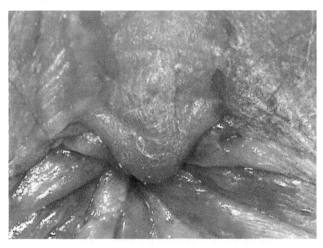

FIGURE 13.34. Perianal fissures are present in this individual who was sodomized. The ability of the anal sphincter to stretch usually prevents deep tears.

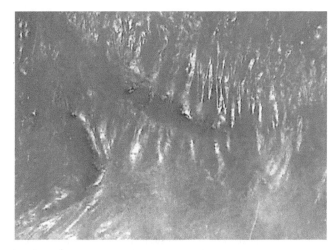

FIGURE 13.35. Minor fissures can be seen in the posterior fourchette of this woman who had consensual intercourse the prior evening.

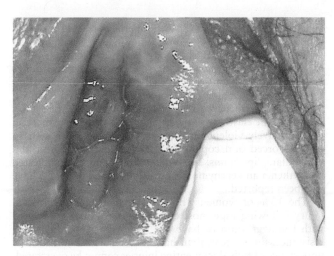

FIGURE 13.36. Erythema in the mucosa of the hymen, introitus, and vagina secondary to vascular engorgement is seen in this woman following consensual intercourse. These findings may be similar to erythema occurring with sexual assault, except that in rape cases other findings of genital trauma are likely.

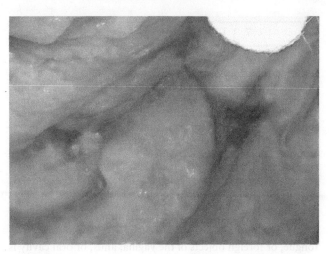

FIGURE 13.38. A tear is noted at the 3 o'clock position of the hymenal ring. This woman also had consensual sexual relations before she was well lubricated. The presenting complaint was localized pain and bright red bleeding during intercourse.

fissures, ecchymoses, or abrasions to occur.[78,79] Women with vulvovaginal candidiasis often present with introital fissures secondary to decreased elasticity resulting from inflammation-induced mucosal edema. Ecchymoses caused by sexual intercourse may be observed in the thinned epithelium of lichen sclerosus. Deep tears in the hymenal ring have been also noted in women who have adjacent thick condylomata.

The second most common site of tears in a woman who has been injured during consensual sexual relations is in the lateral hymenal ring at approximately the 3 o'clock and 9 o'clock positions (Figure 13.38).[9] The presenting complaint is either the sudden onset of coital-induced bleeding or localized searing pain. Once a laceration occurs, it will not heal until the woman abstains from intercourse for 2 to 4 weeks. The duration of healing depends upon the length of time that the laceration has been present. Any woman presenting with a history of introital dyspareunia should be asked whether

the pain is generalized throughout the introitus or localized. Generalized discomfort is most commonly caused by vulvo-vaginal candidiasis, whereas localized pain is usually from an acute or chronically nonhealing tear. A chronic tear will often have a yellow base of granulation tissue and hyperkeratotic ridges that are best identified through the colposcope (Figure 13.39).

Trauma may also result from nonsexual events. The examiner should ask the patient whether she has recently placed tampons, pessaries, contraceptive devices, or other foreign objects in the vagina. A fall onto the horizontal bar of a bicycle or a piece of gymnastic or playground equipment can cause injuries that range from minor tears and abrasions to severe vulvar lacerations. In contrast to injuries sustained during sexual assault, these injuries are almost always located externally. Vigorous foreplay can also result in superficial mucosal trauma.

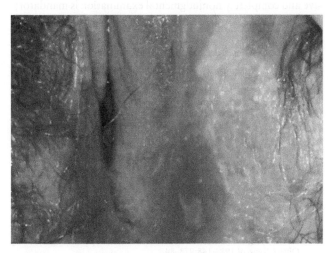

FIGURE 13.37. Introital abrasions are seen in a woman having consensual intercourse without adequate lubrication. Abrasions are usually very shallow and can sometimes be confused with herpes, particularly because they are often very sensitive to touch and to urine.

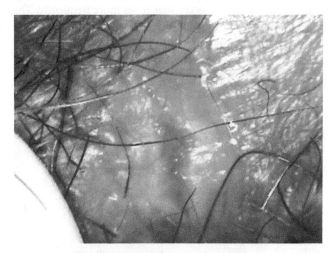

FIGURE 13.39. This 20-year-old woman presented with a complaint of localized dyspareunia of 2 months' duration. A chronic tear was identified on the perineum. Note the elevated hyperkeratotic edges to the tear, indicating that this is not of an acute duration. Resolution occurred following 4 weeks of abstinence with lubrication once intercourse resumed.

13.7.3 Findings in Sexual Assault

Sexual assault is not uncommon.[80] Thirteen percent of adolescent girls have been sexually assaulted, and 10% to 14% of women have been raped by a spouse.[9] Incest is also quite common, reported to happen to more than 25% of women. Unwanted sexual contact is the defining behavior that constitutes sexual assault.[9] Rape is sexual assault involving penetration, whereas sexual contact is sexual assault involving only external contact. In legal terms, sexual assault is considered rape if it meets the following criteria: (1) forced sexual intercourse occurred, (2) psychological coercion, verbal threats, and/or physical force were used, and (3) the person being assaulted did not consent to these actions.[80] Penile penetration is not required to satisfy the legal definition of rape, nor is penetration of the vagina. Any unwanted penetration by fingers, tongue, or foreign objects of the vagina, anus, or oral cavity is considered rape.[9] Also, by definition, rape can be committed by any individual, whether someone of the opposite sex or the same sex, and regardless of his or her relationship to the victim (e.g., spouse, acquaintance, stranger).

When the perpetrator is in the superior position on top of a supine victim, the perpetrator exerts maximum force on the posterior fourchette during the rape. A woman who has been raped while in this position typically will have a combination of erythema, edema, ecchymoses, abrasions, and lacerations (tears) of the introitus from the 5 o'clock to the 7 o'clock position (see Figure 13.40).[9,81,82] Forced penetration from any angle can result in abrasions and ecchymoses on the labia minora and similar findings or lacerations in the hymen. Hymenal swelling is often difficult to document at the time of the initial examination, but it can often be detected by comparing photographs taken at the follow-up examination with those taken initially. Injuries are similar in adults and adolescents, except that hymenal lacerations are more frequent in the latter.[82] In one study of adolescent victims of sexual assault, the most common findings were tears in the posterior fourchette (36%); erythema of the labia minora, hymen, cervix, or posterior fourchette (18% to 32%); and swelling of the hymen (19%).[82] More severe injuries are often seen in elderly female victims of sexual assault because of the increased mucosal atrophy and sexual abstinence in this population.[79] Abrasions and edema occur twice as frequently in sexual assault victims in this age group, and lacerations occur four times more frequently. The most common types of injury resulting from forced digital penetration are erythema (34%,), superficial tears (29%), and abrasions (21%).[83]

Other lower genital sites may be injured during sexual assault. Intense rubbing or sucking on the clitoris may produce swelling and ecchymoses. Cervical ecchymoses and erosions occur in approximately 13% of sexually assaulted women.[9] Vaginal lacerations are rare and found in only 1% of assault victims.[84] The elasticity of the vaginal walls protects against all but excessively violent thrusting or penetration with a sharp object. Forced oral copulation may traumatize the soft and hard palate, lips, gums, and uvula.[9] Oral trauma is manifested by erythema and ecchymoses, but swelling and petechiae have also been reported.

The 13% of women who do not have signs of physical injury following rape most commonly have been penetrated with less aggression or have not fought back with as much resistance, due to fear, than have women with injuries.[9] The importance of fully documenting injuries cannot be overstated. The examiner should be proficient in the colposcopic evaluation of the sexual assault victim. Examination without magnification can result in overlooking important occult findings. Whereas only 10% to 30% of genital injuries will be identified by the naked-eye examination, the detection rate increases to 87% when expert colposcopic evaluation is employed.[9,81,85] Special training in the colposcopic evaluation of the sexual assault victim is now available through many courses taught in the United States. These courses are becoming a prerequisite for those who serve as expert witnesses.

Another reason for not finding genital injuries following sexual assault is failure of the victim to seek medical care in a timely manner. Acute injuries almost always heal within 14 days, and shallow fissures and abrasions may be difficult to identify as early as 3 days after the assault.[9] Many victims are frightened, ashamed, or have other reasons for not seeking medical or legal attention immediately after the assault. Some women only seek medical evaluation after taking time to reflect on the events or at the urging of others. Additionally, whenever physical findings indicative of sexual assault are absent, the possibility that the alleged victim is making false allegations should be considered. False allegations are not common, but occasionally do occur, usually motivated by feelings of anger and/or guilt that are unrelated to the alleged assault.[9] Approximately 4% of sexual assault allegations are false.[9] Even when a false allegation is suspected, a comprehensive and completely nonjudgmental examination is mandatory.

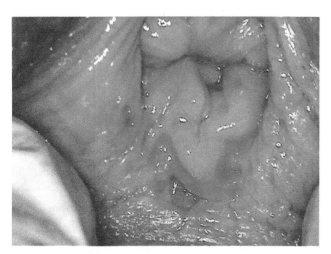

FIGURE 13.40.   Introital tear several days after sexual assault can be seen in consensual intercourse as well.

References

1. Nucci MR. Symposium part III: tumor-like glandular lesions of the uterine cervix. *Int J Gynecol Pathol* 2002;21:347–59.
2. O'Brien PC, Noller KL, Robboy SJ. Vaginal epithelial changes in young women enrolled in the National Cooperative Diethylstilbestrol Adenosis (DESAD) Project. *Obstet Gynecol* 1979;53:300–8.
3. Sherman AI. Cervical-vaginal adenosis after in utero exposure to synthetic estrogens. *Obstet Gynecol* 1974;44:531–45.
4. Herbst AL, Ulfelder H, Poskanzer DC. Adenocarcinoma of the vagina: association of maternal stilbestrol therapy with tumor appearance in young women. *N Engl J Med* 1971;284:878–81.
5. Melnick S, Cole P, Anderson D, et al. Rates and risks of diethylstilbestrol-related clear cell adenocarcinoma of the vagina and cervix. *N Engl J Med* 1987;316:514–6.
6. Kaufman RH, Adam E. Findings in female offspring of women exposed in utero to diethylstilbestrol. *Obstet Gynecol* 2002;99:197–200.
7. Kaufman RH, Noller K, Adam E, et al. Upper genital tract abnormalities and pregnancy outcome in diethylstilbestrol-exposed progeny. *Am J Obstet Gynecol* 1984;148:973–84.
8. Jefferies JA, Robboy SJ, O'Brien PC, et al. Structural anomalies of the cervix and vagina in women enrolled in the diethylstilbestrol adenosis (DESAD) project. *Am J Obstet Gynecol* 1984;148:59–66.
9. Girardin BW, Faugno DK, Seneski PC, Slaughter L, Whelan M. *Color Atlas of Sexual Assault*. St Louis, MO: Mosby Year Book, 1997.
10. Slaughter L, Brown CRV. Colposcopy to establish physical findings in rape victims. *Am J Obstet Gynecol* 1992;166:83.

11. Saunders N, Anderson D, Gilbert L, Sharp F. Unsatisfactory colposcopy and the response to orally administered oestrogen: a randomized double blind placebo controlled trial. *Br J Obstet Gynaecol* 1990;97:731–3.

12. Critchlow CW, Wolner-Hanssen P, Eschenbach DA, et al. Determinants of cervical ectopia and of cervicitis: age, oral contraception, specific cervical infection, smoking, and douching. *Am J Obstet Gynecol* 1995;173:534–43.

13. Taylor HB, Irey NS, Norris HJ. Atypical endocervical hyperplais in women taking oral contraceptives. *JAMA* 1967;202:637.

14. Krumholz BA. What is the significance of microglandular hyperplasia in a post-menopausal woman using hormone replacement therapy? *J Low Gen Tract Dis* 2001;5:187–8.

15. Greeley C, Schroeder S, Silverberg SG. Microglandular hyperplasia of the cervix: a true "pill" lesion? *Int J Gynecol Pathol* 1995;14:50–4.

16. Selvaggi SM, Haefner HK. Microglandular endocervical hyperplasia and tubal metaplasia: pitfalls in the diagnosis of adenocarcinoma on cervical smears. *Diagn Cytopathol* 1997;16:168–73.

17. Witkiewicz AK, Hecht JL, Cviko A, McKeon FD, Ince TA, Crum CP. Microglandular hyperplasia: a model for the de novo emergence and evolution of endocervical reserve cells. *Human Pathol* 2005;36:154–61.

18. Kranl C, Zelger B, Kofler H, Heim K, Sepp N, Fritsch P. Vulvar and vaginal adenosis. *Br J Dermatol* 1998;139:128–31.

19. Kaufman RH, Friedrich EG, Gardner HL. Benign diseases of the vulva and vagina. Chicago, IL: Year Book Medical Publishing, 1989.

20. Emberger M, Lanschuetzer CM, Laimer M, Hawranek T, Staudach A, Hintner H. Vaginal adenosis induced by Stevens-Johnson syndrome. *J Eur Acad Dermatol Venereol* 2006;20:896–8.

21. Sedlacek TV, Riva JM, Magen AB, et al. Vaginal and vulvar adenosis: an unsuspected side-effect of carbon dioxide laser vaporisation. *J Reprod Med* 1990;35:995–1001.

22. Bornstein J, Sova Y, Atad J, Lurie M, Abramovici H. Development of vaginal adenosis following combined 5-fluorouracil and carbon dioxide laser treatments for diffuse vaginal condylomatosis. *Obstet Gynecol* 1993;81:896–8.

23. Dungar CF, Wilkinson EJ. Vaginal columnar cell metaplasia. An acquired adenosis associated with topical 5-fluorouracil therapy. *J Reprod Med* 1995;40:361–6.

24. Goodman A, Zukerberg LR, Nikrui N, Scully RE. Vaginal adenosis and clear cell carcinoma after 5-fluorouracil treatment for condylomas. *Cancer* 1991;68:1628–32.

25. Treffers PE, Hanselaar AG, Helmerhorst TJ, Koster ME, van Leeuwen FE. Consequences of diethylstilbestrol during pregnancy; 50 years later still a significant problem. *Ned Tijdschr Geneeskd* 2001;145:675–80.

26. Hatch EE, Palmer JR, Titus-Ernstoff L, et al. Cancer risk in women exposed to diethylstilbestrol in utero. *JAMA* 1998;280:630–4.

27. Titus-Ernstoff L, Hatch EE, Hoover RN, et al. Long-term cancer risk in women given diethylstilbestrol (DES) during pregnancy. *Br J Cancer* 2001;84:126–33.

28. Swan SH. Intrauterine exposure to diethylstilbestrol: long-term effects in humans. *APMIS* 2000;108:793–804.

29. Palmer JR, Herbst AL, Noller KL, et al. Urogenital abnormalities in men exposed to diethylstilbestrol in utero: a cohort study. *Environ Health* 2009;8:37.

30. Verloop J, van Leeuwen FE, Helmerhorst TJ, van Boven HH, Rookus MA. Cancer risk in DES daughters. *Cancer Causes Control* 2010;21:999–1007.

31. Palmer JR, Hatch EE, Rosenberg CL, et al. Risk of breast cancer in women exposed to diethylstilbestrol in utero: preliminary results (United States). *Cancer Causes Control* 2002;13:753–8.

32. Kurita T, Mills AA, Cunha GR. Roles of p63 in the diethylstilbestrol-induced cervicovaginal adenosis. *Development* 2004;131:1639–49.

33. Tomkova K, Tomka M, Zajac V. Contribution of p53, p63, and p73 to the developmental diseases and cancer. *Neoplasma* 2008;55:177–81.

34. Noller KL. Role of colposcopy in the examination of diethylstilbestrol-exposed women. *Obstet Gynecol Clin North Am.* 1993;20(1):165–76.

35. Troisi R, Hatch EE, Titus-Ernstoff L, et al. Cancer risk in women prenatally exposed to diethylstilbestrol. *Int J Cancer* 2007;121(2):356–60.

36. Hanselaar A, van Loosbroek M, Schuurbiers O, Helmerhorst T, Bulten J, Bernhelm J. Clear cell adenocarcinoma of the vagina and cervix. An update of the central Netherlands registry showing twin age incidence peaks. *Cancer* 1997;79:2229–36.

37. van Dijck JA, Doorduijn Y, Bulten JH, Verloop J, Massuger LF, Kiemeney BA. Vaginal and cervical cancer due to diethylstilbestrol (DES); end epidemic. *Ned Tijdschr Geneeskd* 2009;153:A366.

38. Bachmann GA, Nevadunsky NS. Diagnosis and treatment of atrophic vaginitis. *Am Fam Phys* 2000;61:3090–6.

39. Miller L, Patton DL, Meier A, Thwin SS, Hooton TM, Eschenbach DA. Depomedroxyprogesterone-induced hypoestrogenism and changes in vaginal flora and epithelium. *Obstet Gynecol* 2000;96:431–9.

40. Selvaggi SM. Atrophic vaginitis versus invasive squamous cell carcinoma on ThinPrep(R) cytology: can the background be reliably distinguished? *Diagn Cytopathol* 2002;27:362–4.

41. Acs G, Gupta PK, Baloch ZW. Glandular and squamous atypia and intraepithelial lesions in atrophic cervicovaginal smears. One institution's experience. *Acta Cytol* 2000;44:611–7.

42. Davis GD. Colposcopic examination of the vagina. *Obstet Gynecol Clin N Am* 1993;20:217.

43. Abe C, Simon JA. Vulvovaginal atrophy: current and future therapies (CME). *J Sex Med* 2010;7:1042–50.

44. Society of Obstetricians and Gynaecologists of Canada. SOGC clinical practice guidelines. The detection and management of vaginal atrophy. *Int J Gynaecol Obstet* 2005;88:222–8.

45. Labrie F, Archer D, Bouchard C, et al. High internal consistency and efficacy of intravaginal DHEA for vaginal atrophy. *Gynecol Endocrinol* 2010;26:524–32.

46. Nath A, Sitruk-Ware R. Pharmacology and clinical applications of selective estrogen receptor modulators. *Climacteric* 2009;12:188–205.

47. Bruheim K, Tveit KM, Skovlund E, et al. Sexual function in females after radiotherapy for rectal cancer. *Acta Oncol* 2010;49:826–32.

48. Shield PW. Chronic radiation effects: a correlative study of smears and biopsies from the cervix and vagina. *Diagn Cytopathol* 1995;13:107–19.

49. Anderson M, Jordan JA, Morse AR, Sharp F. *A Text and Atlas of Integrated Colposcopy.* London, UK: Mosby, 1991:80.

50. Valdini A, Vaccaro C, Pechinsky G, Abernathy V. Incidence and evaluation of an AGUS Papanicolaou smear in primary care. *J Am Board Fam Pract* 2001;14:172–7.

51. Wright TC Jr, Cox JT, Massad LS, Twiggs LB, Carlson J, Wilkinson EJ; 2001 ASCCP-Sponsored Consensus Conference. 2001 consensus guidelines for the management of women with cervical intraepithelial neoplasia. *J Low Gen Tract Dis* 2003;7:154–67.

52. Mitchell MF, et al. A randomized clinical trial of cryotherapy, loop electro-surgical excision for treatment of squamous intraepithelial lesions of the cervix. *Obstet Gynecol* 1998;92:737–44.

53. A El-Toukhy S, Mahadevan A E, Davies T. Cold knife cone biopsy—a valid diagnostic tool and treatment option for lesions of the cervix. *J Obstet Gynaecol* 2001;21:175–8.

54. Diakomanolis E, Haidopoulos D, Rodolakis A, et al. Treating intraepithelial lesions of the uterine cervix by laser CO_2. Evaluation of the past, appraisal for the future. *Eur J Gynaecol Oncol* 2002;30:463–8.

55. Schmidt G, Fowler WC Jr. Cervical stenosis following minor gynecologic procedures on DES-exposed women. *Obstet Gynecol* 1980;56:333–5.

56. Kalstone C. Cervical stenosis in pregnancy: a complication of cryotherapy in diethylstilbestrol-exposed women. *Am J Obstet Gynecol* 1992;166:502–3.

57. Spitzer M, Krumholz BA, Seltzer VL. Cervical os obliteration after laser surgery in patients with amenorrhea. *Obstet Gynecol* 1990;76:97–100.

58. Grimbizis GF, Campo R. Congenital malformations of the female genital tract: the need for a new classification system. *Fertil Steril* 2010;94:401–7.

59. Acien P, Acien M, Sanchez-Ferrer M. Complex malformations of the female genital tract. New Types and revision of classification. *Hum Reprod* 2004;19:2377–84.

60. Acien P, Acien M, Sanchez-Ferrer ML. Mullerian anomalies "without a classification": from the didelphys-unicollis uterus to the bicervical uterus with or without septate vagina. *Fertil Steril* 2009;91:2369–75.

61. Deppich LM. Transverse vaginal septum: histologic and embryologic considerations. *Obstet Gynecol* 1972;39:193.

62. Fritz EB, Carlan SJ, Greenbaum L. Pregnancy and transvaginal septation. *J Matern Fetal Neonatal Med* 2002;11:414–6.

63. Ahmed S, Morris LL, Atkinson E. Distal mucocolpos and proximal hematocolpos secondary to concurrent imperforate hymen and transverse vaginal septum. *J Pediatr Surg* 1999;34:1555–6.

64. Rana A, Manandhar B, Amatya A, et al. Mucocolpos due to complete transverse septum in middle third of vagina in a 17-year-old girl. *Obstet Gynaecol Res* 2002;28:86–8.

65. Thabet SM, Thabet AS. Role of new sono-imaging technique 'sonocolpography' in the diagnosis and treatment of the complete transverse vaginal septum and other allied conditions. *J Obstet Gynaecol Res.* 2002;28(2):80–5.

66. Rosenburg HK, Udassin R, Howell C, et al. Duplication of the uterus and vagina, unilateral hydrometrocolpos, and ipsilateral renal agenesis: sonographic aid to diagnosis. *J Ultrasound Med* 1982;1:289–91.

67. Balasch J, Moreno E, Martinez-Roman S, et al. Septate uterus with cervical duplication and longitudinal vaginal septum: a report of three new cases. *Eur J Obstet Gynecol Reprod Biol* 1996;65:241–3.

68. Elam AL, Ray VG. Sexually related trauma:aA review. *Ann Emerg Med* 1986;15:576.

69. Sommers MS, Zink TM, Fargo JD, et al. Forensic sexual assault examination and genital injury: is skin color a source of health disparity? *Am J Emerg Med* 2008;26:857–66.

70. Tjaden P, Thoennes N. Full report of the prevalence, incidence, and consequences of violence against women: findings from the National Violence Against Women Survey. Washington, DC: National Institute of Justice and Centers for Disease Control and Prevention, 2000.

71. Rennison C. Rape and sexual assault: reporting to police and medical attention, 1992–2000. Washington, DC: U. S. Department of Justice, Bureau of Justice Statistics, 2002.

72. Gray-Eurom K, Seaberg D, Wears R. The prosecution of sexual assault cases: correlation with forensic evidence. *Ann Emerg Med* 2002;39:39–46.

73. Logan TK, Cole J, Capillo A. Sexual assault nurse examiner program characteristics, barriers, and lessons learned. *J Forensic Nurs* 2007;3:24–34.
74. Zink, T, Fargo JD, Baker RB, Buschur C, Fisher BS, Sommers MS. Comparison of methods for identifying ano-genital injury after consensual intercourse. *J Emerg Med* 2009. http://www.ncbi.nlm.nih.gov/pubmed/19217245 (accessed 19 June, 2009).
75. Brennan PAW. The medical and ethical aspects of photography in the sexual assault examination: why does it offend? 2006;13:194–202.
76. Keller P, Nelson JP. Injuries to the cervix in sexual trauma. *J Forensic Nurs* 2008;4:130–7.
77. Slaughter L, Brown CR, Crowley S, Peck R. The pattern of genital injury in female sexual assault victims. *Am J Obstet Gynecol* 1997;176:609.
78. Cartwright PS. Factors that correlate with injury sustained by survivors of sexual assault. *Obstet Gynecol* 1987;70:44–6.
79. Cartwright P, Moore A. Elderly victims of rape. *South Med J* 1989;82:988.
80. US Bureau of Justice Statistics. *Violent Crime* (NCI-147486). US Dept of Justice, Washington, DC: US Bureau of Justice Statistics, 1995:51.
81. Slaughter L, Brown CRV. Cervical findings in rape victims. *Am J Obstet Gynecol* 1991;164:528.
82. Slaughter L, Shackelford S. Genital injury in rape. *Adolesc Pediatr Gynecol* 1993;6:175.
83. Rossman L, Jones JS, Dunnuck C, Wynn BN, Bermingham M. Genital trauma associated with forced digital penetration. *Am J Emerg Med* 2004;22:101–4.
84. Geist RF. Sexually related trauma. *Emerg Med Clin N Am* 1988;6:439.
85. Lenahan LC, Ernst A, Johnson B. Colposcopy in evaluation of the adult sexual assault victim. *Am J Emerg Med* 1998;16:183–4.

CHAPTER 14

J. THOMAS COX
MICHAEL A. GOLD

Colposcopy of the Vagina

14.1 INTRODUCTION TO VAGINAL COLPOSCOPY
14.2 INDICATIONS FOR VAGINAL COLPOSCOPY
14.3 TECHNIQUE OF VAGINAL COLPOSCOPY
14.4 BIOPSY OF THE VAGINA
14.5 COLPOSCOPY OF BENIGN VAGINAL EPITHELIAL
     CHANGES
  14.5.1 Inflammation
  14.5.2 Nonbacterial Desquamative Disorders
  14.5.3 Vaginal Papillomatosis
  14.5.4 Congenital Transformation Zone
  14.5.5 Vaginal Adenosis

14.5.6 Traumatic Vaginal Lesions
14.5.7 Miscellaneous Vaginal Colposcopic Findings
14.6 VAGINAL NEOPLASTIC DISORDERS
  14.6.1 Pathology
  14.6.2 Epidemiology and Natural History of VaIN and
         Vaginal Cancer
  14.6.3 Colposcopy of Vaginal Intraepithelial Lesions
  14.6.4 Vaginal High-Grade Intraepithelial Neoplasia
         (VaIN 2,3)
  14.6.5 Vaginal Cancer
  14.6.6 Treatment of Vaginal Neoplasia

14.1 INTRODUCTION TO VAGINAL COLPOSCOPY

For many decades, the colposcope was utilized almost exclusively to evaluate the cervix. Even when a Papanicolaou (Pap) test abnormality remained unexplained by colposcopy of the cervix, the vagina was rarely evaluated. The reasons for this oversight may lie in the rarity of vaginal cancer. Few colposcopists, therefore, had training or experience in detecting vaginal neoplasia colposcopically. Recognizing that residual or recurrent intraepithelial neoplasia may occur in the vagina posthysterectomy and the link between diethylstilbestrol (DES) exposure and vaginal clear-cell adenocarcinoma led to an awareness of the importance of evaluating the vagina as well as the cervix in many clinical situations. While early texts on colposcopy did not mention evaluation of the vagina,[1] colposcopy of the vagina is now included in most colposcopy courses and textbooks. The first description of vaginal intraepithelial neoplasia (VaIN) was published in 1933.[2] Because of the delayed inclusion of vaginal colposcopy in traditional training, VaIN continued to be considered a rare entity. In 1981, Woodruff found that only 300 cases of VaIN carcinoma in situ (CIS) of the vagina were reported in the world's literature.[3]

Once vaginal colposcopy became a more routine procedure, it became evident that VaIN, especially high-grade VaIN, was still rare but more common than previously thought.[4] Increasingly, evaluation of other perplexing clinical problems such as introital pain, profuse chronic leukorrhea, unexplained postcoital spotting, and noncorrelating colposcopy all became less confusing under the gaze of the expert colposcopist. In a short 30 years, vaginal colposcopy has become indispensable for the evaluation of diseases of the lower genital tract.

14.2 INDICATIONS FOR VAGINAL COLPOSCOPY

Some recommend a limited colposcopic evaluation of the upper one-third of the vagina routinely at the time of colposcopic evaluation of the cervix.[5] Most colposcopists, however, reserve intensive vaginal colposcopic appraisal for women with a history of DES exposure, abnormal cervical cytology unexplained by cervical findings, or symptoms remaining unexplained following cervical evaluation.[6,7] The amount of time and thoroughness of the vaginal evaluation will depend on the clinical situation. The reason for this measured approach is the rarity of serious primary vaginal neoplasia and the tedious and time-consuming nature of a comprehensive vaginal colposcopic inspection. The specific indications that demand a more meticulous colposcopic assessment of the entire vagina are shown in Table 14.1.

Recently, vaginal colposcopy has been used as an adjunct to the traditional evaluation of suspected sexual abuse or rape (see Chapter 13). Traumatic genital lesions are not always obvious during a visual clinical examination, underscoring the importance of evaluation with the higher resolution colposcope. Although colposcopy alone may not be sufficient to confirm such cases, colposcopy facilitates a clear, valid, and reproducible description of vaginal trauma. It can also provide photographic documentation of medical findings and helps the peer review process.[8,9]

In addition, colposcopy has become indispensable in the evaluation of intravaginal products and devices.[10,11] Perhaps because of the poor innervation of the vagina, patient-reported symptoms do not correlate well with visual findings. The high sensitivity of vaginal colposcopy has made it a standard in safety evaluations of intravaginal products and devices conducted both premarket and postmarket approval. Studies generally conform to the World Health Organization CONRAD Manual for the Standardization of Colposcopy for the Evaluation of Vaginal Products.[11] Evaluations of tampons and their applicators, vaginal applicators for medication instillation, vaginal lubricants, vaginal spermicides and microbicides, contraceptive vaginal rings, diaphragms, and the effects of oral contraceptives on the vaginal epithelium have all been reported. This has been especially important because mucosal damage may actually adversely alter the efficacy and safety of products by causing discomfort or by

TABLE 14.1	INDICATIONS FOR A THOROUGH COLPOSCOPIC ASSESSMENT OF THE ENTIRE VAGINA

- An abnormal Pap smear following hysterectomy
- An abnormal Pap test after apparently successful treatment for cervical neoplasia
- Any Pap test unexplained by cervical colposcopy or sampling of the endocervical canal
- Any palpable or unexplained grossly visible vaginal lesion
- All women with cervical, vulvar, perianal, or anal HPV disease
- Confirmed cervical neoplasia in the immunosuppressed patient
- Monitoring all women with a history of *in utero* DES exposure
- Any woman with abnormal, unexplained, or recalcitrant vaginal discharge or bleeding
- All women with unexplained introital pain and/or dyspareunia
- Prior to cervical conization for noncorrelating cytology, histology, and colposcopic impression

creating breaches in the mucosal barrier, thereby allowing increased acquisition of pathogens.

14.3 TECHNIQUE OF VAGINAL COLPOSCOPY

Gross assessment of the vagina can be easily performed as the speculum is removed following every cervical colposcopy exam; however, thorough colposcopy permits a more accurate examination of the vaginal epithelium when a thorough clinical assessment is indicated. The vagina is much more difficult to evaluate than the cervix because it includes a much larger surface area and because areas are hidden under speculum blades, between rugae, in the fornices, and in the vaginal reflection proximal of the cul-de-sac (Figure 14.1).[6] Furthermore, the majority of the epithelium is parallel to the plane of visual inspection. Thus, a greater degree of manual dexterity and patience are demanded of the colposcopist. Full colposcopic evaluation of the vagina may add additional discomfort to that imposed by examination of the cervix only. Local anesthesia may be required for biopsies, particularly if in the one-third of the vagina just distal to the hymen.

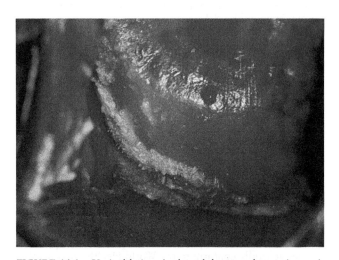

FIGURE 14.1. Vaginal lesions in the cul-de-sac and posterior vaginal wall can be most difficult to detect because the posterior blade of the speculum will cover this area and the cervix will usually drop back into the cul-de-sac as the speculum is removed. Adequate visualization often requires manipulation of the cervix anteriorly with an Ayre spatula or other instrument as the speculum is rotated to expose the posterior vaginal wall. Patience and dexterity are often required. Here the speculum has been manipulated to expose condylomas in the cul-de-sac.

Vaginal colposcopy is usually performed on completion of the cervical examination unless the cervix is absent from previous hysterectomy. The application of both 3% to 5% acetic acid and Lugol's iodine solution (in noniodine allergic patients) is essential for a complete colposcopic evaluation of the vagina, since subtle lesions may be missed with acetic acid but become obvious after application of iodine. When evaluation of the vestibule is warranted, it is best done prior to application of Lugol's solution to the vagina. Prior to insertion of the speculum, a quick gross inspection of the hymeneal ring, the proximal mucosa, the minor and major vestibular gland openings, and urethral meatus should be performed. If an abnormality is identified, then a more detailed assessment can be conducted.

Once inspection of the vestibule is complete, a medium Graves or larger speculum is usually inserted unless the vagina is atrophic or particularly small and requires use of a smaller speculum. The cervix or vaginal vault is visualized prior to the application of acetic acid. If symptoms attributable to the vagina or an abnormal discharge are noted, a sample of this discharge should be collected for vaginal pH, microscopic examination, and appropriate cultures. The cervix should then be evaluated as described in Chapter 7. Following completion of the cervical evaluation, first apply a saline-soaked cotton ball or large swab to the vaginal walls to remove discharge if present. The vagina can then be visualized prior to the application of acetic acid, which may obscure abnormal vaginal vessels, just as it may similarly obscure cervical vasculature. The looser connective tissue of the vagina is more richly vascularized than that of the cervix. Consequently, somewhat more enhanced punctation and atypical vessels are found, grade-for-grade, in vaginal lesions than in cervical lesions. Mosaicism, however, is uncommon in the vagina. The normal vaginal epithelium has a fine terminal capillary network similar to that seen on the cervix (Figure 14.2). The vascular pattern may be diffusely enhanced by inflammation (Figure 14.3A,B), whereas vascular changes in neoplasia will be localized to a circumscribed lesion. Atrophy may also diffusely enhance a vascular pattern by thinning the epithelium overlying the vessels (Figure 14.4A,B). Finally, *in utero* DES exposure often resulted in extensive immature metaplasia with fine mosaic and punctation in islands of adenosis or in areas of columnar ectopy extending beyond the cervix to the vaginal wall.[12]

Once this initial evaluation for vaginal discharge and vascular changes is completed, 3% to 5% acetic acid is applied gently to the upper vagina using a large cotton swab or cotton ball. This is followed by a second acetic acid application. A dry cotton ball or large cotton-tipped applicator is used to remove the excess acetic acid and mucus. Acetowhite changes are slower to occur to the vagina than to the cervix, and a 3 to 5 minute delay is often required before the full acetic acid effect can be seen. The vaginal fornices and vault are then assessed. Because these areas are often difficult to view, manipulation of the cervix with small or large cotton-tipped applicators can aid in visualization.

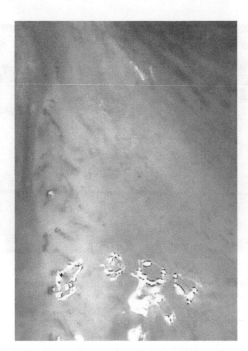

FIGURE 14.2.   Typical network capillaries within the native squamous epithelium of the vagina resemble those seen in similar epithelium of the cervix. The diffuse nature of the vessels and the uniform caliber and shape reassure that the vessels are normal. However, vessels on the ridges of rugae can be accentuated by trauma such as is seen here with overuse of tampons.

To assess the right lateral fornix, press the cotton tip carefully but firmly in the left lateral fornix (Chapter 7, Figure 7.6A,B). This moves the cervix to the left and stretches the rugal folds in the right fornix. After examining the right fornix, transfer the cotton-tipped applicator to the opposite side and press firmly to examine the left fornix. Similarly, anterior and posterior fornices can be assessed by raising or depressing the cervix by firm pressure with the cotton-tipped applicator in the fornix opposite the one to be studied. Alternatively, a wooden or plastic spatula or sponge forceps may be pressed directly against the cervix to gently move it away from each fornix.

If the patient has had a hysterectomy, the folds (corners) or "dog ears" in the lateral aspects of the vaginal vault can be difficult to assess. This is occasionally problematic since recurrent neoplasia may be hidden in these folds. A skin hook or mirror can help to visualize these often obscured sites; however, the hook may cause discomfort and bleeding. The Campion endocervical forceps (modified DesJardins' gallbladder forceps, discussed in Chapter 6), a narrow endocervical speculum, or an empty ring forceps may also be used to better visualize these hidden areas (Figure 14.5). It is wise to apply acetic acid deep into the fold using a small cotton-tipped applicator, since the initial application with a larger swab or cotton ball may not reach to these areas.

The vaginal sidewalls will be exposed to the acetic acid at the time it is applied to the vaginal vault or fornices. After examining these areas, the middle and proximal sidewalls should be evaluated colposcopically, reapplying the acetic acid as necessary. Once completed, the speculum can be collapsed and gently rotated 90 degrees to expose the anterior and posterior vaginal walls. When significant vaginal atypia is present, it is often found on the anterior and posterior walls, which are frequently covered by the blades of the examining speculum. So, it is very important to examine these more inaccessible areas. A degree of dexterity is required in manipulating the speculum and reapplying the acetic acid as necessary. During this time, the exposed areas can be inspected with the colposcope. This can be the most uncomfortable part of the exam, so rotation should be accomplished with care and should not be rushed. Before returning the speculum to the standard anterior-posterior (AP) position, stain the anterior and posterior vaginal walls with half-strength Lugol's iodine solution and inspect fully for nonstaining yellow areas, and then, following return of the speculum to the AP position, do the same for the lateral vaginal walls. Rotation of the speculum after Lugol's iodine application can be difficult, as the dehydrating effect of Lugol's solution on the epithelium often results in considerable resistance to manipulating the speculum. This problem can be avoided by covering the external surface of the speculum blades with a thin film of lubricating jelly prior to insertion.[7]

An alternative to the approach described above is to complete the entire vaginal exam with acetic acid, visualize the anterior and posterior vaginal walls as they fold into view during speculum removal, and then reinsert a lubricated speculum. After applying Lugol's solution to the lateral sidewalls, Lugol's can be applied to the anterior and posterior vaginal walls as the speculum is slowly withdrawn for the second time. Most women prefer that the speculum be introduced only a

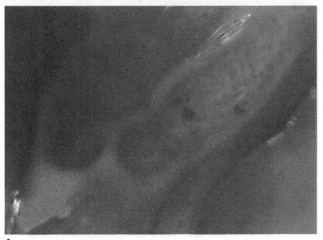

A

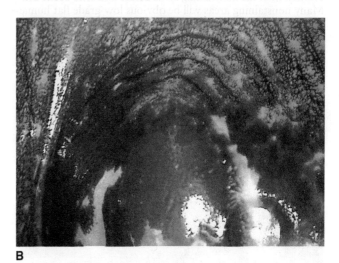

B

FIGURE 14.3.   **A:** Diffuse punctation as demonstrated here with a vaginal streptococcal infection is seen only in inflammatory conditions. In contrast, punctation due to neoplasia is localized within the margins of the lesion. **B:** Application of Lugol's iodine to the vagina of the patient in (**A**) demonstrates diffuse spotty nonstaining.

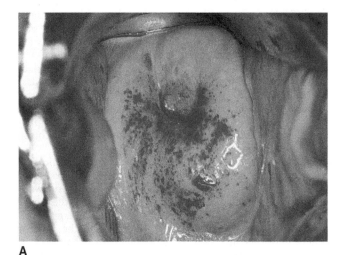 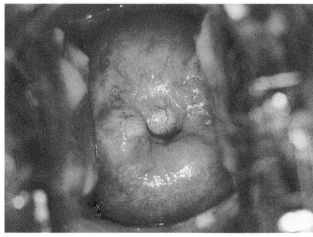

A   B

FIGURE 14.4.   **A:** This postmenopausal woman demonstrates classic findings secondary to the effects of estrogen loss on the vaginal epithelium. **B:** Considerable atrophic changes and multiple nabothian cysts are noted in this 36-year-old woman on Depo-Provera.

single time. So, when possible, try to avoid a second introduction of a speculum into the vagina.

Except for the indications listed in Table 14.1, comprehensive evaluation of the vagina is not standard. For the majority of colposcopy examinations performed for the evaluation of an abnormal Pap test, a more cursory evaluation may be appropriate. The vagina can be effectively evaluated in women at lower risk of having vaginal lesions by closely observing the vaginal walls through the colposcope as the speculum is slowly withdrawn. The speculum can be gently rotated during the removal and Lugol's solution can be applied to the vaginal walls as they fold into view. Sharply demarcated nonstaining areas that may be of concern can be further evaluated in 5 to 10 minutes by reinserting the speculum. The Lugol's effect does not persist beyond this time interval, so the area in question can be more completely evaluated after the staining has dissipated. A nonstaining yellow pattern with sharply demarcated margins is the most reliable and accurate predictor of premalignant vaginal epithelial changes. Once located, however, the severity of the disease process cannot be fully appraised without careful evaluation of the nonstaining areas before and after acetic acid. Many nonstaining areas will be obvious low-grade flat human

papillomavirus (HPV) lesions, often with small asperities that help to confirm the diagnosis without the need to perform this extra step. At completion of the exam, excess iodine should be removed and the patient given a pad to wear to catch residual iodine that could permanently stain clothes.

Among women on progestin-only contraception, and those who are postmenopausal, vaginal mucosal atrophy may prohibit adequate colposcopic evaluation of the vagina. Since inadequate estrogen results in loss of the normal glycogen storage in the vaginal cells, Lugol's uptake may be minimal, and landmarks between normal and neoplastic epithelium may be lost (Figure 14.6). In addition, the epithelium may appear less well affixed to the underlying submucosa and can sometimes be denuded by insertion of the speculum or by swabbing with acetic acid or Lugol's iodine. When inadequate estrogen results in vaginal atrophy precluding the exclusion of important vaginal neoplasia, repeat colposcopy after a course of vaginal estrogen cream may be appropriate.[7] Common regimens include 1 g of estrogen daily or 2 to 3 g twice weekly for

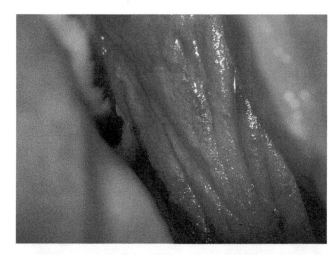

FIGURE 14.5.   Tools for vaginal colposcopy, including (from **top** to **bottom**) skin hook, ring forceps, endocervical speculum, and cotton-tipped swab.

FIGURE 14.6.   Diffuse nonstaining of vaginal epithelium occurs in women with inadequate estrogen priming and compromises evaluation of the vagina for significant lesions. This occurs most frequently in postmenopausal women but is also frequently seen in women on Depo-Provera. Diffuse nonstaining can also occur with excessive tampon use as seen in this young, well-estrogenized woman.

3 to 4 weeks. It is unlikely that any of the usual medical contraindications to estrogen use would place the patient at risk in the use of such a short course of minimally absorbed vaginal estrogen. Therefore, there are few situations in which such a short course of topical estrogen is contraindicated in the interest of excluding or detecting important vaginal neoplasia.

14.4 BIOPSY OF THE VAGINA

Because the colposcopic findings of neoplasia are less specific in the vagina than on the cervix, colposcopists are far less accurate in their evaluation of vaginal findings. Prior to the advent of colposcopy, strip biopsies under anesthesia were often utilized in an attempt to determine the size and distribution of VaIN.[3] Colposcopically directed punch biopsies, however, are more accurate and are best accomplished by a sharp biopsy forceps such as a Burke or Tischler. If disease extends well into the lateral fornices, or into the corners of the vaginal cuff as may be found following hysterectomy, these lateral folds may need to be everted, as far as possible, using a skin hook or tenaculum. The absence of glandular structures or skin appendages in most vaginal mucosa allows biopsy specimens to be only 1.5 to 3.0 mm in depth, while still adequately sampling the mucosa and underlying stromal tissue.

The biopsy should be taken quickly and accurately after warning the patient of a possible "twinge of discomfort." The upper two-thirds of the vagina has less sensation than does the lower third, and many have advocated performing biopsies in this region without local anesthetic, while others prefer to inject a small amount of local anesthetic to ensure that discomfort is minimized. Biopsies should be taken as perpendicular to the vaginal mucosa as possible to ensure an adequate sample. This may be assisted by reducing the tension of the speculum blades to allow the vaginal wall to "bulge" into view or with the use of a small skin hook. Bleeding is usually minimal and is readily stopped by application of silver nitrate or Monsel's solution (Figure 14.7A,B). If multiple biopsies are needed due to the extent or distribution of the lesions, consideration may be given to examination under general or regional anesthesia although the need for this is rare. Each biopsy should be carefully labeled and sent separately for pathologic analysis with the distance from the cervix, vaginal apex, or introitus and with the position on the clock face since treatment is usually site specific.[5]

14.5 COLPOSCOPY OF BENIGN VAGINAL EPITHELIAL CHANGES

The vagina hosts a complex ecosystem and is commonly subjected to trauma from intercourse, lubricants, creams, diaphragms, and tampon insertion. It is, therefore, common that many factors unrelated to neoplasia may alter the vaginal appearance and either obscure normal colposcopic findings or mimic neoplasia. The incidence of benign vaginal colposcopic findings in healthy, sexually active women varies from 7% to 58%, depending upon the population, the definition of "findings," and the interval since last intercourse or tampon use.[13–17] These include abrasions, erythema, increased vascularity, ecchymosis, petechiae, leukoplakia, and acetowhite changes. In a review of 13 previously published trials, O'Neill et al.[18] reported a 17% incidence of benign vaginal lesions among 569 women presenting for baseline colposcopic evaluations prior to participation in safety trials of vaginal products or devices. The most common lesions were petechiae and erythema, but epithelial peeling, abrasions, and lacerations were also seen. The colposcopist must become familiar with the colposcopic patterns presented by these entities; failure to do so will diminish the ability to accurately diagnose both benign and neoplastic vaginal changes. Mastering the following colposcopic appearances will help bridge the gap of diagnostic capability between the "cervical" colposcopist and the expert in diagnosis of all lower genital tract diseases. This section covers the major nonneoplastic situations that may obscure the usual colposcopic findings when neoplasia is present or ensure normalcy when neoplasia is not present (Table 14.2).

14.5.1 Inflammation

Inflammatory conditions may hamper colposcopic evaluation of the vagina by enhancing vascularity, by thinning or denuding epithelium, and by decreasing glycogen storage in the epithelium. This may hamper evaluation for neoplasia or DES sequelae. Specifically identified inflammatory conditions should therefore be treated and the patient should return for colposcopic evaluation after the vaginal mucosa has had time for epithelial regeneration and healing. These inflammatory conditions include infections caused by *Candida*, *Trichomonas vaginalis*, and bacteria-induced desquamative disorders.

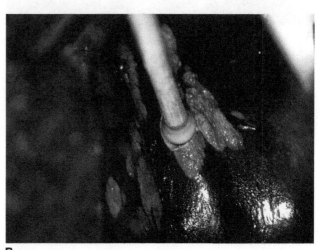

A   B

FIGURE 14.7.   Vaginal biopsies usually bleed very little but when bleeding does occur (**A**), hemostasis can be obtained by applying either Monsel's solution or by using a silver nitrate stick as seen here (**B**).

TABLE 14.2	COLPOSCOPIC APPEARANCES THAT MAY OBSCURE OR MIMIC NEOPLASIA

Inflammation
   Candida
   Trichomonas
   Bacteria-induced desquamative disorders
   DIV
   Erosive LP
Atrophic "vaginitis"
Vaginal papillomatosis
Congenital transformation zone (CTZ)
Vaginal adenosis
Traumatic vaginal lesions
   Endometriosis
   Granulation tissue
   Radiation changes

14.5.1.1 Candida

Vaginal candidiasis is the most common cause of nonneoplastic vaginal colposcopic changes in premenopausal women. Although *Candida* is often present without an associated inflammatory response, when inflammation occurs, it may result in excessive desquamation of the vaginal epithelium, producing thickened areas interspersed with thinned epithelium (Figure 14.8A). These thickened pseudomembranous areas are called "thrush patches" and, if localized, may at first glance mimic hyperkeratotic patches secondary to neoplasia or to trauma. When these patches are removed, the underlying mucosa is frequently denuded, unroofing inflammation-induced increased vascularity (Figure 14.8B,C). The resulting shallow erosions and bleeding may cause diagnostic confusion.

More commonly, "thrush patches" are not present with vaginal candidiasis. Instead, the vaginal epithelium may vary in appearance from normal to diffuse or patchy mild erythema. Application of acetic acid will highlight epithelial regeneration and repair, which will appear as various degrees of enhanced acetowhite epithelium due to the increased nuclear density of epithelial cells undergoing repair and the associated stromal inflammatory process. Lugol's iodine uptake may range from diffuse or patchy yellow to normal brown interspersed with a background of tiny nonstaining spots. Such spots, also termed "reverse punctation," may also be seen with minimal HPV expression and are, therefore, nonspecific (Figure 14.9A,B). When *Candida* causes patchy uptake of Lugol's iodine the borders of the iodine-positive areas are usually vague and diffuse (Figure 14.10A), unlike the sharper borders noted in high-grade VaIN (Figure 14.10B). In low-grade VaIN, the borders may be either sharp or ill defined as observed with *Candida*. In general, however, *Candida*-induced vaginal changes are more commonly diffuse and lack the increased epithelial thickness noted with VaIN.

Some patients will not have symptoms related to *Candida* yet will be found during colposcopy to have findings suggestive of Candida vaginitis. Confirmation of yeast may

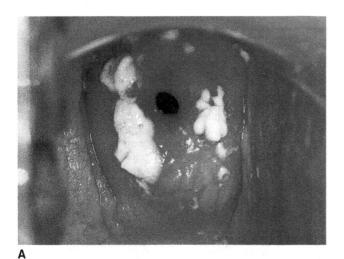

A

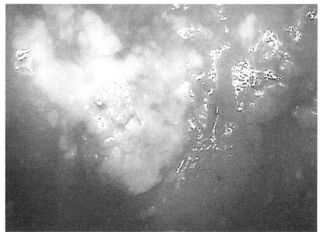

B

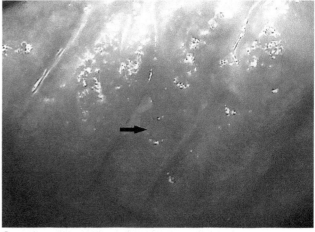

C

FIGURE 14.8.   **A:** Thickened areas of adherent desquamated vaginal cells and mycelia "thrush patches" interspersed with thinned inflamed areas are seen in some women with vulvovaginal candidiasis. **B:** Yeast patches adherent to the vaginal mucosa. **C:** An erosion and erythema (*arrow*) from inflammation noted after the yeast patch was wiped away with a saline-moistened large cotton swab.

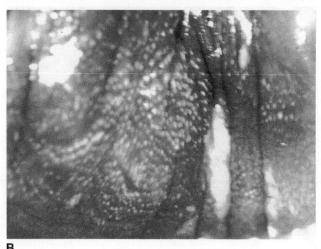

A

B

FIGURE 14.9.   "Reverse punctation" may be seen in several inflammatory conditions and in women with minimal vaginal HPV expression. **A:** This colpophotograph demonstrates tiny nonstaining punctate areas in a woman with vaginal candidiasis. **B:** The likely HPV etiology of "reverse punctation" seen on the cervix and in the left vaginal fornix in this patient is strengthened by the well-circumscribed adjacent VaIN 1.

be compromised by acetic acid and aqueous iodine already applied to the vaginal walls. When this occurs, vaginal scrapings may often be obtained from behind the anterior speculum blade for pH, KOH and saline wet-mount microscopic evaluation. If yeast is confirmed and the colposcopic evaluation of the vagina is compromised by this infection, then the patient will require antifungal treatment before returning for a repeat colposcopic exam. The exam should not be repeated for at least 2 weeks following completion of the treatment in order to allow adequate time for vaginal epithelial regeneration.

14.5.1.2 Trichomonas

Urogenital trichomoniasis is common and is usually diagnosed by visualizing trichomonads on wet mount. In up to 25% of suspected cases, such laboratory evaluation may miss the diagnosis. In such cases, colposcopic evaluation may make the diagnosis.[19] Although many women with Trichomonas vaginitis have only diffuse vaginal erythema, small hemorrhagic papules termed "strawberry spots" frequently dot the

vagina (Figure 14.11A,B). Each of these red spots consists of the tips of a cluster of greatly dilated subepithelial capillaries that reach almost to the surface and are enhanced by desquamation of the overlying vaginal epithelium. Because these papules are denuded of much of the overlying epithelium, only immature, nonglycogenated squamous cells are present. Lugol's staining will, therefore, show a multitude of minute to large nonstaining yellow spots. The larger spots are characteristically so denuded that they do not even stain yellow but instead appear pink on the mahogany background (Figure 14.12).

The colposcopic appearance of "strawberry spots" has been termed colpitis macularis and is virtually classic for Trichomonas cervicitis/vaginitis.[20,21] In one study, colpitis macularis was detected by colposcopy in 52 of 118 *Trichomonas*-infected women. Women with colpitis macularis had more trichomonads on wet mount (mean 18 ± 20 trichomonads/field ×400 magnification) compared with women with *Trichomonas* but without colpitis macularis (7 ± 17).[21] Two other entities may occasionally mimic trichomoniasis.[22] Some women with

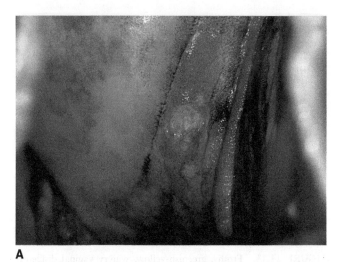

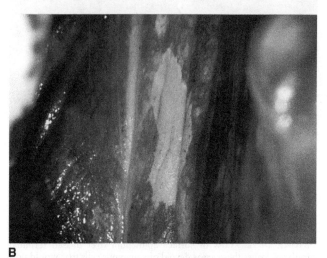

A

B

FIGURE 14.10.   **A:** Diffuse borders to nonstaining areas are seen with inflammatory conditions such as in this woman with vaginal candidiasis. Biopsy (site shown here) demonstrated only inflammation. **B:** Contrast with the sharply nonstaining areas of this VaIN.

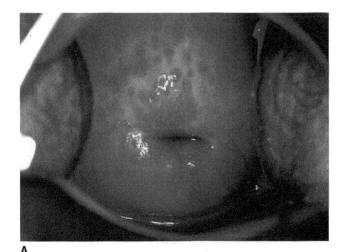
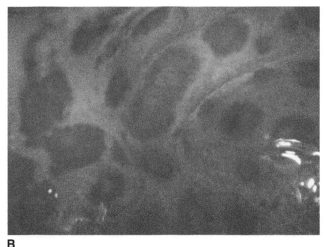

FIGURE 14.11. **A:** Classic "strawberry spots" of vaginal trichomoniasis represent terminal capillary dilation. Similar spots can occasionally be seen in desquamative inflammatory vaginitis (DIV) and in vaginal streptococcal infection. **B:** Terminal capillaries are clearly seen at higher magnification.

desquamative inflammatory vaginitis (DIV) (see below) have a vaginal inflammatory appearance similar to *Trichomonas*-induced "strawberry spots." Additionally, extensive erosion of the vaginal epithelium often noted during treatment of vaginal HPV-induced lesions with 5-fluorouracil (5-FU) causes small diffuse "papules" of vaginal adenosis that may be challenging to discriminate from a *Trichomonas* infection (see below).

More often, "strawberry spots" are caused by *T. vaginalis*. Since they can normally be seen prior to application of acetic acid and aqueous iodine, vaginal secretions for saline and KOH wet mounts and vaginal pH testing can be collected without compromising the specimen. Classic trichomonal discharge is usually described as profuse and watery, with a frothy, greenish-yellow tint and a pH of >4.5. The discharge may, however, be minimal or creamy yellow or ivory in color and without a frothy appearance (Figure 14.13).[21] Other than recognizing the cause of this unusual colposcopic appearance and treating the infection, the primary importance of this finding during the colposcopic examination is that further evaluation may be prohibited until the inflammation is treated and

the epithelium healed. In most cases, however, this infection does not significantly interfere with a diagnostic evaluation for neoplasia. *Trichomonas* is treated effectively with a single 2-g oral dose of oral metronidazole and all sexual contacts should be referred for treatment.[23]

14.5.1.3 Bacteria-Induced Desquamative Disorders

Both excessive *Lactobacillus acidophilus* and the presence of *Leptothrix*, an extremely long anaerobic *Lactobacillus*, have been described as causative agents of cytolysis and desquamation of vaginal epithelium. Cibley[24] named the presence of excessive *Lactobacillus* in symptomatic women "cytolytic vaginosis." The patient usually complains of an excessive vaginal discharge during the 2 weeks before menses, accompanied by mild introital irritation and pruritus. The nature of the symptoms is similar to yeast, and since the symptoms are cyclic, they resolve after menses and after treatment with antifungal medications; the woman is misleadingly reassured that the origin is indeed caused by *Candida*. The nonodorous discharge

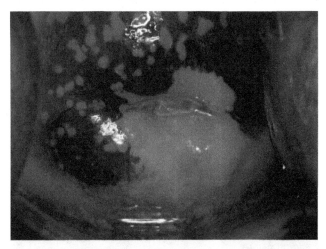

FIGURE 14.12. Loss of surface epithelium over dilated terminal capillaries leaves these areas devoid of squamous cells that would normally stain yellow in the absence of glycogen. This results in complete rejection of aqueous iodine stain and a glistening, pink, almost raw appearance to these "spots" post-Lugol.

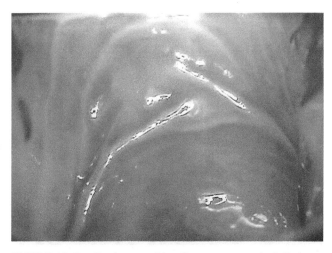

FIGURE 14.13. Frothy, greenish-yellow, watery vaginal discharge commonly seen in *Trichomonas* infections. Many women with this disease will not have such classic findings. Digitalization artifact over areas of glare.

is white and homogeneous with a pH below 4.5. An excessive number of Lactobacilli, nuclei denuded of their cytoplasm ("naked nuclei") and other cellular debris from degeneration of squames are noted in the wet-mount exam. Yeast and other pathogenic organisms are conspicuously absent, and unlike bacterial vaginosis, the "whiff" test is negative. In other instances, the diagnosis may be assisted by a history of "chronic vulvovaginal candidiasis" unresponsive to antifungal therapy. In one series of 210 reproductive age women complaining of abnormal vaginal discharge associated with pruritus, burning, genital irritation, or dyspareunia, 7.1% were diagnosed with cytolytic vaginosis.[25] Treatment consists of suppression of the acid-producing *Lactobacillus* by alkalinizing the vagina by douching with 1-tsp baking soda in 1 pint of water as needed. This resulted in improvement of symptoms in 68% of patients after an average of two cycles of vaginal douches.[26] If the condition interferes with the adequacy of the vaginal examination, the patient may be treated as outlined and brought back for repeat colposcopy; however, this is not usually necessary.

Vaginal lactobacillosis presents with similar symptoms of increased vaginal discharge and introital itching, burning, and irritation occurring in the second half of the menstrual cycle (commonly 2 weeks before menses). Patients will often describe the discharge as thick, white, creamy, or curdy and may also have been treated unsuccessfully in the past for candidiasis. Most patients will report a lengthy history of such complaints, with an average length of symptoms of approximately 2 years.[27] Horowitz attributed these symptoms to the presence of an excessively long (60 to 70 mμ) gram-positive anaerobic *Lactobacillus*, which has previously been named *Leptothrix*.[27] *Leptothrix* has long been considered either a harmless commensal or an organism found in the presence of *Trichomonas*, perhaps as a copathogen. Some symptoms, when present, may be related to coinfection with this known pathogen. This organism has been described in 1% of women of reproductive age, but 78% are asymptomatic. When cyclic introital irritation and dyspareunia occur, and no pathogenic organism can be identified other than these long bacilli, treatment is indicated. Horowitz reported successful treatment with amoxicillin/clavulanic acid 500 mg three times a day for 7 days, doxycycline 100 mg twice a day for 10 days, and mild relief of symptoms in some patients using bicarbonate douches.[27] As in cytolytic vaginosis, inflammatory erythema is absent, but diffuse acetowhitening and patchy Lugol's iodine uptake may obscure colposcopic findings of vaginal neoplasia.

14.5.2 Nonbacterial Desquamative Disorders

14.5.2.1 Desquamative Inflammatory Vaginitis

DIV is an erosive, inflammatory vaginitis of uncertain etiology first described by Herman Gardner in 1969.[28] DIV has been considered by some to be a form of lichen planus (LP),[29] pemphigus vulgaris, or mucous membrane pemphigoid.[30] Others designate it a separate entity that can occur at any age but commonly occurs in perimenopausal and menopausal women. The presenting complaint is usually excessive vaginal discharge, sometimes with postcoital bleeding.[29,31,32] The introitus may be slightly sensitive with mild burning or pruritus suggestive of a candidal infection. Mild dyspareunia may also occur. Dyspareunia, increased vaginal discharge, and a sterile inflammatory infiltrate are considered the classical triad of findings in DIV.[30]

A profuse seropurulent discharge is present, and the vaginal pH tends to be alkalinized above the normal range of 4.0 to 4.4 and even above the usual alkalinity of bacterial vaginosis and *Trichomonas* (5.0 to 5.5) to the more extreme alkalinity of 6 to 7.4.[30,31] Wet-mount microscopic examination

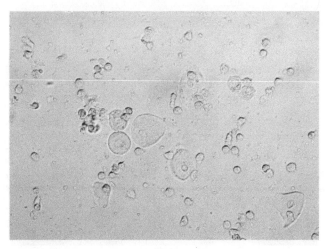

FIGURE 14.14.   Wet mount of profuse vaginal discharge in a woman with DIV shows numerous white blood cells (WBCs) and parabasal cells. More commonly evaluation of the discharge will reveal inflammatory findings more dramatic than seen here.

demonstrates only sheets of leukocytes, parabasal cells, and the absence of *Lactobacillus* or other bacteria (Figure 14.14). No specific infectious etiology can be documented, but an absence of lactobacilli and an overall increase in prevalence of group B streptococci has been demonstrated.[32] Colposcopic evaluation of the vagina may show either diffuse or localized patches of erythema or erosion (Figure 14.15A-C). Other women may present with erythematous spots resembling the "strawberry spots" of a *Trichomonas* infection. Areas of involvement often appear denuded of epithelium, and these areas are occasionally covered by a gray pseudomembrane. Eroded areas are usually shallow but may occasionally present as deep ulcers (Figure 14.16). Application of acetic acid will often cause a diffuse or patchy acetowhite color in areas of involvement that are not eroded, reflecting high-cellular turnover. Lugol's iodine will not stain these areas but the margins between staining and nonstaining areas are not sharp. As with any process involving erosion, biopsy should extend across the margin from noneroded to adjacent eroded epithelium. Histology will show only a dense infiltrate of PMNs, loss of surface epithelium, and thinning and immaturity of adjacent epithelium.[32] Not present are the more classic histologic findings of vulvar LP, particularly the findings obtained from vulvar biopsies through a reticulated area of Wickham's striae.[33] These findings are also not present in other mucous membranes such as the mouth and eyes, common in mucous membrane pemphigoid or the vulvovaginal-gingival syndrome (see Section 14.5.2.2).

Treatment of this condition may be difficult and require long-term therapy. The most successful treatment has been the intravaginal application of 2% clindamycin suppositories or vaginal cream for a minimum of 2 weeks.[32] This results in clinical improvement in >95% of patients, although relapse may occur in 30%.[32] High-potency intravaginal steroids have also been used alone or in combination with clindamycin. Treatment for up to 4 to 6 weeks has been reported.[30] Postmenopausal patients with DIV also may need vaginal or oral estrogen therapy to maintain remission;[31] however, treatment with estrogen alone is likely to be ineffective.[29]

14.5.2.2 Lichen Planus

Mucosal LP (vulvovaginal-gingival syndrome) involves the vagina in addition to other mucous membranes, particularly the mouth. Although LP is most commonly a disease of the

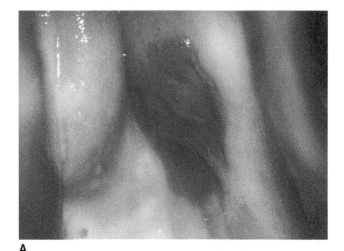

A

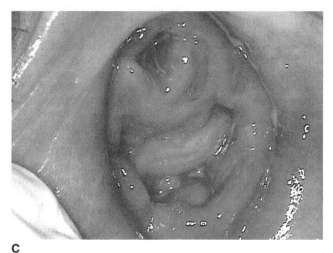

B

FIGURE 14.15. **A:** Shallow erosions are commonly seen in DIV and may present as erythematous patches. **B:** Marked inflammatory changes throughout the vagina, with diffuse punctation and a heavy cream-colored watery discharge with 4+ WBCs on wet mount are classic findings in DIV. **C:** Shallow erosions from DIV extend out to the periurethra, hymen, and introitus of the woman pictured in (**B**).

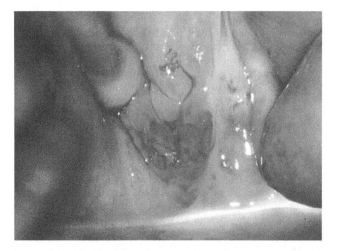

C

skin, about 15% to 25% of patients will have only mucosal involvement.[34] Genital lesions most commonly occur simultaneously with other mucosal lesions but may also precede or follow the oral lesions by up to 2 years.[35] Common symptoms include burning, pruritus, dyspareunia, and a vaginal

discharge that may be bloody. Genital symptoms are generally more severe than those of the oral mucosa.[35]

The diagnosis of LP can be easily established when erosion of the vestibule and/or vagina is accompanied by the characteristic buccal and gingival erythema, desquamation, vesiculation, and erosion. In other patients, white, lacey, reticulated papules and plaques (Wickham's striae) may be seen in both the genital and the oral mucosa.[35] When only genital lesions are seen, the diagnosis depends on eliminating other possible erosive disorders (Figure 14.17A,B). The finding of vestibular erosion makes atrophic vaginitis unlikely since this most commonly affects the vagina only. Otherwise, these two entities can be clinically similar in that they both may cause an excessive seropurulent exudate that is quite alkaline and lacking in *Lactobacillus*. With LP, however, the mucosa is usually more denuded, may have a gray pseudomembrane, and may be gradually obliterated by adhesions, especially in the absence of sexual activity. If the vestibular mucosa is eroded as well, irritation and dyspareunia may be severe. Pemphigus and Behcet's may also present with an eroded vestibular area but usually do not involve the vagina.[31] Behcet's ulcers are usually deep and destructive in comparison with the shallow erosion of LP.

Patients with genital LP may experience brief periods of regression, but spontaneous remission is unlikely. Remissions have been seen with prolonged treatment with topical or systemic corticosteroids with or without cyclosporin, but relapse is almost universal following discontinuation of therapy.[35] Tacrolimus 0.1% ointment, a topical immunosuppressant similar to cyclosporine, has been reported to be effective in the

FIGURE 14.16. Deeper erosions resembling ulcers may occasionally be seen in women with DIV. Secondary infection of shallow erosions may be responsible for these deeper lesions. Differentiation from erosions seen in LP can only be made if the more classic introital and buccal lesions of LP are also present. This cul-de-sac presentation is most common. (Photo courtesy of Dr. Gordon Davis.)

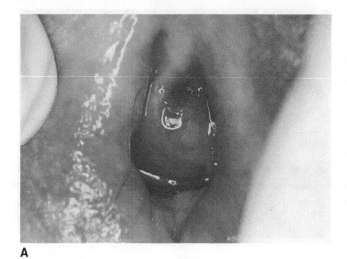

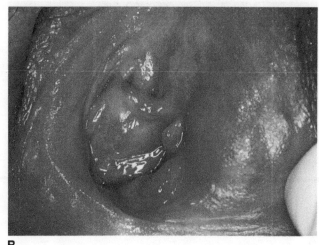

A   **B**

FIGURE 14.17.   Occasionally introital erosions are present without classic signs of LP and the vaginal findings are most consistent with DIV. These findings suggest that the two may be closely related, as seen in these two women with vaginal erosions and minor vestibular erosions (**A and B**).

management of erosive LP.[36] For a more complete discussion of LP, see Chapter 15.

14.5.3 Vaginal Papillomatosis

Localized or diffusely enlarged vaginal papillae are occasionally encountered that may be confused with neoplasia. In DES-exposed women, these are most frequently encountered superior and lateral to the cervix (Figure 14.18).[37] Most women with these findings have not been exposed to DES *in utero*, however, and may have prominent vaginal papillae anywhere in the vagina. Often these papillae may be identified just cephalad to the hymen in the proximal vagina and may be confused with HPV-induced lesions.[38] Although these papillary projections may feel like a mass (or masses) during digital exam, the benign nature of these findings can be easily confirmed by simple inspection after application of aqueous iodine. Since the epithelium covering these papillary structures is normal, application of Lugol's iodine should result in a mahogany-brown staining (Figure 14.19A,B). Colposcopically, these structures are homogeneously pink, just as the surrounding mucosa, with no remarkable vascular structure present. Biopsy is generally not required to establish a diagnosis. In fact, because of the potential for misclassification of normal glycogen-containing cells as koilocytes, biopsy may be incorrectly interpreted as condyloma when it simply represents a normal benign anatomic variant. Garzetti and colleagues evaluated areas of vaginal micropapillary lesions for up to 12 HPV types by *in situ* hybridization and polymerase chain reaction (PCR) and compared them to normal and condylomatous epithelium. In both the micropapillary and normal epithelium, the incidence of HPV positivity was very low (9.4% and 8.3%, respectively) compared to 64.7% among the condylomatous samples.[38]

14.5.4 Congenital Transformation Zone

Approximately 3% to 4% of women have metaplastic epithelium that is persistently arrested in a nonglycogenated, acanthotic phase. Although the congenital transformation zone (CTZ) is most often confined to the cervix, it is mentioned here because this finding extends onto the vaginal wall in

some women.[39] Although the exact etiology of the CTZ is not well established, speculation is that some female fetuses with columnar epithelium on the ectocervix, and occasionally on the upper vagina, develop metaplasia before birth and in the prepubertal years when cervical transformation is usually quiescent.[40] This process may be influenced by maternal estrogen

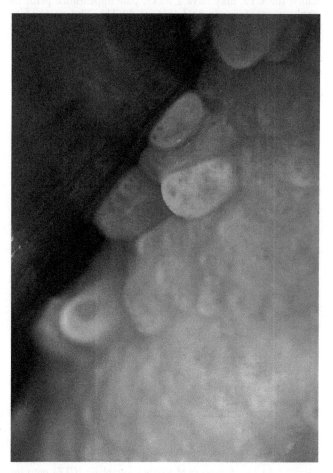

FIGURE 14.18.   A papillary appearance is noted superior and lateral to the cervix in this woman who was not exposed to DES *in utero*.

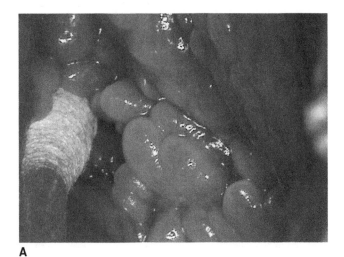

A

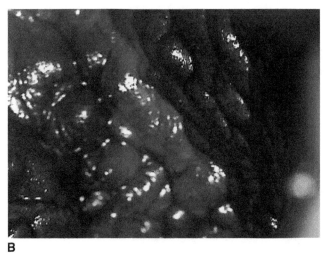

B

FIGURE 14.19. Benign vaginal papillae (**A**) before and (**B**) after application of Lugol's solution. The mahogany-brown staining assures the colposcopist that these papillae are normal.

during the third trimester of fetal life. If this association with timing of the metaplastic process is correct, then the timing must be responsible for the arresting of this process in a perpetual state of nonmaturation.

This benign finding may be localized to the cervix, but when it extends to the vagina, it most commonly extends anteriorly or posteriorly (Figure 14.20),[40] although occasionally extension may be found lateral to the cervix. Colposcopically, the CTZ may have a waxy, pale appearance prior to application of acetic acid (Figure 14.21). The acetowhite response is generally slow to develop and then lingers for some time before fading. A fine, regular-to-irregular mosaic and fine punctation are usually present. The appearance is quite homogeneous throughout, unless a HPV-induced lesion is present within the CTZ. Because the epithelium remains nonglycogenated, Lugol's iodine application is either rejected entirely (yellow staining) or irregularly stained (variegated) (Figure 14.22). The margin is definite but often slightly feathery.

When a large acetowhite area extends from the cervix to the vaginal wall, considerable colposcopic experience is required to differentiate HPV-infected epithelium in the upper vagina from the normal CTZ extending into the anterior and/or posterior vaginal fornices. The primary colposcopic dilemma with vaginal extension of the CTZ is the same dilemma encountered with evaluation of the cervical portion. Because the CTZ has colposcopic features similar to those encountered with intraepithelial neoplasia (particularly a fine mosaic pattern), biopsy may be warranted. The large, uniform nature of the process, symmetry, somewhat smooth margins, and the unusually slow development of the acetowhite effect commonly enable the colposcopist to predict the benign, acanthotic nature of the process. Unfortunately, the occurrence of HPV-induced intraepithelial neoplasia within a benign CTZ may increase the difficulty of detecting the lesion. In this situation, however, a margin, or internal border, with a more prominent colposcopic finding in the lesion should direct the biopsy placement (Figure 14.23A,B).

Colposcopic biopsies from a CTZ can be very difficult to interpret.[39] The characteristic histologic findings are acanthosis, which is frequently misdiagnosed as HPV infection, and subepithelial pearling, which has even been overcalled as indicative of early invasion. The caudal margin of this acanthotic epithelium is sharply demarcated from adjacent normal mature squamous epithelium.

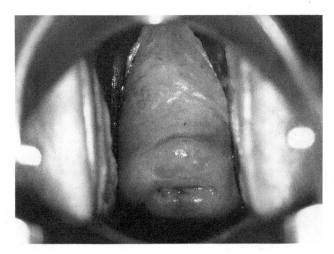

FIGURE 14.20. Extension of arrested metaplasia (CTZ) onto the anterior vaginal wall.

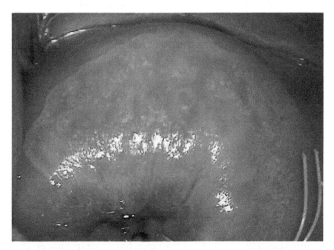

FIGURE 14.21. Before the application of acetic acid, a translucent pale and waxy congenital transformation zone (CTZ) extends over much of the anterior cervix.

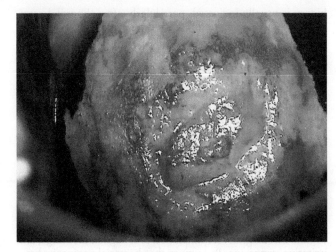

FIGURE 14.22. The CTZ after application of Lugol's solution demonstrates a relatively homogeneous lack of iodine uptake, although some mosaic plates partially stain.

14.5.5 Vaginal Adenosis

Vaginal adenosis is the presence of glandular cells and their products in the vaginal wall.[41] To the naked eye, adenosis may appear as a reddened area. Its colposcopic appearance is varied, commonly presenting as areas of acetowhite epithelium, mosaicism, or both. About half of patients will have varying patterns in different areas of the vagina. The colposcopic appearance of columnar epithelium (same "grapelike" appearance as seen on the cervix) alone is rare, although almost all areas with a columnar appearance represent adenosis.[42] In addition, areas of adenosis do not stain following the application of iodine to the vagina. Vaginal adenosis was initially considered an entirely benign process until the 1971 report on the finding of clear cell adenocarcinoma in a number of women exposed *in utero* to DES.[43] Because DES exposure during fetal life also resulted in structural changes to the cervix and other areas in the genital tract, a complete discussion on DES and vaginal adenosis is included in Chapter 13. Vaginal adenosis has also been reported after intravaginal 5-FU therapy.[44,45]

14.5.6 Traumatic Vaginal Lesions

Sources of vaginal trauma include tampon use, contraceptives such as diaphragm and spermicide, speculum trauma, and even intercourse (consensual or otherwise). Trauma from vaginal speculum insertion occurs on the cervix most commonly, but vaginal trauma may also occur. As with vaginal trauma during intercourse, it is more common in women with atrophic epithelium.

Several effects of vaginal tampons may make vaginal colposcopic evaluation more difficult and may actually mimic changes associated with neoplasia. Recent tampon use, even when not prolonged, causes dehydration of the superficial layers of mucosa and may result in microulcerations and peeling of affected epithelium.[31,46] The resulting regeneration and repair appear colposcopically as patchy acetowhite areas that stain only mustard-yellow after Lugol's iodine application. These areas may be virtually indistinguishable from low-grade HPV-induced vaginal lesions (VaIN 1). Occasionally the tampon-induced nature of the changes can be surmised by a history of recent tampon use and a linear lineup of nonstaining patches on the prominent folds of the vaginal rugae (Figure 14.24). If differentiation is considered important, the patient can be advised to not put a tampon into the vagina for the ensuing 2 weeks and return for repeat staining of the vagina with Lugol's solution. At that time, epithelial regeneration will usually be complete and a mahogany-brown color of the vaginal epithelium will provide reassurance of the non–HPV-related nature of the previous findings.

Tampons, first reported to cause vaginal ulcers in 1977,[47] are now recognized as the most common cause of such ulcers.[31,46,48–50] Short duration use commonly results in microulcerations, which occur more often with superabsorbent compared to conventional tampons.[46] In some instances, however, tampon use may actually lead to minor vaginal erosions, abrasions, and lacerations.[49] These erosions may present as erythematous, superficially denuded areas or as deep ulcers with atypical vessels resembling invasive cancer (Figure 14.25).[46,48,50] They are most commonly found in a limited area of the upper third of the vagina, 2 to 4 cm in diameter, corresponding to the upper resting point of the tampon. Because these lesions may bleed, women often continue to use tampons with the mistaken belief that the bleeding is menstrual in nature, thus prolonging exposure of the denuded area to further irritation. Tampon ulcers have a clean base of granulation tissue and are usually surrounded by a prominent rolled edge. If the history is compatible

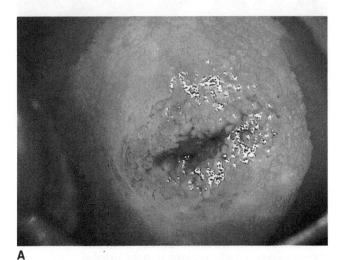

A

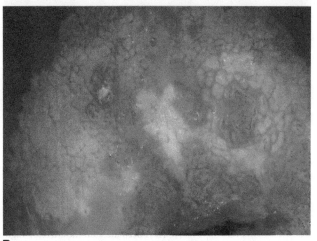

B

FIGURE 14.23. **A:** A large complex transformation zone resembling a CTZ with both immature metaplasia and several foci of CIN 1. **B:** Magnified view of (**A**) shows an internal margin within an area of immature metaplasia.

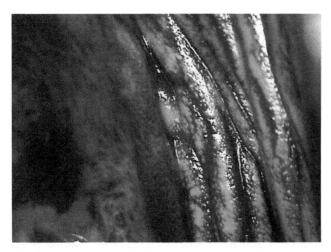

FIGURE 14.24. A linear lineup of nonstaining Lugol's iodine–negative areas is suggestive of tampon-induced epithelial trauma and not intraepithelial neoplasia. Contrast example to the linear lineups of flat vaginal warts/VaIN 1 as seen in Figures 14.34C and 14.38B.

with excessive tampon use, if the patient may be relied upon to return for reevaluation, and if the patient is willing to refrain from using tampons for at least the next 4 weeks, biopsy may not be necessary until a return visit for repeat examination. Since these ulcers most often disappear within 2 to 3 weeks of removal of the offending agent,[31] any persistent lesion should be biopsied. When suspicion is high that a patient may not adhere to follow-up recommendations, a biopsy of the ulcerated area and adjacent rolled edge should be done at the initial visit. The differential diagnosis includes vaginal carcinoma, chancroid, syphilis, and granuloma inguinale. Iatrogenic or sexual blunt trauma and use of a pessary are other possible causes.

Diaphragms will occasionally produce a thickened, hyperplastic epithelium around the margins of contact with the vaginal mucosa that will appear somewhat acetowhite but then rarely cause ulceration. If the diaphragm has been used particularly frequently or had been incorrectly inserted or improperly fitted, an area of leukoplakia may be noted prior to the application of acetic acid (Figure 14.26). Even though diaphragm use may be suspected in the etiology of such leukoplakia, a

biopsy is usually indicated, particularly after abnormal cervical cytology. Similar findings have been reported in association with use of the contraceptive vaginal ring, which may cause colposcopic erythema, raised circular or striated ridges, and intracellular edema.[51] Additional abnormal colposcopic findings such as erythema or bleeding and sloughing of the mucosa of the vaginal fornices may be noted with recent use of spermicides, especially in women sensitive to nonoxynol 9.[52,53] The inflamed tissue may appear erythematous following saline application and very patchy mustard yellow following Lugol's iodine application.

Like diaphragms, vaginal pessaries may produce a thickened epithelium around the contact areas between the pessary and the vaginal mucosa that may appear acetowhite. They may also cause superficial ulceration, especially with prolonged insertions or longer term menopausal state.[54,55] Other common minor side effects that may impede colposcopy include vaginal bleeding, development of a foul vaginal discharge, and irritative symptoms. Presuming that bacterial vaginosis, beta-streptococcal vaginitis, and yeast have been ruled out, these symptoms are more common in the setting of vaginal atrophy and can be treated with low-dose vaginal estrogen cream or a lubricating vaginal buffer preparation.

Vaginal trauma from sexual abuse or rape can also be detected by vaginal colposcopy.[56,57] Findings indicative of blunt force or penetrating trauma include hymenal ecchymosis, laceration, transection, or absence of hymenal tissue. Findings concerning for abuse or trauma, but not clearly demonstrative, include abrasion, laceration, or bruising of the vagina and particularly the posterior fourchette, and a notch or cleft in the posterior hymen >50% of the hymeneal width.[56] Determination of genital trauma using a colposcope is superior to that obtained by gross visual examination alone.[57] Chapter 13 contains a more thorough discussion of this topic.

14.5.7 Miscellaneous Vaginal Colposcopic Findings

14.5.7.1 Vaginitis Emphysematosa

One of the more dramatic, but very rare, colposcopic findings is emphysematous vaginitis, also called vaginitis emphysematosa.[58] In this disorder, the vagina and the cervix present

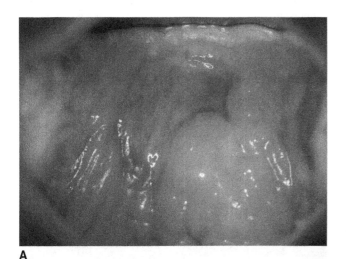

A

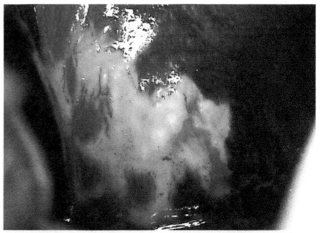

B

FIGURE 14.25. **A:** A deep ulcer on the anterior vaginal wall is secondary to chronic tampon use. **B:** Chronic tampon use due to prolonged spotting resulted in this erosion in the cul-de-sac and adjacent hyperkeratotic area that stained with Lugol's a mustard yellow color. Discontinuation of the use of tampons for a month resulted in healing and resolution of the spotting.

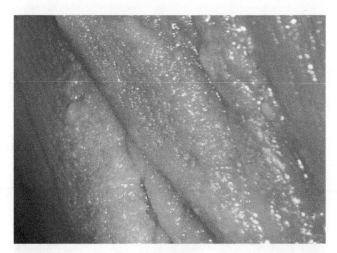

FIGURE 14.26. An area of leukoplakia caused by frequent diaphragm use is seen on the left vaginal wall extending into the cul-de-sac.

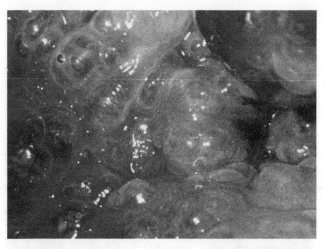

FIGURE 14.27. Extensive gas-filled blebs consistent with a diagnosis of vaginitis emphysematosa are apparent in this woman with a trichomonas infection. (Photo provided courtesy of Duane E. Townsend, MD.)

with diffuse gas-filled "blebs" or cystoid cavities that are most likely caused by bacteria or *Trichomonas* infections. The name "vaginitis emphysematosa" was first given by Zweiful[58] in 1877 following two earlier reports on the subject. Most of these cases have been reported in pregnant or immunosuppressed individuals,[59] although occasionally they appear to be random. The cysts are usually microscopic to a few millimeters in diameter, but some cysts may be as large as 2 cm. Affected patients rarely have symptoms other than an increased vaginal discharge and other symptoms specific for the etiologic agent. Occasionally, the patient will report a "popping" sound during intercourse secondary to rupture of these cysts. Postcoital bleeding has also been reported. The process is self-limited following appropriate treatment of the etiologic agent.

The vagina has been described colposcopically as rough, or "pebbly" (Figure 14.27). The findings are usually most pronounced over the ectocervix and distal vagina.[31] Pressure from a vaginal speculum or examining hand will often rupture some of these tense blebs, with mild bleeding secondarily. Often the diagnosis can be made clinically without biopsy, but when performed, the histology reveals cystoid spaces in the lamina propria, with acute and chronic inflammatory cells, and normal squamous epithelium. Hyperkeratosis and acanthosis, however, may occur in the epithelium. These histologic changes resolve with treatment of the infectious agent responsible for the findings.[31]

14.5.7.2 Gartner's Duct Cysts

The most common vaginal cysts found incidentally during examination of the vagina are called Gartner's duct cysts. While originally believed to be of common mesonephric (wolffian) duct origin, many are derived from the paramesonephric (mullerian) ducts or remnants of the urogenital sinus.[31,60] These cysts usually occur on the lateral to anterolateral vaginal walls. Most cysts do not have a distinctive colposcopic appearance and, unless quite large, are not usually noticed during routine speculum examination. The majority of Gartner's duct cysts are small (1 to 2 cm); however, cysts as large as 2 to 10 cm in diameter are occasionally seen. Large cysts are clinically obvious, with epithelium tensely stretched over the cyst. This results in an almost translucent epithelium, displaying fine but prominent branching blood vessels (Figure 14.28A,B). Large cysts located in the anterolateral vagina may cause urinary urgency during intercourse. Most women with Gartner's duct cysts, however, are asymptomatic.

Most Gartner's duct cysts are incidental findings noted during palpation of the vaginal walls during bimanual examination. The cysts are round, soft, and smooth. These palpable cysts should be easily differentiated from neoplastic nodules. Since the overlying epithelium is normal, application of Lugol's iodine solution will stain the overlying epithelium a mahogany brown, confirming the benign nature of the mass or masses. Large cysts that stretch the overlying epithelium thinly, however, may demonstrate decreased Lugol's iodine uptake without sharp borders. Evaluation of Gartner's duct cysts can usually be accomplished without a colposcope, although magnification may help provide better visualization of the area of concern.

14.5.7.3 Endometriosis

Endometriosis is not commonly found in the vagina but when present is most often found in the cul-de-sac.[60–62] As with cervical endometriosis, vaginal endometriosis may arise from implantation of endometrial fragments shed during childbirth or menstruation that implant into traumatic breaks in the vaginal epithelium.[59,60] Primary extension of pelvic endometriosis through the cul-de-sac, however, is the more common etiology of vaginal endometriotic implants.[31] When endometriosis is this extensive, women most commonly present with symptoms of severe dysmenorrhea and deep dyspareunia. Vaginal endometriosis usually appears colposcopically as brown- to blue-colored spots (Figure 14.29A,B) similar to the "powder burns" visualized laparoscopically on the peritoneum. Occasionally, extension of peritoneal implants through the cul-de-sac will present as larger nodules that may be palpable during bimanual exam. Biopsy will confirm the diagnosis. Excision or destruction with cryotherapy or laser vaporization can effectively treat all but large nodules in the cul-de-sac. Treatment of the pelvic endometriosis, when present, will also be necessary. When nodularity in the rectovaginal septum is pronounced, erosion through the vaginal wall may mimic cancer. Biopsy is important to secure the diagnosis and to exclude the possibility of adenocarcinoma arising in endometrial implants (see Section 14.6.5.2.3).

14.5.7.4 Vaginal Melanosis

Any pigmentation in the vagina is of concern, since the vaginal epithelium is not derived from ectoderm and neural crest tissue does not migrate to this area.[31] Nevertheless, benign pigmented epithelium may occasionally be identified in the vaginal mucosa.[63] More commonly, dark areas in the vagina are due

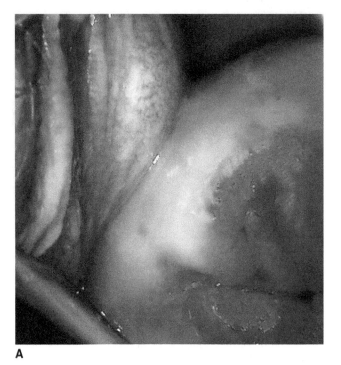

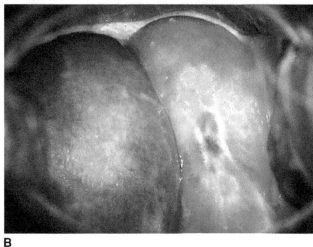

A   **B**

FIGURE 14.28.   **A:** A large vaginal cyst can be seen anterolateral to the cervix. **B:** Marked stretching of the overlying vaginal wall results in thinning of the epithelium and increased visualization of the normal branching vasculature.

to either endometriotic implants or neoplasia. Any melanotic lesion can mimic a vaginal melanoma, and vaginal melanoma has been demonstrated to arise in a large area of melanosis[64] (see Section 14.6.5.3). Therefore, biopsy is always advised to establish the correct diagnosis.[65] If the area of pigmentation is large, multiple biopsies taken from the most darkly pigmented areas will be necessary. If histologic interpretation documents only benign-appearing melanocytes in the basal epithelium, annual colposcopic evaluation may still be prudent despite the rarity of malignant degeneration.[65,66] If, however, atypical melanocytic hyperplasia is identified, it would seem appropriate to resect the lesion since the likelihood of progression to melanoma is unknown.[67]

14.5.7.5 Vaginal Hemangioma and Telangiectasia

Benign vascular changes may be seen during colposcopy of the vagina. These changes are not alarming when found on external skin but are of concern when visualized in the vagina, where their presence is less common. Both hemangiomas and telangiectasias are occasionally noted and have the same etiology as their external counterparts. Most women are asymptomatic, but if present within the rich nerve supply of the introitus, dyspareunia may result. Colposcopically, the vessels may appear atypical, but they are not found within an identifiable lesion (Figure 14.30A,B). Capillary (or "strawberry") hemangiomas are commonly located in the external anogenital

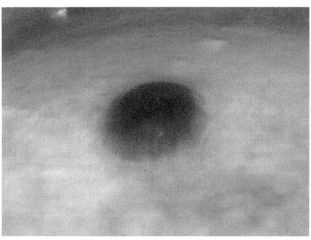

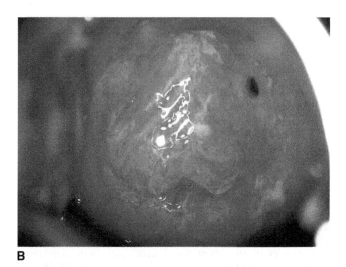

A   **B**

FIGURE 14.29.   **A:** A "powder burn" brown spot is noted near the cervicovaginal margin of this woman with pelvic endometriosis. **B:** Trauma-induced heme deposited at the edge of this large ectopy resembles an endometriotic implant.

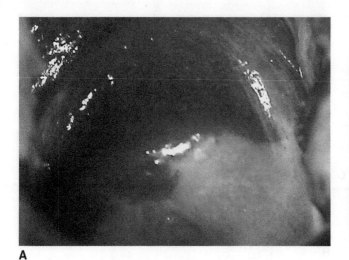

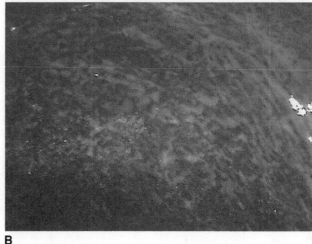

A   **B**

FIGURE 14.30.   **A:** A hemangioma extends from the mid right vagina nearly to the cervical os. **B:** Higher magnification shows the rich vascularity of a vaginal hemangioma. Biopsy was taken at the edge (to reduce the degree of bleeding) to confirm that no element of neoplasia was present. Normal epithelium with enhanced vascularity confirmed a clinical diagnosis of hemangioma.

region, usually appearing at birth or in the first few months of life.[31] They may bleed and should be considered in the differential diagnosis in infants and young children who present with vaginal bleeding.[68] Spontaneous involution, usually by 7 years of age, is common. Most vaginal hemangiomas, when not accompanied by such external anogenital involvement, are discovered as an incidental finding in the vagina during colposcopic evaluation for other indications. They are most commonly small, <1 to 2 cm in diameter, and have the erythematous vascular appearance of those seen externally. Although the overlying epithelium will usually stain brown with aqueous iodine, biopsy may be appropriate to confirm the benign nature of the findings. Histology will show normal epithelium overlying prolific vascular channels.

Telangiectasias are tiny vascular changes of a similar benign nature. Some may be of congenital origin, such as seen in Osler-Weber-Rendu syndrome,[69] although the etiology of most is not clear. Cavernous hemangiomas are occasionally seen on the external genitalia and may extend into the vagina,

where they may be palpated beneath the vaginal mucosa (Figure 14.31A,B).[31] They are larger vascular spaces that usually appear in the first few months of life and then may spontaneously involute. Because cavernous hemangiomas may result in severe hemorrhage if torn during childbirth, their presence on the vulva or vagina frequently requires delivery by cesarean section or resection prior to delivery.

14.5.7.6 Granulation Tissue

Granulation tissue is a fairly common occurrence after surgery involving the vagina, and is the result of a foreign body reaction. Most commonly, it is seen along the vagina cuff following hysterectomy (Figure 14.32A,B) but may occur anywhere in the vagina following vaginal procedures for pelvic organ prolapse, urinary incontinence,[70] or even episiotomy.[71] In a retrospective cohort study involving 312 women who underwent vaginal surgery for prolapse with, and without, graft augmentation, the incidence of granulation tissue was

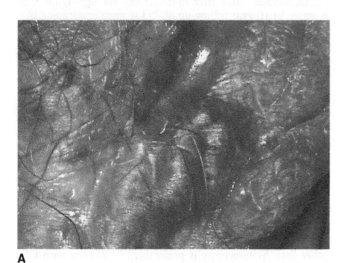

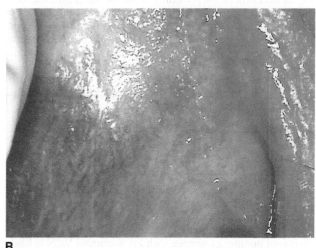

A   **B**

FIGURE 14.31.   A hemangioma extends from the groin to the labia minora (**A**) and into the right vestibule (**B**). The patient had always had some degree of insertion dyspareunia, which may have been secondary to the vascular abnormality.

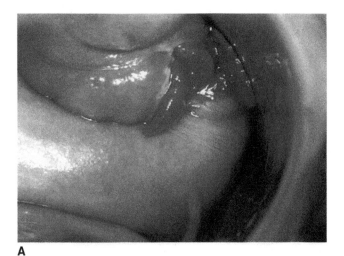

A

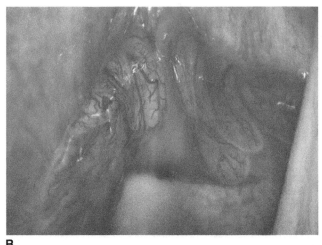

B

FIGURE 14.32. **A:** Granulation tissue 6 months posthysterectomy is noted at the vaginal cuff. **B:** Granulation tissue of the vaginal vault after hysterectomy for benign disease. The vessel pattern is classic in form and distribution. (Reproduced with permission from Wright VC. *Color Atlas of Colposcopy—Cervix, Vagina and Vulva*. Houston: Biomedical Communications, 2000.)

38.8% versus 17.3%, respectively ($p < 0.001$). On multivariate analysis, graft use and the use of braided suture were most associated with the development of granulation tissue.[72] The reddish brown mass may be friable, raising concern for cancer. Biopsy readily establishes the diagnosis. While most women are asymptomatic, some may notice vaginal bleeding or spotting, particularly with intercourse. Small lesions are likely to regress spontaneously, while lesions >5 mm will usually require treatment.[73] Cauterization with silver nitrate will most commonly result in resolution, but occasionally excision or laser vaporization may be necessary.

14.5.7.7 Radiation Changes

Colposcopy of the previously irradiated vagina is particularly difficult and requires considerable colposcopic experience and skill.[74,75] Because of the time required for a complete colposcopic evaluation of the irradiated vagina, it is most commonly reserved for those with abnormal cytology, previous history of cervical or vaginal cancer, or unexplained symptoms such as pain, vaginal bleeding, or discharge. When radiation was administered for cervical cancer, the proximity of the vagina caused the vaginal mucosa to receive maximal radiation doses and thus show marked radiation changes. Chronic changes can be seen in the vaginal stroma (edema and the presence of calcifications and multinucleated giant cells), vessels (sclerosis, nuclear atypia, intimal proliferation of endothelial cells, and infiltration with lymphocytes and plasma cells), and squamous epithelium (atrophy).[76] For a description of the colposcopic changes associated with radiation therapy, see Section 13.3.

14.6 VAGINAL NEOPLASTIC DISORDERS

Squamous cell carcinoma of the vagina was first described in 1826,[77] but the first case of vaginal carcinoma *in situ* was not reported until 1933.[2] Since that time, there has been a noticeable increase in the incidence of VaIN of all grades. The increased number of women with HPV-induced VaIN is likely to be the result of both increased awareness of the need to evaluate the vagina colposcopically and of an absolute increase in incidence. Women with VaIN are asymptomatic, and therefore the presence of VaIN is detected only by colposcopic examination, usually following referral for abnormal cytology.

The incidence of VaIN has been reported to be between 0.2 and 2 cases per 100,000 women,[78–80] significantly less than the incidence of cervical intraepithelial neoplasia (CIN). However, in the prophylactic quadrivalent HPV vaccine trials, 16 cases of VaIN 2,3 were seen among 17,925 women aged 13 to 26 (89 cases per 100,000 women!).[81] These data question older study estimates that VaIN 3 is rare in young women.

VaIN may be identified independent of, or in conjunction with, cervical neoplasia. In fact, as many as 65% of women with VaIN have either concomitant or prior CIN.[39] VaIN may, however, be found in women after hysterectomy for benign conditions.[82–86] Among women with CIN, 2.5%[85] to 9.2%[86] will have coexisting VaIN. In one series, 67% of the vaginal lesions appeared to be confluent with one on the cervix, while in 18.5%, the vaginal lesion was discovered only after treatment of the cervix failed to clear the cytologic abnormalities.[85] More commonly, however, VaIN is diagnosed following a hysterectomy for CIN or invasive cervical cancer.[87–90] While somewhere between 25% and 57%[82–84,90] of women with VaIN 3 have had a prior hysterectomy for CIN, the risk of developing high-grade VaIN after hysterectomy for high-grade CIN is small. In 10-year follow-up of 793 women undergoing hysterectomy for CIN, 41 (5%) developed VaIN, 54% of which occurred in the vaginal suture line and vault angles.[91] For invasive cervical cancer survivors, however, recent analyses estimate the risks of subsequently developing vaginal carcinoma *in situ* and invasive vaginal cancer to be 53.8 and 29.9 times higher than expected, respectively.[92] Long-term follow-up after hysterectomy is therefore important, since the mean latency period between hysterectomy and the development of VaIN is reported to be between 4 and 13 years.[84,89,93,94]

The upper 1/3 of the vagina is where 83% to 100% of VaIN is found.[82–85,90,95] Approximately one-half of VaIN is multifocal, while the other half is solitary.[2,82,90] When VaIN presents following hysterectomy, it may be difficult to detect since it may be mostly hidden within the vaginal cuff or in the recessed areas of the lateral vaginal corners.[96] Since it is much easier to monitor women for posttreatment recurrence of disease when the cervix is left intact, treatment of CIN by means other than hysterectomy is preferable.[86,97] Women with CIN who require hysterectomy for other coexistent gynecologic problems should have colposcopic verification of the distal margin of cervical disease or negative cone margins prior to surgery. This should reduce the possibility that extension of a cervical lesion into the vaginal cuff will be overlooked.

Previous radiation therapy to the cervix or vagina, and immunosuppression, increase the risk of acquiring high-grade VaIN.[84,85,98,99] Immunosuppressed women are more likely to have persistent, multifocal lesions. Risk factors for persistence or progression of VaIN include multifocal lesions within the vagina or throughout the lower genital tract, which has been termed "anogenital neoplasia syndrome."

14.6.1 Pathology

As with CIN, VaIN is divided into three grades: VaIN 1, VaIN 2, and VaIN 3. VaIN 1 and 2 are diagnosed when histologic atypia occupies only the bottom one-third to two-thirds of the epithelium, respectively.[96] If neoplastic cells occupy more than two-thirds of the vaginal epithelium, VaIN 3 is diagnosed. Except for the absence of glandular elements, the histologic features of nuclear pleomorphism, abnormal mitoses, and loss of polarity are identical with that seen in CIN. Recently, some pathologists have adopted nomenclature for VaIN that is consistent with the Bethesda System for cervical cytology, with VaIN 1 reported as low-grade VaIN/ squamous intraepithelial lesion (SIL) and VaIN 2 and 3 as high-grade VaIN/SIL. Vaginal cancer is diagnosed when atypical cells are noted histopathologically beneath the basement membrane.

14.6.2 Epidemiology and Natural History of VaIN and Vaginal Cancer

VaIN 1 and 2 are most commonly detected in young women in whom recent infection with HPV may produce proliferative lesions in the vagina, as well as on the cervix and vulva. The median age for squamous vaginal cancer is 68 to 71 years,[79,100] however, indicating that a very long time is required between the initial exposure to HPV and oncogenesis. Additionally, because vaginal HPV lesions are common and vaginal squamous cell cancer is rare, most women with low-grade vaginal lesions are at minimal risk for cancer. Much is still not known about the natural history of VaIN, but one thing is certain: VaIN 3 definitely increases the risk for vaginal squamous cancer.

Multiple series have reported a direct relationship between age and grade of vaginal dysplasia, with VaIN 3 most commonly occurring in women 15 years older than those with VaIN 1 or 2.[87,102] For example, in one series, the mean ages of women with VaIN 1, 2, and 3 were 44.5, 47.8, and 61.8 years, respectively.[87] While this demonstrates an age-related progression, more recent US data would place the burden of the lower grades of VaIN in much younger women.[81] Other series demonstrate similar trends in progression from carcinoma *in situ* to invasive carcinoma, with median ages 58 and 68 years, respectively.[83] As noted earlier, reports from the prophylactic quadrivalent HPV vaccine trials demonstrated that young women can also develop VaIN 2,3 and sometimes in a rapid fashion—Kjaer et al.[81] reported 16 cases of VaIN 2,3 developing among 17,925 women aged 13 to 26. Ten of these cases occurred in women initially naïve to HPV 16 and 18 and followed for a median of 42 months.

The majority of VaIN 1 and 2 appears to regress spontaneously.[4,101-104] The rate of progression is probably far less than for CIN. As with CIN 3, VaIN 3 may be a true cancer precursor. Spontaneous regression of various degrees of VaIN has been reported in 78% of women followed for 5 years, although 13% had persistent VaIN and 9% developed invasive vaginal cancer.[102] Progression from documented VaIN 3 to vaginal cancer has been for oncogenic HPV by PCR.[105] In a meta-analysis of previously published reports, De Vuyst et al.[106] reported oncogenic HPV in 100% of 107 cases of VaIN 1, 90.1% of

191 cases of VaIN 2,3 and 69.9% of 136 vaginal cancers. In all cases, HPV 16 was the most common type, occurring in 23.4%, 57.6%, and 53.7% of VaIN 1, VaIN 2,3 and vaginal cancer, respectively. Adenocarcinomas are less commonly HPV positive, often arising as a result of DES exposure[106] or without an obvious etiology. Despite this, HPV testing has shown a higher sensitivity for detecting VaIN than vaginal cytology, but because of the large number of vaginal HPV infections without cytologic or histologic abnormality, its specificity is lower.[99,104]

14.6.3 Colposcopy of Vaginal Intraepithelial Lesions

Because VaIN is usually subtle, colposcopy with application of acetic acid and Lugol's solution is necessary to detect these lesions. Abnormal cervical cytology generally initiates the discovery process. Nevertheless, simple use of the colposcope even with acetic acid and Lugol's iodine applications does not ensure recognition of VaIN. Women with various inflammatory conditions of the vagina lack consistent glycogen storage in the vaginal epithelium necessary for Lugol's iodine uptake, so treatment of inflammatory conditions is most often necessary prior to colposcopic evaluation. Once potentially obscuring inflammation is resolved, the following colposcopic features associated with vaginal neoplasia will become more evident.

14.6.3.1 VaIN 1/Low-Grade HPV Expression

HPV infection of the vagina is common.[104] The majority of lesions are located in either the proximal or the distal one-third of the vagina. The moist, rugose, mucosal surfaces of the vagina readily permit acquisition and expression of HPV. Frequently, however, extensive HPV-induced changes affect the entire vagina. Although HPV infection of the vagina may pose minimal clinical consequences, it represents a significant reservoir of infection for HPV types associated with condylomata acuminata, subclinical HPV infection, and genital neoplasia in both sexes. One study found that non–cancer-associated HPV types, especially types 61, 71, and 72, were detected more frequently in the vaginal specimens from hysterectomized women (23.7%) than in the cervical specimens from nonhysterectomized women (16.7%) but no difference between the prevalence of cancer-associated HPV types in the two groups.[104]

The colposcopic features of low-grade VaIN are in most cases identical to those of low-grade disease of the native epithelium of the cervix, except that spiky surface changes (asperities), common in vaginal lesions, are not common in cervical transformation zone lesions. Other vaginal colposcopic signs include punctation, acetowhite epithelium, leukoplakia, changes in the contour of the vaginal wall, and iodine-negative epithelium.[95] Mosaic vessels are not normally seen in the vagina unless a CTZ or cervical neoplasia extends into the vagina, or in areas of active metaplasia within vaginal adenosis. Low-grade vaginal HPV lesions may have varied morphologic appearances including condyloma acuminata, tiny diffuse punctate spots, small nonstaining asperities, and flat warts or VaIN 1.

14.6.3.1.1 Vaginal Condylomata Acuminata

Among women presenting with vulvar condylomata acuminata, as many as 30% will also have similar lesions in the vagina. Although many vaginal condylomata will be large and clinically apparent, many are small and thus best detected using the magnified illumination of the colposcope after applying acetic acid. Occasionally the lateral vaginal walls will be devoid of HPV lesions, while lesions on the anterior and posterior walls may lie hidden behind the speculum blades. This may occur even with the presence of extensive and large

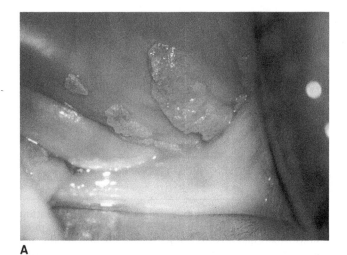

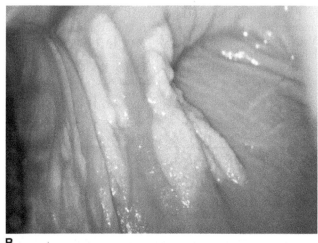

FIGURE 14.33. **A:** Extensive low-grade lesions are seen in the cul-de-sac only when the cervix is elevated and the speculum retracted slightly. **B:** Maneuvering the cervix to the patient's left enabled colposcopic visualization of extensive flat vaginal warts/VaIN 1 in the right vaginal fornix.

condylomata acuminata on the anterior and posterior walls (Figure 14.33A,B). Hence, careful assessment of the vaginal fornices and the rugose vaginal anterior, posterior, and lateral walls, as discussed earlier, is required for detection and accurate diagnosis.

Condyloma acuminata may be exuberant in the vagina, even in women with normal immune systems. Extensive

condylomata, however, are particularly common in immunosuppressed patients and in pregnant women. Women with extensive vaginal condylomata may have a particularly thick white vaginal discharge and mild introital pruritus that mimics yeast vaginitis (Figure 14.34A). Occasionally, bleeding with intercourse may occur as a result of trauma to large or vascular vaginal condyloma (Figure 14.34B,C). Pregnant women with massive

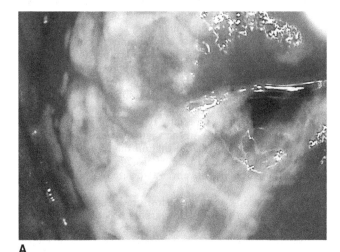

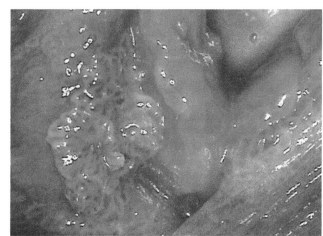

FIGURE 14.34. **A:** Extensive low-grade HPV-associated lesions often exfoliate excessive squamous epithelial cells creating a profuse, thick vaginal discharge resembling a yeast infection. Wet mount was negative for fungal elements. **B:** Nonkeratinized papillary condyloma at the hymen was responsible for the bleeding with intercourse this patient had for 2 months prior to being seen. Flat vaginal warts were also seen on colposcopy of the vagina (**C**) but are not susceptible to trauma and not a source of the bleeding. Nor was her large ectopy (seen to the patient's left) friable.

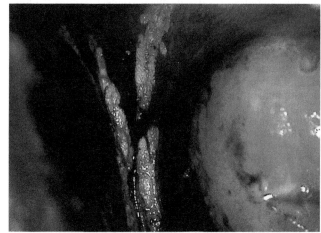

vaginal condylomata acuminata notably risk hemorrhage secondary to tearing of these lesions during vaginal delivery, and the high quantitative HPV level may place the baby at risk for developing laryngeal papillomatosis (see Chapter 12).[108,109]

Vaginal condylomata acuminata are similar in appearance to condyloma seen elsewhere in the lower genital tract. They usually present as raised, papillary structures with central capillaries in each papilla (Figure 14.35A,B). Hyperkeratosis is a common finding, however, and may hide the vessels and result in a rougher surface. Application of 5% acetic acid will usually produce a dense, snow-white response. Following Lugol's iodine application, condylomata assume a yellow color if considerable hyperkeratosis is present. It is not unusual for multiple condylomata acuminata to be in the vagina. Similar HPV-induced lesions may be present on the cervix (Figure 14.35C).

Vaginal condylomata acuminata are caused by low-risk HPV types 6 and 11, as are similar lesions elsewhere in the genital tract. The natural history tends to be one of spontaneous regression, but the length of time over which regression occurs is extremely variable. Women are presumed to be contagious to a susceptible consort when clinical lesions are present. Successful treatment of cervical or vulvar HPV-induced disease may be followed by spontaneous regression of vaginal HPV lesions, which may in part be due to an increase in the effectiveness of the immune response secondary to decreasing HPV viral load.

14.6.3.1.2 SUBCLINICAL HPV INFECTION OF THE VAGINA

Most cervical and vaginal HPV infections are subclinical and time limited. Although there are public health implications for the sexual transmissibility of vaginal and cervical subclinical HPV infections, considering its incidence, the disease is of minimal importance from a cancer perspective. Therefore, aggressive management of subclinical vaginal HPV lesions must be tempered by the realization that these lesions pose little cancer risk. The following discussion is a comprehensive review of the clinical profile of vaginal colposcopic atypia secondary to HPV but is not intended to suggest that the atypia requires aggressive management. Nonetheless, the frequent association of vaginal HPV infection with low-grade SIL Pap reports does foster anxiety for both the patient and her clinician. Resolution of this anxiety demands knowledge about the various colposcopic appearances of subclinical HPV infection. Subclinical HPV infection of the vagina can be manifested in different ways. Some lesions are completely unapparent to the naked eye and are detected only by colposcopy after application of 3% to 5% acetic acid (Figure 14.36A-E). These lesions may appear as flat acetowhite epithelium or as small acetowhite spots. Other lesions consist of tiny micropapillary asperities.

14.6.2.1.2.1 Condylomatous Vaginitis

Both micropapillary asperities, which are tiny epithelial projections from the vaginal walls, and punctate acetowhite spots

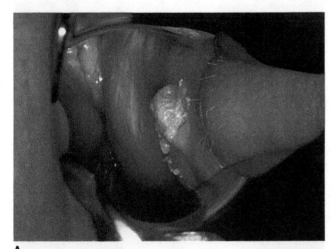

A

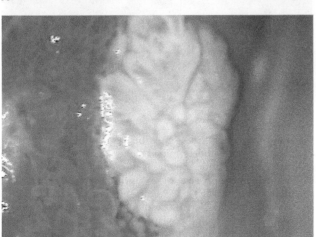

C

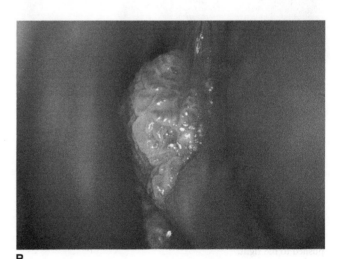

B

FIGURE 14.35.   Typical exophytic condylomas on the right vaginal wall are seen at (**A**) low and (**B**) high power. **C:** Application of 5% acetic acid highlighted this papillary, snow-white condyloma at the squamocolumnar junction of the cervix. Condyloma was also present in the vagina. Note the typical vascular pattern of condyloma in each location.

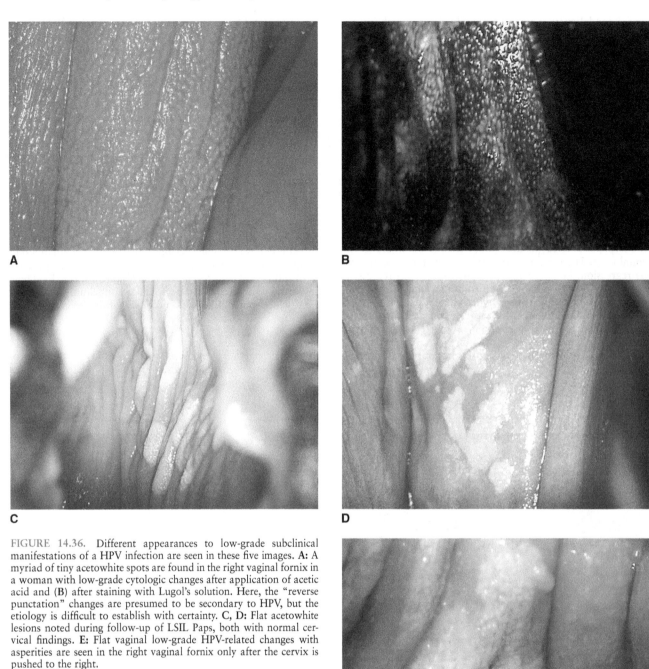

FIGURE 14.36. Different appearances to low-grade subclinical manifestations of a HPV infection are seen in these five images. **A:** A myriad of tiny acetowhite spots are found in the right vaginal fornix in a woman with low-grade cytologic changes after application of acetic acid and **(B)** after staining with Lugol's solution. Here, the "reverse punctation" changes are presumed to be secondary to HPV, but the etiology is difficult to establish with certainty. **C, D:** Flat acetowhite lesions noted during follow-up of LSIL Paps, both with normal cervical findings. **E:** Flat vaginal low-grade HPV-related changes with asperities are seen in the right vaginal fornix only after the cervix is pushed to the right.

that do not stain with Lugol's solution may diffusely cover the entire vaginal vault. They are most common, however, in the upper one-third of the vagina.[110] These manifestations have been termed "condylomatous colpitis or vaginitis."[110,111] Similar involvement of the cervix is called "condylomatous cervicitis." Micropapillary asperities are virtually diagnostic of HPV infection (see Chapter 8), but the tiny punctate dots, which have been called "reverse punctuation," are much more nonspecific and should not be considered a definitive finding of the presence of this virus.

These vaginal entities may be responsible for atypical squamous cells of undetermined significance (ASC-US) HPV-positive and low-grade squamous intraepithelial lesion (LSIL) Pap reports in the absence of an obvious cervical lesion. The dilemma of an inability to explain the source of a HPV-positive ASC-US or LSIL Pap test result at colposcopy will often be resolved when the colposcopist looks for these subtle vaginal manifestations of HPV infection. Tall spiked papillary projections may occasionally be detected without the aid of the colposcope, whereas detection of reverse punctation requires magnification and epithelial contrast agents. Reverse punctation has also been called minimally expressed papillomavirus infection (MEPI). Colposcopically, MEPI, or reverse punctation, presents as a myriad of tiny acetowhite pinpoint dots on the cervix and vagina, highlighted against the flat pink vaginal mucosa. The name "reverse punctation" comes from the resemblance of these tiny round dots to vascular punctation in size and random distribution, but their dissimilarity in being white rather than red. Each of these white dots corresponds to a pinpoint elevation of parakeratotic epithelium capping a prominent intraepithelial capillary. Even after application of 5% acetic acid and inspection using the colposcope, these dots can be quite subtle. They are better visualized as yellow dots against the normal mahogany brown squamous epithelium following the staining of the vagina and cervix with Lugol's iodine (Figure 14.36B). MEPI is simply a transient manifestation of HPV infection and does not require treatment. Additionally, it is a very nonspecific finding, as other inflammatory conditions of the vagina, such as vulvovaginal candidiasis, may produce a similar colposcopic appearance. Therefore, reverse punctation should not be considered definitive proof of HPV infection unless other more specific HPV findings are also present.

Abnormal histologic findings are extremely focal as they are limited to the tiny pinpoint areas of parakeratosis. Histologic interpretations, therefore, may range from normal to condyloma, depending upon whether any of these tiny areas of abnormality are noted in the histologic sections. When abnormalities are found, focal areas of minimal basal hyperplasia, mild koilocytosis, variable dyskeratosis, acanthosis, parakeratosis, prominent intraepithelial capillary growth, and mild nuclear pleomorphism can be identified.

Although micropapillary asperities are commonly found within flat vaginal warts (VaIN 1), they are also common in the vagina outside of circumscribed lesions, where this finding is called condylomatous vaginitis. Prior to application of acetic acid, multiple small pink micropapillary asperities may be seen projecting from the vaginal mucosa. These small lesions are usually multiple and diffuse but may be confined to smaller areas. Most commonly, the micropapillae arise from completely normal surrounding vaginal mucosa (Fig. 14.37A,B), but occasionally they may be found atop slightly hyperkeratotic, acetowhite epithelia that individually do not stain with Lugol's. When viewed through a colposcope, a fine caliber central capillary loop is usually identified in each papilla. If the papillae are poorly developed, they will appear short, blunt with a granular surface contour.

Histologic evaluation of colposcopically directed biopsies may show cytopathic effects of HPV infection, but the manifestations are so tiny that they are often not histologically documented. When present, the histologic features may vary from more subtle changes such as basal hyperplasia and dyskeratosis to florid koilocytotic atypia. A central capillary will be found within each papillary excrescence.

14.6.3.1.2.2 Flat Vaginal Warts/VaIN 1

Subclinical vaginal warts and VaIN 1 are flat to slightly raised, moderately well circumscribed lesions of a few millimeters to several centimeters in diameter. Flat vaginal warts are often difficult to identify even following application of 5% acetic acid and colposcopic evaluation. Following Lugol's iodine application, however, these lesions are usually readily detected. The margins may be distinct, or indistinct, and sharply circumscribed, or irregular and feathered. The surface of a flat vaginal wart is either smooth, slightly elevated and plaque-like, or slightly "spiky" with fine overlying asperities (Figure 14.36E). It is often described as "granular" in appearance. Usually no vascular patterns are apparent, but if present, the vessels are usually fine, nondilated punctation of uniform caliber. The intercapillary distance is narrow but regular, in contrast to the more widely irregularly spaced punctation that may be seen in some high-grade VaIN.

Flat acetowhite lesions are most frequently detected in the upper one-third of the vagina (Figure 14.38A,B). These lesions may be a direct extension from cervical atypia onto the vaginal fornix or they may arise de novo within the vagina. Lugol's iodine stains the surrounding uninvolved vaginal epithelium a dark mahogany brown, usually contrasting sharply with the lesion, which may appear beige to yellow in color. The lesions may also appear a mixed yellow brown variegated color.

Histology of colposcopically directed biopsies will show classic cytopathic effects of HPV infection, including basal hyperplasia and nuclear atypia in the bottom one-third of the epithelium and koilocytes in the upper layers. Flat vaginal warts and VaIN 1 are the same entity; however, some pathologists require the presence of abnormal mitotic figures for the latter diagnosis. From the therapeutic standpoint, there is no true cytologic, histologic, or biologic difference between "flat vaginal warts" and VaIN 1 (mild dysplasia).

Low-grade acetowhite HPV-induced lesions of the vagina are often multifocal. The lesions may be present diffusely within the vagina and may extend to the cervix and vulva. Variegated staining with Lugol's is also indicative of the likelihood of a low-grade lesion (Figure 14.39A,B). However, since both low- and high-grade lesions may stain similarly

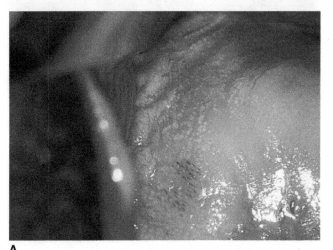
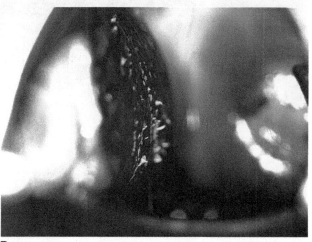

A   B

FIGURE 14.37.   Micropapillary asperities in which (A) diffuse epithelial "spikes" are seen surrounded by normal mucosa. B: Isolated diffuse nonstaining micropapillary aspirates arise from normal glycogen-rich mucosa.

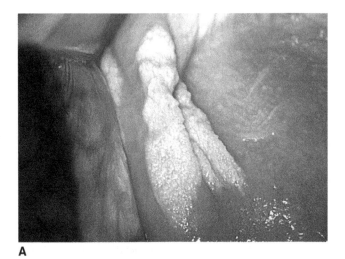 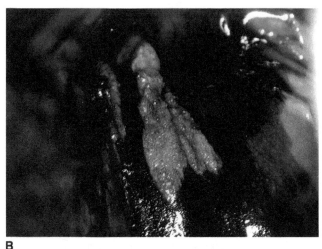

A   **B**

FIGURE 14.38.   Multiple flat vaginal warts/VaIN 1 as seen (**A**) after application of acetic acid and (**B**) after staining with Lugol's iodine solution.

(a mustard yellow color), Lugol's application is most useful to identify and locate lesions and evaluate their margins rather than differentiating between low- and high-grade lesions. Liberal use of colposcopically directed biopsy is required in areas of flat vaginal warts, since a higher grade lesion may coexist similar to that seen in the transformation zone. The most frequently detected HPV types associated with flat vaginal warts and VaIN 1 are the "high-risk" types 16, 31, 33, and 35.

Because most vaginal low-grade HPV lesions are the manifestations of benign, transitory HPV infections, even when high-risk types, management options should always weigh potential benefits against the risk of complications. Lesions are usually asymptomatic and pose minimal to no risk of cancer. The natural history of flat vaginal warts/VaIN 1 has not been studied prospectively; however, VaIN 1 must be less of a risk for cancer than CIN 1, which itself carries little risk. Over time, most of these lesions resolve spontaneously provided the host has a competent immune system. Based upon the relatively rare occurrence of high-grade VaIN and vaginal cancer, it can be deduced that progression of VaIN 1 is extremely infrequent. A histologic continuum of epithelial abnormality from HPV infection to VaIN 2,3 exists. As with the cervix, however, development of VaIN 3

is most likely a monoclonal event and a distinct disease process from VaIN 1. The relative rarity of high-grade vaginal neoplasia suggests that the occurrence of these monoclonal events in the mature epithelium of the vagina is uncommon.

The major implications of vaginal low-grade lesions are the potential for transmission of HPV to others and the association with development of minor or low-grade atypia noted on cervical or vaginal vault cytology. A major concern is the belief that all vaginal papillae, acetowhite patches, and Lugol's non-staining areas are HPV related. Benign papillations of congenital origin are commonly found in the vagina of many women. They may mimic the papillae of HPV-induced condylomatous vaginitis except that non–HPV-related papillae stain positive (brown) when exposed to Lugol's iodine solution. Histology can also be misleading as papillary features and the clinical impression of "rule out HPV" often places the pathologist in the difficult position of discerning whether minor cellular changes, otherwise not diagnostic, are sufficient to support a diagnosis of HPV-related change. Subjectivity in histologic diagnosis may result in overdiagnosis but also in underdiagnosis. Overdiagnosis may prompt management that is not otherwise indicated. Careful expert colposcopic assessment is

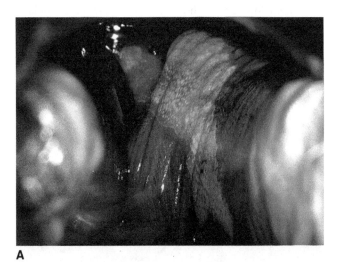 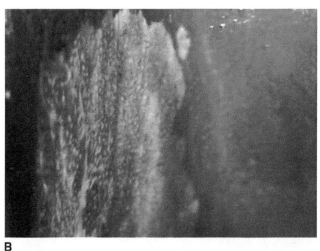

A   **B**

FIGURE 14.39.   The "tortoise shell" variegated staining pattern noted in lesions (**A**) and (**B**) is indicative of low-grade vaginal HPV lesions.

therefore critical if overdiagnosis of normal papillae and other potential low-grade changes is to be minimized.

14.6.4 Vaginal High-Grade Intraepithelial Neoplasia (VaIN 2,3)

Because the vaginal mucosa usually appears clinically normal to the unaided eye, colposcopic examination with application of acetic acid and Lugol's iodine is essential for detecting VaIN of any grade. VaIN 2,3 has essentially the same colposcopic characteristics as cervical high-grade intraepithelial neoplasia CIN 2,3 except that a mosaic vascular pattern is not usually seen unless the lesion arises in vaginal epithelium that was initially an extension of a CTZ or in an area of adenosis. VaIN 2,3 is usually flat, with varying degrees of surface irregularity that cannot be well appreciated without colposcopic magnification (Figure 14.40).[101] When hyperkeratosis is present, raised white leukoplakic lesions may be seen during colposcopic examination prior to applying 5% acetic acid or rarely may be palpated during vaginal examination. More rarely, slightly raised pink lesions may be found. As with CIN 2,3, intercellular desmosomes in VaIN 3 are loosened, diminishing intercellular cohesion. Therefore, peeling or abrasions of the epithelium may occur within high-grade VaIN lesions, particularly in the perimenopausal or postmenopausal women. The margins of VaIN 3 tend to be well circumscribed and regular or smooth, which may be the most consistent finding in vaginal high-grade intraepithelial neoplasia. Furthermore, these lesions may be elevated above the surrounding normal epithelium.

After 5% acetic acid is applied, VaIN of all grades becomes acetowhite. The acetic acid reaction that accompanies VaIN is often subtle and less easily detected than with CIN. The reaction takes longer to develop and the contrast with normal vaginal epithelium is less distinctive. Additionally, the rugose nature of the vaginal epithelium may compromise detection of the changes. An acetowhite color may predominate as the major colposcopic finding in most high-grade VaIN, as the epithelium is often fairly opaque, preventing transillumination of the underlying vasculature (Figure 14.41). Even with dense acetowhitening, however, a fine to coarse capillary punctation may be detected at greater colposcopic magnification when the acetic acid reaction fades. The more prominent vascular patterns associated with VaIN 3 develop late in the neoplastic process (Figure 14.42A-C). A well-developed, varicose, widely spaced capillary

punctation or, more rarely, a mosaic pattern in an area of high-grade VaIN may be seen.[90] An exaggeration of the coarse caliber vessel arrangement is highly suspicious for invasive cancer.

Vaginal high-grade intraepithelial neoplasia may be unifocal or multifocal. VaIN 3 is usually unifocal, although it may be found in association with multifocal lesions of lesser grade. VaIN 1 and VaIN 2 lesions are often multifocal, as they are more likely to represent a diffuse "field effect" of HPV infection. Sometimes lesions appear clinically to be condyloma acuminata but are found to contain high-grade dysplastic morphology on biopsy. These occasional nonspecific colposcopic features, and the difficulty of gaining visual access to the entire vagina, make colposcopy of the vagina a challenge. The need for thorough expert examination and liberal biopsy of any lesion suspicious of high-grade VaIN is critical if noteworthy lesions, including rare cancers, are to be detected and treated appropriately. Examination by colposcopy under regional or general anesthesia may be necessary if disease is very extensive or if the patient is not able to relax enough for adequate evaluation of the vagina and symptoms, or cytology, is of enough concern.

The subtle acetic acid reaction of VaIN coupled with the technical difficulties in colposcopic assessment of the vagina render examination after application of aqueous iodine solution invaluable in vaginal colposcopy. Half- or quarter-strength Lugol's iodine will provide adequate staining and minimize the patient's discomfort often noted with the full-strength solution. Poorly differentiated vaginal epithelium does not contain glycogen. Therefore, high-grade VaIN rejects iodine, resulting in a mustard yellow color that is in sharp contrast with the mahogany brown staining of the normal vaginal mucosa or the variegated, partial uptake of iodine noted in some partially glycogenated low-grade VaIN. This simple test permits clear demarcation of areas of high-grade epithelial atypia, allows for accurate colposcopically directed biopsy, and helps determine disease extent and distribution. The use of Lugol's iodine solution is invaluable for delineation of treatment margins. Iodine staining will not compromise histologic assessment of the biopsy specimen.

14.6.5 Vaginal Cancer

Vaginal cancers constitute only 1% to 4% of all gynecologic cancers, and primary vaginal malignancies are among the rarest of cancers in women, affecting only six women per million annually.[100] More than 95% of primary vaginal cancers are of squamous cell origin, and the remainder are most commonly

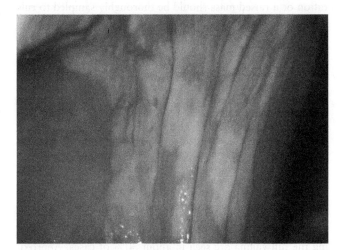

FIGURE 14.40.   Diffuse flat vaginal HPV-induced lesions appear to be low grade. However, the acetowhite effect is more oyster-white. Biopsy revealed VaIN 2,3, illustrating the value of histologic sampling prior to treatment decisions.

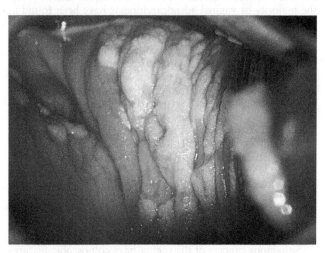

FIGURE 14.41.   Dense acetowhite vaginal intraepithelial lesion that demonstrated VaIN 2 on biopsy.

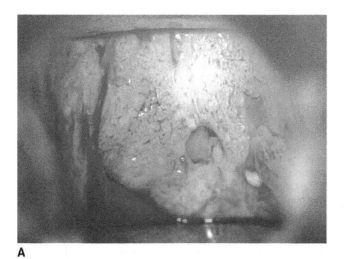

A

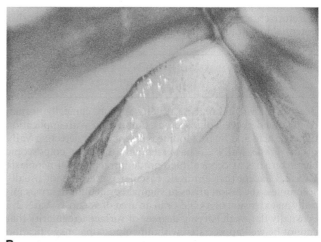

B

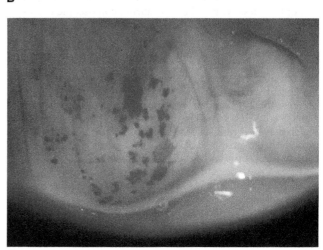

C

FIGURE 14.42.   **A:** Atypical vessels and erosion within a sharply defined lesion are seen in this VaIN 3 raising concern for invasion. **B:** VaIN 3 is seen with the green filter enhancement of abnormal vascular findings. **C:** VaIN 3, slightly raised and with atypical vascular findings and adjacent acetowhite.

clear cell or other adenocarcinomas. Rarely, sarcomas and melanomas are encountered. The age of the patient helps predict the cancer cell type. Endodermal sinus tumor and botryoid embryonal rhabdomyosarcoma are the most commonly seen vaginal cancers of infancy.[112,113] Botryoid cancers and adenocarcinomas may appear during adolescence. Leiomyosarcoma is the most common vaginal cancer in late reproductive years. Squamous carcinoma and melanoma are most common in the seventh and eighth decades of life.[114] During the last 40 years, the majority of vaginal adenocarcinomas have been found in young women exposed to DES *in utero*,[115] whereas adenocarcinomas of the vagina found in non–DES-exposed women have primarily occurred in women over the age of 60 to 70.[116] Secondary vaginal cancers occur occasionally, usually arising by direct spread from the cervix or, less commonly, from the endometrium, ovary, and rectum. Metastasis from cancers distant to the vagina has been reported but is exceedingly rare.

Women with vaginal cancer most commonly present with bleeding or a vaginal discharge that is malodorous, blood tinged, and foul smelling. Urinary distress and pain have also been reported. Although usually appearing as a mass or palpable nodule on examination, flat, infiltrating, superficially spreading or ulcerating carcinomas have also been reported. A rectovaginal exam is often helpful in delineating submucosal extension, paravaginal infiltration, and rectal involvement. Deep involvement of the anterior vaginal wall can spread to the bladder and produce urinary symptoms.

Squamous cancers of the vagina have colposcopic features similar to those seen in cervical squamous cancers, namely, atypical vessels, papillary excrescences, ulcerations, irregular topography, and friability (Figure 14.43A,B). As with early invasive carcinoma of the cervix, tumor angiogenesis factor produced by the neoplastic process stimulates vascular proliferation that presents as bizarre, varicose blood vessels often described as "corkscrew" or "spaghetti-like." Wide intercapillary distances occur secondary to expanding tumor volume. Epithelial and vascular changes associated with palpable induration or a raised mass should be thoroughly sampled to rule out a malignancy.

14.6.5.1 Squamous Cell Carcinoma of the Vagina

Approximately 40% of squamous cell carcinomas of the vagina arise from the upper vagina, often in the posterior fornix where the cervix obscures the lesion. Invasive squamous cell carcinoma of the vagina most commonly presents in older women (average age 68 to 71 years);[79,100] however, it has been reported as early as the fourth decade of life. Approximately 10% of vaginal squamous cancers are found in women with a previous history of invasive squamous cell cancer of the cervix. Some of these lesions arise from cervical cancer that has extended into the vagina, while some distal lesions near the introitus evolve secondary to metastasis from cervical lesions. Vaginal cancers may also develop as asynchronous primary lesions initiated by oncogenic HPV. Advanced lesions involving the full vagina are seen in about 30% of cases. Approximately 40% occur on the anterior wall, 30% on the posterior wall, and 28% on the lateral walls. Early spread occurs primarily by direct extension; however, the abundant lymphatics of the vagina also allow metastatic spread to the inguinal

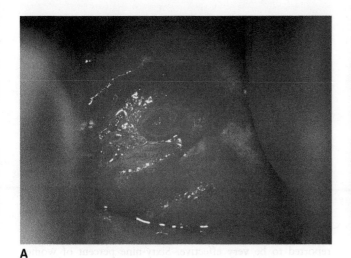 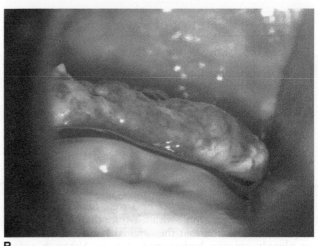

FIGURE 14.43. **A:** Anterior vaginal wall cancer. **B:** This primary squamous cell carcinoma of the vagina displays bizarre atypical vessels and irregular topography. Upon examination, the lesion was noted to be friable.

lymph nodes (for lesions near the introitus) and to the pelvic lymph nodes (for lesions in the upper vagina).

14.6.5.2 Adenocarcinoma of the Vagina

Adenocarcinoma of the vagina may be of primary, metastatic, or endometriotic origin. Metastatic sites of origin include extension of glandular tumors of the endocervix or endometrium or distant sites such as breast, ovary, or bowel. Primary adenocarcinomas of the vagina are far less frequent than metastatic spread from local or distant glandular tumors. Therefore, the diagnosis of adenocarcinoma in the vagina should always raise suspicion of the possibility of a primary elsewhere. Treatment of vaginal adenocarcinoma is similar to treatment of squamous cell types.

14.6.5.2.1 PRIMARY CLEAR CELL ADENOCARCINOMA

Primary clear cell adenocarcinoma has been found primarily in young women between the ages of 7 and 22 exposed *in utero* to DES, although cases have been diagnosed in women up to and in their 40s.[43,107,117,118] Among the DES cohort, the incidence of clear cell adenocarcinoma is estimated to be between 1 and 14 cases per 10,000 exposed persons.[117] In non–DES-exposed women, this is a very rare cancer occurring in much older women and may arise in areas of adenosis.[119] Clear cell adenocarcinomas most likely arise from glandular elements of mullerian origin in the vaginal wall. These foci of glandular cells, or adenosis, are most commonly found in women exposed to DES *in utero*. Vaginal adenocarcinoma, typically of endometrioid type, can arise in foci of vaginal endometriosis[120–122] (see Section 14.6.5.2.3). However, for several decades leading up to the beginning of the 21st century, primary clear cell adenocarcinoma has been the most common vaginal adenocarcinoma of young women. Because of the aging of the population of women exposed to DES, adenocarcinoma of this cell type is becoming less common. Both polypoid and ulcerative clear cell adenocarcinomas occur. Atypical vessels predominate as the most identifiable colposcopic sign in lesions that are less developed. (For more on DES-induced clear cell adenocarcinoma, see Chapter 13.)

14.6.5.2.2 METASTATIC ADENOCARCINOMA TO THE VAGINA

Adenocarcinoma metastatic to the vagina is uncommon but has been reported from primary cancers of the endocervix, ovary, fallopian tube, endometrium, breast, kidney, pancreas, colon, and other distant sites. Metastatic adenocarcinoma cannot be differentiated colposcopically from primary adenocarcinoma since it does not have any features that would distinguish it from a primary invasive malignancy.

14.6.5.2.3 MALIGNANT TRANSFORMATION OF ENDOMETRIOSIS

Any histologic type of tumor that can arise from the endometrium can arise in endometriosis, but endometrioid adenocarcinoma is the most common type. Most cases of malignant transformation of endometriosis occur on the ovaries, but the vagina is a common site of extragonadal transformation, particularly in women with a prior hysterectomy and bilateral salpingo-oophorectomy.[120,123,124] When occurring in the vagina, the apex is the most common location; however, it occurs in other sites including the anterior, posterior, and lateral vaginal walls and in previous episiotomy sites.[121,123] In some cases, there is a history of unopposed estrogen.[120,123,124]

14.6.5.3 Malignant Melanoma

Malignant melanoma is an extremely rare cancer in the vagina; however, any pigmented vaginal lesion should be suspected and biopsied. Until recently, melanocytes were not considered to occur in the vagina, and therefore, vaginal melanoma was considered a metastatic lesion. However, many primary vaginal melanomas have now been reported,[114,125,126] and primary melanocytes have now been documented in this area.[63–65] Melanomas of the vagina have been reported in women between the ages of 22 and 83, with an average age of 55. Most are detected after the onset of postcoital bleeding or with light blood-tinged vaginal discharge that is often purulent and foul smelling.

Colposcopically, vaginal melanomas are similar to melanomas occurring externally, except that their hidden location usually results in much larger, necrotic lesions before they are recognized. Vaginal melanomas are commonly described as polypoid, pedunculated, papillary, or fungating. Ulceration is common. Most vaginal melanomas are brown or black, although red and yellow (necrotic), and amelanotic types (5%) have been reported. Adjacent spread of pigment is less common than with external lesions. Women with vaginal melanomas have a very poor prognosis because detection is frequently late and the lesions aggressive.

14.6.6 Treatment of Vaginal Neoplasia

14.6.6.1 Low-Grade VaIN and Condyloma

Realizing that most low-grade vaginal HPV-related lesions spontaneously resolve has influenced most clinicians to take a less aggressive approach to management; observation has become accepted practice in many cases.[101] Lesions reported as VaIN 1 are almost invariably episomal HPV lesions, with little potential of progression to high-grade VaIN or vaginal squamous cell cancer.[102] In fact, the progressive potential of VaIN 1 to high-grade precursors has not been established, nor has a cancer potential been definitively documented. In our limited experience, the few cases of VaIN 1 subsequently found to have VaIN 2 or 3 were found to have this high-grade "progression" within 6 months of the VaIN 1 diagnosis, suggesting that the original biopsy likely missed an already existing higher grade lesion. Although reducing viral load by eliminating some lesions may theoretically reduce the potential for sexual transmission, in reality the possibility of eliminating all low-grade vaginal lesions with presently available therapies is virtually nonexistent. It is not surprising, therefore, that treatment of VaIN 1, compared to conservative management, may not affect the likelihood of future abnormalities.[89] Therefore, from a cancer perspective, treatment of VaIN 1 is unnecessary and observation is recommended.

The reduction of endogenous estrogen in postmenopausal women may cause confusing cellular changes that mimic atypia, and the general lack of glycogen storage makes colposcopy difficult. Therefore, before treating vaginal lesions in women with vaginal mucosal atrophy, consider first treating the vagina as previously described with topical estrogen therapy[101,127] and reevaluating following estrogen therapy. This will often lead to resolution of the vaginal cytologic and colposcopic changes and clarify their non–HPV-related origins.

When treatment of vaginal low-grade HPV lesions is elected, the most common modality used is trichloroacetic acid (TCA). Treatment of vaginal lesions with TCA is best accomplished under colposcopic guidance. To minimize the amount of TCA used in the vagina, many clinicians apply 50% to 85% TCA on the wooden end of a cotton-tipped applicator to each lesion. However, broad lesions may be treated more efficiently by applying the cotton end of an applicator stick soaked with TCA to the lesion. Success rates vary and appear to be related to the grade of VaIN. In one series, TCA was successful in treating 100% of VaIN 1 cases but only 53% of VaIN 2,3.[128] Caution, however, must be taken to prevent excess TCA from reaching and damaging normal adjoining tissue. Reported side effects include a burning sensation in the vagina and vaginal discharge.[128] The primary difficulties of this therapeutic modality are the imprecise depth of tissue destruction, the diffuse nature of vaginal low-grade lesions, and the occurrence of new lesions between patient visits.

The diffuse nature of low-grade vaginal HPV disease prompted widespread use of vaginal 5-FU in the late 1980s.[129,130] Many treatment protocols were developed for both low- and high-grade VaIN and vaginal condylomata. Successful eradication of vaginal condyloma occurs in approximately 90% of patients after a single application and 97% after a second application. The reported recurrence rate is 7.4%.[131] Treatment of flat condyloma appears to be somewhat less successful, with complete eradication occurring in only 50% and a recurrence rate of 25%.[131] Because of significant complications, including the common occurrence of extensive vaginal ulcerations, the difficulty in subsequent healing of these lesions, often with adenosis subsequently found in previously ulcerated areas,[132] and rare cases of clear cell carcinoma arising from post-5FU adenosis,[133] this treatment approach is now rarely used and its use in treatment of low-grade disease should be discouraged.

Podophyllin, a topically applied toxin commonly used to treat vulvar condyloma, should not be used in the vagina. Systemic toxicity, including bone marrow suppression, peripheral neuropathy, and even death, has been reported with excessive vulvar application.[134] Vaginal absorption of the drug is significantly greater than absorption of the keratinized skin of the vulva and has been reported to result in coma and hemorrhage. There is also some data on the intravaginal use of imiquimod[135] and loop electrosurgical excision procedure (LEEP)[136] for treatment of vaginal condyloma and VaIN, but limited outcome data limit their use. Additionally, difficulty in ensuring shallow excision of vaginal lesions with the loop electrode risks vaginal perforation with this procedure.

Laser ablation of low-grade VaIN and condyloma is also reported to be very effective. Sixty-nine percent of women with vaginal condyloma treated with a single laser procedure will achieve complete eradication of their condyloma, and 97% will do so after a second procedure. The recurrence rate after a 9-month disease free interval is approximately 10%.[131] Flat condyloma is successfully treated with laser ablation in 83.4% of cases, with a recurrence rate of 20%.[131] However, the cost of the CO_2 laser procedure and the skill required of the operator have made this an uncommonly elected option for treatment of vaginal lesions, particularly if low grade.

Extensive vaginal condylomata acuminata can be a cosmetic and aesthetic nuisance. They are infectious to an unexposed host, and most women desire adequate and prompt eradication. Even though this can usually be achieved over time by observation, treatment with simple chemotherapeutic regimens or laser ablation for more extensive lesions may achieve a more rapid result. Extensive recalcitrant disease may require more aggressive and repeated treatments. The patient must be advised, however, that even laser surgery is no guarantee against recurrence. A rescue strategy of topical chemotherapy or repeat ablative treatment may be necessary to control disease. Excision of pedunculated condyloma may also be an appropriate form of therapy.

14.6.6.2 High-Grade VaIN

VaIN 2 and VaIN 3 are grouped as high-grade intraepithelial neoplasia of the vagina. VaIN 3 is a potential cancer precursor, yet the transit time is thought to be greater and the progressive potential less than for CIN 3. Nevertheless, the potential for progressing dictates that treatment is indicated. Three treatment options are presently available for high-grade VaIN: vaginal 5-FU, CO_2 laser ablation, and surgical excision.[134] Other investigational topical agents, such as immune response modifiers, may be used in the future. Although intracavitary radium has been used in the past with good success,[90,137,138] the expense and potential complications have led to the discontinuation of this treatment.

Vaginal 5-FU: As discussed above, 5-FU is now rarely used to treat genital HPV lesions. There may, however, be an occasional indication for its use in treating extensive, multifocal VaIN 2 or 3. Clearance of lesions is reported in approximately 29% to 87% of high-grade VaIN treated by 5-FU.[134,139–141] In the only study comparing 5-FU with and without, surgical resection, Sillman et al.[140] demonstrated greater success with the combined therapy (75%) than with 5-FU alone (29%). As discussed previously, reported severe, chemical vulvovaginitis, erosions, vaginal adenosis, and rare clear cell adenocarcinoma detected following the use of 5-FU reduced the enthusiasm for this approach to treatment of even high-grade VaIN. However, more conservative, less frequent application regimens have proven to be equally effective, yet less prone to complications, making treatment of VaIN 2,3 with 5-FU a reasonable option. The safest regimen has been application of 1/4 to 1/3 of an applicator of 5% 5-FU cream, equivalent to 1 to 1.5 g, vaginally once per week before bedtime for 10 consecutive weeks, and rinsing the medication out in the morning.[130] To prevent introital irritation, application of zinc oxide or petroleum jelly to the vulva is advised before 5-FU insertion.[142] When lesions are present only in the upper vagina, insertion of a small tampon into the lower vagina may further reduce the risk of introital symptoms. Because of marked variability in patient response and potential for serious complications, frequent colposcopic monitoring of the vagina every 3 to 4 weeks is required. Any erosion or excessive erythema should serve as a warning. Treatment should be stopped if erosions are noted. Because 5-FU is contraindicated during pregnancy, women of childbearing age should use an appropriate contraceptive.

Vaginal lesions may be treated without significant discomfort because of the absence of certain sensory receptors in most of the vagina. Nevertheless, introital irritation and burning are not uncommon side effects, and vestibulitis has been reported (Figure 14.44).[139] Significant vaginal erosion and ulceration may result in dyspareunia and postcoital bleeding.[132] When using a once-a-week regimen, however, such symptoms are rarely severe enough to stop treatment. In a follow-up study 2 to 4 weeks after a single 5-day course of vaginal 5-FU therapy, 42% of women were found to have signs of a chemical vaginitis and/or cervicitis and 11.4% had an acute ulcer. Most vaginal 5-FU ulcers occur in the apex of the vagina secondary to pooling of the medication in this area. Women treated with one-time weekly 5-FU had fewer complications, with only 5.7% developing ulcers. Unfortunately, 5-FU–induced ulcers may persist chronically for more that 6 months in many women.[132] These ulcers vary in size from 0.5 to 7 cm in diameter with a mean diameter of 2.5 cm. Eighty percent of women with 5-FU–induced ulcers have symptoms, which include serosanguineous or watery vaginal discharge, postcoital or irregular bleeding, or dyspareunia. These ulcers only rarely (<50%) heal without treatment.[132] Vaginal erosions or ulcers usually heal more quickly following vaginal acidification for 3 to 6 weeks with an acid-based gel. 5-FU treatment may also induce adenosis in the vagina.

CO$_2$ Laser Ablation: The use of carbon dioxide (CO_2) laser for treatment of lower genital tract intraepithelial neoplasia has steadily declined during the past 15 years. However, the inaccessibility of vaginal lesions and the need for exact control of the depth of destruction support the continued use of CO_2 laser for treating high-grade VaIN.[143–149] Physicians skilled in the use of the CO_2 laser can safely and effectively treat high-grade lesions. Healing is generally excellent and laser surgery is usually accepted very well by patients. A greater degree of operator skill is required by the vaginal laser surgeon, however, than for laser surgery in most other lower genital tract locations.

Even with the introduction of efficient, modern electrosurgical equipment (LEEP), the CO_2 laser still remains a more common treatment for VaIN. The vaginal wall is thinner (~0.27 to 0.5 cm thick) relative to other genital sites and vital organs are in close proximity. In addition, surgical access is more difficult. Misdirected electrosurgical excision may place adjacent organs at risk, and delayed healing responses occur more commonly. Despite the impact of LEEP in the management of CIN, ensuring maintenance of laser skills to manage challenging high-grade vulvar and vaginal disease is important (Figure 14.45).

The first report of the use of the CO_2 laser to treat VaIN was by Stafl in 1977.[143] Epithelial involvement with VaIN is <2 mm deep because the vaginal epithelium does not have crypts as in the cervix, nor appendages as in the vulva.[145,147] Hence, maintaining a vaporization depth of 2 to 3 mm will successfully eliminate most VaIN with low risk of adjacent injury. A laser beam spot size and watts of power are chosen, which meets the criteria for effective laser ablation versus cutting.[148,149] The size of the area to be ablated dictates the choice of anesthetic (local vs. general). Generally, the lateral margin of the vaporization should extend 5 to 10 mm beyond disease margins.[101,145] The postoperative care after laser surgery includes insertion of a vaginal cream nightly (if no contraindication) into the vagina three times a week until healed to prevent coaptation (i.e., healing together of the anterior and posterior vaginal walls).[149] Such preparations include estrogen vaginal cream or an antibiotic cream. The vagina is examined visually through a bivalve speculum every 7 to 10 days to assure healing and no coaptation. Cure rates for CO_2 vaporization of VaIN range from 43% to 100%, with the majority 75% to 80% with one treatment.[82,101,145,146,150,151] More than three treatments will be required in 5% to 10% to achieve permanent clearance.[145,146,150] Mean time to relapse of VaIN

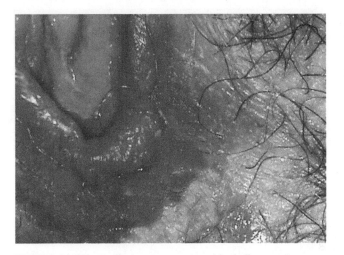

FIGURE 14.44. Erythematous mucosa with shallow erosions can be seen in the vestibule in this young woman treated vigorously with 5-FU. Symptoms of severe dyspareunia persisted after healing of the erosions. The patient was subsequently diagnosed with vulvar vestibulitis syndrome, probably secondary to treatment with 5-FU.

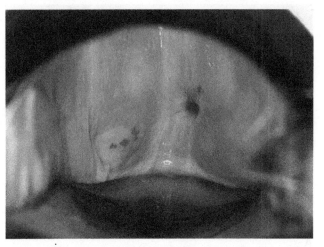

FIGURE 14.45. This patient presented with a high-grade squamous intraepithelial lesion (HSIL) Pap 1 year post-LEEP for CIN 2. In the right vaginal fornix adjacent to the colposcopically normal but now diminished cervix is a small VaIN 3. This lesion would be easily vaporized with the CO_2 laser.

after treatment with CO_2 laser is 9 to 12 months,[146] so patients should be followed every 6 months for at least a year after treatment. Extension of VaIN into the corners of the vaginal cuff, where it is more difficult to effectively reach with the laser, increases the risk of persistent disease.[146,152] Higher failure rates are also reported for multifocal compared to unifocal disease (35.2% vs. 25%)[146] and widespread low- and high-grade HPV disease (Figure 14.46A,B). Persistent HPV positivity is also associated with increased risk of relapse.[93]

When a hysterectomy is performed and the patient is known to have CIN or VaIN, it is imperative that the entire extent of the intraepithelial neoplasia be treated. The cuff is usually best visualized from below in order to determine the extent of removal of the CIN and any remaining vaginal extension. Multifocal disease present at the time of hysterectomy should be treated by laser vaporization or, if localized, by excision. If the vaginal lesion is small and contiguous with, or in close proximity to, the cervical disease, extending the vaginal cuff to remove the vaginal lesion may be possible. If the vaginal lesion is more extensive, surgical excision will inevitably shorten the vagina. Vaporizing the vaginal part of the lesion and proceeding to hysterectomy is possible in this situation. The vaginal vault closure must leave the vault and angles available for adequate postoperative assessment and accessible to treatment if VaIN were to recur at this site.

Skilled application of conservative laser surgery is imperative in the treatment of high-grade VaIN. Delayed healing and scarring of the vagina may occur following unskilled or over-enthusiastic destruction of vaginal mucosa, and postoperative vesicovaginal fistulas have been reported.[151] Posttreatment complications can have serious implications for sexuality and postoperative monitoring.

Excisional and Other Surgical Methods: Because the depth of tissue destruction has been more difficult to control when cryotherapy and electrocautery have been used to treat VaIN, these modalities have been less commonly used for this purpose. The surrounding tissue damage may be excessive and risk of bowel or bladder damage may increase. The potential for iatrogenic injury has become particularly relevant as LEEPs have gained more widespread acceptance for management of CIN and other genital HPV-induced lesions. Although laser ablation is well suited for the treatment of multifocal VaIN, surgical excision is a good option for unifocal lesions and indicated when VaIN recurs at the vaginal cuff following

hysterectomy for high-grade CIN, and when invasive cancer within an area of high-grade VaIN cannot be ruled out.

Surgical excision usually consists of wide local excision, or partial or total vaginectomy. Excision of vaginal lesions may be performed either by scalpel or by CO_2 laser. CO_2 laser has the advantage of securing hemostasis at the time of the excision and potentially reducing the amount of tissue removed, but does require greater skill in using the CO_2 laser to prevent damage to underlying organs such as bladder and bowel. If concerned about ruling out invasion, excising the lesion with a scalpel will eliminate the possibility that the burned excisional margin does not preclude making the diagnosis when present. Sherman reported that injecting fluid under a high-grade VaIN lesion, thereby elevating the lesion and providing a buffer from underlying organs, increased the safety of CO_2 laser excision.[151] Scalpel excision of VaIN has most often been in the form of a partial vaginectomy of the area involved when the possibility of occult invasive cancer is of concern. Overall success ranges between 78% and 88%[82,90,153] and is dependent upon margin status. When complete excision has occurred, the recurrence rate is only 12% compared to 34% with equivocal or positive surgical margins ($p = 0.02$).[90] For those that do recur, mean time to recurrence approximates 24 months.[153] Disadvantages, however, include the risk of hemorrhage, injury to bladder or rectum, and vaginal shortening or stenosis. Depending upon the size of the area removed, split-thickness skin grafts may be needed to restore normal vaginal length.[95]

Laser treatment of VaIN in the vaginal vault of women posthysterectomy was initially considered a very satisfactory treatment. However, studies with longer follow-up intervals, documented 75% recurrence rates. There is also an increased risk of subsequent development of invasive cancer in the vault[154] secondary to high-grade intraepithelial neoplasia epithelium buried in the suture line during hysterectomy. Because of this risk, high-grade VaIN detected in the vaginal vault posthysterectomy is usually best excised.[96,155]

The ability to diagnose occult malignancy with excision has caused many authorities to recommend this modality for the treatment of high-grade VaIN. Elfrink et al.[89] described 161 women with vaginal dysplasia, 9% of whom were ultimately found to have invasive vaginal cancer. Indermaur et al.[153] reported on 105 patients undergoing excision for VaIN lesions contained in the upper one-third of the vagina. Thirteen patients (12%) were diagnosed with squamous cell carcinoma.

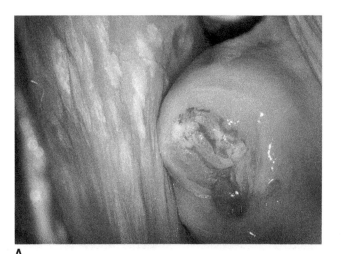

A

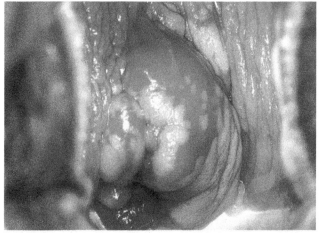

B

FIGURE 14.46. **A:** Vaginal HPV-induced lesions can often be found with cervical lesions, such as seen in this woman with both CIN 1 and VaIN 1 and **(B)** in another patient with CIN 2 and VaIN 2 on the left anterolateral vaginal wall. CO_2 laser vaporization would be an ideal treatment option for the extensive high-grade cervical and VaIN seen here.

References

1. Coppleson M, Pixley E, Reid B. *Colposcopy: A scientific and Practical Approach to the Cervix in Health and Disease*. Springfield, IL: Charles Thomas Publisher, 1971.
2. Hummer WK, Mussey E, Decker DG, Docherty MB. Carcinoma in situ of the vagina. *Am J Obstet Gynecol* 1970;108:1109–16.
3. Woodruff JD. Carcinoma in situ of the vagina. *Clin Obstet Gynecol* 1981;24:485–99.
4. Micheletti L, Zanotto VMC, Barbero M, Preti M, Nicolaci P, Canni M. Current knowledge about the natural history of intraepithelial neoplasms of the vagina. *Minerva Ginecol* 1994;46:195–204.
5. Gagne HM. Colposcopy of the vagina and vulva. *Obstet Gynecol Clin North Am* 2008;35:659–69.
6. Townsend GE. Colposcopy: how to examine the vulva and vagina. *Contemp Obstet Gynecol* 1984;23:161.
7. Davis GD. Colposcopic examination of the vagina. *Obstet Gynecol Clin North Am* 1993;20:217–29.
8. Cheung PCH, Ko CH, Lee HYM, Ho LMC, To WWK, Ip PLS. Correlation of colposcopic anogenital findings and overall assessment of child sexual abuse: prospective study. *Hong Kong Med J* 2004;10:378–83.
9. Mancino P, Parlavecchio E, Melluso J, Monti M, Russo P. Introducing colposcopy and vulvovaginoscopy as routine examinations for victims of sexual assault. *Clin Exp Obstet Gynecol* 2003;30:40–2.
10. Mauck CK, Baker JM, Birnkrant DB, Rowe PJ, Gabelnick HL. The use of colposcopy in assessing vaginal irritation in research. *AIDS* 2000;14:2221–7.
11. WHO/CONRAD. Manual for the standardization of colposcopy for the evaluation of vaginal products, update 2000. Geneva, Switzerland: CONRAD/WHO, 2000.
12. Welch WR, Robboy SJ, Townsend DE, et al. Comparison of histologic and colposcopic findings in DES-exposed females. *Obstet Gynecol* 1978;52:457–61.
13. Fraser IS, Lahteenmaki P, Elomaa K, Lacarra M, et al. Variations in vaginal epithelial surface appearance determined by colposcopic inspection in healthy, sexually active women. *Hum Reprod* 1999;14:1974–8.
14. Van Damme L, Wright A, Depraetere K, et al. A phase I study of a novel potential intravaginal microbicide, PRO2000, in healthy sexually inactive women. *Sex Transm Infect* 2000;76:126–30.
15. Norvell MK, Benrubi GI, Thompson RJ. Investigation of microtrauma after sexual intercourse. *J Reprod Med* 1984;29:269–71.
16. Fraser IS, Lacarra M, Mishell DR, et al. Vaginal epithelial surface appearance in women using vaginal rings for contraception. *Contraception* 2000;61:131–8.
17. Harwood B, Meyn LA, Ballagh SA, et al. Cervicovaginal colposcopic lesions associated with 5 nonoxynol-9 vaginal spermicide formulations. *Am J Obstet Gynecol* 2008;198:32.e1–7.
18. O'Neill EO, Reeves MF, Creinin MD. Baseline colposcopic findings in women entering studies on female vaginal products. *Contraception* 2008;78:162–6.
19. Bataillard P. The laboratory and colposcopy in the diagnosis of urogenital trichomoniasis. *Rev Fr Gynecol Obstet* 1984;79:9–10.
20. Krieger JN, Wolner-Hanssen P, Stevens C, Holmes KK. Characteristics of *Trichomonas vaginalis* isolates from women with and without colpitis macularis. *J Infect Dis* 1990;161:307–11.
21. Wolner-Hanssen P, Krieger JN, Stevens CE, et al. Clinical manifestations of vaginal trichomoniasis. *JAMA* 1989 27;261:571–6.
22. Sonnex C. Colpitis macularis and macular vaginitis unrelated to *Trichomonas vaginalis* infection. *Int J STD AIDS* 1997;8:589–91.
23. CDC. Sexually transmitted diseases treatment guidelines, 2010. *MMWR* 2010;59:RR-12.
24. Cibley LJ, Cibley LJ. Cytolytic vaginosis. *Am J Obstet Gynecol* 1991;165:1245–9.
25. Cerikcioglu N, Beksac S. Cytolytic vaginosis: misdiagnosed as candidal vaginitis. *Infect Dis Obstet Gynecol* 2004;12:13–6.
26. Shopova E, Tiufekchieva E, Karag'ozov I, Koleva V. Cytolytic vaginosis—clinical and microbiological study. *Akush Ginekol* 2006;45(suppl 2):12–3.
27. Horowitz BJ, Mardh PA, Nagy E, Rank EL. Vaginal lactobacillosis. *Am J Obstet Gynecol* 1994;170:857–61.
28. Gardner HL Desquamative inflammatory vaginitis. A newly defined entity. *Am J Obstet Gynecol* 1969;102:1102–4.
29. Oates JK, Rowen D. Desquamative inflammatory vaginitis. A review. *Genitourin Med* 1990;66:275–9.
30. Murphy R. Desquamative inflammatory vaginitis. *Dermatol Ther* 2004;17:47–9.
31. Kaufman RH, Friedrich EG, Gardner HL. *Benign Diseases of the Vulva and Vagina*. Chicago, IL: Year Book Medical Publisher, 1989.
32. Sobel JD. Desquamative inflammatory vaginitis: a new subgroup of purulent vaginitis responsive to topical 2% clindamycin therapy. *Am J Obstet Gynecol* 1994;171:1215–20.
33. Wilkinson EJ, Stone IK. *Atlas of Vulvar Disease*. Baltimore, MD: Williams and Wilkins, 1995.
34. Ridley CM. Chronic erosive vulval disease. *Clin Exp Dermatol* 1990;15:245–52.
35. Eisen D. The vulvovaginal-gingival syndrome of lichen planus. The clinical characteristics of 22 patients. *Arch Dermatol* 1994;130:1379–82.
36. Lotery HE, Galask RP. Erosive lichen planus of the vulva and vagina. *Obstet Gynecol* 2003;101:1121–5.
37. Jefferies JA, Robboy SJ, O'Brien PC, et al. Structural anomalies of the cervix and vagina in women enrolled in the Diethylstilbestrol Adenosis (DESAD) Project. *Am J Obstet Gynecol* 1984;148:59–66.
38. Garzetti GG, Ciavattini A, Goteri G, et al. Vaginal micropapillary lesions are not related to human papillomavirus infection: in situ hybridization and polymerase chain reaction detection techniques. *Gynecol Obstet Invest* 1994;38:134–9.
39. Jordan J. Colposcopy of the abnormal transformation zone. *Obstet Gynecol Clin North Am* 1993;20:69–81.
40. McDonnell JM, Emens JM, Jordan JA. The congenital cervicovaginal transformation zone in sexually active young women. *Br J Obstet Gynaecol* 1984;91:580–4.
41. Kranl C, Zelger B, Kofler H, Heim K, Sepp N, Fritsch P. Vulval and vaginal adenosis. *Br J Dermatol* 1998;139:128–31.
42. Burke L, Antonioli D. Vaginal adenosis—factors influencing detection in a colposcopic evaluation. *Obstet Gynecol* 1976;48:413–21.
43. Herbst AL, Ulfelder H, Poskanzer DC. Adenocarcinoma of the vagina: association of maternal stilbestrol therapy with tumor appearance in young women. *N Engl J Med* 1971;284:878–81.
44. Dungar CF, Wilkinson EJ. Vaginal columnar cell metaplasia. An acquired adenosis associated with topical 5-fluorouracil therapy. *J Reprod Med* 1995;40:361–6.
45. Bornstein J, Sova Y, Atad J, Lurie M, Abramovici H. Development of vaginal adenosis following combined 5-fluorouracil and carbon dioxide laser treatments for diffuse vaginal condylomatosis. *Obstet Gynecol* 1993;81:896–8.
46. Friedrich EG, Siegesmund KA. Tampon-induced vaginal ulcerations. *Obstet Gynecol* 1980;55:149–56.
47. Barrett KF, Bledsoe S, Greer BE, et al. Tampon induced vaginal or cervical ulceration. *Am J Obstet Gynecol* 1977;127:332–3.
48. Friedrich EG. Tampon effects on vaginal health. *Clin Obstet Gynecol* 1981;24:395–406.
49. Shehin SE, Jones MB, Hochwalt AE, Sarbaugh FC, Nunn S. Clinical safety-in-use study of a new tampon design. *Infect Dis Obstet Gynecol* 2003;11:89–99.
50. Raudrant D, Frappart L, De Haas P, Thoulon JM, Charvet F. Study of the vaginal mucous membrane following tampon utilization; aspect on colposcopy, scanning electron microscopy, and transmission electron microscopy. *Eur J Obstet Gynecol Reprod Biol* 1989;31:53–65.
51. Bounds W, Szarewski A, Lowe D, et al. Preliminary report of unexpected local reactions to progesterone-releasing contraceptive vaginal ring. *Eur J Obstet Gynecol Reprod Biol* 1993;48:123–5.
52. Stafford MK, Ward H, Flanagan A, et al. Safety study of nonoxynol-9 as a vaginal microbicide: evidence of adverse effects. *J Acquir Immune Defic Syndr* 1998;17:327–31.
53. Niruthisard S, Roddy RE, Chutivongse S. The effects of frequent nonoxynol-9 use on the vaginal and cervical mucosa. *Sex Transm Dis* 1991;18:176–9.
54. Clemons JL, Aguilar VC, Tillinghast TA, et al. Risk factors associated with an unsuccessful pessary fitting trial in women with pelvic organ prolapse. *Am J Obstet Gynecol* 2004;190:345.
55. Hanson LA, Schulz JA, Flood CG, et al. Vaginal pessaries in managing women with pelvic organ prolapse and urinary incontinence: patient characteristics and factors contributing to success. *Int Urogynecol J Pelvic Floor Dysfunct* 2006;17:155.
56. Adams JA. Evolution of a classification scale: medical evaluation of suspected child sexual abuse. *Child Maltreat* 2001;6:31–6.
57. Lenahan LC, Ernst A, Johnson B. Colposcopy in evaluation of the adult sexual assault victim. *Am J Emerg Med* 1998;16:183–4.
58. Zweiful P. Die vaginitis emphasematosa, oder colpohyperplasia cystica nach Winlel. *Arch Gynecol* 1877;12:39.
59. Tjugum J, Jonassen F, Olsson JH. Vaginitis emphasematosa in a renal transplant patient. *Acta Obstet Gynecol Scan* 1986;65:377–8.
60. Evans DMD, Hughes H. Cysts of the vaginal wall. *Br J Obstet Gynecol* 1947;53:335.
61. Gardner HL. Cervical and vaginal endometriosis. *Clin Obstet Gynecol* 1966;9:358–72.
62. Gardner HL. Cervical endometriosis, a lesion of increasing importance. *Am J Obstet Gynecol* 1962;84:170–3.
63. Tsukada Y. Benign melanosis of the vagina and cervix. *Am J Obstet Gynecol* 1976;124:211–2.
64. Kerley SW, Blute ML, Keeney GL. Multifocal malignant melanoma arising in vesicovaginal melanosis. *Arch Pathol Lab Med* 1991;115:950–2.
65. Karney MY, Cassidy MS, Zahn CM, Snyder RR. Melanosis of the vagina. A case report. *J Reprod Med* 2001;46:389–91.
66. Lee RB, Buttoni L Jr, Dhru K, Tamimi H. Malignant melanoma of the vagina: a case report of progression from preexisting melanosis. *Gynecol Oncol* 1984;238–45.
67. Bottles K, Lacey CG, Miller TR. Atypical melanocytic hyperplasia of the vagina. *Gynecol Oncol* 1984;19:226–30.
68. Cook CL, Sanfilippo JS, Verdi GD, Pietsch JB. Capillary hemangioma of the vagina and urethra in a child; response to short-term steroid therapy. *Obstet Gynecol* 1989;73:883–5.

69. Humphries JE, Frierson HF Jr, Underwood PB Jr. Vaginal telangiectasias: unusual presentation of the Osler-Weber-Rendu syndrome. *Obstet Gynecol* 1993;81:865–6.

70. Myers DL, LaSala CA. Conservative surgical management of Mersilene mesh suburethral sling erosion. *Am J Obstet Gynecol* 1998;179:1424–9.

71. Atia WA, Tidbury PJ. Persistent episiotomy granulation polyps; a polysymptomatic clinical entity. *Acta Obstet Gynecol Scand* 1995;74:361–6.

72. Vakili B, Huynh T, Loesch H, Franco N, Chesson RR. Outcomes of vaginal reconstructive surgery with and without graft material. *Am J Obstet Gynecol* 2005;193:2126–32.

73. Marzieh G, Soodabeh D, Narges IM, Saghar SS, Sara E. Vaginal reconstruction using no grafts with evidence of squamous epithelialization in neovaginal vault: a simple approach. *Obstet Gynaecol Res* 2011;37:195–201.

74. Blythe JG. The value of colposcopy in follow-up care of the treated gynecologic oncology patient. *Gynecol Oncol* 1983;15:186–9.

75. Arbitol MM, Davenport JH. The irradiated vagina. *Obstet Gynecol* 1974;44:249–56.

76. Shield PW. Chronic radiation effects: a correlative study of smears and biopsies from the cervix and vagina. *Diagn Cytopathol* 1995;13:107–19.

77. Cruveilhier J. Varices des veines du ligament rond, stimulant une hernie inguinale: anomalie remarquable dans la disposition general du peritoine: cancer ulcere de la paroi ante-rieure du vagin et du bas-sond de la vessie. *Bull Soc Anat Paris* 1826;1:199.

78. Cramer DW, Cutler SJ. Incidence and histology of malignancies of the female genital organ in the US. *Am J Obstet Gynecol* 1974;118:443–60.

79. Wu X, Matanoski G, Chen VW, et al. Descriptive epidemiology of vaginal cancer incidence and survival by race, ethnicity, and age in the United States. *Cancer* 2008;113(10 suppl):2873–82.

80. Audet-Lapointe P, Body G, Vauclair R, Drouin P, Ayoub J. Vaginal intraepithelial neoplasia. *Gynecol Oncol* 1990;36:232–9.

81. Kjaer SK, Sigurdsson K, Iversen OE, et al. A pooled analysis of continued prophylactic efficacy of quadrivalent human papillomavirus (types 6/11/16/18) vaccine against high-grade cervical and external genital lesions. *Cancer Prev Res* 2009;2:868–78.

82. Lenehan PM, Meffe F, Lickrish GM. Vaginal intraepithelial neoplasia: biologic aspects and management. *Gynecol Oncol* 1986;68:333–7.

83. Mao CC, Chao KC, Lian YC, Ng HT. Vaginal intraepithelial neoplasia: diagnosis and management. *Chung Hua I Hsueh Tsa Chih* 1990;46:35–42.

84. Ruiz-Morena JA, Garcia-Gomez R, Vargas-Solano A, Alonso P. Vaginal intraepithelial neoplasia. Report of 14 cases. *Int J Gynaecol Obstet* 1987;25:359–62.

85. Townsend DE. Intraepithelial neoplasia of the vagina. In: Coppleson M, ed. *Gynecologic Oncology*. Edinburgh, UK: Churchill Livingston, 1991:493.

86. Spuhler S, De Grandi P. Hysterectomy and intraepithelial neoplasia of the lower genital tract. *J Gynecol Obstet Biol Reprod* 1992;21:903–7.

87. Diakomanolis E, Stephanidis K, Rodolakis A, et al. Vaginal intraepithelial neoplasia: report of 102 cases. *Eur J Gynaecol Oncol* 2002;23:457–9.

88. Dodge JA, Eltabbakj GH, Mount SL, et al. Clinical features and risk of recurrence among patients with vaginal intraepithelial neoplasia. *Gynecol Oncol* 2001;83:363–9.

89. Elfrink SH, Gold MA, Walker JL, Moore KN. Vaginal intraepithelial neoplasia: evaluation, management, and outcome. Abstract Presentation 2008 ASCCP Biennial Meeting, Las Vegas, NV.

90. Benedet JL, Sanders BH. Carcinoma in situ of the vagina. *Am J Obstet Gynecol* 1984;148:695–700.

91. Kalogirou D, Antoniou G, Karakitsis P, et al. Vaginal intraepithelial neoplasia (VaIN) following hysterectomy in patients treated for carcinoma in situ of the cervix. *Eur J Gynaecol Oncol* 1997;18:188–91.

92. Balamurugan A, Ahmed F, Saraiya M, et al. Potential role of human papillomavirus in the development of subsequent primary in situ and invasive cancers among cervical cancer survivors. *Cancer* 2008;113(10 suppl):2919–25.

93. Frega A, French D, Piazze J, et al. Prediction of persistent vaginal intraepithelial neoplasia in previously hysterectomized women by high-risk HPV DNA detection. *Cancer Lett* 2007;249:235–41.

94. Gonzalez Bosquet E, Torres A, Busquets M, et al. Prognostic factors for the development of vaginal intraepithelial neoplasia. *Eur J Gynaecol Oncol* 2008;29:43–5.

95. Singer A, Monaghan JM, eds. Vaginal intraepithelial neoplasia. In: *Lower Genital Tract Precancer: Colposcopy, Pathology and Treatment*. Oxford, UK: Blackwell Science, 2000:214–32.

96. Hoffman MS, de Cesare SL, Roberts WS. Upper vaginectomy for in situ and occult superficially invasive carcinoma of the vagina. *Am J Obstet Gynecol* 1992;166:30–3.

97. Wright TC Jr, Cox JT, Massad LS, Carlson J, Twiggs LB, Wilkinson EJ; American Society for Colposcopy and Cervical Pathology. 2001 consensus guidelines for the management of women with cervical intraepithelial neoplasia. *Am J Obstet Gynecol* 2003;189(1):295–304.

98. Bowen-Simpkins PB, Hull MG. Intraepithelial vaginal neoplasia following immunosuppressive therapy treated with topical 5-FU. *Obstet Gynecol* 1975;46:360–2.

99. Barzon L, Pizzighella S, Corti L, et al. Vaginal dysplastic lesions in women with hysterectomy receiving radiotherapy are linked to high-risk human papillomavirus. *J Med Virol* 2002;67:401–5.

100. Di Saia P, Creaseman WT. Invasive cancer of the vagina and urethra. In: DiSaia P, Creaseman W, eds. *Clin Gynecol Oncol*. St Louis, MO: CV Mosby and Co., 33.

101. Lopes A, Monaghan JM, Robertson G. Vaginal intraepithelial neoplasia. In: Luesley D, Jordan J, Richart R, eds. *Intraepithelial Neoplasia of the Lower Genital Tract*. New York: Churchill Livingston, 1995:169–76.

102. Aho M, Vesterinen E, Meyer B, et al. Natural history of vaginal intraepithelial neoplasia. *Cancer* 1991;68:195–7.

103. Sillman FH, Fructer RC, Chen Y-C et al. Vaginal intraepithelial neoplasia: risk factors for persistence, recurrence, and invasion and its management. *Am J Obstet Gynecol* 1997;176:93–9.

104. Castle PE, Schiffman M, Bratti MC, et al. A population-based study of vaginal human papillomavirus infection in hysterectomized women. *J Infect Dis* 2004;190(3):458–67.

105. Dahling JR. Madeleine MM, Sherman KJ, et al. Anogenital tumors associated with human papillomavirus. In: Fortner JG, Rhoads JE, eds. *Accomplishments in Cancer Research*. Philadelphia, PA: JB Lippincott, 1993:280–7.

106. De Vuyst H, Clifford GM, Nascimento MC, et al. Prevalence and type distribution of human papillomavirus in carcinoma and intraepithelial neoplasia of the vulva, vagina, and anus: a meta-analysis. *Int J Cancer* 2009;124:1626–36.

107. Verloop J, van Leeuwen FE, Helmerhorst TJ, van Boven HH, Rookus MA. Cancer risk in DES daughters. *Cancer Causes Control* 2010;21:999–1007.

108. Aaltonen LM, Rihkanen H, Vaheri A. Human papillomavirus in larynx. *Laryngoscope* 2002;112:700–7.

109. Syrjanen S, Puranen M. Human papillomavirus infections in children: the potential role of maternal transmission. *Crit Rev Oral Biol Med* 2000;11:259–74.

110. Schneider A, de Villiers EM, Schneider V. Multifocal squamous neoplasia of the female genital tract: significance of human papillomavirus infection of the vagina after hysterectomy. *Obstet Gynecol* 1987;70:294–8.

111. Rylander E, Eriksson A, von Schoultz B. Wart virus infection of cervix uteri and vagina in women with atypical cervical cytology. *Scand J Urol Nephrol Suppl* 1984;86:223–6.

112. Hilgers RD, Malkasian GD Jr, Soule EH. Embryonal rhabdomyosarcoma (botryoid type) of the vagina. A clinicopathologic review. *Am J Obstet Gynecol* 1970;107:484–502.

113. Leuschner I, Harms D, Mattke A, Koscielniak E, Treuner J. Rhabdomyosarcoma of the urinary bladder and vagina: a clinicopathologic study with emphasis on recurrent disease: a report from the Kiel Pediatric Tumor Registry and the German CWS Study. *Am J Surg Pathol* 2001;25:856–64.

114. Gupta D, Malpica A, Deavers MT, Silva EG. Vaginal melanoma: a clinicopathologic and immunohistochemical study of 26 cases. *Am J Surg Pathol* 2002;26:1450–7.

115. O'Brien PC, Noller KL, Robboy SJ. Vaginal epithelial changes in young women enrolled in the National Cooperative Diethylstilbestrol Adenosis (DESAD) Project. *Obstet Gynecol* 1979;53:300–8.

116. Trimble EL, Rubinstein LV, Menck HR, Hankey BF, Kosary C, Giusti RM. Vaginal clear cell adenocarcinoma in the United States. *Gynecol Oncol* 1996;61:113–5.

117. Melnick S, Cole P, Anderson D, et al. Rates and risks of diethylstilbestrol-related clear cell adenocarcinoma of the vagina and cervix. An update. *N Engl J Med* 1987;316:514–6.

118. Troisi R, Hatch EE, Titus-Ernstoff L, et al. Cancer risk in women prenatally exposed to diethylstilbestrol. *Int J Cancer* 2007;121(2):356–60.

119. Stafl A, Mattingly RF. Vaginal adenosis: a precancerous lesion? *Am J Obstet Gynecol* 1974;120:666–77.

120. Grainai CO, Walters MD, Safaii H et al. Malignant transformation of vaginal endometriosis. *Obstet Gynecol* 1984;64:592–5.

121. Kwon YS, Nam JH, Choi G. Clear cell adenocarcinoma arising in endometriosis of a previous episiotomy site. *Obstet Gynecol* 2008;112:475–7.

122. Shah C, Pizer E, Veljovich DS, et al. Clear cell adenocarcinoma of the vagina in a patient with vaginal endometriosis. *Gynecol Oncol* 2006;103:1130–2.

123. Staats PN, Clement PB, Young RH. Primary endometrioid adenocarcinoma of the vagina. A clinicopathologic study of 18 cases. *Am J Surg Pathol* 2007;31:1490–1501.

124. Leiserowitz GS, Gumbs JL, Oi R, et al. Endometriosis-related malignancies. *Int J Gynecol Cancer* 2003;13:466–71.

125. Saito T, Takehara M, Tanaka R, Sato K, Fujita M, Kudo R. Usefulness of silver intensification of immunostaining for cytologic diagnosis of primary melanoma of the female genital organs. *Acta Cytol* 2002;46:1075–80

126. Liu LY, Hou YJ, Li JZ. Primary malignant melanoma of the vagina: a report of seven cases. *Obstet Gynecol* 1987;70:569–72

127. Kaminski PF, Sorosky JI, Wheelock JB, Stevens CW Jr. The significance of atypical cervical cytology in an older population. *Obstet Gynecol* 1989;73:13–5

128. Lin H, Huang E-Y, Chang H-Y, ChangChien C-C. Therapeutic effect of topical application of trichloroacetic acid for vaginal intraepithelial neoplasia after hysterectomy. *Jpn J Clin Oncol* 2005;35:651–4.

129. Krebs HB. Treatment of vaginal condylomata acuminata by weekly topical application of 5-fluorouracil. *Obstet Gynecol* 1987;70:68–71.

130. Kirwin P, Naftalin NJ. Topical 5-fluorouracil in the treatment of vaginal intraepithelial neoplasia. *Br J Obstet Gynecol* 1985;92:287–91.

131. Ferenczy A. Comparison of 5-fluorouracil and CO2 laser treatment of vaginal condylomata. *Obstet Gynecol* 1984;64:773–8.

132. Krebs HB, Helmkamp F. Chronic ulcerations following topical therapy with 5-fluorouracil therapy for vaginal human papillomavirus associated lesions. *Obstet Gynecol* 1991;78:205–8.

133. Goodman A, Zukerberg LR, Nikrui N, Scully RE. Vaginal adenosis and clear cell carcinoma after 5-fluorouracil treatment for condylomas. *Cancer* 1991;68(7):1628–32.

134. Rome RM, England PG. Management of vaginal intraepithelial neoplasia: a series of 132 cases with long-term follow-up. *Int J Gynecol Cancer* 2000;10:382–90.

135. Buck HW, Guth KJ. Treatment of vaginal intraepithelial neoplasia (primarily low grade) with imiquimod 5% cream. *J Low Genit Tract Dis* 2003;7(4):290–3.

136. Powell JL, Asbery DS. Treatment of vaginal dysplasia: just a simple loop electrosurgical excision procedure? *Am J Obstet Gynecol* 2000;182(3):731–2.

137. Hernandez-Linares W, Puthawala A, Nolan JF, Jernstrom PH, Morrow P. Carcinoma in situ of the vagina: past and present management. *Obstet Gynecol* 1980;56:356–60.

138. Ogin I, Kitamura T, Okajima H, et al. High-dose-rate intracavitary brachytherapy in the management of cervical and vaginal intraepithelial neoplasia. *Int J Radiat Oncol Biol Phys* 1998;40:881–7.

139. Gonzalez Sanches JL, Flores Murrieta G, Chavez Brambila J, Deolarte Manzano JM, Andrade Manzano AF. Topical 5-fluorouracil for treatment of vaginal intraepithelial neoplasms. *Ginecol Obstet Mex* 2002;70:244–7.

140. Sillman FH, Sedlis A, Boyce JG. 5-FU/chemosurgery for difficult lower genital intraepithelial neoplasia. *Contemp Obstet Gynecol* 1985;27:79–101.

141. Petrilli ES, Townsend DE, Morrow CP, Nakao CY. Vaginal intraepithelial neoplasia: biologic aspects and treatment with topical 5-fluorouracil and the carbon dioxide laser. *Am J Obstet Gynecol* 1980;138:321–8

142. Daly JW, Ellis GF. Treatment of vaginal dysplasia and carcinoma in situ with topical 5-fluorouracil. *Obstet Gynecol* 1980;55:350–2.

143. Stafl A, Wilkinson EJ, Mattingly RF. Laser treatment of cervical and vaginal neoplasia. *Am J Obstet Gynecol* 1977;128:136.

144. Jobson VW, Homesley HD. Treatment of vaginal intraepithelial neoplasia with the carbon dioxide laser. *Obstet Gynecol* 1983;62:90–3.

145. Stuart GCE, Flagler EA, Nation JG et al. Laser vaporization of vaginal intraepithelial neoplasia. *Am J Obstet Gynecol* 1988;158:240–3.

146. Diakomanolis E, Rodolakis A, Boulgaris Z, Blachos G, Michalas S. Treatment of vaginal intraepithelial neoplasia with laser ablation and upper vaginectomy. *Gynecol Obstet Invest* 2002;54:17–20.

147. Benedet JL, Wilson PS, Matisic JP. Epidermal thickness measurements I vaginal intraepithelial neoplasia: a basis for optimal CO2 laser vaporization. *Reprod Med* 1992;37:809–12.

148. Townsend DE. Laser treatment of the vagina. In: Baggish, ed. *Basic and Advanced Laser Surgery in Gynecology*. Norwalk, CT: Appleton-Century-Crofts, 1995:152–9.

149. Wright VC. CO_2 laser surgery for vaginal intraepithelial neoplasia. In: Wright VC, Fisher JC, eds. *Laser Surgery in Gynecology: A Clinical Guide*. Philadelphia, PA: W. B. Saunders, 1993:152–9.

150. Townsend DE, Levine RU, Crum CP, Richart RM. Treatment of vaginal carcinoma in situ with carbon dioxide laser. *Am J Obstet Gynecol* 1982;143:565–8.

151. Sherman AI. Laser therapy for vaginal intraepithelial neoplasia after hysterectomy. *J Reprod Med* 1990;35:941–4.

152. Volante R, Pasero L, Saraceno L, Magurano M, Ribaldone R. Carbon dioxide laser surgery in colposcopy for cervicovaginal intraepithelial neoplasia treatment. 10 years experience and failure analysis. *Eur J Gynaecol Oncol* 1992;13(1 suppl)78–81.

153. Indermaur MD, Martino MA, Fiorica JV, Roberts WS, Hoffman MS. Upper vaginectomy for the treatment of vaginal intraepithelial neoplasia. *Am J Obstet Gynecol* 2005;193:577–81.

154. Woodman CB, Jordan JA, Wade-Evans T. The management of vaginal intraepithelial neoplasia after hysterectomy. *Br J Obstet Gynaecol* 1984;91:707–11.

155. Monaghan JM. Vaginal cancer. In: Burghardt E, ed. *Surgical Gynecologic Oncology*. Stuttgart, Germany: George Thieme Verlag, 1993:171–84.

Vulvar Abnormalities

15.1 NORMAL ANATOMY AND HISTOLOGY
15.2 EXAMINATION AND BIOPSY TECHNIQUES
15.3 DIFFERENTIATION OF DEFINITE DISEASE FROM
      NORMAL
      15.3.1 Micropapillations
      15.3.2 Acetowhitening
      15.3.3 Vascular Ectasia
      15.3.4 Fordyce's Spots
15.4 VULVAR INFECTIONS
      15.4.1 Viruses
      15.4.2 Bacteria
      15.4.3 Chlamydia
      15.4.4 Fungi
15.5 VULVODYNIA
      15.5.1 Historical Information
      15.5.2 Terminology

15.5.3 Etiologic Theories
15.5.4 Treatment of Vulvodynia
15.6 VULVAR NONNEOPLASTIC EPITHELIAL CONDITIONS
      15.6.1 Lichen Sclerosus
      15.6.2 Squamous Cell Hyperplasia (Lichen Simplex
            Chronicus)
      15.6.3 Other Dermatoses
15.7 VULVAR NONINVASIVE NEOPLASTIC
      ABNORMALITIES
      15.7.1 Vulvar Intraepithelial Neoplasia (Squamous and
            Nonsquamous)
      15.7.2 Other Noninvasive Neoplastic Abnormalities
15.8 VULVAR INVASIVE CARCINOMA
      15.8.1 Squamous Cell Carcinoma
      15.8.2 Melanocytic Carcinoma (Melanoma)
      15.8.3 Adenocarcinoma

15.1 NORMAL ANATOMY AND HISTOLOGY

Vulvar embryology, normal anatomy, and histology are discussed in detail in Chapter 2. Some important comments are reiterated here for correlation with the different pathophysiologies, clinical presentations, and histopathologies of the various vulvar disorders. The vulva encompasses an area between the genitocrural folds laterally and between the mons pubis anteriorly and the anus posteriorly (Figure 15.1).[1-4] This area includes the mons pubis, labia minora and majora, clitoris, vestibule, Skene's glands and ducts, hymen, Bartholin's glands and ducts, urethral meatus, and vestibulovaginal bulbs. The *vestibule* is defined as that portion located between the hymen and Hart's line. It is medial to the labia minora extending from the clitoral region to the posterior fourchette.

The majority of the vulva is covered by keratinized skin. The exception is the vestibule, which is partially covered by a nonkeratinized surface that is flush with the vagina. The junction of keratinized squamous epithelium on the posterior fourchette and labia minora with the mucosa of the vestibule is *Hart's line*. Hart's line reflects the derivation of these two structures during embryonic development, as the vulva arises from ectoderm and the inner vestibule arises from the endodermally derived urogenital sinus.[2]

The vestibule has numerous gland openings. Skene's ducts are directly inferior and lateral to the urethra. Bartholin's glands and ducts (the major vestibular glands and ducts) are located along the vestibule at the 5 and 7 o'clock positions. The minor vestibular glands are located in a semicircular area of the vestibule. The vestibule also contains numerous micropapillary structures (micropapillomas) (Figure 15.2). These small papillary projections have been previously confused with vulvar condylomas or subclinical human papillomavirus (HPV) infections; however, HPV has not been consistently identified in these structures.[5]

The hymenal ring represents the boundary between the vulvar vestibule and the vagina. Prior to intercourse, the hymen is a plate-like structure with some degree of perforation. An imperforate hymen, in which the hymenal plate is solid, can lead to an accumulation of menstrual efflux and vaginal material known as a *hematocolpos*.[6]

Histologically, the keratinized squamous epithelial surface or epidermis is divided into layers or strata. The entire epidermis is known as the *stratum Malpighi*. The keratinized surface is the *stratum corneum epidermidis*. The epithelial cells containing basophilic keratohyaline granules are located directly beneath the keratin layer and compose the *stratum granulosum epidermidis*. The *stratum spinosum epidermidis* represents the majority of the squamous cells. The *stratum basale epidermidis* is made up of the least mature squamous cells and is located adjacent to the basement membrane. The individual squamous cells that compose the keratinized surface are also known as *keratinocytes* (Figure 15.3).[2]

The epidermis has undulating extensions into the underlying dermis, which are known as *rete pegs*. The superficial, loose dermis located between the rete pegs is known as the *papillary dermis*. The dense collagenous dermis below the papillary layer is the *reticular dermis*. The deepest layer beneath the dermis is the subcutaneous fat.

The adnexal structures found in the reticular dermis include eccrine (sweat) glands, apocrine glands (pheromone glands), specialized nerve receptors, and hair structures or pilosebaceous units. The free nerve endings, sensory structures that register itching and pain, are located in the superficial dermis directly beneath the stratum basalis.

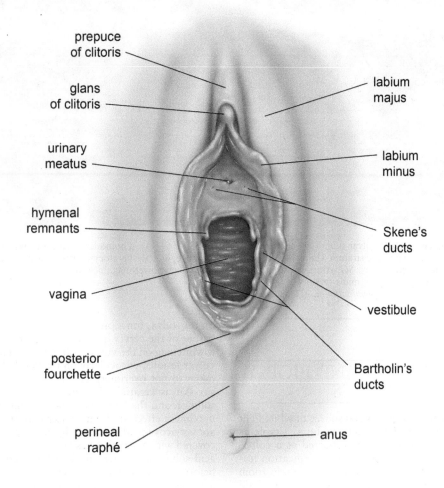

prepuce
of clitoris

glans
of clitoris

urinary
meatus

hymenal
remnants

vagina

posterior
fourchette

perineal
raphé

labium
majus

labium
minus

Skene's
ducts

vestibule

Bartholin's
ducts

anus

FIGURE 15.1.   Illustration of a normal vulva. The labia minora are opened to reveal the vestibule.

Numerous dermatological changes and diseases can occur in the keratinized portion of the vulva. It is important that the colposcopist understands the following terms and their definitions.

The term *acantholysis* refers to the abrupt separation of epidermal cells resulting from dissolution of the intercellular cement substance, leading to loss of cellular cohesion. There is localized clearing and bullous formation, with detached cells within the cavity. The term *acanthosis* is used to describe thickening in the epidermal layer, predominately through enlargement of the rete pegs (Figure 15.4). *Dyskeratosis* is faulty and premature keratinization of individual squamous cells. When seen in vulvar dysplasia, individual dyskeratocytes are also known as *corps ronds* (Figure 15.5). *Exocytosis* refers to the presence of inflammatory cells in the epidermis. *Hyperkeratosis* refers to an increase in the thickness of the stratum corneum or keratin layer. This is a subjective observation made by comparing the skin surface in question to skin that appears to have a normal keratin thickness. Lentiginous or *lentigo formation* is a linear pattern of melanocytic cell proliferation within the basal layer (Figure 15.6). *Lichenoid change* refers to the development of a plaque-like lesion with a flattened appearance of the epidermis or adjacent chronic inflammatory cells. *Parakeratosis* is the presence of nuclei within the keratin layer that, along with hyperkeratosis and dyskeratosis, implies a rapid and excessive keratinization of squamous epithelial cells (Figure 15.7). *Papillomatosis* refers to elongation of the papillary

dermis and the associated extension of the adjacent epidermis. *Spongiosis* is intercellular edema that results in separation of individual epithelial cells. A mononuclear infiltrate is typically present with this condition (Figure 15.8).[7]

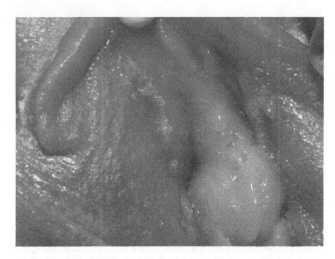

FIGURE 15.2.   Vulvar vestibule demonstrating papules with single papillary projections (micropapillomas). These are a normal finding.

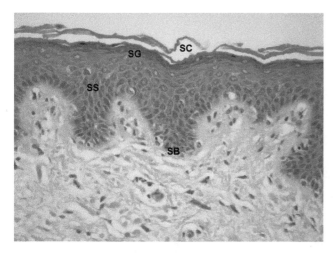

FIGURE 15.3. Photomicrograph of vulvar skin. The entire epidermal surface of the vulva is known as the stratum Malpighi. *SC*, stratum corneum epidermidis (keratin layer); *SG*, stratum granulosum epidermidis; *SS*, stratum spinosum epidermidis or *prickle cell layer*; *SB*, stratum basale epidermidis or *germinativum*. (Hematoxylin-eosin stain; high power magnification.)

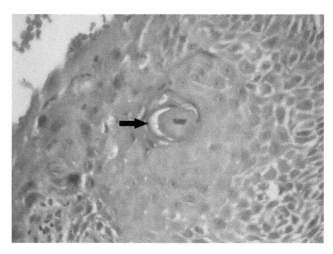

FIGURE 15.5. Photomicrograph of dyskeratocytosis. A single orangeophilic dyskeratocyte (*arrow*) is present. (Hematoxylin-eosin stain, high power magnification.)

15.2 EXAMINATION AND BIOPSY TECHNIQUES

The vulva is best examined using a good source of white light and a magnification device. The latter can be as simple as a handheld magnifying lens or as sophisticated as a colposcope. If a colposcope is used, the lower magnification levels of a fixed magnification system or the wide-angle zoom on a variable magnification system is recommended to aid in identification of vulvar landmarks. Examination should be systematic and deliberate, incorporating all aspects of the vulvar surface. Any abnormality that is not clearly benign or is ambiguous should be biopsied before any treatment is instituted.[8]

Dilute acetic acid (vinegar, 3% to 5%) can occasionally be helpful in clarifying the etiology of some ambiguous lesions on the vulva, functioning in much the same way as it affects tissues of the cervix and vagina (Figure 15.9). However, acetowhitening on the vulva is often nonspecific for HPV-induced vulvar lesions, particularly on the vestibule, and care must be taken to not overinterpret this finding. The majority of vulvar skin is keratinized; therefore, the amount of acetic acid solution and the length of exposure time required to achieve maximum effect are both greater than that required to evaluate cervicovaginal mucosa. To accomplish this, the vulva is covered with gauze that has been soaked in a 3% to 5% acetic acid solution. It is left in place for approximately 5 minutes before the examination is started. Liberal amounts of acetic acid are then reapplied as the inspection continues. Use of acetic acid on fissured, ulcerated, or denuded epithelium can be quite painful and is discouraged. Potassium iodide (Lugol's solution) is not helpful in the evaluation of lesions on keratinized epithelium.

The choice of a biopsy instrument is dependent on the type of abnormality or area to be sampled. Kevorkian or Tischler forceps can be used to sample raised or warty lesions. Macular

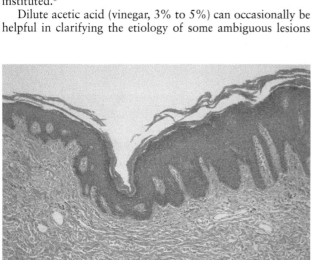

FIGURE 15.4. Photomicrograph of epidermal acanthosis. The epidermis at the right of the microscopic field is thickened. In addition, the rete pegs are lengthened and focally confluent. (Hematoxylin-eosin stain; medium power magnification.)

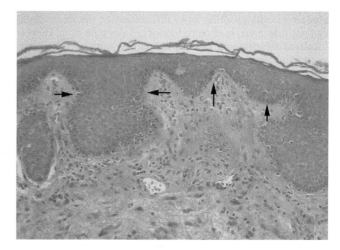

FIGURE 15.6. Photomicrograph of epidermal lentigo. Note the increase in the number of melanocytes and basal pigmentation (*arrows*). (Hematoxylin-eosin stain; medium power magnification.)

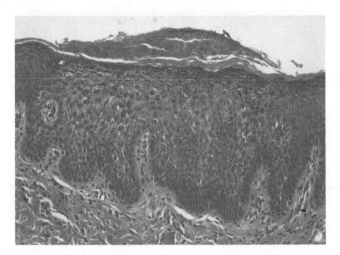

FIGURE 15.7. Photomicrograph of parakeratosis. Note the pyknotic nuclei scattered throughout the keratin layer. (Hematoxylin-eosin stain; high power magnification.)

lesions are best sampled by making an elliptical excision using a small knife blade or performing a Keyes punch biopsy (Figure 15.10). The latter, when twisted into the skin until it penetrates through the dermis, creates a circular cookie-cutter incision. The central portion can then be raised and the specimen cut off at the base. A punch with a diameter of at least 4 mm is recommended to remove an adequate amount of tissue. Areas of ulceration, blistering, atrophy, or scaring should be sampled along the edge in order to remove an area of surface epithelium. Biopsies performed at the center of these areas may only demonstrate necrosis, granulation tissue, fibrin, and inflammation. Papular lesions, especially pigmented lesions, should be biopsied at the most abnormal part. When biopsying the labia minora, take care to keep the punch or incision from penetrating through both sides of the structure creating a hole. As with any skin biopsy, applying local anesthesia is necessary. This is easily accomplished a couple of minutes before the procedure by injecting 1 to 2 mL of a 1% lidocaine with epinephrine 1:200,000 solution into the dermis of the area to be sampled. The addition of sodium bicarbonate is often beneficial in reducing the injection pain. A ratio of 1 mL of

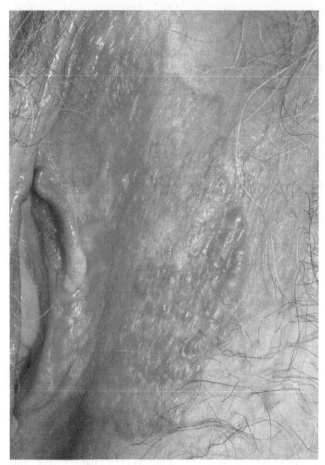

FIGURE 15.9. The clinical application of 3% to 5% acetic acid assists in visualizing tissue abnormalities. Tissue that has an increased nuclear to cytoplasmic ratio stains white in color.

sodium bicarbonate to 9 mL of lidocaine with epinephrine is used. A tuberculin syringe with a 30-gauge needle is ideal for this purpose. The epinephrine is useful in reducing the bleeding that occurs after the biopsy. Particularly, sensitive areas

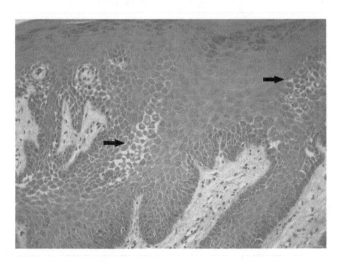

FIGURE 15.8. Photomicrograph of spongiosis. Individual keratinocytes are separated from each other (arrows). (Hematoxylin-eosin stain; medium power magnification.)

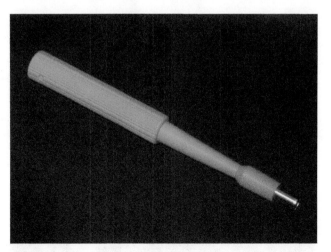

FIGURE 15.10. Keyes punch biopsy instrument. The round sharp end at the base is rotated into the skin and superficial dermis. Once the dermis is transected, the core of tissue is removed, being careful not to crush the sample.

may require the application of an additional topical anesthetic prior to anesthesia injection. For clitoral biopsies, it is generally recommended that lidocaine without epinephrine be utilized. Also, consider performing a 3-mm-size biopsy on the clitoris, rather than a 4-mm-size biopsy. Once the biopsy is accomplished, small defects at the biopsy site can be cauterized using silver nitrate sticks or Monsel's solution; larger defects can be approximated with interrupted suture.

15.3 DIFFERENTIATION OF DEFINITE DISEASE FROM NORMAL

Using colposcopy in the evaluation and management of vulvar diseases has opened uncharted waters for many clinicians unfamiliar with both normal and abnormal colposcopic findings. The two most important decisions facing any colposcopist in evaluating the vulva are, first, to define whether there is definite disease present and, second, to decide whether treatment will provide specific and definable benefits that are greater than the risk of the procedure. The most common normal vulvar findings that have been misdiagnosed as disease are micropapillations, acetowhitening, vascular ectasia, and sebaceous hyperplasia (Fordyce's spots).

15.3.1 Micropapillations

Micropapillae of the inner labia minora and acetowhite changes anywhere in the lower genital tract have commonly been misinterpreted as being secondary to HPV.[9]

Micropapillae consist of papillary projections, each having a single base (Figure 15.11), whereas HPV changes have multiple papillae on a broad base (Figure 15.12). It was the presumed association of micropapillae with HPV that led to the erroneous theory that vestibulodynia was secondary to HPV.[10]

In *Micropapillomatosis*, the vestibular papillae are prominent.[5] The papillae are usually small (1 to 3 mm) and are best detected with magnification but can be seen with the naked eye. The papillae may be few or cover the majority of the mucosal surface of the labia minora. Visualization is enhanced by application of 3% to 5% acetic acid, which results in a nonspecific acetowhitening of these papillae. Biopsies of micropapillae have often been reported to have koilocytes, but

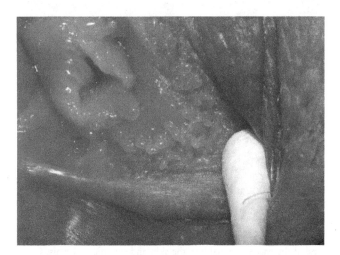

FIGURE 15.11. *Micropapillomatosis* of the vulva is characterized by small papillae, each having a single base.

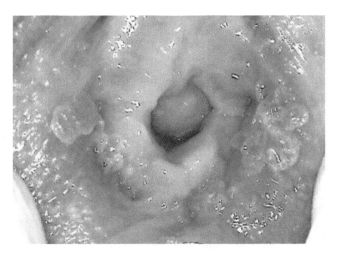

FIGURE 15.12. The papillae of these HPV lesions have multiple projections from a broad base. They are patchy and acetowhite.

up to 90% of such biopsy specimens have been determined to be normal when reevaluated by a panel of expert pathologists with expertise in interpreting HPV changes.[5] Although biopsies of areas of micropapillomatosis will contain papillomatosis, acanthosis, and sometimes parakeratosis, they uniformly lack true koilocytes with nuclear atypia, multinucleated cells, or dyskeratosis necessary to make a firm diagnosis of HPV-related disease.[5,11] Instead, these equivocal interpretations are made on the basis of papillomatosis and a misinterpretation of glycogen within the cytoplasm as koilocytotic vacuoles. More importantly, HPV-DNA is not more commonly found in these specimens than in specimens from women not having micropapillations.[12,13] The modern colposcopist must be able to differentiate between these normal findings and those that are an expression of HPV disease without relying on biopsy to make the diagnosis. Avoidance of biopsy when vulvar micropapillations have colposcopic findings most consistent with *micropapillomatosis* offers the best chance of avoiding overdiagnosis and overtreatment.

15.3.2 Acetowhitening

Areas of acetowhitening may also be found in the absence of micropapillations in the fossa navicularis and on the vestibule (Figure 15.13). Acetowhite changes are also frequently misinterpreted as being secondary to HPV. Vulvar acetowhite changes may occur from the trauma of intercourse, from yeast infections, from other inflammatory conditions of the vulva, as well as from subclinical HPV changes,[9] and therefore should always be considered to be nonspecific. Acetowhite changes from trauma or inflammation are likely to be diffuse and flat and may be either symptomatic or asymptomatic. In contrast, acetowhite changes from HPV are more likely to be slightly raised and may have colposcopically visible asperities (small papillations) or satellite lesions (Figure 15.14). Such areas may be slightly pruritic or asymptomatic. Colposcopic visualization prior to application of acetic acid will often show punctation or looped blood vessels that are classic for condyloma (Figure 15.15).

15.3.3 Vascular Ectasia

Depending upon the thickness of the mucosal epithelium, the vestibule may normally exhibit various degrees of erythema

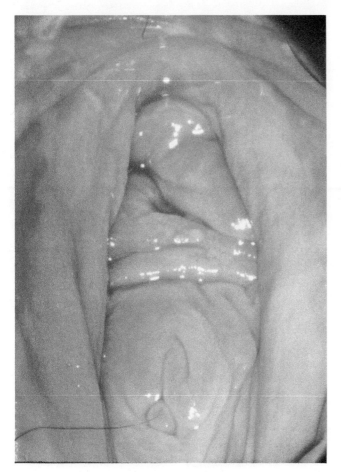

FIGURE 15.13. Acetowhite changes are seen here in the absence of micropapillations in the fossa navicularis and at the junction of this inferior part of the vestibule with the perineum. This represents a normal finding most likely seen in this patient because of increased cell turnover secondary to friction from intercourse.

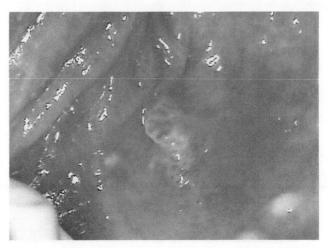

FIGURE 15.15. Another clue that the acetowhitening represents HPV changes is the colposcopic detection of localized punctation prior to application of acetic acid.

In contrast, erythema of the labia majora usually signifies an enhancement of the underlying vasculature by inflammation or neoplasia (Figure 15.18).

15.3.4 Fordyce's Spots

Sebaceous glands are normally found in association with a hair follicle. Fordyce's spots are a form of ectopic sebaceous glands. These glands may create a cobblestone appearance (Figures 15.19 and 15.20). Age and inflammation may both result in hypertrophy of these glands, but such hypertrophy should never be interpreted as a primary disease process.[8] Biopsies of these areas may be interpreted as "sebaceous hyperplasia" and should be considered a variant of normal.

15.4 VULVAR INFECTIONS

The vulva is susceptible to a number of infectious agents including viral, bacterial, and fungal organisms. These organisms can result in discharge, surface irritation, papule formation, and ulceration. A complete description of the wide

as the color of the underlying vasculature transmits through the nonkeratinized epithelium. While vestibulodynia is typically manifested by increased erythema in the vestibule (Figure 15.16), marked individual variation in normal color makes this a difficult sign to interpret (Figure 15.17).

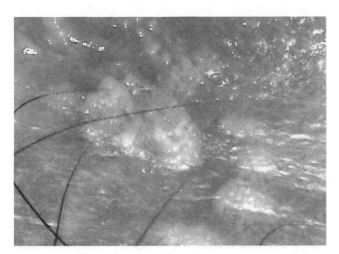

FIGURE 15.14. Here the acetowhite changes are typical of HPV-induced lesions as they are raised from the surrounding skin with colposcopically visible asperities.

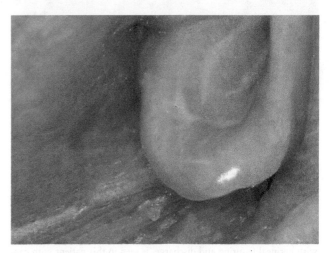

FIGURE 15.16. Localized erythema is noted in this patient with vestibulodynia.

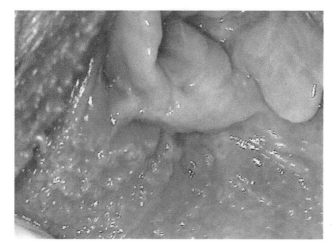

FIGURE 15.17.   This woman has severe symptoms of vestibulodynia yet has no increased erythema and outwardly appears to be entirely normal.

variety of vulvar infections is beyond the scope of this chapter, and the reader should refer to more detailed sources for additional information.[1,8,14-16] The Web site for the Centers for Disease Control and Prevention (CDC) *www.cdc.gov/std/treatment/* contains the most up-to-date information on various antibiotic regimens, dosages, and treatment durations for these infections.[17] Brief discussions of the more common and unique abnormalities are included here.

15.4.1 Viruses

15.4.1.1 Herpes Simplex Virus

The herpes simplex virus (HSV) is the most common cause of infectious vulvar ulcers. The herpes viruses are double-stranded DNA viruses. There are two types of HSVs that affect the vulva: herpes 1 and 2. HSV type 2 (HSV-2) has traditionally been associated with genital lesions and HSV-1 with oral lesions. However, over the past several decades, genital lesions secondary to HSV-1 have become increasingly common, with

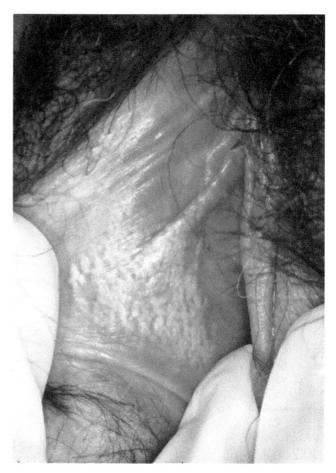

FIGURE 15.19.   Fordyce's spots with fine to moderately coarse changes.

up to 50% of first-episode cases of genital herpes now caused by HSV-1.[17] However, recurrences and subclinical shedding are much less frequent with genital HSV-1 infection than infection with genital HSV-2.[17] Genital HSV lesions are usually contracted through sexual contact, which may be either oral-genital (HSV-1) or genital-genital (HSV-1 or 2). Transmission

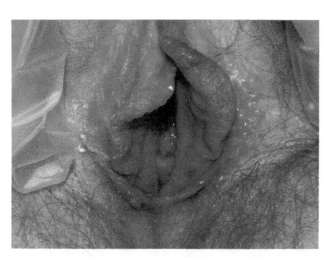

FIGURE 15.18.   Erythema of the labia majora and perineum, along with perineal fissuring and discharge, is seen in this patient with candida vulvovaginitis.

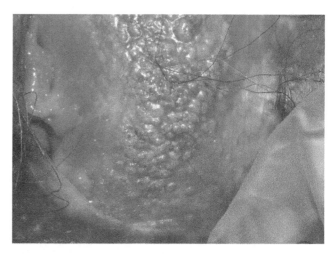

FIGURE 15.20.   A closer view demonstrates the cobblestone appearance of Fordyce's spots.

most commonly occurs during periods of asymptomatic viral shedding from partners unaware that they are infectious. Primary herpes simplex lesions most commonly occur within 1 week following exposure and usually present with initial burning, followed by the formation of small vesicles. These vesicles rupture to form erosions and, on occasion, shallow ulcers that are extremely painful and vary in width and depth (Figures 15.21 and 15.22). Patients may complain of a paresthesia for 2 to 3 days, and some will have fever, malaise, headache, and myalgia. Pain can vary from moderate to severe. After initial infection, particularly with HSV-2, recurrent outbreaks are common and may be frequent. The majority of patients present with nonprimary recurrent disease. In recurrent infections, tingling, itching, and burning before the onset of vesiculation may be noted but are typically less prominent than with initial infection.

A variety of methods to diagnose herpes exist including culture, direct immunofluorescence, and polymerase chain reaction (PCR). A culture should be obtained to confirm the diagnosis; however, false-negative results are common. In order to minimize false-negative results, the culture should be taken from lesions in the vesicular or early ulcerative stage, as these contain the highest concentration of viral particles.

Tzanck smears are only helpful on fresh vesicles. Microscopically, look for multinucleated giant epithelial cells with opaque "ground glass" nuclei. Multinucleated giant cells are classic for herpes.[18]

Although both type-specific and non–type-specific antibodies develop in the first few weeks after infection, serology is typically not helpful in the initial evaluation of acute first-episode herpes lesions. Type-specific HSV assays are most helpful when (1) HSV cultures are negative and genital symptoms are recurrent or atypical, (2) a clinical diagnosis of genital herpes was made without laboratory confirmation, or (3) clarifying whether the partner of a person having genital herpes is at risk of acquiring the infection.[17]

Treatment is symptomatic, for example, sitz baths (warm water baths that cover the vulva, buttocks, and hips) to relieve burning, pain relievers, and loose underclothes. The use of antiviral agents such as acyclovir, famciclovir, or valacyclovir can reduce the duration and frequency of recurrences of the infection and should be started as soon as HSV lesions are suspected clinically.[17,19,20] Intravenous acyclovir therapy should be provided for patients who have severe disease or complications that necessitate hospitalization, such

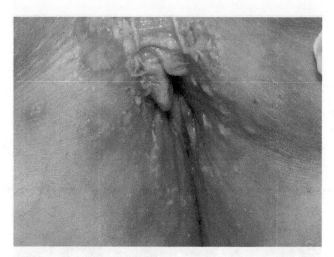

FIGURE 15.22. Herpes. Extremely tender perianal herpes lesions in a patient experiencing a primary infection with herpes.

as disseminated infection, pneumonitis, hepatitis, or complications of the central nervous system (e.g., meningitis or encephalitis).

15.4.1.2 Genital Herpes in Pregnancy

Women who acquire genital herpes near the time of infant delivery have a high risk for transmission of herpes to the (30% to 50%). It is low (<1%) among women with histories of recurrent herpes at term or who acquire genital HSV during the first half of pregnancy. Pregnancy recommendations for the evaluation and management of women with genital herpes are available in the Morbidity and Mortality Weekly Report.[17] Women without known genital herpes should be counseled to avoid intercourse during the third trimester with partners known or suspected of having genital herpes. In addition, pregnant women without known orolabial herpes should be advised to avoid receptive oral sex during the third trimester with partners known or suspected to have orolabial herpes. Some specialists believe that type-specific serologic tests are useful to identify pregnant women at risk for HSV infection and to guide counseling regarding the risk for acquiring genital herpes during pregnancy. Testing should be offered to women without genital herpes whose sex partner has HSV infection.

Pregnant women should be asked whether they have a history of genital herpes. When labor begins, women should be questioned carefully about symptoms of genital herpes, including prodromal symptoms. All women should be examined carefully for herpetic lesions. Women without symptoms or signs of genital herpes or its prodrome can deliver vaginally. The majority of specialists recommend that women with recurrent genital herpetic lesions at the onset of labor deliver by cesarean section to prevent neonatal herpes. Unfortunately, cesarean section does not completely eliminate the risk for HSV transmission to the infant.

15.4.1.3 Molluscum Contagiosum

Molluscum contagiosum is caused by the DNA poxvirus, molluscum contagiosum virus (MCV). The disease is most commonly transmitted by direct skin contact and is more prevalent in children than adults. In children, the lesions may involve the face, trunk, and extremities and is usually transmitted through nonsexual means. In the adult population, MCV is usually transmitted sexually, particularly when found on the genital area and inner thighs. They appear as a single or

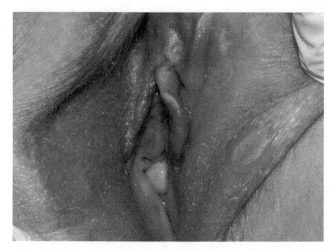

FIGURE 15.21. Herpes. Numerous erosions classic for herpes are demonstrated on the vulva. The inferior lesions are starting to coalesce into an ulcer.

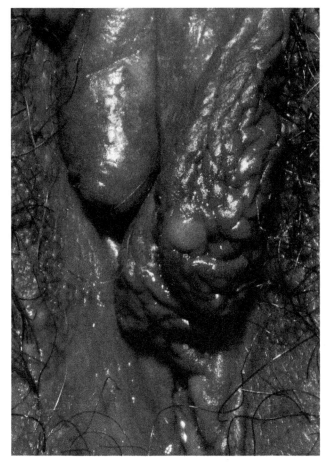

FIGURE 15.23.   Vulvar molluscum contagiosum with a small raised nodule with a central umbilicated dimple.

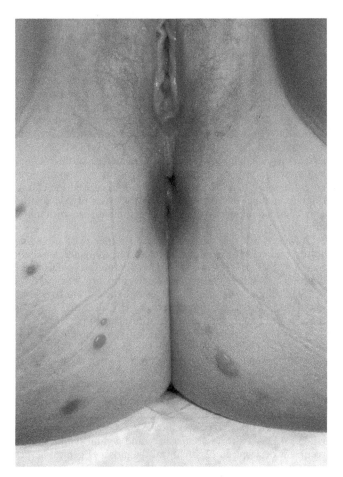

FIGURE 15.24.   Numerous lesions of molluscum contagiosum.

multiple isolated small papules (Figure 15.23) with a central umbilicated core that contains a cheesy material. Extensive body-wide papules may be present in patients with immunosuppression (Figure 15.24).

MCV is generally diagnosed by its clinical appearance, though it can be examined histologically by curetting or biopsying a lesion. On microscopic examination, the papule consists of focally hyperplastic squamous cells. The squamous cells near the center are filled with numerous eosinophilic inclusions known as molluscum bodies (Figure 15.25). These cells contain large numbers of viral particles that lyse as they enter the center and move upward. *In situ* hybridization for MCV DNA has also been performed.[21]

15.4.1.3.1 TREATMENT OF MOLLUSCUM CONTAGIOSUM

Molluscum contagiosum is a self-limited disease, which will most commonly resolve in immunocompetent hosts. In children, the lesions are generally left alone and given time to resolve.[22] However, the time to resolution can be quite long. Treatment of molluscum contagiosum is advisable in healthy adults to prevent autoinoculation or transmission. A variety of treatments for molluscum contagiosum exist including physical destruction of the lesions and topical treatments (Table 15.1).[23–25] Most authorities recommend physical destruction as the preferred method for treatment of MCV lesions. On rare occasions, systemic therapy is required.[26]

15.4.1.4 Condyloma

Warts are caused by HPV, of which more than 150 subtypes exist, 30 that are found on the genital area. Although

the most prevalent HPV type in genital warts is HPV type 6, approximately one-fourth of all condylomas contain HPV 11. Although external genital warts are commonly accompanied by cervical and/or vaginal HPV-expression, these lesions are most commonly low grade and likely to resolve spontaneously. Hence, the presence of external genital warts is not an indication for either colposcopy or accelerating the schedule for cervical screening (2006 ASCCP Guidelines).[1,8,26]

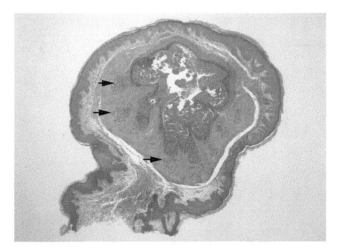

FIGURE 15.25.   Eosinophilic molluscum bodies that contain the viral particles (*arrows*). Acanthosis of the epidermis is present. (Hematoxylin-eosin stain; low power magnification.)

TABLE 15.1	COMMON TREATMENTS FOR MOLLUSCUM

Evisceration (scalpel, needle)
Curettage with dermal curette
Cantharidin—a single application that may need to be
  repeated once or twice every 3–4 wk
Tretinoin cream (0.1%) or gel (0.025%)—applied daily
Cryosurgery (liquid nitrogen, dry ice)
Tape stripping
Podophyllin, podofilox
Imiquimod 5% cream (best if applied under occlusion)
Trichloroacetic acid
Tincture of iodine
Silver nitrate or liquefied phenol
KOH
Cidofovir

Adapted from http://emedicine.medscape.com/article/1132908-
overview. Accessed November 30, 2009.

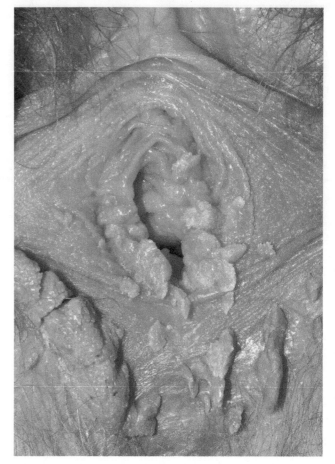

FIGURE 15.27. Vulvar condyloma. Multiple raised, papillary projections are demonstrated.

Vulvar condylomas may present as flat lesions (Figure 15.26) or exophytic lesions (Figure 15.27). Exophytic condylomas, or condylomata acuminata (genital warts), are typically papillary or verrucous in appearance. Although they can arise singly, condylomas usually occur in clusters and in many instances are confluent. External genital warts can be found at any site of the lower genital tract, including the vestibule, labia minora and majora, perineum, and perianal region. Clinical identification of condyloma is usually straightforward because of their characteristic appearance. They are often white in color but can be flesh colored, gray, brown (Figure 15.28), or multicolored (Figure 15.29). Soaking the affected area with a 5% acetic acid solution can help identify small lesions.

Histologically, exophytic condylomas demonstrate papillomatosis, acanthosis, and hyperkeratosis (Figure 15.30). The granular cell layer is prominent (granulosis). Occasional dyskeratocytes are seen. Multinucleation and the presence of koilocytes (cells with hyperchromasia, irregular nuclear borders, and perinuclear clearing) differentiate condylomas from other benign papillary skin tumors.[8]

Flat condylomas are indistinguishable from low-grade vulvar intraepithelial neoplasia (VIN). Histologically, they demonstrate some basal epithelial hyperplasia and cells with features consistent with koilocytosis. Mitotic activity and multinucleation also are present.

A variety of treatments exist for condyloma that can be divided into those that are patient applied and those provider applied.[27–29] Provider-applied treatments include local

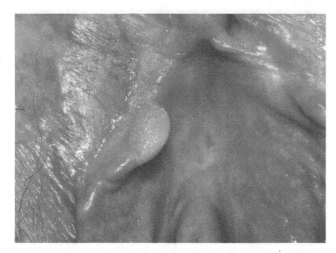

FIGURE 15.26. Flat vulvar condyloma. Punctation and early mosaicism are noted on the labium minus.

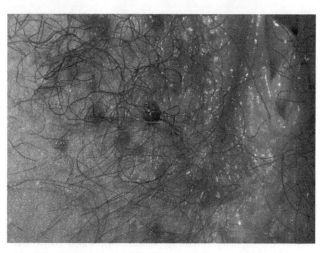

FIGURE 15.28. Vulvar condyloma with brown discoloration in multiple locations are present.

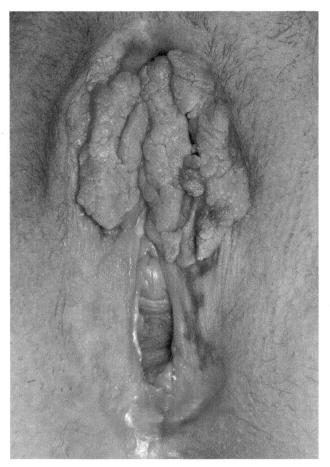

FIGURE 15.29.   Extensive vulvar condyloma with a variety of color changes are noted.

ablation using astringents such as bichloracetic or trichloracetic acid (50% to 90%)[30] and cryotherapy with either liquid nitrogen or a nitrous oxide tank with appropriate cryoprobe. Topical anesthesia may be applied before freezing the area. Podophyllin, which has mutagenic and systemic side effects,

is no longer in common use. Patient-applied therapies include podofilox 0.5% solution or gel, which are a safer alternative to podophyllin. The immunomodulator, imiquimod 5% cream, and Sinecatachins 15% ointment applied topically are successful in treating condyloma.[31] Interferon has been used to reduce intractable condylomas; however, interferon is very expensive and the long-term success from the use of this agent is not well established. Hence, the CDC sexually transmitted disease treatment guidelines do not recommend this therapy.[17]

Surgical excision, wire loop excision, and laser therapy[32] can also be used for larger lesions. It is often helpful in extensive disease to use a fine tip electrocautery pencil to debulk the condylomatous tissue (Figure 15.31) prior to laser treatment. Once this tissue is ablated and hemostasis achieved (Figure 15.32), a topical antibiotic is applied (Figure 15.33). Vigilant long-term observation is also acceptable for managing small isolated lesions. Nevertheless, lesions that enlarge, persist, or fail to respond to treatment require a biopsy to exclude VIN or carcinoma.[8]

15.4.2 Bacteria

15.4.2.1 Syphilis

Syphilis is associated with the spirochete organism *Treponema pallidum*. Primary syphilis usually appears 3 weeks after exposure and is characterized by the formation of a single ulcer, which is indurated ("hard chancre") and nontender (Figure 15.34). Inguinal adenopathy may be present. The ulcer regresses after 1 to 2 months. About one-third of untreated individuals with syphilis will develop secondary syphilis, which most commonly occurs 2 to 8 weeks after the appearance of the chancre but in some may not occur for many months. The primary presentation of secondary syphilis is a generalized skin rash that often involves the palms and soles. Mucous patches may also be found on the oral or vaginal mucosa. The characteristic genital lesions often found in secondary syphilis are the gray plaque-like lesions known as condyloma lata (Figure 15.35). A biopsy of a syphilitic lesion will demonstrate numerous perivascular and dermal plasma cells. Dark-field examinations and direct fluorescent antibody tests of lesion exudate or tissue are the definitive methods for diagnosing early syphilis. A presumptive diagnosis is possible with the use of two types of serologic tests: (1) nontreponemal tests (e.g.,

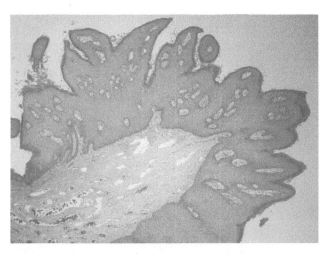

FIGURE 15.30.   Vulvar condyloma. There is acanthosis and extension of the papillary dermis (papillomatosis), which forms small spikes. Hyperkeratosis is also present. (Hematoxylin-eosin stain; low power magnification.)

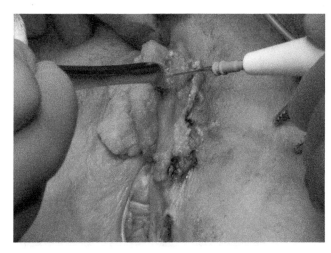

FIGURE 15.31.   A fine electrocautery tip is used to remove extensive condyloma, followed by CO_2 laser treatment.

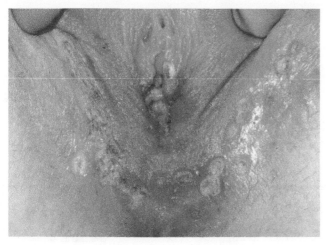

FIGURE 15.32. The procedure is completed and hemostasis is obtained.

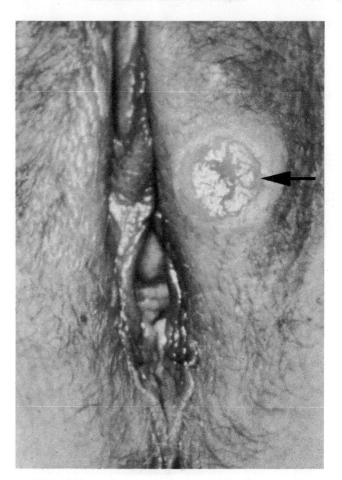

FIGURE 15.34. In this patient, primary syphilis characterized by a single large round indurated ulcer (chancre) occupying the center of the left labium majus (*arrow*). Note the relative lack of bleeding and discharge.

Venereal Disease Research Laboratory and reactive protein reagent) and (2) treponemal tests (e.g., fluorescent treponemal antibody absorbed and *T. pallidum* particle agglutination). The use of only one type of serologic test is insufficient for diagnosis because false-positive nontreponemal test results are sometimes associated with various medical conditions unrelated to syphilis.[17] Some clinical laboratories and blood banks now screen samples using treponemal enzyme immunoassay.[33] This strategy will identify both persons previously treated and persons with untreated or incompletely treated syphilis. False-positive results can occur, particularly among populations with a low prevalence of syphilis. These organisms can also be identified on biopsy material by applying silver stains.

Penicillin G, administered parenterally, is the preferred drug for treatment of all stages of syphilis. The preparation(s) used (i.e., benzathine, aqueous procaine, or aqueous crystalline), the dosage, and the length of treatment depend on the stage and clinical manifestations of the disease. For the primary syphilis seen with the vulvar chancre(s), benzathine penicillin G (50,000 units/kg up to the adult dose of 2.4 million units intramuscular [IM]) is given in a single dose. Neither combinations of benzathine penicillin and procaine penicillin nor oral penicillin preparations are considered appropriate for

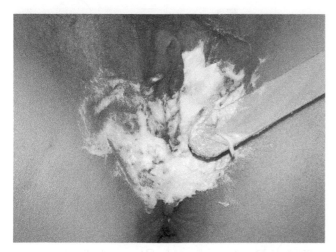

FIGURE 15.33. A topical antibiotic is applied to the surface of the vulva.

the treatment of syphilis. Reports have indicated that inappropriate use of combination benzathine-procaine penicillin (Bicillin C-R®) instead of the standard benzathine penicillin product widely used in the United States (Bicillin L-A®) has occurred.[17] Practitioners, pharmacists, and purchasing agents should be aware of the similar names of these two products and avoid use of the inappropriate combination therapy agent for treating syphilis.[17,34,35]

For nonpregnant patients who have primary or secondary syphilis, and allergies to penicillin, several therapies might be effective. Doxycycline (100 mg orally twice daily for 14 days) and tetracycline (500 mg four times daily for 14 days) are regimens that have been used for many years.[17] Adherence is likely to be better with doxycycline than tetracycline because of less frequent dosing and tetracycline can cause gastrointestinal side effects. It has been suggested that ceftriaxone is effective for treating early syphilis; however, the optimal dose and duration of ceftriaxone therapy have not been defined. Additionally, some patients who are allergic to penicillin also might be allergic to ceftriaxone; in these circumstances, use of an alternative agent might be required. Close follow-up of persons receiving alternative therapies is essential.[17] Patients with penicillin allergy whose compliance with therapy or follow-up cannot be ensured should be desensitized and treated with benzathine penicillin as described above.[17]

Additional screening for coinfection with other sexually transmitted diseases such as human immunodeficiency virus (HIV), *Neisseria gonorrhoeae,* and *Chlamydia trachomatis* is

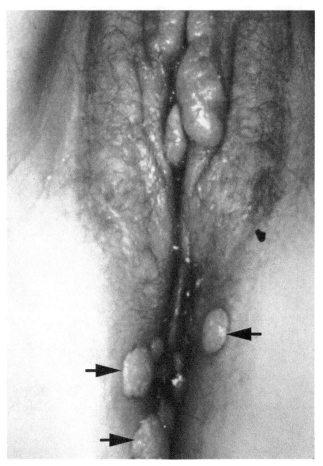

FIGURE 15.35. Secondary syphilis is characterized in this patient by raised broad-based papules (condyloma lata) along the posterior fourchette and perianal region (*arrows*). Note the similarity in appearance to genital warts (condyloma acuminatum) and fibroepithelial polyps. (Photos courtesy of the Armed Forces Institute of Pathology.)

prudent.[1,8,36] The CDC recommends that all women be screened serologically for syphilis during the early stages of pregnancy. For communities and populations in which the prevalence of syphilis is high, or for patients at high risk, serologic testing should be performed twice during the third trimester, at 28 to 32 weeks' gestation and at delivery.[17]

15.4.2.2 Granuloma Inguinale

Granuloma inguinale is a genital ulcerative disease caused by the intracellular gram-negative bacterium *Klebsiella granulomatis* (formerly known as *Calymmatobacterium granulomatis*).[17,37,38] While the disease occurs rarely in the United States, it is endemic in some tropical and developing areas, including India; Papua, New Guinea; central Australia; and southern Africa. Clinically, small red lesions appear on the vulva from 3 weeks to 3 months after exposure. These evolve into erosive ulcerations resulting in fibrosis and loss of superficial labial structures. Due to the extent of damage, fistula formation may occur. Inguinal lymphadenopathy also develops, but the degree is less than that seen with lymphogranuloma venereum (LGV) and chancroid (Figure 15.36). The causative organism is difficult to culture. Diagnosis requires visualization of dark-staining Donovan bodies on tissue crush preparation or biopsy (Figure 15.37).

Treatment consists of doxycycline 100 mg orally twice a day for at least 3 weeks and until all lesions have

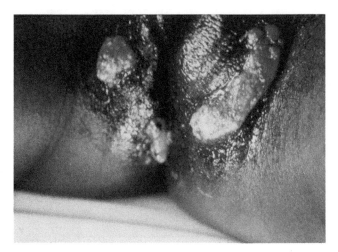

FIGURE 15.36. Vulvar granuloma inguinale. Large, irregularly shaped ulcerations erode the labia majora bilaterally and the perianal region (Photo courtesy of the Armed Forces Institute of Pathology, used with permission.)

completely healed. Several alternative treatment regimens exist utilizing azithromycin, ciprofloxacin, erythromycin, or trimethoprim-sulfamethoxazole.[17]

Therapy should be continued at least 3 weeks and until all lesions have completely healed. Some specialists recommend the addition of an aminoglycoside (e.g., gentamicin 1 mg/kg IV every 8 hours) to these regimens if improvement is not evident within the first few days of therapy. Relapse can occur 6 to 18 months after apparently effective therapy.

15.4.2.3 Chancroid

Chancroid is caused by *Haemophilus ducreyi*, a gram-negative anaerobic facultative bacillus. After an incubation period of 3 to 5 days, infected women will develop small papules that evolve into ulcers. Chancroid presents as a single or, more often, multiple ulcer with a necrotic base and purulent exudate.[39] These ulcers enlarge over time and become tender yet do not indurate ("soft chancres") (Figure 15.38). Sinus tracts may develop. Adenopathy also occurs and may eventually enlarge to form a bubo (an inflamed, purulent

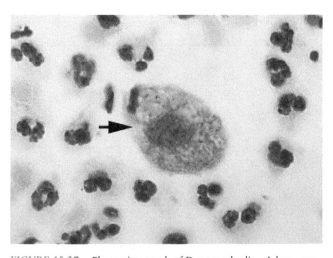

FIGURE 15.37. Photomicrograph of Donovan bodies. A large macrophage (*arrow*) contains numerous small organisms, many of which show a characteristic halo (Giemsa stain; high power magnification).

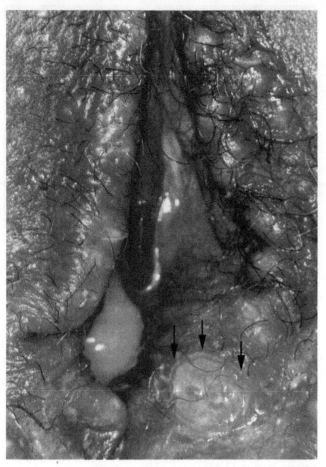

FIGURE 15.38.   Vulvar chancroid. An ulcer is present on the left posterior labium majus (*arrows*). In contrast to a syphilitic chancre, the shape is less round and symmetrical. (Photo courtesy Wilkinson EJ, Stone IK. *Atlas of Vulvar Diseases* (2nd ed.). Baltimore, MD: Lippincott Williams & Wilkins, 2008, used with permission.)

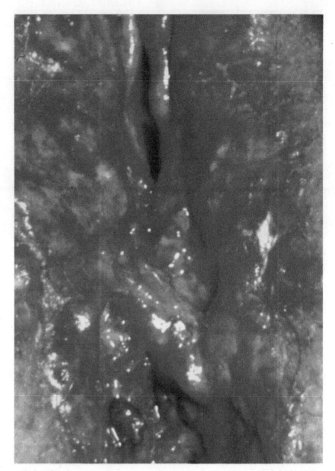

FIGURE 15.39.   Vulvar lymphogranuloma venereum. Large erosive areas replace a portion of the mons and the labia majora. Surface hemorrhage is present.

lymph node). In its late stage, a chancroid resembles other erosive vulvar conditions such as Crohn's disease, granuloma inguinale, and LGV. In Crohn's disease, however, ulcerations occur along labial or inguinal skin folds and most often involves the bowel. In cases of LGV, the ulcers rapidly resolve into inguinal adenopathy with large draining buboes.

A definitive diagnosis of chancroid requires the identification of *H. ducreyi* on special culture media. This test is not widely available from commercial sources. No Food and Drug Administration (FDA)-approved PCR test for *H. ducreyi* is available in the United States, but such testing can be performed by clinical laboratories that have developed their own PCR test and conducted a Clinical Laboratory Improvement Amendments (CLIA) validation analysis.[17] The combination of a painful genital ulcer and tender suppurative inguinal adenopathy suggests the diagnosis of chancroid. A probable diagnosis of chancroid can be made if the following criteria are met: (1) the patient has one or more painful genital ulcers; (2) the patient has no evidence of *T. pallidum* infection by dark-field examination of ulcer exudate or by a serologic test for syphilis performed at least 7 days after onset of ulcers; (3) the clinical presentation, appearance of genital ulcers, and, if present, regional lymphadenopathy are typical for chancroid; and (4) a test for HSV performed on the ulcer exudate is negative.[17]

Treatment consists of a variety of antibiotics including azithromycin, ceftriaxone, ciprofloxacin, or erythromycin base.[17] Azithromycin and ceftriaxone offer the advantage of single-dose therapy.

15.4.3 Chlamydia

15.4.3.1 Lymphogranuloma Venereum

LGV is an ulcerative vulvar lesion that is associated with the Chlamydial organism. *C. trachomatis* are intracellular bodies that are associated with a number of mucosal abnormalities (trachoma, genital lesions), depending on the serotype. Serotypes L1, L2, and L3 are associated with LGV. Recent outbreaks have been reported from numerous countries.[40] The most common clinical manifestation of LGV among heterosexuals is tender inguinal and/or femoral lymphadenopathy that is typically unilateral. A self-limited genital ulcer or papule sometimes occurs at the site of inoculation. However, by the time patients seek care, the lesions might have disappeared. The small painless ulcers on the vulva, rectum, and perineum appear 1 to 3 days after inoculation (Figure 15.39). These ulcers quickly heal, and a lymphangitis develops over the ensuing months. The disease extends bilaterally into multiple inguinal nodes, which enlarge, coalesce, and form draining abscesses or buboes (Figure 15.40). These buboes can be found above and below the inguinal ligament. Due to obstructed lymphatic drainage, elephantiasis of the vulva has been observed.

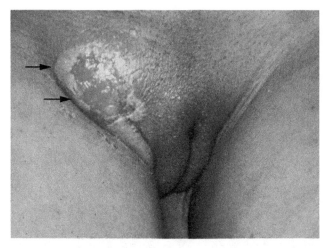

FIGURE 15.40.   A large bubo (*arrows*) is located in the right inguinal region. (Photos courtesy of the Armed Forces Institute of Pathology, used with permission.)

The microscopic features are nonspecific but can include a mixed inflammatory response and severe fibrosis. A culture or a complement fixation assay using a titer greater than 1:64 can confirm the presence of chlamydial organisms. Diagnosis is based on clinical suspicion, epidemiologic information, and the exclusion of other etiologies of proctocolitis, inguinal lymphadenopathy, or genital or rectal ulcers, along with *C. trachomatis* testing, if available.

Swabs or bubo aspirates from genital and lymph node specimens may be tested for *C. trachomatis* by culture, direct immunofluorescence, or nucleic acid detection. Nucleic acid amplification tests (NAAT) for *C. trachomatis* are not cleared by the FDA for testing rectal specimens. Additional procedures (e.g., genotyping) are required for differentiating LGV from non-LGV *C. trachomatis*. However, these tests are not widely available.[17]

Chlamydia serology (complement fixation titers >1:64) can support the diagnosis. However, serologic test interpretation for LGV is not standardized, tests have not been validated for clinical proctitis presentations, and *C. trachomatis* serovar–specific serologic tests are not widely available.

In the absence of specific LGV diagnostic testing, patients with a clinical syndrome consistent with LGV, including proctocolitis or genital ulcer disease with lymphadenopathy, should be treated with the same regimen as those with a definitive diagnosis for LGV. The recommended treatment is oral administration of doxycycline 100 mg PO bid for 21 days. An alternative regimen is erythromycin base 500 mg qid for 21 days. Doses of both drugs should be doubled in severe infections. An alternate treatment regimen is azithromycin.[17,41,42] Fluctuant buboes should be aspirated to prevent rupture. Incision or biopsy of buboes is not recommended, as sinus tracts may form.

15.4.4 Fungi

15.4.4.1 Candidiasis

15.4.4.1.1 Vulvovaginal Candidiasis

Despite therapeutic advances, vulvovaginal candidiasis (VVC) remains a common problem worldwide.[43] The incidence of mycotic vulvovaginitis is rising dramatically in the United States. There are over 13 million cases of VVC annually in the United States. Seventy-five percent of all women will have at least one episode of VVC. About half of those infected experience more than one episode. Five percent of women with VVC

TABLE 15.2	RISK FACTORS FOR RVVC
Antibiotic use	Receptive oral genital sex
Estrogen excess (oral contraceptive pills, hormone replacement, local estrogens)	Glucose excess (uncontrolled diabetes, refined sugar excess)
Immune suppression (lupus, HIV, corticosteroids)	Vulvar dermatoses (LS, eczema, atopic dermatitis)
Intrauterine device use	Sponge for contraception
Stress	

Adapted from Sobel JD. Pathogenesis of recurrent vulvovaginal candidiasis. *Curr Infect Dis Rep* 2002;4:514–9.

will develop recurrent episodes. Predisposing factors are listed in Table 15.2.[44,45] Additionally, immune system alterations such as HIV/AIDS may be associated with a higher incidence and greater persistence of yeast infections.

The majority of vulvovaginal yeast infections are caused by the organism *Candida albicans*. However, over the past two decades, an increasing trend in the number of vaginal infections attributable to yeasts other than *C. albicans* has emerged. Recently, there has been an increase in the number of Candida infections caused by *Candida glabrata*.

The most common presentation, particularly with *C. albicans*, is vulvar itching and burning. A white "cottage cheese" discharge is often present (Figure 15.41). However, *C. glabrata* may present primarily with introital sensitivity and burning during intercourse, little discharge, and the sensation of introital dryness. Erythema of the vulva is common, but not always present (Figure 15.42).

A wet mount preparation (a small amount of discharge placed on a glass slide with a saline solution) reveals spores of *C. albicans*, which are uniform in size, isolated, and almost always associated with hyphae filaments. The spores of *C. glabrata* are of variable size (2 to 8 □m), spherical or ovoid, and usually smaller than a red cell. They are often grouped in clusters, although they may appear alone. Potassium hydroxide (KOH) (10% to 20%) preparation is often used to evaluate for yeast when they are not seen on saline prep. In this solution, white blood cells and red blood cells dissolve. The branching, budding, and cell walls of *C. albicans* are easily visualized. Rapid antigen testing is also available for Candida. A positive test is very helpful, but a negative test does not rule out infection.

In biopsy specimens, special stains such as periodic acid-Schiff stain or Gomori's stain are necessary to localize these organisms.[1,8] The presence of persistent budding forms may indicate the presence of *C. glabrata*. Accurate diagnosis depends on culture techniques that will yield correct identification of the fungal species.

Cultures should be obtained when symptoms are not explained on the wet prep or when patients present with recurrent candidiasis. Some yeast forms may require as long as a month of incubation for detection (particularly with a small inoculum). Sabouraud's dextrose agar on modified Sabouraud's Difco mycobiotic media and Nickerson's media are satisfactory for growing Candida in an incubator or at room temperature, although identification of the species is not possible. The most reliable differentiation of the species is provided by sugar fermentation reactions.

15.4.4.1.2 Treatments

It is necessary to consider removal or improvement of predisposing factors, such as uncontrolled diabetes mellitus and vaginal douching, in the treatment of candidiasis. Numerous

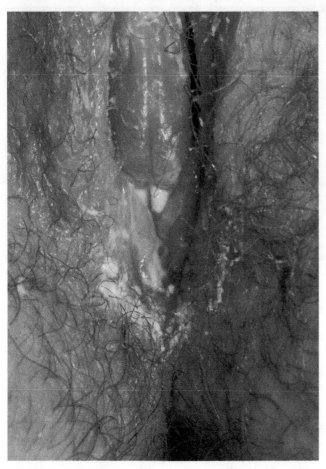

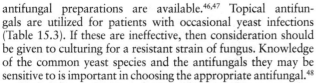

FIGURE 15.41.   Vulvar candidiasis. Thick, curd-like white discharge is present on a patient complaining of pruritus, classic for *Candida albicans*.

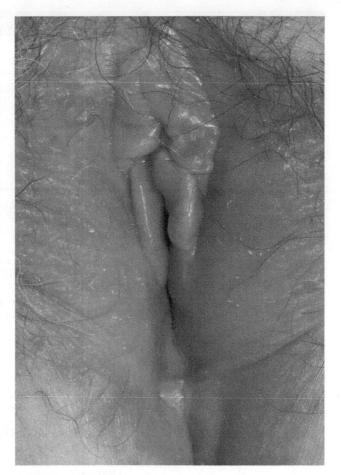

FIGURE 15.42.   Vulvar candidiasis. An erythematous, irritated vulva is seen in the patient with *C. glabrata*.

antifungal preparations are available.[46,47] Topical antifungals are utilized for patients with occasional yeast infections (Table 15.3). If these are ineffective, then consideration should be given to culturing for a resistant strain of fungus. Knowledge of the common yeast species and the antifungals they may be sensitive to is important in choosing the appropriate antifungal.[48]

With failure of topical therapies or recurrent yeast infections, oral preparations should be considered. Oral azoles are also used for short-term treatment, having the same spectrum of activity as topical azoles. The most common oral antifungal is fluconazole, 150 mg one time orally for a patient with occasional yeast infections. Other agents such as ketoconazole and itraconazole have been utilized.[49]

15.4.4.1.3 MANAGEMENT OF CHRONIC AND RECURRENT VVC

Recurrent vulvovaginal candidiasis (RVVC) is defined as four or more episodes of symptomatic Candida vaginitis in a 12-month period. To maintain clinical and mycologic control, some specialists recommend a longer duration of initial therapy (e.g., 7 to 14 days of topical therapy or a 100 mg, 150 mg, or sequential therapy).[50] One regimen consists of 150 to 200 mg oral dose of fluconazole every third day for a total of three doses (day 1, 4, and 7) to attempt mycologic remission before initiating a maintenance weekly oral antifungal regimen. Most patients with recurrent yeast prefer the oral antifungals. Side effects occur infrequently. Hepatotoxicity, such as is seen with ketoconazole, occurs far less often with fluconazole but is a known complication. In a patient with no known

liver function abnormalities, consider checking liver function tests after 6 months of treatment with fluconazole.

15.4.4.1.4 MAINTENANCE REGIMENS

Oral fluconazole (i.e., 100-, 150-, or 200-mg dose) weekly for 6 months is the first line of treatment.[51,52] If this regimen is not feasible, some specialists recommend topical clotrimazole, 200 mg twice a week, or clotrimazole (500-mg dose vaginal suppositories once weekly), or other topical treatments used intermittently.

Suppressive maintenance antifungal therapies are effective in reducing RVVC. However, 30% to 50% of women will have recurrent disease after maintenance therapy is discontinued. Routine treatment of sex partners is controversial. *C. albicans* azole resistance is rare in vaginal isolates, and susceptibility testing is usually not warranted for individual treatment guidance.

A variety of other topical treatments are utilized dependent on the yeast species. These include boric acid suppositories (per vagina), topical gentian violet, and topical 5-flucytosine (Table 15.4).[53–58] Many of the above agents are not to be recommended in pregnancy. Generally topical azole therapies, applied for 7 days, are recommended for use among pregnant women.[17]

15.4.4.2 Tinea Cruris

Tinea cruris is a superficial fungal infection of the groin and adjacent skin. Clinically, tinea cruris presents as a reddened area with raised sharp borders (Figure 15.43) occurring along

TABLE 15.3   TOPICAL ANTIFUNGAL AGENTS (FIRST-LINE THERAPY) FOR THE PRIMARY TREATMENT OF VVC

■ DRUG	■ FORMULATION	■ DOSAGE
Butoconazole (Gynazole-1®)	2% vaginal cream	1 applicator (5 g) vaginally × 1 d
Butoconazole (Femstat 3®, Mycelex-3®)	2% vaginal cream	1 applicator (5 g) vaginally × 3 d
Butoconazole 1 sustained release (Gynazole 1)	2% vaginal cream	1 applicator (5 g) vaginally once
Clotrimazole vaginal (Mycelex 7®, Gyne-Lotrimin 7)	1% cream	1 applicator (5 g) vaginally × 7 d
Clotrimazole vaginal tablet (Gyne-Lotrimin, Mycelex®)	100-mg vaginal tablet	1 tablet vaginally daily for 7 days or 2 tablets vaginally daily for 3 days
Clotrimazole (Gyne-Lotrimin 3®)	2% vaginal cream	1 applicator vaginally for 3 d
Clotrimazole (Lotrimin)*	Cream 1% Lotion 1% Solution 1%	Apply cream topically to vulva twice daily
Clotrimazole (Lotrisone®)	Clotrimazole.1% topical cream with betamethasone 0.5%	Apply cream topically to vulva BID (maximum use 2–4 wk)
Miconazole (Monistat 7®)	2% vaginal cream	1 applicator (5 g) vaginally × 7 d
Miconazole (Monistat 7®)	100 mg vaginal suppository	1 suppository vaginally daily for 7 d
Miconazole (Monistat 7® Combination pack)	100 mg vaginal suppository and 2% topical cream	1 suppository vaginally × 7 days; apply cream twice daily (maximum use 2–4 wk)
Miconazole (Monistat 7® Combination pack)	2% vaginal and 2% topical cream	1 applicator of 2% cream for 7 days; apply topically twice daily (maximum use 2–4 wk)
Miconazole (Monistat 3®)	200 mg ovule	Insert 1 ovule vaginally × 3 d
Miconazole (Monistat 3®)	4% vaginal cream	1 applicator (5 g) vaginally × 3 d
Miconazole (Monistat 3®)	200 mg vaginal suppository	1 suppository vaginally × 3 d
Miconazole (Monistat 3® Combination pack)	200 mg vaginal suppository and 2% topical cream	1 suppository vaginally for 3 nights; 2% cream bid topically
Miconazole (Monistat 3® Combination pack)	4% cream and 2% topical cream	1 applicator of 4% cream for 3 nights; 2% cream bid topically
Monistat 1 Combination Pack®	Ovule insert (miconazole nitrate 1200 mg) for vagina plus miconazole nitrate cream 2% for vulva	Insert 1 ovule vaginally × 3 days; 2% cream bid topically
Miconazole (Monistat 1®)	1200 mg vaginal suppository	1 suppository vaginally once
Tioconazole (Vagistat-1®, Monistat 1®)	6.5% vaginal cream	1 applicator (5 g) vaginally once
Terconazole (Terazol 7®)	0.4% vaginal cream	1 applicator (5 g) vaginally × 7 d
Terconazole (Terazol 3®)	0.8% vaginal cream	1 applicator (5 g) vaginally × 3 d
Terconazole (Terazol 3®)	80 mg vaginal suppository	1 suppository vaginally × 3 d
Econazole nitrate (Spectazole®)	1% topical cream	Apply cream to vulva twice daily
Polyene nystatin	100,000-unit vaginal tablet	1 tablet daily for 14 d (best choice for 1st trimester of pregnancy)
Nystatin powder	100,000 units/g	Apply to vulva bid × 14 d
Nystatin topical (Mycostatin topical®)	100,000 units/g cream, ointment, powder	Apply to vulva bid × 14 d
Nystatin/triamcinolone topical	100,00 units/1 mg cream, ointment	Apply to vulva bid × 14 d

the inner aspect of the thigh. It often extends into the perianal and perineal region. Tinea cruris may be very itchy. It is three times more common in men than in women. Adults are affected much more commonly than children.[59] The organisms responsible for this type of tinea are the dermatophytes, *Trichophyton rubrum* and *Epidermophyton floccosum* (most common), and *Trichophyton mentagrophytes* and *Trichophyton verrucosum* (less common).

The diagnosis of tinea cruris is made by KOH preps and fungal staining for fungal elements from scrapings of scaly lesions. Adding dimethyl sulfoxide (DMSO) to the KOH speeds the destructions of keratocytes in the sample, and inexpensive premixed KOH, DMSO, and fungal stain (such as Swartz-Lampkin stain) combinations are commercially available. Specific instructions for this procedure have been previously described.[60] Growth on Mycosel or Sabouraud agar plates usually is sufficient within 3 to 6 weeks to allow specific fungal identification.

A punch biopsy is diagnostic but has a low sensitivity and a low specificity. A Wood lamp examination may help to exclude erythrasma, which usually will glow red in color.[60]

Treatment involves application of topical antifungal creams or powders medications (Table 15.5).[61] With follicular or extensive disease, a combination of topical and systemic therapy is often used.

15.5 VULVODYNIA

Vulvodynia is a condition that is challenging for patients and health care providers. The pain and discomfort of vulvodynia affects the quality of life of women with this condition. Pain can be continuous or intermittent and is most often aggravated by activities such as sitting at a desk, bicycle riding, and sexual intercourse.

TABLE 15.4	OTHER TOPICAL MEDICATIONS UTILIZED FOR VVC	
■ AGENT	**■ DOSAGE**	**■ NOTES**
Boric acid suppositories (per vagina)	Fill a gel capsule halfway (600 mg). For the initial treatment, a 600-mg capsule is inserted per vagina nightly for 14 d. For long-term maintenance, insert into vagina twice weekly.	Especially useful with *C. glabrata*
Gentian violet	0.25% or 0.5% aqueous solution is applied at home daily or it may be given in the health care providers' office as a 1.0% solution (once weekly for up to three times).	Permanent purple staining on clothing may occur. Some patients develop a vulvar irritation following application of gentian violet.
5-flucytosine	500 mg/5 g compounded in hydrophilic cream base. Insert 5 g per vagina qhs × 14 nights.	Pyrimidine developed for use as an anticancer drug. Though not effective against cancer, it is fungicidal and is apparently deaminated within the yeast cell to 5-fluorouracil, which is incorporated into RNA and interferes with cell development. Extremely expensive.
Amphotericin B	50-mg amphotericin B vaginal suppositories nightly × 14 days	Can be combined with flucytosine if needed.

15.5.1 Historical Information

A discussion of vulvar pain first appeared in the literature in the late 1800s. Dr. Theodor G. Thomas described a patient with "excessive sensibility of the nerves supplying the mucous membrane of some portion of the vulva..."[62] In 1889, Dr. Alexander Skene commented on a condition characterized by "a supersensitiveness of the vulva. When, however, the examining finger comes in contact with the hyperaesthetic part, the patient complains of pain, which is sometimes so great as to cause her to cry out...."[63] The topic was not readdressed until 1928, when Dr. Howard Kelly mentioned "exquisitely sensitive deep red spots in the mucosa of the hymeneal ring are a fruitful source of dyspareunia."[64] In 1983, Dr. Eduard G. Friedrich, Jr., reported on 13 patients with "vestibular adenitis."[65]

15.5.2 Terminology

The International Society for the Study of Vulvovaginal Disease (ISSVD) popularized a definition of vulvar pain in the 1980s (essential or dysesthetic vulvodynia) describing patients with a chronic discomfort, burning, stinging, irritation, and rawness of the vulva. In 1987, Friedrich developed the term "vulvar vestibulitis syndrome."[66] The most recent terminology changes are described in Table 15.6.[67]

Patients with pain localized to the vestibule have a normal-appearing vulva, other than occasional erythema. Although erythema in the posterior part of the vestibule (especially at the 4 and 8 o'clock location near the major vestibular duct openings) is felt to be classic for vestibulodynia (Figure 15.44), erythema in the vestibule is quite variable. There are two major forms of vulvar pain, hyperalgesia (low pain thresholds) and allodynia (pain to light touch).

15.5.3 Etiologic Theories

The exact etiology of vulvodynia is unknown and is most likely due to multiple causes. Etiologic theories proposed include abnormalities of embryologic development, infection, inflammation, genetic/immune factors, and nerve pathways. Table 15.7 summarizes the various theories on the potential etiologies of vulvodynia.[68-80] Since this disorder may occur in postmenopausal women, it is imperative that atrophic vaginitis be considered in the differential diagnosis of vulvodynia.

15.5.3.1 Vaginismus

Vaginismus is an involuntary *spasm* of the *pelvic floor* muscles affecting the introitus. It is important to evaluate for vaginismus in the patients with vulvodynia, particularly if the pain is localized vulvodynia.[81] It can make penetration painful or even impossible. One of the main causes is fear or anticipation of pain. When painful penetration has been experienced, this pain may be expected in further sexual intercourse attempts. The degree of vaginismus may then increase the amount of pain, and a vicious circle is established.

15.5.4 Treatment of Vulvodynia

15.5.4.1 Treatment of Localized Vulvar Pain (Vestibulodynia)

Many treatment regimens exist for localized vulvodynia. Patients often combine a variety of the following regimens:

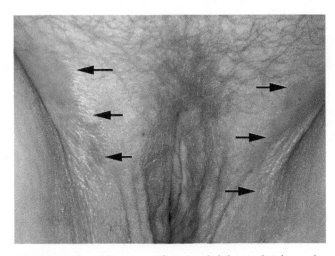

FIGURE 15.43. Vulvar tinea. Glistening slightly raised pink macular areas are located in the right and left inguinal regions (*arrows*). (Photo courtesy Dr. Gordon Davis, used with permission.)

TABLE 15.5   TOPICAL ANTIFUNGAL AGENTS (FIRST-LINE THERAPY) FOR THE PRIMARY TREATMENT OF TINEA CRURIS

DRUG	FORMULATION	DOSAGE
Butenafine (Mentax)	Cream 1%	Apply topically once per day
Ciclopirox (Loprox)	Cream 1%, lotion 1%, topical suspension 0.77%	Apply topically twice per day
Clotrimazole (Lotrimin, Mycelex)*	Cream 1%, lotion 1%, solution 1%	Apply topically twice per day
Clotrimazole with betamethasone (Lotrisone)	Clotrimazole 1% with betamethasone 0.5% cream	Apply topically twice per day (maximum use 2–4 wk)
Econazole (Spectazole)	Cream 1%	Apply topically once per day
Haloprogin (Halotex)	1% cream, 1% solution, 1% spray	Apply topically three times per day
Ketoconazole (Nizoral)	Cream 2%	Apply topically once per day
Miconazole (Micatin, Monistat-Derm)*	Cream 2%	Apply topically twice per day
Naftifine (Naftin)	Cream 1% Gel 1%	Apply topically once per day (cream) Apply twice per day (gel)
Oxiconazole (Oxistat)	Cream 1%, lotion 1%	Apply topically once or twice per day
Sertaconazole (Ertaczo)	Cream 2%	Apply topically twice per day
Sulconazole (Exelderm)	Cream 1%, solution 1%	Apply topically once or twice per day
Terbinafine (Lamisil)	Cream 1%, gel 1%	Apply topically once or twice per day
Tolnaftate (Tinactin)*	Cream 1%, gel 1%, powder 1%, topical aerosol, liquid (1%), powder (1%), solution 1%	Apply topically twice per day

*Also available in over-the-counter preparations.

15.5.4.1.1 VULVAR CARE MEASURES

Cotton underwear is recommended. No underwear should be worn at night. If the patient is sweating with exercise, Wicking underwear has been used by some patients. Vulvar irritants such as perfumes, washes, and over-the-counter anesthetics, as well as douching should be avoided. The patient should be advised to use mild soaps for bathing, to not apply soaps to the vulva, to not use fabric softeners on underclothes, and to fully rinse underwear after washing. If menstrual pads are irritating, 100% cotton pads may be helpful. Adequate lubrication for intercourse is recommended. Cool gel packs are helpful in some patients.

15.5.4.1.1.0 Topical Medications

The use of lubricants should be discussed with the patient. For minor degrees of vulvar pain, consider lidocaine ointment. Doxepin 5% cream can be applied to skin daily with gradual increase not to exceed four times daily. Topical amitriptyline 2% with Baclofen 2% in a water-washable base (squirt 1/2 mL from syringe onto finger and apply to affected area daily for three times a day) has also been used for point tenderness. Topical estrogens have been used by some for treatment of vulvar pain. Estrogen is applied to the vulva twice daily, with a gradual decrease to daily use, then every other day use. Topical nitroglycerin has been used for the treatment of localized vulvar pain.[82] Unfortunately, a significant number of patients developed headaches with its use.

15.5.4.1.1.0 Tricyclic Antidepressants

A common treatment for vulvar pain is the use of a tricyclic antidepressant. This group of drugs (e.g., amitriptyline [Elavil®], nortriptyline [Pamelor®], desipramine [Norpramin®]) has been used to treat many chronic pain conditions where a cause cannot be found. Information on the medication dosages

TABLE 15.6   ISSVD TERMINOLOGY AND CLASSIFICATION OF VULVAR PAIN (2003)

(A) Vulvar pain related to a specific disorder
  (1) Infectious (e.g., candidiasis, herpes, etc.)
  (2) Inflammatory (e.g., lichen planus, immunobullous disorders, etc.)
  (3) Neoplastic (e.g., Paget's disease, squamous cell carcinoma, etc.)
  (4) Neurologic (e.g., herpes neuralgia, spinal nerve compression, etc.)
(B) Vulvodynia
  (1) Generalized
    (a) Provoked (sexual, nonsexual, or both)
    (b) Unprovoked
    (c) Mixed (provoked and unprovoked)
  (2) Localized (vestibulodynia, clitorodynia, hemivulvodynia, etc.)
    (a) Provoked (sexual, nonsexual, or both)
    (b) Unprovoked
    (c) Mixed (provoked and unprovoked)

Reprinted from Moyal-Barracco M, Lynch PJ. 2003 ISSVD terminology and classification of vulvodynia: a historical perspective. *J Reprod Med* 2004;49(10):772–7, with permission.

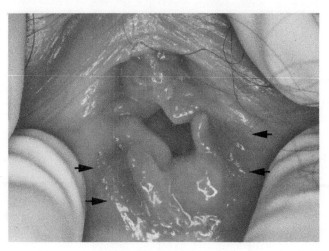

FIGURE 15.44. Marked vestibular erythema in the posterior vestibule at the 4 and 8 o'clock positions *(arrows)* are classic for vestibulodynia. (Photo courtesy of Dr. Gordon Davis, used with permission.)

utilized for vulvodynia can be obtained at: http://www.med.umich.edu/obgyn/cvd/ref_phys.htm

Published and presented reports indicate about a 60% response rate for various pain conditions. Currently, a National Institutes of Health trial is analyzing antidepressants in patients with vulvar pain. While traditionally this treatment has been used for generalized vulvodynia, recent reports have found it to be helpful in treating vestibular pain as well. The mechanism of action is believed to be associated with blockage of reuptake of transmitters, specifically norepinephrine and serotonin. Yet, the mechanism may actually be from the anticholinergic effects of the medication by affecting sodium channels and N-methyl-D-aspartate receptors. When recommending a tricyclic antidepressant, consider emphasizing to the patient that the primary effect of the drug, when used for the treatment of vulvodynia, is in altering the sensation of pain rather than its effect on depression. Understanding this difference may aid adherence to the regimen. Patients should not be pregnant or intend to become pregnant or breast-feed while using tricyclic antidepressants. These medicines will add to the effects of alcohol and other CNS depressants. Other antidepressants have been used for vulvodynia including duloxetine (Cymbalta) and Effexor XR (Venlafaxine). Anticonvulsants are helpful in treating vulvodynia. Gabapentin (Neurontin®) has been used to treat chronic pain conditions.[83,84] Another anticonvulsant utilized for chronic pain is pregabalin (Lyrica®).

Biofeedback and physical therapy are also currently used in the treatment of vulvar pain.[85-90] Biofeedback aids in developing self-regulation strategies for confronting and reducing pain. Patients with vestibular pain in general have an increased resting tone and a decreased contraction tone. With the aid of an electronic measurement and amplification system or biofeedback machine, an individual can view a display of numbers on a meter or colored lights to assess nerve and muscle tension. In this way, it is possible to develop voluntary control over those biological systems involved in pain, discomfort, and disease. The time required for biofeedback and the frequencies of visits will vary with each person. Success rates in the 60% to 80% range have been reported. Physical therapists with experience in vulvar pain can frequently be helpful.

Trigger point steroid and bupivacaine injections have been successful for some patients with localized vulvodynia.[91,92] This regimen can be repeated monthly. Generally patients do not tolerate more than three or four injections. Consider using a topical anesthetic prior to the injection. Interferon has also been studied and utilized for vestibular pain.[93-100] It has a varied

■ TABLE 15.7	VARIOUS THEORIES ON THE ETIOLOGIES OF VULOVDYNIA
■ THEORY	**■ DESCRIPTIONS**
Embryologic development	It has been noted that tissues from these two distinct anatomic sites have a common embryologic origin and therefore are predisposed to similar pathologic responses when challenged.
Infection	Candida infections in patients with vestibular pain have been studied. The exact association is difficult to determine since many patients report candida infections without verified testing for yeast. Bazin et al. found little association of infection and pain on the vestibule.
Inflammation	"-itis" (as in vestibulitis) has been excluded from the recent ISSVD terminology since studies found a lack of association between excised tissue and inflammation. Bohm-Starke et al. found a low expression of the inflammatory markers cyclooxygenase 2 and inducible nitric oxide synthase in the vestibular mucosa of women localized vestibular pain as well as in healthy control subjects.
Genetic/immune factors	Goetsch was one of the first researchers to question a genetic association of localized vulvar pain. Fifteen percent of patients questioned over a 6-month period were found to have localized vestibular pain. Thirty-two percent had a female relative with dyspareunia or tampon intolerance, raising the issue of a genetic predisposition. Another genetic connection was found in a study evaluating gene coding for interleukin 1 receptor antagonist.
Neuropathways	Kermit Krantz examined the nerve characteristics of the vulva and vagina. The region of the hymenal ring was richly supplied with free nerve endings. No corpuscular endings of any form were observed. Only free nerve endings were observed in the fossa navicularis. A sparsity of nerve endings were noted in the vagina as compared to the region of the fourchette, fossa navicularis, and hymenal ring. More recent studies have analyzed the nerve factors, thermoreceptors, and nociceptors in women with vulvar pain.

response long term and is used less frequently today. Botulinum toxin (Botox) type A is used as a treatment for many chronic pain disorders.[101,102] Recent studies have been done on injectable Botox for vulvar pain, many with positive outcomes.[103–106] Further studies are being performed.

Few studies have evaluated the use of acupuncture for vulvar pain.[107–109] A recent article by Kandyba and Binik describes successful use of hypnotherapy as a treatment for pain localized to the vestibule.[110]

Surgical excision of the vulvar vestibule has met with success in up to 80% of reported cases but should be reserved for women with long-standing and localized vestibular pain where other management has failed.[111] The patient should undergo cotton swab testing to outline the areas of pain prior to anesthesia while in the operating room. Often the incision will need to extend to the opening of Skene's ducts onto the vestibule. It is carried down laterally along Hart's line to the perianal skin. The mucosa should be undermined above the hymenal ring. The specimen should be excised superior to the hymenal ring. The vaginal tissue is further undermined and brought down to close the defect. The defect should be closed in two layers using absorbable 3-0 and 4-0 sutures.[112] On microscopic examination, inflammatory cells may be seen in the stroma surrounding the minor vestibular glands (Figure 15.45). However, this finding is not specific as inflammation may also be seen in normal tissue. The vulvodynia algorithm summarizes the diagnosis and treatment of vulvodynia (Figure 15.46).

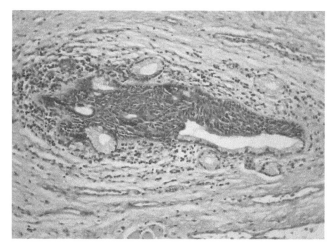

FIGURE 15.45. Photomicrograph of a biopsy from a patient with (or showing) histologic features underlying vestibulodynia. Chronic inflammatory cells surround a cluster of minor vestibular glands. There is also focal squamous metaplasia. (Hematoxylin-eosin stain; medium power magnification.)

15.6 VULVAR NONNEOPLASTIC EPITHELIAL CONDITIONS

Lichen sclerosus (LS), lichen planus, and squamous cell hyperplasia (lichen simplex chronicus) are the most common nonneoplastic epithelial disorders of the vulva.[113] Historically, there has been a long-standing uncertainty regarding the classification of the so-called nonneoplastic and preneoplastic vulvar lesions. Various specialties have had an interest in identifying and categorizing vulvar abnormalities. In some cases, this led to an overlapping of terms representing the same clinical entity and considerable confusion among clinicians about the significance and management of these lesions.

In 1976, the ISSVD proposed a categorization of the *vulvar dystrophies*, dividing them into two general groups, atrophic dystrophy and hyperplastic dystrophy. Because of continued misunderstanding regarding terminology and definitions as new terms were introduced, ISSVD, in conjunction with the International Society for Gynecologic Pathologists modified the original two categories into three categories. Table 15.8 summarizes the reclassification.[114,115]

Patients with these conditions frequently complain of itching.[116] Treatment regimens for the nonneoplastic abnormalities usually include topical steroid ointments. Table 15.9 lists the different steroid potency levels and examples of various medications for each category.

15.6.1 Lichen Sclerosus

In the dermatologic literature, LS was previously referred to as *lichen sclerosus et atrophicus*. Vulvar LS also has been labeled *kraurosis vulvae*. The term *lichen sclerosus* is preferred because the surface epithelial cells are metabolically active and not truly "atrophic."[117]

The disorder tends to occur among postmenopausal women but can occur at any age. The etiology of the condition is unknown, although there is some indication that the disease represents an autoimmune phenomenon.[118] Various autoantibodies such as antithyroid, gastric parietal cell, intrinsic factor, and antinuclear and anti–smooth-muscle antibodies have been identified in patients with LS. There is an association of hypothyroidism and LS.[119] An analysis of 84 patients with LS found an increase in the HLA antigens DQ7, DQ8, and DQ9.[120] Other etiologies that have been considered include familial associations and hypoestrogenism.

The clinical appearance and pathology of LS are very characteristic. Grossly, these lesions present as white patch–like areas overlying both labia (Figure 15.47). In some cases, affected areas may resemble a butterfly wing or an hourglass pattern (Figure 15.48). As the disease progresses, there may be a shrinkage and fusion of the labia minora and clitoris. The overlying skin becomes thinned and has a "cigarette paper" appearance (Figure 15.49). Areas of ecchymoses and erosion (Figure 15.50) may be present from chronic rubbing and scratching. The skin splits easily due to loss of elasticity. Microscopically, hyperkeratosis is seen on the surface with epithelial thinning. There is disruption of the basal layer and the rete pegs are lost. Directly beneath the epithelial surface, the superficial dermis is transformed into a homogenous, collagenized hypocellular matrix, and beneath this matrix is a band of chronic inflammatory cells (Figure 15.51). However, only minimal changes such as mild epithelial thinning and superficial chronic inflammation may be visible in the early transformation of the epithelium in LS. Focal hemorrhage and spongiosis may be seen in the epidermal/dermal border. With advanced lesions, marked sclerosus is present within the underlying dermis.[14]

The true incidence of LS is unknown with the care of patients being fragmented among various specialties.[121] Between 3% and 6% of women with LS will develop vulvar squamous cell carcinoma. Patients with LS can also have associated epithelial hyperplasia. In a series of 33 women with a mixture of LS and squamous cell hyperplasia, 3 (10%) developed squamous cell carcinoma of the vulva.[122] Thus, patients with LS, and particularly those with a combination of LS and squamous cell hyperplasia, need to be followed carefully. The carcinoma associated with these lesions is usually keratinizing and not commonly associated with HPV.

In the past, LS was treated with limited success with the topical application of testosterone cream.[123] Currently, the treatment of choice is topical fluorinated steroids such as clobetasol 0.05% ointment. Treatment of non–LS-affected

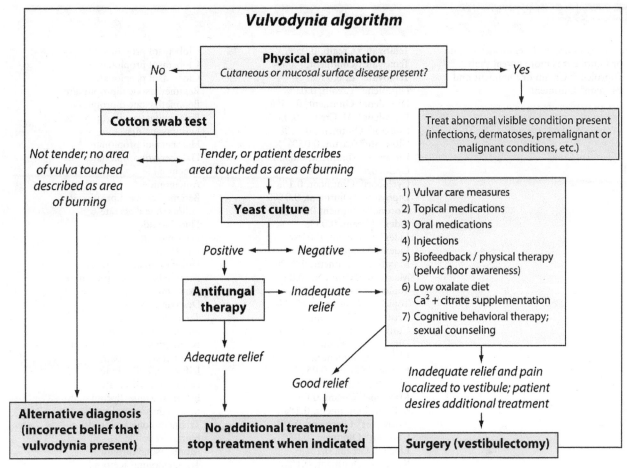

FIGURE 15.46. The vulvodynia algorithm summarizes the diagnosis and treatment of vulvodynia. (Reprinted from Haefner H, Collins ME, et al. The Vulvodynia Guideline. *J Low Gen Tract Dis* 2005;9(1):40–51, with permission. Copyright © 2005 ASCCP.)

genital skin with high-potency corticosteroids, such as clobetasol, may quickly result in steroid-induced epithelial atrophy. However, skin affected by LS is far less susceptible to the adverse effects of high-potency corticosteroids. Nevertheless, adjacent normal skin may be particularly susceptible to repeated application over a prolonged period of time.[124] Therefore, treatment should be limited to involved areas. The general recommendation is to use a class 1 topical steroid (clobetasol propionate 0.05% ointment) twice daily for 1 month and then once daily for 2 months. Debate exists about whether or not patients should then use twice weekly clobetasol propionate 0.05% ointment long-term versus decreasing to a mid-dose topical steroid (triamcinolone acetonide ointment 0.01%) as a daily regimen. Careful follow-up by a clinical provider is recommended.[125]

15.6.2 Squamous Cell Hyperplasia (Lichen Simplex Chronicus)

Squamous cell hyperplasia is characterized by epithelial changes that represent a surface thickening from constant rubbing and scratching on an irritated area of vulvar skin. Another term for this condition is lichen simplex chronicus. The degree to which this diagnosis is made depends on the experience of the pathologist with dermatopathologic conditions.[126]

On gross physical examination, the vulva has areas of surface thickening and often includes scratch marks (Figure 15.52). Histologically, mild to moderate hyperkeratosis is present (Figure 15.53). There is acanthosis with deepening of the rete pegs. The rete pegs are also broadened and the papillary dermis is narrowed. The squamous epithelial cells show normal maturation without atypia. Parakeratosis may be found. Mitotic figures are infrequent but can be present. A mild superficial perivascular inflammation is present.[8] The squamous alterations adjacent to invasive cancers often encompass a form of squamous cell hyperplasia reflecting a reactive change to chronic irritation.[122,127]

The recommended treatment for lichen simplex chronicus is application of topical corticosteroids and oral antipruritics and avoidance of agents that cause surface irritation.[128] At times, with severe disease, antibiotics, antifungals, and oral intralesional or intramuscular steroids are required to break the itch scratch cycle.[8,129]

TABLE 15.8	ISSVD CLASSIFICATION OF VULVAR NONENOPLASTIC EPITHELIAL DISORDERS OF THE VULVA
■ 1976–1988	■ 1989–PRESENT
Lichen sclerosus et atrophicus	Lichen sclerosis
Hyperplastic dystrophy	Squamous cell hyperplasia/ lichen simplex chronicus
Mixed dystrophy	Other dermatoses

TABLE 15.9 CLASSIFICATION OF STEROIDS BY POTENCY

Super-high Potency I Temovate® Cream or Ointment is more potent than Diprolene® Cream or Ointment and Psorcon® Ointment	Temovate® Cream, 0.05%	Clobetasol propionate
	Temovate® Ointment, 0.05%	Clobetasol propionate
	Temovate® E, 0.05%	Clobetasol propionate
	Diprolene® Cream, 0.05%	Betamethasone dipropionate
	Diprolene® Ointment, 0.05%	Betamethasone dipropionate
	Diprolene® AF Cream, 0.05%	Betamethasone dipropionate
	Psorcon® Ointment, 0.05%	Diflorasone diacetate
	Ultravate® Cream, 0.05%	Halobetasol propionate
	Ultravate® Ointment, 0.05%	Halobetasol propionate
II	Cyclocort® Cream, 0.1%	Amcinonide
	Cyclocort® Ointment, 0.1%	Amcinonide
	Diprosone® Ointment, 0.05%	Betamethasone dipropionate
	Florone® Ointment 0.05%	Diflorasone diacetate
	Lidex® Cream, 0.05%	Fluocinonide
	Lidex® Ointment, 0.05%	Fluocinonide
	Lidex-E® Cream, 0.05%	Fluocinonide
	Maxiflor® Ointment, 0.05%	Diflorasone diacetate
	Maxivate®, Ointment 0.05%	Betamethasone dipropionate
	Topicort® Cream, 0.25%	Desoximetasone
	Topicort® Ointment, 0.25%	Desoximetasone
III	Aristocort A® Cream 0.5%	Triamcinolone acetonide
	Cutivate® Ointment, 0.05%	Fluticasone propionate
	Diprosone® Cream, 0.05%	Betamethasone dipropionate
	Elocon® Ointment 0.1%	Mometasone furoate
	Florone® Cream, 0.05%	Diflorasone diacetate
	Maxiflor® Cream, 0.05%	Diflorasone diacetate
	Maxivate® Cream, 0.05%	Betamethasone dipropionate
	Valisone® Ointment, 0.1%	Betamethasone valerate
IV	Aristocort® Ointment, 0.1%	Triamcinolone acetonide
	Cordran® Ointment, 0.05%	Flurandrenolide
	Elocon® Cream, 0.1%	Mometasone furoate
	Kenalog® Ointment, 0.1%	Triamcinolone acetonide
	Synalar® Ointment, 0.025%	Fluocinolone acetonide
	Topicort LP® Cream, 0.05%	Desoximetasone
V	Aristocort® Cream, 0.1%	Triamcinolone acetonide
	Cordran® Cream, 0.05%	Flurandrenolide
	Cutivate® Cream, 0.05%	Fluticasone propionate
	Dermatop® Emollient Cream, 0.05%	Prednicarbate
	Kenalog® Cream, 0.1%	Triamcinolone acetonide
	Kenalog Ointment, 0.025%	Triamcinolone acetonide
	Locoid® Cream, 0.1%	Hydrocortisone butyrate
	Synalar® Cream, 0.025%	Fluocinolone acetonide
	Valisone® Cream, 0.1%	Betamethasone valerate
	Uticort® Cream 0.025%	Betamethasone benzoate
	Westcort® Cream, 0.2%	Hydrocortisone valerate
	Westcort® Ointment, 0.2%	Hydrocortisone valerate
VI	Aclovate® Cream, 0.05%	Alclometasone dipropionate
	Aclovate® Ointment, 0.05%	Alclometasone dipropionate
	Tridesilon® Cream, 0.05%	Desonide
VII Low potency	Numerous preparations exist	Dexamethasone, flumethasone, hydrocortisone
		Methylprednisolone, prednisolone

It is best to use ointments on the vulva.

15.6.3 Other Dermatoses

This category encompasses a wide range of dermatopathologic conditions, including lichen planus and psoriasis. Depending on the experience of the pathologist, many of these lesions will be given descriptive interpretations ("hyperkeratosis," "acanthosis," "superficial perivascular inflammation"). The pathologist must be careful to identify the histopathologic changes unique to these dermatoses so that proper categorization and clinical management is accomplished.

15.6.3.1 Lichen Planus

Lichen planus is an inflammatory dermatosis with an autoimmune association.[130] Oral (Figure 15.54) and vulvovaginal lichen planus often coexist.[131] The vestibule, labia minora, and vagina undergo marked erosion and desquamation (Figures 15.55 and 15.56). The vulvar vestibule will show reticular striae. Over time the vestibule and vagina may undergo scarring and retraction. Vaginal dilation is important to prevent the scarring.

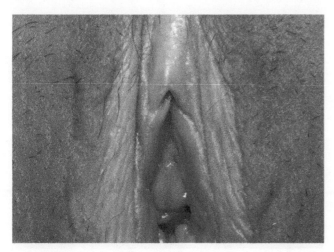

FIGURE 15.47.   LS with classic vulvar whitening and some loss of the labia minora.

Microscopically, lichen planus demonstrates marked destruction of the basal cells and erosion of the rete pegs by an underlying band-like chronic inflammatory infiltrate (Figure 15.57). The rete pegs often contain apoptotic bodies (Civatte bodies).

A variety of treatments exist for lichen planus.[132,133] The initial treatment is application of topical corticosteroid ointment (clobetasol propionate 0.05% ointment). For advanced lichen

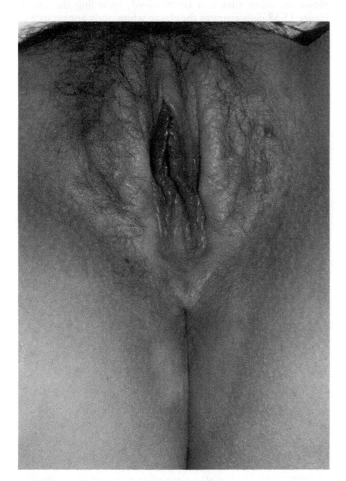

FIGURE 15.48.   Often patients will have an hour glass configuration or figure of eight pattern with LS.

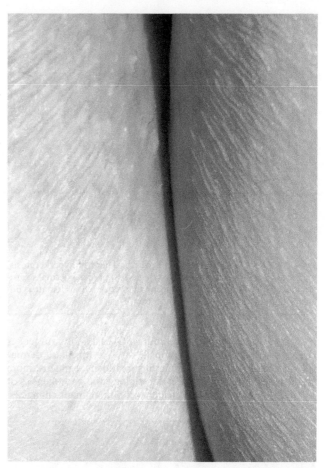

FIGURE 15.49.   A crinkled texture is noted in the LS present on this vulva. This appearance is also described as a "cigarette paper" appearance.

planus, multiple treatments exist including anti-inflammatory antibiotics, topical tacrolimus ointment, oral steroids, hydroxychloroquine, cyclosporine, cyclophosphamide, azathioprine, etanercept, mycophenolate mofetil, and methotrexate. Vulvovaginal agglutination may result in difficulty with urination

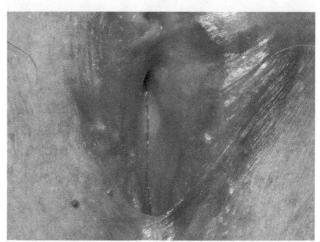

FIGURE 15.50.   Erosions can be associated with vulvar LS. A low threshold for biopsy at the edge of the erosion should be present to rule out VIN or cancer.

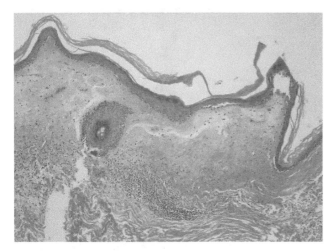

FIGURE 15.51. Photomicrograph of LS. There is hyperkeratosis, epidermal thinning with loss of the rete pegs, superficial dermal sclerosis, and a lichenoid band of chronic inflammatory cells. (Hematoxylin-eosin stain; medium power magnification.)

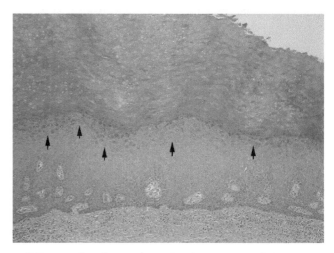

FIGURE 15.53. Photomicrograph of squamous cell hyperplasia (lichen simplex chronicus). There is acanthosis with marked broadening and confluence of the rete pegs. There is also hyperkeratosis and an increase in the granular cell layer, or granulocytosis (arrows). The individual keratinocytes, however, are not atypical. (Hematoxylin-eosin stain; medium power magnification.)

as well as difficulty with intercourse. Occasionally, surgery is required to release the adhesions.[134,135] As with many dermatologic conditions having numerous treatment regimens, more studies are needed to establish the etiology and pathogenesis of LP and to identify those at greater risk of malignant change.[136]

15.6.3.2 Psoriasis

Psoriasis is a plaque-like dermatosis of unknown etiology. Clinically, the condition consists of pink or silver-white plaques that commonly cover the elbows, knees, scalp, and back. However, other sites can be involved, including the vulva. Figure 15.58 demonstrates the classic white, scaly appearance of psoriasis. However, Figure 15.59 shows a frequent appearance of psoriasis on the vulva that is erythematous and less scaly than the classic psoriasis. Associated findings that help confirm the presence of psoriasis include the *Koebner phenomenon*, the occurrence of new lesions at a site of skin injury, and *Auspitz's sign*, the presence of small bleeding sites on the underside of an area where a plaque has been removed. Symptoms consist of pruritus and burning.[137] Microscopically, there is hyperkeratosis and exocytosis. Acute inflammatory cells will aggregate in the surface (Munro abscess). There is acanthosis and deepening of the rete pegs. The superficial dermis will contain scattered foci of inflammatory cells (Figure 15.60). Mitoses are commonly seen; however, there is no cytological atypia.

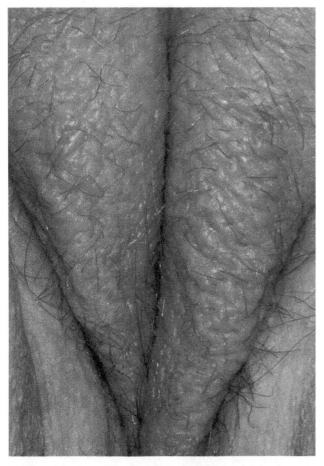

FIGURE 15.52. Vulvar squamous cell hyperplasia (lichen simplex chronicus). Grossly, the labial surface is raised, roughened, and slightly erythematous. There are areas where tissue loss on the labia majora has occurred secondary to scratching.

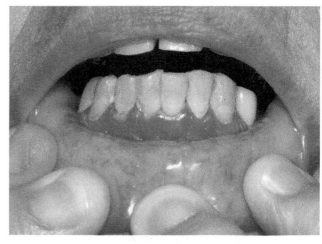

FIGURE 15.54. Lichen planus can affect the mouth on the gingivae or side walls. The gums have significant erythema and tissue erosion.

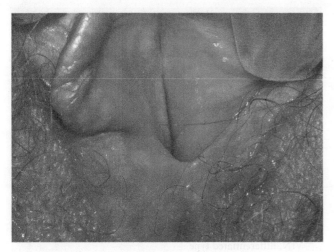

FIGURE 15.55. Vulvar lichen planus. Grossly, there is marked erythema involving the vestibule.

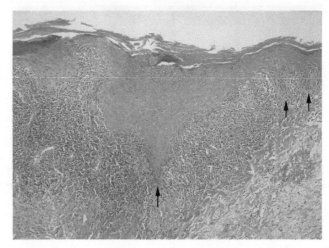

FIGURE 15.57. Microscopically, a band-like inflammatory infiltrate erodes and blunts the rete pegs, which become pointed (*arrows*). (Hematoxylin-eosin stain; medium power magnification.)

Treatment consists of stopping vulvar irritants, treating infection (cefadroxil or cephalexin × 10 days), and the use of a topical steroid ointment. For mild to moderate psoriasis of the vulva, a low-dose topical ointment is generally adequate. For moderate to severe disease, a high-dose topical steroid such as clobetasol 0.05% ointment nightly for 2 weeks and then every other night is used. Calcipotriene (Dovonex) ointment, tacrolimus 0.1%, or pimecrolimus 1% topically may also be added to the regimen. For unresponsive disease, systemic medications are required at times.

15.7 VULVAR NONINVASIVE NEOPLASTIC ABNORMALITIES

15.7.1 Vulvar Intraepithelial Neoplasia (Squamous and Nonsquamous)

There are two categories of noninvasive neoplastic vulvar abnormalities consisting of squamous and nonsquamous tissue changes.[138] The squamous abnormalities are more common than the nonsquamous abnormalities. Historically, squamous intraepithelial neoplasia has had numerous names including *Bowen's disease, Erythroplasia of Queyrat, Bowenoid papulosis* or *Bowenoid dysplasia, atypical hyperplastic dystrophy, carcinoma* in situ *simplex,* and squamous cell carcinoma *in situ.* The categorization of these abnormalities, including the proposed new ISSVD classification of VIN, is summarized in Table 15.10.[139]

15.7.1.1 Vulvar Intraepithelial Neoplasia—Squamous

The incidence of VIN is difficult to determine because it depends on the persistence with which colposcopists search for and biopsy these lesions in asymptomatic patients so that a definitive diagnosis can be made. It is generally assumed, however, that the incidence of VIN usual has increased in recent decades and is now more common in younger women. Specifically, the incidence of VIN in women under age 35 years has nearly tripled over time.[140,141] Before 1970, VIN was found most often in women in the fifth or sixth decade of life; currently about half of the patients are less than 40 years old. A recent study evaluated the incidence of VIN and found that it increased until ages 40 to 49 and then declined gradually, in contrast to the rate of invasive squamous cell carcinoma of

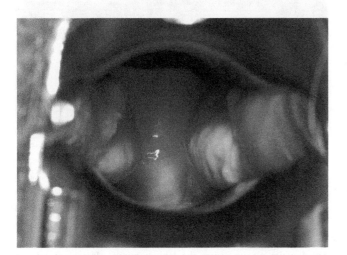

FIGURE 15.56. Vaginal lichen planus. Erosion is noted at the apex of the vagina.

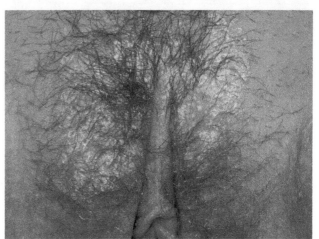

FIGURE 15.58. Vulvar psoriasis. Grossly, multiple slightly raised patches are present with a characteristic silver color.

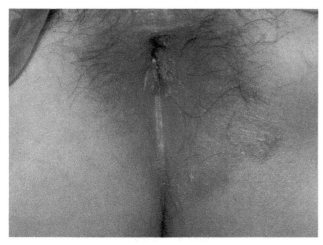

FIGURE 15.59.   A more common appearance than the silver scale that is seen on the elbows and knees, vulvar psoriasis will have an erythematous appearance. Moisture and friction in the area limit the amount of scales. Secondary changes of excoriation and crusting may occur.

TABLE 15.10	VIN OLD TERMINOLOGY

1. Squamous type (with or without HPV change)
   a. VIN I
   b. VIN II
   c. VIN III (squamous cell carcinoma in situ (CIS), Bowen's disease, Erythroplasia of Queyrat, CIS simplex)
2. Nonsquamous type
   Paget's disease
   Melanoma in situ

NEW TERMINOLOGY FOR SQUAMOUS-TYPE VIN

Squamous VIN Terminology (ISSVD 2004)
   VIN, usual type
       VIN, warty type
       VIN, basaloid type
       VIN, mixed (warty/basaloid) type
   VIN, differentiated type

NOTE: The occasional example of VIN that cannot be classified into either of the above VIN categories (usual type and differentiated type) may be classified as VIN, unclassified type (or VIN, NOS). The rare VIN of pagetoid type may be classified as such, or placed in this category.

the vulva, which gradually increased until ages 60 to 69.[142] The prevalence of VIN and its association with HPV has been evaluated. Insinga et al.[143] found that following multitype adjustment, HPV 16 was estimated to contribute to more than three-fourths (77.7%) of VIN lesions. VIN in young women is frequently in multiple locations and is associated with HPV. Currently, approximately 80% of patients with VIN are HPV positive. Patients may be asymptomatic or complain of pruritus or burning.

15.7.1.1.1 CLINICAL APPEARANCE

The lesions associated with VIN often appear as raised plaques and papules on the surface of the vulva and/or perineum. The lesions can be white (50%) (Figure 15.61) or become acetowhite after soaking the vulva and perineum with dilute acetic acid, brown (approximately 25%) (Figure 15.62), or red in color (Figure 15.63). Many patients will have a combination of color changes. The lesions are often multifocal and can be located throughout the vulvar surface, anus, and

surrounding perineum. VIN can appear warty; therefore, it is prudent to perform a biopsy on any lesion originally diagnosed as a condyloma that does not respond to conservative therapy.

15.7.1.1.2 HISTOLOGY

The histologic features seen in Figure 15.64 are characteristic of typical VIN usual. There is an increase in cell number extending from the basal layer to a point at least two-thirds above the basement membrane and usually to the surface. The cells lose their orderly arrangement and show a lack of maturation. The nuclei vary in size, shape, and chromatin distribution. Mitotic activity is abundant and this activity can be seen throughout the epithelium. Abnormal mitotic figures are common and are the result of aneuploidy and polyploidy.[15,16]

Commonly, VIN can involve the skin appendages. Although acanthosis, broadening of the rete pegs, and adnexal involvement are common, the basement membrane remains intact. VIN usual can also be subcategorized into different histologic

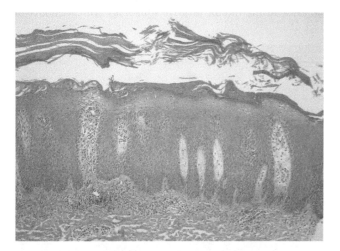

FIGURE 15.60.   Photomicrograph of vulvar psoriasis. The rete pegs are uniformly elongated. There is hyperkeratosis and superficial dermal inflammation. (Hematoxylin-eosin stain; medium power magnification.)

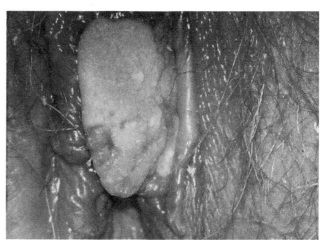

FIGURE 15.61.   Vulvar intraepithelial neoplasia (usual). A broad-based white plaque covers the labium minus. (Photo courtesy of Dr. Gordon Davis, used with permission.)

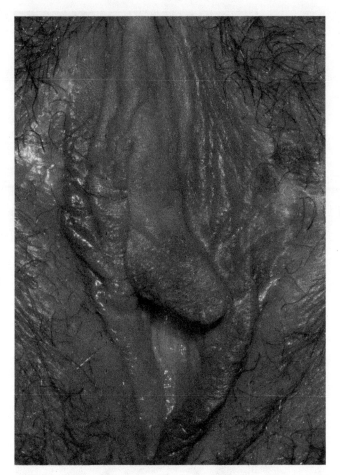

FIGURE 15.62. Vulvar intraepithelial neoplasia (usual). Areas of brown discoloration are diffusely present on the vulva.

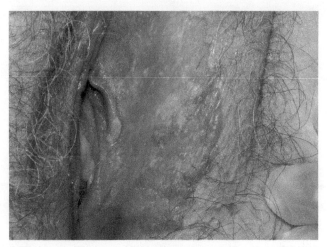

FIGURE 15.63. Vulvar intraepithelial neoplasia (usual). Reddened areas are present in some areas with whitening in extensive VIN.

types. The most common are the warty VINs (Figure 15.65). The warty type of VIN contains mature squamous cells with large nuclei and peripheral chromatin clumping. Multinucleation and perinuclear cytoplasmic clearing reminiscent of koilocytes are present. The basaloid type of VIN usual consists of cells similar in appearance to epidermal basal cells, which are found throughout the epithelial surface (Figure 15.66). Total lack of maturation is present. The warty and basaloid VINs are related to HPV infection, most commonly type 16, and are often seen in younger women who are sexually active and smoke. The risk of invasive carcinoma of the vulva with basaloid and warty VIN is low to moderate. The least common form of VIN is the differentiated VIN (previously termed simplex type) (Figure 15.67).[144,145] The differentiated type of VIN occurs in older women, usually at a site that has been chronically irritated. It is most often seen in association with LS. There is often no association with HPV exposure or tobacco use. Differentiated VIN has an epidermis with squamous cells that have markedly pleomorphic nuclei. The chromatin is peripherally clumped and there are large nucleoli present. Keratin pearls are prominent within the rete pegs (Figure 15.68). The differentiated VIN has an extremely high association with vulvar squamous cell cancer. Table 15.11 summarizes the features of the different morphologic types of VIN.

15.7.1.1.3 VIN Treatment

Prior to any form of treatment for VIN, a biopsy to confirm the diagnosis is indicated. If the biopsy reveals only condyloma (or the old terminology, VIN 1), either observation or treatment with topical antiviral medications or surgical treatments are choices. As with cervical and vaginal HPV infection, if the patient is asymptomatic, observation of the low-grade disease is often the preferred treatment. Treatment of VIN usual (VIN 2,3) has traditionally been accomplished surgically (wide local excision or laser), but more recently the treatment has included administration of topical immunomodulating agents.[146] While it is acceptable to treat the usual basaloid and warty VINs with ablation, the differentiated VINs should always be excised initially to rule out a cancer. Additionally, lesions in hair-bearing areas are generally treated with a wide local excision. The standard procedure is as follows: An inked margin around the lesion is made providing gross clearance of 0.5 to 1 cm around the site of resection. The depth of resection is to the subcutaneous fat but not deeper. Closure depends on the size of resection but is often by primary approximation. Smaller resections may not require closure and larger lesions may require local advancement skin flaps or grafts. It is important to realize that vulvar skin thickness varies considerably by its location. Particular care must be taken at the clitoris,

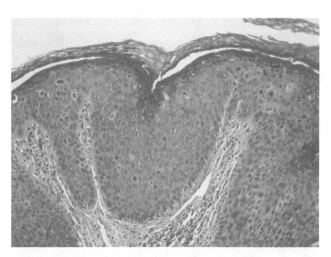

FIGURE 15.64. Photomicrograph of VIN (usual). There is proliferation of atypical basaloid cells over as much as two-thirds of the epidermal surface. Mitotic figures are also present. The basement membrane, however, remains intact. (Hematoxylin-eosin stain; low power magnification.)

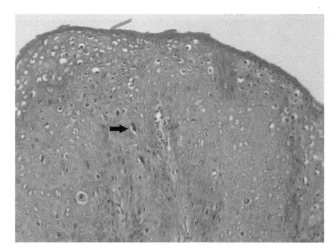

FIGURE 15.65. Photomicrograph of VIN (usual). Warty-type VIN. In this case, there are large numbers of koilocytic cells. Multinucleation is also seen (*arrow*). (Hematoxylin-eosin stain; medium power magnification.)

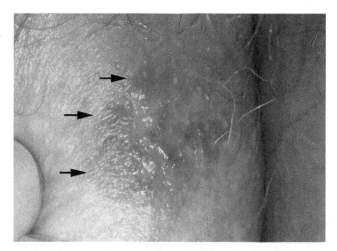

FIGURE 15.67. Vulvar intraepithelial neoplasia (differentiated). The area is broad, slightly raised with alternating red and white coloration (*arrows*), consistent with chronic irritation. (Photo courtesy of Dr. Gordon Davis, used with permission.)

urethra, anus, and labia minora as the squamous epithelium is very thin. CO_2 laser is generally performed in the non–hair-bearing areas, provided there is no concern for invasion. Some providers perform loop electrosurgical excision procedure for VIN.

Recently, a topical treatment for VIN usual has been introduced in women in whom invasive cancer has been ruled out. Imiquimod (Aldara®) has reported to be effective for VIN usual (off-label use).[146–149]

The association of invasive carcinoma with VIN ranges from 2% to 20% for the basaloid and warty types, and greater than 95% for the differentiated types.[150,151] Immunocompromised women also appear to have a greater risk of VIN progressing to invasive disease.

Resected VIN specimens should be examined closely by the pathologist for completeness of excision and potential areas of superficial squamous cell carcinoma. Reporting microscopic diagnoses of VIN should include the histologic type to assist in treatment decisions.

Long-term follow-up of patients with VIN is very important.[152] In a study by Park et al.[153], 21% of the women with

vulvar disease had abnormal anal cytology. Those patients who smoke tobacco should be counseled that smoking cessation is critical for the various treatments to succeed. Consider screening patients with VIN by taking anal Pap tests. A moistened Dacron swab or Cytobrush can be used to obtain

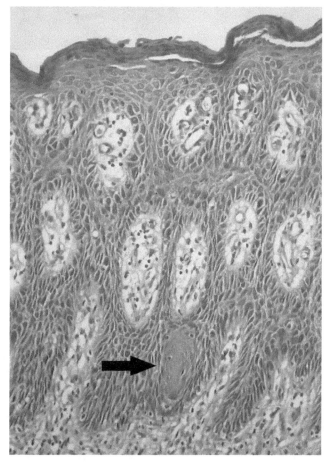

FIGURE 15.68. Photomicrograph of VIN (differentiated). The keratinocytes are atypical, but they continue to resemble mature squamous cells. A squamous pearl is present in a rete peg (*arrow*). (Hematoxylin-eosin stain; medium power magnification.)

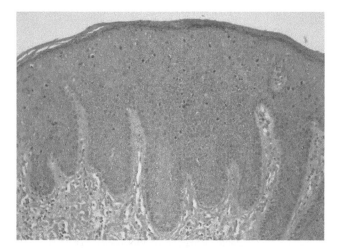

FIGURE 15.66. Photomicrograph of VIN (usual). Basaloid-type VIN. The predominant dysplastic cells are similar in appearance to the basaloid cells from the stratum germinativum. (Hematoxylin and eosin, medium power magnification.)

■ MORPHOLOGIC TYPE	■ AGE	■ SMOKING HISTORY	■ ASSOCIATION WITH HPV	■ INVASIVE CANCER RISK
Warty VIN	Younger	Smoker	Common	Low-intermediate
Basaloid VIN	Younger	Smoker	Common	Low-intermediate
Differentiated VIN	Older	Nonsmoker	Uncommon	High

TABLE 15.11 COMPARISON OF THE THREE MORPHOLOGIC TYPES OF VIN

these smears. Insert the swab or brush into the canal approximately 5 to 6 cm above the anal verge to the rectum. Rotate the swab or brush, applying pressure to the walls of the canal while removing the sampling device.

15.7.1.2 Vulvar Intraepithelial Neoplasia— Nonsquamous

15.7.1.2.1 PAGET'S DISEASE

Paget's disease of the vulva is the nonsquamous form of VIN, which may be associated with an underlying carcinoma.[154] In 1874, Sir James Paget originally observed that excoriation of the areola could represent "a chronic affliction of the nipple succeeded by scirrhous carcinomas of the breast." He also suggested that this characteristic change could result in a "similar sequence of events in other sites." Dubreuilh described the first case of extramammary Paget's disease of the vulva in 1901 in a 51-year-old woman.[155]

The significance of Paget's disease of the nipple is well known. It represents the surface extension of an underlying ductal carcinoma of the breast. The association of vulvar Paget's disease and other neoplastic processes is less clear. The most common is apocrine gland neoplasia; however, it can involve other sites, including the bladder and colorectal region.[8,156,157] Up to 25% of vulvar extramammary Paget's disease are associated with an underlying adenocarcinoma of an adnexal tissue. Less commonly it is associated with a distant carcinoma of breast, GI, GU, or the genital tract. Perianal extramammary Paget's has a higher degree of association with underlying colorectal adenocarcinoma than Paget's located on the vulva. In view of the possible coexistence of sweat gland carcinoma of the vulva or another adjacent internal carcinoma, the overall prognosis for Paget's disease is less favorable than for squamous VIN. Rarely, Paget's disease may present as surface extension of a ductal carcinoma arising from vulvar ectopic breast tissue that forms along the mammary ridge.

The mean age for Paget's disease of the vulva is 65 years. Almost all of the patients are white. Clinically, the lesions present on the vulva as geographic red macular areas that can appear excoriated (Figure 15.69). Often small white patches will cover this region. They often appear as soft velvety papules that are slowly growing into crusty scaly plaques. The area may be asymptomatic but can be pruritic (in over 50% of patients) or cause a burning sensation.

The diagnosis is made by identifying the so-called pagetoid cells that occupy the epidermis. These cells are round in shape and considerably larger than the surrounding keratinocytes or melanocytes. The cytoplasm is pink but often retracts; the nuclei are large, round, and have prominent nucleoli. The pagetoid cells tend to cluster and form small nests in the rete pegs. Single cells spread into the superficial epidermis (Figure 15.70). The appearance is similar to superficial melanoma. In some

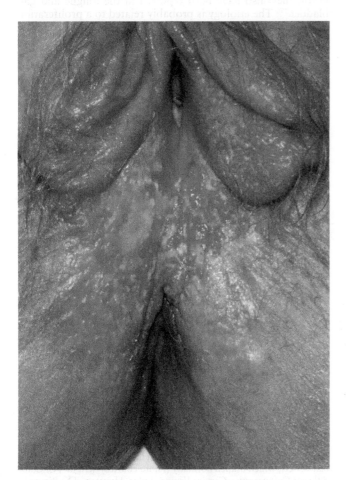

FIGURE 15.69.   Extramammary Paget's disease of the vulva. A red, velvety appearance is classic for Paget's disease.

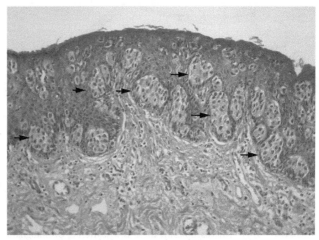

FIGURE 15.70.   Vulvar Paget's disease. As viewed microscopically, nests and individual pagetoid cells are scattered throughout the epidermis (*arrows*). (Hematoxylin-eosin stain; medium power magnification.)

cases, immunostaining using markers that separate malignant melanocytes from adenocarcinoma *in situ* (pagetoid) cells may be necessary to identify the correct tumor.[1,8,158–160] A panel of stains may be helpful in uncertain cases including CK-7, Mart-1, and D-PAS. Other potentially helpful stains in uncertain cases include carcinoembryonic antigen, gross cystic disease fluid protein-15 (GCDFP-15), HMB-45, S-100 protein, Alcian blue, and mucicarmine.[161]

Once diagnosed, a patient with vulvar Paget's disease should undergo a workup to identify any associated invasive carcinoma. Depending on where the disease is located, the evaluation should include cervical cytology, cystoscopy, colonoscopy, breast examination, and mammography. The treatment of Paget's disease of the vulva is wide local excision. Depending on the size of the lesion, simple vulvectomy may be necessary. At times skin grafts or flaps are required for closure. The tissue excised should include the reticular dermis so that adnexal structures, particularly apocrine glands, can be examined microscopically. Complete excision of Paget's disease can be difficult.[162] Examination of frozen sections of the margin is often frustrating and is not recommended, as the lesion usually extends beyond any recognizable border.[1,8]

Laser therapy has been used on recurrent Paget's disease. Treatment with topical imiquimod cream has also been reported to be effective for both primary and recurrent vulvar Paget's disease.[163–165]

15.7.1.2.2 MELANOMA *IN SITU*

Melanoma *in situ* consists of melanin containing carcinoma cells that spread along the epidermis but do not extend into the papillary dermis. As such, the lesion is considered a "melanoma *in situ*" and is included in the noninvasive neoplastic abnormalities.

Malignant melanocytes spread across the superficial epidermis in a "scattered buckshot" pattern and occupy the rete pegs (Figure 15.71). As the pattern may resemble extramammary Paget's disease, special stains may be necessary to confirm the melanocytic origin of these cells.[166]

15.7.2 Other Noninvasive Neoplastic Abnormalities

Numerous additional benign vulvar neoplasms are found occasionally on routine examination. These lesions rarely develop a subsequent carcinoma; however, excision is usually necessary for a definitive diagnosis. The following are examples of other common noninvasive abnormalities seen by the colposcopist.

15.7.2.1 Papillary Hidradenoma

Also known as *hidradenoma papilliferum*, a *papillary hidradenoma* is a benign neoplasm thought to arise in specialized sweat glands. While its exact origin is unknown, evidence of derivation from an apocrine-type cell includes the presence of occasional hidradenomas in the areola and the ability to identify apocrine gland proteins in these neoplasms. Clinically, these tumors present as small dermal nodules, usually in the labial sulci. They can, however, occur in any site including the mons. They are hard, mobile, nontender, and about 0.5 to 1.0 cm in size (Figure 15.72). Ulceration is uncommon. Histologically, the neoplasm is circumscribed with a pushing border. The gland pattern is complex and suggests an adenocarcinoma; however, there is no cytologic atypia and no mitoses (Figure 15.73). On high-power microscopic examination, two cell layers are seen: an inner layer of acinar cells surrounded by contractile myoepithelial cells. The treatment is surgical removal. On occasion, an adenocarcinoma *in situ* or an adenocarcinoma is found on histopathology.[167–169]

15.7.2.2 Granular Cell Tumor

Formerly known as *granular cell myoblastomas, granular cell tumors* are benign neoplasms that originate from the peripheral nerve sheath. While these rare tumors can occur on the vulva, they also have been reported in the tongue and gall bladder.[170] The etiology is probably related to a proliferation of malformed lysosomes in Schwann cells. The most common vulvar site is the labium majus (Figure 15.74); however, they can occur at other sites on the vulva.[171] The initial presentation is a local swelling. Granular cell tumors are intradermal, although thickening or ulceration of the overlying skin can sometimes occur. Microscopically, the reticular dermis is infiltrated by large round cells with eosinophilic granular cytoplasm. The nuclei are small and dark with few mitoses (Figure 15.75). The tumor margins are indistinct. The granular cells' origin from the peripheral nerve sheath can be confirmed by the presence of cytoplasmic neural markers. The treatment is wide local excision. Although granular cell

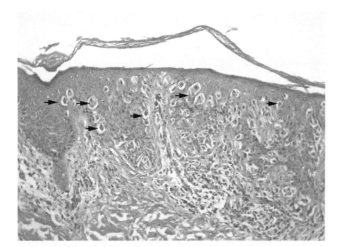

FIGURE 15.71. Microscopically, there is a scattering of malignant melanocytic cells throughout the epidermis in a "scattered buckshot" pattern (*arrows*). Melanin pigment is present in the superficial dermis, which helps differentiate this entity from Paget's disease. (Hematoxylin-eosin stain; medium power magnification.)

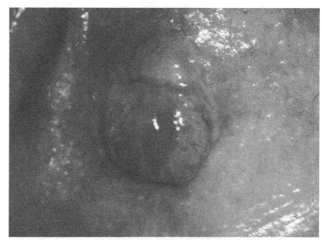

FIGURE 15.72. Papillary hidradenoma of the vulva. Grossly, a round, raised intradermal lesion is present. Note the dilated superficial vessels, which branch normally (Photo courtesy Wright VC. *Color Atlas of Colposcopy—Cervix, Vagina, Vulva.* Houston, TX: Biomedical Communications, 2003, used with permission).

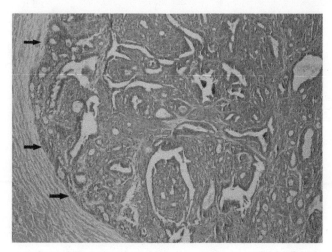

FIGURE 15.73. Microscopically, the tumor contains numerous irregularly shaped gland-like cystic spaces. Note the pushing border between the tumor and the surrounding dermis (*arrows*). (Hematoxylin-eosin stain; medium power magnification.)

tumors at other sites have shown malignant potential, recurrences and metastases from vulvar neoplasms are extremely rare.[172] Treatment consists of a wide local excision for the benign lesions.[173]

15.7.2.3 Nevi

Nevi are skin tumors that arise from melanocytic-type cells derived from the neural crest that are located in the epidermis and superficial dermis. Although occasionally congenital, they are more often seen in sun-exposed areas of the skin after birth. Nevi are divided into three types. *Junctional nevi* are characterized by nevus cells in the dermal epidermal junction; microscopically, the nevus cells cluster in the rete pegs. A *compound nevus* has nevus cells along the basal epidermis as well as the superficial dermis. The *intradermal nevus* contains nevus cells located exclusively in the superficial dermis. The evolution of these lesions starts with junctional activity. Over time, the nevus cells start to migrate into the superficial dermis. Continued migration results in loss of the epidermal nevus cells, resulting in the mature, intradermal nevus.

Nevi are benign pigmented tumors. Colors range from tan to black, although the most common are different shades of brown. The border is usually distinct. Junctional nevi are flat, while compound and intradermal nevi may be raised (papules) (Figure 15.76). The latter can be rubbed and become irritated. Atypical genital nevi are rare melanocytic lesions that most commonly arise on the vulva of young women.[174] Melanomas have irregular contours and variegated coloration. However, it can be difficult to grossly differentiate pigmented lesions and it is best to remove any vulvar pigmented lesion that is at all suspicious.

Microscopically, nevus cells are somewhat larger than melanocytes; the cells contain large oval nuclei and little cytoplasm. They can occasionally elongate and resemble neural elements. Melanin pigment may or may not be present. The location of the nevus cell in the epidermis of superficial dermis dictates the type of tumor (junctional, compound, or intradermal) (Figure 15.77).

Nevi are benign and shave or narrow-margin full-thickness excision is usually all the treatment that is needed if they are symptomatic or a tissue abnormality needs to be excluded. Malignant degeneration into a melanoma is rare (and difficult to document) but can occur. Differentiating a melanoma from a benign or dysplastic nevus can require careful

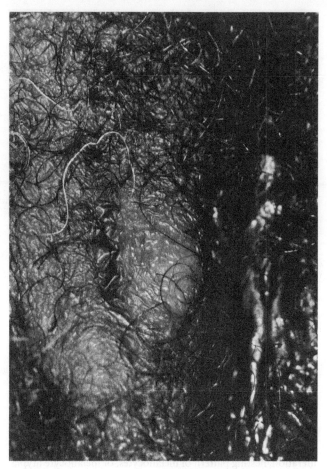

FIGURE 15.74. Granular cell tumor of the vulva. Grossly, a slightly raised area of dermal expansion is present. Although occasionally pigmented, the epidermis in this case is normal. (Photo courtesy Wilkinson EJ, Stone IK. *Atlas of Vulvar Diseases* (2nd ed.). Baltimore, MD: Lippincott Williams & Wilkins, 2008, used with permission.)

microscopic examination. Melanomas will have atypical melanocytic cells that extend into the middle and superficial epidermis, while nevus cells tend to remain at the base of the epidermis.[8]

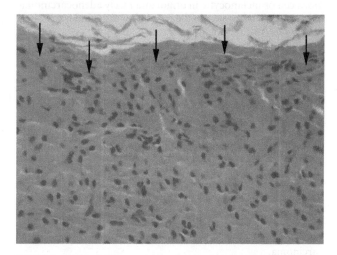

FIGURE 15.75. Microscopically, sheets of pink neoplastic cells are present (*arrows*). The cytoplasm demonstrates a fine granular appearance. (Hematoxylin-eosin stain; high power magnification.)

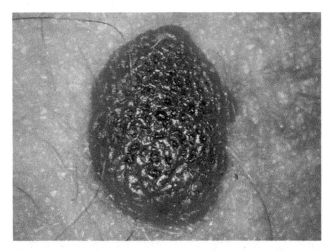

FIGURE 15.76. Vulvar nevus. Grossly, a symmetrical, slightly raised tan-brown macule is present. (Photo courtesy Wright VC. *Color Atlas of Colposcopy—Cervix, Vagina, Vulva.* Houston, TX: Biomedical Communications, 2003, used with permission.)

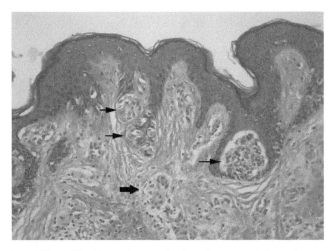

FIGURE 15.77. Photomicrograph of a vulvar nevus. Nests of nevus cells are present in the rete pegs (*small arrows*), indicating junctional activity, as well as in the superficial dermis (*large arrow*). These changes are diagnostic of a compound nevus. (Hematoxylin-eosin stain; medium power magnification.)

15.7.2.4 Melanosis

Benign vulvar melanosis (lentigo) consists of a brown discoloration. It is usually asymptomatic. Often, there will be more than one area of melanosis present. Margins may vary from smooth to jagged. Melanosis of the vulva may mimic melanoma on visual appearance with intensely pigmented irregular macules. While on visual inspection of the vulva, it can be difficult to differentiate melanosis from melanoma, it is not difficult on histologic grounds. Melanosis lacks a substantial melanocytic proliferation, nesting pattern of melanocytes, or melanocyte atypia. Dendritic melanocytes are normal in number or only slightly increased along the basal layer of the epidermis in association with hyperpigmentation. On occasion, the melanin pigment is also located in the upper dermis. Melanosis is a benign process, and thus no treatment is needed once the diagnosis is made.

15.8 VULVAR INVASIVE CARCINOMA

The majority of vulvar invasive carcinomas are either squamous cell or melanocytic in origin and rarely adenocarcinoma, in contrast to other sites in the female lower genital tract where primary adenocarcinomas are more common.

15.8.1 Squamous Cell Carcinoma

Vulvar squamous cell carcinomas are similar in appearance and histology to squamous cell cancers that occur in the vagina and cervix. The most common histologic type is a well-differentiated keratinizing squamous carcinoma, although variants such as nonkeratinizing squamous, warty (condylomatous), verrucous, and basaloid carcinomas can occur on the vulva. Although the incidence of VIN has been rising in recent decades, the incidence of invasive keratinizing squamous carcinoma has remained relatively stable.[134] The cause for this may be related to the unique histologic types and the disparate etiologies of VIN and vulvar keratinizing squamous cell carcinoma.

Squamous cell carcinoma of the vulva occurs in older women often at a site that has been chronically irritated because of prolonged itching or burning. Antecedent or adjacent lesions

include squamous cell hyperplasia variants or differentiated VIN. HPV is generally not found in these cancers. The common VINs (warty and basaloid) occur in younger women who are sexually active and often use tobacco. The cancers associated with these VINs are also warty and basaloid. HPV, usually type 16, is consistently identified in these intraepithelial lesions and cancers.[175,176]

Women often delay seeking medical attention after discovering a vulvar tumor. By the time care is sought, these tumors are often quite large and may be exophytic or ulcerative (Figure 15.78). Enlarged inguinal or femoral lymph nodes may be identified. Ideally, regular examinations will result in early recognition of vulvar cancers. In 1984, the ISSVD defined *superficially invasive carcinoma of the vulva* as a unifocal lesion measuring 2 cm or less in diameter with a depth of invasion no greater than 1 mm.[177] The term "microinvasive carcinoma of the vulva" should not be used since the term "microinvasive" refers to early invasive carcinomas of the cervix that have

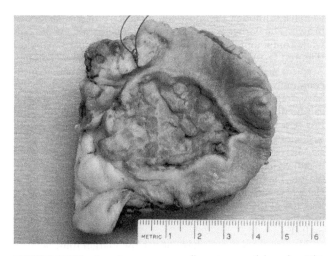

FIGURE 15.78. Invasive squamous cell carcinoma of the vulva. This pathologic specimen represents a radical resection of a large ulcerative lesion. Residual labial structures are difficult to identify but are toward the left.

specific diagnostic criteria. The clinical appearance of lesions that represent early or superficially invasive carcinoma of the vulva is similar to that of VIN. They often present as red and white plaques or as small ulcers (Figures 15.79–15.81). Extremely small lesions may only appear after the application of acetic acid. In contrast to cervical colposcopic abnormalities, different degrees of whiteness or vascular patterns are not useful criteria to differentiate early carcinomas from intraepithelial lesions. Because of this, tissue samples for histologic examination should be taken of any unexplained lesion on the vulva. Solid lesions can be sampled centrally at the most abnormal appearing areas, while ulcers should have tissue removed along the lesion edge. The biopsy should extend far enough into the reticular dermis to document invasion.

In 1988, International Federation of Gynecology and Obstetrics (FIGO) Committee on Gynecologic Oncology adopted a surgical staging system for vulvar cancer. In 1991, the Gynecologic Oncology Group reported a survival analysis of 588 patients with stage I to stage IV disease. Problems with previous staging were addressed in a recently revised FIGO staging for carcinoma of the vulva.[178,179]

Histologically, invasive squamous cell carcinomas of the vulva are similar to squamous cancers of the vagina and cervix (Figures 15.82 and 15.83). Infiltrating nests of malignant squamous cells extend beyond the basement membrane into the surrounding dermis and subcutaneous tissues. A desmoplastic response, characterized by fibrosis and inflammation, usually occurs around these nests and can help in identification. Histologically, the keratinocytic malignant cells are characterized by large irregularly shaped nuclei, prominent nucleoli, and abundant eosinophilic cytoplasm. Mitoses, including abnormal forms, are present. The keratinizing squamous cancers will contain squamous pearls. Extension into lymphatic or vascular spaces can occur. Although the significance of this finding is not clear in vulvar cancers, its presence or absence should be reported.[177]

The depth of invasion is an important prognostic variable and it should be measured on all excised specimens. Information that should be included in the final report is the tumor's thickness, lateral dimensions, and depth of invasion as measured from the nearest papillary dermis basement membrane. By convention, the tumor thickness is determined by measuring from the surface of the squamous epithelium if nonkeratinized or the stratum granulosum (granular cell layer) if keratinized,

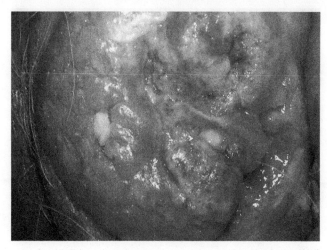

FIGURE 15.80.   A broad-based, raised lesion representing vulvar invasive squamous cell carcinoma. Note the irregular (undulating) surface and the root-like atypical vessels. (Reprinted from Wright VC. *Color Atlas of Colposcopy—Cervix, Vagina and Vulva.* Houston, TX: Biomedical Communications, 2003, with permission.)

to the deepest extent of tumor invasion. The depth of invasion is determined by subtracting the normal epidermal thickness, which is measured from the surface or stratum granulosum to the papillary dermal junction, from the tumor thickness. When reporting the various measurements of tumor size and depth, it is important to describe the method used to determine the measurements (Figure 15.84).[1]

The present treatment for vulvar squamous cell cancer includes wide and deep resection of the primary tumor with unilateral regional (inguinal and femoral) lymph node dissection; bilateral regional nodes are removed for midline lesions.[180,181] Recently, sentinel node mapping has been used among women with vulvar squamous cell cancer.[182] The sentinel nodes are the most superficial draining nodes in the inguinal region. If they are positive, then a full superficial and deep lymph node dissection is performed. Patients who have tumors of less than 1 mm have minimal risk for regional lymph node metastasis, and local excision may be all that is necessary.[183,184] The outlook for women with vulvar squamous cell carcinoma is dependent on the tumor's size, depth of invasion, and extension into regional lymph nodes or surrounding structures.[16,185]

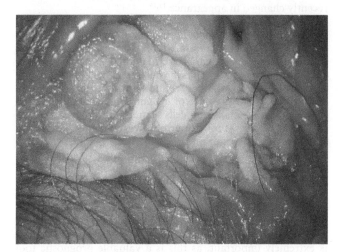

FIGURE 15.79.   Colpophotographs of vulvar invasive squamous cell carcinoma. There is an exophytic, round, pink lesion present in the periphery of a large area of leukoplakia. (Reprinted from Wright VC. *Color Atlas of Colposcopy—Cervix, Vagina and Vulva.* Houston, TX: Biomedical Communications, 2003, with permission.)

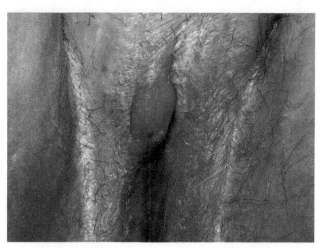

FIGURE 15.81.   A discrete raised hemorrhagic lesion that is vulvar invasive squamous cell carcinoma. Numerous small coiled atypical vessels are present.

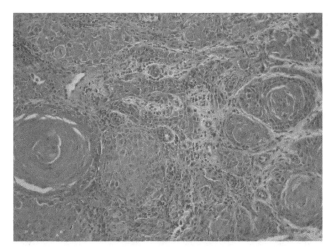

FIGURE 15.82. Photomicrograph of vulvar invasive keratinizing squamous cell carcinoma. Irregular nests of malignant squamous cells are present beneath the epidermis, surrounded by a fibrotic response (desmoplasia). (Hematoxylin-eosin stain; medium power magnification.)

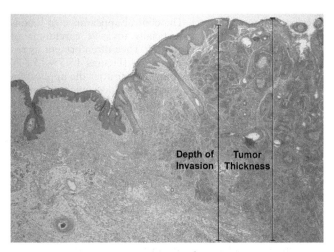

FIGURE 15.84. Measuring the depth of invasion in a squamous cell carcinoma of the vulva. The tumor invasion depth is determined by measuring from the nearest normal dermal papilla to the deepest invasion point. It can also be determined by subtracting the normal epidermal thickness (*white bracket*) from the tumor thickness. The latter is measured from the tumor surface to the deepest point of invasion. (Hematoxylin-eosin stain; medium power magnification.)

Verrucous carcinomas are squamous cell carcinoma variants that make up approximately 1% of vulvar carcinomas. Verrucous carcinomas occur as large exophytic wart–like tumors that occupy considerable surface area. In the past, they have been classified as giant condylomas or Buschke-Lowenstein condylomas (Figure 15.85). Histologically, these neoplasms are composed of large papillae containing bland keratinocytes. The invasive component, consisting of nests of invading tumor cells, can only be noted at the broad tumor base. These tumors are associated with HPV, particularly subsets of type 6. Verrucous carcinomas are locally erosive tumors that grow into surrounding structures, including bone. The treatment is wide excision. Microscopic examination should pay particular attention to the base where the small invasive foci will be found.[1]

Condylomatous or warty carcinomas are also squamous cell variants that histologically will show cytologic features of HPV (koilocytosis, multinucleation). These tumors probably represent the invasive counterpart of warty VIN. Basaloid carcinomas consist of small, immature cells similar to abnormal

basal cells and probably represent the invasive counterpart to basaloid VIN. Condylomatous and basaloid carcinomas both contain HPV, usually type 16.[1]

15.8.2 Melanocytic Carcinoma (Melanoma)

Melanomas make up approximately 5% of vulvar malignancies. They occur in older women and are more common in Caucasian than black women. Melanomas present as pigmented areas that are usually flat or slightly raised (Figure 15.86). Their appearance is similar to other benign pigmented lesions, and excision is necessary to make a definitive diagnosis. Features that suggest melanoma are large pigmented areas with irregular borders and satellite lesions. However, amelanotic melanomas of the vulva are also seen.[186]

Any pigmented lesion of questionable etiology should be removed for histologic examination, especially if it is new or it recently changed in appearance.[15,16]

Histologically, melanomas demonstrate three growth patterns: (1) superficial spreading, with a predominant lateral spread; (2) nodular, with a predominant vertical spread; and (3) acral lentiginous, with mixed lateral and vertical spread patterns. The hallmark cell is the malignant melanocyte, which is typically round with large, round to oval nuclei, and prominent nucleoli. The presence of melanin pigment varies. Initial tumors will have malignant cells scattered throughout the epidermis in a "buckshot" pattern; however, continued growth will result in extension into the superficial (papillary) dermis and eventually into the subcutaneous tissues (Figure 15.87). The distribution of nonpigmented malignant melanocytes in the epidermis may resemble the intraepithelial adenocarcinoma cells of Paget's disease. Those arising in large tumors can resemble epithelioid cells seen in poorly differentiated carcinomas. Markers are occasionally required to document a melanocytic origin.[16] Determining the depth of invasion is extremely important, as this is a valuable prognostic tool and will dictate the method of treatment. Because of this, it is better to completely excise a pigmented lesion suspicious for melanoma, than just biopsy it. The resultant crush artifact and scarring from biopsy may render measurements inaccurate. However, for large lesions, a biopsy is acceptable.

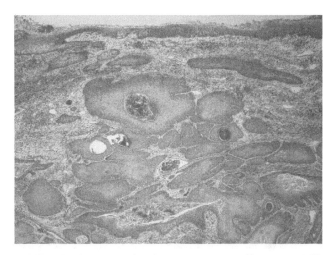

FIGURE 15.83. Nests of malignant squamous cells are seen infiltrating throughout the dermis. Numerous keratin pearls are present. (Hematoxylin-eosin stain; medium power magnification.)

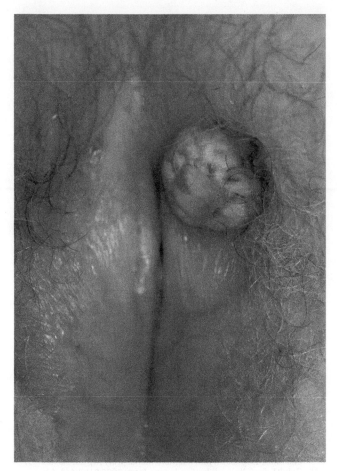

FIGURE 15.85.   Verrucous carcinoma of the vulva in a patient with coexisting LS.

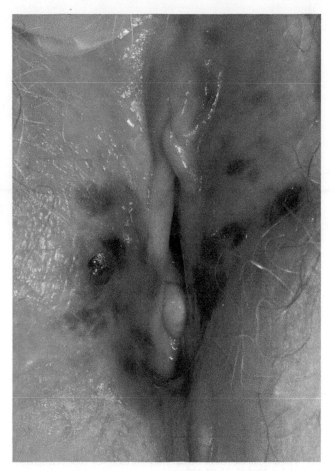

FIGURE 15.86.   Malignant melanoma of the vulva. Irregular asymmetric pigmented lesions are present.

Traditionally, Clark's levels were used to classify these tumors, but these could be highly variable due to the background morphology of the epidermis and dermis. Precise measurements extending from the stratum granulosum into the underlying dermis (Breslow's depth) are presently the preferred method (Figure 15.88).[182]

The treatment for superficial melanoma is wide local excision, including enough lateral skin to ensure the entire lesion is removed.[8,187,188] Small tumors that are minimally invasive can be treated by local excision with a 1- to 2-cm-wide margin. Large tumors and those that invade into the reticular dermis or subcutaneous fat are usually treated by excision and regional lymphadenectomy.[1,16,189] Grafts and/or flaps are required at times.[190] Sentinel lymph node studies are currently ongoing in the evaluation of patients with vulvar melanoma.[191] Positron emission tomography and computed tomography scans for staging and evaluation of response, and adjuvant chemo or biochemotherapy require further investigation before they are routinely utilized.[192]

15.8.3 Adenocarcinoma

Vulvar adenocarcinomas can be metastatic or arise from glandular structures that comprise the skin adnexae and the vestibular glands, the most common site being Bartholin's glands.[193] Clinically, these carcinomas often present as raised irregular firm nodules or erosive ulcerations. Microscopically, the histology is typical of other glandular cancers, with nests of malignant cells that form irregular gland lumens. The degree of differentiation is dependent on the ability of the adenocarcinoma cells to recapitulate gland structures. Poorly differentiated neoplasms consist mostly of solid sheets of malignant cells with only an occasional gland structure.[15] The recommended treatment for adenocarcinoma is similar to that for squamous carcinomas of the vulva and includes radical excision of the tumor and regional lymph node sampling.

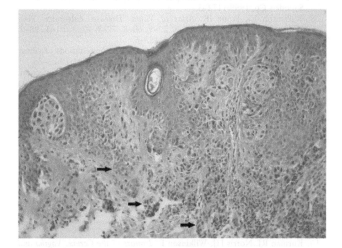

FIGURE 15.87.   Photomicrograph of malignant melanoma. Nests of malignant melanocytes, many of which contain brown pigment, are found in the epidermis and the superficial dermis (arrows). (Hematoxylin-eosin stain; medium power magnification.)

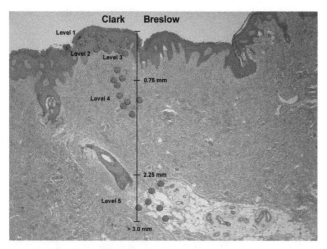

FIGURE 15.88.   Measuring the depth of invasion in malignant melanoma of the vulva. Traditionally, the depth was marked by different levels (Clark): *1* indicates confinement to the epidermis, *2* indicates extension into the papillary dermis, *3* indicates malignant cells filling the dermal papillae, *4* indicates extension into the reticular dermis, and *5* indicates extension into the subcutaneous fat. Because the actual depths of these levels vary depending on the skin morphology, absolute measurements are now used (Breslow). (Hematoxylin-eosin stain; medium power magnification.)

References

1. Wilkinson EJ. Benign diseases of the vulva. In: Kurman RJ, ed. *Blaustein's Pathology of the Female Genital Tract* (4th ed.). New York, NY: Springer-Verlag, 1994:31–87, 93–108.
2. Wilkinson EJ, Hart NS. Vulva. In: Sternberg SS, ed. *Histology for Pathologists*. New York, NY: Raven Press, 1992:865–81.
3. O'Connell HE, Sanjeevan KV, Hutson JM. Anatomy of the clitoris. *J Urol* 2005;174(4, pt 1):1189–95.
4. Martin-Alguacil N, Schober JM, Sengelaub DR, Pfaff DW, Shelley DN. Clitoral sexual arousal: neuronal tracing study from the clitoris through the spinal tracts. *J Urol* 2008;180(4):1241–8.
5. Bergeron C, Ferenczy A, Richart RM, Guralnick M. Micropapillomatosis labialis appears unrelated to human papillomavirus. *Obstet Gynecol* 1990;76:281–6.
6. Edgardh K, Ormstad K. The adolescent hymen. *J Reprod Med* 2002;47(9):710–4.
7. Murphy GM, Mihm MC. The skin. In: Cotran RS, Kumar V, Collins T, eds. *Robbins Pathologic Basis of Disease* (6th ed.). Philadelphia, PA: WB Saunders Co, 1999:1172–3.
8. Wilkinson EJ, Stone IK. *Atlas of Vulvar Disease*. Baltimore, MD: Williams and Wilkins, 1995:5–8, 27–9, 60–8, 77–8, 82–3, 91–3, 98–9, 122–4, 137–8,141–3, 154–5, 171–6, 183–6.
9. Cone R, Beckmann A, Aho M, et al. Subclinical manifestations of vulvar human papillomavirus infection. *Int J Gynecol Pathol* 1991;10:26–35.
10. di Paola GR, Rueda NG. Deceptive vulvar papillomavirus infection. A possible explanation for certain cases of vulvodynia. *J Reprod Med* 1986;31(10):966–70.
11. Julian TM. Vulvar pain: diagnosis, evaluation and management. *J Low Genit Tract Dis* 1997;1:185–94.
12. Wilkinson EJ, Guerrero E, Daniel R, et al. Vulvar vestibulodynia is rarely associated with human papillomavirus infection types 6, 11, 16, or 18. *Int J Gynecol Pathol* 1993;12(4):344–9.
13. Origoni M, Rossi M, Ferrari D, Lillo F, Ferrari AG. Human papillomavirus with co-existing vulvar vestibulodynia syndrome and vestibular papillomatosis. *Int J Gynecol Pathol* 1999;64:259–63.
14. Lever WF, Schaumburg-Lever G. *Histopathology of the Skin* (6th ed.). Philadelphia, PA: Lippincott, 1990:156–61, 168–74, 308–12, 364–8.
15. Wilkinson EJ. Premalignant and malignant tumors of the vulva. In: *Blaustein's Pathology of the Female Genital Tract* (4th ed.). New York, NY: Springer-Verlag, 1994:87–93, 117–21.
16. Kurman RJ, Norris HJ, Wilkinson E. *Tumors of the Cervix, Vagina and Vulva. Atlas of Tumor Pathology* (Third Series: Fascicle 4). Washington, DC: American Registry of Pathology, Armed Forces Institute of Pathology, 1992:191–202.
17. Department of Health and Human Services Centers for Disease Control and Prevention 2010 STD Treatment Guidelines http://www.cdc.gov/std/treatment/default.htm. Accessed August 1, 2011.
18. Arduino PG, Porter SR. Herpes simplex virus type 1 infection: overview on relevant clinico-pathological features. *J Oral Pathol Med* 2008;37(2):107–21.
19. Cernik C, Gallina K, Brodell RT. The treatment of herpes simplex infections: an evidence-based review. *Arch Intern Med* 2008;168(11):1137–44.
20. Martinez V, Caumes E, Chosidow O. Treatment to prevent recurrent genital herpes. *Curr Opin Infect Dis* 2008;21(1):42–8.
21. Watanabe T, Tamaki K. Detection of molluscum contagiosum virus gene transcripts by in situ hybridization. *J Dermatol Sci* 2009;54(3):209–12.
22. Gould D. An overview of molluscum contagiosum: a viral skin condition. *Nurs Stand* 2008;22(41):45–8.
23. Guirguis-Blake J. Interventions for molluscum contagiosum. *Am Fam Physician* 2006;74(9):1504.
24. van der Wouden JC, Menke J, Gajadin S, et al. Interventions for cutaneous molluscum contagiosum. *Cochrane Database Syst Rev* 2006;(2):CD004767.
25. Kauffman CL. Molluscum Contagiosum. http://emedicine.medscape.com/article/1132908-overview. Accessed May 25, 2010.
26. Wright TC, Massad S, Dunton CJ, Spitzer M. Wilkinson EJ, Solomon D. 2006 consensus guidelines for the management of women with abnormal cervical cancer screening tests. *Am J Obstet Gynecol* 2007;197(4):346–55.
27. Brownell I, CK. Treatments for genital warts. *J Drugs Dermatol* 2008;7(8):801–7.
28. Kennedy CM, Boardman LA. New approaches to external genital warts and vulvar intraepithelial neoplasia. *Clin Obstet Gynecol* 2008;51(3):518–26.
29. Mayeaux EJ Jr, Dunton C. Modern management of external genital warts. *J Low Genit Tract Dis* 2008;12(3):185–92.
30. Taner ZM, Taskiran C, Onan AM, Gursoy R, Himmetoglu O. Therapeutic value of trichloroacetic acid in the treatment of isolated genital warts on the external female genitalia. *J Reprod Med* 2007;52(6):521–5.
31. Dede M, Kubar A, Yenen MC, et al. Human papillomavirus-type predict the clinical outcome of imiquimod therapy for women with vulvar condylomata acuminata. *Acta Obstet Gynecol Scand* 2007;86(8):968–72.
32. Aynaud O, Buffet M, Roman P, Plantier F, Dupin N. Study of persistence and recurrence rates in 106 patients with condyloma and intraepithelial neoplasia after CO$_2$ laser treatment. *Eur J Dermatol* 2008;18(2):153–8.
33. Pope V. Use of treponemal tests to screen for syphilis. *Infect Med* 2004;21:399–402.
34. CDC. Inadvertent use of Bicillin® C-R to treat syphilis infection—Los Angeles, California, 1999–2004. *MMWR Morb Mortal Wkly Rep* 2005;54:217–9.
35. Goh BT. Syphilis in adults. *Sex Transm Infect* 2005;81(6):448–52.
36. Nnoruka EN, Ezeoke AC. Evaluation of syphilis in patients with HIV infection in Nigeria. *Trop Med Int Health* 2005;10(1):58–64.
37. Rashid RM, Janjua SA, Khachemoune A. Granuloma inguinale: a case report. *Dermatol Online J* 2006;12(7):14.
38. Richens J. Donovanosis (granuloma inguinale). *Sex Transm Infect* 2006;82(suppl 4):iv21–2.
39. Kaliaperumal K. Recent advances in management of genital ulcer disease and anogenital warts. *Dermatol Ther* 2008;21(3):196–204.
40. Kapoor S. Re-emergence of lymphogranuloma venereum. *J Eur Acad Dermatol Venereol* 2008;22(4):409–16.
41. White J, Ison C. Lymphogranuloma venereum: what does the clinician need to know? *Clin Med* 2008;8(3):327–30.
42. McLean CA, Stoner BP, Workowski KA. Treatment of lymphogranuloma venereum. *Clin Infect Dis* 2007;44(suppl 3):S147–52.
43. Sobel JD. Vulvovaginal candidiasis. *Lancet* 2007;369:1961–71.
44. Xu J, Schwartz K, Bartoces M, Monsur J, Severson RK, Sobel JD. Effect of antibiotics on vulvovaginal candidiasis: a MetroNet study. *J Am Board Fam Med* 2008;21(4):261–68.
45. Ehrstrom SM, Kornfeld D, Thuresson J, Rylander E. Signs of chronic stress in women with recurrent candida vulvovaginitis. *Am J Obstet Gynecol* 2005;193(4):1376–81.
46. Faro S, Apuzzio J, Bohannon N, et al. Treatment considerations in vulvovaginal candidiasis. *Female Patient* 1997;22:39–56.
47. Pappas PG, Rex JH, Sobel JD, et al. Infectious Diseases Society of America. Guidelines for treatment of candidiasis. *Clin Infect Dis* 2004;38:161–89.
48. Richter SS, Galask RP, Messer SA, Hollis RJ, Diekema DJ, Pfaller MA. Antifungal susceptibilities of Candida species causing vulvovaginitis and epidemiology of recurrent cases. *J Clin Microbiol* 2005;43(5):2155–62.
49. Urunsak M, Ilkit M, Evruke C, Urunsak I. Clinical and mycological efficacy of single-day oral treatment with itraconazole (400 mg) in acute vulvovaginal candidosis. *Mycoses* 2004;47:422–7.
50. Sobel JD, Kapernick PS, Zervos M, et al. Treatment of complicated Candida vaginitis: comparison of single and sequential doses of fluconazole. *Am J Obstet Gynecol* 2001;185:363–9.
51. Bauters TG, Dhont MA, Temmerman MI, Nelis HJ. Prevalence of vulvovaginal candidiasis and susceptibility to fluconazole in women. *Am J Obstet Gynecol* 2002;187:569–74.
52. Sobel JD, Wiesenfeld HC, Martens M, et al. Maintenance fluconazole therapy for recurrent vulvovaginal candidiasis. *N Engl J Med* 2004;351:876–83.
53. Thai L, Hart LL. Boric acid vaginal suppositories. *Ann Pharmacother* 1993;27:1355–7.

54. Guaschino S, De Seta F, Sartore A, et al. Efficacy of maintenance therapy with topical boric acid in comparison with oral itraconazole in the treatment of recurrent vulvovaginal candidiasis. *Am J Obstet Gynecol* 2001;184:598–602.

55. Ray D, Goswami R, Banerjee U, et al. Prevalence of *Candida glabrata* and its response to boric acid vaginal suppositories in comparison with oral fluconazole in patients with diabetes and vulvovaginal candidiasis. *Diabetes Care* 2007;30(2):312–7.

56. Khan ZU, Ahmad S, Al-Obaid I, Al-Sweih NA, Joseph L, Farhat D. Emergence of resistance to amphotericin b and triazoles in *Candida glabrata* vaginal isolates in a case of recurrent vaginitis. *J Chemother* 2008;20(4):488–91.

57. Phillips AJ. Treatment of non-albicans Candida vaginitis with amphotericin B vaginal suppositories. *Am J Obstet Gynecol* 2005;192(6):2009–12; discussion 2012–3.

58. Sobel JD, Chaim W, Nagappan V, Leaman D. Treatment of vaginitis caused by *Candida glabrata*: use of topical boric acid and flucytosine. *Am J Obstet Gynecol* 2003;189:1297–300.

59. Wiederkehr M. Tinea cruris. http://emedicine.medscape.com/article/1091806-overview. Accessed May 25, 2010.

60. Wiederkehr M. Tinea cruris: differential diagnoses & workup. http://emedicine.medscape.com/article/1091806-diagnosis. Accessed May 25, 2010.

61. Nadalo D, Montoya C, Hunter-Smith D. What is the best way to treat tinea cruris? *J Fam Pract* 2006;55(3):256–8.

62. Thomas TG. *Practical Treatise on the Diseases of Women* (4th ed.). Henry C. Philadelphia, PA: Lea's Son & Co., 1874:114–6.

63. Skene AJC. *Treatise on the Diseases of Women*. New York, NY: D Appleton and Co, 1889:93–4.

64. Kelly HA. Gynecology. New York, NY: D. Appleton and Co., 1928:235–9.

65. Friedrich EG Jr. The vulvar vestibule. *J Reprod Med* 1983;28(11):773–7.

66. Friedrich EG Jr. Vulvar vestibulitis syndrome. *J Reprod Med* 1987;32(2):110–4.

67. Moyal-Barracco M, Lynch PJ. 2003 ISSVD terminology and classification of vulvodynia: a historical perspective. *J Reprod Med* 2004;49(10):772–7.

68. McCormack WM. Two urogenital sinus syndromes. Interstitial cystitis and focal vulvitis. *J Reprod Med* 1990;35(9):873–6.

69. Fitzpatrick CC, DeLancey JO, Elkins TE, McGuire EJ. Vulvar vestibulitis and interstitial cystitis: a disorder of urogenital sinus-derived epithelium. *Obstet Gynecol* 1993;81(5):860–2.

70. Bohm-Starke N, Falconer C, Rylander E, Hilliges M. The expression of cyclooxygenase 2 and inducible nitric oxide synthase indicates no active inflammation in vulvar vestibulitis. *Acta Obstet Gynecol Scand* 2001;80:638–44.

71. Meana M, Binik YM, Khalif S, Cohen DR. Deconstructing dyspareunia: description, classification and biopsychosocial correlates of a pain disorder (Thesis). Montreal, Canada: McGill University, 1995.

72. Mann MS, Kaufman RH, Brown D Jr, Adam E. Vulvar vestibulitis: significant clinical variables and treatment outcome. *Obstet Gynecol* 1992;79(1):122–5.

73. Bazin S, Bouchard C, Brisson J, Morin C, Meisels A, Fortier M. Vulvar vestibulitis syndrome: an exploratory case-control study. *Obstet Gynecol* 1994;83(1):47–50.

74. Goetsch MF. Vulvar vestibulitis: prevalence and historic features in a general gynecologic practice population. *Am J Obstet Gynecol* 1991;164(6, pt 1):1609–14; discussion 1614–6.

75. Jeremias J, Ledger WJ, Witkin SS. Interleukin 1 receptor antagonist gene polymorphism in women with vulvar vestibulitis. *Am J Obstet Gynecol* 2000;182(2):283–5.

76. Witkin SS, Gerber S, Ledger WJ. Differential characterization of women with vulvar vestibulitis syndrome. *Am J Obstet Gynecol* 2002;187(3):589–94.

77. Foster DC, Piekarz KH, Murant TI, LaPoint R, Haidaris CG, Phipps RP. Enhanced synthesis of proinflammatory cytokines by vulvar vestibular fibroblasts: implications for vulvar vestibulitis. *Am J Obstet Gynecol* 2007;196(4):346.e1–8.

78. Krantz KE. Innervation of the human vulva and vagina. *Obstet Gynecol* 1958;12:382–96.

79. Bohm-Starke N, Hilliges M, Brodda-Jansen G, Rylander E, Torebjork E. Psychophysical evidence of nociceptor sensitization in vulvar vestibulitis syndrome. *Pain* 2001;94(2):177–83.

80. Tympanidis P, Terenghi G, Dowd P. Increased innervation of the vulval vestibule in patients with vulvodynia. *Br J Dermatol* 2003;148:1021–7.

81. Abramov L, Wolman I, David MP. Vaginismus: an important factor in the evaluation and management of vulvar vestibulitis syndrome. *Gynecol Obstet Invest* 1994;38(3):194–7.

82. Walsh KE, Berman JR, Berman LA, Vierregger K. Safety and efficacy of topical nitroglycerin for treatment of vulvar pain in women with vulvodynia: a pilot study. *J Gend Specif Med* 2002;6:21–7.

83. Ben-David B, Friedman M. Gabapentin therapy for vulvodynia. *Anesth Analg* 1999;89:1459–62.

84. Scheinfeld N. The role of gabapentin in treating diseases with cutaneous manifestations and pain. *Int J Dermatol* 2003;42(6):491–5.

85. Bergeron S, Binik YM, Khalife S, et al. A randomized comparison of group cognitive—behavioral therapy, surface electromyographic biofeedback, and vestibulectomy in the treatment of dyspareunia resulting from vulvar vestibulitis. *Pain* 2001;91:297–306.

86. Glazer HI, Rodke G, Swencionis C, Hertz R, Young AW. Treatment of vulvar vestibulitis syndrome with electromyographic biofeedback of pelvic floor musculature. *J Reprod Med* 1995;40:283–90.

87. Glazer HI, Marinoff SC, Sleight IJ. Web-enabled Glazer surface electromyographic protocol for the remote, real-time assessment and rehabilitation of pelvic floor dysfunction in vulvar vestibulitis syndrome. A case report. *J Reprod Med* 2002;47(9):728–30.

88. McKay E, Kaufman RH, Doctor U, Berkova Z, Glazer H, Redko V. Treating vulvar vestibulitis with electromyographic biofeedback of pelvic floor musculature. *J Reprod Med* 2001;46:337–42.

89. Bergerson S, Brown C, Lord MJ, Oala M, Binik YM, Khalife S. Physical therapy for vulvar vestibulitis syndrome: a retrospective study. *J Sex Marital Ther* 2002;28(3):183–92.

90. Hartmann EH, Nelson C. The perceived effectiveness of physical therapy treatment on women complaining of chronic vulvar pain and diagnosed with either vulvar vestibulitis syndrome or dysesthetic vulvodynia. Section Womens Health 2001;25:13–8.

91. Segal D, Tifheret H, Lazer S. Submucous infiltration of betamethasone and lidocaine in the treatment of vulvar vestibulitis. *Eur J Obstet Gynecol Reprod Biol* 2003;107(1):105–6.

92. Calvillo O, Skaribas IM, Rockett C. Computed tomography-guided pudendal nerve block. A new diagnostic approach to long-term anoperineal pain: a report of two cases. *Reg Anesth Pain Med* 2000;25(4):420–3.

93. Marinoff SC, Turner ML, Hirsch RP, Richard G. Intralesional alpha interferon. Cost-effective therapy for vulvar vestibulitis syndrome. *J Reprod Med* 1993;38(1):19–24.

94. Horowitz BJ. Interferon therapy for condylomatous vulvitis. *Obstet Gynecol* 1989;73(3, pt 1):446–8.

95. Sonnendecker EW, Sonnendecker HE, Wright CA, Simon GB. Recalcitrant vulvodynia. A clinicopathological study. *S Afr Med J* 1993;83(10):730–3.

96. Kent HL, Wisniewski PM. Interferon for vulvar vestibulitis. *J Reprod Med* 1990;35(12):1138–40.

97. Umpierre SA, Kaufman RH, Adam E, Woods KV, Adler-Storthz K. Human papillomavirus DNA in tissue biopsy specimens of vulvar vestibulitis patients treated with interferon. *Obstet Gynecol* 1991;78(4):693–5.

98. Larsen J, Peters K, Petersen CS, Damkjaer K, Albrectsen J, Weismann K. Interferon alpha-2b treatment of symptomatic chronic vulvar vulvodynia associated with koilocytosis. *Acta Derm Venereol* 1993;73(5):385–7.

99. Gerber S, Bongiovanni AM, Ledger WJ, Witkin SS. A deficiency in interferon-alpha production in women with vulvar vestibulitis. *Am J Obstet Gynecol* 2002;186(3):361–4.

100. Bornstein J, Abramovici H. Combination of subtotal perineoplasty and interferon for the treatment of vulvar vestibulitis. *Gynecol Obstet Invest* 1997;44(1):53–6.

101. Argoff CE. A focused review on the use of botulinum toxins for neuropathic pain. *Clin J Pain* 2002;18(6 suppl):S177–81.

102. Lang AM. Botulinum toxin type A therapy in chronic pain disorders. *Arch Phys Med Rehabil* 2003;84(3 suppl 1):S69–73; quiz S74–75.

103. Gunter J, Brewer A, Tawfik O. Botulinum toxin a for vulvodynia: a case report. *J Pain* 2004;5(4):238–40.

104. Brown CS, Glazer HI, Vogt V, Menkes D, Bachmann G. Subjective and objective outcomes of botulinum toxin type A treatment in vestibulodynia: pilot data. *J Reprod Med* 2006;51(8):635–41.

105. Dykstra DD, Presthus J. Botulinum toxin type A for the treatment of provoked vestibulodynia: an open-label, pilot study. *J Reprod Med* 2006;51(6):467–70.

106. Graziottin A. Botulinum neurotoxin type A injections for vaginismus secondary to vulvar vestibulitis syndrome. *Obstet Gynecol* 2009;114(5):1008–16.

107. Danielsson I, Sjoberg I, Ostman C. Acupuncture for the treatment of vulvar vestibulitis: a pilot study. *Acta Obstet Gynecol Scand* 2001;80:437–41.

108. Powell J, Wojnarowska F. Acupuncture for vulvodynia. *J R Soc Med* 1999;92:579–81.

109. Aung SKH. Sexual dysfunction: a modern medical acupuncture approach. Medical Acupuncture online Journal. http://www.medicalacupuncture.org/aama_marf/journal/index.html. Accessed May 25, 2010.

110. Kandyba K, Binik YM. Hypotherapy as a treatment for vulvar vestibulitis syndrome: a case report. *J Sex Marital Ther* 2003;29:237–42.

111. McCormack WM, Spence MR. Evaluation of the surgical treatment of vulvar vestibulitis. *Eur J Obstet Gynecol Reprod Biol* 1999;86:135–8.

112. Haefner HK. Critique of new gynecologic surgical procedures: surgery for vulvar vestibulitis. *Clin Obstet Gynecol* 2000;43:689–700.

113. O'Connell TX, Nathan LS, Satmary WA, Goldstein AT. Non-neoplastic epithelial disorders of the vulva. *Am Fam Physician* 2008;77(3):321–6.

114. Wilkinson EJ. The 1989 presidential address: International Society for the Study of Vulvar Disease. *J Reprod Med* 1989;35:981–91.

115. Wilkinson EJ, Ridley CM, McKay M, Lynch P, Kaufman RH. What is the ISSVD classification of vulvar nonneoplastic epithelial disorders and intraepithelial neoplasia? *Am J Dermatopathol* 1991;13(4):428–9.

116. Bohl TG. Overview of vulvar pruritus through the life cycle. *Clin Obstet Gynecol* 2005;48(4):786–807.

117. van Hoeven KH, Kovatich AJ. Immunohistochemical staining for proliferating cell nuclear antigen, BCL-2, and Ki-67 in vulvar tissues. *Int J Gynecol Pathol* 1996;15:10–6.

118. Cooper SM, Ali I, Baldo M, Wojnarowska F. The association of lichen sclerosus and erosive lichen planus of the vulva with autoimmune disease: a case-control study. *Arch Dermatol* 2008;144(11):1432–5.

119. Birenbaum DL, Young RC. High prevalence of thyroid disease in patients with lichen sclerosus. *J Reprod Med* 2007;52(1):28–30.
120. Marren P, Yell F, Charnock M, Bunce M, Welsh K, Wojnarowska F. The association between lichen sclerosus and antigens of the HLA system. *Br J Dermatol* 1995;132:197–203.
121. van de Nieuwenhof HP, van der Avoort IA, de Hullu JA. Review of squamous premalignant vulvar lesions. *Crit Rev Oncol Hematol* 2008;68(2):131–56.
122. Rodke G, Friedrich EG, Wilkinson EJ. Malignant potential of mixed vulvar dystrophy. (Lichen sclerosus associated with squamous cell hyperplasia.) *J Reprod Med* 1988;33:545–50.
123. Paslin D. Treatment of lichen sclerosus with topical dihydrotestosterone. *Obstet Gynecol* 1991;78:1046–9.
124. Dalziel KL, Wojnarowska F. Long-term control of vulval lichen sclerosus after treatment with a potent topical steroid cream. *J Reprod Med* 1993;38:25–7.
125. Jones RW, Scurry J, Neill S, MacLean AB. Guidelines for the follow-up of women with vulvar lichen sclerosus in specialist clinics. *Am J Obstet Gynecol* 2008;198(5):496.e1–3.
126. Ambros RA, Malfetano JH, Carlson JA, Mihm MC. Non-neoplastic epithelial alterations of the vulva: recognition and comparisons terminologies used among the various specialties. *Mod Pathol* 1997;10:401–8.
127. Toki T, Kurman RJ, Park JS, Kessis T, Daniel RW, Shah KV. Probable non-papillomavirus etiology of squamous cell carcinoma of the vulva in older women; a clinicopathologic study using in situ hybridization and polymerase chain reaction. *Int J Gynecol Pathol* 1991;10:107–25.
128. Lichon V, Khachemoune A. Lichen simplex chronicus. *Dermatol Nurs* 2007;19(3):276.
129. Cattaneo A, Bracco GL, Maestrini G, Carli G, Colafranceschi M, Marchionini M. Lichen sclerosus and squamous hyperplasia: a clinical study of medical treatment. *J Reprod Med* 1991;36:301–5.
130. Cooper SM, Ali I, Baldo M, Wojnarowska F. The association of lichen sclerosus and erosive lichen planus of the vulva with autoimmune disease: a case-control study. *Arch Dermatol* 2008;144(11):1432–5.
131. Belfiore P, Di Fede O, Cabibi D, et al. Prevalence of vulval lichen planus in a cohort of women with oral lichen planus: an interdisciplinary study. *Br J Dermatol* 2006;155(5):994–8.
132. Cooper SM, Haefner HK, Abrahams-Gessel S, Margesson LJ. Vulvovaginal lichen planus treatment: a survey of current practices. *Arch Dermatol* 2008;144(11):1520–1.
133. Kennedy CM, Galask RP. Erosive vulvar lichen planus: retrospective review of characteristics and outcomes in 113 patients seen in a vulvar specialty clinic. *J Reprod Med* 2007;52(1):43–7.
134. Stalburg CM, Haefner HK. Vaginal stenosis in lichen planus: surgical treatment tips for patients in whom conservative therapies have failed. *J Pelvic Med Surg* 2008;14:193–8.
135. Kortekangas-Savolainen O, Kiilholma P. Treatment of vulvovaginal erosive and stenosing lichen planus by surgical dilatation and methotrexate. *Acta Obstet Gynecol Scand* 2007;86(3):339–43.
136. Neill SM, Lewis FM. Vulvovaginal lichen planus: a disease in need of a unified approach. *Arch Dermatol* 2008;144(11):1502–3.
137. Zamirska A, Reich A, Berny-Moreno J, Salomon J, Szepietowski JC. Vulvar pruritus and burning sensation in women with psoriasis. *Acta Derm Venereol* 2008;88(2):132–5.
138. van de Nieuwenhof HP, van der Avoort IA, de Hullu JA. Review of squamous premalignant vulvar lesions. *Crit Rev Oncol Hematol* 2008;68(2):131–56.
139. Sideri M, Jones RW, Wilkinson EJ, et al. Squamous vulvar intraepithelial neoplasia: 2004 modified terminology, ISSVD Vulvar Oncology Subcommittee. *J Reprod Med* 2005;50(11):807–10.
140. Sturgeon SR, Brinton LA, Devesa SS, Kurman RJ. In situ and invasive vulvar cancer incidence trends (1973 to 1987). *Am J Obstet Gynecol* 1992;166:1482–5.
141. Hart WR. Vulvar intraepithelial neoplasia: historical aspects and current status. *Int J Gynecol Pathol* 2001;20:16–30.
142. Saraiya M, Watson M, Wu X, et al. Incidence of in situ and invasive vulvar cancer in the US, 1998–2003. *Cancer* 2008;113(10 suppl):2865–72.
143. Insinga RP, Liaw KL, Johnson LG, Madeleine MM. A systematic review of the prevalence and attribution of human papillomavirus types among cervical, vaginal, and vulvar precancers and cancers in the United States. *Cancer Epidemiol Biomarkers Prev* 2008;17(7):1611–22.
144. Yang B, Hart WR. Vulvar intraepithelial neoplasia of the simplex (differentiated) type: a clinicopathological study including analysis of HPV and p53 alterations. *Am J Surg Pathol* 2000;24:429–41.
145. Park BS, Jones RW, McLean MR, et al. Possible etiologic heterogeneity of vulvar intraepithelial neoplasia: a correlation of pathologic characteristics with human papillomavirus detection by in situ hybridization and polymerase chain reaction. *Cancer* 1991;67:1599–1607.
146. Davis G, Wentworth J, Richard J. Self-administered topical imiquimod treatment of vulvar intraepithelial neoplasia. *J Reprod Med* 2000;45:619–23.
147. Mathiesen O, Buus SK, Cramers M. Topical imiquimod can reverse vulvar intraepithelial neoplasia: a randomised, double-blinded study. *Gynecol Oncol* 2007;107(2):219–22.
148. van Seters M, van Beurden M, ten Kate FJ, et al. Treatment of vulvar intraepithelial neoplasia with topical imiquimod. *N Engl J Med* 2008;358(14):1465–73.

149. Kennedy CM, Boardman LA. New approaches to external genital warts and vulvar intraepithelial neoplasia. *Clin Obstet Gynecol* 2008;51(3):518–26.
150. Rouzier R, Haie-Meder C, Lhomme C, Avril MF, Duvillard P, Castaigne D. Prognostic significance of epithelial disorders adjacent to invasive vulvar carcinomas. *Gynecol Oncol* 2001;81:414–6.
151. Barbero M, Micheletti L, Preti M, et al. Biologic behavior of vulvar intraepithelial neoplasia. Histologic and clinical parameters. *J Reprod Med* 1993;38:108–12.
152. Athavale R, Naik R, Godfrey KA, Cross P, Hatem MH, de Barros Lopes A. Vulvar intraepithelial neoplasia—the need for auditable measures of management. *Eur J Obstet Gynecol Reprod Biol* 2008;137(1):97–102.
153. Park IU, Ogilvie JW Jr, Anderson KE, et al. Anal human papillomavirus infection and abnormal anal cytology in women with genital neoplasia. *Gynecol Oncol* 2009;114:399–403.
154. Bakalianou K, Salakos N, Iavazzo C, et al. Paget's disease of the vulva. A ten-year experience. *Eur J Gynaecol Oncol* 2008;29(4):368–70.
155. Dubreuilh W. Paget's disease of the vulva. *Br J Dermatol* 1901;13(11):407–13.
156. Turner AG. Pagetoid lesions associated with carcinoma of the bladder. *J Urol* 1980;123–6.
157. Fanning J, Lambert HCL, Hale TM, Morris PC, Schuerch C. Paget's disease of the vulva: prevalence of associated vulvar adenocarcinoma, invasive Paget's disease, and recurrence after surgical excision. *Am J Obstet Gynecol* 1999;180:24–7.
158. Roth LM, Lee SC, Ehrlich CE. Paget's disease of the vulva: a histogenetic study of five cases including ultrastructural observations and review of the literature. *Am J Surg Pathol* 1977;1:193–206.
159. Mai KT, Alhalouly T, Landry D, Stinson WA, Perkins DG, Yazdi HM. Pagetoid variant of actinic keratosis with or without squamous cell carcinoma of sun-exposed skin: a lesion simulating extramammary Paget's disease. *Histopathology* 2002;41(4):331–6.
160. Plaza JA, Torres-Cabala C, Ivan D, Prieto VG. HER-2/neu expression in extramammary Paget disease: a clinicopathologic and immunohistochemistry study of 47 cases with and without underlying malignancy. *J Cutan Pathol* 2009;36(7):729–33.
161. Shaco-Levy R, Bean SM, Vollmer RT, et al. Paget disease of the vulva: a histologic study of 56 cases correlating pathologic features and disease course. *Int J Gynecol Pathol* 2009;29:69–78.
162. Black D, Tornos C, Soslow RA, Awtrey CS, Barakat RR, Chi DS. The outcomes of patients with positive margins after excision for intraepithelial Paget's disease of the vulva. *Gynecol Oncol* 2007;104(3):547–50.
163. Hatch KD, Davis JR. Complete resolution of Paget disease of the vulva with imiquimod cream. *J Low Genit Tract Dis* 2008;12(2):90–4.
164. Geisler JP, Manahan KJ. Imiquimod in vulvar Paget's disease: a case report. *J Reprod Med* 2008;53(10):811–2.
165. Hatch KD, Davis JR. Complete resolution of Paget disease of the vulva with imiquimod cream. *J Low Genit Tract Dis* 2008;12(2):90–4.
166. Estrada R, Kaufman R. Benign vulvar melanosis. *J Reprod Med* 1993;38:5–8.
167. Obaidat NA, Awamleh AA, Ghazarian DM. Adenocarcinoma in situ arising in a tubulopapillary apocrine hidradenoma of the peri-anal region. *Eur J Dermatol* 2006;16(5):576–8.
168. Shah SS, Adelson M, Mazur MT. Adenocarcinoma in situ arising in vulvar papillary hidradenoma: report of 2 cases. *Int J Gynecol Pathol* 2008;27(3):453–6.
169. Biedrzycki OJ, Rufford B, Wilcox M, Barton DP, Jameson C. Malignant clear cell hidradenoma of the vulva: report of a unique case and review of the literature. *Int J Gynecol Pathol* 2008;27(1):142–6.
170. Cheewakriangkrai C, Sharma S, Deeb G, Lele S. A rare female genital tract tumor: benign granular cell tumor of vulva: case report and review of the literature. *Gynecol Oncol* 2005;97(2):656–8.
171. Laxmisha C, Thappa DM. Granular cell tumour of the clitoris. *J Eur Acad Dermatol Vereol* 2007;21(3):392–3.
172. Majmudar B, Castellano PZ, Wilson RW, Siegel RJ. Granular cell tumors of the vulva. *J Reprod Med* 1990;35:1008–14.
173. Levavi H, Sabah G, Kaplan B, Tytiun Y, Braslavsky D, Gutman H. Granular cell tumor of the vulva: six new cases. *Arch Gynecol Obstet* 2006;273(4):246–9.
174. Gleason BC, Hirsch MS, Nucci MR, et al. Atypical genital nevi. A clinicopathologic analysis of 56 cases, *Am J Surg Pathol* 2008;32(1):51–7.
175. Anderson WA, Franquemont DW, Williams J, Taylor PT, Crum CP. Vulvar squamous cell carcinoma and papillomavirus: two separate entities? *Am J Obstet Gynecol* 1991;165:329–35.
176. Rusk D, Sutton GP, Look KY, Roman A. Analysis of invasive squamous cell carcinoma of the vulva and vulvar intraepithelial neoplasia for the presence of human papillomavirus DNA. *Obstet Gynecol* 1991;77:918–22.
177. Scully RE, Bonfiglio TA, Silverberg SG. *Histologic Typing of Female Genital Tract Tumours. World Health Organizaiton International Histological Classification of Tumours* (2nd ed.). New York, NY: Springer-Verlag, 1994:64–70;74–5.
178. Pecorelli S. Revised FIGO staging for carcinoma of the vulva, cervix, and endometrium. *Int J Gynaecol Obstet* 2009;105(2):103–4.
179. Hacker NF. Revised FIGO staging for carcinoma of the vulva. *Int J Gynaecol Obstet* 2009;105(2):105–6.
180. Asjoe FMT, van Bekkum E, Ewing P, Burger CW, Ansink AC. Sentinel node procedure in vulvar squamous cell carcinoma: a histomorphologic

review of 32 cases. The significance of anucleate structures on immunohistochemistry. *Int J Gynecol Cancer* 2008;18(5):1032–6.

181. Johann S, Klaeser B, Krause T, Mueller MD. Comparison of outcome and recurrence-free survival after sentinel lymph node biopsy and lymphadenectomy in vulvar cancer. *Gynecol Oncol* 2008;110(3):324–8.

182. Levenback C, Coleman RL, Burke TW, Bodurka-Bevers D, Wolf JK, Gershenson DM. Intraoperative lymphatic mapping and sentinel node identification with blue dye in patients with vulvar cancer. *Gynecol Oncol* 2001;83:276–81.

183. Hicks ML, Hempling RE, Piver MS. Vulvar carcinoma with 0.5 mm of invasion in associated inguinal lymph node metastasis. *J Surg Oncol* 1993;54:271–3.

184. Atamdede F, Hoogerland D. Regional lymph node recurrence following local excision for microinvasive vulvar carcinoma. *Gynecol Oncol* 1989;34:125–8.

185. Hacker NF. Vulvar cancer. In: Berek JS, Hacker NF, eds. *Practical Gynecologic Oncology* (3rd ed.). Philadelphia, PA: Williams and Wilkins, 2000:563–76.

186. Baderca F, Cojocaru S, Lazar E, et al. Amelanotic vulvar melanoma: case report and review of the literature. *Rom J Morphol Embryol* 2008;49(2):219–28.

187. Sugiyama VE, Chan JK, Shin JY, Berek JS, Osann K, Kapp DS. Vulvar melanoma: a multivariable analysis of 644 patients. *Obstet Gynecol* 2007;110(2, pt 1):296–301.

188. Suwandinata FS, Bohle RM, Omwandho CA, Tinneberg HR, Gruessner SE. Management of vulvar melanoma and review of the literature. *Eur J Gynaecol Oncol* 2007;28(3):220–4.

189. El-Ghobashy AE, Saidi SA. Sentinel lymph node sampling in gynaecological cancers: techniques and clinical applications. *Eur J Surg Oncol* 2009;35(7):675–85.

190. Staiano JJ, Wong L, Butler J, Searle AE, Barton DP, Harris PA. Flap reconstruction following gynaecological tumour resection for advanced and recurrent disease—a 12 year experience. *J Plast Reconstr Aesthet Surg* 2009;62(3):346–51.

191. Dhar KK, Das N, Brinkman DA, Beynon JL, Woolas RP. Utility of sentinel node biopsy in vulvar and vaginal melanoma: report of two cases and review of the literature. *Eur J Surg Oncol* 2007;17(3):720–3.

192. Sugiyama VE, Chan JK, Kapp DS. Management of melanomas of the female genital tract. *Curr Opin Oncol* 2008;20(5):565–9.

193. Sahincioglu O, Berker B, Gungor M, Kankaya D, Sertcelik A. Adenoid cystic carcinoma of the Bartholin's gland: a rare tumor unmarked by persistent vulvar pain in a postmenopausal woman. *Arch Gynecol Obstet* 2008;278(5):473–6.

CHAPTER 16

HPV Infections in Adolescents

16.1 INTRODUCTION
16.2 EPIDEMIOLOGY AND THE NATURAL HISTORY OF HPV AND CERVICAL SQUAMOUS NEOPLASIA IN ADOLESCENTS
16.3 RISKS FOR HPV AMONG ADOLESCENTS
16.4 NATURAL HISTORY OF HPV AND SIL
16.5 CERVICAL CANCER SCREENING

16.6 COLPOSCOPIC FINDINGS IN ADOLESCENTS
16.7 HISTOLOGY
16.8 MANAGEMENT
    16.8.1 Treatment Decisions
    16.8.2 Treatment of CIN 1
    16.8.3 Treatment of CIN 2,3
16.9 CONCLUSION

16.1 INTRODUCTION

Most cervical cancer evidence-based screening guidelines define adolescents as persons before their 21st birthday. Adolescents have a unique niche in the world of human papillomavirus (HPV). They appear to be highly vulnerable to HPV infections, resulting in high rates of HPV detection, yet have extremely low rates of cervical cancer. Whether HPV infection during adolescence is a greater risk factor for high-grade precursor disease or cancer than the risk with HPV infection at other ages is yet to be determined. However, it is clear that detection of HPV in an adolescent is not a marker of current cancer risk. The risk for future cancer, that is, those who end up being at risk, is usually decades away. The high rates of HPV detection go hand in hand with high rates of abnormal cytology, raising the question, "How do we care for adolescents with abnormal cytology?" or, better, "Do we care about abnormal cytology in adolescents?"

Numerous studies document that adolescents have high rates of repeated HPV acquisition with equally high rates of clearance for each of these acquisitions. Since the cytologic description of squamous intraepithelial lesion (SIL) is a reflection of HPV infection, it is not surprising that the same effect is seen for SILs in adolescents. On the other hand, there is no question that HPV is the cause of cervical cancer—so scientists ask, "Is there a relationship between first infection, which usually occurs under the age of 21 years, and the development of cervical cancer several decades later?" Adolescence is a time of biologic and psychological development, and both may contribute to high HPV prevalence and incidence. But, it remains questionable whether or not these factors also contribute to the vulnerability of developing cancer in the far future. It has become increasingly clear that numerous events, besides exposure to HPV, are required for cancer to develop, underscoring the point that HPV is necessary but not sufficient in cancer development. This chapter discusses the epidemiology of HPV and squamous neoplasia in sexually active adolescents, biologic changes unique to the adolescent cervix, current screening strategies, management of abnormal cytology, and preferred treatments of abnormal histology diagnoses.

16.2 EPIDEMIOLOGY AND THE NATURAL HISTORY OF HPV AND CERVICAL SQUAMOUS NEOPLASIA IN ADOLESCENTS

The acquisition of cervical HPV is common shortly after the onset of intercourse, with over 50% of adolescents having a positive cervical HPV test within 3 to 4 years of reporting first sex.[1-4] HPV infections in adolescents are also rapidly cleared, with 50% clearing within 6 months and 90% clearing within 2 to 3 years.[5-8] The natural history of abnormal cytology parallels these figures. Low-grade squamous intraepithelial lesion (LSIL) cytology reports are most common in women aged 10 to 19 years of age[9] with prevalence of 2% to 14% and 90% showing LSIL clearance within 3 years.[10] Due to the insensitivity of cervical cytology, it is likely that most LSILs remain undetected. In a prospective study, only 25% of HPV-infected adolescents developed LSIL cytology.[2] Risks for HPV acquisition in these women included having a recent new sexual partner and evidence of Herpes simplex virus (HSV) infections. In the same cohort, risks for development of LSIL were different when controlling for HPV—new sexual partners and HSV were no longer significant risks but smoking cigarettes was. This may be interpreted to suggest that certain risks result in LSIL development and can be distinguished from those associated with HPV acquisition. On the other hand, risks such as smoking may allow the altered epithelium to become prominent enough to be detected by cytology. Certainly, smoking cigarettes has long been shown to be an independent risk for cervical cancer.[11] Proposed mechanisms for cigarette smoking include suppression of host immune responses to HPV.[12] In contrast, HSV and new sexual partners remain risks for HPV infection itself. HSV can result in inflammation and disruption of epithelia, allowing access to basal epithelial cells.

Repeated HPV infections are also common in adolescents. This likely contributes to the high prevalence rates ranging from 12% to 56% in women under 21 years of age. This is six- to eightfold higher than rates in women 30 years of age and older, suggesting that the rate of new infection declines over time.[1,3,13–15] A meta-analysis by de Sanjose[14] showed a peak HPV prevalence of 23% for women <20 years of age and a rapid decline to around 10% by 30 years of age. This decline is thought to be due to a robust immune response in most women clearing the infection and probably protecting the majority.

Most of this decrease in acquisition is thought to be associated with sexual behavior, in that older women tend to be more monogamous than young women.[16] Increasing rates of monogamy by both men and women would decrease transmission rates. In one study, incidence of HPV was highest in the adolescent group with a cumulative incidence of 35.7% by 3 years of observation. In comparison, the incidence rate among the 20- to 24-year-old group was 24.1% and only 8.1% among women 45 years and older. However, this pattern is not always present. In Hanoi, Vietnam, prevalence rates for all ages was <5%, whereas in Nigeria, rates were high among all ages.[15] The reasons for these observations are intriguing and may have to do with cultural norms and the degree of sexual mixing or may result from simple testing biases.

In comparison to HPV and LSIL cytology detection rates, high grade intraepithelial lesion (HSIL) is much less common in adolescents. As mentioned above, there is around a 5:1 ratio of HPV:LSIL detection in adolescents. In women 30 years of age and older, the HPV:LSIL detection ratio is around 10:1.9.[17–19] The pattern for HSIL detection also is somewhat different. Although adolescent rates of HSIL cytology are much lower than LSIL, the rate of HSIL cytology in adolescents is similar to other age groups. The prevalence of HSIL is around 0.7% in women aged 15 to 19, 20 to 29, and 30 to 39 years. The natural history of HSIL appears to be different in young women in that it regresses more often. Reasons for this are unclear but may be due to the fact that these are relatively new lesions rather than persistent lesions found in older women.[20,21]

16.3 RISKS FOR HPV AMONG ADOLESCENTS

As in all age groups, sexual exposure is the predominant risk for acquiring genital HPV in adolescents. Numerous studies show that having a new sexual partner within the past 4 to 8 months is the greatest and most consistent risk for HPV acquisition.[2,4,22,23] Having a sexually transmitted disease also poses a risk. Whether the STI reflects epithelial trauma, and therefore easy access to the basal cells, or partner risk remains to be explained. No other risk factors are as consistently associated with acquisition. The question often raised is "are adolescents particularly biologically vulnerable to HPV, or is the risk all linked to sexual behavior?" Several studies suggest that there may be some type of biologic vulnerability regarding adolescents and acquisition. National survey data in the United States report that by 19 years of age, 75% to 77% of females report having had sexual intercourse, and 50% report having had four or more partners with a median of 4.[16,24] Data indicate that adolescents have more "new" partners—22% of the 15- to 19-year-old females and 26% of 20- to 24-year-old-females report two or more partners in the past 12 months compared to 12% of the 25- to 44-year-olds.[16] The reports also indicate that adolescents do not have regular sexual exposure, so frequency of sex is less than among older age groups. Forty-three percent of adolescent females reported no sexual partners in the past 12 months compared to only 13% of 20- to 24-year-olds and 7.4% of 25- to 44-year-olds.[16]

We return to the question, "Are adolescents biologically vulnerable?" Several studies have shown that the age of first intercourse is a risk factor for future development of cervical cancer.[25–28] Some interpret this as "more time" to develop cancer rather than "a time" of vulnerability. However, a recent collaborative study of over 4500 women with CIN 3 and nearly 11,000 with cervical cancer showed the age of first intercourse to be an important risk factor for developing cervical cancer, but it was not the same as for CIN 3.[28] The relative risk (RR) for cervical cancer was 3.52 for age at first intercourse ≥14 versus ≥25 years, when taking into account number of lifetime partners and other sexual risk factors. This may parallel the most dramatic changes in the transformation zone developmentally.[29] Certainly, the topography of the adolescent cervix differs from the adult cervix in most young women.[29]

During embryologic development, the cervix is initially lined by müllerian columnar epithelium and later replaced by urogenital squamous epithelium from the vagina toward the endocervical os (see Chapter 2). This replacement is incomplete with an abrupt squamous–columnar junction occurring on the ectocervix in the majority of neonates. The squamocolumnar junction remains quiescent until puberty, when the position of the squamocolumnar junction returns, in most cases, to the ectocervix. Hormonal influences result in cervical and uterine growth. With the cervix–vaginal junction, a fixed entity, there is a downward and outward growth of the glandular columnar epithelium; hence, there appears to be an eversion of the squamocolumnar tissue resulting in placement of the junction even further onto the ectocervix. Estrogen also influences retention of fluid, which may also contribute to the eversion phenomenon. Consequently, most non–sexually active adolescents appear to have relatively large areas of columnar epithelium on the outer surface of their cervix (Figure 16.1A–E). As the adolescent continues through puberty, the cervix begins to undergo more rapid changes due to cell transformation. It is believed that these changes are triggered by increasing estrogen levels and increasing acidity of the cervicovaginal milieu due to the increasing presence of lactobacilli and lactate production. Now, uncommitted generative cells of the columnar epithelium begin a process called squamous metaplasia, which is the transformation of columnar epithelium into squamous epithelium (Figure 16.2A–E). This process results in changing the single cuboidal cell layer of columnar epithelium into a 60- to 80-cell-layer-thick squamous epithelium. Cells are undergoing rapid cellular proliferation (Figure 16.3A–G). This process appears to occur in spurts with episodes of quiescence.[30] Eventually, a new squamocolumnar junction occurs in the older women that is now located well into the os and not visible by simple speculum examination (Figure 16.4A–D). So, in cross-sectional view, the predominant cell type in adults is the mature squamous cell seen colposcopically as homogeneous pink mucosal epithelium, whereas in an adolescent, both columnar and metaplastic cells have a greater presence (Figure 16.5A–D). It is postulated, though not proven, that one of the vulnerabilities to HPV may be the thinness of columnar epithelium compared to the thick squamous epithelium, so that with intercourse, the columnar epithelium is at greater risk for trauma, leading to easier access to the basal epithelial cells by HPV.

No study to date has shown that ectopy is a risk for HPV. Therefore, more important than the presence of columnar epithelium is the presence of metaplastic epithelium. The importance of the transformation zone is well known since all squamous cell cancers of the cervix appear to arise within this area. HPV replication is dependent on its host cell replication and differentiation. Similarly, replication and differentiation are hallmarks of squamous metaplasia; hence, the process of metaplasia is a fertile ground for establishing HPV infections. Other than puberty, triggers of squamous metaplasia are not well defined. Most studies of ectopy have been cross-sectional. These cross-sectional studies reported that sexually active adolescents have more tissue maturity (greater squamous epithelium) than non–sexually active adolescents, and similarly,

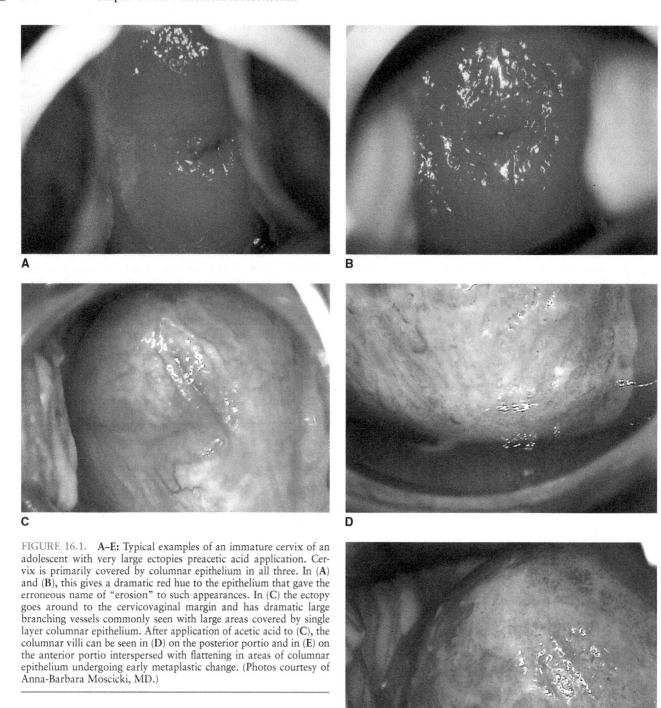

FIGURE 16.1.   A–E: Typical examples of an immature cervix of an adolescent with very large ectopies preacetic acid application. Cervix is primarily covered by columnar epithelium in all three. In (**A**) and (**B**), this gives a dramatic red hue to the epithelium that gave the erroneous name of "erosion" to such appearances. In (**C**) the ectopy goes around to the cervicovaginal margin and has dramatic large branching vessels commonly seen with large areas covered by single layer columnar epithelium. After application of acetic acid to (**C**), the columnar villi can be seen in (**D**) on the posterior portio and in (**E**) on the anterior portio interspersed with flattening in areas of columnar epithelium undergoing early metaplastic change. (Photos courtesy of Anna-Barbara Moscicki, MD.)

adolescents with multiple sexual partners appear to have even greater levels of tissue maturation.[31,32] It may imply, however, that women with multiple partners or those sexually active with few partners are exposed to other environmental factors such as sexually transmitted infections, which induce inflammation, repair, and metaplasia, or semen that may itself induce metaplasia.[33] The only longitudinal study about metaplasia using logistic regression analysis showed that oral contraceptives and smoking were both independent risk factors for accelerated maturation, but the number of sexual partners and STIs were not.[30]

This underscores the importance of longitudinal analyses in defining factors associated with epithelial maturation. Certainly, estrogen and progesterone are known to enhance cell proliferation; hence, the association seems plausible. However, this refutes previous assumptions that oral contraceptives cause eversion and increased ectopy. This assumption may have been associated with analysis of older data from a time when higher estrogen levels were present in the available oral contraceptives. Smoking may result in DNA damage, which is repaired through other mechanisms. Several compounds from cigarette smoke, nicotine, cotinine, and the potent carcinogen NNK have been

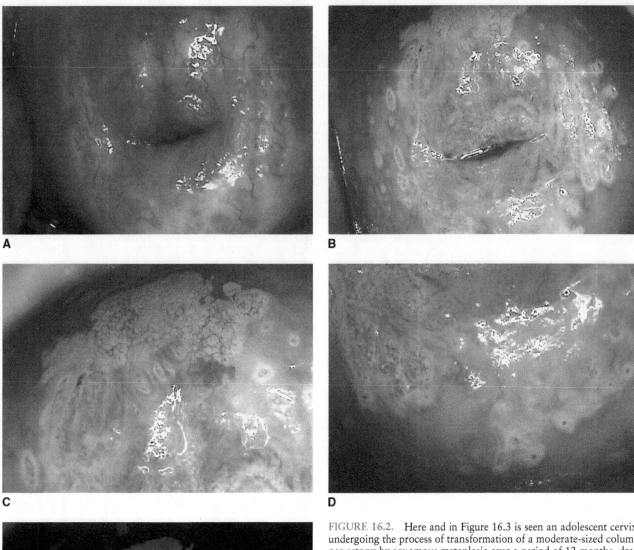

A

B

C

D

E

FIGURE 16.2.   Here and in Figure 16.3 is seen an adolescent cervix undergoing the process of transformation of a moderate-sized columnar ectopy by squamous metaplasia over a period of 12 months, dramatically decreasing the size of the ectopy over this relatively short period of time. Figure 16.2 shows the cervix at the initial visit and Figure 16.3 shows it 6 and 12 months later. A: Prior to the application of acetic acid, many branching blood vessels under what appears to be a large red ectopy can be seen. B: Acetic acid clarifies the normal appearance of villi, metaplasia surrounding gland openings, and delineates the true size of the ectopy, which is smaller than it appears to be preacetic acid, and the squamocolumnar junction. C: The anterior portio has an area of mosaic and punctation common in both immature metaplasia and in CIN. D: The posterior portio with acetowhite rings of metaplasia surrounding gland openings demonstrate how far out the ectopy originally went before the metaplastic process began its march toward the portio. E: Lugol's application defines the junction between mahogany-staining mature squamous epithelium and immature metaplasia. (Photos courtesy of Anna-Barbara Moscicki, MD.)

identified in cervical mucus, and the occurrence of smoking-related DNA damage in the cervical epithelium has been documented.[30] Interestingly, both oral contraceptives and smoking have been implicated in the development of cervical cancer.[11,34] These data imply that one of the mechanisms may be through enhancing cellular proliferation and consequent DNA damage.

The high rates of LSIL in adolescents may also be explained by these high rates of metaplasia. A study of serial colpophotographs from adolescents showed that those with evidence of rapid acceleration in the metaplastic process were more likely to develop LSIL cytology if infected with HPV than adolescents with a relatively quiescent cervix (no changes in the area of metaplasia).[35] This confirms evidence that squamous metaplasia may support viral replication and its pathologic consequences are basal cell proliferation induced by E6 and E7 and cytoskeletal koilocytosis induced by E4 (see Chapter 5).[36]

A second reason adolescents may be more vulnerable to HPV acquisition than adults is the lack of immune memory. With time (and clearance), it would be expected that women would develop immunologic memory to HPV protecting them from

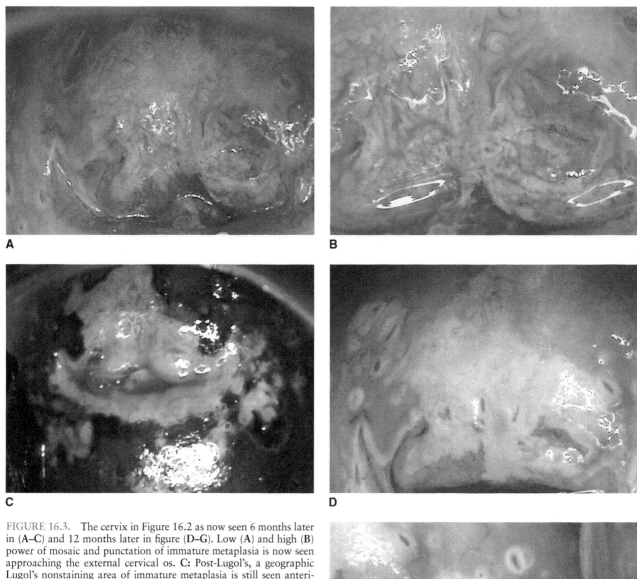

FIGURE 16.3. The cervix in Figure 16.2 as now seen 6 months later in (**A–C**) and 12 months later in figure (**D–G**). Low (**A**) and high (**B**) power of mosaic and punctation of immature metaplasia is now seen approaching the external cervical os. **C:** Post-Lugol's, a geographic Lugol's nonstaining area of immature metaplasia is still seen anteriorly, but the posterior portio now is mostly mahogany-stained mature metaplasia. **D:** The anterior portio 12 months from first visit now has denser acetowhite that could represent CIN or maturing metaplasia. Most of the mosaic is no longer present except at the distal 12:00 o'clock position. **E:** Denser acetowhite is also seen around gland openings at 3:00 o'clock.

future infections if reexposed to the same HPV types. Moscicki observed a population of adolescents and young women who were enrolled at the ages of 12 to 22 years and who acquired HPV 16.[37] Among those women who cleared HPV 16, approximately 18% had HPV 16 redetected over 8 years. Redetection was strongly associated with new sexual partners and reporting more than 1 recent sexual partner. Most impressive is that virtually all of the redetected HPV 16 infections cleared rapidly. These data suggest that some protection may develop over time and also document the repeated nature of HPV infections in young women and their association with sexual risk behaviors.

A third reason for HPV acquisition vulnerability may be that epithelial cells have a certain predilection to specific HPV types. Castle et al.[38] found that infections with alpha nine HPV types such as 16, 31, 33, 35, 52, 58, and 67 were more common in women with large areas of ectopy, whereas these types were not as common in women with a mature cervix. This again might be related to age and immunologic memory that goes hand in hand with cervical maturation.

In summary, adolescents' vulnerability to HPV acquisition is very likely due to multiple factors. These include, but are not

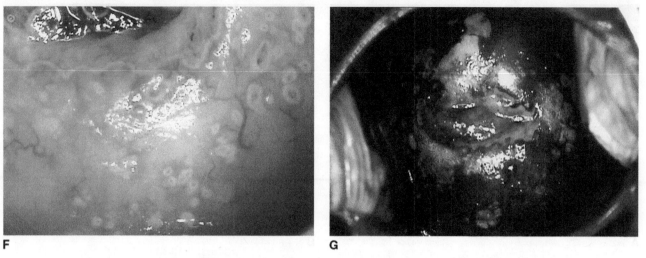

F

G

FIGURE 16.3. *(Continued)* F: The squamocolumnar junction is migrating closer to the cervical os posteriorly, with clearly mature squamous epithelium. Less dramatic gland openings and branching blood vessels reassure that the posterior portio is normal. G: Lugol's staining further demonstrates the maturation process of metaplasia with much more of the portio staining mahogany brown, areas less mature partially staining "tortoise shell" and one area completely nonstaining Lugol's at 12:00 o'clock. Biopsy of this area was read as metaplasia. (Photos courtesy of Anna-Barbara Moscicki, MD.)

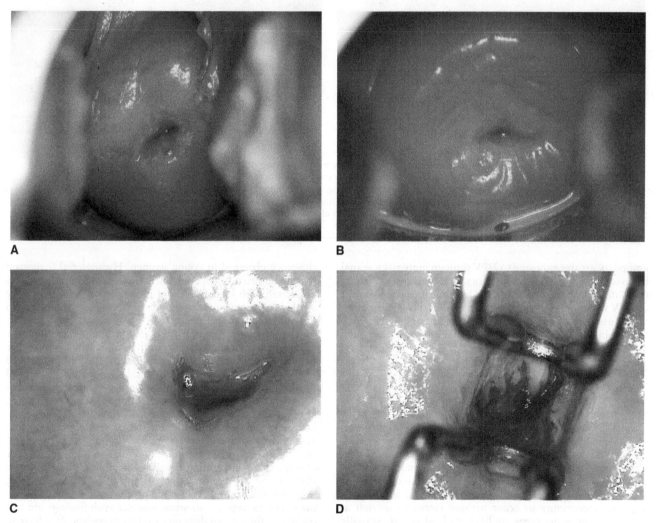

A

B

C

D

FIGURE 16.4.   A,B: Typical examples of a mature cervix with little to no columnar epithelium visible. The entire cervix is covered by mature squamous epithelium. C: In this patient, the SCJ is right at the external cervical os posteriorly but cannot be seen anteriorly. D: An endocervical speculum is introduced to see the SCJ within the canal anteriorly, revealing a small area of acetowhitening. (Photos courtesy of Anna-Barbara Moscicki, MD.)

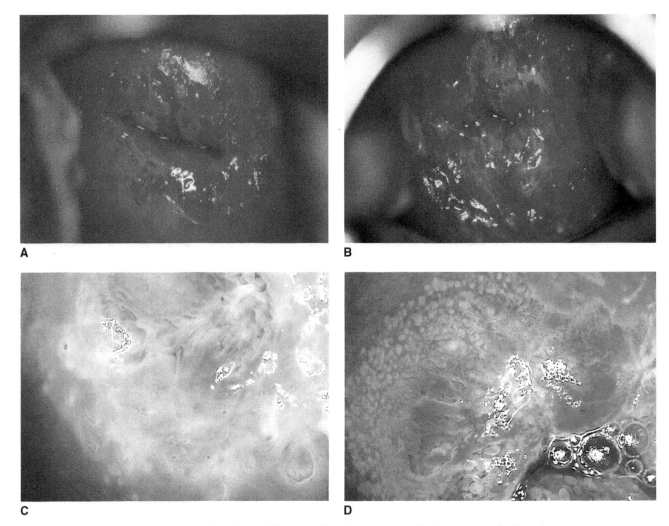

FIGURE 16.5. **A,B:** Examples of an adolescent cervix with a mixture of columnar, metaplastic, and squamous epithelium. The process of squamous metaplasia can be somewhat random and often occurs in patches. **C:** Transparent acetowhite gland openings and adjacent flattening within columnar epithelium illustrate metaplastic transformation. **D:** Fine mosaic and punctation so often seen in immature metaplasia interspersed with islands of villous columnar epithelium and flattening columnar epithelium characteristic of the beginning of metaplastic transformation. (Photos courtesy of Anna-Barbara Moscicki, MD.)

limited to, greater exposure to HPV through more risky sexual behavior, a lack of immune memory, and high rates of squamous metaplasia, which are fertile grounds for establishment of HPV infections. HPV detection in adolescents is most commonly associated with normal cytology; approximately 75% of HPV-infected adolescents have normal cytology.[2]

16.4 NATURAL HISTORY OF HPV AND SIL

Factors known to influence clearance or immune suppression of HPV are few. Plummer et al.,[39] showed that the longer HPV persists, the less likely it will be cleared. Infections with multiple types are reported to clear slowly in some patients.[7,10] The presence of multiple HPV types likely reflects a defect in the immune response to HPV in some adolescents. Hence, acquisition continues to occur without clearance so that at any one point, more types are likely to be detected. Sexually transmitted diseases such as *Chlamydia trachomatis*, common in adolescents, may also influence persistence.[40,41] The mechanism of this association is not clear. Of note is the high rate of

clearance observed in young women. Hwang et al.[42] showed that immature cervical epithelium often seen in adolescents is associated with higher levels of inflammatory and regulatory cytokines; hence, innate immune responses may be inherent to this vulnerable epithelium.

The important role of HPV persistence in the development of invasive cervical cancer has been established. On the other hand, how long persistence is required for the development of CIN 3 or cancer remains controversial. LSIL and HSIL cervical cytology reports in adolescents have been shown to develop within months to years after infection.[2,43] As noted earlier, approximately 25% of adolescents will have a LSIL Pap report within 3 years of an infection; the risk of developing abnormal cytology diminishes after 3 years.[2,43,44] In one study, the development of high-grade lesions was similar to that reported for low-grade lesions, noting that 7% of adolescents developed HSIL within 19 months of acquiring HPV. However, finding low-and high-grade CIN in equal proportions at any age is not the norm, raising the question whether such findings are secondary to the known difficulty that pathologists often have in differentiating CIN 1 and CIN 2 lesions, thereby inflating the high-grade category.[45] If CIN 2 and CIN 3 are read as separate entities, the time to CIN 3 appears to be somewhat longer than to CIN 2. This is represented by prevalence data that demonstrate the rate of CIN 3 peaking in women aged 27 to 30 years, 7 to 10 years after peak rate for HPV infections.[46] Although most women appear not to develop CIN 3 shortly after infection, individual cases have been reported.[44] Additionally, small numbers of CIN 3 were found within 36 months in the initially "HPV-naïve" population of women in the HPV vaccine trials, indicating that newly acquired hrHPV (within 3 years) can cause CIN 3 within that short period of time.[47,48] Such rapid development of CIN 3 is most commonly associated with HPV 16 infection. In one study, 20% of young women 18 to 22 years of age with incident HPV16 or HPV18 infection developed CIN 2 within 36 months and 6.7% developed CIN 3.[44]

The natural history of LSIL in adolescents parallels that of HPV with 92% of adolescents showing regression within 36 months and only 3% going onto HSIL.[10] These progression rates significantly differ from that in older women, which, in the ASCUS/LSIL Triage Study (ALTS), with a median age of 29, was closer to 13%.[49] Differences are likely due to two reasons: (1) Prevalent low-grade lesions as HPV, in older women, are likely to reflect a persistent infection increasing the chance of development of CIN 2,3.[2] (2) LSIL cytology is more likely to harbor an undiagnosed CIN 3 in the older women than in the adolescent. It is well known that the majority of CIN 3 is diagnosed in women referred for LSIL cytology, and the rates of CIN 3 are higher in older women than adolescents.[20,46] The natural history of HSIL cytology is less well defined than that of LSIL mostly because all HSIL are referred immediately for colposcopy and biopsy, and those with CIN 2,3 are treated, unlike CIN 1 and simple HPV findings that are observed. Two studies of CIN 2 in adolescents show high rates of regression (approximately 60%)[20,50] with no progression to cancer. SEER statistics show that between 2003 and 2006, the incidence rate of cervical cancer was 0.1 per 100,000 in women aged 15 to 19 years.[51] Despite extensive screening of adolescents under the previous standard to begin screening at first intercourse or age 18, whichever came first, this rate remained basically unchanged from the time period 1973 to 1977 when the rate of cervical cancer in 15- to 19-year-olds also was 0.1 per 100,000 adolescents. During this time, screening in adolescent populations went from no screening to considerable screening of sexually active adolescents. This underscores the likelihood that cervical cancer in adolescents is not prevented by cytology screening alone.[52,53]

16.5 CERVICAL CANCER SCREENING

These natural history studies have highly influenced recent strategies in the guidelines for cervical cancer screening in adolescents. Older guidelines in the United States recommended that all adolescents begin screening at age 18 or once sexually active, whichever came first.[54,55] The data available during the past decade suggest that this type of screening results in considerable numbers of unnecessary referrals for follow-up and management and are associated with potential harm associated with ablation or excisional treatments that may result in premature delivery and low birth weight infants.[56–61] The evidence is clear that the majority of LSIL and HSIL cytology in adolescents will regress and that cancer in this age group is extremely rare. The data also suggest that screening this age group does not decrease cancer rates among 20- to 30-year-olds.[61,62] The 2002 American Cancer Society guidelines moved away from screening all sexually active adolescents by constructing a framework that was based on sexual risk (time from initiation of sex) and allowed for a time frame for regression to occur if disease occurred.[62] Recently, several groups

recommended that screening for cervical cancer in the United States begin at the age of 21 years and not before.[63–67] Although many countries have chosen a higher screening age, 21 years of age was considered a realistic age for adherence and access to patients, particularly since the United States has no organized screening program. The cap also allows for women who were unwilling or unable to report sexual activity. These recommendations are regardless of when sexual activity begins or of history of STI or pregnancy. (see Chapter 18.4.1, When to Begin Screening). In comparison, some countries with organized screening, such as the United Kingdom, start screening at 25 years.[68] In contrast, Australia begins screening at the age of 18 years, or 1 to 2 years after first sexual intercourse, whichever is later.[69]

16.6 COLPOSCOPIC FINDINGS IN ADOLESCENTS

Although the colposcopic appearance of CIN and cancer is identical in adolescents and adult women, many lesions are smaller and more difficult to diagnose in the adolescents. Several studies document normal histology in loop electrosurgical excision procedure (LEEP) specimens in young women with CIN 2,3 on initial biopsy.[20,70–72] Either the lesion regressed before LEEP or the biopsy for diagnoses removed the entire lesion. In addition to small lesions, adolescents often have large immature transformation zones colposcopically similar to CIN. The appearance is often termed "atypical metaplasia" (Figure 16.6A–D).

Singer and Jordan[73] divide the squamous metaplastic process colposcopically into five stages, which have been demonstrated in the many colpophotos in this chapter. Stage 1 consists of columnar epithelium demonstrating grape-like villi. In stage 2, the new squamous epithelium begins to grow down the sides of the villi, and the colposcopic appearance is that of attachment of adjacent villi. In stage 3, the fusion is completed, and the new epithelium appears smooth and pink. Stage 4 reflects continuing maturation with capillary networks appearing near the surface giving the appearance of coarse punctation and mosaicism often associated with CIN. Finally, in stage 5, these capillary structures are compressed forming a network under the epithelium, resulting in tissue indistinguishable from original squamous epithelia. Since the process is erratic, all four stages can be present on the cervix at any point with islands of villi adjacent to mature epithelium (Figure 16.7A–C). It is stage 4 that is frequently confused with CIN and referred to as atypical squamous metaplasia (Figure 16.6). These changes make colposcopy even more challenging in adolescents, which often results in low specificity for CIN 3.

16.7 HISTOLOGY

As with adult women, the reproducibility of CIN lesions is low, specifically for CIN 2.[21] Different than in adults, CIN 3 also has poor reproducibility in adolescents.[74] The presence of immature squamous metaplasia can occasionally be misinterpreted as CIN 3 by pathologists of all levels of experience as evidenced by interobserver variability in this interpretation in the ALTS trial.[75] Early features of squamous metaplasia include undifferentiated sheets of cells toward the top of the villi with degeneration of the original basement membrane.[73] Within the newly formed squamous epithelium, there are often residual columnar-lined surfaces with endocervical cells. It is not uncommon to see patches of smooth-surfaced epithelium with stromal papillae projecting into the epithelium representing the original stromal cores of the fused villi. Occasionally,

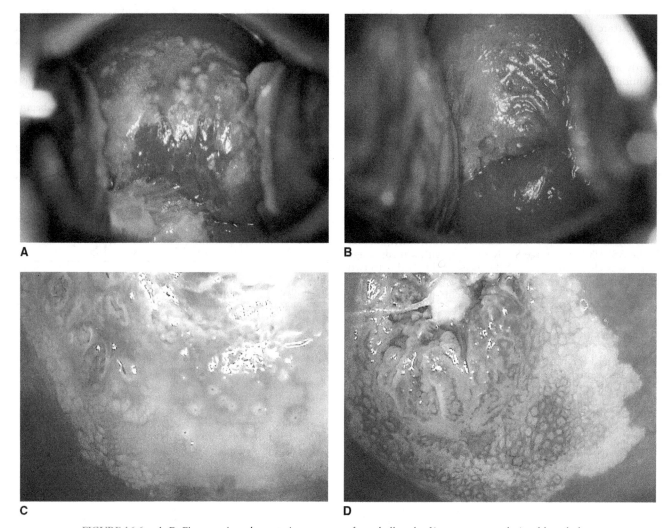

FIGURE 16.6.   A–D: Fine mosaic and punctation are most often a hallmark of immature metaplasia, although they also can be seen in congenital transformation zones (see Chapter 13) and in low-grade HPV lesions (CIN 1). **A:** Area at 10:00 to 11:00 o'clock demonstrates white epithelium, fine punctation, and mosaicism after the application of 3% to 5% acetic acid. This area is often also referred to as atypical squamous metaplasia, and this is often confused with CIN. **B:** Fine punctation in a large transformation zone with immature metaplasia. **C:** Very fine punctation and mosaic with gland openings and villi of columnar epithelium. **D:** More dramatic mosaic and punctation in large areas of immature metaplasia, with fingers of translucent acetowhite metaplasia fusing over flattened areas of columnar epithelium. (Photos courtesy of Anna-Barbara Moscicki, MD.)

columnar epithelium lies under the new metaplastic epithelium, and metaplastic epithelium is seen within clefts of columnar epithelium. These bizarre changes can sometimes be interpreted as neoplastic.

16.8 MANAGEMENT

Although screening for cervical cancer in adolescent populations is no longer recommended in the United States, some adolescents will likely continue to be screened for the near future.[64] Consequently, adolescents having abnormal cervical cytology should be managed according to the guidelines outlined for women 21 to 24 years of age detailed in Chapter 19. This is consistent with the prior management guidelines for adolescents because the 2013 guidelines for women aged 21 to 24 years were adopted from prior adolescent recommendations.[76–78] Under no circumstance should HPV testing be used in adolescents because HPV is so common at this age and significant risk from HPV so minimal.[78,79]

16.8.1 Treatment Decisions

The decision to treat should be the exception, not the norm, in adolescent populations. Also, histologically proven CIN 2,3 should be the absolute minimum criteria, not cytology (see Chapter 20).

16.8.2 Treatment of CIN 1

As in adults, treatment of CIN 1 among adolescents is considered unwarranted.[76,78,80] Follow-up of histologically diagnosed CIN 1, like with ASC-US/LSIL cytology reports, is with repeat cytology at 12-month intervals as outlined in Chapter 19 for women aged 21 to 24 years. Progression to a HSIL cytology report at any time during the 2-year follow-up warrants rereferral. If CIN 1 remains the histologic diagnosis, continued observation is warranted. (For more discussion see Chapter 20, on Management of CIN 1 in Women Age 21 to 24.)

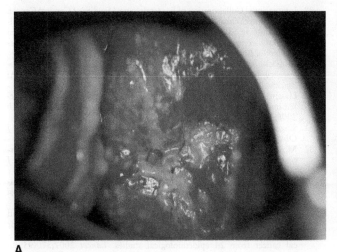

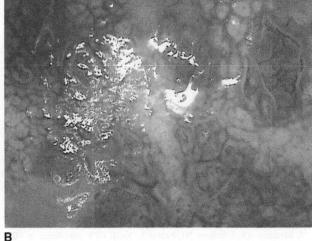

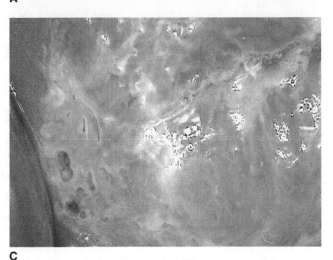

FIGURE 16.7. **A:** Adolescent cervix with several types of epithelium present. After the application of 3% to 5% acetic acid, mature squamous epithelium (*smooth pink areas*), mature metaplastic epithelium (*thicker white areas*), early metaplasia (*more translucent white areas*), and columnar (*red areas*) and trapped columnar epithelium forming small nabothian cysts (*yellow spots*) can all be visualized. **B:** Patchy acetowhite weaving though islands of columnar villi. **C:** Many of the elements of early metaplasia can be seen here. (Photos courtesy of Anna-Barbara Moscicki, MD.)

16.8.3 Treatment of CIN 2,3

Current recommendations for managing CIN 2,3 in adolescents depend on colposcopic findings and are identical to that of women aged 21 to 24 years of age.[78] CIN 2 and CIN 3 are often not distinguished by the pathologist, resulting in a diagnosis of CIN 2,3. Because CIN 2 lesions are more common than CIN 3 in adolescents, it is recommended that CIN 2,3 be managed by observation similar to CIN 2, although treatment is acceptable. Management of CIN 2 by observation is preferred. If adherence to follow-up is doubtful, treatment may be the better option. When colposcopy is inadequate or the lesion is specified as CIN 3, treatment is recommended. When observation is elected for CIN 2 or CIN 2,3, colposcopy and cytology are recommended at 6-month intervals.[78] Treatment is recommended if the lesion progresses to CIN 3, or if CIN 2 or CIN 2,3 persists for 24 months. Because high rates (9%) of pelvic inflammatory disease have been reported in adolescents after treatment,[81] screening for *C. trachomatis* and *Neisseria gonorrhoeae* prior to treatment is ideal and should be strongly considered. Some propose that cryotherapy be used rather than LEEP for suitable cases in adolescents because of the lower rate of complications and less loss of cervical mass. Alternatively, in large transformation zones, LEEP can be targeted to the lesion itself, avoiding excision of the entire transformation zone with less deep ablation peripherally.

16.9 CONCLUSION

In summary, although HPV infections are extremely common in adolescents, spontaneous clearance of these infections occurs in the majority. These high rates of infection are due to sexual behavior, biologic vulnerability, or a combination of both. Because regression rates of HPV infections, CIN 1, and CIN 2 are common in this age group and invasive cervical cancer is rare, postponement of screening until 21 years of age is now recommended. In adolescents accidentally screened and having abnormal findings, the 2013 guidelines recommend that they be managed according to the guidelines for women aged 21 to 24 years.[78] Even more so, observation is preferred over intervention because, despite the risky sexual behavior among adolescents, the risk of progression to cancer in the adolescent years is miniscule.

With the availability of HPV vaccines, it is essential to vaccinate children prior to the onset of sexual activity. By insuring vaccination prior to acquisition of HPV, it will be possible to prevent a majority of high-grade precancer and to gain maximal protection from the vaccine, and for adolescents who have already initiated sexual activity, administration of the vaccine may still have benefit and is recommended, for they may not have yet acquired any of the HPV types protected by the vaccine. All adolescents vaccinated must be counseled about the importance of regular cervical cancer screening once they reach an age appropriate to begin screening.

References

1. Moscicki AB, Ellenberg JH, Vermund SH, et al. Prevalence of and risks for cervical human papillomavirus infection and squamous intraepithelial lesions in adolescent girls: impact of infection with human immunodeficiency virus. *Arch Ped Adolesc Med* 2000;154:127–34.

2. Moscicki AB, Hills N, Shiboski S, et al. Risks for incident human papillomavirus infection and low-grade squamous intraepithelial lesion development in young females. *JAMA* 2001;285(23):2995–3002.

3. Moscicki AB, Palefsky J, Gonzales J, Schoolnik G. Human papillomavirus infection in sexually active adolescent females: prevalence and risk factors. *Pediatr Res* 1990;28:507–13.

4. Winer RL, Lee SK, Hughes JP, Adam DE, Kiviat NB, Koutsky LA. Genital human papillomavirus infection: incidence and risk factors in a cohort of female university students. *Am J Epidemiol* 2003;157(3):218–26.

5. Evander M, Edlund K, Gustaffson A, et al. Human papillomavirus infection is transient in young women: a population-based cohort study. *J Infect Dis* 1995;171:1026–30.

6. Ho GY, Bierman R, Beardsley L, Chang CJ, Burk RD. Natural history of cervicovaginal papillomavirus infection in young women. *N Engl J Med* 1998;338(7):423–8.

7. Moscicki AB, Ellenberg JH, Farhat S, Xu J. HPV persistence in HIV infected and uninfected adolescent girls: risk factors and differences by phylogenetic types. *J Infect Dis* 2004;190(1):37–45.

8. Moscicki AB, Shiboski S, Broering J, et al. The natural history of human papillomavirus infection as measured by repeated DNA testing in adolescent and young women. *J Pediatr* 1998;132:277–84.

9. Mount SL, Papillo JL. A study of 10,296 pediatric and adolescent Papanicolaou smear diagnoses in northern New England. *Pediatrics* 1999; 103(3):539–46.

10. Moscicki AB, Shiboski S, Hills NK, et al. Regression of low-grade squamous intraepithelial lesions in young women. *Lancet* 2004;364(9446):1678–83.

11. International Collaboration of Epidemiological Studies of Cervical Cancer. Comparison of risk factors for invasive squamous cell carcinoma and adenocarcinoma of the cervix: collaborative reanalysis of individual data on 8,097 women with squamous cell carcinoma and 1,374 women with adenocarcinoma from 12 epidemiological studies. *Int J Cancer* 2007;120(4):885–91.

12. Scott M, Nakagawa M, Moscicki AB. Cell-mediated immune response to human papillomavirus infection. *Clin Diagn Lab Immunol* 2001;8(2):209–20.

13. Burchell A, Winer R, de Sanjose S, Franco E. Epidemiology and transmission dynamics of genital human papillomavirus infection. *Vaccine Monogr* 2006;24(suppl 3):52–62.

14. de Sanjose S. La investigacion sobre la infeccion por virus del papilloma human y el cancer de cuello uterino en Espana. In: de Sanjose S, Garcia A, eds. *El Virus del Papiloma Human y Cancer: Epidemiologia y Prevencion.* Madrid, Spain: EMISA, 2006.

15. Franceschi S, Herrero R, Clifford GM, et al. Variations in the age-specific curves of human papillomavirus prevalence in women worldwide. *Int J Cancer* 2006;119(11):2677–84.

16. Mosher WD, Chandra A, Jones J. Sexual behavior and selected health measures: men and women 15–44 years of age, United States, 2002. *Adv Data* 2005;362:1–55.

17. Bjorge T, Gunbjorud AB, Langmark F, Skare GB, Thoresen SO. Cervical mass screening in Norway—510,000 smears a year. *Cancer Detect Prev* 1994;18(6):463–70.

18. Sadeghi SB, Hsieh EW, Gunn SW. Prevalence of cervical intraepithelial neoplasia in sexually active teenagers and young adults. *Am J Obstet Gynecol* 1984;148:726–9.

19. Schydlower LTM, Greenberg MH, Patterson CPH. Adolescents with abnormal cervical cytology. *Clin Pediatr* 1981;20(11):723–6.

20. Moore K, Cofer A, Elliot L, Lanneau G, Walker J, Gold MA. Adolescent cervical dysplasia: histologic evaluation, treatment, and outcomes. *Am J Obstet Gynecol* 2007;197(2):141, e141–6.

21. Moscicki AB, Ma Y, Wibbelsman C, et al. Risks for cervical intraepithelial neoplasia 3 among adolescents and young women with abnormal cytology. *Obstet Gynecol* 2008;112(6):1335–42.

22. Brown DR, Shew ML, Qadadri B, et al. A longitudinal study of genital human papillomavirus infection in a cohort of closely followed adolescent women. *J Infect Dis* 2005;191(2):182–92.

23. Munoz N, Mendez F, Posso H, et al. Incidence, duration, and determinants of cervical human papillomavirus infection in a cohort of Colombian women with normal cytological results. *J Infect Dis* 2004;190(12):2077–87.

24. Santelli JS, Brener ND, Lowry R, Bhatt A, Zabin LS. Multiple sexual partners among U.S. adolescents and young adults. *Fam Plan Perspect* 1998;30(6):271–5.

25. Green J, Berrington de Gonzalez A, Sweetland S, et al. Risk factors for adenocarcinoma and squamous cell carcinoma of the cervix in women aged 20–44 years: the UK National Case–control Study of Cervical Cancer. *Br J Cancer* 2003;89(11):2078–86.

26. Herrero R, Brinton LA, Reeves WC, et al. Sexual behavior, venereal diseases, hygiene practices, and invasive cervical cancer in a high-risk population. *Cancer* 1990;65(2):380–6.

27. Sierra-Torres CH, Tyring SK, Au WW. Risk contribution of sexual behavior and cigarette smoking to cervical neoplasia. *Int J Gynecol Cancer* 2003;13(5):617–25.

28. International Collaboration of Epidemiological Studies of Cervical Cancer. Cervical carcinoma and sexual behavior: collaborative reanalysis of individual data on 15,461 women with cervical carcinoma and 29,164 women without cervical carcinoma from 21 epidemiological studies. *Cancer Epidemiol Biomarkers Prev* 2009;18(4):1060–9.

29. Moscicki AB, Singer A. The cervical epithelium during puberty and adolescence. In: Jordan JA, Singer A, eds. *The Cervix* (2nd ed.). Malden, MA: Blackwell, 2006:81–101.

30. Hwang LY, Ma Y, Moscicki AB. Factors that influence the rate of epithelial maturation in the cervix of healthy young women. *J Adolesc Health* 2008;42(2 suppl 1):2.

31. Singer A. The uterine cervix from adolescence to the menopause. *Br J Obstet Gynaecol* 1975;82(2):81–99.

32. Moscicki AB, Ma Y, Holland C, Vermund SH. Cervical ectopy in adolescent girls with and without human immunodeficiency virus infection. *J Infect Dis* 2001;183(6):865–70.

33. Schachter J, Hill EC, King EB, Coleman VR, Jones P, Meyer KF. Chlamydial infection in women with cervical dysplasia. *Am J Obstet Gynecol* 1975;123(7):753–7.

34. Appleby P, Beral V, Berrington de Gonzalez A, et al. Cervical cancer and hormonal contraceptives: collaborative reanalysis of individual data for 16,573 women with cervical cancer and 35,509 women without cervical cancer from 24 epidemiological studies. *Lancet* 2007;370(9599): 1609–21.

35. Moscicki AB, Grubbs-Burt V, Kanowitz S, Darragh T, Shiboski S. The significance of squamous metaplasia in the development of low grade squamous intraepithelial lesions in young women. *Cancer* 1999;85:1139–44.

36. Solomon D, Davey D, Kurman R, et al. The 2001 Bethesda System: terminology for reporting results of cervical cytology. *JAMA* 2002; 287(16):2114–9.

37. Moscicki AB, Ma Y, Farhat S, et al. Redetection of cervical human papillomavirus type 16 (HPV16) in women with a history of HPV16. *J Infect Dis* 2013;208(3):403–12.

38. Castle PE, Jeronimo J, Schiffman M, et al. Age-related changes of the cervix influence human papillomavirus type distribution. *Cancer Res* 2006; 66(2):1218–24.

39. Plummer M, Schiffman M, Castle PE, Maucort-Boulch D, Wheeler CM. A 2-year prospective study of human papillomavirus persistence among women with a cytological diagnosis of atypical squamous cells of undetermined significance or low-grade squamous intraepithelial lesion. *J Infect Dis* 2007;195(11):1582–9.

40. Silins I, Ryd W, Strand A, et al. *Chlamydia trachomatis* infection and persistence of human papillomavirus. *Int J Cancer* 2005;116(1):110–5.

41. Samoff E, Koumans EH, Markowitz LE, et al. Association of *Chlamydia trachomatis* with persistence of high-risk types of human papillomavirus in a cohort of female adolescents. *Am J Epidemiol* 2005;162(7):668–75.

42. Hwang LY, Scott ME, Ma Y, Moscicki AB. Higher levels of cervicovaginal inflammatory and regulatory cytokines and chemokines in healthy young women with immature cervical epithelium. *J Reprod Immunol* 2011;88(1):66–71.

43. Woodman CB, Collins S, Winter H, et al. Natural history of cervical human papillomavirus infection in young women: a longitudinal cohort study. *Lancet* 2001;357(9271):1831–6.

44. Winer RL, Kiviat NB, Hughes JP, et al. Development and duration of human papillomavirus lesions, after initial infection. *J Infect Dis* 2005;191(5):731–8.

45. Heatley MK. How should we grade CIN? *Histopathology* 2002;40(4):377–90.

46. Bosch FX, de Sanjose S. Chapter 1: Human papillomavirus and cervical cancer burden and assessment of causality. *J Natl Cancer Inst Monogr* 2003;31:3–13.

47. The FUTURE II Study Group. Quadrivalent vaccine against human papillomavirus to prevent high-grade cervical lesions. *N Engl J Med* 2007;356:1915.

48. Paavonen J, Naud P, Salmeron J, et al. Efficacy of human papillomavirus (HPV)-16/18 AS04-adjuvanted vaccine against cervical infection and precancer caused by oncogenic HPV types (PATRICIA): final analysis of a double-blind, randomised study in young women. *Lancet* 2009;374:301.

49. Cox JT, Schiffman M, Solomon D, ASCUS-LSIL Triage Study (ALTS) Group. Prospective follow-up suggests similar risk of subsequent cervical intraepithelial neoplasia grade 2 or 3 among women with cervical intraepithelial neoplasia grade 1 or negative colposcopy and directed biopsy. *Am J Obstet Gynecol* 2003;188(6):1406–12.

50. Moscicki AB, Ma Y, Wibbelsman C, et al. Rate of and risks for regression of cervical intraepithelial neoplasia 2 in adolescents and young women. *Obstet Gynecol* 2010;116(6):1373–80.

51. Surveillance, Epidemiology and End Results (SEER) Program. http://seer.cancer.gov (Accessed December 12, 2009).

52. Chan PG, Sung HY, Sawaya GF. Changes in cervical cancer incidence after three decades of screening US women less than 30 years old. *Obstet Gynecol* 2003;102(4):765–73.

53. Sasieni P, Castanon A, Parkin DM. How many cervical cancers are prevented by treatment of screen-detected disease in young women? *Int J Cancer* 2009;124(2):461–4.

54. American College of Obstetrics and Gynecology. Recommendations on Frequency of Pap Test Screening. Washington, DC: Committee Opinion No. 152, March 1995.

55. American Medical Association. Guidelines for adolescent preventive services. Chicago, IL: American Medical Association, 1992.

56. Albrechtsen S, Rasmussen S, Thoresen S, Irgens LM, Iversen OE. Pregnancy outcome in women before and after cervical conisation: population based cohort study. *BMJ* 2008;337:a1343.

57. Kyrgiou M, Koliopoulos G, Martin-Hirsch P, Arbyn M, Prendiville W, Paraskevaidis E. Obstetric outcomes after conservative treatment for intraepithelial or early invasive cervical lesions: systematic review and meta-analysis. *Lancet* 2006;367(9509):489–98.

58. Norman JE. Preterm labour. Cervical function and prematurity. *Best Pract Res Clin Obstet Gynaecol* 2007;21(5):791–806.

59. Sadler L, Saftlas A, Wang W, Exeter M, Whittaker J, McCowan L. Treatment for cervical intraepithelial neoplasia and risk of preterm delivery. *JAMA* 2004;291:2100–6.

60. Samson S-L, Bentley JR, Fahey TJ, McKay DJ, Gil GH. The effect of loop electrosurgical excision. *Obstet Gynecol* 2005;105:325–32.

61. Sasieni P, Castanon A, Cuzick J. Effectiveness of cervical screening with age: population based case–control study of prospectively recorded data. *BMJ* 2009;339:b2968.

62. Saslow D, Runowicz CD, Solomon D, et al. American Cancer Society guideline for the early detection of cervical neoplasia and cancer. *CA Cancer J Clin* 2002;52(6):342–62.

63. Moscicki AB, Cox JT. Practice improvement in cervical screening and management (PICSM): symposium on management of cervical abnormalities in adolescents and young women. *J Low Gen Tract Dis* 2010;14(1):73–80.

64. ACOG Practice Bulletin No. 109. American College of Obstetricians and Gynecologists. *Obstet Gynecol* 2009;114:1409–20.

65. Saslow D, Solomon D, Lawson HW, et al. American Cancer Society, American Society for Colposcopy and Cervical Pathology, and American Society for Clinical Pathology screening guidelines for the prevention and early detection of cervical cancer. *Am J Clin Pathol* 2012;137(4):516–42.

66. Moyer VA. Screening for cervical cancer: U.S. Preventive Services Task Force recommendation statement. *Ann Intern Med* 2012;156(12):880–91. Erratum in: *Ann Intern Med* 2013;158(11):852.

67. American College of Obstetricians and Gynecologists (ACOG). Screening for cervical cancer. Washington, DC: American College of Obstetricians and Gynecologists (ACOG); November 2012. (Practice Bulletin No. 131).

68. NHS Cancer Screening Programmes. NHS Cervical Screening Programme. http://www.cancerscreening.nhs.uk/cervical/index.html#invited (Accessed April 21, 2011).

69. National Health and Medical Research Council. www.nhmrc.gov.au/publications. November 23, 2006 (Accessed December 28, 2009).

70. Castle PE, Schiffman M, Wheeler CM, Solomon D. Evidence for frequent regression of cervical intraepithelial neoplasia-grade 2. *Obstet Gynecol* 2009;113(1):18–25.

71. Castle PE, Stoler MH, Solomon D, Schiffman M. The relationship of community biopsy-diagnosed cervical intraepithelial neoplasia grade 2 to the quality control pathology-reviewed diagnoses: an ALTS report. *Am J Clin Pathol* 2007;127(5):805–15.

72. Stoler MH, Wright TC Jr, Sharma A, Apple R, Gutekunst K, Wright TL; the ATHENA (Addressing THE Need for Advanced HPV Diagnostics) HPV Study Group. High-risk human papillomavirus testing in women with ASC-US cytology: results from the ATHENA HPV study. *Am J Clin Pathol* 2011;135:468–75.

73. Singer A, Jordan JA. The functional anatomy of the cervix, the cervical epithelium and the stroma. In: Jordan JA, Singer A, eds. *The Cervix* (2nd ed). Malden, MA: Blackwell, 2006:13–37.

74. Moscicki AB, Powers A, Ma Y, Wibbelsman C, Shaber R, Clayton C. Years sexually active and oral contraceptives are a risk for CIN 3 in adolescents and young women. Paper presented at: 23rd International Papillomavirus Conference 2006, September, 2006, Prague.

75. Stoler MH, Schiffman M. Atypical Squamous Cells of Undetermined Significance-Low-grade Squamous Intraepithelial Lesion Triage Study (ALTS) Group. Interobserver reproducibility of cervical cytologic and histologic interpretations: realistic estimates from the ASCUS-LSIL Triage Study. *JAMA* 2001;285(11):1500–5.

76. ACOG Practice Bulletin No. 99. Management of abnormal cervical cytology and histology. *Obstet Gynecol* 2008;112:1419–44.

77. Wright TC Jr, Massad LS, Dunton CJ, Spitzer M, Wilkinson EJ, Solomon D. 2006 consensus guidelines for the management of women with abnormal cervical screening tests. *J Low Genit Tract Dis* 2007;11:201–22.

78. Massad LS, Einstein MH, Huh WK, et al. 2012 updated consensus guidelines for the management of abnormal cervical cancer screening tests and cancer precursors. *J Low Genit Tract Dis* 2013;17(5 suppl 1):S1–S27. Jointly published without algorithm figures as Massad LS, Einstein MH, Huh WK, et al.; 2012 ASCCP Consensus Guidelines Conference. 2012 updated consensus guidelines for the management of abnormal cervical cancer screening tests and cancer precursors. *Obstet Gynecol* 2013;2121(2014):829–46.

79. Cox JT, Moriarty AT, Castle PE. Commentary on statement on human papillomavirus test utilization. *Arch Pathol Lab Med* 2009;133(8):1192–94.

80. Wright TC Jr, Massad LS, Dunton CJ, Spitzer M, Wilkinson EJ. 2006 consensus guidelines for the management of women with cervical intraepithelial neoplasia or adenocarcinoma in situ. *J Low Genit Tract Dis* 2007;11:223–39.

81. Hillard PA, Biro FM, Wildey L. Complications of cervical cryotherapy in adolescents. *J Reprod Med* 1991;36:711–6.

The Anal Canal and Perianus: HPV-Related Disease

17.1 EPIDEMIOLOGY OF ANAL HPV INFECTION, ANAL INTRAEPITHELIAL NEOPLASIA, AND ANAL CANCER IN MEN AND WOMEN
   17.1.1 Epidemiology of Anal HPV Infection in Men and Women
   17.1.2 Epidemiology of AIN in Men and Women
17.2 ANAL CANCER SCREENING
17.3 PATHOLOGY OF HPV-RELATED DISEASE OF THE ANAL CANAL AND PERIANUS
   17.3.1 Anal Cytology
   17.3.2 Histopathology of HPV-Related Disease of the Anal Canal and Perianus
17.4 EVALUATION OF THE ANUS AND PERIANUS
   17.4.1 Assessment of New Patients
   17.4.2 The Anal and Perianal Examination
   17.4.3 Anal Cytology Collection
   17.4.4 Digital Anorectal Examination
   17.4.5 High-Resolution Anoscopy
   17.4.6 Differences between HRA and Cervical Colposcopy
   17.4.7 Anal and Perianal Biopsies

   17.4.8 HRA Terminology
   17.4.9 Normal Anal Transformation Zone
   17.4.10 Abnormal Anal Transformation Zone
   17.4.11 Perianal Examination
17.5 MANAGEMENT AND TREATMENT OF ANAL CANAL AND PERIANAL LESIONS
   17.5.1 Rationale for Treating HGAIN or Condyloma
   17.5.2 Role of HRA in Management and Treatment of Anal Neoplasia
   17.5.3 Office-Based Treatment of AIN
   17.5.4 Approach to Patients in the Operating Room: UCSF Experience
   17.5.5 Specific Management Scenarios If Cancer Is Identified or Suspected
   17.5.6 Specific Recommendations for Management and Treatment of HGAIN and Condyloma
   17.5.7 Management of Anal Cancer
17.6 SUMMARY AND CONCLUSIONS
   17.6.1 Primary Prevention: Hope for the Future

17.1 EPIDEMIOLOGY OF ANAL HPV INFECTION, ANAL INTRAEPITHELIAL NEOPLASIA, AND ANAL CANCER IN MEN AND WOMEN

Most anal cancers are classified histologically as squamous cell carcinoma (SCC) with a smaller proportion classified as adenocarcinoma and small cell/neuroendocrine carcinoma.[1] While most studies have not distinguished among these histologic types when identifying risk factors, given the predominance of squamous cell cancer, most of the data available reflect risk factors associated with it.

Like cervical cancer, most anal cancers are associated with human papillomavirus (HPV).[2] The HPV types associated with anal cancer are similar to those found in cervical cancer, but HPV 16 may be even more dominant in anal cancers than it is in cervical cancer. Approximately 90% of anal cancers are associated with HPV, and it is possible that this number will increase even further with future studies. As with other HPV-associated cancers, the proportion of anal cancers associated with HPV has varied from study to study,[2] with the more recent studies tending to show a higher prevalence, most likely due to improvements in molecular detection techniques. Overall, the evidence suggests that the relationship between HPV and anal cancer is the same for both men and women;[2] however, one study showed a lower prevalence of HPV infection in anal cancers obtained from men.[3]

As in the cervix, anal cancer is likely preceded by anal intraepithelial neoplasia (AIN), which is morphologically analogous to cervical intraepithelial neoplasia (CIN), and like CIN, AIN is strongly associated with HPV infection. Both cervical and anal cancers commonly develop in regions of metaplastic squamous epithelium of the transformation zones. Given the concordance between their histology, association with HPV, and similarity of their precursor lesions, anal cancer and cervical cancer are very similar diseases.

While anal cancer strongly resembles cervical cancer, there are substantial biologic differences between the anus and the cervix, including their physiologic functions and hormonal and microflora environments. As described later, anal HPV infection is very common in some populations of men and women, and among some female populations, anal HPV infection is more common than cervical HPV infection. Given the relatively lower incidence of anal cancer compared with cervical cancer, the incidence of anal cancer on a per-HPV infection basis is substantially lower than that of the cervix. It would thus appear that the anal epithelium is less susceptible to HPV-associated oncogenic transformation than the cervix. The reason for this discrepancy is not clear but may reflect differences in hormonal influences and other differences in the microenvironment such as microflora, and pH.

The overall incidence of anal cancer in the United States between 1998 and 2003 was 1.52/100,000, with the incidence of squamous cell cancer, adenocarcinoma, and small cell/neuroendocrine cancer being 1.28/100,000, 0.22/100,000, and 0.02/100,000, respectively.[1] In the general population, anal squamous cell cancer is more common among women than men, while adenocarcinomas are more common among men.[1] During this time period, the average annual incidence among males in the United States was 1.0/100,000 and among females was about 50% higher.[4] Among men, the median age of diagnosis of anal cancer was 57 years and among women, 68 years. The incidence of anal cancer increased with age among men, with the highest incidence (3.1/100,000) among those over 70 years of age. The incidence of anal cancer among women followed the same age-related pattern with a peak incidence of 5.2/100,000 among those over 70 years of age.[4] In 2010, there were an estimated 2000 cases of anal cancer among men and 3260 cases among women in the United States.[5] In comparison, in 2010 there were an estimated 12,200 cases of cervical cancer in women in the United States[6] or an age-adjusted incidence of 6.7/100,000.[7]

While the incidence of anal cancer is relatively low compared with cervical cancer, the incidence of this disease has been increasing among both men and women by about 2% per year (Figure 17.1).[8] Thus in the 2003 to 2007 time period, the incidence of anal cancer was 1.8/100,000 in women and 1.4/100,000 in men. The reason for this increase is not well understood.

Prior to the human immunodeficiency virus (HIV) epidemic, the main risk factors identified for anal cancer were smoking, history of male homosexual contact, and history of genital warts and other sexually transmitted infections (presumably reflecting exposure to HPV).[9] Other risk factors found include chronic irritation in the form of hemorrhoids, fissures, and fistulas.[10]

Men who have sex with men (MSM) have been shown to be one of the populations at highest risk for anal cancer, with an estimated incidence as high as 36.9/100,000 prior to the onset of the HIV epidemic.[11] Although the exact reasons for this high incidence in MSM are not fully understood, it likely reflects high rates of receptive anal intercourse that expose them to anal HPV infection, as well as risk of other sexually transmitted infections and chronic anal irritation. Overall,

the incidence of anal cancer among HIV-uninfected MSM is greater than the incidence of cervical cancer in the general population of women. In the United States, most women are screened for cervical cancer. MSM remain largely unscreened for anal cancer and its precursor, AIN.

While it is clear that having receptive anal intercourse is a risk factor, many men and women diagnosed with anal cancer report no history of anal intercourse. Other sexual practices such as exposure to HPV-infected skin surfaces without anal penetration could lead to HPV inoculation of the anal canal. Theoretically, shedding from other genital surfaces could also lead to autoinoculation. Consistent with this, a history of HPV-associated lesions at genital sites other than the anus is associated with anal cancer, presumably reflecting common exposure to HPV.[12,13]

Finally, an increasingly important risk factor for anal cancer is immunosuppression. At least some of the population-based increase in anal cancer, described above, may reflect growing numbers of immunosuppressed individuals. Solid organ transplant recipients, including kidney, heart, and lung transplants, are at increased risk of anal cancer.[14-16]

Individuals with HIV-associated immunosuppression are also at increased risk of anal cancer. This was true prior to the availability of highly active antiretroviral therapy (HAART),[17] and there is evidence that the incidence of anal cancer has not declined since HAART became widely available. On the contrary, in some HAART-treated populations, the incidence of anal cancer may be continuing to increase. Several reports describe a higher incidence of anal cancer post-HAART compared with pre-HAART.[18-22] One recent report showed that the incidence of anal cancer increased from the pre-HAART era to the early post-HAART era, but that the incidence did not continue to increase beyond that in the later post-HAART era.[23] In another report, however, the incidence of anal cancer has continued to rise into the later post-HAART era, with the incidence among HIV-infected MSM on HAART as high as 128/100,000.[24] The risk of anal cancer may correlate with duration of immunodeficiency and high viral load prior to initiation of HAART.[25] Given that most HIV-positive individuals currently do not undergo screening or treatment for high-grade AIN (HGAIN), the longer survival time afforded by HAART gives an untreated HGAIN lesion more time to potentially progress to cancer. Notably, the incidence of anal

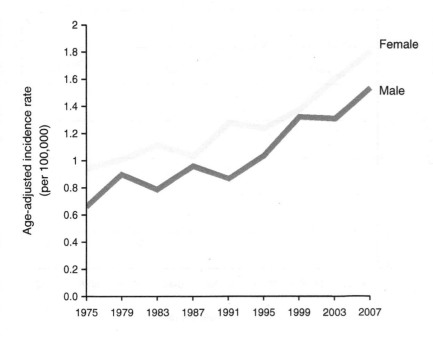

FIGURE 17.1. Age-adjusted incidence rate of anal cancer by gender and year of diagnosis, adapted from http://seer.cancer.gov/statfacts/html/anus.html (accessed 2/8/2011).

cancer reported in these studies exceeds some of the highest reported incidences of cervical cancer anywhere in the world.[26]

In summary, anal cancer is very similar biologically to cervical cancer with its strong association with HPV infection. The incidence of anal cancer is low in the general population, but is rising steadily among both men and women; it is particularly high among MSM and both men and women immunosuppressed due to transplantation or HIV. Risk factors for anal cancer largely reflect exposure to HPV, chronic irritation, and immunosuppression and are similar among men and women. Anal intercourse is likely an efficient mode of acquisition of anal HPV infection but is clearly not the only mode of transmission of HPV to the anal canal.

17.1.1 Epidemiology of Anal HPV Infection in Men and Women

Given that the underlying cause of anal cancer is HPV, it is important to understand the epidemiology of anal HPV infection. Given the particularly high incidence of anal cancer in both HIV-infected and HIV-uninfected MSM, many of the earliest studies of anal HPV infection were performed in these populations.

Most studies show a very high prevalence of anal HPV in MSM regardless of HIV status.[27–31] The largest study of HIV-uninfected sexually active MSM, performed in four cities in the United States, showed that the prevalence of anal HPV ranged between 50% and 60% over a wide age range, from <20 years of age to over 55 years of age.[32] Interestingly, in contrast to the steep age-related decline in the prevalence of cervical HPV infection in most studies in women over the age of 30 years, the age-related anal HPV prevalence curve was flat over this age range in MSM (Figure 17.2). The reasons for this difference are unknown but may partially reflect a larger number of new sexual partners after the age of 30 years among MSM compared with women in the general population. In that study, anal HPV infection was independently associated with receptive anal intercourse during the preceding 6 months and with having more than five sex partners during the preceding 6 months.

Most studies of HIV-infected MSM show that a very high proportion (>90%) have detectable anal HPV infection.[27,31,33,34] Most of the men have at least one oncogenic HPV type, and many have multiple HPV types; this is also true for men on HAART.[35] Detection of HPV and number of HPV types correlated with lower CD4+ level in the pre-HAART era, but the relationship with CD4+ level in the post-HAART era is not as clear, most likely due to HAART-associated increases in CD4+ level. In one study, the highest incidence rates among HIV-infected MSM were found for HPV 16, HPV 52 and HPV 53, with cumulative incidences at 36 months of approximately 30%.[31]

In the recently reported Study to Understand the Natural History of HIV/AIDS in the Era of Effective Therapy (SUN) study of HIV-infected individuals from the United States, the prevalence of anal HPV infection among HIV-infected MSM was 96%.[36] The prevalence of anal HPV was also high among HIV-infected men who only have sex with women, with 59% having anal HPV infection.[36] In an earlier study from France of HIV-infected men who only have sex with women, nearly half had anal HPV infection.[37]

Risk factors for anal HPV infection in HIV-infected MSM have been difficult to determine since the proportion infected with HPV is so high. One report showed that oncogenic anal HPV infection was associated with receptive anal intercourse.[35] It is clear, however, that as with anal cancer, having receptive intercourse is not necessary to acquire anal HPV infection, as shown in studies of men who have sex only with women.[38] In that study, which included men who were presumably HIV uninfected, the overall prevalence of anal HPV infection was

FIGURE 17.2. Prevalence of HPV DNA in the anal canals of HIV-negative men who have sex with men, by age group and by cancer-associated risk type. High-risk (HR) types include 16, 18, 31, 33, 35, 39, 45, 51, 52, 56, 58, 59, 68, and 73; low-risk (LR) types include 6, 11, 53, 54, 55, 66, Pap 155, and Pap 291. (Reprinted from Chin-Hong P, et al. Age-specific prevalence of anal human papillomavirus infection in HIV-negative sexually active men who have sex with men: The EXPLORE Study. *J Infect Dis* 2004;190:2070–76.)

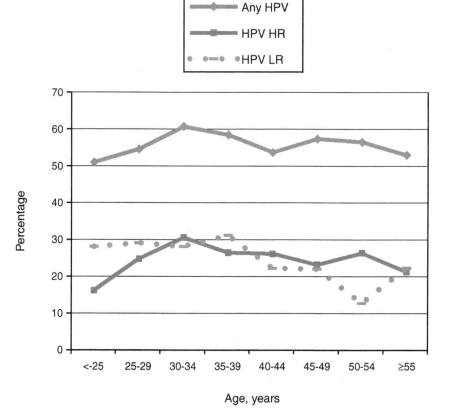

25%, and about one-third of the HPV-infected men had an oncogenic HPV type.[38] Risk factors for anal HPV infection in this population included lifetime number of female sex partners and frequency of sex with females during the preceding month.

The prevalence of anal HPV infection in women is lower than in MSM yet still surprisingly high; in several studies, it was similar to or higher than the prevalence of cervical HPV infection. Studies from a cohort of healthy, presumably HIV-uninfected Hawaiian women show that 27% were positive for anal HPV DNA compared with 29% with cervical HPV DNA.[39] Women with cervical HPV infection had greater than a threefold increased risk of concurrent anal infection. Concurrent anal and cervical HPV infection was most prevalent among the youngest women and steadily decreased through age 50 years. However, similar to results described above for HIV-uninfected MSM, the prevalence of anal infection alone remained relatively steady in all age groups. The overall distribution of HPV genotypes in the anus was more heterogeneous than in the cervix and included a greater proportion of nononcogenic types. The investigators reported a high degree of genotype-specific concordance among women with concurrent anal and cervical infections, consistent with a common source of infection through sexual activity or spread from one site to the other. Among women followed prospectively, half had an incident anal HPV infection and of these, 58% cleared during a follow-up period of approximately 1 year.[40] The median duration of an incident infection was 150 days, with factors associated with persistence being douching, long-term tobacco smoking, and anal intercourse.

Among HIV-infected women and women at high risk for HIV infection, anal HPV infection is even more common than cervical HPV infection.[41] In one study among HIV-infected women in San Francisco, anal HPV infection was detected in 79%, compared with cervical HPV infection in 53%.[41] Among HIV-uninfected, high-risk women, anal HPV infection was found in 43%, compared with cervical HPV infection in 24%. Among the HIV-infected women, anal HPV infection was associated with lower CD4+ level, cervical HPV infection, and younger age. Receptive anal intercourse was not associated with anal HPV infection in the HIV-infected women in this study. In the SUN study from the United States, the prevalence of anal HPV among HIV-infected women was 90%.[36]

Transplant recipients also have a high prevalence of anal HPV infection. In one recent study,[42] anal HPV infection was found in 21% of male and female renal transplant recipients with a mean age of 58.1 years.

Overall, these data indicate that anal HPV infection is common even among those with no history of receptive anal intercourse. Among women, anal infection is associated with cervical infection, consistent with the relationship between anal and cervical cancer. Clearly, however, as with cervical HPV and cervical cancer, most anal HPV infections do not lead to anal cancer, and as described above, it is likely that the anus is less susceptible to malignant transformation on a per-HPV infection basis than is the cervix. In contrast, the prevalence of anal HPV infection is even higher among HIV-uninfected MSM, and higher still among HIV-infected MSM. Given the very high prevalence of anal HPV infection in these two groups, the incidence of anal cancer on a per-HPV infection basis in these groups is relatively low. However, the incidence of anal cancer in MSM and HIV-infected men and women is high enough to warrant consideration of screening programs to detect and treat the anal cancer precursor, HGAIN, to reduce the risk of progression to cancer.[43]

17.1.2 Epidemiology of AIN in Men and Women

Similar to cervical cancer which is preceded by high-grade CIN (CIN 2,3), anal cancer is preceded by AIN, with HGAIN (AIN 2,3), specifically, being the cancer precursor. Several reports describe progression of HGAIN to anal cancer, often in the setting of immunosuppression among transplant recipients.[44,45] There is also long-standing experience with perianal HGAIN, in the form of perianal intraepithelial neoplasia, grade 3 (PAIN 3) or Bowen's disease, progressing to anal cancer.[46] Consistent with its role as a cancer precursor, HGAIN has a profile of HPV types similar to that of CIN 2,3.[2]

Although many individuals in research studies have undergone anal cytology testing as a measure of AIN prevalence or incidence, anal cytology screening has limited sensitivity and specificity.[47] Consequently, like CIN, the diagnosis of HGAIN requires histologic confirmation. This is accomplished using high-resolution anoscopy (HRA) with treatment based on HRA-guided biopsy (discussed later in this chapter). Optimal performance of HRA requires a lengthy training process, and many studies that report prevalence or incidence of anal neoplasia rely solely on cytology, due to the difficulties in performing HRA and biopsy, particularly in the setting of prospective cohorts. As a result, many studies that use anal cytology without HRA-guided biopsy may substantially underestimate the true prevalence or incidence of AIN.

Overall, the prevalence of AIN and risk of HGAIN, specifically, mirrors that of anal HPV prevalence in various populations. The prevalence of AIN is highest among HIV-infected MSM, followed by HIV-uninfected MSM. The effect of HAART on the prevalence and incidence of HGAIN has varied in different studies. In studies performed in the pre-HAART era, the prevalence and incidence of HGAIN were very high.[33,48] A study of San Francisco HIV-infected MSM conducted after the introduction of HAART showed that 81% had AIN of any grade and 52% had HGAIN.[34] These figures were even higher than those seen in pre-HAART era studies, suggesting that HAART had little or no beneficial effect in reducing the incidence of HGAIN.[49] Risk factors for detection of HGAIN included having more than six HPV types and using HAART. In a study from New York, the investigators reported that 40% of participants had AIN on biopsy.[35] Risk factors included history of receptive anal intercourse and lower nadir CD4+ cell counts, and in contrast to the San Francisco findings, being on HAART was associated with lower risk of AIN. In the only population-based data reported, a post-HAART study in San Francisco showed that the prevalence of any grade of AIN was 57% in HIV-infected MSM and the prevalence of HGAIN was 43%.[50] Among HIV-uninfected MSM, the prevalence of any grade of AIN was 35% and the prevalence of HGAIN was 25%. Overall, it is clear that the prevalence of AIN, including HGAIN, is very high in both HIV-uninfected and HIV-infected MSM, and if HAART is reducing the incidence of HGAIN or accelerating its regression, its effect is very limited.

There is one report on the prevalence of AIN in HIV-infected men who have sex only with women, and in this study from Paris, the prevalence of HGAIN (18%) was similar to that seen in a cohort of HIV-infected MSM.[37] To date, there are no published reports of the prevalence or incidence of AIN in HIV-uninfected men who only have sex with women.

Consistent with the detection of anal HPV infection at frequencies similar to or higher than in the cervix, AIN is also common in high-risk women in the post-HAART era. In a multisite study from the Women's Interagency HIV Study

(WIHS) from the United States, AIN 1 was found in 12% of HIV-infected and 5% of HIV-uninfected women.[51] HGAIN was present in 9% of HIV-infected and 1% of HIV-uninfected women. In multivariable analyses among HIV-infected women, the only significant risk factor for HGAIN was anal HPV infection. The prevalence of AIN was similar to the prevalence of CIN in both groups of women.

In the SUN study of HIV-infected women, using anal cytology to measure anal disease, squamous intraepithelial lesion (SIL) was found in 21% of women; this is similar to the prevalence of SIL on cervical cytology in the same group.[52] A history of anal intercourse was not associated with abnormal anal cytology.

There is comparatively little information published on the prevalence of AIN in the general population of healthy women. A recent analysis of healthy women with CIN or vulvar or vaginal intraepithelial neoplasia showed that 12% had biopsy-proven AIN.[53] In that study, 8% of women had HGAIN. Among renal transplant recipients in London, using anal cytology to assess disease, anal SIL was found in only 6% of patients.[42]

In summary, anal HPV is common in a wide range of populations, including healthy women and men. Populations at particularly high risk include MSM and men and women immunosuppressed due to HIV infection or organ transplantation. Relatively little is known about AIN in other populations. The incidence of anal cancer tracks closely with those populations at risk for anal HPV infection and AIN. With high incidences of anal cancer in high-risk populations, and the growing incidence of anal cancer in the general population, it is clear that more information is needed about the natural history of anal HPV infection and AIN in all of these populations. To date, no prospective, randomized studies comparing treatment of HGAIN to observation have been conducted, demonstrating that treatment prevents the development of anal cancer. However, since the populations at highest risk of anal cancer are well known, initial efforts to screen and treat HGAIN to prevent anal cancer should be focused to these populations. Additional evidence supporting the treatment of HGAIN will be presented in a following section on the rationale for treating HGAIN.

17.2 ANAL CANCER SCREENING

Anal cancer screening is in its infancy. There are no national screening guidelines for anal cancer, and no randomized clinical trials have been conducted to validate the efficacy of any type of screening. Anal cancer screening is not yet a standard of care in the United States. However, given the similarities between HPV-related cervical and anal disease and the increasing incidence of anal cancer and high-grade precursor lesions in the populations at risk, focusing anal cancer screening to these populations has been proposed.[54] The program of cervical cancer screening and management of abnormal cervical cytology is used as the model for cancer prevention and is based on the triad of cytologic screening, colposcopy, and directed biopsy. In an analogous manner, anal cytology is used in combination with HRA and HRA-directed biopsy, to identify HGAIN and early cancer. As with cervical disease, treatment of HGAIN aims to prevent invasive anal SCC, thus reducing its morbidity and mortality.

An integral addition to the anal evaluation, which differs from routine cervical cancer screening, is the regular use of the digital anorectal examination (DARE) to detect palpable masses and areas of pain, induration, or thickening that may reflect early invasive disease.[55] DARE is used in conjunction with cytologic screening or may be used alone. Particularly if resources are not available for anal cytology or HRA, using

DARE alone to potentially detect early invasive cancers, even in the absence of clinical symptoms, is a low-cost, low-resource tool that is underutilized for anal cancer screening in high-risk populations.[55]

A proposed algorithm for triage of anal cytology and DARE results, used in the context of anal cancer screening in high-risk populations, is presented in Figure 17.3. This is based on the authors' experience with anal screening and HRA, but has not been validated. Cytologic screening is inappropriate unless triage using HRA and treatment options for HGAIN are available.

The role of high-risk HPV testing in anal cancer screening and triage of abnormal cytology is controversial. The prevalence of HPV is high in the populations at risk, making the contribution of HPV testing to screening and triage of anal cytology with mild abnormalities problematic.[55,56]

17.3 PATHOLOGY OF HPV-RELATED DISEASE OF THE ANAL CANAL AND PERIANUS

The morphologic changes, caused by HPV infection in either the cervix or the anus, are similar on both cytology and histopathology. The spectrum of HPV-related cutaneous perianal disease is essentially identical to vulvar neoplasia. The basic morphologic manifestations of HPV infection on anal mucosa and perianal skin are described below.

17.3.1 Anal Cytology

The goal of anal cytology is to sample the surface epithelium of the entire anal canal—from the distal rectal vault to the anal verge. Due to the normal resting tone of the anal sphincters, the epithelium of the anal canal is apposed, with much of its surface hidden inside the folds and invaginations of the canal. For an adequate cytologic specimen, all these areas need to be sampled. The technique for collecting anal cytologic samples is detailed in a section below. In the laboratory, either liquid-based cytology or direct smears are prepared and stained in a manner analogous to cervical Pap tests.

Modified Bethesda System terminology is used to report the findings on anal cytology.[57,58] Anal cytology is evaluated using criteria similar to a cervical Pap test. The interpretive categories, morphologic criteria, and terminology parallel cervical cytology and are discussed in brief below.

17.3.1.1 Sensitivity and Specificity

In experienced hands, anal cytology has operational characteristics similar to the Pap test.[47] However, since these samples are collected without direct visualization of the anal canal, sampling errors may play a larger role than in cervical cytology. In addition, the interpretation of anal cytology often underrepresents the grade of disease ultimately found on HRA-guided biopsy.[58,59]

The sensitivity of anal cytology for biopsy-proven HGAIN in HIV-positive patients ranges from 69% to 93%, and the specificity ranges from 32% to 59% using atypical squamous cells of undetermined significance (ASC-US) or worse as the threshold for triage to HRA.[59,60] In a 2010 study reported by Salit et al.,[61] anal cytology had a sensitivity of 84% and a specificity of 39% using ASC-US or worse as the threshold; high-grade squamous intraepithelial lesion (HSIL) on anal cytology had 91% specificity for high grade AIN but a correspondingly lower sensitivity. Overall, these test statistics are comparable to those for cervical Pap tests.

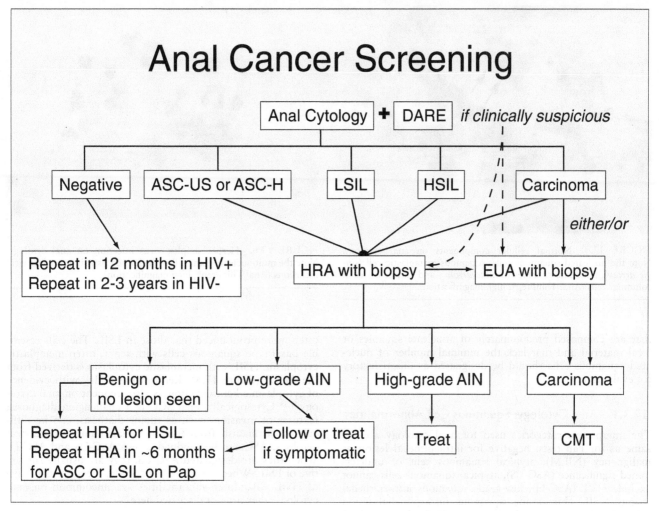

FIGURE 17.3. Anal cancer screening algorithm. AIN, anal intraepithelial neoplasia; ASC-US,. atypical squamous cells of undetermined significance; ASC-H, atypical squamous cells cannot exclude high-grade SIL; CMT, combined modality therapy; DARE, digital anorectal examination; EUA, examination under anesthesia; HRA, high-resolution anoscopy; HSIL, high-grade intraepithelial lesions; LSIL, low-grade squamous intraepithelial lesions. (Adapted from Park IU, Palefsky JM. Evaluation and management of anal intraepithelial neoplasia in HIV-negative and HIV-positive men who have sex with men. *Curr Infect Dis Rep* 2010;12(2):126–33.)

The sensitivity of anal cytology for the detection of HGAIN is highest in HIV-infected MSM, presumably due to the larger lesion size and burden of disease frequently seen in this population. In studies of both HIV-positive and HIV-negative MSM,[47,56] the sensitivity of ASC-US or greater for the detection of HGAIN on conventional smear cytology was 87% in HIV-positive MSM and 55% in HIV-negative MSM; specificity was 42% and 81%. The sensitivity, using low-grade squamous intraepithelial lesion (LSIL) or greater as the threshold, was 77% and 50% in HIV-positive and HIV-negative MSM, respectively; the specificity was 53% and 85%, respectively. In HIV-positive MSM, the specificity and positive predictive value (PPV) of HSIL cytology was high at 93% and 89%.

17.3.1.2 Anal Cytology: Benign Findings and Specimen Adequacy

An anal cytology test samples surface epithelial cells from the entire anal canal—the distal rectal vault to the anal verge; this includes the anal transformation zone (AnTZ) and the non-keratinized and keratinized portions of the canal. As such, rectal columnar cells, squamous metaplastic cells, nucleated

squamous cells, and anucleated squames are normal components of anal cytology (Figure 17.4). Similar to cervical-vaginal cytology, a variety of organisms can be identified on anal cytology; these may be pathogenic or nonpathogenic. As with the Pap test, clinical correlation is needed to determine whether or not evaluation or treatment is warranted. Some of these organisms detected on anal cytology are similar to those seen on Pap tests: for example, *Candida* and herpes virus infection (Figures 17.5 and 17.6). Others, such as ameba and pinworm eggs, are more common to the gastrointestinal tract and are rarely encountered on cervical-vaginal cytology.

Per the 2001 Bethesda System, the minimal cellularity for an adequate anal cytology is approximately 2000 to 3000 cells, or 1 to 2 nucleated squamous cells per high-power field (hpf) for ThinPreps® and 3 to 6 nucleated squamous cells per hpf for SurePath™ preparations.[57] Little is known about how cellularity influences sensitivity and specificity of anal cytology. Some studies have indicated that more cellular specimens have better performance characteristics.[62] The presence or absence of transformation zone components (rectal columnar cells and squamous metaplastic cells) is reported as a quality indicator. When no abnormal cells are identified, samples

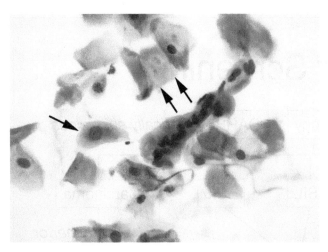

FIGURE 17.4. Normal cellular components on anal cytology. Note the nucleated squamous cells, squamous metaplastic cell (*single arrow*), anucleate squames (*double arrow*), and cluster of rectal columnar cells (Anal ThinPrep®, high magnification).

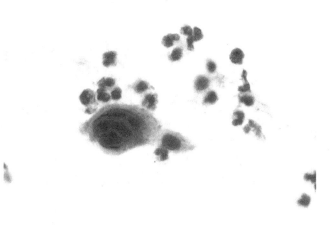

FIGURE 17.6. Herpes simplex virus infection on anal cytology. Note the multinucleate giant cell with characteristic intranuclear viral inclusions (Anal ThinPrep®, high magnification).

that are composed predominately of anucleate squames or fecal material and that lack the minimal number of nucleated squamous cells should be designated as unsatisfactory for evaluation.

17.3.1.3 Anal Cytology: Squamous Cell Abnormalities

The interpretive categories used for anal cytology are the same as for Pap tests: negative for intraepithelial lesion or malignancy (NILM), atypical squamous cells of undetermined significance (ASC-US), atypical squamous cells cannot exclude HSIL (ASC-H), low-grade squamous intraepithelial lesions (LSIL), high-grade squamous intraepithelial lesion (HSIL), and squamous cell carcinoma (SCC). The alterations seen in squamous cells of the anal canal caused by HPV are remarkably similar to those seen in cervical cytology and are summarized here.

LSIL is characterized by dysplastic nuclear changes (enlargement, hyperchromasia, chromatin, and contour abnormalities) in mature squamous cells with abundant cytoplasm (Figure 17.7). In HSIL, the nuclear changes are

often more pronounced that those in LSIL. The cells resemble basal-type squamous cells with scant, often metaplastic cytoplasm. HSIL with metaplastic cytoplasm is derived from the AnTZ (Figure 17.8). Keratinizing HSIL, with evidence of cytoplasmic keratinization, is also frequent on anal cytology.[57,58] Cytologically, anal SCC is a challenging diagnosis; features of invasion, such as tumor diathesis, can be difficult to distinguish from fecal material. Similar to cervical cytology, ASC can be subdivided into ASC-US and ASC-H. When they are designated ASC-US, they are usually suggestive of LSIL. When designated as ASC-H, they are suggestive of HSIL. Glandular abnormalities are uncommon on anal cytology; they are not discussed here.

17.3.2 Histopathology of HPV-Related Disease of the Anal Canal and Perianus

There are a variety of classification schemes used to describe HPV-related disease of lower anogenital mucocutaneous

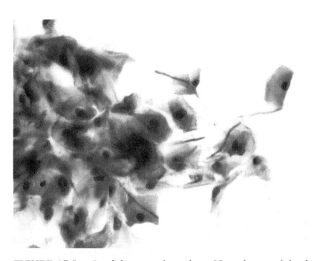

FIGURE 17.5. *Candida* on anal cytology. Note the pseudohyphae 'spearing' the squamous cells (Anal ThinPrep®, high magnification).

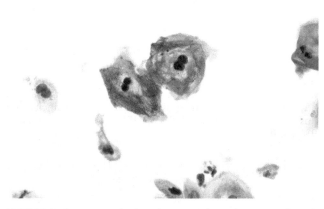

FIGURE 17.7. LSIL on anal cytology. Binucleate squamous cells with HPV-cytopathic effect or koilocytosis are present (Anal ThinPrep®, high magnification).

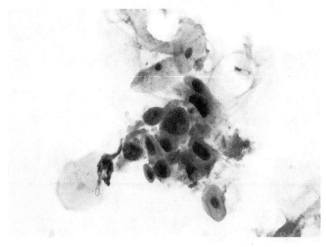

FIGURE 17.8.   HSIL on anal cytology. Note the cells with enlarged, hyperchromatic nuclei and scant, dense cytoplasm characteristic of HSIL arising in immature squamous metaplasia of the AnTZ (Anal ThinPrep®, high magnification).

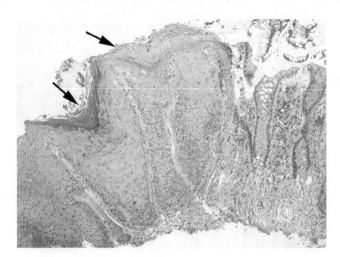

FIGURE 17.10.   Low-grade AIN. This biopsy at the anal SCJ shows surface hyperkeratosis and parakeratosis at *arrows* (H&E, low magnification).

squamous epithelia. Here, for the anus and perianus, AIN will be categorized as either low-grade (LGAIN) or high-grade (HGAIN). LGAIN is considered the histopathologic manifestation of HPV infection; it can be caused by either low-risk or high-risk HPV types. It consists of the low-grade spectrum of lesions: condyloma and mild dysplasia or AIN 1. These appear to have little if any potential for cancer and do not require therapy unless symptomatic or cosmetically troubling. HGAIN is a potential cancer precursor and, like HSIL on anal cytology, is usually associated with high-risk HPV types. It is also referred to as moderate dysplasia, severe dysplasia, carcinoma *in situ*, and AIN 2, AIN 2,3, or AIN 3. On perianal skin, clinical terms such as Bowen's disease or bowenoid papulosis are sometimes used; morphologically, these are high-grade squamous intraepithelial neoplasms.

The squamous epithelium of the anal canal is stratified (Figure 17.9). The distal canal is a keratinized mucosa, devoid of epidermal appendages. LGAIN and HGAIN may be either keratinized or nonkeratinized. Mucosal lesions with prominent keratinization are more commonly encountered in the anal canal than on the cervix (Figure 17.10). The morphologic features of HPV infection are identical to those of other anogenital mucosal and cutaneous surfaces. Architecturally, LGAIN

can be flat or have a warty profile. In LGAIN, abnormal cells are seen throughout the epithelial thickness, though cells in the superficial layer have appreciable cytoplasm, often with the prominent cytoplasmic cavitation or koilocytosis associated with HPV. Many HPV-related lesions, particularly HGAIN, arise in the metaplastic squamous epithelium of the AnTZ near the squamocolumnar junction (SCJ) (Figure 17.11). In HGAIN, the immature-appearing dysplastic cells fill even the upper levels of the epithelium; mitotic figures can be seen well above the basal layers (Figure 17.12).

The vast majority of anal canal cancers are squamous (Figure 17.13); histologic subclassification of anal SCC has little clinical value.[63] Currently, about 93% are associated with high-risk HPV types, particularly HPV 16 and 18, with type 16 predominating.[1] The equivalent of cervical microinvasion, with its specific histologic depth and lateral spread measurements and management and prognostic implications, is not defined for minimally invasive anal SCC. The role, if any, of HPV in glandular neoplasia in the anus is not known. Approximately 10% of anal canal cancers are adenocarcinomas[63]. Most have a colorectal phenotype and probably arise from the distal rectum or glandular epithelium of the AnTZ.[63]

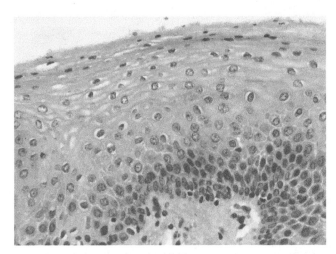

FIGURE 17.9.   Benign nonkeratinized squamous mucosa of the anal canal (H&E, medium magnification).

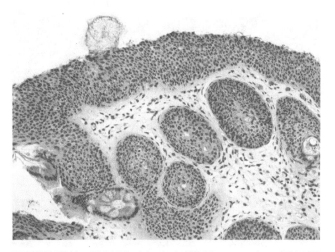

FIGURE 17.11.   HGAIN arising in AnTZ. Note extension of HGAIN down the rectal glands (H&E, low magnification).

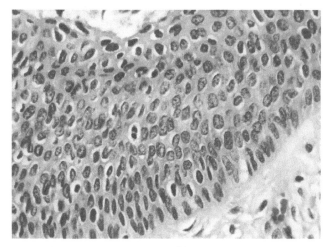

FIGURE 17.12.   High-grade AIN. Note the mitotic figure in the midportion of the epithelium, above the basal layer (H&E, medium magnification).

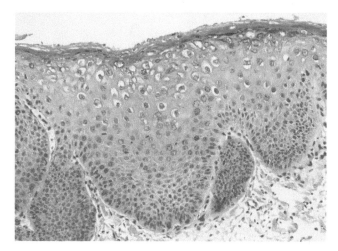

FIGURE 17.14.   Low-grade PAIN. Prominent HPV-cytopathic effect is seen (H&E, medium magnification).

The histopathology of perianal disease mirrors vulvar disease. HPV-related cytopathic changes are frequently not prominent on keratinized squamous epithelium but may be seen, particularly in low-grade PAIN (Figure 17.14). High-grade perianal lesions are characterized by abnormal maturation with dysplastic keratinocytes occupying the majority of the epithelial thickness. Morphologically, Bowen's disease and bowenoid papulosis are high-grade PAIN (Figure 17.15).

17.4 EVALUATION OF THE ANUS AND PERIANUS

17.4.1 Assessment of New Patients

The first step in evaluating a new patient is to obtain a HPV-focused history (see Table 17.1 for the new patient questionnaire used in the University of California San Francisco [UCSF] Anal Neoplasia Clinic). The questions are designed to elicit information about specific anal symptoms such as painful bowel movements, pain during sex, irritation, or bleeding. It is important to ask whether the patient has ever been treated for HPV-related lesions and if so, how they were treated.

Questions are designed to identify recognized risk factors, contraindications for invasive procedures, and likelihood of response to therapy.

The history should contain an assessment of overall health; prior surgical procedures, particularly anal surgery; presence of any bleeding tendencies such as thrombocytopenia, hemophilia or medications such as warfarin, aspirin, and platelet inhibitors; and risk of infection due to leukopenia. The key role of the immune system in controlling HPV infection has been discussed earlier. Therefore, it is important to ask questions regarding HIV status or the presence of other immune compromising conditions such as solid organ transplantation, bone marrow transplantation, autoimmune disease, and prolonged treatment with corticosteroids and other biologic response modifiers, or chemotherapeutic drugs. For HIV-infected patients, it is useful to know duration of seropositivity, CD4 lymphocyte count nadir and current CD4 lymphocyte count, HIV viral load, and treatment for opportunistic infections.

A sexual history should be included routinely: ask about sexual preference (sex with men, women, or both), lifetime and current number of partners, whether there are any sexual problems, history of sexually transmitted infection and screening, condom use, and history of ever having receptive anal

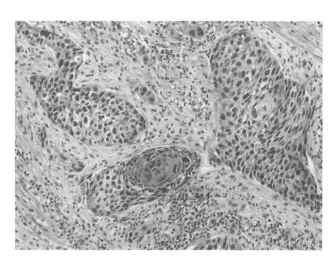

FIGURE 17.13.   Invasive SCC with nests of pleomorphic squamous cells invading stroma (H&E, medium magnification).

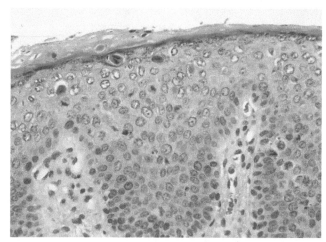

FIGURE 17.15.   High-grade PAIN. Note the disorderly maturation of the keratinocytes and individual dyskeratotic cells (H&E, medium magnification).

TABLE 17.1   UCSF ANAL NEOPLASIA CLINIC NEW PATIENT QUESTIONNAIRE

UCSF Helen Diller Family
Comprehensive
Cancer Center

Affix Patient Label Here

Anal Neoplasia Questionnaire

Please answer the following questions as accurately as you can.

What is the reason for your visit today? _____

How are you feeling in general today? _____

Are you having any anal symptoms such as:

❑ itching   ❑ discomfort, pain, difficult or painful or uncomfortable bowel movements

❑ diarrhea   ❑ bleeding when you have a bowel movement

❑ feel a lump or bumps   ❑ blood on the toilet paper when wiping

❑ inability to have receptive sex due to pain or discomfort

Have you had any anal warts?   ❑ YES   ❑ NO   If Yes, where were these treated?

   ❑ Office Procedure   ❑ Surgery in the operating room   ❑ Other_____

Have you ever been diagnosed with potentially pre cancerous lesions in the anus (also referred to as moderate to severe dysplasia, AIN, high-grade lesions, carcinoma in situ, or Bowen's disease)?

❑ YES   ❑ NO   If yes, when? _____ How were they treated?_____

If you are a woman, have you even had an abnormal cervical Pap? ❑ YES   ❑ NO

Ever been treated for cervical pre cancerous lesions or lesions on your vulva? ❑ YES   ❑ NO
If yes, when? _____ How were they treated?_____

Have you ever been diagnosed with anal cancer? ❑ YES   ❑ NO
If yes, when? _____ How were they treated?_____

Did you receive radiation and chemotherapy? ❑ YES   ❑ NO
If yes, when was the last day of your radiation treatment?_____

Have you ever been diagnosed or treated for any other anal problems including hemorrhoids, fissures, fistulas, perianal abscess, or incontinence? ❑ YES   ❑ NO
If yes, please document and explain when and how it was treated? _____

_____

Has your sexual partner(s) even been treated for HPV (human papilloma virus) related pre cancerous changes or warts? ❑ YES   ❑ NO

Anal Neoplasia Questionnaire   Page 1 of 2

(continued)

TABLE 17.1   UCSF ANAL NEOPLASIA CLINIC NEW PATIENT QUESTIONNAIRE *(continued)*

UCSF Helen Diller Family
Comprehensive
Cancer Center

Affix Patient Label Here

Have you been treated with any of the following drugs?

❑ Aldara (5% imiquimod)   ❑ Veregen   ❑ Condylox

❑ Efudex (5% fluorouracil cream)   ❑ Other_____

If yes, please give details as to when, for how long, did it help, and if you experienced any side effects?

_____

_____

Are you HIV positive? ❑ YES   ❑ NO

If yes, what was your lowest CD4 lymphocyte or t-cell count ever? _____

When was that? _____

What was your most recent CD4+ count? _____ When was that test done? _____

Are you taking antiretroviral drugs for HIV , also known as HAART? ? ❑ YES   ❑ NO

How long have you been taking HAART? _____

What was your highest HIV viral load? _____ When? _____

What was your most recent HIV viral load? _____ When was that test done? _____

Have you ever had any opportunistic infections, KS (Kaposi Sarcoma), HD or NHL (Hodgkin or non-Hodgkin lymphoma)? ❑ YES   ❑ NO

If yes, please specify which_____

Are you immunocompromised for any other reason? ❑ YES   ❑ NO

If yes, please explain _____

Have you had an organ transplant? ❑ YES   ❑ NO

If yes, when _____ Have you had any rejection episodes? _____

**   **   **   ****

For Office Use Only
Provider Documentation

Instructions to Attending Physician: Your signature below indicates that you have reviewed the information contained in the <u>entire</u> questionnaire and that you have reviewed the pertinent or key finding(s) with the patient and/or family. Key finding(s) must be summarized in your progress note, however the questionnaire may be referenced for additional details.

_____

Attending Provider Signature   **Date**

Anal Neoplasia Questionnaire   Page 2 of 2

intercourse. Routinely ask about tobacco, drug, and alcohol use. Smoking may play a role in facilitating progression of lesions as well as hindering treatment response by increasing the likelihood of recurrent or persistent disease.[64] It is imperative that these questions be asked in a nonjudgmental manner. Assisting patients to create a plan for tobacco cessation, in addition to the obvious health benefits, makes them active participants in their treatment. An educated and motivated patient is more likely to adhere to follow-up recommendations and tolerate treatment-related side effects, both of which are necessary parts of effective therapy regimens.

17.4.1.1 Key Questions to Answer during HRA Examination

Does the patient have signs or symptoms suggestive of cancer? If a diagnosis or an evaluation cannot be made in the office, then patients should be examined under anesthesia by a clinician experienced in the management of AIN. Although not specific for cancer, hallmarks of cancer include pain, irritation, and bleeding; patients with these symptoms should be evaluated appropriately. When no cancer is identified on the examination, the presence or absence of symptoms is one of the most important factors in deciding how aggressively to manage an individual patient, since treatment may provide symptomatic relief. For instance, the following patients with AIN are usually *not* treated aggressively: asymptomatic patients with significant coexisting medical problems, asymptomatic patients with extensive lesions and poor or marginal immune function,

and patients with poor functional status or limited life expectancy. Do the patients understand the potential risk for cancer and are they motivated to decrease that risk? Given the relatively high recurrence rate with any therapeutic modality, it is important that patients clearly understand the importance of regular, careful, and prolonged follow-up.

17.4.2 The Anal and Perianal Examination

Distinction is made between the anus (or anal canal) and the perianus (or anal margin). The basic anatomic landmarks of the anal canal are indicated in Figure 17.16. The anal canal is approximately 4 to 6 cm long, but varies in length from individual to individual; it tends to be shorter in women. The proximal end of the anal canal begins anatomically where the rectum enters the puborectalis sling at the internal edge of the anal sphincter complex. This is palpable as the anorectal ring on DARE. The resting tone of the sphincter muscles keeps the walls of the anal canal apposed. The anal canal extends distally to the point where the squamous mucosa blends with the perianal skin of the anal verge. The anal verge is the opening to the anus as seen on external examination and roughly coincides with the band of cutaneous tissue over the external sphincter at the anal opening. The palpable intersphincteric groove or the outermost boundary of the internal sphincter muscle is the proximal edge of the verge. The anal canal is divided by the undulating dentate line, a macroscopically visible landmark that marks the transition from anodermal

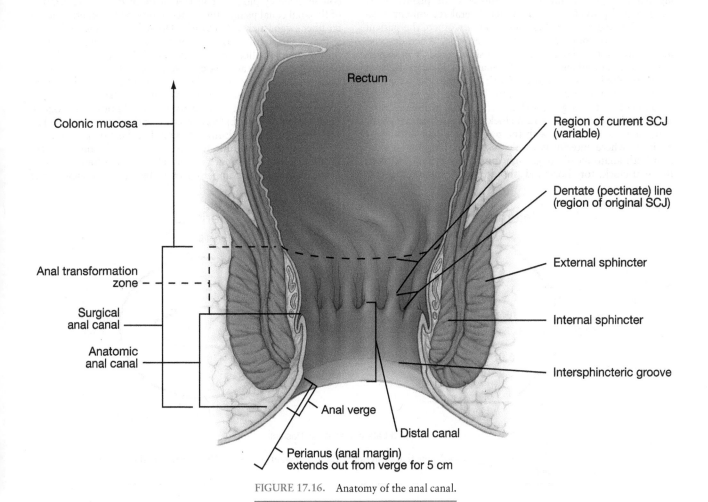

FIGURE 17.16.   Anatomy of the anal canal.

squamous mucosa, which is firmly attached to the underlying fibromuscular tissue of the distal canal, from the anal mucosa that loosely overlies the internal hemorrhoidal plexus. The anal transformation (or transition) zone and anal SCJ are proximal to the dentate line. The SCJ is located approximately 1 to 2 cm above the dentate line; its location varies. The perianus or anal margin is the circumferential region extending laterally 5 cm from the anal verge.

The goal of evaluating the anus and perianus is to determine the presence, extent, or absence of HPV-associated disease by systematically examining the entire SCJ, anal canal including AnTZ, and perianal skin. A complete examination includes cytology collection, a thorough DARE, HRA using the colposcope with vinegar and Lugol's solution to visualize lesions, and biopsies to determine the extent and grade of disease. A thorough examination, requiring biopsies of both intra-anal and perianal areas, typically will take 20 to 30 minutes to complete. New patients, unfamiliar with the procedures, will require additional time for teaching and counseling.

The equipment for HRA is similar to that used for evaluation of the cervix with the following differences: synthetic polyester fiber swabs are recommended for anal cytology collection, not cytobrushes or spatulas; metal or disposable plastic anoscopes instead of specula; and smaller biopsy forceps with bites that are ≤3 mm, such as the baby Tischler or ENT laryngeal forceps. HRA also requires higher magnification than cervical colposcopy. The colposcope should magnify to at least 25×. Colposcopes that only magnify to 10× are not adequate for HRA. It is also important to have angled eyepieces, as the straight-on view colposcopes are ergonomically difficult to use for HRA (Figure 17.17).

Patients can be examined in any of several positions including left or right lateral, dorsal lithotomy, or prone. Most patients and providers prefer the left lateral recumbent position. Following a cervical examination in women, the patient is repositioned from lithotomy to her left side. When describing the location of lesions and the position used, it is important to be clear and consistent. The anal clock is different from the gynecologic clock (Figure 17.18); note that the patient is in the left lateral decubitus position. Based on the convention used in colorectal surgery, with patients in the prone position, the posterior anal aspect is 12 o'clock; this is in contrast to the gynecologic convention, with the patient in dorsal lithotomy position, where anterior is 12 o'clock. Describing lesion location both anatomically (e.g., right posterior-lateral) and with the anal clock, for shorthand, should reduce communication

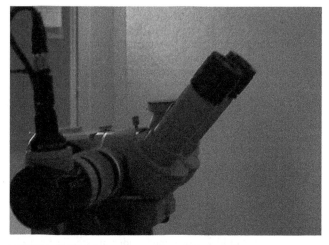

FIGURE 17.17.   Colposcope with angled eyepieces.

errors regarding lesion location between clinicians of various disciplines.

17.4.3 Anal Cytology Collection

Collection of anal cytology is a simple procedure and is done first, before any lubrication is used, to increase the yield of cell collection. In addition, patients are instructed to refrain from inserting anything per anus for 24 hours before the procedure; this includes no enemas, douching, or receptive anal intercourse. Anal cytology is collected without direct visualization of the anal canal using a tap-water–moistened synthetic polyester fiber swab, such as Dacron™. Do not use a prescored swab; it may snap at the score line when using adequate pressure during sample collection. The cytobrush is uncomfortable and unnecessary since adequate sampling can be obtained using synthetic swabs. Cotton swabs should not be used; cells adhere more to the cotton and are not as easily transferred to the glass slide or vial for liquid-based cytology. In addition, the wooden handle of cotton swabs may fracture and splinter with the lateral pressure applied during the sample collection process.

To collect the sample for anal cytology, the buttocks are gently separated; patients in the left lateral recumbent position can retract their upper cheek to facilitate the view of the

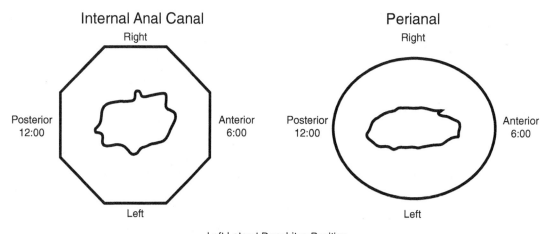

FIGURE 17.18.   The anal "clock;" note that posterior is 12:00 and anterior is 6:00. The patient is in the left lateral decubitus position.

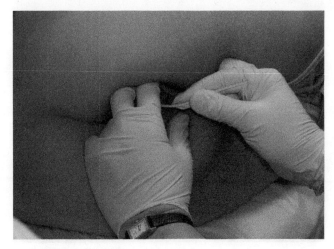

FIGURE 17.19.   Anal cytology collection.

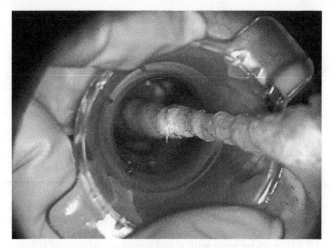

FIGURE 17.20.   The cotton-tipped swab, wrapped in 4 × 4 gauze and soaked in vinegar, is inserted through the anoscope.

anal opening. Premoisten the swab with tap water and gently insert into the anal canal until it bypasses the internal sphincter and abuts the distal wall of the rectum. In most patients, this will be 2 to 3 inches (~5 to 7 cm). Initial resistance (at <1 inch) is sometimes caused by a hemorrhoid or prolapsed mucosa. If this occurs, reinsert the swab at a different angle or position, until it can be inserted without force. Once fully inserted, rotate the swab 360 degrees in a circular fashion, applying firm lateral pressure against the walls of the canal, while slowly retracting the swab. The swab should bend slightly with the pressure applied. The collection procedure typically takes 10 to 20 seconds. Counting slowly to 10 before removing the swab helps ensure that enough cells are collected (Figure 17.19).

Transfer the cell sample to a liquid-based cytology vial or smear on a glass slide for conventional cytology. Place the swab in the liquid medium and agitate vigorously to transfer cells. If using conventional cytology slides, quickly fix the slides once smeared; air-drying artifacts easily occur. Patients can also provide self-collected samples for liquid-based cytology, although home kits are not currently available.[50,65]

For patients referred for HRA after an abnormal anal cytology result, repeating it at the time of examination is suggested if the results are (1) older than 3 months, (2) not available, or (3) the previous result was unsatisfactory (insufficient) or equivocal (ASC-US or ASC-H).

17.4.4 Digital Anorectal Examination

The DARE is an essential part of anal cancer screening. It is performed after the collection of the anal cytology and before HRA. The goal of the DARE is to detect any palpable abnormalities; it may help guide further evaluation, including the anoscopic examination and biopsies.

Using a mixture of water-soluble lubricant gel and 2% to 5% lidocaine gel (3/4 lube to 1/4 lidocaine gel) for lubrication, insert a gloved finger slowly into the anus. Apply firm pressure on the external sphincter, allowing it to relax before advancing into the rectum. Systematically palpate the entire circumference and length of the anal canal, beginning in the rectum. Palpate the mucosa over the internal sphincter and the walls of the distal anal canal. Palpate for warts, masses, and areas of induration, discomfort, or pain. Once completed, also examine the prostate in men. Finally, palpate the perianal region in its entirety. Areas that are hard, firm, indurated or immobile are suspicious for cancer. Warts are typically soft, mobile, and nodular or gritty

to palpation. Document the location and size of any palpated abnormalities and correlate these with the visual exam.

17.4.5 High-Resolution Anoscopy

To begin the HRA, lubricate the anoscope with additional lubricant/lidocaine gel mixture and insert it into the anus. Either disposable or nondisposable anoscopes can be used. Remove the anoscope's obturator and insert a cotton-tipped swab wrapped in gauze previously soaked in 3% to 5% acetic acid (Figure 17.20). Medical grade acetic acid (not glacial acetic acid) can be used, but commercially available white table vinegar is 5% acetic acid, and it can be used or diluted to 3%. Remove the anoscope, leaving the gauze-wrapped cotton-tipped swab in place (Figure 17.21). Allow the vinegar to saturate the epithelium of the anal canal for 1 to 2 minutes. Remove the cotton-tipped swab and gauze, and reinsert the anoscope with the obturator in place; remove the obturator again for the exam itself.

Begin using a colposcope on low magnification; a larger area in the field of vision aids in establishing anatomic landmarks. With the anoscope fully inserted, the first area visualized is the distal rectum. Observing through the colposcope,

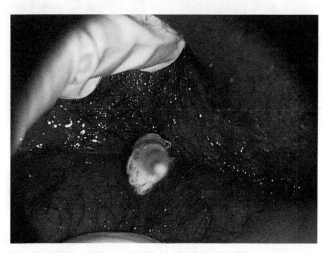

FIGURE 17.21.   The cotton-tipped swab and gauze is left in the anal canal for 1 minute.

slowly withdraw the anoscope until the anal SCJ and/or AnTZ come into focus. Refocus the colposcope continually while the anoscope is repositioned and withdrawn. The anal canal varies from 2 to 5 cm in length.[66] In some patients, the SCJ, the most proximal aspect of the AnTZ, is viewed immediately with the anoscope completely inserted. In other patients, the SCJ is not seen until the anoscope is withdrawn nearly to the anal verge. The first landmark to identify is the anal SCJ. The SCJ, the junction between the rectal columnar epithelium and anal squamous epithelium, is located where the darker red colonic epithelium abuts the lighter pink anal squamous epithelium (Figure 17.22). Once the SCJ is identified, additional vinegar is applied, using a cotton-tipped swab, to examine the entire circumference of the transformation zone. The AnTZ is distal to the SCJ; it is the region of squamous metaplasia. As with the cervix, its appearance varies: it may appear as a thin-white line of metaplasia (Figure 17.22), a wider zone with gland openings, islands of columnar epithelium within the mature squamous epithelium, or a more diffuse region of faint acetowhite epithelium (AWE) (Figure 17.23A,B).

After locating the SCJ and AnTZ, continue to reapply vinegar throughout the exam. Use higher magnification (e.g., 16×

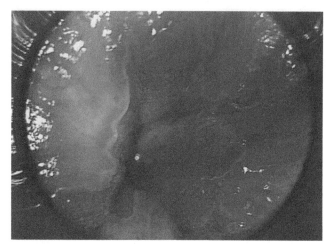

FIGURE 17.22. Rectal columnar epithelium and anal squamous epithelium abut at the SCJ. Note that the rectal mucosa is dark red compared to the lighter pink color of the anal epithelium. The AnTZ here is seen as a thin, white line of metaplasia.

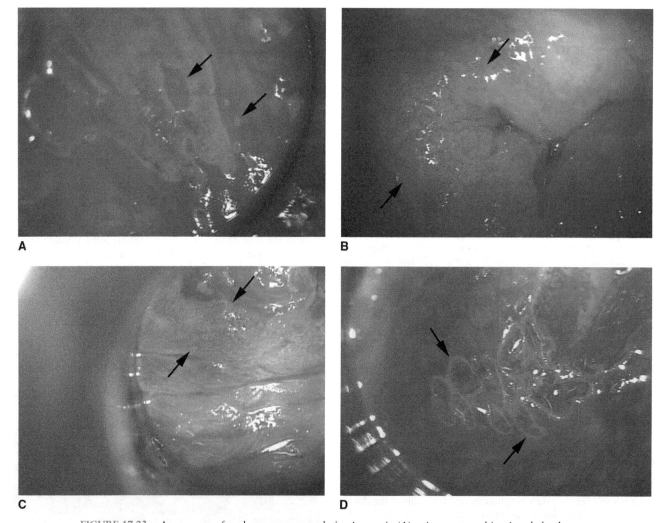

FIGURE 17.23. Appearance of anal squamous metaplasia. *Arrows* in (A) point to acetowhite-ringed gland openings and an island of mature squamous epithelium surrounded by columnar epithelium. B: Diffuse acetowhitening in early metaplasia, between *arrows*. Mid metaplasia is shown in (C) with acetowhite ringed glands noted between the *arrows*. D: Islands of columnar epithelium and coalesced glands indicative of early metaplasia.

to 25×) for better visualization of specific regions. To view all aspects of the SCJ and AnTZ, manipulate the anoscope or use cotton-tipped swabs to visualize areas hidden by folds, hemorrhoids, normal anal papillae, or prolapsed mucosa. An adequate HRA requires that the entire SCJ and AnTZ are visualized. With proper manipulation of the mucosa, it is rare for an exam to be inadequate.

After completely examining the SCJ and AnTZ, begin withdrawing the anoscope to examine the distal anal canal. Continue to move the colposcope to maintain focus as the anoscope is withdrawn. Although most HGAIN arises in the AnTZ, it can also be found in the distal canal, especially in patients who have had prior treatment. Low-grade lesions may be found anywhere in the anal canal.

Application of Lugol's iodine solution helps to distinguish lesions more likely to be high-grade from those that are low-grade. Most high-grade lesions will be negative staining. Low-grade AIN may be Lugol's negative, show partial Lugol's uptake, or occasionally be Lugol's positive. Complete the entire vinegar exam prior to applying Lugol's stain. Lugol's stain can obscure the margins of a lesion previously identified with acetic acid. Columnar epithelium, scar tissue from prior treatments, and keratinized epithelium will not stain. These nonstaining areas need to be distinguished from true Lugol's-negative lesions.

Continue withdrawing the anoscope until the anal verge comes into view. The anal verge is where the epithelium of the distal anal canal transitions to the epidermal epithelium of the perianus. The anal margin begins at the anal verge, proximally, and extends onto the perianal skin. The anal verge is viewed through the anoscope or visualized directly, by gentle retraction of the buttocks. Visualize the remainder of the perianus using the colposcope; the anoscope is not needed. The perianus (anal margin) extends out to approximately 5 cm from the anal verge (see Figure 17.24). The 10× magnification typically allows adequate viewing of the perianus. Switch to higher magnification for better viewing of specific lesions or other abnormal findings.

A complete HRA includes evaluation of the entire anal canal including the SCJ, AnTZ, distal anal canal, anal verge, and perianus. An adequate HRA indicates that these areas are seen in their entirety. Documentation should include whether or not the HRA was adequate and, if not, the reasons noted. Reasons for inadequate exams include mucosal swelling, obscuring stool, condyloma, large hemorrhoids, or the patient's inability to tolerate the procedure. Whenever possible, repeat an inadequate exam at another visit.

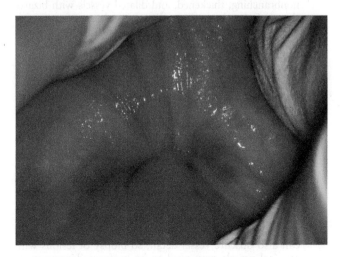

FIGURE 17.24.   A view of the anal verge and perianus.

17.4.6 Differences between HRA and Cervical Colposcopy

The principles of cervical colposcopy have been instrumental in the development of HRA. While there are many similarities, compared with cervical colposcopy, HRA can be more challenging. In many ways, HRA is more similar to vaginal and vulvar colposcopy. Clinicians familiar with cervical colposcopy may be surprised by the difficult transition. During HRA, one hand continually holds and manipulates the anoscope; only the alternate hand is available for adjusting the colposcope and other tasks. HRA is physically more challenging for the colposcopist; the hand holding the anoscope is extended for long periods, often applying significant pressure to keep the anoscope in place. Ergonomically, angled lenses on the colposcope are preferred; few tables can be raised high enough to comfortably use a colposcope with straight-on lenses for HRA. As noted earlier, colposcopes with only low magnification settings will be inadequate for evaluating anal lesions. Colposcopes with zoom lenses can be used but may be more difficult to keep in focus with the frequent repositioning during HRA, although a zoom controlled by a foot pedal can be helpful.

With HRA, once the anoscope is in place, it is more difficult to locate the SCJ and AnTZ. The mucosa needs to be manipulated to view the entire SCJ to have an adequate exam. Vinegar needs to be regularly reapplied. In general, more vinegar is needed than with the cervical exam to adequately visualize lesions. Locating lesions and distinguishing HGAIN from LGAIN are all more challenging. The similarities and differences in terminology and lesion characteristics were noted previously.

Clean technique is more difficult to maintain with HRA than with cervical colposcopy. Using disposable covers on parts of the colposcope touched during the exam (e.g., the magnification dials, fine focus knobs, or stand) will help keep the instrument clean. Use disinfectant wipes or other nonabrasive cleansers to disinfect the colposcope between patients.

Another difference between cervical colposcopy and HRA is the length of the learning curve. Expertise develops in both fields with time and experience. However, becoming an expert HRA provider takes more time, even for those experienced in cervical colposcopy. As it is a young field with a paucity of providers, novice learners will rarely have the benefit of an expert to proctor or provide observation experience. Maintaining logbooks, correlating with cytology and histology results, exam adequacy, and clinical impression, will provide feedback on the adequacy of the cytology specimens as well as a record of discordant cytology/histology results. A discordant result is considered one in which the histology result indicates a lower grade disease than the cytology. In these cases, it is assumed that the higher-grade disease was missed, as a false-positive HSIL on anal cytology is rare in our experience.[56,67] As expertise with HRA develops, there should be fewer discordant results. Logbooks will help document and determine improvement over time.

A complete HRA is one in which all anatomic landmarks are seen and all lesions identified, using adequate amounts of vinegar and Lugol's solution. Documentation should indicate the adequacy of the exam, or if inadequate, the reasons for this. Rarely, patients may require a mild sedative prior to examination. Novice HRA providers may take longer than those with more experience to perform the exam; the anal mucosa can swell and obscure parts of the anal canal with prolonged examination. A reasonable balance between the time needed to visualize the entire canal and the exam's length is needed.

Dedicating a sufficient amount of clinic time is necessary for clinicians wanting to develop expertise in HRA. Minimally, a half-day or 4 to 6 exams weekly is recommended. This should ensure an adequate number and frequency of exams to develop the skill set used for HRA. A consistent clinical practice will enable the novice provider, with patience, to become an expert HRA provider.

17.4.7 Anal and Perianal Biopsies

Histology results are the gold standard for determining the patient's diagnosis. All lesions with significant colposcopic abnormalities should be biopsied. For anal canal biopsies, use small biopsy forceps to reduce risk of bleeding and infection. Anal biopsies taken from above the dentate line do not require anesthesia. Distal canal and perianal biopsies require local anesthesia. Perianal biopsies require topical lidocaine gel or spray followed by injection of 1% to 2% lidocaine. For the anal canal, biopsy the lower or more dependent lesions first as bleeding may obscure the field of vision for subsequent biopsies. Once all biopsies are complete, use Monsel's solution or silver nitrate for hemostasis; however, the pressure of the anal walls, which are apposed at rest, is usually sufficient to stop bleeding once the anoscope is removed.

Generally, patients can expect to feel a sensation of pressure, but not pain, after intra-anal biopsies. Mild bleeding with bowel movements is common and may persist for several days. Complications such as infection or severe bleeding are extremely rare. Patients should also be advised to avoid receptive anal intercourse for at least 1 week and then only if bleeding has ceased.

17.4.8 HRA Terminology

The terminology for HRA is adapted from cervical colposcopy.[68] The SCJ in the anus is the area where anal squamous epithelium abuts colonic-type rectal glandular epithelium. The original SCJ is located near the dentate line. The current SCJ is the proximal edge of the AnTZ adjacent to the glandular epithelium of the distal rectum. The AnTZ is the region of squamous metaplasia that extends from the current SCJ to the original SCJ (Figure 17.25). The AnTZ has similar features to the cervical transformation zone. These features, although not as common in the anus, include acetowhite ringed gland openings (Figure 17.23A,C), islands of columnar epithelium (Figure 17.23D), and acetowhite accentuation of the current SCJ (Figure 17.23A).

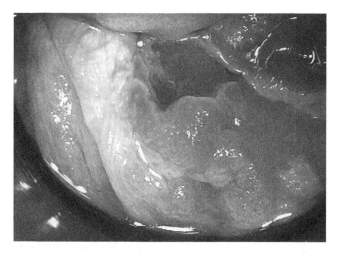

FIGURE 17.26.   The acetowhite coloring is distinct and shiny in this LGAIN lesion.

On HRA, lesions are described using terms similar to cervical colposcopy: color, contour, margins, vascular patterns, and Lugol's staining. Exceptions, unique to HRA, are termed epithelial honeycombing (EH) and a vascular pattern termed striated vessels.

■ Color: Acetowhite changes occur after the application of vinegar. The acetowhitening may be barely visible or distinct. AWE can be snowy white or have a gray hue. The sheen can be flat or shiny (Figures 17.26 and 17.27).
■ Contour: Lesions can be flat or raised. Slightly raised lesions reflect thickening of the epithelium. Papillae and micropapillations can be seen (Figures 17.28 and 17.29).
■ Margins: Determine the size and borders of the lesions. The borders may be distinct or indistinct. Identify lesions within lesions or internal margins; they may indicate HGAIN. The border of a lesion adjacent to the rectum at the SCJ is often indistinct and can be difficult to distinguish from the rectal mucosa (Figures 17.30 and 17.31A,B).
■ Vascular patterns: These are similar to cervical patterns with some exceptions. Punctation and mosaic patterns are usually coarse; fine mosaic and punctate patterns are rarely seen in the anus. Mosaic patterns are infrequent in LGAIN. Looped warty vessels are typical in raised LGAIN and are associated with warty papillae. Atypical or abnormal vessels can be seen with both HGAIN and cancer. They include nonbranching, thickened, and dilated vessels with bizarre shapes. Striated patterns or linear vessels are often seen in patients who have had prior ablative procedures, but can also be seen associated with AIN (Figures 17.32 to 17.37).
■ Lugol's staining: Also similar to cervical staining patterns; normal squamous epithelium picks up the stain completely, turning a dark mahogany brown color. Warts and other LGAIN may partially or completely stain with iodine. Negative or nonstaining epithelium is yellow in color. Normal rectal mucosa is also nonstaining and is typically pale yellow. Lugol's can be especially helpful at demarcating the squamous-squamous borders of a lesion. Lugol's negative lesions at the SCJ may be difficult to distinguish from the normal rectal mucosa. Partial staining patterns show varying uptake of the stain or a mottled appearance. It is important to continue looking through the colposcope while applying the Lugol's so that the lesion can still be located. (Figure 17.38). Lugol's can also obscure vessel detail, so biopsy of lesions with atypical vessels may need to be performed prior to its application.

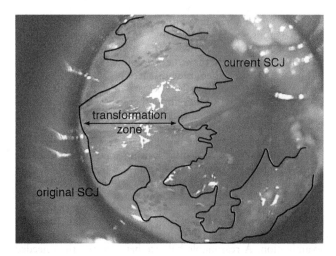

FIGURE 17.25.   A partial view of the AnTZ indicating the transformation zone between the original and current anal SCJ.

(Text continuous on page 503)

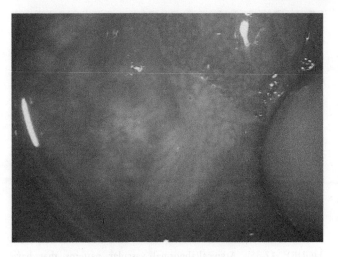

FIGURE 17.27. The acetowhite coloring has a grey hue and flat sheen in this HGAIN lesion.

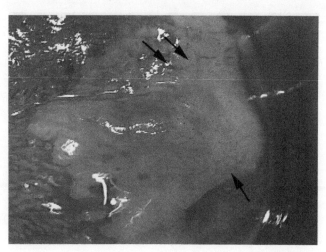

FIGURE 17.30. Example of a distinct margin in an acetowhite HGAIN lesion with coarse punctation and striated vessels. *Single arrow* points to lower border of lesion; *double arrows*, near upper edge.

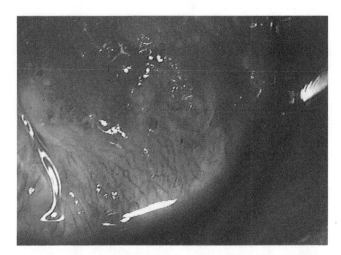

FIGURE 17.28. Example of flat contour in HGAIN lesion. Faint acetowhite with coarse punctation and mosaic pattern.

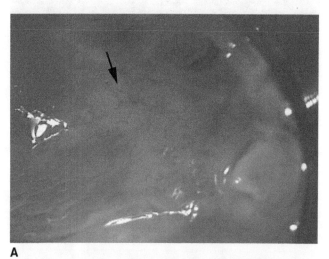

A

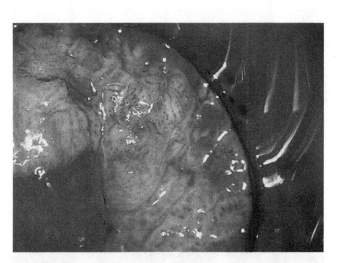

FIGURE 17.29. Example of a raised contour in HGAIN lesion. Acetowhite with coarse punctation and mosaic pattern.

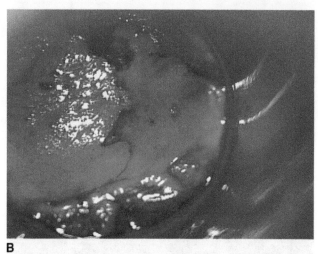

B

FIGURE 17.31. **A:** Example of an indistinct margin in an acetowhite HGAIN lesion at *arrow*. **B:** The lesion margins are better defined with application of Lugol's seen in this lower powered view.

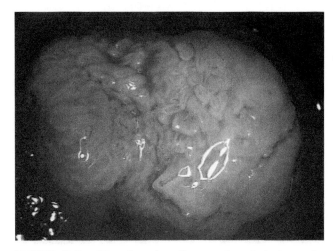

FIGURE 17.32.   Warty looped capillary vessels typical of a condyloma (LGAIN).

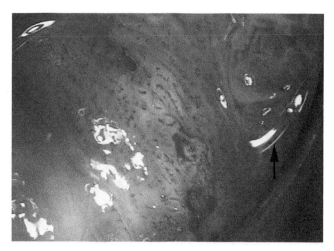

FIGURE 17.35.   Atypical/abnormal vascular patterns that have bizarre patterns and irregular dilations. This lesion was HGAIN and is adjacent to a typical-appearing condyloma (*arrow*).

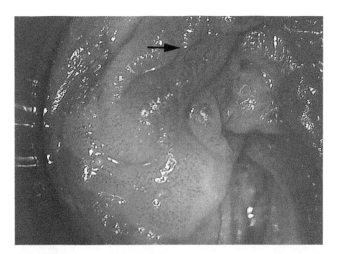

FIGURE 17.33.   An example of coarse punctation in a HGAIN lesion. Note the mosaic pattern at *arrow*.

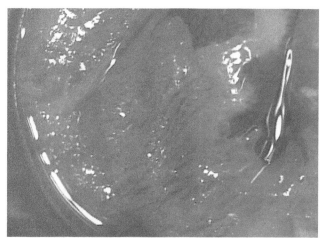

FIGURE 17.36.   Striated vascular pattern can be considered a variation of punctation. It can frequently be seen following treatment, such as IRC, but can be found in AIN. It should be biopsied regardless of treatment history.

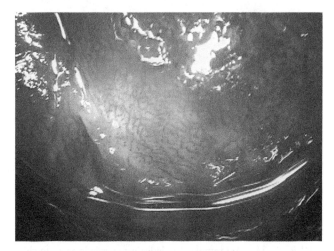

FIGURE 17.34.   An example of mosaic pattern in a HGAIN lesion. There is also diffuse coarse punctation in this lesion.

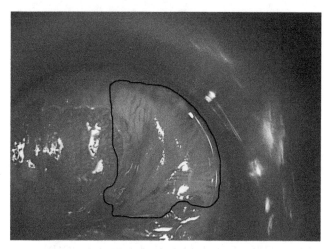

FIGURE 17.37.   Striated vessels; biopsy showed HGAIN.

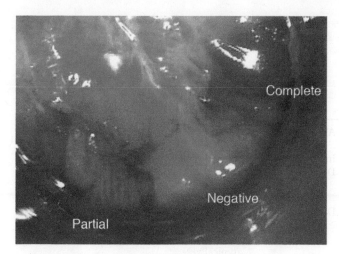

Complete

Negative

Partial

FIGURE 17.38. Lugol's staining patterns: complete, partial, and negative.

EH is an additional pattern sometimes seen in the AnTZ. It refers to an epithelial pattern resembling a honeycomb. This is not a vascular change and may indicate reactive or atypical metaplasia, or HGAIN (Figure 17.39).

17.4.9 Normal Anal Transformation Zone

Like the cervix, the AnTZ has colposcopic features such as squamous metaplasia and gland openings to help identify its location. These are best visualized with the colposcope's magnification and lighting and continued application of vinegar. Most AIN is found at or near the SCJ of the AnTZ. Therefore, identification of the AnTZ and SCJ helps to locate areas at highest risk for disease. Unlike the cervix, the anal SCJ and AnTZ are more subtle and difficult to visualize.

Anal squamous metaplasia is a normal process whereby the surface of the columnar epithelium of the distal rectum is replaced by stratified squamous epithelium. The triggers of squamous metaplasia in the anus are unknown; local trauma to the anorectal epithelium likely plays a role. There are different stages of maturation of the metaplastic squamous epithelium, termed early, mid, and late (Figure 17.23A). In early or immature metaplasia, coalescence and clustering of the columnar epithelium is just beginning; it is barely acetowhite. The grapelike clustering of the coalesced columnar epithelium, seen in the cervical transformation zone, is not as pronounced in the AnTZ (Figure 17.23B). In mid metaplasia, coalescence is more advanced, and acetowhite changes are more prominent (Figure 17.23C). Late or mature metaplastic changes are more pronounced with nearly complete coalescence of the columnar epithelium that can mimic the appearance of a true lesion. In the AnTZ, gland openings and islands of columnar epithelium within fully mature squamous epithelium can be seen (Figure 17.23D). They help identify the region of the original SCJ. The zone between them and the current SCJ constitute the active AnTZ.

17.4.10 Abnormal Anal Transformation Zone

Typical patterns encountered on HRA are summarized in Table 17.2. As with cervical colposcopy, the features associated with the abnormal AnTZ overlap with benign changes of squamous metaplasia, AIN, and sometimes, even cancer. Biopsy remains the mainstay for grading of lesions.

Low- and high-grade lesions in the immature AnTZ can be subtle; it is often difficult to distinguish between normal and abnormal changes. Areas of AWE in the AnTZ (Figure 17.40), even with the absence of vascular changes, are often high-grade lesions. EH is nonspecific and can be associated with either squamous metaplasia or AIN in the AnTZ (Figures 17.39, 17.41 to 17.43). Isolated ringed gland openings are normal and indicate mature squamous metaplasia surrounding the opening to a gland in the mucosa. In the AnTZ, a preponderance of ringed glands clustered in an acetowhite lesion may, however, indicate HGAIN (see Figure 17.44).

17.4.10.1 HRA: Low-Grade Anal Intraepithelial Neoplasia

Typical low-grade lesions are acetowhite. Condylomas often have contour changes such as micropapillae or delicate papillae with central looped capillary vessels (Figures 17.32, 17.45 and 17.46). They frequently have a cauliflower-like profile

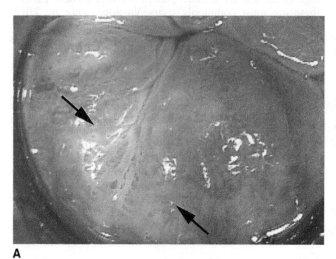

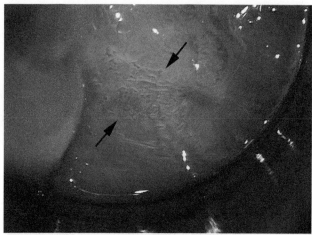

A **B**

FIGURE 17.39. Epithelial honeycombing designated by *arrows*. This pattern is seen both in HGAIN (A) and with reactive squamous metaplasia (B).

TABLE 17.2   TYPICAL SQUAMOUS PATTERNS ON HRA

TYPICAL SQUAMOUS PATTERNS ON HRA	COLOR (AWE)	SURFACE ARCHITECTURE (CONTOUR)	MARGINS (BORDERS)	VASCULAR CHANGES	LUGOL'S STAINING
Benign AnTZ	+ translucent	Flat	AWE edge or line at SCJ	None	Mature AnTZ = positive Immature AnTZ = negative
Posttreatment changes	+	Flat	Indistinct	Striated vessels	Negative, partial, positive
Low-grade lesions	++ to +++	Variable flat or raised	Distinct or indistinct	Punctation, looped capillaries	Negative, partial, positive
High-grade lesions	+ to +++	Flat, slightly raised or thickened	Distinct or indistinct	Coarse punctation and mosaic, atypical vessels, or none	Negative
Cancer	Variable	Irregular, raised or ulcerated	Poorly defined, peeling edges	Atypical vessels, often friable	Negative

AWE, acetowhite epithelium; AnTZ, anal transformation zone; SCJ, squamocolumnar junction; + to +++: faint to distinct.

(Figure 17.46). Condyloma with cerebriform contour can mimic high-grade vascular changes and particularly when also Lugol's negative should be biopsied to exclude high-grade disease (Figure 17.49). The Lugol's staining pattern is variable with LGAIN; it may be positive, show partial staining, or be Lugol's negative. Lugol's staining is particularly helpful in defining the squamous-squamous border of the lesion (Figure 17.50).

Flat low-grade lesions can be subtle, with minor acetowhitening and Lugol's-negative staining (Figures 17.51 and 17.52). Biopsy is essential to confirm the colposcopic impression of lesion grade and truly distinguish these lesions from benign squamous metaplasia of the AnTZ.

17.4.10.2 HRA: High-Grade Anal Intraepithelial Neoplasia

Similar to cervical colposcopy, the classic appearance of HGAIN on HRA is a flat or thickened area of AWE associated with vascular changes including punctation and a mosaic pattern (Figure 17.53). High-grade lesions are frequently located in the AnTZ near the SCJ (Figures 17.54 and 17.55). In high-risk populations, high- and low-grade lesions often coexist; examining around the base of condyloma will often yield HGAIN on biopsy (Figures 17.56 and 17.57). Vinegar must be regularly reapplied to the entire SCJ and AnTZ and distal canal during the exam for adequate visualization of lesions.

Acetowhitening, particularly in the AnTZ, is an important clue for identifying high-grade lesions (Figures 17.54 and 17.55). HGAIN can have a variety of appearances and be quite subtle with only faint AWE (Figure 17.58). Although HGAIN is frequently flat or plaque-like, high-grade lesions with other surface contours can be seen (Figure 17.59); biopsy is needed for confirmation. Reapplying vinegar to the entire AnTZ is crucial during HRA in order to visualize lesions.

Since vinegar causes vasoconstriction, vessels will appear more prominent prior to the application of vinegar and after the vinegar effect diminishes. Vessel changes associated with high-grade lesions include punctation and mosaic pattern; these are most commonly coarse in appearance on HRA. Examples of punctation are seen in Figures 17.59 and 17.60. A more subtle presentation of punctation, unique to HRA, is termed striated vessels and although this finding is nonspecific, it is frequently associated with HGAIN (Figure 17.61). Mosaic patterns are similar to those seen with cervical colposcopy (Figures 17.62 and 17.63). Whenever atypical vessels are seen or focal areas of atypical vessels are seen within an acetowhite lesion, these areas should be targeted for biopsy to evaluate for possible occult invasion (Figure. 17.64 to 17.66).

Most HGAIN will be negative staining with Lugol's solution. It can be helpful during HRA to help identify lesions (Figures 17.52, 17.59 and 17.67). Care must be taken to correlate with the appearance on vinegar exam; lesions at the SCJ may be difficult to differentiate from rectal mucosa after Lugol's is applied.

17.4.10.3 HRA: Invasive Squamous Cell Carcinoma

DARE is an essential part of the examination of the anal canal. Palpable hard masses or thickening is pathognomonic for invasive cancer (Figures 17.68 to 17.70). On HRA, cancers are often friable or ulcerated lesions with atypical vessels

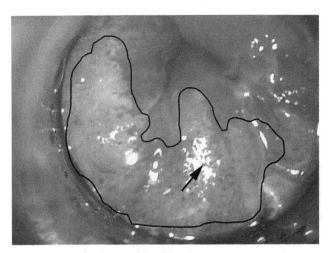

FIGURE 17.40.   Atypical-appearing metaplasia: AWE with "lacey" pattern designated by *arrow*; biopsy showed HGAIN.

(Text continuous on page 511)

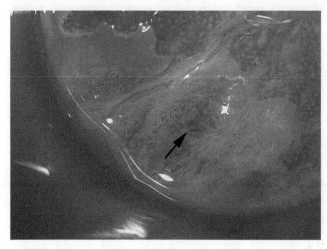

FIGURE 17.41. Epithelial honeycombing; biopsy (*arrow*) showed HGAIN.

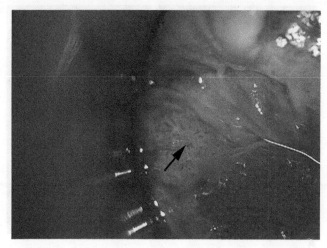

FIGURE 17.42. Biopsy of another area of honeycombing (*arrow*), in same patient as Figure 17.41, showed immature and reactive squamous metaplasia.

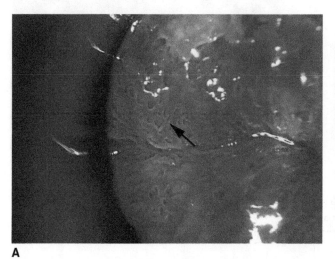

A

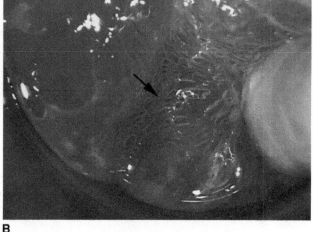

B

FIGURE 17.43. Epithelial honeycombing. Both images are from the same patient. *Arrows* indicate biopsy sites. **A:** Biopsy showed HGAIN. **B:** Biopsy showed immature and reactive squamous metaplasia.

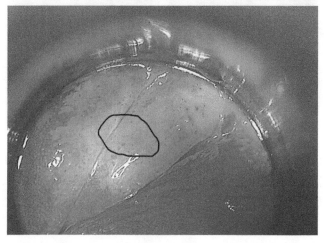

FIGURE 17.44. Atypical metaplasia with ringed glands; biopsy (*designated by circle*) showed HGAIN.

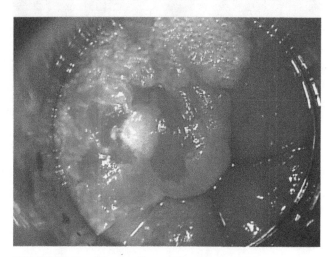

FIGURE 17.45. Micropapillae seen in typical LGAIN.

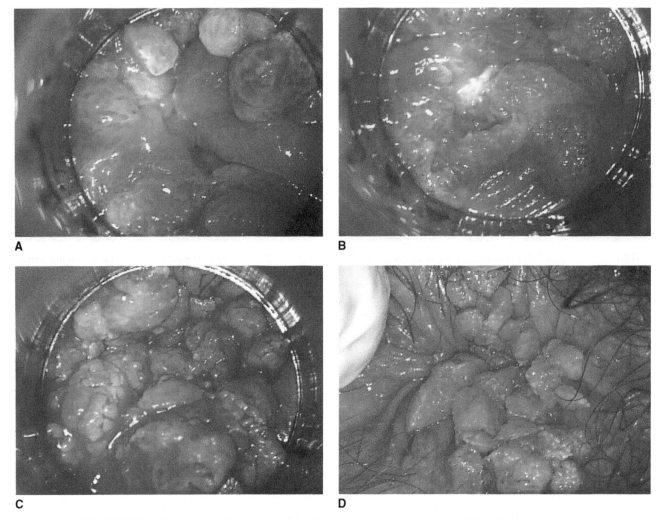

FIGURE 17.46. Extensive condyloma; patient required surgical treatment. **A:** At SCJ, **B:** mid-canal near dentate line, **C:** distal canal near verge, and **D:** perianal condyloma.

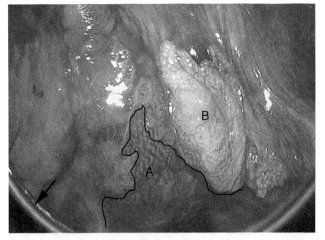

FIGURE 17.47. Intraoperative HRA. *Arrow* points to Hill-Ferguson anal retractor. *Black line* outlines SCJ. (*A*, Normal rectal glandular openings. *B*, Condyloma.)

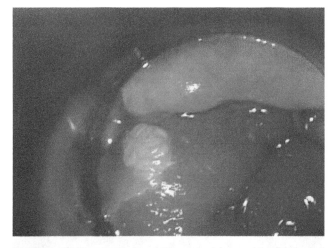

FIGURE 17.48. Atypical-appearing condyloma, biopsy showed LGAIN.

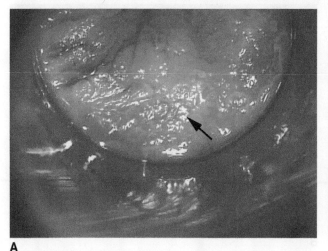

A

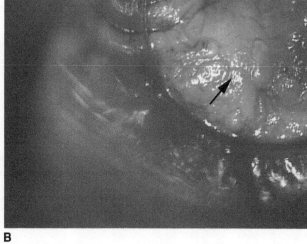

B

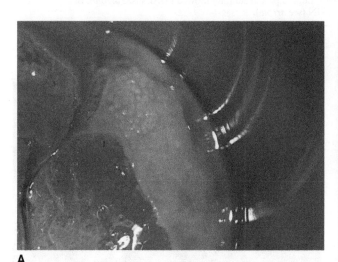

C

FIGURE 17.49.   **A:** AWE with cerebriform appearance and mosaic pattern, low-power view. **B:** Lugol's negative staining; biopsy (*arrow*) showed LGAIN. **C:** Magnified view prior to application of Lugol's to lesion.

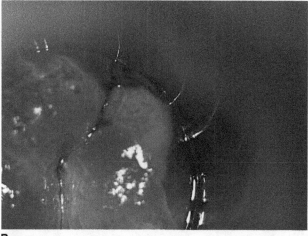

A

B

FIGURE 17.50.   **A:** Micropapillae. **B:** Lugol's negative staining; biopsy showed LGAIN.

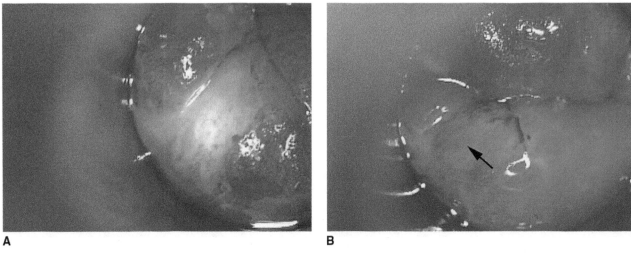

FIGURE 17.51.   **A:** Faint AWE. **B:** Lugol's negative staining; biopsy at *arrow* showed LGAIN.

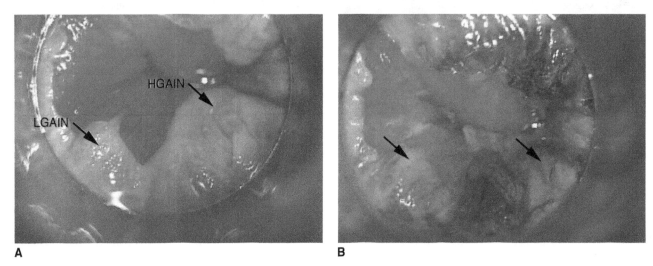

FIGURE 17.52.   **A:** Biopsy of the more granular lesion with Lugol's partial staining showed LGAIN (see *arrow*). **B:** Biopsy of flat AWE that was Lugol's negative showed HGAIN (see *arrow*).

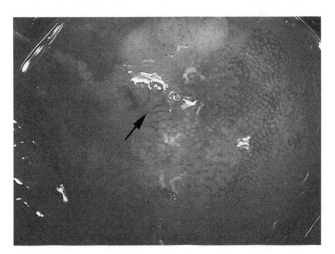

FIGURE 17.53.   AWE with punctation and mosaic pattern. Biopsy at *arrow* showed HGAIN. Additional biopsies (e.g., toward the top of the image) are also appropriate.

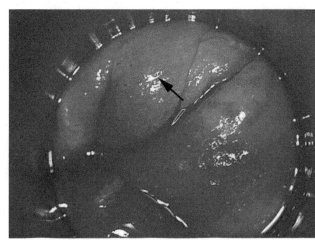

FIGURE 17.54.   Biopsy of this dense acetowhite lesion with abnormal ringed glands, at *arrow*, showed HGAIN.

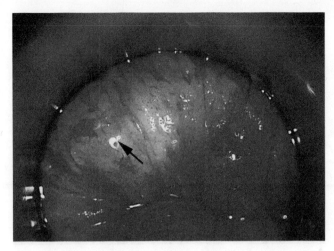

FIGURE 17.55. Thickened, dense acetowhite lesion. Biopsy at *arrow* showed HGAIN.

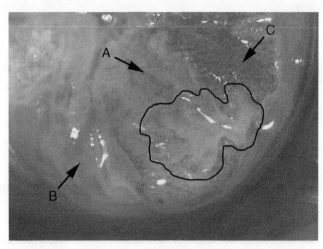

FIGURE 17.58. AWE extends over the rectal mucosa and is outlined in *black line*; biopsy showed HGAIN. (*Arrows: A,* AWE of immature AnTZ adjacent to lesion. *B,* Translucent normal squamous mucosa. C, Normal rectal mucosa.)

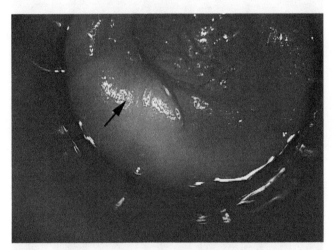

FIGURE 17.56. Punctation off the SCJ and adjacent to a condyloma; biopsy at *arrow* showed HGAIN.

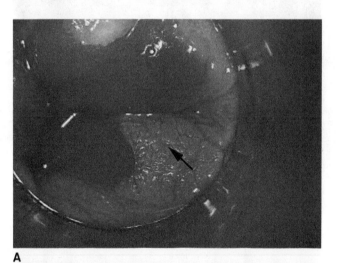

A

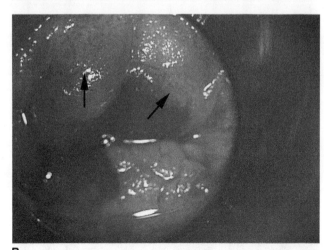

B

FIGURE 17.59. The lower lesion is cerebriform and Lugol's negative (*arrow* in [**A**]). The other two areas show punctation (*arrows* in [**B**]). *Arrows* also indicate biopsy sites; all showed HGAIN.

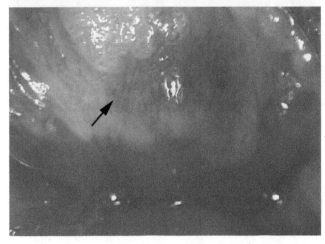

FIGURE 17.57. Punctation and mosaic pattern at base of condyloma (*arrow*); biopsy showed HGAIN.

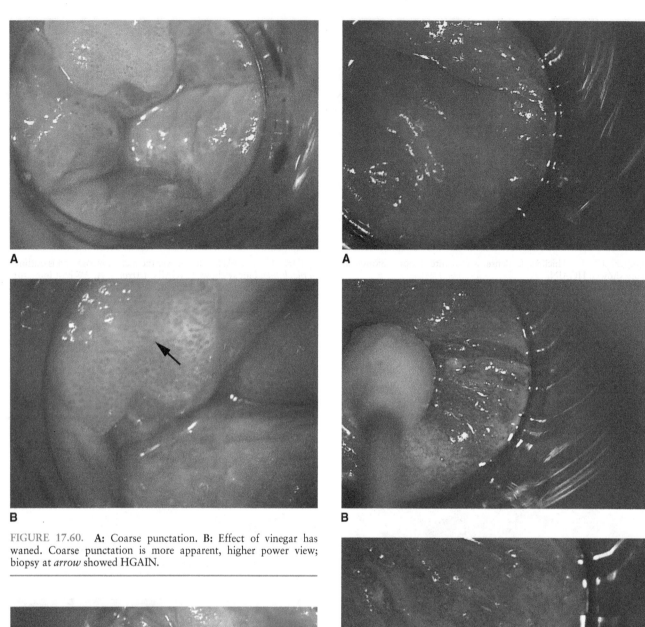

FIGURE 17.60. **A:** Coarse punctation. **B:** Effect of vinegar has waned. Coarse punctation is more apparent, higher power view; biopsy at *arrow* showed HGAIN.

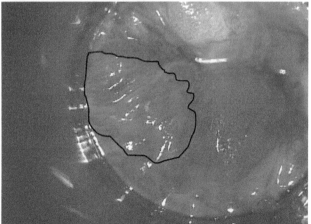

FIGURE 17.61.   AWE with striated vessels, outlined in *black line*; biopsy showed HGAIN.

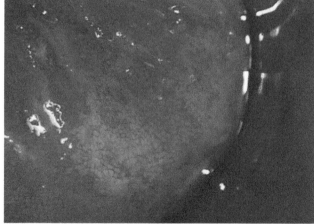

FIGURE 17.62.   Reapplying acetic acid is essential to visualize lesions. **A:** Area prior to reapplication of vinegar. **B:** Coarse mosaic pattern demonstrated after reapplying vinegar. **C:** Higher magnification after vinegar. Biopsy showed HGAIN.

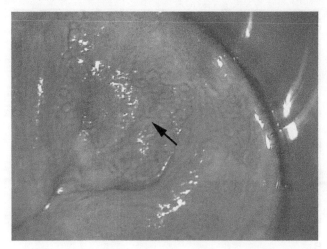

FIGURE 17.63. Mosaic pattern and punctation and in the distal canal; biopsy designated by *arrow* showed HGAIN.

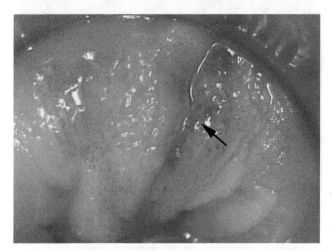

FIGURE 17.64. Coarse punctation and atypical vessels causing concern for occult invasion; biopsy designated by *arrow* showed HGAIN. Lesion was successfully ablated using IRC.

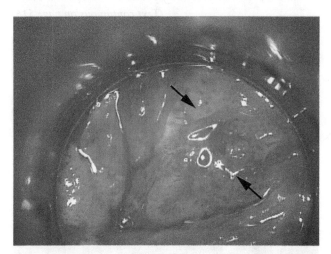

FIGURE 17.65. Thickened, friable, dilated, abnormal vessels clinically suspicious for occult invasion denoted between arrows; biopsy multiple areas to rule out invasion; here, however, biopsy showed HGAIN, and lesion was ultimately treated in-office with good results.

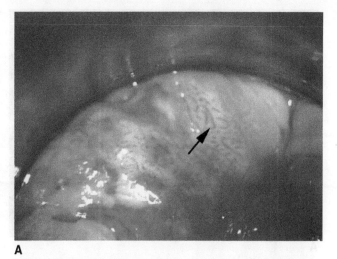

A

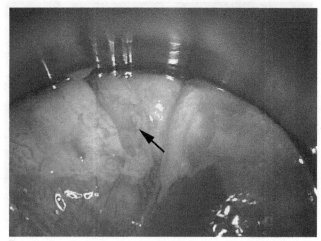

B

FIGURE 17.66.   **A:** Coarse mosaic pattern; biopsy (*arrow*) showed HGAIN. **B:** Adjacent area with atypical vessels; biopsy (*arrow*) read as suspicious for superficial invasion. The lesion in (**B**) was subsequently excised in the OR and because of the complex growth pattern; superficial invasion was still suspected but not confirmed.

(Figures 17.71 and 17.72). The diagnosis of anal cancer can sometimes be technically challenging. The patient in Figure 17.68 had a 3-cm palpable mass, but a biopsy in the office was superficial and only showed HGAIN. She was referred for additional surgical biopsies under anesthesia which confirmed invasive cancer. The patient depicted in Figure 17.73 had a similar presentation and required an examination under anesthesia (EUA) to definitely diagnose invasive cancer.

With advanced anal cancer, patients may present with a mass or symptoms of pain or unexplained bleeding. At presentation, the patient in Figure 17.74 had an obvious advanced cancer that extended from the SCJ through the entire anal canal to the verge. The patient in Figure 17.75 had previously been treated with radiation and chemotherapy for anal cancer, but never returned for surveillance until he developed pain, bleeding, and an obvious mass.

Often cancer is obvious, but in its earliest stages, there may be only subtle changes on DARE and it can be detected only after careful HRA. When patients have lesions that are clinically or colposcopically concerning for invasion and a

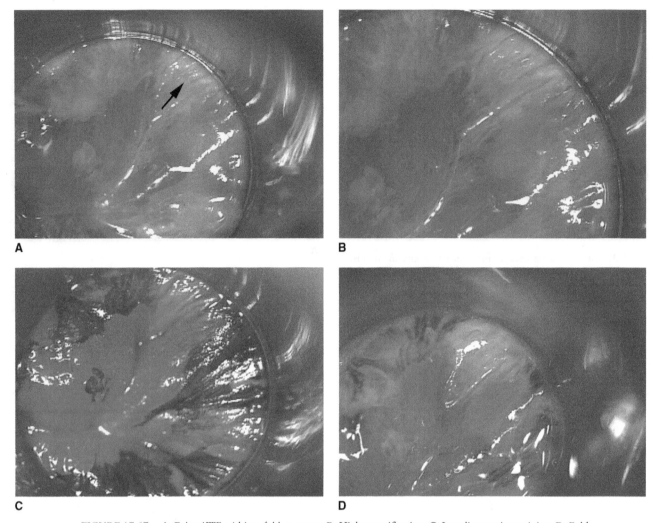

FIGURE 17.67. **A:** Faint AWE within a fold at *arrow*. **B:** High magnification. **C:** Lugol's negative staining. **D:** Fold opened up better displaying the entire lesion. *Arrow* in (A) indicates biopsy site: HGAIN.

diagnosis of invasive cancer cannot be made in the office, then EUA, with larger or multiple biopsies, is indicated.

17.4.11 Perianal Examination

The perianal exam begins at the anal verge, the distal end of the anal canal, which is just visible with gentle retraction of the buttocks. The anal verge is where the squamous mucosal epithelium transitions to true skin of the perianus. The exam includes all aspects of the perianus. By convention, the perianus extends distally approximately 5 cm from the anal verge (Figure 17.76).

HRA of the perianus is similar to colposcopy of the vulva. Perianal disease often presents in diffuse or circumferential patterns and may be hard to distinguish from perianal excoriation. Visually, differentiation of abnormal from benign changes or LGAIN from HGAIN may be difficult. HPV-associated changes present in patterns similar to the vulva and are often contiguous with vulvar disease. Compared with intra-anal disease, there are fewer lesion characteristics to help distinguish between high-grade and low-grade lesions. Biopsy of all abnormal areas determines the extent and grade of disease.

Examine the perianus prior to applying vinegar. Look for fissures, ulcerations, and generalized excoriation, which may result from excessive wiping after bowel movements. Fissures and other skin breaks can be sensitive when vinegar is applied;

however, the lidocaine-lubricant mixture used at the beginning of the HRA generally provides adequate anesthesia even if skin breaks are present. Make note of areas of leukoplakia. This is

(Text continuous on page 516)

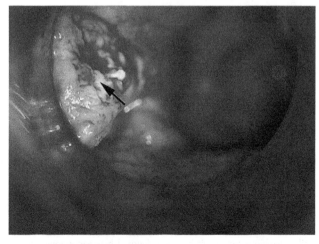

FIGURE 17.68. Patient had a 3-cm palpable mass. HRA showed friable papillary lesion; EUA with biopsy (*arrow*) revealed invasive cancer.

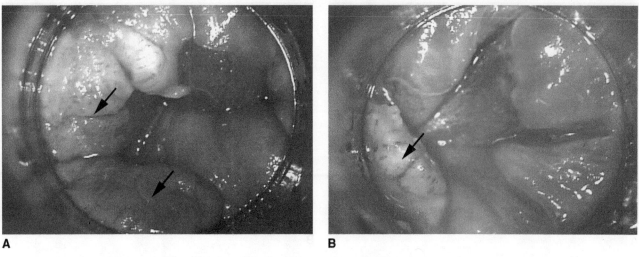

FIGURE 17.69.   **A,B:** Patient had palpable thickening on DARE. HRA showed a mass with atypical vessels. *Arrows* indicate biopsy sites taken in office; biopsies showed invasive SCC.

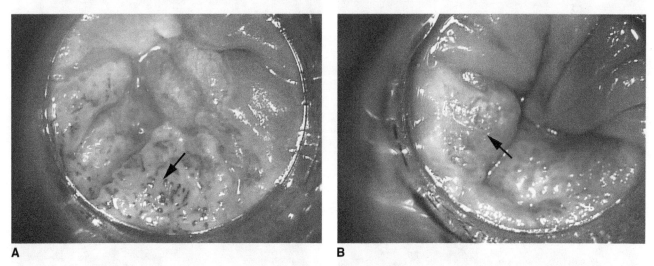

FIGURE 17.70.   Patient had palpable thickening on DARE. HRA showed the mass with atypical vessels consistent with cancer. **A:** At SCJ. **B:** In distal canal, at *dentate line*. *Arrows* indicate biopsy sites performed in the office; biopsies showed invasive SCC.

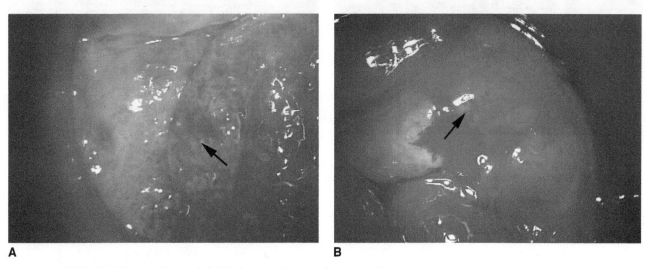

FIGURE 17.71.   **A:** Ulcerated, friable lesion with atypical vessels; office biopsy (*arrow*) was suggestive of superficial invasion. **B:** Ulcerated, friable lesion with atypical vessels; biopsy of this site (*arrow*) showed superficially invasive SCC.

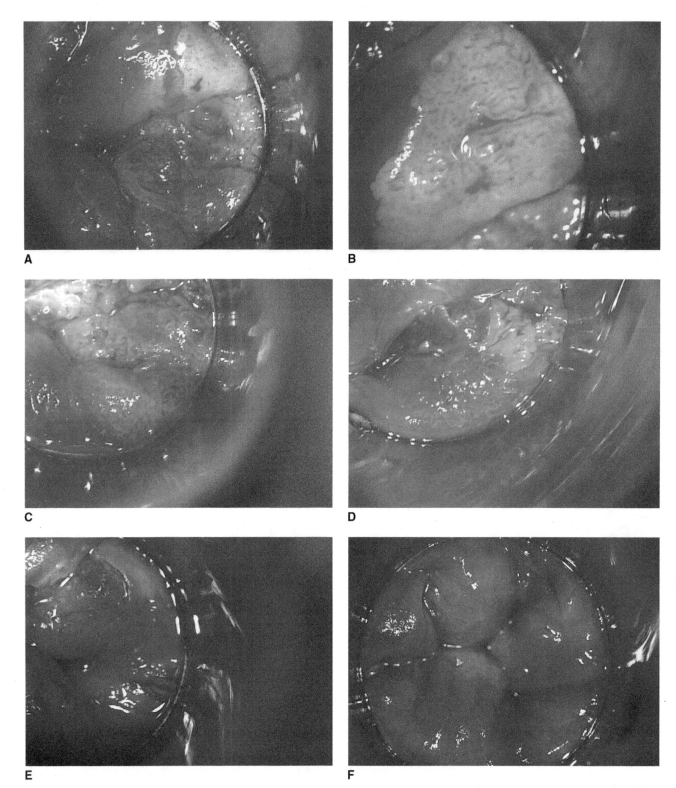

FIGURE 17.72.   A–D: Obvious cancer extending from the SCJ to the distal canal with thickened area palpated in the anterior midline. Biopsy showed superficially invasive SCC. The lesion was adherent to the sphincter clinically; he was referred for CMT. **E,F:** 15 months after completion of CMT showing a complete response.

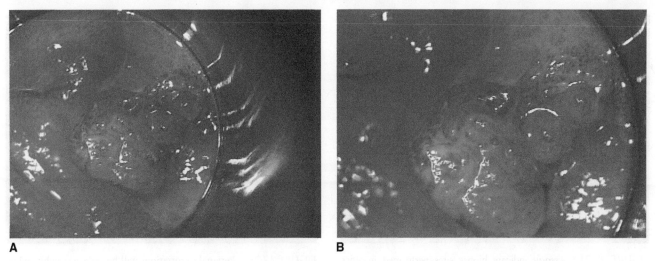

FIGURE 17.73.   Patient with palpable mass that was initially difficult to visualize during HRA until correlated with the DARE. In-office biopsy showed HGAIN; due to the clinical concern for invasive cancer, the patient was referred for EUA that confirmed the diagnosis of invasive SCC. **A:** Low magnification. **B:** Same lesion, higher magnification.

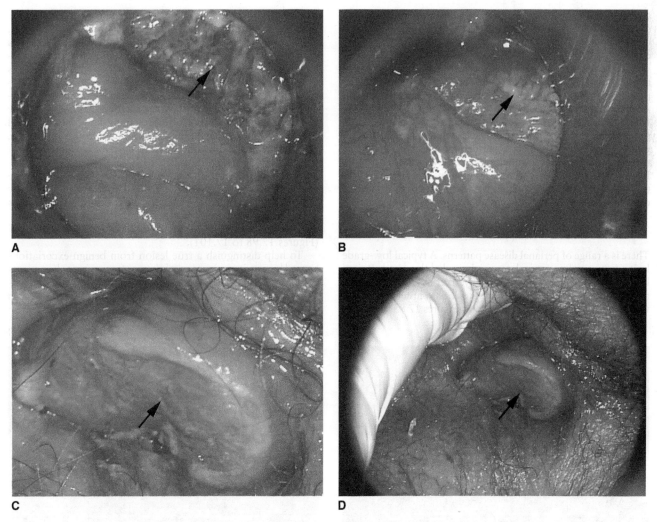

FIGURE 17.74.   **A–D:** Advanced cancer with friable mass that extended throughout the anal canal to the verge denoted by *arrows*.

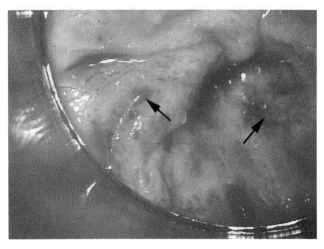

FIGURE 17.75. *Arrows* indicate biopsy sites performed in-office that confirmed recurrent SCC s/p radiation and chemotherapy for anal cancer. The patient was subsequently successfully treated with an APR and colostomy.

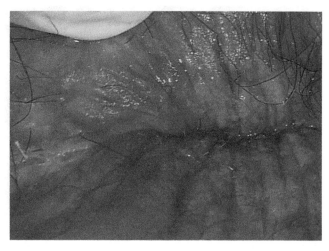

FIGURE 17.77. Perianal excoriations will become acetowhite when vinegar is applied. While some AIN presents as diffuse acetowhitening, excoriations, as seen here, will be both generalized and diffuse with no other lesion characteristics.

a reflection of hyperkeratosis; it can be a reactive change or associated with disease. Examine perianal skin tags and hemorrhoids. Note if any findings are associated with focal discomfort or pain (Figures 17.77 to 17.82).

The perianal examination continues with the additional application of vinegar. Use several 4 × 4 gauze pads soaked in 5% acetic acid. Apply the gauze for 1 minute or longer. Acetic acid takes longer to absorb into keratinized epithelium. After removing the gauze, observe the entire perianus with low magnification. Make note of any acetowhite changes. Distinguish diffuse patterns of acetowhitening consistent with excoriation from focal acetowhitening that may indicate a lesion. Evaluate all potential perianal lesions on higher magnification. Continue applying vinegar with scopettes or Q-tips while examining each area. Document all abnormal findings.

17.4.11.1 Features of Perianal Disease

There is a range of perianal disease patterns. A typical low-grade lesion is acetowhite, granular, raised, or slightly raised. Raised lesions often have warty papillae or a verrucous contour. Similar to the vulva, perianal LGAIN may present as clusters of lesions with similar patterns or discrete lesions (Figures 17.83 to 17.86).

A typical high-grade lesion is acetowhite or grey, with or without hyperpigmentation. Perianal HGAIN may be flat, slightly raised, or raised. On the perianus, vascular changes are less common than on nonkeratinized squamous epithelium, but if present, the lesion is often high-grade. The findings may also be subtle; an ulcer in the center of a granular warty-type lesion may indicate high-grade changes or cancer. Ulcerations can present as shallow, denuded epithelium or can be deep. Perianal HGAIN can also present as discrete or clustered lesions. Bowen's disease and bowenoid papulosis, respectively, are clinical terms sometimes used to describe these patterns of perianal HGAIN (Figures 17.87 to 17.97).

A painful, hard, friable mass is likely to be a cancer. Large warts may be painful and may bleed, but are not typically hard to palpation. Early cancers may present as subtle areas of focal discomfort with fissures, ulcerations, or small abnormal growths within a lesion that looks otherwise like LGAIN (Figures 17.98 to 17.101).

To help distinguish a true lesion from benign excoriations caused by pruritus, vigorous wiping, or frequent stools, patients should be advised to use moist wipes, apply a cream such as hydrocerin gel, Califlora gel or aloe vera gel daily, and return for a repeat exam in 1 month. If there is no improvement in

(Text Continuous on Page 521)

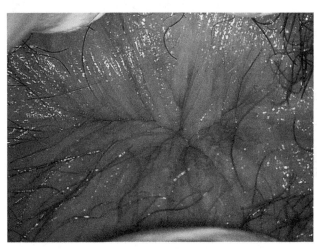

FIGURE 17.76. Perianus, a normal view.

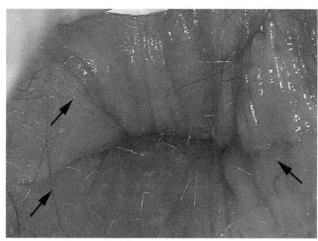

FIGURE 17.78. Perianal fissures (*arrows*).

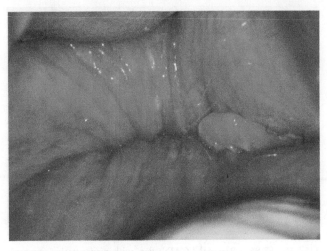

FIGURE 17.79. Redundant perianal tissue or skin tag.

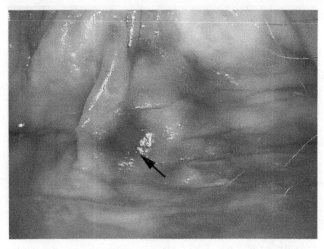

FIGURE 17.82. Perianal hyperpigmentation in a field of AWE in a woman with a history of treated HGAIN. The pigmented area shown by *arrow* was LGAIN.

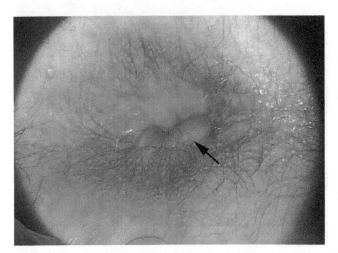

FIGURE 17.80. Perianal hemorrhoid (*arrow*).

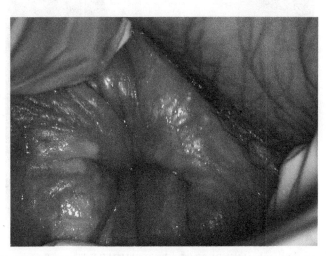

FIGURE 17.83. Perianal LGAIN: cluster of three granular, flat acetowhite lesions.

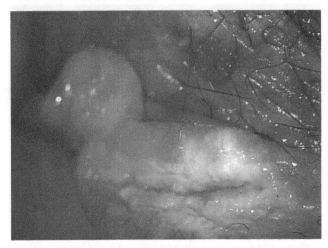

FIGURE 17.81. Perianal hyperkeratosis occurs with excessive wiping or as fissures heal. It is difficult to distinguish from AIN (see Figure 17.83).

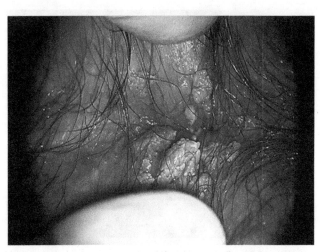

FIGURE 17.84. Perianal LGAIN: cluster of verrucous condyloma with papillae.

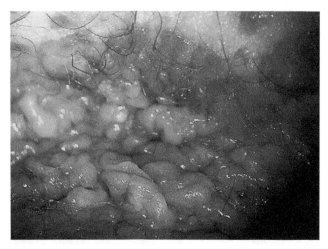

FIGURE 17.85. Perianal LGAIN: circumferential raised granular lesions with areas of hyperpigmentation.

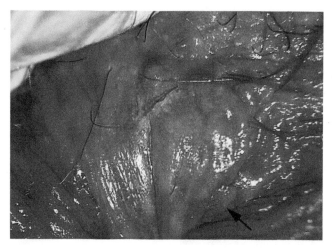

FIGURE 17.86. Perianal LGAIN: flat, with pigmentation, acetowhitening, and an area of coarse punctation at the base of the lesion (*arrow*).

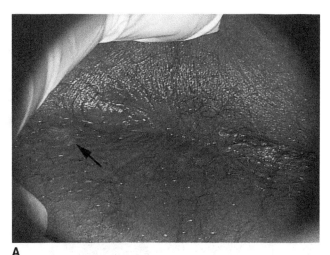

A

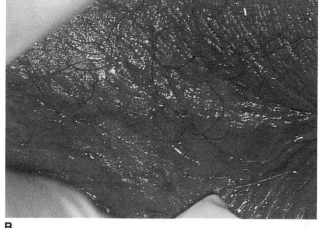

B

FIGURE 17.87.   Perianal HGAIN: discrete, flat, acetowhite lesion with jagged edges. Viewed at low power denoted by *arrow* (**A**) and high power (**B**).

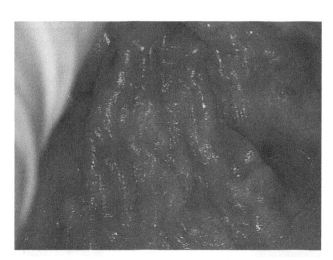

FIGURE 17.88. Perianal HGAIN: faint, barely visible lesion with granularity, small fissure, and indistinct margins.

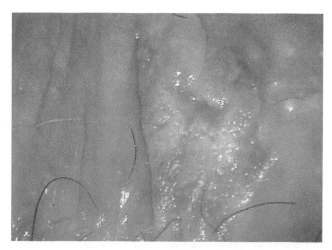

FIGURE 17.89. Perianal HGAIN: acetowhite, slightly raised, and granular with a shallow ulceration at the base where the epithelium is peeling.

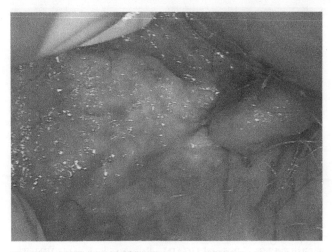

FIGURE 17.90. Perianal HGAIN: acetowhite, flat, granular, and thickened.

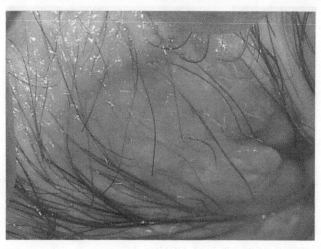

FIGURE 17.93. Perianal HGAIN: extensive lesion with flat and slightly raised areas at the base and center, and a raised thickened area with defined margins at the superior aspect of the lesion.

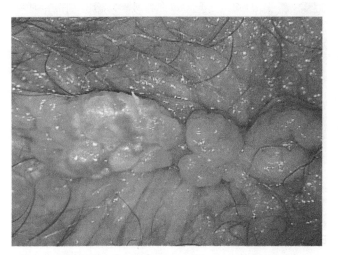

FIGURE 17.91. Perianal HGAIN: thickened and raised lesion with ulcerations. Adjacent to benign perianal tags.

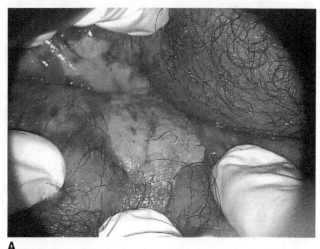

A

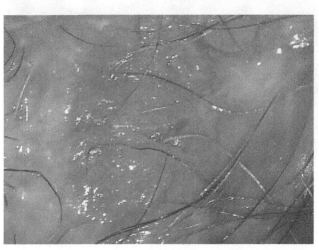

FIGURE 17.92. Perianal HGAIN: erythematous barely acetowhite lesion with a discrete margin, slightly raised or thickened, course punctation, and several fissured areas.

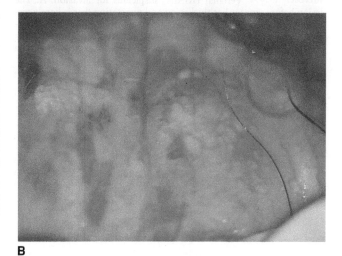

B

FIGURE 17.94. **A:** Perianal HGAIN: thickened, acetowhite and hyperpigmented lesion with shallow ulcerations. **B:** Mosaic patterns can be seen adjacent to the ulcerations in the high-power image.

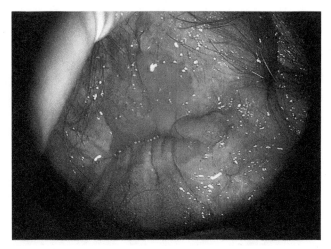

FIGURE 17.95. Perianal HGAIN: diffuse but well-demarcated denuded epithelium. Thickening is seen at the base of the lesion.

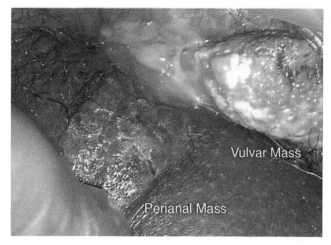

FIGURE 17.96. Perianal HGAIN adjacent to high-grade VIN. The perianal mass is thickened and hyperpigmented.

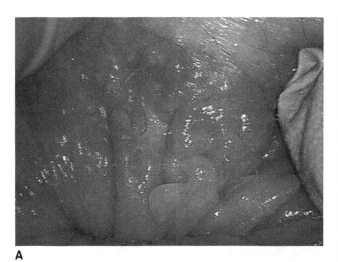

A

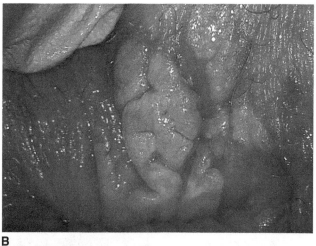

B

FIGURE 17.97. Perianal HGAIN, suspicious for invasion. **A:** The lesion before vinegar has thickening and punctation that is barely visible. **B:** After soaking the perianus with vinegar, the thick acetowhitening, punctation, and fissuring are more apparent. **C:** Three months later, the lesion has progressed; abnormal vascular changes are more prominent. It showed SCC on excision.

C

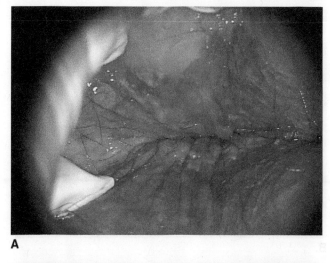

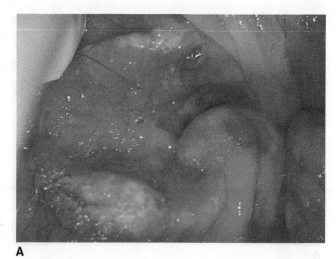

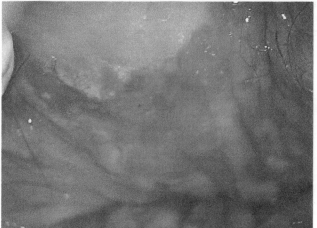

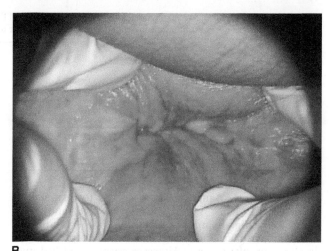

FIGURE 17.98. Perianal superficially invasive SCC at low power (**A**) and high power (**B**). The epithelium is diffusely ulcerated with small protruding polyploid growths.

FIGURE 17.100. Perianal cancer associated with a fistula tract. **A:** The mass before treatment. **B:** The normal epithelial changes after radiation therapy.

1 month, biopsy the abnormal-appearing areas. A gentle scraping of the perianal skin for a wet mount smear can be done if a fungal infection is suspected; if positive, the patient can be directed to use an over-the-counter antifungal agent. There are various dermatologic conditions that can cause pruritus; refer patients to a dermatologist for perianal pruritus that is longstanding and unresponsive to treatment.

Because perianal lesions are harder to grade clinically, it is important to biopsy representative areas to ascertain the extent and grade(s) of disease. Once the region is anesthetized, these biopsies are generally well tolerated. There is little bleeding from perianal biopsies and hemostasis can easily be managed by applying a silver nitrate stick to the biopsy site.

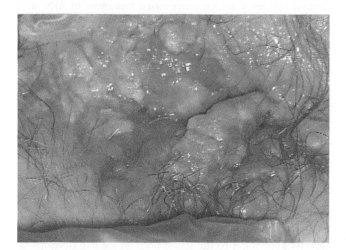

FIGURE 17.99. Perianal SCC with polyploid growths emanating from ulcerated areas in the mass. These growths are a hallmark of perianal cancer.

17.5 MANAGEMENT AND TREATMENT OF ANAL CANAL AND PERIANAL LESIONS

Once AIN is biopsy-confirmed, a management strategy is individually designed to reduce the potential risk for progression of HGAIN to cancer, to relieve symptoms if present, and by factoring in underlying health conditions, such as immune

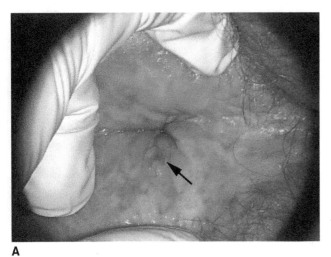

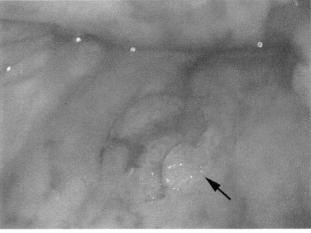

A   **B.**

FIGURE 17.101.   Perianal cancer recurred post-CMT. **A:** The low power image shows diffuse telangiectasias, common postradiation-induced changes. *Arrows* point to the cancer in both the low- and high-power image (**B**).

status and medical conditions that predispose to bleeding and/or infection.

17.5.1 Rationale for Treating HGAIN or Condyloma

Since HGAIN is considered precancerous, it is treated to prevent progression to anal cancer, analogous to treatment of high-grade CIN (CIN 3). To date, no prospective, randomized studies comparing treatment of HGAIN to observation have been conducted demonstrating that treatment prevents the development of anal cancer. However, several published studies indirectly suggest that treatment of HGAIN may prevent progression to cancer. In a retrospective review of 246 patients treated surgically at UCSF using HRA to guide therapy, 3 patients progressed to cancer for a progression rate of 1.2%.[69] This compares to a rate of 7.5% (3 of 40) in patients with HGAIN progressing to cancer who were managed expectantly by physical exam every 6 months with biopsy of any new masses or ulcerations.[70] In a German study following 156 HIV-positive men with HGAIN, five subjects (3.2%) who refused ablative therapy progressed to cancer. None of the remaining subjects who had HGAIN treated progressed to cancer.[71]

Warts are not thought to progress directly to cancer. However, once diagnosed with anal warts, most patients want them treated to reduce symptoms if present, increase their sense of well-being, decrease shame, reduce the risk of transmission to partners, and to feel more sexually attractive. Medical reasons supporting the treatment of condyloma include recently published papers documenting an increased prevalence of unsuspected HGAIN in surgically removed anal warts ranging from 47% to 52% in HIV-positive MSM and 20% to 26% in HIV-negative MSM.[72,73]

17.5.2 Role of HRA in Management and Treatment of Anal Neoplasia

The simple statement: "If you can't see it, you can't treat it"—being able to adequately visualize and biopsy lesions—is a fundamental tenet of treatment. However, it is more than knowing the anal biopsy result: the clinician must be able to define the proximal, distal, and lateral borders of lesions and

must do a thorough exam to detect any additional lesions. HRA should be performed prior to treatment to identify all of the lesions present and determine the extent of disease. Biopsies of multiple lesions should be performed, especially if they have differing appearances on HRA. Even to an experienced eye, it may not be possible to distinguish reactive metaplasia from HGAIN. Careful HRA with biopsies of any abnormal acetowhite areas guides treatment planning and facilitates targeted destruction of lesions.

If there is a clinical suspicion of underlying cancer and a diagnosis of cancer has not been made in the office, patients should be examined under anesthesia and larger biopsies obtained for diagnosis. Providers should avoid simple ablation in this situation since it does not provide tissue for pathologic analysis. Clinically suspicious signs of cancer include a firm submucosal bulge, a frank mass, focally tender high-grade lesions, ulcerated lesions with heaped-up borders, indurated areas, and lesions with grossly abnormal vessels.

17.5.3 Office-Based Treatment of AIN

Several options exist for office-based treatment of AIN, and office-based treatment is preferred whenever possible. Each of the options will be briefly discussed along with the best application for treatment of AIN. See Table 17.3 for an overview of treatment options.

17.5.3.1 Provider-Applied Therapy: Cryotherapy and 85% Trichloroacetic Acid

Cryotherapy is generally not useful for the treatment of intra-anal lesions; however, it is very useful for small to moderate-sized perianal lesions, including condyloma and HGAIN in the clinical experience of the author (JMB). It is difficult to use intra-anally because the vapors produced obscure visualization, making it difficult to determine if a lesion has been adequately frozen. It can be used on multiple perianal lesions measuring up to 2 cm. Cryotherapy can be easily applied by soaking a cotton-tipped wooden swab in liquid nitrogen and directly applying it to the lesion until an ice ball develops or using a probe to spray the liquid nitrogen directly on the lesion. It is common to do three freeze-thaw cycles. Some providers will apply 85% trichloroacetic acid (TCA) after freezing without problems reported; however, there are no published data

TABLE 17.3	AN OVERVIEW OF TREATMENT OPTIONS FOR CONDYLOMA AND HGAIN*			
■ GENERIC NAME	■ PERIANAL CONDYLOMA	■ PERIANAL HGAIN	■ INTRA-ANAL CONDYLOMA	■ INTRA-ANAL HGAIN
0.5% Podofilox gel	Yes	No	No	No
5% Imiquimod	Yes	Possibly	Possibly	Possibly
5% Fluorouracil	Possibly	Possibly	Possibly	Possibly
15% Sinecatechins	Yes	No	No	No
Trichloroacetic acid[†]	Yes	Yes	Yes	Yes
Cryotherapy	Yes	Yes	No	No
Ablation[‡]	Yes	Yes	Yes	Yes
Excision	Yes	Yes	Yes	Yes

*Only FDA-approved indications are designated as "yes" in the table; otherwise use is non–FDA-approved or "off-label."
[†]Best for smaller nonbulky lesions.
[‡]IRC, hyfrecation, electrocautery, laser ablation, and argon beam coagulation.

using this approach. Cryotherapy is somewhat uncomfortable, but anesthesia is usually not required. Erythema and blistering may occur fairly quickly and there may be burning for several days. The area usually heals in 7 to 14 days. The process can be repeated every 2 to 3 weeks until clearance of lesions.[74] If the lesions do not resolve, then other topical therapies or ablative methods can be used (see Section 17.5.3.3). If lesions progress or there is hyperpigmentation or ulceration unrelated to the treatment, then lesions should be biopsied.

Eighty-five percent TCA is most useful for small perianal or intra-anal lesions or in combination with cryotherapy.[75] Two or fewer thin, flat areas of HGAIN comprising <25% of the perianal circumference tend to respond well to TCA treatment. Thicker lesions and bulky warts do not respond as well. The wooden end of a cotton-tipped swab is placed in a small amount of TCA, the excess is shaken off to prevent dripping, and the stick is directly applied to the lesions (Figure 17.102). Treatments are repeated at 3- to 4-week intervals for up to four treatments.[75] In a retrospective analysis of patients treated in the UCSF Anal Neoplasia Clinic, complete clearance of HGAIN was found in 9 of 28 patients (32%); however, the response rate per HGAIN lesion was 64%. Recurrence of AIN was common and occurred in 15 of 21 patients (72%).[75] Clearance rates were higher in HIV-negative compared with

HIV-positive men, but the difference was not statistically significant.

17.5.3.2 Patient-Applied Topical Treatments: 0.5% Podofilox Gel, 5% Imiquimod Cream, 5% Fluorouracil Cream, 15% Sinecatechins

Given appropriate instructions, most patients can self-apply podofilox gel (Condylox®), to perianal condyloma. The gel is applied in a thin film twice daily for 3 consecutive days followed by 4 days off; this cycle can be repeated for up to four courses. Patients often experience transient erythema, burning, or shallow erosions, which resolve in about a week. Clearance rates have been reported between 37% and 83%.[76] Unpurified podophyllin is no longer used based on its theoretical potential toxicity and mutagenicity.

Imiquimod cream (Aldara®) is rubbed into the affected cutaneous areas thoroughly at bedtime and then rinsed off in the morning. It is applied on alternating days three times a week, until the lesion disappears. Frequency of application can be reduced if perianal inflammation, erosion, and pain secondary to the treatment impede compliance. Imiquimod is dispensed in a box of 12 packets and prescribed for up to 16 weeks of treatment. It is an immune modulator and induces production

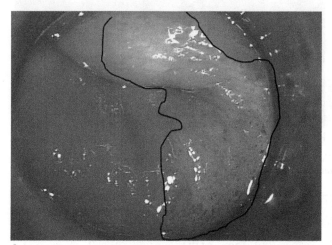

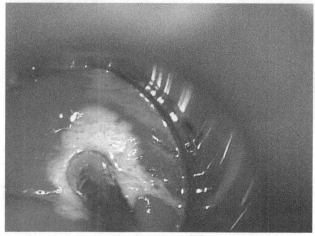

A   **B**

FIGURE 17.102.   Example of treatment of a thin flat high-grade lesion with TCA. **A:** Appearance of HGAIN on HRA. **B:** Application of TCA using wooden end of cotton-tipped swab.

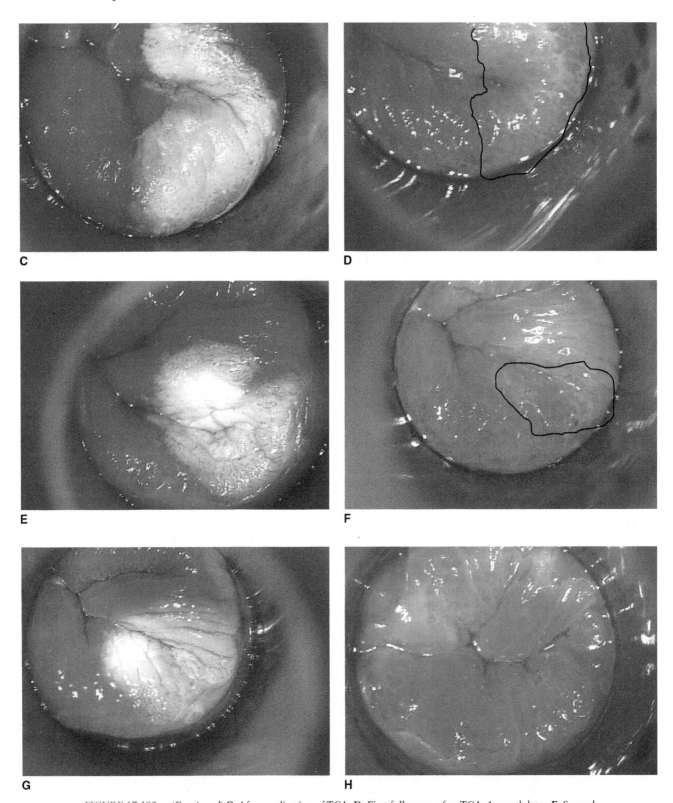

FIGURE 17.102. *(Continued)* C: After application of TCA. D: First follow-up after TCA, 1 month later. E: Second application of TCA. F: Follow-up after TCA, 3 weeks later. G: Third application of TCA and, (H) no lesions are seen 4 months later.

of cytokines and stimulates dendritic cells locally. In immunocompetent patients evaluated in placebo-controlled studies, complete response rates of 40% to 70% were seen; these differences were statistically significant from placebo response rates of 0% to 34%.[77] Better efficacy has been reported against

genital warts in HIV-negative compared with HIV-positive patients, with 62% of HIV-negative patients having complete clearance compared with 31% of HIV-positive patients. In another study, podofilox and imiquimod were directly compared in 45 nonimmunocompromised patients with anogenital warts; there were no statistical differences between associated side effects or response rates at 72% and 75%, respectively.[76]

There are limited reports of efficacy using imiquimod for treatment of intra-anal HGAIN in cohort studies and case reports.[78] In one study, 14 of 19 (74%) HIV-positive MSM had complete regression of either intra-anal or perianal AIN after treatment with imiquimod and 5 developed recurrent HGAIN. A decrease in the number of HPV types and HPV viral load was also seen following treatment.[79] The results from a randomized, double-blind placebo-controlled study of imiquimod for anal canal HGAIN were reported in 53 patients. In the treatment arm, 4 resolved and 8 were downgraded to AIN 1 versus only 1 of 25 in the placebo arm who spontaneously regressed. Patients from both arms were treated with open-label imiquimod after completing the study; 29 of 47 (61%) had sustained regression of HGAIN with imiquimod. Interestingly, patients were instructed to use only half a packet per application three times per week, applied no more than 2 cm into the canal; they were treated for 4 months, and the dosage was reduced if significant symptoms developed.[80]

There are limited data evaluating 5% fluorouracil (5FU, Efudex®) for genital warts; however, a Cochrane review suggests that despite the paucity and heterogeneity of the literature, there is evidence for a therapeutic effect against genital warts.[81] A randomized study evaluated 5FU as maintenance therapy to decrease recurrence of high-grade CIN following loop electrosurgical excision procedure (LEEP) in HIV-positive women. Recurrence of CIN was 47% in the observation arm compared with 28% in the 5FU group. In addition, time without recurrence was significantly prolonged, and the likelihood of high-grade CIN recurrence was decreased from 31% to 8%.[82]

Published literature describing the specific use of 5FU for anal lesions is also limited. In one study, evaluating treatment of patients with perianal HGAIN, 7 of 8 patients treated with 5% fluorouracil cream, applied twice a week for 16 weeks, had no evidence of Bowen's disease on follow-up biopsies 1 year later.[83] An open-label study has been reported in 46 patients with intra-anal lesions; multifocal lesions were seen in 76%, and 74% had HGAIN. All were HIV positive. In this study, 1 g of 5FU cream was inserted into the anus using an applicator two nights a week for 16 weeks. Complete responses were seen in 12 of 34 patients and partial responses, with a decrease in HGAIN to LGAIN, were seen in an additional 8 subjects.

Moderate to severe side effects of redness, swelling, pain, irritation, erosion, and ulceration were reported in 48%.[84] Results were recently reported in 11 patients using a slightly different dosing schedule inserting approximately 0.25 g of 5FU intra-anally each night, as tolerated, for a median treatment time of 20 weeks. One patient discontinued therapy due to side effects, and 73% of patients experienced some amount of irritation. Six patients had improvement in their disease including one with extensive condyloma who had no lesions on follow-up HRA.[85]

Sinecatechins 15% (Veregen®) ointment is FDA approved for the treatment of genital warts and is an extract of green tea leaves. The pooled results of two randomized, placebo-controlled trials demonstrate complete clearance of all warts defined at baseline and new warts in 54.9% of subjects compared with 35.4% treated with placebo.[86] The ointment is self-applied three times daily for a total of 16 weeks. Subjects had normal immune function and either genital or perianal warts, but not vaginal or "rectal" warts that required treatment. Erosion, ulceration, or erythema was associated with response and often occurred with greatest intensity between weeks 2 and 4. Subjects treated with active ointment were more likely to have a local skin reaction than those treated with vehicle alone, 85.9% versus 60.4% respectively. Overall, sinecatechins 15% ointment is an effective and well-tolerated treatment for external genital warts. It has not been evaluated for treatment of HGAIN, for treatment of intra-anal lesions, or in immunocompromised patients.

17.5.3.3 Surgical Excision and Ablative Techniques

Surgical excision is the preferred treatment method when additional histopathologic analysis is required to rule out cancer. There are multiple techniques for physically ablating HGAIN and condyloma, including infrared coagulation (IRC), hyfrecation, electrocautery, laser ablation, and argon beam coagulation. To date, there are no published studies comparing effectiveness or morbidity of each of the various methods. See Table 17.4 for a comparison of equipment costs and feasibility for office-based treatment associated with various methods of ablation. In the absence of comparative effectiveness, the choice of ablation primarily relates to availability of equipment and to the provider's training, experience, and comfort in using a particular method. All ablative methods, except for IRC, require a smoke evacuator. For more extensive perianal lesions, IRC may be more difficult because the unit tends to overheat in this situation. Judging depth of ablation using laser and electrocautery is required; significant problems can occur if providers are not properly trained.

There is a paucity of literature describing treatment of HGAIN and very few articles in which HRA was used to guide treatment. At UCSF, HRA is used in the operating room to guide surgical treatment of HGAIN. We performed over 550 HRA-guided operations for treatment of anal lesions between 2001 and 2010, and published two reports describing our experience.[69,87] The first, published in 2002, described outcomes and morbidity for HRA-guided surgical ablation of HGAIN in 29 HIV-positive and 8 HIV-negative patients.[87] In this report, among HIV-negative patients, no recurrence of HGAIN was seen, but in 79% (23 of 29) of HIV-positive patients recurrence of HGAIN was seen within 12 months. Uncontrolled pain was reported in 16 of 29 patients lasting a mean of 2.9 weeks. No stenosis, incontinence, infection, or significant bleeding occurred postoperatively.

TABLE 17.4	COMPARISON OF OFFICE-BASED ABLATION METHODS INCLUDING APPROXIMATE EQUIPMENT COSTS			
	■ PUBLISHED RESULTS	■ SMOKE EVACUATOR	■ OFFICE-BASED	■ EQUIPMENT EXPENSE
Infrared coagulation	Yes	No	Yes	$8395
Hyfrecation	No	Yes	Yes	$825*
Electrocautery	Yes	Yes	Yes	$2600*
Laser ablation	Yes	Yes	Yes	$75,000
Argon plasma coagulation	Abstract	Yes	Yes	$38,000
Surgical excision	Yes	Yes	Yes	$25,000†

*Smoke evacuator separate ~$2600.
†Operating Microscope.

Two factors mitigate the apparently poor results seen in the HIV-positive patients. First, some patients had lesions too extensive to be treated in a single operation. For purposes of this analysis, they were scored as recurrences, when in fact they had not completed their planned treatment. Second, this study was completed prior to the introduction of IRC as an office-based treatment. The only option for treatment of recurrences was to return to the operating room. These results indicate that, particularly in HIV-positive patients, surgical treatment alone is insufficient to control HGAIN. If surgical ablation is not guided by HRA, less favorable results will likely occur since many lesions will potentially be missed. The lack of efficacy of ablative therapy has often been cited based on the results of this paper.

In October 2002, we began using IRC in the office at UCSF to treat patients with HGAIN. Collectively, our group performed over 2500 IRC procedures. Based on our clinical experience, IRC demonstrates good efficacy and mild to moderate morbidity that is well tolerated. Retrospective studies, initially published by Goldstone[88,89] and subsequently by Cranston,[90] confirm the efficacy and minimal morbidity of IRC. Combining results from these studies, the individual lesion eradication rate was 64% to 81% with 35% to 47% having a per-subject complete response.

As with other modalities, 60% developed metachronous lesions; however, with successive treatments, the likelihood of recurrence decreased. Results from a prospective multicenter pilot study conducted by the AIDS Malignancy Consortium showed a complete response at 1 year in 10 of 16 (63%) HIV-positive persons with an eradication rate of 66% per lesion.[91] Treatment efficacy is better in HIV-negative patients than in HIV-positive patients. In all of these studies, HRA was used to guide treatment.

Nathan et al. published their results using HRA-guided office-based laser ablation of both high-grade and low-grade AIN in 181 patients.[92] No evidence of disease at 12 months was seen in 114 of 181 (63%) patients, and they experienced minimal morbidity. Kreuter et al. in Germany prospectively followed a cohort of 446 HIV-positive men. HGAIN was diagnosed in 156 (35%), LGAIN in 163 (36.5%), and 11 (2.5%) were diagnosed with anal cancer. Subjects were followed with HRA, and lesions were treated with electrocautery. Progression to invasive cancer was seen only in the five subjects who refused treatment of their lesions.[71]

Our 10-year results treating 246 patients with HGAIN using HRA-guided surgical ablation combined with office-based treatment of recurrences using IRC demonstrates the feasibility of treating HGAIN (Figure 17.103).[69] In this study, 192 of 246 (78%) had no evidence of HGAIN at their last follow-up.

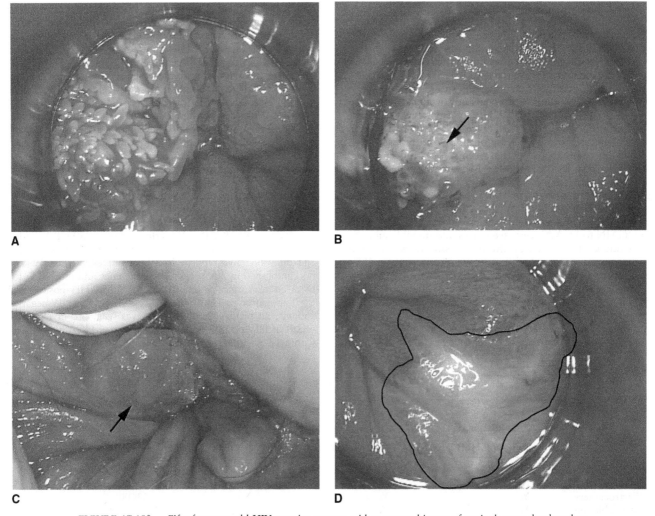

A   **B**   **C**   **D**

FIGURE 17.103. Fifty-four-year-old HIV-negative woman with a remote history of vaginal warts developed an external perianal lump and bleeding with bowel movements. **A:** Friable atypical condyloma in anal canal. **B:** *Arrow* indicates biopsy site somewhat more distal to image (A); histology was HGAIN. **C:** Palpable firm, ulcerated but not indurated perianal lesion; histology showed HGAIN. She was successfully treated with HRA-guided ablation. **D:** She had a small recurrence of intra-anal HGAIN detected at her 4-month postoperative visit that was easily treated with IRC in the office. Image is after infiltration of lidocaine prior to IRC. One year later she remains disease free.

Only nine patients developed complications of note: one had bleeding requiring reoperation, two developed anal stenosis, four developed anal fissures, one had a myocardial infarction on post-op day 3, and one developed cellulitis at the local anesthetic injection site. Overall, three patients progressed to invasive cancer despite treatment: two were lost to follow-up after treatment until they presented 14 and 19 months later with symptomatic masses; the third patient had preexisting anal stenosis that complicated treatment and had multiple recurrences of HGAIN prior to progressing to invasive cancer.

Guidelines for treatment of HGAIN were published by Chin-Hong and Palefsky[93] and recently updated by Park and Palefsky.[54] What conclusions can be drawn based on our clinical experience and these published studies regarding treatment of HGAIN? The majority of patients, who present to the UCSF Anal Neoplasia Clinic and are diagnosed with HGAIN, are treated in the office. Whenever clinically appropriate, we treat patients in the office because recovery is quicker, postprocedure pain associated with office-based treatment is less, and it is a more pragmatic and economical way to treat HGAIN, particularly if lesions are likely to recur and additional treatments are needed. It is also similar to the rationale for office-based management of CIN. Not surprisingly, most patients prefer office-based treatment to surgical treatment. However, when lesions are too extensive or there is a clinical suspicion that cancer may be present, patients are referred for surgical consultation.

Currently, for patients with circumferential intra-anal or perianal lesions and who have relatively intact immune function (here defined as a CD4+ lymphocyte count >200/mm³), and are otherwise healthy, we routinely offer staged surgery followed by office-based treatment with good results. In staged surgery, approximately 60% of the lesions are ablated at the first operation. Patients are then evaluated 8 to 10 weeks after surgery and scheduled for their second procedure 2 to 4 weeks later. In addition to surgical ablation, almost all require additional in-office ablation. Ultimately, the majority of these patients have no HGAIN identified on subsequent follow-up. HGAIN can be successfully eradicated in almost all patients who are medically fit and motivated. However, patients with significant comorbidities or severely compromised immune function are usually observed carefully with regular DARE with the goal of early detection of cancer should it develop.

Successful eradication of HGAIN requires close patient follow-up using HRA and treatment of persistent or recurrent HGAIN. Recurrence and persistence of HGAIN are common, particularly in HIV-positive persons, and some of these lesions may progress to cancer.[69,71] We have seen progression to superficially invasive cancer in as little as 3 months postoperatively. However, based on the experience in the UCSF Anal Neoplasia Clinic, in the absence of HRA, regular follow-up every 4 to 6 months with anal cytology, DARE, and simple anoscopy should be performed. Close follow-up facilitates the early detection of cancer. Additionally, early recognition and treatment of persistent or recurrent HGAIN maximizes the likelihood of eliminating HGAIN. Whether treatment of HGAIN ultimately succeeds in preventing progression to invasive cancer is still unknown.

17.5.3.3.1 Office-Based Infrared Coagulation

Prior to IRC, patients have HRA with biopsy to confirm HGAIN, rule out occult invasion, and identify areas of metaplasia that do not require treatment. Immediately prior to IRC, 5% anorectal lidocaine cream is applied topically for 10 to 15 minutes; it does not affect the appearance of the lesions. HRA is repeated to visualize all areas that need to be treated; these areas are then infiltrated with local anesthetic, such as 1% lidocaine with epinephrine buffered with sodium bicarbonate (1 mL bicarbonate added to 5 mL lidocaine). Injections are usually performed via the anoscope using a 25-gauge spinal needle attached to a 10-mL control syringe. Small volumes are infiltrated beginning proximally, at the SCJ, and working out distally towards the dentate line. Papillae that extend proximally from the dentate line and the portion of the canal distal to it are cutaneously innervated and highly sensitive. A 1-inch 30-gauge needle is used for injection in these areas and for the verge and perianal region. Once all areas in the canal are anesthetized, the anoscope is removed to allow bleeding secondary to the injections to stop.

For the IRC, the anoscope is replaced and lesions reidentified with the application of vinegar. The light guide of the IRC machine is placed in contact with the lesional mucosa and the trigger fired. The IRC machine is set for 1.5 seconds; this corresponds to approximately 1.5-mm depth of burn, which is sufficient for most lesions. Immediate blanching of the mucosa is observed. The ablated tissue can easily be debrided down to the level of the submucosal vessels. Following debridement, the base of the lesion is usually retreated both for hemostasis and for control of disease. Figures 17.104 to 17.106 show examples of in-office IRC from identification of lesions using HRA to final debridement. Patients are instructed to maintain

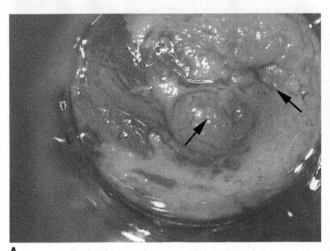
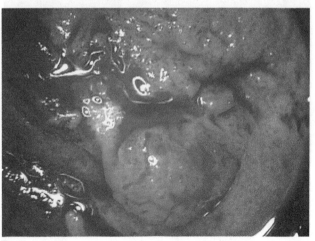

A   **B**

FIGURE 17.104.   Large lesion occupying the anterior midline. Multiple deep biopsies of the raised friable area were taken, indicated by *arrows* in (**A**); biopsies showed HGAIN. The patient had a medical contraindication to surgery, so was offered treatment in the office using IRC. **B**: Higher power view.

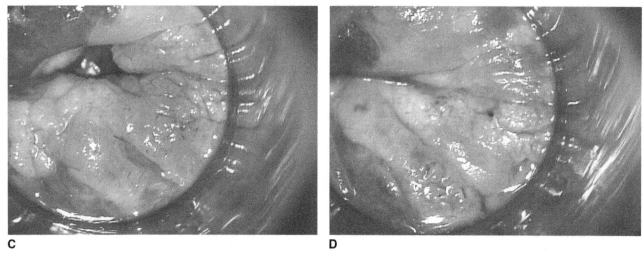

FIGURE 17.104.   *(Continued)* **C,D:** Distal margins of lesion.

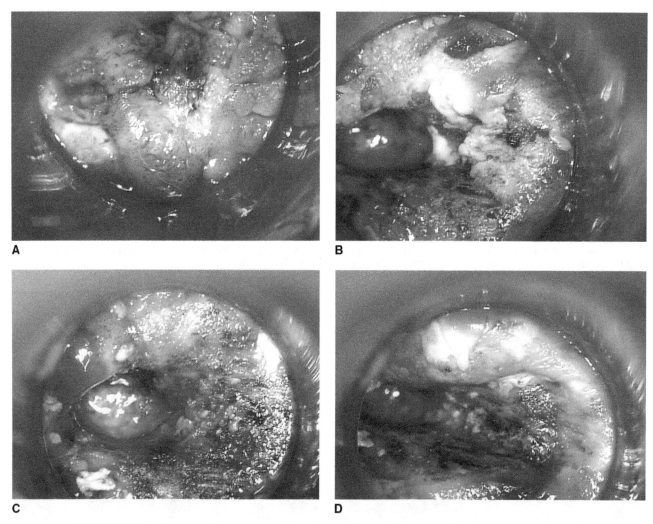

FIGURE 17.105.   Panels **(A–D)** show progressive ablation of lesion, followed by debridement down to the level of the submucosal vessels. In **(D)**, the lesion extends into the distal canal, so this area was anesthetized and ablated.

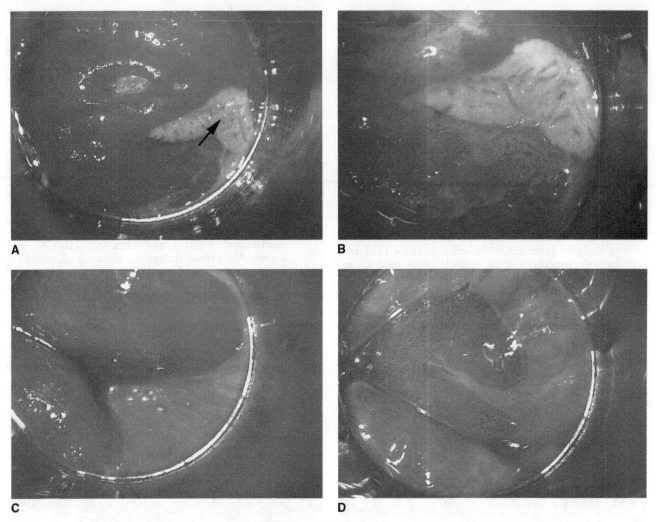

FIGURE 17.106.   Three months following IRC, a small persistent area of AIN 2 was biopsied (*arrow*) and ablated with IRC seen in (**A**) and (**B**). In (**C**) and (**D**), 4 months later, he had no evidence of HGAIN.

soft bowel movements and avoid constipation using fiber supplements, stool softeners, increased hydration, and intake of fresh fruits and vegetables. For pain control, patients are given 5% anorectal lidocaine cream, instructed to take nonsteroidal anti-inflammatory drugs for the first few days, and to soak in hot water several times per day. Following treatment of extensive lesions, patients are cautioned against heavy workouts or other activity to avoid bleeding associated with increased intra-abdominal pressure. They are also instructed to refrain from receptive anal sex for 6 to 8 weeks. It is important to remind patients to practice safe sex, particularly during this time, because of the increased likelihood of bleeding that may facilitate transmission of HIV. They return for reexamination and ongoing follow-up in 3 to 4 months.

17.5.4 Approach to Patients in the Operating Room: UCSF Experience

Patients are placed in the prone jackknife position, buttocks taped apart, and prepped with antiseptic solution. Some providers prefer to treat patients in the dorsal lithotomy position. Usually patients are heavily sedated, but not given general or a spinal anesthetic. Once the patient is sedated, a perianal block is placed using a combination of a short- and long-acting anesthetic such as lidocaine and bupivacaine. DARE is repeated by the surgeon to palpate for masses and areas of induration. The anus is saturated with 5% acetic acid, and HRA is repeated by the surgeon, if trained in this technique. Alternatively, the surgeon exposes or everts the anal mucosa so that it can be examined using the operating microscope. Areas clinically suspicious for cancer are excised; the remaining lesions are ablated using electrocautery. Treatment of circumferential lesions that extend from the distal canal to the verge and perianal area are staged to avoid anal stenosis.

17.5.5 Specific Management Scenarios If Cancer Is Identified or Suspected

1. If an intra-anal or perianal mass or indurated area is felt that is associated with obvious high-grade vascular changes, the most worrisome-appearing areas should be biopsied. If invasive cancer is found, then refer for combined modality therapy (CMT). If cancer is not diagnosed or the biopsy is only suspicious, or has features suggestive of cancer, then patients should be referred for an EUA and surgical biopsy (Figure 17.107).
2. If superficially invasive cancer in found in perianal or anal margin lesions, patients may be candidates for

local excision. To determine who is a suitable candidate, patients should be carefully evaluated by an expert in anal neoplasia to rule out simultaneous intra-anal HGAIN or cancer. Please see discussion below regarding treatment of superficially invasive cancer (Figure 17.108).

3. If a submucosal mass without a mucosal component is palpated, it is best to refer the patient for an incisional biopsy in the operating room; these are difficult to biopsy in the office. DARE is an essential part of the anal exam; when a mass is palpated and there is no clear underlying cause, patients should be referred for a surgical evaluation. Refer again to Figure 17.108.

4. If a patient has known HGAIN, extensive perianal lesions, or areas that are focally tender, or if ulcerated areas with atypical vessels are seen during HRA, and HRA-guided biopsies do not show cancer, then EUA with biopsy should be considered. If the clinical suspicion of cancer is high and the patient is not able to easily be examined in the office, refer for EUA and biopsy, particularly since multiple areas need to be sampled to determine whether or not cancer is present (Figures 17.109 to 17.111).

5. If a large firm papillary lesion, not typical for condyloma, is identified and biopsy reveals HGAIN, refer for EUA and additional biopsies; these patients are at high risk of occult cancer and must have adequately sized biopsies or excision under anesthesia (Figure 17.112).

6. If a biopsy in the office is interpreted as having features suggestive of invasion, the patient should be referred for EUA and HRA-guided surgical biopsies.

17.5.6 Specific Recommendations for Management and Treatment of HGAIN and Condyloma

17.5.6.1 Extensive Circumferential Lesions

1. If a patient is in good medical condition and has circumferential perianal and intra-anal HGAIN with lesions that extend though the distal canal, or >25% involvement of distal canal, he or she is best managed with surgery as described above. An alternative is to use

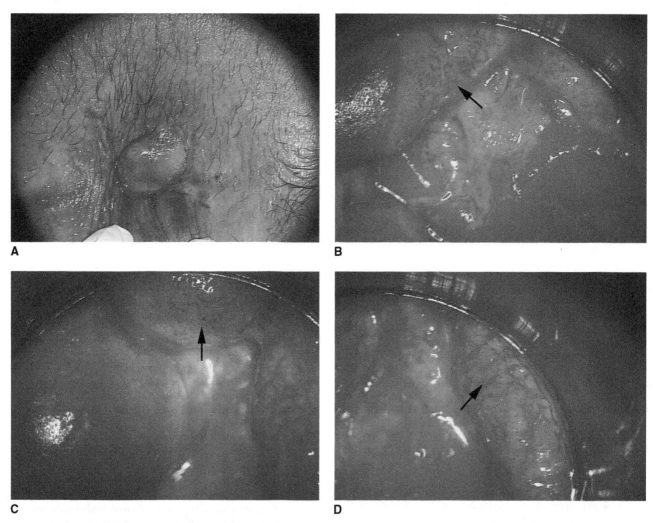

A   **B**

C   **D**

FIGURE 17.107.   **A:** Forty-six-year-old HIV-positive MSM with obvious mass at anal verge and absence of perianal mucosal changes. **B:** HRA-guided biopsy (*arrow*) of very coarse punctation in anal canal showed AIN 3. **C:** Histology of this area of abnormal vessels distally (*arrow*) also was AIN 3; however, biopsy was superficial, and invasion could not be excluded. **D:** Histology of this area of mosaic pattern and abnormal vessels (*arrow*) was superficially invasive SCC (<1 mm depth of invasion). Clinically, there was invasion of the sphincter and therefore, the mass was not resectable, and the patient was referred for radiation and chemotherapy.

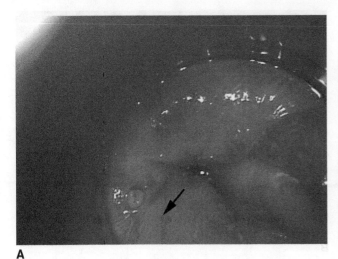

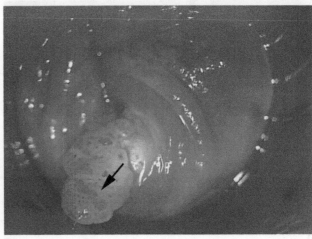

A

B

FIGURE 17.108. **A:** Sixty-two-year-old HIV-positive man presented for screening. On DARE, firm nodularity was palpated. **A:** During HRA, there appeared to be a submucosal bulge with mass effect. Biopsy adjacent to it as indicated by the *arrow* was AIN 3. **B:** Biopsy of this friable lesion (*arrow*) with blunted papillae and abnormal vessels showed superficially invasive SCC. Because there appeared to be a deeper submucosal component, the patient was not considered a candidate for conservative management and was successfully treated with CMT.

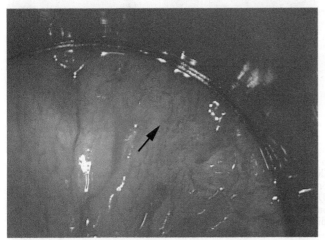

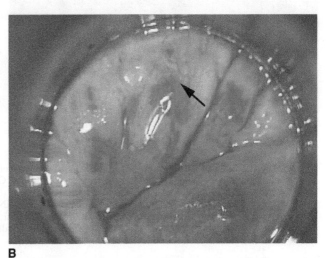

A

B

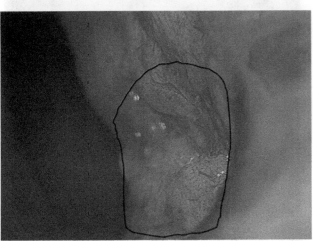

C

FIGURE 17.109. This is a 44-year-old woman, s/p liver transplant 20 years ago for autoimmune hepatitis. In November 2009, she had excision of two anal masses, thought to be hemorrhoids, which showed superficially invasive carcinoma. She was referred for further evaluation to the UCSF Anal Neoplasia Clinic. Subsequent cervical evaluation showed high-grade CIN. **A:** On initial HRA, biopsy at *arrow* showed HGAIN with foci suspicious for invasion. However, a larger surgical excisional biopsy of this area showed only HGAIN. **B:** Patient returned for follow-up 5 months later, and exam had worsened clinically, and anal cytology was HSIL with features suspicious for invasion. The *arrow* indicates the area of primary concern corresponding to previous suspicious biopsy. **C:** Subsequent intraoperative excision showed superficially invasive SCC.

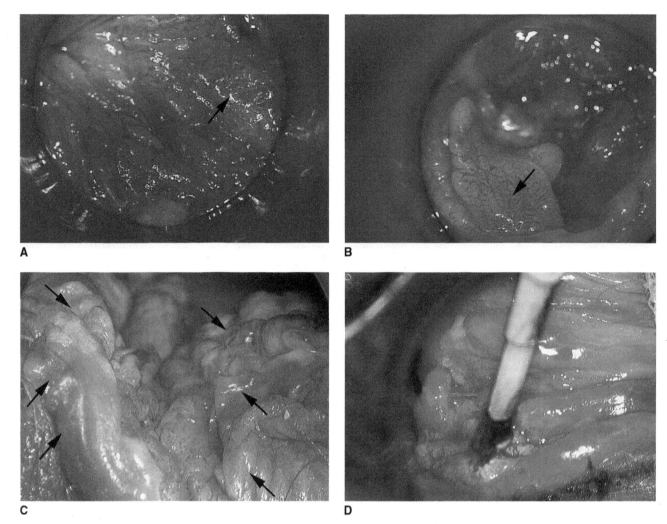

FIGURE 17.110. This is a 57-year-old HIV-positive man who presented with a year of anal irritation. He was seen by a local surgeon and biopsy of an anal verge ulcer showed HGAIN. Clinically, the lesion was highly suspicious for cancer. **A:** On his initial evaluation, multiple biopsies were taken of this area (one site designated by *arrow*); histology was HGAIN. **B:** Note coarse mosaic pattern and punctation; histology again HGAIN. **C:** Because of the concern for occult invasion, the patient was taken to the operating room. *Arrows* indicate margin of excision. Histology was focally invasive SCC associated with HGAIN. **D:** Additional intraoperative image showing fulguration of additional adjacent areas of HGAIN.

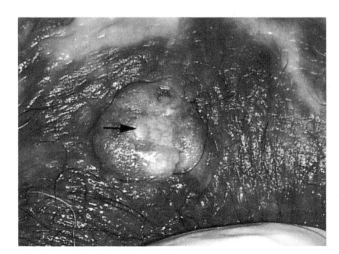

FIGURE 17.111. Fifty-four-year-old HIV-positive man, with suspicious perianal lesion. Excision showed a superficially invasive well-differentiated SCC (*arrow*) arising in condyloma acuminatum.

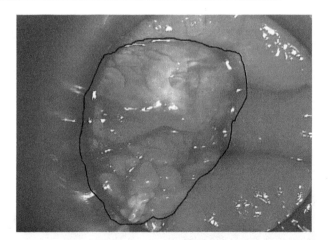

FIGURE 17.112. Fifty-one-year-old HIV-positive man who presented with a 5-cm distal rectal mass and bleeding. Colonoscopic biopsy was highly suspicious for invasion. He was taken to the operating room for biopsy, which showed superficial stromal invasion. Perirectal nodes were present on endoanal ultrasound and on CT scan; therefore, he was staged as a T3N1M0 and referred for CMT. He had an initial complete response, but developed a local recurrence and pulmonary metastases within 10 months after completing therapy.

intra-anal and perianal 5FU twice a day for 5 days on and 9 days off for 8 to 16 weeks. Using this approach, many patients have significant reduction in the volume and extent of their lesions, permitting an office-based IRC. This approach can be used in patients who are reluctant or unable to have surgery.

2. If a patient has nearly circumferential intra-anal HGAIN with lesions that extend distally to the verge in some areas, some providers may treat in the office using IRC. A procedure to treat lesions that are this extensive may take up to 90 minutes. Again 5FU could be used to decrease the volume of lesions to be treated.

3. If nearly circumferential intra-anal HGAIN exists, but lesions only extend to the dentate line focally, these patients can be treated by experienced providers using IRC in the office.

4. Patients with large bulky condyloma involving the distal canal are also more easily managed surgically because adequate local anesthesia of large areas distal to the dentate line is challenging and time-consuming in most patients. Ideally, these lesions should be excised to rule out occult invasion. We do not generally use 5FU for these patients.

17.5.6.2 Medium and Small-Volume Disease

1. HGAIN occupying 25% to 50% of circumference, some lesions relatively thick. Thicker lesions covering a greater extent are probably better managed with IRC than TCA.

2. A thin HGAIN lesion occupying <25% of circumference can be treated easily with TCA.

3. LGAIN occupying 25% to 50% of intra-anal circumference. Treat using IRC or observe with repeat HRA every 6 months and treat if HGAIN develops.

4. Several small condyloma occupying <25% of circumference can be treated easily with TCA or observation.

17.5.7 Management of Anal Cancer

17.5.7.1 Staging and Management of Invasive Anal Cancer

Invasive anal cancer is curable in many patients, particularly when diagnosed early while tumors are small. A distinction is made with regard to staging and treatment between cancers of the anal canal and perianal or anal margin cancers. The anal canal begins at the anorectal junction where the rectum enters the puborectalis sling; this can be palpated as the anorectal ring and is where the AnTZ is located. Histologically, this is nonkeratinized squamous epithelium that continues distally to the dentate line. Distal to the dentate line, the squamous mucosal epithelium is keratinized but devoid of hair follicles and apocrine and sweat glands; it lines the distal anal canal continuing to the mucocutaneous junction at the anal verge. The palpable intersphincteric groove, at the distal border of the internal sphincter muscle, is located in this portion of the canal. The anal canal is usually about 4 cm long (Figure 17.16). Tumors beyond the verge and continuing for 5 cm radially are classified as perianal or anal margin cancers.[63,94]

Anal canal cancer is clinically staged according to the T, N, and M (TNM) (Table 17.5). In the current American Joint Committee on Cancer (AJCC) Staging Manual, perianal cancers are staged using the same criteria as cutaneous squamous cell cancers.[95] Specific adaptation for perianal cancers will likely need to be created, since much of the staging is related to skin cancers of the head and neck region and does not readily apply to perianal cancers. Most anal cancers are located within the anal canal (71% to 87%), while only 13%

to 29% are described as anal margin cancers.[96–99] However, in one study comparing outcomes in HIV-positive versus HIV-negative patients, anal margin cancers comprised 65% of the cancers in HIV-positive patients.[100]

Once a diagnosis of anal cancer is made, consultation with a cancer specialist is recommended. Appropriate staging studies are performed to determine whether it is localized or has metastasized either to nearby lymph nodes or to distant organs. The recommended staging workup for patients diagnosed with anal cancer is DARE to evaluate tumor size and location, HRA or standard anoscopy with biopsy to confirm diagnosis, palpation of inguinal nodes with biopsy or fine needle aspiration if clinically suspicious, chest x-ray or chest CT scan, abdominal and pelvic CT scan or MRI. A PET-CT can be considered, but its routine use has not been validated. HIV testing is indicated with CD4 lymphocyte count. Women should have a gynecologic exam including screening for cervical cancer.[101]

Prior to the 1970s, the standard treatment for anal cancer was an abdominoperineal resection (APR) with colostomy. Currently, the standard of care for treatment of anal cancer is CMT: mitomycin and 5-fluorouracil combined with radiation. The exception may be a small T1 (<2 cm) intra-anal tumor that is not deeply invasive, if it can be excised without compromising sphincter function. This is based on review of older surgical literature prior to the advent of CMT as the standard of care for treatment of anal cancer and represents a very small proportion of patients.[102–104] CMT results in complete tumor regression in 80% to 90% of patients, but with significant morbidity.[105] Stage of cancer provides prognostic information; overall survival rates according to stage are listed in Table 17.6.[106] Prognostic factors associated with poorer disease-free outcomes and lower overall survival include tumor size >5 cm, clinically positive nodes, male versus female gender, older age, and longer treatment duration outcome.[99,107,108] Regular screening of patients at risk for anal cancer with DARE may detect cancers at an earlier stage. Based on the above data, these patients would be expected to have less morbidity and better outcomes.

The management of perianal cancers is primarily surgical with use of nonoperative modalities based on tumor size and invasion of adjacent structures (Figure 17.113).[95] There is little literature regarding CMT for perianal cancers. In the first UKCCCR trial, which demonstrated a beneficial effect of combining chemotherapy with radiation, patients with anal margin cancers were included.[109] Long-term results have been reported, and there is no specific mention of site having a differential outcome. Other studies that have focused on anal margin cancers did not uniformly treat patients with CMT; they used primarily radiation alone and had outcomes comparable to treatment of anal canal cancers.[110,111] Excellent outcomes were reported in a small series from the University of Florida in which 24 of 26 patients achieved a complete response when treated with radiation alone. The two patients who did not achieve a complete response had AIDS. One additional patient who did not receive inguinal node irradiation subsequently died of recurrent anal cancer. This study also provides an excellent review of the available literature with guidelines for treatment that mirror the National Comprehensive Cancer Network (NCCN) treatment guidelines.[112]

A series from Germany, however, reported inferior results among those with only anal margin involvement; overall survival was 54% compared to 75% in anal canal cancers. One speculation for this imbalance was an excess of patients with larger tumors and nodal involvement.[98] Many perianal cancers are noticed at less advanced stages because they are more likely to be symptomatic earlier. According to NCCN Guidelines, local excision is recommended for well-differentiated T1, N0 tumors if adequate margins can be achieved without compromising sphincter function. All other perianal cancers are treated in the same fashion as anal canal cancer, with CMT.[101]

TABLE 17.5	STAGING OF ANAL CANAL CANCER

▪ STAGING OF ANAL CANAL CANCER

Primary tumor (T):
Tx: primary tumor cannot be assessed
T0: no evidence of primary tumor
Tis: carcinoma *in situ* (Bowen's disease, HSIL, AIN II–III)
T1: tumor is 2 cm or less in greatest dimension
T2: tumor is more than 2 cm but not more than 5 cm in greatest dimension
T3: tumor is more than 5 cm in greatest dimension
T4: tumor of any size that invades adjacent organs, such as the vagina, urethra, or bladder
   (involvement of the sphincter muscle alone is not classified as a T4)

Regional lymph nodes (N):
Nx: regional lymph nodes cannot be assessed
N0: no regional lymph node metastasis
N1: metastasis in perirectal lymph node or nodes
N2: metastasis in unilateral internal iliac and/or inguinal lymph node or nodes
N3: metastasis in perirectal and inguinal lymph nodes and/or bilateral internal iliac and/or
   inguinal lymph node or nodes

Distant metastasis (M):
Mx: metastasis cannot be assessed
M0: no distant metastasis
M1: distant metastasis

Stage grouping:

Stage 0: Tis	N0	M0	
Stage I:	T1	N0	M0
Stage II: T2	N0	M0	
	T3	N0	M0
Stage IIIA:	T1	N1	M0
	T2	N1	M0
	T3	N1	M0
	T4	N0	M0
Stage IIIB:	T4	N1	M0
	any T	N2	M0
	any T	N3	M0
Stage IV:	any T	any N	M1

Based on the *American Joint Committee on Cancer (AJCC) Cancer Staging Manual*, 7th edition (2010) published by Springer-Verlag, New York.

17.5.7.2 Conservative Management of Superficially Invasive Squamous Cell Carcinoma of the Anus

According to NCCN guidelines, well-differentiated T1 (<2 cm) SCCs of the anal margin can be excised if clear margins can be achieved (Figure 17.110).[101] If, with re-excision, margins remain positive, patients should be referred for standard CMT. Outside of this specific recommendation for anal margin cancers, CMT is the standard of care for all other invasive anal cancers regardless of depth of invasion. The pathologic equivalent to microinvasive cervical carcinoma, which is treated with cold knife cone excision and has a low incidence of nodal metastases, has not been validated in the anus. As high-risk patients are more frequently being screened and followed, an increasing number of patients with asymptomatic, superficially invasive squamous cell carcinomas of the anus (SISCCA) are being identified. Although not part of the formal recommendation, based on our clinical experience, patients with SISCCA of the anal margin need careful evaluation by providers experienced in managing anal neoplasia, preferably who perform HRA. In patients referred for conservative management, other areas of invasion were occasionally found intra-anally that had been unrecognized; these patients are not good candidates for simple excision. The histologic diagnosis of superficially invasive cancer must be put in clinical context. Often it is challenging to get representative biopsy samples of suspected anal cancers that are large enough for diagnosis, so if a patient has a mass or mass effect and a diagnosis of SISCCA, these patients should be referred for CMT (Figures 17.107, 17.108, and 17.112). Therefore, anal margin cancers that are superficially invasive can be managed with local excision, which is consistent with NCCN guidelines. With the exception of clinical trials, all other superficially invasive cancers should be managed with CMT.

TABLE 17.6	PREVALENCE AND OUTCOME OF ANAL CANCER ACCORDING TO STAGE IN 19,199 PATIENTS FROM THE NATIONAL CANCER DATA BASE

▪ STAGE	▪ PERCENTAGE OF PATIENTS AT DIAGNOSIS	▪ FIVE-YEAR OVERALL SURVIVAL (%)
Stage I	25.3	69.5
Stage II	51.8	59.0
Stage III	17.1	40.6
Stage IV	5.7	18.7

Source: Bilimoria KY, Bentrem DJ, Rock CE, Stewart AK, Ko CY, Halverson A. Outcomes and prognostic factors for squamous-cell carcinoma of the anal canal: analysis of patients from the National Cancer Data Base. *Dis Colon Rectum* 2009;52(4):624–31.

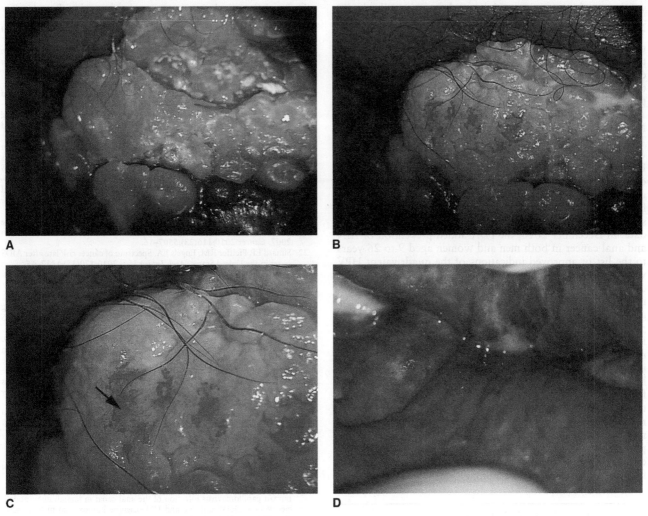

FIGURE 17.113.   **A:** Fifty-one-year-old HIV-positive man presented with locally advanced perianal cancer measuring 8 to 9 cm. **B:** After application of acetic acid. **C:** *Arrow* indicates site with grossly abnormal vessels; biopsy showed invasive SCC. **D:** 1 year after completing CMT with no evidence of disease.

17.6 SUMMARY AND CONCLUSIONS

The treatment of anal cancer is one of the success stories of modern cancer care, and many patients will be cured with surgery or CMT. However, the side effects of therapy can be substantial, and not all patients respond well to treatment. Early diagnosis will help improve outcome, and small tumors can be treated more effectively and with fewer side effects. There is little doubt that the best way to treat anal cancer is to prevent it from occurring. Patients with an increased risk of anal cancer may benefit from screening with anal cytology and DARE followed by eradication of identified HGAIN, the precursor of anal cancer. It is our hope that with screening, rates of anal cancer will decline similar to the success seen with cervical cancer screening.

17.6.1 Primary Prevention: Hope for the Future

In 2009, the U.S. Food and Drug Administration approved the quadrivalent HPV vaccine for use in boys aged 9 to 26 years for the prevention of external genital warts associated with HPV 6 or 11. The Advisory Committee on Immunization Practice (ACIP) subsequently issued a permissive recommendation for the quadrivalent vaccine, indicating that it may be given to males aged 9 through 26 years to reduce their likelihood of acquiring genital warts. Although it does not carry the same "routine recommendation" as in similarly aged girls and women, the ACIP did recommend that the vaccine be covered for boys under the Vaccines for Children program; thus the vaccine is also provided free of charge to eligible boys between 9 and 18 years of age.

The FDA's approval of the quadrivalent vaccine was based on data recently published from the Merck 020 protocol.[113] The Merck 020 protocol was a double-blinded, placebo-controlled randomized clinical trial of the quadrivalent vaccine. The study included 3463 heterosexual men and 602 MSM. The data from this study showed that the vaccine was well tolerated and immunogenic in boys aged 16 to 26 years old with no more than five reported lifetime partners. The data also showed that it was effective in preventing persistent penile/scrotal/perianal infection with each of HPV 6 (84%), 11 (91%), 16 (100%) and 18 (100%) in vaccine recipients naïve to these four vaccine HPV types throughout the vaccination period (the per-protocol [PP] population). In the intent to treat (ITT) population of all trial participants, whether or not naïve to the four vaccine HPV types, the vaccine was less effective, with lower, but statistically significant efficacies for HPV 6 (45%), 11 (59%), 16 (47%), and 18 (56%). In this age group, most of the incident external genital lesions would be expected to be condyloma acuminatum, and thus almost all of the lesions that were prevented compared with the placebo group were condyloma acuminatum, with an 89% efficacy in the PP population and 67% in the ITT population.

A substudy in the Merck 020 protocol evaluated 602 MSM for prevention of intra-anal HPV infection and AIN. The data showed prevention of 95% of intra-anal infection with HPV 6/11/16/18 in the PP population and 59% in the ITT population.[114] The data also showed prevention of 75% of HGAIN related to vaccine types. These results may not be generalizable to older individuals and those with more than five lifetime partners, as they have a higher risk of prior exposure to vaccine-targeted HPV types. Based on these and other data, in December 2010, the FDA added prevention of AIN and anal cancer in both men and women aged 9 to 26 years to the list of approved indications of the quadrivalent HPV vaccine. The ACIP is reviewing these data and is expected to decide whether to retain the current permissive recommendation for boys and men, or recommend that the vaccine be given on a routine basis as it is for girls. Since this is a prophylactic vaccine, optimal efficacy will be achieved with the lowest number of prevaccination sexual partners, hence the recommendation that boys (and girls) be vaccinated prior to initiation of sexual activity, if possible. The bivalent vaccine has not yet been studied in males and is not currently approved for use in this population. However, the demonstration that the quadrivalent HPV vaccine prevents most cases of HGAIN related to the most important HPV types causing anal cancer means that HPV vaccination should be an important tool for primary prevention of anal cancer in the long term. This is especially important given the absence of routine screening for AIN and challenges in treating HGAIN when diagnosed.

References

1. Joseph D, Miller J, Wu X, et al. Understanding the burden of human papillomavirus-associated anal cancers in the US. *Cancer* 2008;113(S10):2892–900.
2. Hoots BE, Palefsky JM, Pimenta JM, Smith JS. Human papillomavirus type distribution in anal cancer and anal intraepithelial lesions. *Int J Cancer* 2009;124(10):2375–83.
3. Frisch M, Glimelius B, van den Brule AJ, et al. Sexually transmitted infection as a cause of anal cancer [see comments]. *N Engl J Med* 1997;337(19):1350–8.
4. Watson M, Saraiya M, Ahmed F, et al. Using population-based cancer registry data to assess the burden of human papillomavirus-associated cancers in the United States: overview of methods. *Cancer* 2008;113(10 suppl):2841–54.
5. *http://www.cancer.org/Cancer/AnalCancer/DetailedGuide/anal-cancer-what-is-key-statistics* (last accessed on 6/12/2011).
6. *http://www.cancer.org/Cancer/CervicalCancer/DetailedGuide/cervical-cancer-key-statistics* (last accessed on 6/12/2011).
7. *http://seer.cancer.gov/csr/1975_2005/results_merged/sect_05_cervix_uteri.pdf* (last accessed on 6/12/2011).
8. Johnson LG, Madeleine MM, Newcomer LM, Schwartz SM, Daling JR. Anal cancer incidence and survival: the surveillance, epidemiology, and end results experience, 1973–2000. *Cancer* 2004;101(2):281–8.
9. Daling JR, Weiss NS, Hislop TG, et al. Sexual practices, sexually transmitted diseases, and the incidence of anal cancer. *N Engl J Med* 1987;317(16):973–7.
10. Holly EA, Whittemore AS, Aston DA, Ahn DK, Nickoloff BJ, Kristiansen JJ. Anal cancer incidence: genital warts, anal fissure or fistula, hemorrhoids, and smoking. *J Natl Cancer Inst* 1989;81(22):1726–31.
11. Daling JR, Weiss NS, Klopfenstein LL, Cochran LE, Chow WH, Daifuku R. Correlates of homosexual behavior and the incidence of anal cancer. *JAMA* 1982;247(14):1988–90.
12. Melbye M, Sprogel P. Aetiological parallel between anal cancer and cervical cancer. *Lancet* 1991;338(8768):657–9.
13. Rabkin CS, Biggar RJ, Melbye M, Curtis RE. Second primary cancers following anal and cervical carcinoma: evidence of shared etiologic factors. *Am J Epidemiol* 1992;136(1):54–8.
14. Penn I. Cancer in the immunosuppressed organ recipient. *Transplant Proc* 1991;23(2):1771–2.
15. Patel HS, Silver AR, Northover JM. Anal cancer in renal transplant patients. *Int J Colorectal Dis* 2005;22:1–5.
16. Collett D, Mumford L, Banner NR, Neuberger J, Watson C. Comparison of the incidence of malignancy in recipients of different types of organ: a UK Registry audit. *Am J Transplant* 2010;10(8):1889–96.
17. Frisch M, Biggar RJ, Goedert JJ. Human papillomavirus-associated cancers in patients with human immunodeficiency virus infection and acquired immunodeficiency syndrome. *J Natl Cancer Inst* 2000;92(18):1500–10.
18. Patel P, Hanson DL, Sullivan PS, et al. Incidence of types of cancer among HIV-infected persons compared with the general population in the United States, 1992–2003. *Ann Intern Med* 2008;148(10):728–36.
19. Piketty C, Selinger-Leneman H, Grabar S, et al. Marked increase in the incidence of invasive anal cancer among HIV-infected patients despite treatment with combination antiretroviral therapy. *AIDS* 2008;22(10):1203–11.
20. D'Souza G, Wiley DJ, Li X, et al. Incidence and Epidemiology of Anal Cancer in the Multicenter AIDS Cohort Study. *J Acquir Immune Defic Syndr* 2008;48(4):491–9.
21. Seaberg EC, Wiley D, Martinez-Maza O, et al. Cancer incidence in the multicenter aids cohort study before and during the HAART era: 1984 to 2007. *Cancer* 2010;116(23):5507–16.
22. Simard EP, Pfeiffer RM, Engels EA. Spectrum of cancer risk late after AIDS onset in the United States. *Arch Intern Med* 2010;170(15):1337–45.
23. Franceschi S, Lise M, Clifford GM, et al. Changing patterns of cancer incidence in the early- and late-HAART periods: the Swiss HIV Cohort Study. *Br J Cancer* 2010;103(3):416–22.
24. Crum-Cianflone NF, Hullsiek KH, Marconi VC, et al. Anal cancers among HIV-infected persons: HAART is not slowing rising incidence. *AIDS* 2010;24(4):535–43.
25. Guiguet M, Boue F, Cadranel J, Lang JM, Rosenthal E, Costagliola D. Effect of immunodeficiency, HIV viral load, and antiretroviral therapy on the risk of individual malignancies (FHDH-ANRS CO4): a prospective cohort study. *Lancet Oncol* 2009;10(12):1152–9.
26. Ferlay J, Shin HR, Bray F, Forman D, Mathers C, Parkin DM. Estimates of worldwide burden of cancer in 2008: GLOBOCAN 2008. *Int J Cancer* 2010;127(12):2893–917.
27. Critchlow CW, Holmes KK, Wood R, et al. Association of human immunodeficiency virus and anal human papillomavirus infection among homosexual men. *Arch Intern Med* 1992;152(8):1673–6.
28. Palefsky J. Anal cancer in HIV-positive individuals: an emerging problem. *AIDS* 1994;8:283–95.
29. Palefsky J, Barasso R. HPV infection and disease in men. *Obstet Gynecol Clin North Am* 1996;23:895–916.
30. Palefsky JM, Holly EA, Ralston ML, Jay N. Prevalence and risk factors for human papillomavirus infection of the anal canal in human immunodeficiency virus (HIV)-positive and HIV-negative homosexual men. *J Infect Dis* 1998;177(2):361–7.
31. de Pokomandy A, Rouleau D, Ghattas G, et al. Prevalence, clearance, and incidence of anal human papillomavirus infection in HIV-infected men: the HIPVIRG cohort study. *J Infect Dis* 2009;199(7):965–73.
32. Chin-Hong PV, Vittinghoff E, Cranston RD, et al. Age-specific prevalence of anal human papillomavirus infection in HIV-negative sexually active men who have sex with men: the EXPLORE study. *J Infect Dis* 2004;190(12):2070–6.
33. Critchlow CW, Surawicz CM, Holmes KK, et al. Prospective study of high grade anal squamous intraepithelial neoplasia in a cohort of homosexual men: influence of HIV infection, immunosuppression and human papillomavirus infection. *AIDS* 1995;9(11):1255–62.
34. Palefsky JM, Holly EA, Efirdc JT, et al. Anal intraepithelial neoplasia in the highly active antiretroviral therapy era among HIV-positive men who have sex with men. *AIDS* 2005;19(13):1407–14.
35. Wilkin TJ, Palmer S, Brudney KF, Chiasson MA, Wright TC. Anal intraepithelial neoplasia in heterosexual and homosexual HIV-positive men with access to antiretroviral therapy. *J Infect Dis* 2004;190(9):1685–91.
36. Conley L, Bush T, Darragh TM, et al. Factors associated with prevalent abnormal anal cytology in a large cohort of HIV-infected adults in the United States. *J Infect Dis* 2010;202(10):1567–76.
37. Piketty C, Darragh TM, Da Costa M, et al. High prevalence of anal human papillomavirus infection and anal cancer precursors among HIV-infected persons in the absence of anal intercourse. *Ann Intern Med* 2003;138(6):453–9.
38. Nyitray A, Nielson CM, Harris RB, et al. Prevalence of and risk factors for anal human papillomavirus infection in heterosexual men. *J Infect Dis* 2008;197(12):1676–84.
39. Hernandez BY, McDuffie K, Zhu X, et al. Anal human papillomavirus infection in women and its relationship with cervical infection. *Cancer Epidemiol Biomarkers Prev* 2005;14(11 pt 1):2550–6.
40. Shvetsov YB, Hernandez BY, McDuffie K, et al. Duration and clearance of anal human papillomavirus (HPV) infection among women: the Hawaii HPV cohort study. *Clin Infect Dis* 2009;48(5):536–46.
41. Palefsky JM, Holly EA, Ralston ML, Da Costa M, Greenblatt RM. Prevalence and risk factors for anal human papillomavirus infection in human immunodeficiency virus (HIV)-positive and high-risk HIV-negative women. *J Infect Dis* 2001;183(3):383–91.

42. Patel HS, Silver AR, Levine T, Williams G, Northover JM. Human papillomavirus infection and anal dysplasia in renal transplant recipients. *Br J Surg* 2010;97(11):1716–21.

43. Palefsky JM. Anal cancer prevention in HIV-positive men and women. *Curr Opin Oncol* 2009;21(5):433–8.

44. Scholefield JH, Castle MT, Watson NF. Malignant transformation of high-grade anal intraepithelial neoplasia. *Br J Surg* 2005;92(9):1133–6.

45. Watson AJ, Smith BB, Whitehead MR, Sykes PH, Frizelle FA. Malignant progression of anal intra-epithelial neoplasia. *ANZ J Surg* 2006;76(8):715–7.

46. Rickert RR, Brodkin RH, Hutter RV. Bowen's disease. *CA Cancer J Clin* 1977;27(3):160–6.

47. Palefsky JM, Holly EA, Hogeboom CJ, Jay N, Berry M, Darragh TM. Anal cytology as a screening tool for anal squamous intraepithelial lesions. *J Acquir Immune Defic Syndr* 1997;14:415–22.

48. Palefsky JM, Holly EA, Ralston ML, Jay N, Berry JM, Darragh TM. High incidence of anal high-grade squamous intraepithelial lesions among HIV-positive and HIV-negative homosexual/bisexual men. *AIDS* 1998;12:495–503.

49. Palefsky JM, Holly EA, Hogeboom CJ, et al. Virologic, immunologic, and clinical parameters in the incidence and progression of anal squamous intraepithelial lesions in HIV-positive and HIV-negative homosexual men. *J Acquir Immune Defic Syndr* 1998;17(4):314–9.

50. Chin-Hong PV, Berry JM, Cheng SC, et al. Comparison of patient- and clinician-collected anal cytology samples to screen for human papillomavirus-associated anal intraepithelial neoplasia in men who have sex with men. *Ann Intern Med* 2008;149(5):300–6.

51. Hessol NA, Holly EA, Efird JT, et al. Anal intraepithelial neoplasia in a multisite study of HIV-infected and high-risk HIV-uninfected women. *AIDS* 2009;23(1):59–70.

52. Kojic EM, Cu-Uvin S, Conley L, et al. Human papillomavirus infection and cytologic abnormalities of the anus and cervix among HIV-infected women in the study to understand the natural history of HIV/AIDS in the era of effective therapy (The SUN Study). *Sex Transm Dis 2011*;38(4):253–9.

53. Santoso JT, Long M, Crigger M, Wan JY, Haefner HK. Anal intraepithelial neoplasia in women with genital intraepithelial neoplasia. *Obstet Gynecol* 2010;116(3):578–82.

54. Park IU, Palefsky JM. Evaluation and management of anal intraepithelial neoplasia in HIV-negative and HIV-positive men who have sex with men. *Curr Infect Dis Rep* 2010;12(2):126–33.

55. Darragh TM, Winkler B. Anal cancer and cervical cancer screening: key differences. *Cancer Cytopathol* 2011;119(1):5–19.

56. Berry JM, Palefsky JM, Jay N, Cheng SC, Darragh TM, Chin-Hong PV. Performance characteristics of anal cytology and human papillomavirus testing in patients with high-resolution anoscopy-guided biopsy of high-grade anal intraepithelial neoplasia. *Dis Colon Rectum* 2009;52:239–47.

57. Darragh TM, Birdsong GG, Luff RD, Davey DD. Anal-rectal cytology. In: Solomon D, Nayar R, eds. *The Bethesda System for Reporting Cervical Cytology: Definitions, Criteria and Explanatory Notes* (2nd ed.). New York, NY: Springer, 2004:169–75.

58. Darragh TM. Anal cytology. In: Wilbur DC, Henry MR, eds. *College of American Pathologists Practical Guide to Gynecologic Cytopathology: Morphology, Management and Molecular Methods*. Northfield, IL: CAP Press, 2008:177–81.

59. Bean SM, Chhieng DC. Anal-rectal cytology: a review. *Diagn Cytopathol* 2010;38(7):538–46.

60. Chiao EY, Giordano TP, Palefsky JM, Tyring S, El Serag H. Screening HIV-infected individuals for anal cancer precursor lesions: a systematic review. *Clin Infect Dis* 2006;43(2):223–33.

61. Salit IE, Lytwyn A, Raboud J, et al. The role of cytology (Pap tests) and human papillomavirus testing in anal cancer screening. *AIDS* 2010;24(9):1307–13.

62. Arain S, Walts AE, Thomas P, Bose S. The anal Pap smear: cytomorphology of squamous intraepithelial lesions. *CytoJournal* 2005;2:4.

63. Shia J. An update on tumors of the anal canal. *Arch Pathol Lab Med* 2010;134(11):1601–11.

64. Daling JR, Madeleine MM, Johnson LG,. Human papillomavirus, smoking, and sexual practices in the etiology of anal cancer. *Cancer* 2004;101(2):270–80.

65. Cranston RD, Darragh TM, Holly EA, et al. Self-collected versus clinician-collected anal cytology specimens to diagnose anal intraepithelial neoplasia in HIV-positive men. *J Acquir Immune Defic Syndr* 2004;36(4), 915–20.

66. Salerno G, Sinnatamby C, Branagan G, Daniels IR, Heald RJ, Moran BJ. Defining the rectum: surgically, radiologically and anatomically. *Colorectal Dis* 2006;8(suppl 3):5–9.

67. Berry JM, Palefsky JM. Invited Commentary to Screening anal dysplasia in HIV-infected patients: is there an agreement between anal Pap smear and high resolution anoscopy-guided biopsy? *Dis Colon Rectum* 2009;52(11):7–10.

68. Jay N, Berry M, Hogeboom CJ, Holly EA, Darragh TM, Palefsky JM. Colposcopic appearance of anal squamous intraepithelial lesions: relationship to histopathology. *Dis Colon Rectum* 1997;40:919–28.

69. Pineda CE, Berry JM, Jay N, Palefsky JM, Welton ML. High-resolution anoscopy targeted surgical destruction of anal high-grade squamous intraepithelial lesions: a ten-year experience. *Dis Colon Rectum* 2008;51(6):829–35; discussion 35–7.

70. Devaraj B, Cosman BC. Expectant management of anal squamous dysplasia in patients with HIV. *Dis Colon Rectum* 2006;49(1):36–40.

71. Kreuter A, Potthoff A, Brockmeyer NH, et al. Anal carcinoma in HIV-positive men: results of a prospective study from Germany. *Br J Dermatol* 2010;162(6):1269–77.

72. McCloskey JC, Metcalf C, French MA, Flexman JP, Burke V, Beilin LJ. The frequency of high-grade intraepithelial neoplasia in anal/perianal warts is higher than previously recognized. *Int J STD AIDS* 2007;18(8):538–42.

73. Schlecht HP, Fugelso DK, Murphy RK, et al. Frequency of occult high-grade squamous intraepithelial neoplasia and invasive cancer within anal condylomata in men who have sex with men. *Clin Infect Dis* 2010;51(1):107–10.

74. Scheinfeld N, Lehman DS. An evidence-based review of medical and surgical treatments of genital warts. *Dermatol Online J* 2006;12(3):5. Review.

75. Singh JC, Kuohung V, Palefsky JM. Efficacy of trichloroacetic acid in the treatment of anal intraepithelial neoplasia in HIV-positive and HIV-negative men who have sex with men. *J Acquir Immune Defic Syndr* 2009;52(4):474–9.

76. Komericki P, Akkilic-Materna M, Strimitzer T, Aberer W. Efficacy and safety of Imiquimod versus Podophyllotoxin in the treatment of anogenital warts. *Sex Transm Dis* 2011;38(3):216–8.

77. Wagstaff AJ, Perry CM. Topical imiquimod: a review of its use in the management of anogenital warts, actinic keratoses, basal cell carcinoma and other skin lesions. *Drugs* 2007;67(15):2187–210.

78. Mahto M, Nathan M, O'Mahony C. More than a decade on: review of the use of imiquimod in lower anogenital intraepithelial neoplasia. *Int J STD AIDS* 2009;21(1):8–16.

79. Kreuter A, Potthoff A, Brockmeyer NH, et al. Imiquimod leads to a decrease of human papillomavirus DNA and to a sustained clearance of anal intraepithelial neoplasia in HIV-infected men. *J Invest Dermatol* 2008;128(8):2078–83.

80. Fox PA, Nathan M, Francis N, et al. A double-blind, randomized controlled trial of the use of imiquimod cream for the treatment of anal canal high-grade anal intraepithelial neoplasia in HIV-positive MSM on HAART, with long-term follow-up data including the use of open-label imiquimod. *AIDS* 2010;24(15):2331–5.

81. Batista CS, Atallah AN, Saconato H, da Silva EM. 5-FU for genital warts in non-immunocompromised individuals. *Cochrane Database Syst Rev* 2010;4:CD006562.

82. Maiman M, Watts DH, Andersen J, Clax P, Merino M, Kendall MA. Vaginal 5-fluorouracil for high-grade cervical dysplasia in human immunodeficiency virus infection: a randomized trial. *Obstet Gynecol* 1999;94(6):954–61.

83. Graham BD, Jetmore AB, Foote JE, Arnold LK. Topical 5-fluorouracil in the management of extensive anal Bowen's disease: a preferred approach. *Dis Colon Rectum* 2005;48(3):444–50.

84. Richel O, Wieland U, De Vries HJ, et al. Topical 5-fluorouracil treatment of anal intraepithelial neoplasia in human immunodeficiency virus-positive men. *Br J Dermatol* 2010;163(6):1301–7.

85. Snyder SM, Siekas L, Aboulafia DM. Initial experience with topical fluorouracil for treatment of HIV-associated anal intraepithelial neoplasia. *J Int Assoc Physicians AIDS Care (Chic)* 2011;10(2):83–8.

86. Tatti S, Stockfleth E, Beutner KR, et al. Polyphenon E: a new treatment for external anogenital warts. *Br J Dermatol* 2009;162(1):176–84.

87. Chang GJ, Berry JM, Jay N, Palefsky JM, Welton ML. Surgical treatment of high-grade anal squamous intraepithelial lesions: a prospective study. *Dis Colon Rectum* 2002;45(4):453–8.

88. Goldstone SE, Kawalek AZ, Huyett JW. Infrared coagulator: a useful tool for treating anal squamous intraepithelial lesions. *Dis Colon Rectum* 2005;48(5):1042–54.

89. Goldstone SE, Hundert JS, Huyett JW. Infrared coagulator ablation of high-grade anal squamous intraepithelial lesions in HIV-negative males who have sex with males. *Dis Colon Rectum* 2007;50(5):565–75.

90. Cranston RD, Hirschowitz SL, Cortina G, Moe AA. A retrospective clinical study of the treatment of high-grade anal dysplasia by infrared coagulation in a population of HIV-positive men who have sex with men. *Int J STD AIDS* 2008;19(2):118–20.

91. Stier EA, Goldstone SE, Berry JM, et al. Infrared coagulator treatment of high-grade anal dysplasia in HIV-infected individuals: an AIDS malignancy consortium pilot study. *J Acquir Immune Defic Syndr* 2008;47(1):56–61.

92. Nathan M, Hickey N, Mayuranathan L, Vowler SL, Singh N. Treatment of anal human papillomavirus-associated disease: a long term outcome study. *Int J STD AIDS* 2008;19(7):445–9.

93. Chin-Hong PV, Palefsky JM. Natural history and clinical management of anal human papillomavirus disease in men and women infected with human immunodeficiency virus. *Clin Infect Dis* 2002;35(9):1127–34.

94. Ryan DP, Willett CG. Clinical features, staging and treatment of anal canal cancer. *www.uptodatecom*. 2010; Accessed January 15, 2011.

95. Edge SB, Byrd DR, Compton CC, Fritz AG, Greene FL, Andy Trotti I. *American Joint Committee on Cancer (AJCC) Staging Manual* (7th ed.). New York, NY: Springer-Verlag, 2010.

96. Dillard BM, Spratt JS Jr, Ackerman LV, Butcher HR Jr. Epidermoid cancer of anal margin and canal. Review of 79 cases. *Arch Surg* 1963;86:772–7.

97. Glynne-Jones R, Meadows H, Wan S, et al. EXTRA—a multicenter phase II study of chemoradiation using a 5 day per week oral regimen of capecitabine and intravenous mitomycin C in anal cancer. *Int J Radiat Oncol Biol Phys* 2008;72(1):119–26.

98. Grabenbauer GG, Kessler H, Matzel KE, Sauer R, Hohenberger W, Schneider IH. Tumor site predicts outcome after radiochemotherapy in squamous-cell carcinoma of the anal region: long-term results of 101 patients. *Dis Colon Rectum* 2005;48(9):1742–51.

99. Nilsson PJ, Svensson C, Goldman S, Ljungqvist O, Glimelius B. Epidermoid anal cancer: a review of a population-based series of 308 consecutive patients treated according to prospective protocols. *Int J Radiat Oncol Biol Phys* 2005;61(1):92–102.

100. Seo Y, Kinsella MT, Reynolds HL, Chipman G, Remick SC, Kinsella TJ. Outcomes of chemoradiotherapy with 5-Fluorouracil and mitomycin C for anal cancer in immunocompetent versus immunodeficient patients. *Int J Radiat Oncol Biol Phys* 2009;75(1):143–9.

101. Engstrom PF, Arnoletti JP, Benson AB III, et al. NCCN clinical practice guidelines in oncology. Anal carcinoma. *J Natl Compr Canc Netw* 2010;8(1):106–20.

102. Boman BM, Moertel CG, O'Connell MJ, et al. Carcinoma of the anal canal. A clinical and pathologic study of 188 cases. *Cancer* 1984;54(1):114–25.

103. Eby LS, Sullivan ES. Current concepts of local excision of epidermoid carcinoma of the anus. *Dis Colon Rectum* 1969;12(5):332–7.

104. Schraut WH, Wang CH, Dawson PJ, Block GE. Depth of invasion, location, and size of cancer of the anus dictate operative treatment. *Cancer* 1983;51(7):1291–6.

105. Eng C, Abbruzzese J, Minsky BD. Chemotherapy and radiation of anal canal cancer: the first approach. *Surg Oncol Clin N Am* 2004;13(2):309–20, viii.

106. Bilimoria KY, Bentrem DJ, Rock CE, Stewart AK, Ko CY, Halverson A. Outcomes and prognostic factors for squamous-cell carcinoma of the anal canal: analysis of patients from the National Cancer Data Base. *Dis Colon Rectum* 2009;52(4):624–31.

107. Ajani JA, Winter KA, Gunderson LL, et al. Prognostic factors derived from a prospective database dictate clinical biology of anal cancer: the intergroup trial (RTOG 98-11). *Cancer* 2010;116(17):4007–13.

108. Ben-Josef E, Moughan J, Ajani JA, et al. Impact of overall treatment time on survival and local control in patients with anal cancer: a pooled data analysis of Radiation Therapy Oncology Group trials 87-04 and 98-11. *J Clin Oncol* 2010;28(34):5061–6.

109. UKCCCR Anal Cancer Trial Working Party. UK Coordinating Committee on Cancer R. Epidermoid anal cancer: results from the UKCCCR randomised trial of radiotherapy alone versus radiotherapy, 5-fluorouracil, and mitomycin. *Lancet* 1996;348(9034):1049–54.

110. Chapet O, Gerard JP, Mornex F, et al. Prognostic factors of squamous cell carcinoma of the anal margin treated by radiotherapy: the Lyon experience. *Int J Colorectal Dis* 2007;22(2):191–9.

111. Khanfir K, Ozsahin M, Bieri S, Cavuto C, Mirimanoff RO, Zouhair A. Patterns of failure and outcome in patients with carcinoma of the anal margin. *Ann Surg Oncol* 2008;15(4):1092–8.

112. Balamucki CJ, Zlotecki RA, Rout WR, et al. Squamous cell carcinoma of the anal margin: The University of Florida Experience. *Am J Clin Oncol* 2011;34(4):406–10.

113. Giuliano AR, Palefsky JM, Goldstone SE, et al. The efficacy of the quadrivalent vaccine in preventing HPV 6/11/16/18-related external genital disease and anogenital infection in young men. *N Engl J Med* 2011;364:401–11.

114. Palefsky JM, Giuliano AR, Goldstone S, et al. Quadrivalent HPV vaccine efficacy against anal HPV 6/11/16/18 infection and anal intraepithelial neoplasia. Provisional acceptance, *N Engl J Med* (in press).

Primary and Secondary Prevention: HPV Vaccination and Cervical Cancer Screening

18.1 INTRODUCTION
18.2 PRIMARY PREVENTION OF CERVICAL CANCER
    18.2.1 Abstinence
    18.2.2 Condoms
    18.2.3 HPV Vaccination
18.3 SECONDARY PREVENTION THROUGH CERVICAL CANCER SCREENING
    18.3.1 Cervical Screening Technologies
    18.3.2 Impediments to Screening
18.4 PRIMARY CERVICAL CANCER SCREENING GUIDELINES
    18.4.1 When to Begin Screening
    18.4.2 When to Discontinue Screening

18.4.3 Screening after Hysterectomy
18.4.4 Screening Interval
18.4.5 Will HPV Testing as a Stand-Alone Become the Primary Screen?
18.4.6 Screening in the Era of HPV Vaccination
18.5 ADDITIONAL OBSERVATIONS ON CERVICAL CANCER SCREENING
    18.5.1 Considerations and Precautions Regarding HPV Testing
    18.5.2 Psychological Effects of Testing Positive for HPV and Counseling Messages
18.6 PROSPECTS FOR THE FUTURE OF CERVICAL CANCER PREVENTION

18.1 INTRODUCTION

Prior to the late 1940s, cervical cancer was the second most common malignancy in women in the United States in both incidence and mortality. By 2005, incidence had fallen to 11th place and mortality to 13th.[1] The American Cancer Society (ACS) estimated that 12,340 cervical cancers would occur in 2013 and approximately 4030 deaths.[2] The decrease in both cervical cancer incidence and mortality began prior to the introduction of widespread Papanicolaou (Pap) screening in the 1950s and 1960s, perhaps partly due to the change from subtotal hysterectomies to total hysterectomies in the late 1930s, reducing the proportion of women at risk for cervical cancer. However, the majority of this decrease has been attributed to the diagnosis and treatment of intraepithelial neoplasia, which only became possible following the implementation of cervical cancer screening with the Pap test.[3,4] Incidence rates have declined over most of the past several decades in white women of all ages and for African American women under the age of 50.[5] Since 2004, rates have decreased by 2.1% per year in women younger than 50 years of age and by 3.1% per year in women 50 and older. Mortality rates also declined rapidly in past decades but have plateaued in recent years for white women. In contrast, mortality rates for African American women decreased by 2.6% per year during the period from 2004 to 2008.[5]

Within the last 30 years, the confirmation of human papillomavirus (HPV) as a necessary cause of high-grade cervical intraepithelial neoplasia (CIN) and cervical cancer[6-9] has led research down two separate pathways with the goal of further reducing cervical cancer incidence and mortality. One pathway led to the potential for primary prevention of cervical cancer by blocking infection through vaccination for oncogenic HPV types.[10,11] The other led to the development and evaluation of sensitive tests for HPV DNA detection now included in guidelines for both primary cervical cancer screening and management of women with abnormal cervical cancer screening tests and cancer precursors.[11-16] This chapter discusses detailed strategies for reducing the burden of cervical cancer by both primary prevention of infection with HPV and secondary prevention with cervical cancer screening and treatment of cancer precursors. Chapter 19 reviews the guidelines for the management of equivocal and abnormal cervical screening tests and Chapter 20, the management of HPV-induced benign and neoplastic lesions.

18.2 PRIMARY PREVENTION OF CERVICAL CANCER

The three options for the primary prevention of cervical cancer are lifelong abstinence from sexual intercourse, barrier protection during sexual activity in the use of male and female condoms, and use of vaccines to prevent infection.[11] The timeline of the natural history of HPV and development of cervical cancer is shown in Figure 18.1, with overlay of age-appropriate primary and secondary cervical cancer prevention strategies.

18.2.1 Abstinence

The first description of cervical cancer is attributed to Hippocrates around 400 BC in the writings titled *Corpus Hippocraticum*. However, it was not recognized that cervical cancer might be secondary to a sexually transmitted agent until the 1842 publication by a physician in Florence, Italy, of his observation that married women and prostitutes died of cervical cancer but that nuns professing lifelong abstinence rarely developed this cancer. The virtual absence of cervical cancer in virginal women suggests that HPV rarely infects the cervix in the absence of sexual intercourse, even though HPV is

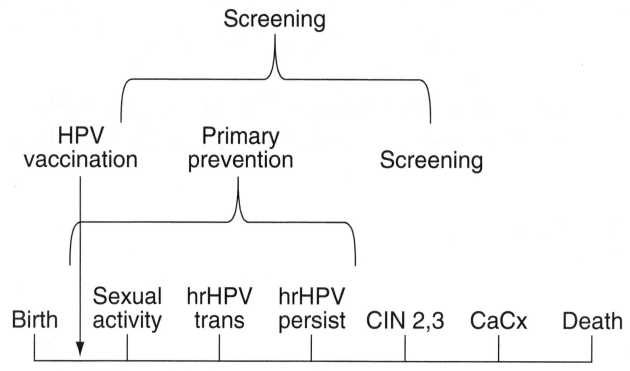

FIGURE 18.1.   Natural history of cervical cancer with overlay of primary prevention and secondary screening and treatment. The primary message is to ideally administer the vaccine before sexual activity typically may begin in order to prevent transmission of high-risk (hr)HPV, which can lead in some women to hrHPV persistence and the cascade of disease progression demonstrated in this timeline. (Adapted from Lynge E, Antilla A, Arbyn M, Segnan N, Ronco G. What's next? Perspectives and future needs of cervical screening in Europe in the era of molecular testing and vaccination. *Eur J Cancer* 2009;45(15):2714–21, with permission.)

easily transmitted to the introitus and external genitalia with external genital contact.[17,18] A number of studies support this presumption. In one, HPV DNA was detected on sampling the vulva in 20% of virginal women, whereas cervical sampling on the same women did not detect any HPV.[19] Thus, it would appear that cervical HPV infection most likely requires direct cervical exposure to this virus.[18] Winer et al.[20] did detect genital HPV types in the fingertips of women with genital HPV infection. However, the rarity of repeat detection of HPV in the fingertips suggested that true infection under the fingernails was uncommon, and although finger–genital transmission is plausible, it is unlikely to be a significant source of genital HPV infection.[20]

Of course, the most definitive protection against getting cervical and other HPV-induced lower genital tract cancers is lifelong abstinence. However, for the vast majority of the population, this is not a viable option, although abstinence until after the age of 20 appears to reduce the lifetime risk of cervical cancer to some degree.[21] Lifetime commitment by two individuals without prior sexual exposure would also be protective but is also not the path taken by the majority of the population.

18.2.2 Condoms

Whether condoms protect the cervix remains controversial, and many individuals who claim to use condoms use them inconsistently and often not during foreplay.[18] Reliable condom use reduces the risk of acquiring cervical HPV by about 70%, but faithful use over a lifetime is uncommon.[22] A meta-analysis of 20 studies concluded that condom use provides some level of protection against the development and/or persistence of HPV-associated disease but does not completely protect against getting HPV infection.[23] Evidence of long-term cervical protection with consistent condom use was demonstrated in a study of Danish prostitutes. Those using condoms consistently were 80% less likely to test positive for cervical HPV than those who did not.[24] Clearly, HPV infections outside the areas protected by the condom will still transmit HPV, so patients should be informed that condoms may provide some level of protection against infection of the cervix but do not fully protect against infection of other external anogenital areas, and that condoms may break and expose the cervix to infection.[18] In a recent European study, about one-third of girls did not use condoms at sexual debut.[25] Once HPV was known to be the cause of cervical cancer, development of a vaccine to prevent infection became a realistic option for primary prevention.

18.2.3 HPV Vaccination

18.2.3.1 General Principles of Human Papillomavirus–Like Particle Vaccination

Vaccination against a number of diseases that historically caused immense suffering and death has proved to be the most effective means of reducing morbidity and mortality from these diseases. Prominent examples of the success of prophylactic vaccines are found in the 72% reduction in hepatitis B, the 99.9% reduction in measles, diphtheria, and rubella, and the almost complete eradication of polio and smallpox.[18] Many of these vaccines have used live attenuated virus, but because HPV is a DNA virus capable of causing cancer, the development of a live attenuated HPV vaccine was never considered.

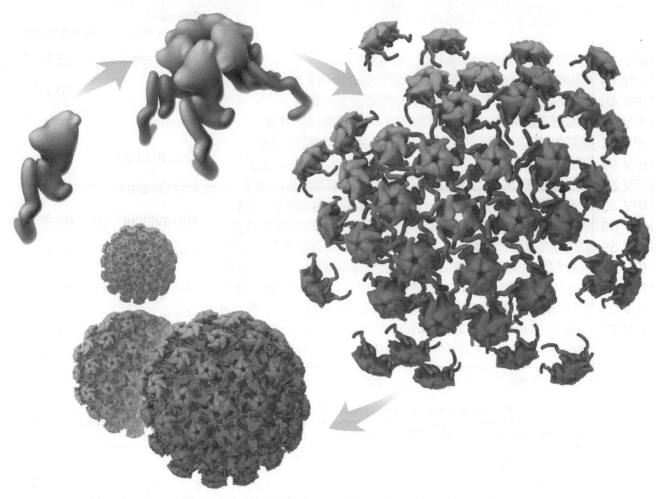

FIGURE 18.2.   VLP self-assembly: L1 proteins produced in yeast cells self-assemble into five L1 protein groups. These then assemble into a single L1 pentamer. Seventy-two pentamers then self-assemble into a full, noninfectious HPV VLP almost identical in structure and antigens to that assembled by the virus, but not containing any infectious HPV DNA.

Hence, the goal was to develop a noninfectious HPV vaccine that did not contain any genetic material capable of inducing HPV manifestations, including cancer.[11] In the early 1990s, Ian Frazer and colleagues in Australia began the search for a way to produce HPV 16 L1 capsid proteins that serve as the building blocks for the virus-like particles (VLPs) used in the prophylactic HPV vaccines (Figure 18.2).[11,26] Because the capsid surrounding the HPV genome must first come into contact with epithelium for infection to occur, stimulating production of antibodies to these capsid proteins to block this attachment appeared to be an ideal mechanism for prophylaxis against HPV.[27] Additionally, a protein-only vaccine would not include HPV DNA that could be potentially infectious. Discovery that HPV capsids could be produced by splicing the HPV L1 genome into yeast or a plasmid initiated the race to develop the bivalent (HPV 16 and 18) and quadrivalent (HPV 6,11,16,18) vaccines and the potential that a vaccine against all oncogenic HPV types might eventually be available (Figure 18.3).

18.2.3.2 Proof of Principle: Demonstration of Type-Specific Antibody Secondary to HPV 16 Vaccination

The first VLP vaccines were single HPV–type (monovalent) vaccines containing VLPs for either HPV 11 or HPV 16, evaluated in studies designed to provide "proof of principle" for safety and immunogenicity of recombinant VLPs in humans.[18,28] By month 7 after the first of three injections, both vaccines induced 100% seroconversion with high titers of type-specific antibodies, and antibody levels remained detectable at month 36 in 98.6% (HPV 11) and 93.5% (HPV 16) of women vaccinated.[28] No vaccine-related serious adverse events were reported, with pain at the injection site reported as the most common adverse event.

The first double-blind efficacy trial utilizing HPV VLPs as a vaccine evaluated the HPV 16 monovalent vaccine versus the placebo adjuvant in 2000 women 16 to 23 years of age. There were no persistent HPV 16 infections in the women receiving the vaccine against HPV 16 VLPs in comparison to 41 of the placebo recipients, for 100% efficacy against vaccine type-specific persistent infection.[29] Additionally, the anti–HPV 16 antibody titers were 50-fold higher than those produced as a response to natural HPV 16 infection, 99.7% were seroconverted, and the vaccine was well tolerated with no reported vaccine-related serious adverse events. The results from this proof-of-principle study confirmed the safety and immunogenicity of VLPs as vaccines and strongly suggested that VLP vaccines can prevent persistent infection, the most important risk factor for developing HPV-associated cervical lesions.[18] Long-term follow-up of this study group has demonstrated nearly complete protection against HPV 16 infection for at least 8.5 years after HPV 16 vaccination.[30]

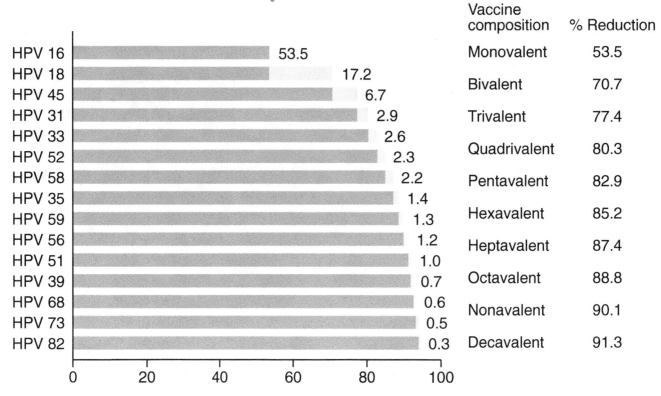

FIGURE 18.3.   Predicted reductions in cervical cancer with increasing number of types in HPV vaccines. (From Frazer IH, Cox JT, Mayeaux EJ Jr, et al. Advances in prevention of cervical cancer and other human papillomavirus-related diseases. *Pediatr Infect Dis J* 2006;25(2 suppl):S65–81, with permission.)

18.2.3.3 The HPV Vaccine Safety and Efficacy Trials

The "proof-of-principle" studies paved the way for the bivalent HPV 16, 18 (Cervarix; GlaxoSmithKline, Rixensart, Belgium) and the quadrivalent HPV 6, 11, 16, 18 (Gardasil; Merck & Co., Inc., Whitehouse Station, New Jersey) vaccine safety and efficacy trials. Both were evaluated in double-blind, randomized placebo-controlled phase III trials. The bivalent HPV 16, 18 vaccine is administered at 0, 1, and 6 months and the quadrivalent HPV 6, 11, 16, 18 vaccine at 0, 2, and 6 months. Both vaccines target HPV genotypes 16 and 18, which cause approximately 70% of cervical cancers and over 50% of the precancerous lesions (CIN 2,3). The quadrivalent vaccine also targets HPV 6 and HPV 11, the two types responsible for over 90% of genital warts.

Neither antibody titers to the HPV types in the vaccine nor prevention of cervical cancer could be used as the primary end point efficacy standard.[18] Antibody titers are not a useful end point because there is no established correlate between a titer level and protection against HPV infection or the development of CIN/cancer. Reduction in the rate of cervical cancer is the ultimate goal of vaccination against oncogenic HPV types but could not be a primary efficacy end point because the typically slow natural history from HPV infection to the development of cervical cancer would delay proof of efficacy for decades. Therefore, HPV vaccine efficacy was defined for several natural history events that serve as surrogate markers for the development of cervical cancer.[18] These are the development of incident HPV infection for the vaccine HPV types, persistence of these types for >6 or >12 months, abnormal cervical cytology, and cervical intraepithelial neoplasia grades 1, 2, and 3 (CIN 1,2,3) and adenocarcinoma in situ (AIS). Of these, the most important primary end point was reduction in the incidence of CIN 2, CIN 3, and AIS lesions type specific

for either HPV 16 or HPV 18, the two oncogenic HPV types in both vaccines.[18] The primary efficacy end point for HPV 6 and HPV 11 in the quadrivalent vaccine was the reduction in external genital warts.

There are no published head-to-head studies available comparing the bivalent and quadrivalent vaccines for effectiveness or duration of protection against cervical neoplasia and precancerous lesions.[31] There is one direct comparison of antibody levels that demonstrated significantly higher serum neutralizing antibody titers in all age strata ($p < 0.0001$) to HPV 16/18 following vaccination with the bivalent vaccine than that detected following quadrivalent vaccination.[32] However, the clinical relevance of this finding has yet to be demonstrated, as the level of antibody needed for protection against infection is unknown, as is the duration of protection.

18.2.3.3.1 The Quadrivalent HPV 6, 11, 16, 18 Vaccine Efficacy Trials

The quadrivalent HPV 6, 11, 16, 18 vaccine has been evaluated in two large, randomized clinical trials named FUTURE I and II (females united to unilaterally reduce endo-/ectocervical disease). The FUTURE I trial was a phase III placebo-controlled trial to assess the efficacy of the quadrivalent vaccine to prevent HPV-related anogenital disease in 5455 women aged 16 to 24 years.[33] Women with greater than four lifetime sexual partners or a history of any genital warts or abnormal cytology were excluded from the study. Because most women in this age group are already sexually active, evidence of past or current infection with one or more of the vaccine genotypes (HPV 6, 11, 16, and/or 18) as measured by serology and DNA detection in cervical specimens was found among 38% of the women in the vaccine arm and in 42% in the placebo arm as measured at enrollment and through 1-month follow-up

TABLE 18.1   FUTURE I: PRIMARY AND SECONDARY END POINTS

Efficacy in the "HPV-susceptible" population
- Efficacy in reducing the incidence of anogenital warts, VIN 1–3, VaIN 1–3, of cancer associated with HPV 6,11,16, or 18
  - 100% effective in preventing anogenital disease
  - Zero cases in women receiving the vaccine vs. 60 cases in women receiving the placebo
- Efficacy in reducing the incidence of CIN 1–3 or AIS associated with HPV 6,11,16, or 18
  - 100% effective in preventing CIN 1–3 disease
  - Zero cases in women receiving the vaccine vs. 65 cases in women receiving the placebo

Efficacy in the entire population (ITT)
- Efficacy in reducing the incidence of anogenital warts, VIN 1–3, VaIN 1–3, of cancer associated with HPV 6,11,16, or 18.
  - 20% effective in preventing anogenital disease

From Garland SM, Hernandez-Avila M, Wheeler CM, et al. Quadrivalent vaccine against human papillomavirus to prevent anogenital diseases. *N Engl J Med* 2007;356:1928.

after the third (and final) vaccine dose. The primary end point evaluated among vaccine recipients was reduction in the rate of HPV 6–, 11–, 16–, and 18–related anogenital warts, vulvar intraepithelial neoplasia grades 1, 2, and 3 (VIN1,2,3), vaginal intraepithelial neoplasia grades 1, 2, and 3 (VaIN1,2,3), or cancer. Reduction in CIN grades 1 to 3, AIS, or cancer associated with a vaccine-type HPV was a secondary end point. The mean follow-up was 3 years. Efficacy for preventing all of these vaccine type-specific noncervical HPV lesions was 100% for the primary efficacy group (According-To-Protocol [ATP] analysis group), defined as those study participants without evidence of HPV 6, 11, 16, or 18 infection as measured by HPV DNA or HPV serologic testing through 1 month after the third vaccine dose and receiving all three doses of the vaccine per protocol. These patients were referred to as "HPV susceptible."[33] The results of the FUTURE I trial are in Table 18.1.

When vaccine efficacy is evaluated for all participants in the vaccine trials (the Intention-to-Treat [ITT] analysis), it is always significantly lower than in the ATP analysis. This is because the ITT group includes all trial participants regardless of whether they initially test positive for vaccine-type HPV DNA or serology and whether they completed the series of three HPV vaccine doses. Because the majority of participants were already sexually active, with the potential of prior exposure to one or more of the vaccine HPV types, the ITT group represents the "real-world" experience with vaccinating young women in this age group. In contrast, the ideal target age for HPV vaccination is prior to the onset of sexual activity. Efficacy for young girls receiving all three vaccine doses prior to coitarche would be expected to attain efficacy levels found in the ATP group. In FUTURE I, efficacy in the ITT group for prevention of all anogenital lesions of any HPV type was only 20% (Table 18.1).[33]

The FUTURE II trial was also a phase III, prospective, double-blind, placebo-controlled trial with more than 12,000 women, aged 15 to 26 years randomly assigned to receive a three-dose regimen of vaccine or placebo (aluminum hydroxyphosphate sulfate adjuvant).[34] As with the FUTURE I trial, the primary efficacy analysis was on the ATP group of "HPV-susceptible" women. An additional exclusion in this group was a history of any prior abnormal cervical cytology. Approximately one-quarter of the trial participants had evidence of past or current infections with HPV 16 and/or HPV 18 as measured by serology and/or DNA detection in cervical specimens through 1-month follow-up after vaccination. The primary efficacy end point was the development of CIN 2 or 3, AIS, or cervical cancer related to HPV 16 or HPV 18 among the "HPV-susceptible" women during a mean follow-up of 3 years. Vaccine efficacy for prevention of all HPV 16/18–related CIN 2,3 and AIS was 98%, and even when study participants either did not receive all three doses in the series or received all but were not on the trial schedule, there was still a 95% reduction in this composite end point. Although more data on the impact on efficacy of the timing of administration and the number of doses are needed, these data suggest possible flexibility in each.[31]

As with the FUTURE I trial, efficacy fell in the FUTURE II trial significantly when all trial participants were evaluated, whether or not they had evidence of prior HPV infection (the ITT population). The overall efficacy of the quadrivalent HPV vaccine for preventing HPV 16 or 18 CIN 2,3+ or AIS was approximately 44%.[34] This low level of efficacy for the majority of participants already sexually active highlights the importance of immunizing girls and young women before they become sexually active. The results are summarized in Table 18.2. A subpopulation of 1512 vaccinated women were

TABLE 18.2   FUTURE II: EVALUATION OF THE QUADRIVALENT HPV VACCINE

Efficacy for the prevention of CIN 2,3 and AIS in the "HPV-susceptible" group (ATP group)
- For women receiving the entire series of 3 shots
  - 98% reduction in HPV 16/18 CIN 2,3 and AIS
- For women not receiving all doses
  - 95% reduction in the women who did not receive all doses of vaccine ATP
  - This high success rate suggests some flexibility in the timing of the vaccine schedule

Efficacy for the prevention of CIN 2,3 and AIS for all women in the trial whether they were "HPV naïve" or not (ITT group)
- 44% reduction in HPV 16/18 CIN 2,3 and AIS

From The FUTURE II Study Group. Quadrivalent vaccine against human papillomavirus to prevent high-grade cervical lesions. *N Engl J Med* 2007;356:1915.

evaluated at 24 months for detectable antibodies to the four types in the vaccine, with 96% still positive for antibodies to HPV 6, 97% positive for HPV 11, 99% positive for HPV 16, but only 68% positive for HPV 18.[34] At 44 months, antibody levels were again evaluated, and even though there had been further decline in detection of antibodies to HPV 18 to 60%, vaccine efficacy for preventing HPV 18–related CIN 2,3 and AIS remained at near 100%, suggesting that immune memory for HPV 18 is still present even when antibodies are no longer detectable.[35] To date, no commercially available HPV type–specific antibody tests are available to measure antibody levels, and there is no indication that the information would be clinically useful even if available.

18.2.3.3.2 THE BIVALENT HPV 16, 18 VACCINE EFFICACY TRIALS

The bivalent HPV 16, 18 vaccine protects against the two HPV types that cause the majority of cervical and other HPV-associated anogenital and head and neck cancers. It does not protect against genital warts. The bivalent HPV vaccine has been evaluated in two large trials: PATRICIA (Papilloma Trial Against Cancer in Young Adults), a phase III, multinational prospective, double-blind, placebo-controlled trial with more than 18,000 women, aged 15 to 25 years[36] and a U.S. National Cancer Institute (NCI)–sponsored trial in Guanacaste, Costa Rica.[37] Participants in PATRICIA were randomly assigned to receive a three-dose regimen of vaccine or a control hepatitis A vaccine.[36] Excluded from the study were women with a history of greater than six lifetime sexual partners or of colposcopy. As with the quadrivalent HPV vaccine trials, approximately one-quarter of the trial participants had evidence of current or past HPV 16 and/or HPV 18 infections.[35,36]

The primary efficacy analysis was the development of HPV 16 or 18 CIN 2 or 3, AIS, or cancer in the group of women naïve to these two HPV types at enrollment and through 1 month following the third vaccine dose (ATP analysis).[36] The primary composite end point was the development of CIN 2 or 3, AIS, or cervical cancer related to HPV 16 or HPV 18. After a mean follow-up of 3 years, 93% of these high-grade lesions in the ATP group had been prevented compared to the control group receiving the Hep A vaccine, with a reduction of 94% in incident HPV 16 or 18 infections at 6 months and 91% of persistent infections at 12 months, when compared to the control group.[36] Vaccine efficacy for CIN 2+ was reduced to 30% for CIN 2,3 or AIS due to all HPV types in the overall study population (ITT) regardless of HPV status at enrollment and through month 7, similar to the quadrivalent vaccine (Table 18.3).

18.2.3.4 Evidence of Cross-Protection with Closely Related HPV Types

Both vaccines have evidence of some cross-protection against closely related HPV types. In the HPV-naïve population, the number of CIN 1–3 and AIS lesions due to nonvaccine HPV types closely related to HPV 16 or 18 was 29% less in the Gardasil recipients than in the placebo group, and persistent infections with these types was 25% less.[38] This includes HPV 31, 33, and 52, closely related to HPV 16, and HPV 45 and 58, closely related to HPV 18. As might be expected among a cohort of mostly sexually active women with opportunities for prior exposure to these types, cross-protection in the ITT population was lower at 18% and 19%.[39] Partial cross-protection in the HPV-naïve population was also demonstrated for the bivalent HPV vaccine against acquisition of these same closely related types, with a reduction in persistent infection of 30% at 6 months, 24% at 12 months, and 53% of CIN 2+ lesions associated with these types.[36]

18.2.3.5 HPV Vaccine Safety

The safety of the quadrivalent HPV vaccine was studied in seven clinical trials in over 21,000 females aged 9 to 26 before it was licensed; it was deemed to be very safe. Similar conclusions were reached regarding safety in the over 18,000 females aged 15 to 25 evaluated in the bivalent HPV vaccine trials. The primary reactions for both vaccines were pain, erythema, pruritus, and/or swelling at the injection site that was greater in the vaccine recipients than in those receiving the placebo adjuvant (the quadrivalent vaccine trial) and Hep A vaccine (the bivalent HPV vaccine trial) (Table 18.4). The most common systemic events were fever and malaise. There were no differences in serious adverse events by study arm in any of the trials.[33–37]

The quadrivalent HPV vaccine is the only HPV vaccine to have been available and widely used in the United States long enough to have postlicensure safety data by the beginning of 2011. There are three systems used to monitor the safety of any vaccine after licensing and marketing in the United States: (1) the

---

TABLE 18.3	PATRICIA: EVALUATION OF THE BIVALENT HPV VACCINE

Efficacy for the prevention of CIN 2,3 and AIS in the "HPV-susceptible" group (ATP group)
- For women receiving the entire series of 3 shots
  - 93% reduction in HPV 16/18 CIN 2,3 and AIS
  - 94% reduction in incident HPV 16/18 infection at 6 months and in persistent infections at 12 months

Efficacy for the prevention of CIN 2,3 and AIS for all women in the trial whether they were "HPV naïve" or not (ITT group)
  - 30% reduction in HPV 16/18 CIN 2,3 and AIS

From Paavonen J, Naud P, Salmeron J, et al. Efficacy of human papillomavirus (HPV)-16/18 AS04-adjuvanted vaccine against cervical infection and precancer caused by oncogenic HPV types (PATRICIA): final analysis of a double-blind, randomized study in young women. *Lancet* 2009;374:301–14.

TABLE 18.4	LOCAL AND SYSTEMIC SYMPTOMS REPORTED IN THE BIVALENT HPV 16, 18 TRIAL

	VACCINE GROUP ($n = 3077$)	CONTROL GROUP ($n = 3080$)
Injection Site Symptoms[*]		
Pain	90.5%	78.0%
Redness	43.8%	27.6%
Swelling	42.0%	19.8%
General Symptoms[*]		
Fatigue	57.6%	53.6%
Headache	54.1%	51.3%
Myalgia	52.2%	44.9%
Gastrointestinal	27.6%	27.3%
Arthralgia	20.6%	17.9%
Raised temperature[†]	12.4%	10.9%
Rash	10.1%	8.4%
Urticaria	9.7%	7.9%

[*]Participants who reported a specified symptom within 7 days of vaccine injection.
[†]Defined as axillary or oral temperature ≥37.5°C.
Adapted from Paavonen J, et al. *Lancet* 2007;369:2161–70.

Vaccine Adverse Event Reporting System (VAERS), (2) the Vaccine Safety Datalink (VSD) project, and (3) the Clinical Immunization Safety Assessment (CISA) network. The VSD and CISA projects are Centers for Disease Control and Prevention (CDC) collaborations with health care organizations and academic centers that evaluate side effects reported in the VAERS to determine whether they are caused by the vaccine. The VAERS is a passive reporting system open to the public, and hence collects data without verification of its relationship with the vaccine other than proximity of timing. It is administered jointly by the U.S. Food and Drug Administration (FDA) and the CDC. The first review of adverse events following HPV4 immunization was reported in December 2008.[40] At that time, the VAERS had received 12,424 reports of adverse events in the 2 years following licensure distribution, or 53.9 reports per 100,000 doses distributed. The proportion of adverse events per vaccine dose was similar to those observed for other vaccines, except for an increased reporting of syncope and a small increase in venous thromboembolic events (VTEs). Because of the increased risk of vasovagal syncope, the CDC recommends that patients receive the HPV vaccine in either a sitting or a supine position and be observed for 15 minutes postinjection before being released.[40] Hence, it is important for the HPV vaccine to be given in a setting where the patient can be observed for syncope and ideally, as for any vaccine administration, where facilities are available for management of rare anaphylactic reactions.

VTE was the only adverse event to meet the CDC screening criteria for "signal detection" and will continue to be closely monitored, but the rate of VTE was not increased among those without predisposing risk factors when compared to age-matched recipients of other vaccines. Anaphylaxis has also been reported at a rate of 0.1 case per 100,000 doses. There was no increased risk of Guillain-Barré syndrome.[40]

The most recent review of the safety of the HPV vaccine comes from a report on the side effects recorded in the VSD on 600,558 quadrivalent doses administered to women and girls aged 9 to 26 years between 2006 and 2009.[41] There was no statistically significant increased risk for any of the following adverse outcomes: Guillain-Barré syndrome (GBS), stroke, venous thromboembolism (VTE), appendicitis, seizures, syncope, allergic reactions, and anaphylaxis. A nonstatistically significant relative risk (RR) for VTE of 1.98 was detected among females aged 9 to 17 years. However, review of the medical records of all eight potential VTE cases showed that only five met the standard case definition for VTE and all five had known risk factors for VTE (oral contraceptive use, coagulation disorders, smoking, obesity, or prolonged hospitalization). The question of potential risk of VTE with HPV vaccination will continue to be studied.[41]

18.2.3.6 Recommendations for Administration of the HPV Vaccines

The quadrivalent HPV vaccine was approved by the FDA in June 2006 for use in females 9 to 26 years of age, and in October 2009 for males of the same age distribution. The bivalent HPV vaccine was also approved in October 2009 by the FDA for use in females 9 to 26 years of age. Both have been approved for use in approximately 100 countries worldwide. For maximum benefit, the HPV vaccine should ideally be administered before onset of sexual activity; hence, the Advisory Committee on Immunization Practices (ACIP) recommended that HPV vaccination (with either vaccine) be routinely offered to females aged 11 to 12 years to prevent cervical and anal intraepithelial neoplasia (AIN) and cervical and anal cancer.[42,43] It can be given as young as age 9 years. Catch-up vaccination is recommended for females aged 13 to 26 years not previously vaccinated or with a previously

interrupted vaccine series.[42,43] Females who are sexually active should still be vaccinated consistent with the age-specific recommendations above, but immunization is less beneficial for females already infected with one of more of the vaccine's included HPV types.

The American College of Obstetricians and Gynecologists (ACOG) guidelines on HPV vaccination are consistent with the ACIP guidelines, with the added suggestion that clinicians seeing girls and young women of this age range routinely inquire about prior receipt of the HPV vaccine and whether the entire series of three shots was completed.[44] If she has not received all three doses, encouraging "catch-up" vaccination is recommended. The ACS HPV vaccination guidelines differ in that the routine recommendation for HPV vaccination is limited to girls and young women aged 11 to 18 years, but HPV vaccination may begin at as early as 9 years of age.[45] Because review of data for clinical trials associated with both vaccine trials demonstrated far less effectiveness for the women already sexually active, many already exposed to a vaccine HPV type, the ACS did not recommend "catch-up" vaccination in women 19 to 26 years. The ACS concluded that at the time of the FDA approval, there was insufficient evidence for, or against, the vaccination of women aged 18 to 26 years.[45] The World Health Organization also emphasizes that the primary target population is girls within the age range of 9 through 13 years.[46] No analyses have shown catch-up vaccination to be cost-effective, as vaccine efficacy decreases significantly following the onset of sexual activity. This has been confirmed by a number of studies. Analysis of the Swedish national cohort study demonstrated that HPV4 vaccine effectiveness against genital warts was 93% for girls vaccinated with all three doses before age 14 years, declining to 76% for those starting the three-dose series before age 20, and then to 48% among women vaccinated between age 20 and 22 years and decreasing to 21% among women aged 23 to 26 years.[47] HPV prevalence for vaccine types is falling in the United States despite suboptimal vaccination rates in the youngest women but has not fallen for women over 20.[48] These studies confirm that every effort should be made to target young women for vaccination.

Both vaccines are given in a three-shot series. The bivalent HPV vaccine schedule is 0, 1, and 6 months, and the quadrivalent HPV vaccine is 0, 2, and 6 months. The CDC recommends that when the series is interrupted for any length of time, it can be resumed without restarting the series.[42] It also recommends staying with the same vaccine through the entire series, however, acknowledging that the patient may not always know which HPV vaccine she previously received.[42]

18.2.3.7 HPV Vaccination Recommendations for Special Populations

19.2.3.7.1 PREGNANT WOMEN

Both HPV vaccines have been classified by the FDA as a category B drug. In the FUTURE II trial, pregnancy occurred in 1053 women in the vaccine group and 1106 in the placebo group, with no obvious congenital anomalies attributable to the vaccine observed.[34] Evaluation of VAERS has also not demonstrated increased risk to the fetus from quadrivalent HPV vaccination during pregnancy.[40] However, until more data on safety in pregnancy are available, use of either vaccine in pregnancy is not recommended.[42,43]

Some women will receive the HPV vaccine before knowing that they are pregnant. If so, the patient should be reassured that there is no evidence that the vaccine will harm the pregnancy, but that further shots in the series should be postponed until the postpartum period.[42,43] The same recommendation is made to resume the series postpartum for women who started the series but become pregnant before completion of the three-shot series. Both HPV vaccine manufacturers maintain pregnancy registries to monitor fetal outcomes of pregnant women exposed to their HPV vaccine, and pregnancies should be reported.[42,43] Lactating women can receive the immunization series, as VLP vaccines have not been shown to affect the safety of breast-feeding.[42]

18.2.3.7.2 Immunosuppressed

The ACIP guidelines state that HPV vaccination of individuals with immunosuppression can be considered since it is not a live vaccine,[31,49] and the immunogenicity and safety of the quadrivalent HPV vaccine have been established in adult HIV-seropositive men as well as in HIV-seropositive boys and girls aged 7 to 12.[50,51]

18.2.3.7.3 Women with a History of Preexisting Precancer or Cancer

The ACIP, ACOG, and the ACS all state that a history of genital warts, abnormal cervical cytology, positive HPV DNA test result, or prior treatment for cervical dysplasia is not definitive evidence that the patient would not receive benefit from HPV vaccination, as none are specific evidence of prior infection with any or all of the vaccine HPV types.[42,44,45] Therefore, the ACIP recommends that women with a history of preexisting HPV-related changes who are within the recommended age range for immunization could still be vaccinated and gain some benefit, with an acknowledgment that their potential for benefit from HPV vaccination may be less.[42]

18.2.3.7.4 HPV Immunization of Males

Studies evaluating efficacy and safety of HPV vaccination in boys and men have been done. The primary focus has been on prevention of genital warts, and penile and AIN, but there is also enthusiasm for the potential to reduce transmission of vaccine-type HPV to unimmunized females through "herd immunity." Studies with both the quadrivalent HPV vaccine and the bivalent HPV vaccine show seroconversion rates similar to those of females (99% to 100%) with similar adverse event profiles.[52,53,54] A randomized, placebo-controlled, double-blind trial of the efficacy and safety of the quadrivalent vaccine enrolling 4065 healthy boys and men 16 to 26 years of age demonstrated 66% reduction in external genital lesions related to HPV 6, 11, 16, or 18 in the entire population receiving the vaccine. Efficacy was higher (90%) for those naïve to these four types through month 7 following vaccination and receiving all three shots as per schedule.[55] There are at this time no published data on efficacy of the bivalent HPV vaccine in the prevention of HPV-related disease in males. On the basis of the data on safety and efficacy in preventing genital warts in males, in 2009, the FDA approved the use of the quadrivalent vaccine in males.[56] In 2010, the ACIP added a statement to the previous recommendations for women that "the quadrivalent vaccine may be given to males aged 9 through 26 years to reduce their likelihood of acquiring genital warts."[31,57] In 2011, the ACIP replaced the language of "permissive" use of the vaccine for males with "recommendation for routine use" of quadrivalent HPV vaccine (HPV4) in males aged 11 or 12 years.[58] The ACIP also recommended vaccination with HPV4 for males aged 13 through 21 years who have not been vaccinated previously or who have not completed the three-dose series. The permissive use recommendation remains only for males aged 22 through 26 years who "may be vaccinated." The stronger recommendation was based on newer data on prevention of grade 2 or 3 anal intraepithelial neoplasia [AIN2/3], and on vaccine safety, estimates of disease and cancer resulting from HPV, cost-effectiveness, and programmatic considerations.[57] This is also supported by a mathematical model of HPV transmission indicating that the planned extension of the Australian National HPV Vaccination Program to

males will lead to the near elimination of genital warts in both the female and male heterosexual populations in this country.[59]

Males who have sex with males (MSM) have a high rate of both AIN and anal cancer, and women have a risk of HPV-induced anal cancer that is twice that of the general male population.[60] Since nearly 90% of anal cancer is caused by HPV, and approximately 90% of that is caused by HPV 16, prevention of HPV 16 acquisition by HPV vaccination is also a priority for the prevention of this cancer (see Chapter 17). HPV vaccination of males could also potentially prevent oral cancers associated with HPV 16 and 18. One large US study demonstrated that 6.9% of men and women aged 14 to 69 years tested positive for oral HPV infection and 1.0% for HPV 16.[61] The prevalence was higher among men than among women, consistent with the gender discrepancy in the prevalence of oral–pharyngeal cancers.

18.2.3.8 Cost-Effectiveness of HPV Vaccination

Several cost-effectiveness evaluations of HPV vaccination have demonstrated that vaccination of the primary target age group of 11- to 12-year-old girls is cost-effective, but that vaccination becomes increasingly less cost-effective as the age of vaccination increases.[62-64] One modeling study concluded that if all 12-year-old girls in the United States were vaccinated for HPV, 200,000 HPV infections, 100,000 abnormal cervical cytology examinations, and 3300 cases of cervical cancer would be prevented within the lifetime of that cohort.[62] Another modeling study did not show the vaccine to be cost-effective unless cervical cancer screening onset was delayed to age 24 and performed every 2 years rather than annually.[64] Cervical cancer screening in the age of vaccination will be discussed in greater detail at the end of this chapter, but certainly will need to continue for some time as not all HPV types responsible for cervical cancer are in the vaccine, and women already exposed to one or more of these types, or not receiving the vaccine, will continue to be at risk. Combining HPV vaccination prior to the age of onset of sexual intercourse with routine cervical screening beginning later than presently recommended would be most cost-effective and have the greatest impact on cervical cancer incidence and mortality.

Vaccinating both boys and girls prevents more disease but is less cost-effective.[65,66] Estimating cost-effectiveness is limited by the information available and the uncertainty of the duration of protection, the effect of herd immunity, the level of vaccine uptake among both females and males, the age of uptake, the level of continued participation in cervical cancer screening, and the prevalence of vaccine-specific HPV types circulating in age-specific populations.[67,68] Additionally, most cost-effectiveness modeling has not taken into account the impact of HPV vaccination on the prevention of HPV 16/18–associated cancers of the oropharynx, penis, anus, vulva, and vagina. When these are factored in, cost-effectiveness improves.[69]

18.2.3.9 Success of HPV Vaccination But Concern About Uptake

All national cohort studies on the target population for HPV vaccination have demonstrated remarkable success in reducing the prevalence of vaccine HPV types and genital warts.[47,48,70] Large declines in genital warts have been reported within 5 years after introduction of near-universal (80%+) free HPV4 vaccination of girls and young women in Sweden and in Australia. As in Sweden, success in preventing genital warts in the Australian cohort was dependent on the age of vaccination.[47,70] Less than 1% of women aged under 21 years presenting at Australian sexual health clinics were found to have genital warts in 2011, compared with 10.5% in 2006 before the vaccination program started, a 93% reduction in this age group. By 2011, no genital warts were diagnosed in women under 21 who reported being vaccinated.[70] A significant but lesser 73% decline also occurred in genital wart diagnoses in 21- to 30-year-old women, a trend not observed in women older than this age, indicating that the decline in genital warts was not due to factors other than the vaccine.[70] A similar pattern of declining diagnoses, but of a lesser magnitude, seen in young heterosexual men was probably due to herd immunity.

Unfortunately, HPV vaccination uptake in the United States has been far less. In 2010, the vaccination coverage rates in the Australian school-based program were reported to be 83% for the first dose, 80% for the second dose, and 73% for the third dose in 12- to 13-year-olds, with coverage rates decreasing with increasing age.[70] In contrast, three-dose vaccine coverage in 2010 in the United States was only 32% among 13- to 17-year-olds.[48] However, despite low-coverage vaccine-type HPV prevalence decreased 56% among female teenagers 14 to 19 years of age, probably due to the high effectiveness of the vaccine and to herd immunity.[48] Among other age groups, vaccine-type HPV prevalence did not fall significantly. The vaccine effectiveness of at least one dose was 82%. This definitive demonstration of the effectiveness of the HPV4 vaccine prompted Dr. Thomas Frieden, Director of the CDC, to state "This report shows that HPV vaccine works well, and the report should be a wakeup call to our nation to protect the next generation by increasing HPV vaccination rates."[71] He noted that 50,000 girls alive today will develop cervical cancer over their lifetime that would have been prevented if we reach 80% vaccination rates and that for every year we delay in doing so, another 4400 girls will develop cervical cancer in their lifetime.[71]

18.3 SECONDARY PREVENTION THROUGH CERVICAL CANCER SCREENING

It is currently estimated that systematic screening can reduce death rates from invasive cervical cancer (ICC) by 70%.[4] The ability to detect and treat precursor lesions before progression to invasion was responsible for the continuing decline in cervical cancer rates from 14 per 100,000 women in 1973 to approximately 8 per 100,000 in 1994.[72] This decline continued at a much slower rate through the late 20th century, although a rise in incidence in the past decade, particularly in young women, has been reported in some countries despite cervical cancer screening programs.[73] Additionally, although cervical cancer rates have decreased for all races, significant differences by race and/or ethnicity persist. Hispanic and Black women continue to be at higher risk of developing ICC than White women.[74] However, disparities in cervical cancer incidence rates were recently shown to be eliminated for black women less than age 50 in comparison with similarly aged white women, but persisted for blacks aged 50 years and older.[5] In countries without cervical cancer screening, ICC continues to rank first or second among all cancers in women.[72] These differences in cervical cancer rates, both within racial/ethnic groups in the United States and in developing countries, are primarily due to differences in quality of, and access to, screening.

Even though HPV infection is common, the lifetime risk of cervical cancer for US women is estimated to be only 0.68%, primarily because most women in the United States receive cervical cancer screening.[75,76] Although screening with the Pap test has been very successful in lowering the rate of cervical cancer, 40% to 50% of women who get cervical cancer have had screening, and some have had screening as recommended.[75] Failures in screening occasionally occur because cervical cytology is relatively insensitive for the detection of cervical neoplasia and must be repeated frequently to achieve programmatic effectiveness.[4] The relatively greater risk of

missing important glandular lesions on cytology heightens concern.[77–79] Given that about half of the US women in whom cervical cancer develops have never been screened,[76] efforts aimed at encouraging women to be screened hold the most promise for reducing the incidence of, and mortality from, cervical cancer.[75,76] This is even more urgent considering that about half of cervical cancers detected in women with inadequate or no screening are not detected until late stage.[80] Unfortunately, women not receiving screening are most often those least likely to obtain preventative health care. However, clinicians can help increase screening attendance by offering a Pap test to women who are being seen for other reasons. For example, in one study of a large prepaid health plan with few barriers to access, most of the women with ICC had not had a Pap test in the 3 years before their diagnosis, even though most had attended the medical facility one or more times for other health issues, and had not received cervical screening.[81] Despite barriers to coverage, the Pap test is the most widely used cancer-screening tool in the United States, with more than 80% of women undergoing screening in any 2-year period and more than 90% having been screened at least once.[82]

By the 1960s, annual screening became the standard in the United States, partly to minimize the risk of missing any abnormal lesion and partly because it became equated with the "annual" gynecologic exam. Analyses of outcomes associated with annual screening have shown that in most instances it is excessive.[75,83] This is particularly true among women who have had multiple consecutive negative screens.[83,84] In 2007, Solomon et al.[85] estimated that if the screening strategy of annual cervical cytology did not change by 2010, approximately 75 million Pap tests would be done each year—a nearly 50% increase from the estimated 50 million performed in the mid-1990s (Figure 18.4). While part of this increase is due to a growing population, a considerable part is overscreening.

Beginning in the late 1990s and through the first decade of the 21st century, randomized screening trials and large cross-sectional observational studies comparing cervical cytology and HPV testing, separately and in combination, were conducted to determine whether a HPV DNA test, with or without cervical cytology, might increase sensitivity of screening and provide a more powerful risk-based approach to predicting adverse outcomes than cytology alone.[86–93] If so, safely extending the screening interval could reduce screening costs, better protect women screened irregularly, and reduce the number of transient HPV-induced cell changes detected when screening is annual. In 2003, the FDA approved HPV testing (Hybrid Capture 2 [hc2] High-risk HPV DNA Test, Qiagen, Gaithersburg, MD) as an adjunct to the Pap for primary cervical cancer screening of women aged 30 and over. This FDA approval subsequently resulted in the inclusion of HPV testing with the Pap (cotesting) for women ≥30 in the primary cervical screening guidelines issued in 2002 by the ACS,[94] in 2003[95] and 2009[96] by the ACOG, and in 2012 by the ACS/ASCCP/ASCP,[97] USPSTF,[98] and ACOG.[99] The 2012 guidelines all recognize cotesting as an alternative to screening by cytology alone as an option for extending the screening interval, but the ACS/ASCCP/ASCP and ACOG guidelines state that cotesting is *preferred*.[97,99]

18.3.1 Cervical Screening Technologies

18.3.1.1 Cytology-Based Cervical Screening Technologies

18.3.1.1.1 CONVENTIONAL CERVICAL CYTOLOGY

The reduction in cervical cancer incidence and mortality following the introduction of cervical cytologic screening[100] provided indirect proof of the value of screening with conventional

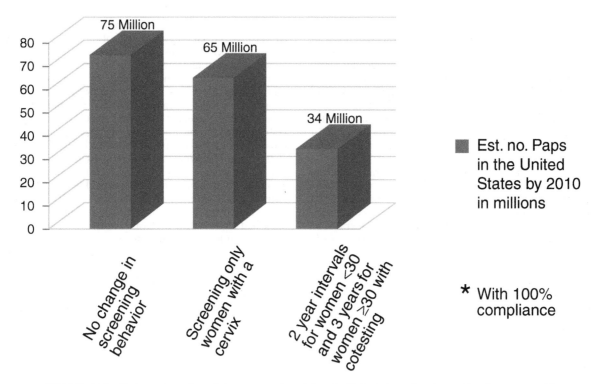

FIGURE 18.4. Estimated number of Pap tests projected for the United States in 2010 with adherence to different screening recommendations. (Adapted from Solomon D, Breen N, McNeel T. Cervical cancer screening rates in the United States and the potential impact of implementation of screening guidelines. *CA Cancer J Clin* 2007;57(2):105–11, with permission.)

cervical cytology (CC) despite the absence of any randomized trial on its effectiveness.[4] The average annual age-adjusted rate of cervical cancer among women before screening was introduced was estimated to be about 35/100,000, declining each decade[94,95] to the 8.1/100,000 incidence reported by the NCI in the most recent Surveillance, Epidemiology, and End Results (SEER) publication covering the years 2005 to 2009.[74,101,102] However, implementation of CLIA'88,[103] the Bethesda System,[104] and the CDC's National Breast and Cervical Cancer Early Detection Program[105] were all, to some degree, secondary to recognition of problems with the cervical cancer screening program.[106–108] Until the late 1990s, the sensitivity of cervical cytology was significantly overestimated. In 1999, the Agency for Health Care Policy and Research sponsored an analysis of the best 85 studies evaluating Pap sensitivity.[109] That review concluded that a single CC detected cervical cancer precursor lesions with only 51% sensitivity, overturning the conventional wisdom that the sensitivity of CC was approximately 80%.[109,110] Similar poor sensitivity of cervical cytology has been reported in other meta-analyses[111,112] and in RTCs.[94] Despite cervical cytology's mediocre sensitivity, its use has resulted in the dramatic reduction in cervical cancer incidence and mortality discussed previously. The success of all cervical cancer prevention programs is attributable to repeated screening of women during the relatively slow progression from incident HPV infection to precancer (typically approximately 10 years) and from precancer to cancer (typically 10 or more years) (Figure 18.5).[4,113,114] This long precursor phase provides room for "missed" lesions most commonly detected at some point prior to invasion.

18.3.1.1.2 LIQUID-BASED CYTOLOGY

During the 1990s, several technologic innovations revolutionized cervical cytologic screening, particularly the development of improved sampling devices, liquid-based collection systems, and computer-assisted screening.[115] Following the

1996 FDA approval of the first liquid-based cytology (LBC) (ThinPrep, CYTYC, Boxsborough, MA) and in 1999 the second (SurePath, TriPath, Burlington, NC), there have been two very different modalities used to prepare cervical cytology slides: conventional dry slide Pap tests (CC) and liquid-based Pap tests (LBC). By 2006, only a decade after the first FDA approval, nearly 90% of Pap tests done in the United States were liquid based.

LBC has a number of theoretical advantages over conventional cytology. These include more complete collection of exfoliated cells, random and presumably more representative transfer of exfoliated cells to slides, and improved microscopic visualization attributable to reduced overlapping, obscuring blood, and inflammation.[116-119] LBC also provides residual cells to test for HPV, *Chlamydia*, gonorrhea,[120,121] and other histochemical markers such as p16 and ProEXc once they, or others, become available. However, despite early studies that appeared to demonstrate superiority of LBC over CC, most of the studies conducted more recently failed to confirm improvement in sensitivity with LBC but have shown reduction in specificity. The 2008 meta-analysis of Arbyn et al. using the strictest criteria did not show a significant difference in either sensitivity or specificity, although there was a slight drop in specificity for LBC when atypical squamous cells of undetermined significance (ASC-US) were the threshold for colposcopy.[122] Two prior meta-analyses based on less stringent criteria concluded that LBC is more sensitive but possibly less specific than conventional cytology.[119,123] In the largest randomized controlled trial (RTC) of LBC compared to CC, LBC did not perform better than CC in relative sensitivity or positive predictive value (PPV) for detection of cervical cancer precursors.[124,125] However, LBC resulted in significantly fewer unsatisfactory tests. While specimen adequacy of LBC is generally improved,[126] identification of endocervical cells as a marker for sampling of the transformation zone is often more

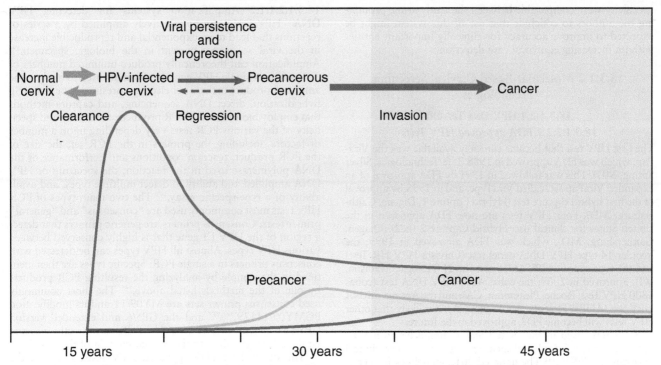

FIGURE 18.5. The peak prevalence of transient infections with carcinogenic types of HPV (*blue line*) occurs among women during their teens and 20s, after the initiation of sexual activity, and coincides with a high rate of ASC-US and LSIL Pap results. The peak prevalence of cervical precancerous conditions occurs approximately 10 years later (*green line*) and the peak prevalence of invasive cancers at 40 to 50 years of age (*red line*). (The peaks of the curves are not drawn to scale.) (From Schiffman M, Castle PE. The promise of global cervical-cancer prevention. *N Engl J Med* 2005;353(20):2101–4.)

difficult than with conventional Paps.[116,127,128] Several studies have shown that detection of glandular lesions by LBC is improved compared to detection rates noted with CC,[118,129,130] and specificity for glandular abnormality, including more accurate subcategorization of atypical glandular cytology (AGC) results, is also increased.[118,131] One study reported a 50% decline in the AGC rate with LBC, yet a fivefold increase in the PPV for AIS.

One clear advantage of LBC that has promoted widespread conversion to this technique is that the slides are markedly less fatiguing to read and can be read in far less time. One study demonstrated that time spent in reading LBC slides was half that spent on reading CC, at 4 minutes per slide compared to 8.[132] At the time of the deliberations on the 2002 ACS guidelines, the data on improved sensitivity of LBC appeared to support increasing the screening interval on women under the age of 30 for women screened with this technology but not for women screened with CC.[94] Clearly, further study did not support this differential. However, the improved visualization of the cells, decreased reading time, decreased unsatisfactory Pap tests, and the logistical advantage of having a representative specimen for ancillary testing have made LBC the dominant technology for cervical screening in the United States.[119,132,133]

The two dominant LBP technologies in the United States appear to have equivalent performance in PPV, atypical predictive value, and total predictive value.[134] One advantage of the SurePath system is the elimination of the problem of reduced cell recovery that can occur with ThinPrep technology secondary to lubrication and excessive mucus.[135] The 2009 College of American Pathologists (CAP) Interlaboratory Comparison Program survey found the most common reason for unsatisfactory Paps to be too few squamous cells.[133] One disadvantage of SurePath is that, as of 2013, HPV testing out of the SurePath liquid media has not been FDA approved.

One option to ameliorate this problem is to collect the HPV sample in a separate STM viral transport medium when the LBP is SurePath.

18.3.1.1.3 AUTOMATED SCREENING

The development of automated screening devices was originally driven more by the need to reduce the labor required for manual screening than by improvement in sensitivity.[136] Automated devices classify a set percentage of Paps as being so normal (negative) that they do not need to be reviewed by human eyes. One study of automated screening used a slide set highly enriched with abnormal thin-layer Paps, yet the automated screener was able to sort out 837/1275 (66%) as being so normal that they did not need human review and still detected 98% of the slides classified as high-grade squamous intraepithelial lesion (HSIL).[137] In contrast, 100% manual reading by cytopathologists of the same set of 1275 slides detected only 91% of the slides classified as HSIL. Such results suggest that automated cytology provides more rapid, accurate, standardized screening, while reducing labor and costs.[138] Automated screening instruments are now available that save digital images of cells appearing to be most abnormal. Sherman predicted in 2003 that eventually computer-assisted automated screening would permit expert cytologic reviews without microscopic reexamination of glass slides.[138] A more recent prospective, two-armed, masked clinical trial of the BD Focal-Point GS Imaging System (BD Diagnostics-TriPath, Burlington, NC) using SurePath slides comparing routine manual screening and quality control rescreening with computer-assisted, field-of-view screening, and device-directed quality control rescreening appears to substantiate this prediction.[139] The detection sensitivity for HSIL+ was increased by 19.6% and for LSIL+ by 9.8% in the computer-assisted arm, with small statistically significant decreases in specificity.[139] For ASC-US+, sensitivity and specificity were comparable between the study arms, prompting the authors to conclude that use of this system might be expected to improve accuracy for clinically important entities without increasing equivocal case detection.

18.3.1.2 Molecular-Based Cervical Screening Technologies

18.3.1.2.1 HPV Dna Testing

18.3.1.2.1.1 FDA-approved HPV Tests

The first HPV test that became clinically available was the Vira-Pap, which was FDA approved in 1988 (Life Technologies, Silver Spring, MD). This was followed in 1991 by FDA approval of an expanded ViraPap set, called ViraType, and in 1995 by approval of the first hybrid capture test (Hybrid Capture 1, Digene, Gaithersburg, MD). Four HPV tests are now FDA approved in the United States for clinical use: Hybrid Capture 2 (hc2) (Qiagen, Gaithersburg, MD), which was FDA approved in 1999; the Invader 14-type HPV DNA panel test (Cervista HPV HR Test) and the type-specific HPV 16/18 test [Inv2] (Hologic, Madison, WI), approved in 2009; the cobas 4800 HPV DNA test (cobas 4800 HPV Test, Roche, Pleasanton, CA); and the Aptima mRNA HPV test (AHPV, Hologic, San Diego, CA). It is likely that other HPV tests will become FDA approved in the future.

HPV tests used in the United States should be both FDA approved (for validity) and meet specific criteria for clinical performance.[16,97,140,141] The updated 2012 guidelines for cervical cancer screening were developed based on HPV tests with performance characteristics similar to the HPV tests used in the supporting evidence. The guidelines cannot be expected to balance the benefits and harms when using HPV tests with different performance characteristics.[16,97]

18.3.1.2.1.1.1 Hybrid Capture Systems for Detecting HPV The hybrid capture system is based on hybridization in solution of RNA probes complementary to the DNA of common, clinically relevant HPV types. Hybrid Capture 2 (hc2) has two separate test panels: a high-risk panel that tests for 13 high-risk HPV (hrHPV) types associated with cervical cancer (16, 18, 31,33, 35, 39, 45, 51, 52, 56, 58, 59, and 68) and a low-risk panel that tests for five low-risk HPV types (6, 11, 42, 43, and 44) that do not cause cervical cancer. All of the cervical cancer screening and management guidelines clearly state that testing for the low-risk panel is not indicated because these types do not cause cervical cancer.[12,15,16,97-99] If one of the 13 hrHPV types is present in the clinical specimen, the RNA probe that corresponds to that type will hybridize in solution and will then be captured by antibodies specific for the RNA:DNA hybrid. The "captured" hybrid is then detected by a series of reactions that give rise to a luminescence that can be measured in a luminometer.[142] The intensity of light emitted is proportional to the number of genomes present in the sample, providing a semiquantitative measure of the HPV viral load expressed as relative light units (RLU). The test is only semiquantitative for viral load because it does not standardize for the cellularity of the sample being tested. The hc2 test can be taken directly from the LBC sample, as is done for "reflex HPV testing" in ASC-US management, or it can be obtained by taking a separate sample in the manufacturer's proprietary viral transport media (STM).

The FDA-recommended cutoff value for test-positive results is 1.0 RLU (equivalent to 1 pg/mL HPV DNA or 5000 genomes). One issue perplexing to clinicians has been the report of "equivocal" hc2 HPV test results, reported to average 1.6%.[143] The problem of "equivocal" hc2 tests is that samples with a ratio ≥1.0 RLU/CO but <2.5 are retested as "low levels of HPV DNA detected." These "equivocal" values are then reported as positive for hrHPV if either of two subsequent test values equals or exceeds 1.0 RLU/CO. Samples that show <1.0 RLU/CO after two repeat tests are reported as negative for hrHPV.

18.3.1.2.1.1.2 Amplification systems for detecting HPV DNA HPV DNA can be selectively amplified by a series of reactions that lead to an exponential and reproducible increase in the viral sequences present in the biologic specimen.[144] Amplification can theoretically produce unlimited numbers of copies from a single HPV genome. Formats used to analyze the amplified product include gel electrophoresis, dot or line strip hybridization, direct DNA sequencing, and capture methods that employ biotin-labeled PCR products. Sensitivity and specificity of the various PCR tests vary depending upon a number of factors, including the primers in the PCR set, the size of the PCR product, reaction conditions and performance of the DNA polymerase used in the reaction, the spectrum of HPV DNA amplified and ability to detect multiple types, and availability of a type-specific assay.[142] The two main types of PCR HPV tests most commonly used are "consensus" and "general" primer tests. Consensus primers are generic primers that detect a region of the HPV L1 gene that is highly conserved between various HPV types. Almost all HPV types can be detected with consensus primers in a single PCR. Specific types are then identified in the sample by analyzing the resulting PCR products by one of the methods listed above.[145] The most commonly used consensus primer sets are MY09/11 and its modification PGMY09/11129,[146,147] and the GP5/6 and extended version GP5+/6+ general primer sets.[148,149] PCR can directly measure viral load standardized to the cellular content of the sample.[142]

The other three FDA-approved HPV tests, Cervista, the cobas 4800 HPV Test, and the Aptima mRNA HPV test, are amplification diagnostics but differ in important ways. The Cervista HPV DNA test is based on Invader technology, a signal amplification method for detecting specific nucleic acid sequences.[150] The reagents for the HPV HR test are provided as three oligonucleotide mixtures, which altogether detect the 14 types of HPV grouped according to their HPV phylogenetic relatedness. The HPV 16/18 genotyping test is separate from the panel test. A positive hrHPV result indicates that at least 1 of the 14 HR types is present in the DNA sample. For the separately ordered HPV 16/18 genotyping test, a positive result indicates that HPV 16, HPV 18, or HPV 16 and 18 have been detected in the sample. The test also has an internal control to confirm that a negative result is not due to insufficient sample and to ensure that the testing procedure was adequately performed. FDA approval included a statement that the Invader HPV 16, 18 test can be *"used adjunctively with the Cervista HPV HR test in patients with ASC-US cervical cytology results, to assess the presence or absence of specific high-risk HPV types. The results of this test are not intended to prevent women from proceeding to colposcopy."*[151] Appropriately, this was not further defined since there is as yet no consensus and no recommendation on how HPV 16, 18 genotyping would be used in the management of women with ASC-US cytology reports.

The cobas 4800 HPV Test is a real-time PCR test that simultaneously detects in three separate channels a total of 14 HR-HPV types: HPV16 individually, HPV18 individually, and 12 pooled HR-HPV genotypes (31, 33, 35, 39, 45, 51, 52, 56, 58, 59, 66, and 68) in addition to a separate beta-globin control.[152,153] It is reported out as positive or negative for the panel of 12 types that does not include HPV 16 and 18, and positive or negative for 16 and for 18 separately. It runs on a fully automated sample preparation system combined with real-time PCR, plus software that integrates the two components.[152] The test was approved in April 2011 for cotesting of women ≥30 and for triage of cytology specimens categorized as ASC-US and in 2014 for first-line primary cervical screening without initial cytology.[154]

The APTIMA mRNA HPV test is an in vitro nucleic acid amplification test for the qualitative detection of E6/E7 viral messenger RNA (mRNA) from 13 high-risk types of HPV (16, 18, 31, 33, 35, 39, 45, 51, 52, 56, 58, 59, and 68) and one "possible" high-risk type (type 66). The test is reported out as positive or negative for the panel of 14 types. The APTIMA HPV test is run on the fully automated TIGRIS DTS (Hologic, San Diego, CA) system.[155] Because the Aptima test detects increased production of mRNA from the two genetic loci (E6 and E7) most responsible for progression to CIN 3 and cervical cancer, specificity for these lesions has generally been shown to be higher than HPV DNA tests.[156–158] A separate APTIMA HPV 16/ 18/45 genotype assay has recently achieved FDA approval as a "reflex test" to an ASC-US cytology report or to a cytology–/HPV+ cotest result. The genotyping assay can differentiate HPV 16 from HPV 18 and/or HPV 45, but does not differentiate between HPV 18 and HPV 45.[155] As with other FDA-approved HPV tests, the indications for use include the statement that "Test results should be used together with the physician's assessment of cytology history, other risk factors, and professional guidelines that may be used to guide patient management" and that the "results of this test are not intended to prevent women from proceeding to colposcopy."[155]

With these FDA test approvals, clinicians and laboratories now have four HPV platforms to choose from.

18.3.1.2.1.2 Overview of the Clinical Utility of HPV Testing
The primary role of HPV testing initially was in the study of the etiology and natural history of HPV and cervical cancer. Once evidence of HPV involvement in the etiology of CIN and cervical cancer was confirmed, attention turned to using this new technology to improve cervical cancer screening and abnormal Pap management. Five main clinical uses of HPV testing have been delineated: (1) primary screening with, and without, the Pap test; (2) secondary triage of women with ASC-US and postmenopausal women with low-grade squamous intraepithelial lesion (LSIL); (3) follow-up of women with ASC-US or LSIL normal at colposcopy or only found to have CIN 1; (4) follow-up of women with AGC NOS and normal on initial evaluation; and (5) posttreatment test of cure. The use of HPV tests in the management of abnormal cervical screening results is discussed extensively in Chapter 19 and the use in posttreatment "test of cure" in Chapter 20.

18.3.1.2.1.2.1 HPV testing in primary cervical cancer screening
The principle of a cervical cancer screening strategy based on detection of persistent HPV infection was first discussed by Meijer et al. in 1992 following their documentation of increasing HPV prevalence with increasing grades of cervical dysplasia, with up to 100% of cervical carcinomas testing positive.[8] Based on this prevalence study, and on data demonstrating that progression of cervical lesions was always associated with persistent infection with hrHPV types, the potential of cervical cancer screening based on HPV detection was proposed.[8,11] Strong evidence of the predictive value of a hrHPV test was provided by the 10-year follow-up of 20,810 women from the 1992 Kaiser Northwest collaboration with the NCI.[159,160] Combined Pap and HPV testing (cotesting) divided the cohort into two distinctly different risk groups. The cohort with either an abnormal Pap (≥ASC-US) or a positive HPV test, or both, had a cumulative incidence of CIN 3+ at 10 years of nearly 7.0%, compared with 0.8% for women negative on both tests. Results were not greatly different when the results of the HPV test combined with cytology were evaluated, demonstrating that cytology did not add greatly to the predictive power of an HPV test (Figure 18.6).

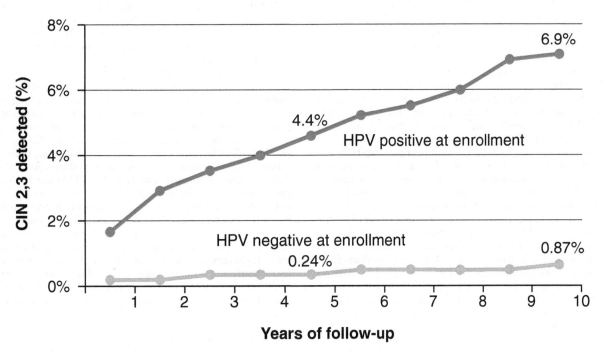

Kaiser Portland NCI Study

FIGURE 18.6.   The 10-year follow-up NCI HPV natural history study from Portland Kaiser has provided information on the risk of testing hrHPV positive at a single point in time compared to testing HPV negative. In this study, a single hrHPV-positive sample at enrollment predicted a risk of 4.4% for detection of CIN 3 by year 4 and nearly 7% by year 10. In contrast, the risk for CIN 3 for women testing negative was negligible despite the likelihood that many of these women must have been newly infected with hrHPV types during the subsequent 10-year follow-up. This clearly demonstrates the long-term reassurance provided by an initial negative HPV result. (Data from Sherman ME, Lorinzc AT, Scott DR, et al. Baseline cytology, human papillomavirus testing, and risk for cervical neoplasia: a ten year cohort analysis. *J Natl Cancer Inst* 2003;95:46–52.)

The combination of a negative Pap and negative HPV test provided strong reassurance that no prevalent disease was present, while a negative HPV test alone provided long-term reassurance that the future risk for disease was low.[11] These principles continue to guide the premise that the most valuable aspect of cotesting women ≥30 years with both cervical cytology and HPV testing is the reassurance provided that little high-grade disease or cancer is being missed, nor likely to occur over the next few years. Most of the available research on cotesting comes from countries with organized screening programs that can facilitate large screening studies, which are more difficult to do in the United States, where screening is opportunistic.[11] The earliest of these studies provided compelling evidence that HPV testing in primary cervical cancer screening, both combined as a cotest with the Pap and as a "stand-alone" test, was likely to provide 96% to nearly 100% reassurance that no CIN 2,3 or cancer was being missed.[161-167] However, randomized control trials (RCTs) and large population screening studies were needed to fully compare different screening strategies. By the start of the 21st century, several large ongoing evaluations of HPV testing and cytology in primary cervical screening were initiated.[11] Cuzick et al. in a 7-year follow-up study of over 2400 women in London reported that a negative HPV test (hc2) offered about twice the predictive value of a negative conventional Pap that CIN 2,3+ would not be found over the subsequent 6 years and was still more predictive of risk status at 9 years than cytology.[168] Additionally, a positive HPV test was far more predictive of increased risk in the follow-up period than a positive Pap, with substantially more CIN 2+ lesions found within 9 years of follow-up in those initially HPV positive than in those HPV negative. Little difference was noted according to initial cytology results.

In a 2008 evaluation of eight studies conducted in North America and Europe that paired hc2 hrHPV testing and cervical cytology, the pooled sensitivity for CIN 2+ of hc2 was 98.1% and the pooled specificity 91.7%.[169] In general, sensitivity of hc2 in primary screening for high-grade CIN was 33% higher than cytology at an ASC-US threshold for referral to colposcopy, but specificity was 6% lower. While Pap/HPV cotesting only marginally increased sensitivity over that of the HPV test alone, specificity was decreased by another 5% over that with hc2 alone. Specificity for CIN 2+ was increased by only sending to colposcopy cytology-negative/HPV-positive (cyto−/HPV+) women found 12 months following the initial screen to have either a repeat positive HPV test or an abnormal Pap, as recommended by current management guidelines.[13,15,16] The primary value of cotesting is the reassurance of the low risk of high-grade disease for several years for the approximately 90% of women who are cyto−/HPV−. In contrast, management of women testing cyto−/HPV+ has been compromised by issues of specificity and lack of an ideal follow-up solution to improve specificity. Therefore, other combinations of screening options needed to be evaluated.[11]

Results of the Swedescreen trial were reported in 2009 on 6257 women aged 32 to 38 screened with both conventional cytology and hc2 in a population-based randomized trial.[170] The trial evaluated the efficacy of 10 different cervical cancer screening strategies based on hrHPV DNA testing alone, cytology alone, and cotesting with both tests. When the threshold for referral to colposcopy for women cyto−/HPV+ was any abnormal Pap (≥ASC-US) or repeat hrHPV+ test at 12 months, cotesting was 35% more sensitive for CIN 3+ than Pap test alone.[170] Reduction in PPV was considered only modest. Of the 10 possible screening combinations, the most effective was screening first with an HPV test followed by a Pap test only among women with a positive HPV test. This increased the sensitivity for CIN 3+ by 30% over that detected in a cytology-only primary screening program, while maintaining a high PPV and increasing the number of screening tests by only 12% over the number presently done in Sweden, where the routine screening interval is every 3 years.[170] The authors concluded that the best screening option for women of this age was primary hrHPV DNA testing, followed by "reflex Pap testing" of hrHPV-positive women, and type-specific HPV testing of persistently Pap−/HPV+ women in 12 months.

18.3.1.2.1.2.2 Will more sensitive screening reduce the number of cervical cancers?

The benchmark for determining success of a cervical cancer screening program has been the incidence of cervical cancer. Heretofore, all such evaluations have been only on populations screened with conventional cytology. Hence, the question remains about whether incorporating LBC or HPV testing will favorably impact cervical cancer incidence and mortality beyond that obtained with conventional cytology. As discussed previously, LBC has some positive characteristics but is unlikely to further reduce the rate of cervical cancer since sensitivity for CIN 3 appears to be similar to that of conventional cytology.[122] A randomized population study of 38,000 women by Anttila et al.[168] supports the findings of other large RTCs, demonstrating increased detection of CIN 3+ when hrHPV testing is incorporated in primary cervical cancer screening.[171] As with the study by Naucler, cost-effectiveness was improved by screening with the hrHPV test alone, followed by "reflex" cytology testing of hrHPV-positive women. This provided nearly the same margin of safety demonstrated with cotesting, while eliminating one of the cotest elements (cytology) for the majority testing HPV negative. In the first 5-year (average 3.3) period of follow-up, 76 CIN 3+ cases (including six cancers) were detected in the HPV arm and 53 (including eight cancers) in the cytology arm. As expected, the incidence of CIN 3 subsequently detected following an HPV-negative test was lower than the incidence of CIN 3 detected following a normal cytology test. Longer-term follow-up will demonstrate whether detection and treatment of more CIN 3 in the initial round by HPV testing than by cytology result in fewer cancers subsequently being found in the women screened with the HPV test.

Ronco et al. demonstrated this clearly, as twice as many CIN 3 cases were detected and treated in their RCT in the women receiving cotesting than in the women receiving cytology alone.[93] At the next screen 3 years after randomization, no cancers were detected in the cotesting group compared to nine among women screened 3 years earlier by cytology alone (Table 18.5). The authors attributed this difference in cervical cancers found to the increased detection and treatment of CIN 3 in the women initially cotested. A 2009 study by Sankaranarayanan et al. demonstrated that a single round of HPV testing reduced both cervical cancer mortality and the number of cases of advanced cervical cancer.[172] In contrast, neither a single Pap test nor a single visual inspection after acetic acid (VIA) significantly impacted either incidence of advanced cervical cancers or mortality during the 9 years of follow-up. Importantly, not a single cancer occurred over this long period of follow-up in the 90% testing negative for HPV at enrollment despite all enrollees having never had a previous cervical cancer screen.

These studies provided the basis of the 2012 ACS/ASCCP/ASCP determination that a screening test or modality that immediately detected more CIN 3, thereby reducing the risk of CIN 3+ in the next screening interval, is of great benefit. Hence, the conclusion that the addition of HPV testing to cytology is beneficial.[97] However, it is also important to recognize that most cancers occur in unscreened and underscreened women. While more sensitive screening may reduce the risk of cervical cancer in underscreened women, a more sensitive screen will not impact the incidence of cancer in women never receiving screening. Getting these women in for any screening

TABLE 18.5	RELATIVE NUMBER OF CASES OF CIN 2, CIN 3, AND CERVICAL CANCER DETECTED AT INITIAL SCREENING OF WOMEN AGE 35–60 WITH HPV TESTING PLUS CYTOLOGY (COTEST) AND CYTOLOGY ALONE AND AT SUBSEQUENT SCREENING (MEDIAN ~3 Y LATER)					
	■ HPV TESTING GROUP			■ CYTOLOGY-ONLY GROUP		
■ SCREENING	■ CIN 2	■ CIN 3/AIS	■ CANCER	■ CIN 2	■ CIN 3/AIS	■ CANCER
Round one	108	98	6	54	47	8
Round two	8	8	0	15	17	7
Total over both rounds	116	106	6	69	64	15

From Ronco G, Giorgi-Rossi P, Carozzi F, et al.; New Technologies for Cervical Cancer screening (NTCC) Working Group. Efficacy of human papillomavirus testing for the detection of invasive cervical cancers and cervical intraepithelial neoplasia: a randomised controlled trial. *Lancet Oncol* 2010;11(3):249–57.

should make a major impact on cervical cancer rates, but more expensive screening or increasingly complex screening might create barriers to getting these women in. Diligence will be required to ensure that this does not occur.

18.3.1.2.1.2.3 Using HPV testing for cervical cancer screening: Pros and cons
The hallmarks of HPV testing are greater sensitivity but lower specificity for CIN 2+ and CIN 3+[94,168–171,173,174] and better reproducibility than cytology.[97,175] The concerns expressed about using HPV testing for cervical cancer screening relate to the lower specificity of the tests and to cost. Sensitivity of any test is improved by lowering the threshold for calling a test "positive." However, because lowered thresholds also bring in more women with normal results for evaluation, specificity almost always suffers as sensitivity increases. Improvement in sensitivity will result in missing few serious lesions, but achieving this success may require evaluation of many more women and, in a normal screening population, even small changes in specificity may require further evaluation of a very large number of normal women due to increases in false-positive results.[94] Whether maximizing sensitivity at the expense of specificity is most valued depends on many issues, not the least of which are societal expectations, costs, and medicolegal risks.[176,177] Although sensitivity of cervical cytology is not optimal, multiple screenings throughout life are highly effective in preventing most cervical cancers. In contrast, while Pap test sensitivity is low, specificity is high, particularly for cytology read as LSIL or HSIL. In contrast, specificity for cytology read as "atypical" is less due to the large number of normal women having this finding. Specificity for both conventional and LBC is reported to be in the range of 76% to 98%,[116,122,178] but rates below 94% are rarely reported in studies in the United States.

The low sensitivity of a single Pap test can be problematic for women receiving only infrequent screening. Additionally, about 30% of all cervical cancers occur among women with one or more prior Pap results read as normal but later found on review to have abnormal cells.[179] Even under ideal screening circumstances, an incidence rate of 2 to 3/100,000 can be expected.[179] Unfortunately, many women do not participate in regular screening. About half of the women with cervical cancer have never had a Pap, and another 10% have had a least one Pap but have not participated in adequate screening.[179] To improve outcomes among this cohort at considerably increased risk of cervical cancer, it is necessary to reduce barriers, to improve access to screening services and, when possible, to provide tests that will be most accurate and cost-effective. Unfortunately, many rarely and never screened women are indigent and underinsured, so that accessing any testing may be a formidable barrier. The potential for increased cost of the cervical cancer screening program secondary to the added cost of new technologies has been widely discussed and continues to be of some concern, particularly among public-funded programs with limited resources.[180,181] However, societal expectations of having a "perfect" test will likely continue to drive the use of tests with highest sensitivity. The advantage of HPV testing in primary screening is that HPV test results predict the risk of cervical cancer and CIN 3 better and longer than the cytologic and colposcopic abnormalities that result from HPV infection.[182] This longer "window" of safety should provide the reassurance clinicians require to extend cervical cancer screening intervals, but will almost inevitably meet with resistance, as current gynecologic and cytology laboratory practices are presently built on frequent screening.[182] If screening and management recommendations for the new technologies are followed, the initial increased cost of these technologies should be more than made up by the savings accrued with screening less frequently. However, excessive costs will accrue if the recommendations are not followed and women are overscreened. Education of clinicians, as well as of the general public, about harms that may occur with excessive screening is crucial.

18.3.2 Impediments to Screening

Clearly, ensuring that women receive risk-appropriate information about cervical cancer screening whenever they access health care is imperative if the rate of cervical cancer is to be further reduced. Several public health studies addressing access to cervical cancer screening concluded that cultural and social barriers and time restraints are more important impediments to access than cost and transportation.[183–185] Country of origin and current US geographic residence are important determinants of women's perspectives and knowledge of anatomy, experiences with the medical system, and access to services essential to developing effective cancer control interventions.[185] Although cervical cancer is considered a women's health issue, it cannot be addressed outside the sociopolitical structures of local communities, especially for immigrant women in the United States for <10 years. Others, however, conclude that economic barriers and lack of insurance also adversely impact access.[186,187] Women with disabilities, as a group, have been underinsured. This is an additional barrier to their accessing cervical cancer screening and other preventive services.[188] Multiple persistent barriers indicate why further reduction in the incidence of cervical cancer has been difficult to achieve. Research continues in this area, with the prospect that improved understanding of how to overcome these barriers will result in increased access to cervical cancer screening and other important health services for groups previously underscreened and without essential health care.[189,190]

18.4 PRIMARY CERVICAL CANCER SCREENING GUIDELINES

In 2012, new primary cervical cancer screening guidelines were published through the combined efforts of the ACS, the American Society for Colposcopy and Cervical Pathology (ASCCP), and the American Society for Clinical Pathology (ASCP).[97] At the same time, the U.S. Preventative Services Task Force (USP-STF) released new primary cervical screening guidelines that were nearly identical.[98] In late 2012, the ACOG joined the consensus agreement with its own release.[99] The new guidelines replace the 2002 ACS, 2003 USPSTF, and 2009 ACOG cervical cancer screening guidelines.[94,96,191] Each of these guidelines incorporates a much broader understanding of the trade-offs of benefits, harms, and opportunities that come with recommendations on when to begin screening, when to end screening, and how often to screen. Understanding the rationale and basic tenets (Table 18.6) for each of the recommendations is imperative since many represent a departure from standards of practice established for over a quarter of a century and widely accepted by providers and by the public. Of note, years after updated primary screening guidelines were published that made changes to recommendations on the age range of screening (when to begin and when to end) and on screening frequency, most surveys show that adherence to these recommendations has been moderate to poor.[192] In the next section, guidelines from each organization that are identical will be discussed together, and the rare differences will be pointed out.

It is also important to recognize that these guidelines only apply to cervical cancer screening in the general population; that is, they do not address screening of women in subpopulations who may need more intensive or alternative screening.[97-99] These subpopulations include women (1) with a history of cervical precancer or cancer; (2) exposed in utero to diethylstilbestrol (DES); and (3) who are immunocompromised (e.g., infection with the human immunodeficiency virus and organ transplant recipients).[97,99,193]

18.4.1 When to Begin Screening

Recommendation: Do not screen women before age 21
Rationale: In 1988, the ACS recommended that screening begin at the onset of vaginal intercourse or at age 18, whichever

came first.[194] Improved understanding of the natural history of cervical cancer and the role played by HPV has provided a far better appraisal of the most appropriate time to begin screening. There is almost no risk of developing cervical cancer within 5 years of first sexual exposure and very little risk during the subsequent 5 years. For this reason, cervical cancer is extremely rare in adolescents, and there continues to be very low risk for cervical cancer through the early 20s. The NCI's SEER program for the years 1998 to 2003 reported a cervical cancer incidence rate of 0.1 per 100,000 annually among girls aged 15 to 19 years (Table 18.7).[1] Based on this report and SEER data from 2002 to 2006, this translates to one to two cases of cervical cancer annually per 1,000,000 females aged 15 to 19 years.[1,96,102] Although one could argue the value of screening for even a few cases, the evidence suggests that screening does not reduce incidence of, and mortality from, cervical cancer in this age group.[97,99,195-197] The incidence rate of cervical cancer for women under age 20 is unchanged from the rate reported in the 1973 to 1977 period, which preceded the recommendation to start screening at age 18 or at first intercourse, whichever occurred first.[196] Because of this change in age to begin screening, adolescent populations went from no screening to considerable screening. A recent study in England showed that screening women aged 20 to 24 years old had no detectable impact on reducing cervical cancer rates, nor in rates of stage 1B cervical cancer or worse, in women under 30 years of age.[195] By contrast, screening older women leads to a substantial reduction in both incidence and mortality from cervical cancer. This is consistent with previous studies demonstrating no, or only modest, change in cervical cancer rates in women under the age of 30 in numerous countries in the decades following introduction of cervical cytology screening, compared to the reduction noted for all other age groups.[198,199] (Figure 18.7). Additionally, although incidence rates for cervical cancer peak at different ages for White, Black and Hispanic women, all ages and races showed significant decreases in incidence between 1995 to 1999 and 2000 to 2004 except among all women ages 15 to 24 and non-Hispanic/other category women ages 25 to 34.[74] This underscores the report that cervical cancer in adolescents and young women may not be prevented by cytology screening.[195]

The reasons that screening appears ineffective in these age groups are not clear, but one possible explanation is that cervical precancer that transits to invasion in adolescents and young women progresses so quickly and is so aggressive that screening does not make a difference.[198] It may also partially

---

TABLE 18.6   BASIC TENETS OF RISK-BASED STRATEGIES

- Preventing all cervical cancer is unrealistic. No screening test has perfect sensitivity, and therefore there will always be a residual cancer risk following any round of screening. More rapidly progressive cervical cancers, such as those occurring in women in their teens and early 20s, may not be preventable through feasible screening strategies.
- Reasonable risk is determined by the strategy of cytology alone as a benchmark. Cytology alone at 3-y intervals is consistently included in current guidelines of major professional societies and is generally accepted as the standard of care in the United States.[95-97] Screening strategies that achieve equivalent or better reductions in cervical cancer incidence and mortality, without an undue increase in harms, compared with cytology, would be acceptable options for consideration. The optimal balance of benefit and harm should be chosen so that equipoise is achieved between screening too frequently and finding mostly benign HPV infections or correlates of HPV infection (e.g., LSILs) or screening too infrequently and thereby exceeding the reasonable interval cancer risk threshold.
- Women at similar cancer risk should be managed independently of how the risk is measured (i.e., screening modality); women with similar cancer risk share the same tradeoffs of benefits and harms from routine screening, increased surveillance, referral to colposcopy, or treatment. It is therefore rational to provide the same care for similar women at similar cancer risk.
- Women at different ages may have different tradeoffs in benefits and harms from screening, which can be addressed through the development of age-specific screening recommendations.

From Saslow D, Solomon D, Lawson HW et al.; for the American Cancer Society; American Society for Colposcopy and Cervical Pathology; American Society for Clinical Pathology. American Cancer Society, American Society for Colposcopy and Cervical Pathology, and American Society for Clinical Pathology screening guidelines for the prevention and early detection of cervical cancer. *Am J Clin Pathol* 2012;137(4):516–42.

TABLE 18.7	ANNUAL COUNTS, AGE-ADJUSTED INCIDENCE RATES AND MEDIAN AGE AT DIAGNOSIS OF INVASIVE CERVICAL CARCINOMA AGE: UNITED STATES, 1998–2003			
■ AGE	■ AVERAGE ANNUAL	■ INCIDENCE RATE (95% CI)	■ PERCENT	■ MEDIAN AGE
All ages	10,846	8.9 (8.8–9)	100	47
Age, y				
0–14	0	0.0		
15–19	14	0.2 (0.1–0.2)	0.1	
20–24	123	1.6 (1.5–1.7)	1.1	
25–29	543	6.9 (6.7–7.2)	5.0	
30–34	1045	12.3 (12–12.6)	9.6	
35–39	1350	14.6 (14.3–14.9)	12.5	
40–44	1534	16.3 (15.9–16.6)	14.1	
45–49	1323	15.4 (15–15.7)	12.2	
50–59	1958	14.5 (14.2–14.7)	18.0	
60–69	1352	14.8 (14.5–15.1)	12.5	
70–79	1008	12.9 (12.6–13.3)	9.3	
≥80	595	11.2 (10.9Y11.6)	5.5	

From Watson M, Saraiya M, Benard V, et al. Burden of cervical cancer in the united States, 1998–2003. *Cancer* 2008;113(10 suppl):2855–64.

reflect an increasing incidence in women under 30 of cervical adenocarcinoma, whose precursor lesion is poorly detected by cytology.[138,200,201]

While cervical cancer is very rare in adolescents and very young women, HPV infections and LSIL are both extremely common and frequently appear shortly after the onset of sexual activity (Figures 18.8 and 18.9).[17,202–205] There is now good evidence that in adolescents ≥90% of HPV infections, LSIL cytology, and CIN 1 lesions will regress within 3 years.[206,207] This epidemiologic evidence strongly supports not screening adolescents and observing rather than treating young women with LSIL cytology and CIN 1 histopathology

results.[198] High rates of new HPV infection (50% will have a repeated or new infection within 3 years), detection of hrHPV in over 70% of adolescents with ASC-US, and the high rate of regression of CIN 2 do not support screening this population.[208–211] It has been estimated that when screening starts at a very young age, approximately 50% of screen detected and treated CIN 2,3 would likely have resolved spontaneously by age 25 if screening had not begun until that age.[195,201] Progression to cancer, even among those with CIN 3, appears to be negligible, as there are no published natural history studies in adolescents showing progression from CIN 2,3 to cancer.[198]

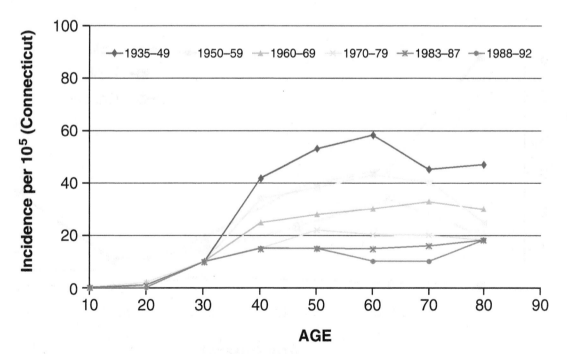

FIGURE 18.7.   Gustaffsson evaluated cervical cancer rates in Connecticut from the period prior to the onset of cervical screening in 1949 to 1992. Dramatic decreases in cervical cancer incidence occurred in all age groups except for women under age 30. For this latter group, no change in cervical cancer incidence could be demonstrated during the 43 years of screening. (From Gustafsson L, Ponten J, Zack M, Adami HO. International incidence rates of invasive cervical cancer after introduction of cytological screening. *Cancer Causes Control* 1997;8:755–63, with permission.)

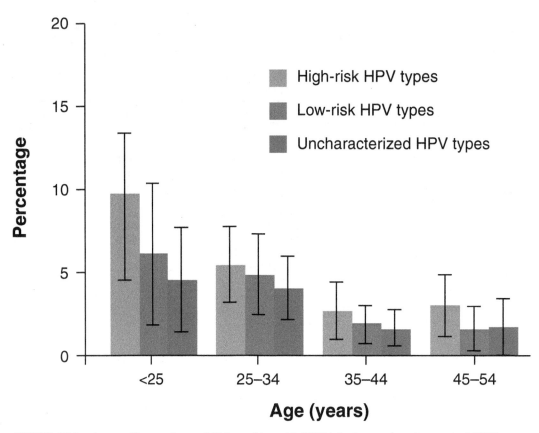

FIGURE 18.8.   Age-specific prevalence of high- and low-risk HPV infections and uncharacterized HPV types. (From Frazer IH, Cox JT, Mayeaux EJ Jr, et al. Advances in prevention of cervical cancer and other human papillomavirus-related diseases. *Pediatr Infect Dis J* 2006;25(2 suppl):S65–81, quiz S82, with permission; data from Herrero R, Hildesheim A, Bratti C, et al. Population-based study of human papillomavirus infection and cervical neoplasia in rural Costa Rica. *J Natl Cancer Inst* 2000;92:464–474.)

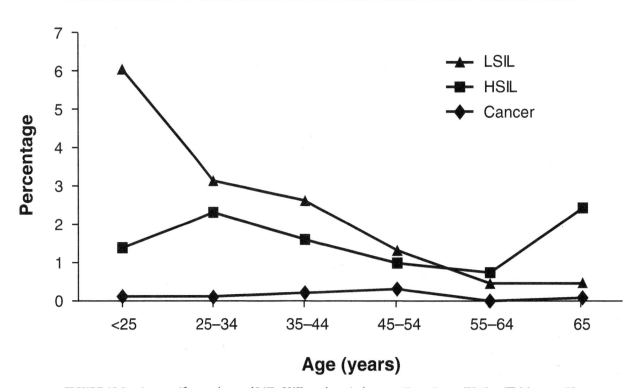

FIGURE 18.9.   Age-specific prevalence of LSIL, HSIL, and cervical cancer. (From Frazer IH, Cox JT, Mayeaux EJ Jr, et al. Advances in prevention of cervical cancer and other human papillomavirus-related diseases. *Pediatr Infect Dis J* 2006;25(2 suppl):S65–81, quiz S82, with permission.)

There are also extensive data that screening adolescents may be harmful. Adverse psychological effects related to cervical cancer screening, evaluation of abnormal cytology results, and treatment of CIN are reported to have adverse consequences, including negative effects on sexual functioning, particularly because adolescence is a time of heightened concern for self-image and emerging sexuality.[96,212-214] Numerous studies show that cervical excision procedures, including LEEP, increase the risk of premature delivery and low birth weight babies.[215-217] The majority of studies on pregnancy outcomes following LEEP demonstrate a two- to threefold increase in adverse pregnancy outcomes.[215,217,218] In studies where the depth of treatment was specified, the risk of preterm delivery was greater if the depth was >10 mm than if it was <10 mm (RR 2.6, 95% CI 1.3 to 5.3)[215,217] and when the patient had more than one excisional procedure.[217] There are no data demonstrating an adverse effect of treatment on fertility.[212] Because adolescents have most or all of their childbearing years ahead of them, it is important to avoid unnecessary excision or ablation of the cervix.[96,219] This overtreatment, and subsequent increased risk of reproductive problems, represents a net harm.[97,198] The best way to prevent unnecessary cervical treatment of adolescents is to avoid screening this age group in the first place.

With all of these issues in mind, all three guidelines (ACS/ASCCP/ASCP, USPSTF, and ACOG) recommend the following based on good and consistent scientific evidence (Level A or Strong Evidence): Cervical cancer screening should begin at age 21 years. Adolescent girls and young women <21 years of age should not be screened regardless of age of initiation of sexual

TABLE 18.8	WHEN TO BEGIN SCREENING

ACS/ASCCP/ASCP and ACOG[96,98]:
- **Age 21:** Women aged younger than 21 y should not be screened.
  - Cervical cancer screening should begin at age 21 y regardless of the age of sexual initiation or other risk factors.

USPSTF[97]:
- **Age 21:** Recommends against screening for cervical cancer in women younger than age 21 y.
  - There is adequate evidence that screening women younger than age 21 y (regardless of sexual history) does not reduce cervical cancer incidence and mortality compared with beginning screening at age 21 y.

activity or other risk factors (Table 18.8).[97-99] ACS stresses that adolescent cervical cancer prevention programs should focus on universal HPV vaccination, which is safe, highly efficacious, and, when used in adolescents before they become sexually active, highly effective and cost-effective.[97] The ACS and ACOG also recommend that adolescents continue to have access to appropriate health care, including assessment of health risks; family planning and contraception; and prevention counseling, screening, and treatment of sexually transmitted infections[97,99,198] (Figure 18.10). These measures may be

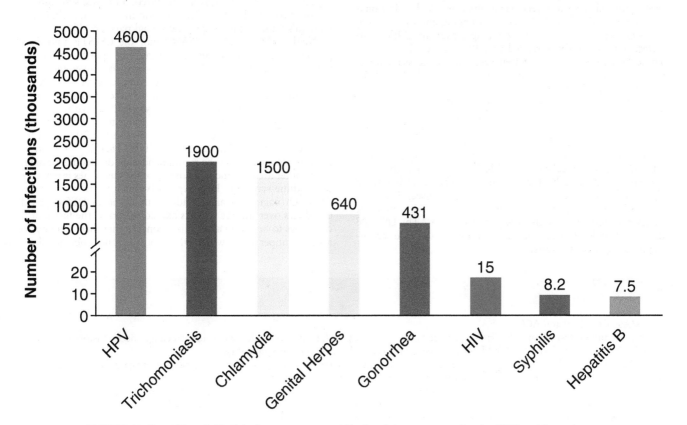

FIGURE 18.10. Although HPV is the most common STD in adolescents, screening for HPV at this age is not helpful because there is no treatment for the virus itself and most HPV infections are transient. In contrast, it is important to screen adolescent sexually active girls and young women for STDs that do have treatments available and can cause considerable harm. Here is demonstrated the annual incidence of common sexually transmitted infections among Americans 15 to 24 years old. (From Frazer IH, Cox JT, Mayeaux EJ Jr, et al. Advances in prevention of cervical cancer and other human papillomavirus-related diseases. *Pediatr Infect Dis J* 2006;25(2 suppl):S65–81, quiz S82, with permission; data from Weinstock H, Berman S, Cates W Jr. Sexually transmitted diseases among American youth: incidence and prevalence estimates, 2000. *Perspect Sex Reprod Health* 2004;36:6–10.)

carried out without cervical cytology and, in the asymptomatic patient, without the introduction of a speculum.

18.4.2 When to Discontinue Screening

Recommendation: No screening after age 65 for women with adequate negative prior screening and no history of CIN 2+ within the last 20 years

Rationale: Women aged 65 years and older represent 14.3% of the US population but have 19.5% of new cases of cervical cancer.[96,102,220] Among white women in the United States, the rate of new-onset cervical cancer decreases following peak incidence in the middle 40s. In Hispanic and Pacific Island women, the peak incidence is in the early 70s and in the late 70s, respectively. Among African American women, the incidence of cervical cancer continues to increase throughout life.[96,102] These statistics would appear to argue for continued cervical screening of older women. However, cervical cancer that occurs in women aged 65 to 70 or over is almost entirely in the rarely or never screened portion of the population, or in women without a history of three recent consecutive normal cytology results.[221] Additionally, the prevalence of CIN 2+ in well-screened women >65 is low,[222] and the long natural history of progression of incident HPV infections to invasive cancer provides reassurance that newly detected CIN 3 after age 65 years would rarely have sufficient time to progress to invasion in the woman's lifetime.[97] Therefore, continuing to screen women in this age group with a history of several recent normal cervical screening results offers little additional protection, and the epithelial effects of aging and of declining estrogen often produce cellular changes that are difficult to differentiate from those related to HPV and neoplasia.[97,99,138] These "misclassified" Paps often result in unnecessary anxiety, overevaluation, and increased costs with little patient benefit.[96] The age to discontinue screening (65) was chosen as the best age to balance the benefits and harms of screening in older women.[97] Guidelines from the ACS, USPSTF, and ACOG are now all in agreement that cervical cancer screening should be discontinued in women older than 65 with evidence of adequate negative prior screening and no history of CIN 2, CIN 3, AIS, or cervical cancer (Table 18.9).[97-99] Adequate prior screening is defined by the ACS and ACOG as either three consecutive negative cytology results or two consecutive negative cotest results within the previous 10 years, with the most recent test performed within the past 5 years.[97,99] The USPSTF does not provide a recommendation on when to cease screening based on cotest results.

18.4.3 Screening after Hysterectomy

Recommendation: No screening after hysterectomy for women with no history within the last 20 years of CIN 2+

Rationale: Vaginal cancer is one of the rarest of gynecologic malignancies, with an incidence of 1 to 7/1,000,000 women per year.[2] However, abnormal Pap test results in women having hysterectomy with removal of the cervix are fairly common, primarily due to minor cytologic changes secondary to estrogen deficiency.[94] High-grade abnormal vaginal cytology is uncommon and rarely identifies clinically important lesions. A systematic literature review of 19 studies with 6543 women post hysterectomy for benign indications (no cervical abnormalities) and 5043 women posthysterectomy for CIN 3 showed that 1.8% of the women with hysterectomy for benign indications had an abnormal cytology result, only 0.12% had VaIN on biopsy, and no cases of cancer were found.[223] In contrast, 14.1% of the women with CIN 3 prehysterectomy had abnormal cytology, 1.7% had VaIN on biopsy, and there was one case of cancer diagnosed within 3 years of the hysterectomy.[223] Therefore, continued vaginal cytology examinations are not cost-effective for women having a hysterectomy for benign indications, in particular because of the very low risk of developing vaginal cancer and the likelihood of causing anxiety and overtreatment.[96,97-99] Therefore, all three guidelines recommend against vaginal cuff screening of women at any age without a history of CIN 2+ following a hysterectomy with removal of the cervix (Table 18.10). Evidence of adequate negative prior screening is not required, and once screening is discontinued, it should not resume for any reason, including a woman's report of having a new sexual partner.[97-99]

Neither the ACS/ASCCP/ASCP nor the USPSTF guidelines provide recommendations for screening posthysterectomy women with a history of CIN 2+. However, because women with a history of CIN 2,3 can develop recurrent precancer or cancer at the vaginal cuff years postoperatively,[223-225] the ACOG guidelines recommend that women with a history of CIN 2+ within the last 20 years, or of cervical cancer ever, continue to be screened after total hysterectomy by cytology every 3 years for 20 years after the initial posttreatment surveillance (Table 18.10).[96,99] HPV testing was not included in the recommendation due to lack of data.

Another area not included in any of the guidelines is whether to continue screening DES-exposed women posthysterectomy. Although vaginal clear cell adenocarcinoma in DES-exposed daughters over the age of 50 is exceedingly rare, the fact that it continues to be found at all raises concern that there may be no absolute upper age at which DES exposure is no longer a risk.[226]

TABLE 18.9	WHEN TO CEASE SCREENING

ACS/ASCCP/ASCP and ACOG[96,98]:
- **Age 65 and no history of CIN 2+:** Women aged older than 65 y with evidence of adequate prior screening and no history of CIN 2+ within the last 20 y should not be screened for cervical cancer with any modality.
  - Adequate negative prior screening is defined as 3 consecutive negative cytology results or 2 consecutive negative cotests within the 10 y before ceasing screening, with the most recent test occurring within the past 5 y.
  - Once screening is discontinued, it should not resume for any reason, even if a woman reports having a new sexual partner.
- **Age 65 with history of CIN 2+:** Following spontaneous regression, or appropriate management of CIN 2, CIN 3, or AIS, routine screening should continue for at least 20 y (even if this extends screening past age 65 y).

USPSTF[97]:
- **Age 65:** There is adequate evidence that screening women older than age 65 y who have had adequate prior screening and are not otherwise at high risk provides little to no benefits.
  - Screening may be clinically indicated in older women for whom the adequacy of prior screening cannot be accurately accessed or documented.
  - Screening in women older than age 65 y who are otherwise considered high risk may be appropriate, such as women with a CIN 2, CIN 3, or AIS or cervical cancer, women with in utero exposure to DES, and women who are immunocompromised.

TABLE 18.10   SCREENING AFTER HYSTERECTOMY

<u>No History of CIN 2+</u>
ACS/ASCCP/ASCP and ACOG[96,98]:
- Women at any age following a hysterectomy with removal of the cervix who have no history of CIN 2+ should not be screened for vaginal cancer using any modality.
  - Evidence of adequate negative prior screening is not required.
  - Once screening is discontinued, it should not resume for any reason, including a woman's report of having a new sexual partner.

USPSTF[97]:
- There is convincing evidence that continued screening after hysterectomy with removal of the cervix for indications other than a high-grade precancerous lesion or cervical cancer provides no benefits.
- The USPSTF recommends against screening for cervical cancer in women who have had a hysterectomy with removal of the cervix and who do not have a history of a high-grade precancerous lesion (CIN grade 2 or 3) or cervical cancer.
- Clinicians should confirm through review of surgical records or direct examination that the cervix was removed.

<u>History of CIN 2+</u>
ACS/ASCCP/ASCP[96]:
- Women who have had a hysterectomy for cervical intraepithelial lesions may be at an increased risk of vaginal cancer, but the data are limited.
- Women who discontinue screening should continue to obtain age-appropriate preventive health care.

ACOG[98]:
- Women should continue to be screened if they have a total hysterectomy and have a history of CIN 2+ in the past 20 y or cervical cancer ever.
  - The role of HPV testing in this population has not been clarified.
  - Therefore, screening with cytology every 3 y for 20 y after the initial posttreatment surveillance period seems reasonable.

USPSTF[97]:
- No recommendation

18.4.4 Screening Interval

18.4.4.1 Screening Women Aged 21 to 29 Years

Recommendation: For women aged 21 to 29 years, screening with cytology alone every 3 years is recommended (Table 18.11).

TABLE 18.11   SCREENING INTERVALS FOR WOMEN AGED 21–29

ACS/ASCCP/ASCP[96]:
- For women aged 21–29 y, screening with cytology alone every 3 y is recommended.
  - For women aged 21–29 y with 2 or more consecutive negative cytology results, there is insufficient evidence to support a longer screening interval (i.e., more than 3 y).
- HPV testing should not be used to screen women in this age group, either as a stand-alone test or as a cotest with cytology.

USPSTF[97]:
- The USPSTF recommends screening for cervical cancer in women aged 21 to 29 y with cytology (Pap smear) every 3 y

ACOG[98]:
- Women aged 21–29 should be tested with cervical cytology alone, and screening should be performed every 3 y. Cotesting should not be performed in women younger than 30 y.

18.4.4.2 Screening Women Aged 30 to 65 Years

Recommendation: For women aged 30 to 65 years, screening with cytology alone every 3 years is *acceptable* or cotesting every 5 years is *preferred*[*97–99] (Table 18.12).

TABLE 18.12   SCREENING INTERVALS FOR WOMEN AGED 30–65

ACS/ASCCP/ASCP[96]:
- Women aged 30–65 y should be screened with cytology and HPV testing ("cotesting") every 5 y (preferred) or cytology alone every 3 y (acceptable).
- There is insufficient evidence to change screening intervals in this age group following a history of negative screens.

USPSTF[97]:
- The USPSTF recommends screening for cervical cancer in women aged 30–65 y with cytology (Pap smear) every 3 y, or for women who want to lengthen the screening interval, screening with a combination of cytology and HPV testing every 5 y.

ACOG[98]:
- In women 30–65 y of age, screening with cytology alone every 3 y is acceptable. Annual screening should not be performed.
- Cotesting with cytology and HPV testing every 5 y is *preferred.*

All Three Screening Guidelines[90–92]:
- Women who have a history of cervical cancer, have HIV infection or otherwise immunocompromised, or were exposed to DES in utero should not follow routine screening guidelines.

---

*The only difference in these recommendations is that the USPSTF does not use the descriptors "acceptable" or "preferred."

18.4.4.3 Rational for Screening Interval Recommendations

18.4.4.3.1 Screening Interval with Cytology

Over time, improved understanding of the natural history of cervical cancer and the harms associated with excessive screening has increased recognition that prior recommendations for annual screening were excessive. Today, there is little evidence to support the annual screening of women at any age by any screening test, method, or modality.[97] The predicted lifetime risk of death from cervical cancer is only 0.05 per 1000 women screened by cytology every 3 years, the same for every 2 years, and only minimally reduced to 0.03 for women screened annually.[227,228] In contrast to the only small reduction in mortality with annual cytology screening, when compared to triennial, colposcopy rates dramatically increase as screening intervals decrease regardless of the modality employed.[97,229,230] While these studies support the conclusion that increasing the cytology screening interval from 1 to 3 years only minimally increases the risk for cervical cancer, the risk of cancer increases significantly when intervals are prolonged beyond 3 years even after controlling for prior negative cytology tests.[96,231–234] From all the data on risks and benefits at each screening interval, the ACS concluded that a 3-year interval for cytology provides an appropriate balance of benefits and harms. Prolonging the screening interval beyond 3 years for cytology only was not supported, even with a screening history of consecutive negative cytology tests.[97] When screening with cytology alone, there was insufficient evidence to recommend different screening intervals for women aged 21 to 29 and women aged 30 to 65 years.[97–99]

Despite reassuring evidence that screening at least every 3 years does not radically increase cervical cancer rates but does radically increase harms and cost, clinicians and their patients have resisted changes in recommended screening intervals. Part of this has been secondary to provider concern that attendance for preventative health exams, that is, the "annual exam," will decline if annual cervical cytology screening does not continue. There is also provider fear that the absence of an organized system to invite women in for screening at guaranteed intervals will likely result in some women postponing screening for 4 or 5 or more years and increase the risk of interval high-grade disease and cancer. Additionally, there is concern that extending the cytology screening interval may increase the risk of missing AIS, already missed by cervical cytologic screening in increased proportion to squamous lesions, and contribute further to an already increasing rate of adenocarcinoma.[200,235]

18.5.4.3.2 Screening Interval with Cotesting

Prior to the 2002 ACS and 2003 ACOG recommendations, increased screening intervals were recommended only for women with three consecutive normal Pap results who were considered at low risk for cervical neoplasia on the basis of the cytology results and mostly nonverifiable patient risk factors such as age of onset of intercourse, number of partners, number of her partner's partners, and history of smoking.[97,236] However, most women had one or more of these "high-risk" factors. Additionally, the partner's history could almost never be verified. The result was that most clinicians did not feel comfortable increasing the screening interval for any woman. The strict association of HPV with CIN 3 and cervical cancer, and numerous evaluations of HPV testing as an adjunct to the Pap, provided the basis for the 2012 recommendations from all three guideline groups that included HPV testing and cervical cytology (cotesting) as an option for screening women aged 30 and older.[97–99] All three groups also recommend that HPV testing should not be used to screen women under the age of 30 because of the high prevalence of transient HPV infection in women <30.[97–99]

The addition of the word "preferred" by the ACS/ASCCP/ASCP and ACOG to the cotesting option will likely make cotesting the standard for primary cervical screening of women in this age group. Insurance and government coverage for HPV testing are now broad and not likely to be a prohibitive factor. Management algorithms have been developed to minimize as much as possible the increase in colposcopy evaluation that comes with using a less specific test, and several studies are reassuring that the number of women added to the follow-up pool of abnormal screening results is not excessively burdensome.[89] Only 3.99% of the 812,596 women aged 30 and above cotested between 2003 and 2008 in the Kaiser Permanente Northern California clinics were cytology−/HPV+.[89] The rate was highest for women ages 30 to 34 (6.76%) and lowest for women ages 60 to 64 (2.56%). Overall, 6.27% of women ages 30 and over were HPV+, and 90% tested cytology negative/HPV negative (Figure 18.11). These results are similar to the findings in the 47,000-patient ATHENA study that found 6.1% of the women ages ≥30 with cytology normal/HPV positive.[237]

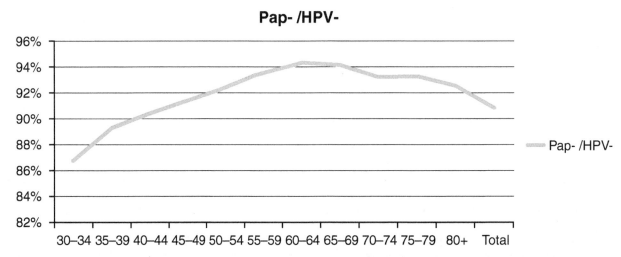

Pap- /HPV-

FIGURE 18.11.   Pap-negative HPV/negative rate per 5-year age groups in over 812,000 women in the Kaiser Permanente Northern California HMO between 2003 and 2008. For these women, the next cervical screen should not be before 3 years, and safety is projected for at least 5 to 6 years. (Adapted from Castle PE, et al. Five-year experience of human papillomavirus DNA and Papanicolaou test cotesting. *Obstet Gynecol* 2009;113:595–600, with permission.)

Cotesting was recommended by the ACS and ACOG as the preferred method of screening women ages 30 and older because, in the majority of studies reviewed, the addition of HPV testing to cytology resulted in increased detection of prevalent CIN 3 when compared to cytology screening alone, and a decrease in CIN 3 and cancer in subsequent screening rounds.[93,97,170,238] HPV testing is, on average, 25% to 40% more sensitive than a single cytology for detecting CIN 3+.[86–88,93,166–171,229,239–241] Additionally, it is relatively easy to standardize the procedure for HPV testing, so that interlaboratory variation is minimal.[175] The 2005 ACOG Practice Bulletin highlighted the reassurance provided by a double-negative test result with the statement, "Because HPV DNA testing is more sensitive than cervical cytology in detecting CIN 2,3, women with negative concurrent test results can be reassured that their risk of unidentified CIN 2,3 or cervical cancer is approximately 1/1000."[14]

The very high protective value of cotesting not only is for present disease but also predicts low risk for a number of years in the future.[87,241] The Joint European Cohort Study demonstrated the margin of safety of a negative HPV test is at least 6 years (Figure 18.12).[87] In this study, the 6-year risk of CIN 3+ was 0.27% following a negative HPV test compared to a 3-year CIN 3+ risk of 0.51% and a 6-year CIN 3+ risk of 0.97% for women screened by cytology alone. In a retrospective observational study of 330,000 women ages 30 years and older cotested at 3-year intervals in routine clinical practice, women with initial dually negative cotest results who were HPV and/or cytology positive 3 years later were at a lower risk

of CIN 3 or cancer than women with an initial HPV and/or cytology positive result at their initial screen.[97,242] This and the preceding data provide additional reassurance of the safety of extending the screening interval after negative cotesting. This is particularly important because the women at highest risk are those screened infrequently or not at all.

Another important advantage of adding HPV testing to cytology in screening is that molecular testing enhances the identification of women with adenocarcinoma of the cervix and its precursors.[171,200,219,242] This is particularly important because of the relative ineffectiveness of cytology in detection of glandular neoplasia and the increasing incidence of adenocarcinoma in countries screened exclusively by cytology.[243–245]

In contrast to the increased sensitivity of cotesting, specificity is decreased. To mitigate at least some of the harms (i.e., increased colposcopies and possible unnecessary treatment) secondary to decreased specificity of the screening test, the interval can be extended as long as such extension does not increase the risk of interval cervical cancer. Hence, the ACS/ASCCP/ASCP guideline development process concluded that if the incident cervical cancer rates associated with cytology at 3-year intervals are acceptable and cotesting at 5-year intervals provides similar or lower cancer risk,[242] then both options for screening women ≥30 are reasonable, but that cotesting is *preferred*.[97,99] All three guideline groups recommend that combined screening be done no more frequently than every 5 years for women testing negative for both cytology and HPV, because overscreening would increase cost without benefit and potentially result in the overtreatment of many women having

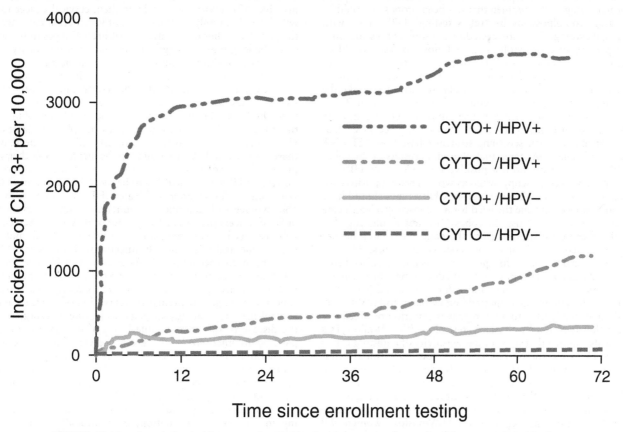

FIGURE 18.12.   Cumulative incidence rate for CIN 3+ for women according to baseline test results in the first 72 months of follow-up in all seven countries demonstrates significant reassurance of safely extending the screening interval for women with both normal cytology and a negative HPV test. Even women with abnormal cytology but negative HPV test had low long-term risk. (Adapted from Dillner J, Rebolj M, Birembaut P, et al.; Joint European Cohort Study. Long term predictive values of cytology and human papillomavirus testing in cervical cancer screening: joint European cohort study. *BMJ* 2008;337:a1754, with permission.)

only transient HPV infections.[97–99] The potential for increased harm due to the decrease in specificity of the HPV test also serves as the basis for the recommendation that cotesting is only for women ages ≥30, as the likelihood of being HPV positive in the absence of disease decreases with increasing age. Even women in this age group have a relatively low likelihood of having CIN 2/3 when they are cytology–/HPV+ and have been previously screened. In the Portland NCI prospective study, the risk of detection of a high-grade lesion over the 3 to 5 years following a cytology–/HPV+ was 4.4% but only 0.24% for women testing cytology–/HPV–.[159] Management of cytology–/HPV+ cotest results is discussed in Chapter 19.

18.4.5 Will HPV Testing as a Stand-Alone Become the Primary Screen?

Recommendation: In most clinical settings, women aged 30 to 65 years should not be screened with HPV testing alone as an alternative to cotesting at 5-year intervals or cytology alone at 3-year intervals.[97]

Rationale: At the time that the 2012 guidelines were written, no HPV test had been FDA-approved as a stand-alone test for primary cervical cancer screening. However, this 2012 recommendation is likely to change secondary to the May 2014 FDA approval of the cobas HPV test as a first-line primary cervical screening test for women aged 25 years and over.[246] Its use in the United States now awaits guideline recommendations for the management of various combinations of results that will occur with this new screening modality. One option for managing HPV+ women that has been proposed would be to triage to colposcopy by "reflex testing" HPV+ tests with cervical cytology.[97,170] However, data to estimate how the clinical performance of cytology (as a follow-up test) would be affected by a priori knowledge of positive HPV status is not yet available. Would knowledge that every cytology being reviewed was accompanied by an HPV-positive test make the reading more accurate, or result in biased overreading? The FDA approval did outline a recommendation that mirrors the algorithm found to be most effective in a recent evaluation of nine cervical screening strategies based on ATHENA data.[246,247] The FDA stated that "Based on results of the cobas HPV test, women who test positive for HPV 16 or HPV 18 should have a colposcopy, whereas women testing positive for one or more of the 12 other high-risk HPV types should have a Pap test to determine the need for a colposcopy. Health care professionals should use the cobas HPV test results together with other information, such as the patient screening history and risk factors, and current professional guidelines."[246]

HPV testing alone for primary screening is also being adopted in some areas in Europe and does appear promising.[97] A recent systematic review and a large observational study have both demonstrated that adding cytology to HPV testing only marginally (3% to 5%) improves detection of precancer over that detected by the HPV test alone.[242,248] While RTCs have also shown that most of the sensitivity of cotesting is due to the HPV test, these trials have been less successful at defining the specificity of HPV testing, and therefore, the potential harms of primary HPV testing are poorly quantified.[97] The algorithm proposed by the FDA appears to best mitigate the potential harms of instigating HPV testing in primary screening, but optimal management for HPV-positive women will need to be further defined by guideline organizations. Additionally, some HPV tests (but not all) do not have an internal cellular control to determine specimen adequacy. Without such a control, false-negative results could be secondary to the absence of cells in the sample, and unlike with cytology screening, the absence of cellularity would not be obvious. Because the cobas HPV test has a cellular control, this is not a concern with the use of this test as a stand-alone screening test.

18.4.6 Screening in the Era of HPV Vaccination

Recommendation: Recommended screening practices should not change on the basis of HPV vaccination status.

Rationale: With the introduction of prophylactic HPV vaccines, and with improved cervical cancer screening and management of abnormal cervical cytology and cancer precursors, we are on the verge of possibly reducing the risk of cervical cancer to negligible levels. However, depending on the level of vaccine uptake, it will be many decades before this becomes a reality. Unfortunately, HPV vaccine uptake in the United States has been lower than expected, with only 32% of eligible girls and women receiving all three doses by 2010.[249] In Australia and in the United Kingdom, countries with publicly funded, school-based vaccination programs, high coverage (80+%) of preadolescents and young women has been achieved.[70,71] However, in the United States, delivery of HPV vaccine is largely opportunistic and does not universally focus on girls and young women before the onset of sexual activity, and distribution is also affected by geographic and socioeconomic disparities in vaccination coverage.[97,249]

Vaccinating young girls, particularly those before coitarche, will not significantly impact cervical cancer rates until these girls attain the median age of incident microinvasive (42) and invasive (47) cervical cancer. Even then, cervical cancer rates will depend not only on the degree of vaccination coverage in the population but on the number of hrHPV types in the vaccine, the length and strength of vaccine immunogenicity, and whether the medical community and the public adhere closely to recommended screening guidelines.[250] If immune protection falls below a critical clinical threshold over time, booster HPV vaccine doses should provide continuing protection, but immunity will depend upon the percent of the population obtaining the booster. If the population becomes complacent about cervical cancer screening as the risk of cervical cancer decreases, there could actually be a rebound in the incidence of otherwise preventable cancers. VLP vaccines for most of the important oncogenic HPV types will likely be available in the next few years. But until long after multivalent HPV vaccines are available, women will continue to require screening to prevent the 30% of cancers that occur from other hrHPV types. Screening will also need to continue to protect women who do not get the vaccine and those already infected with oncogenic HPV types prior to vaccination.[251] As Franco and Harper stated, "Although the future seems bright on the vaccine front, policy makers are strongly cautioned to avoid scaling back cervical cancer screening. Any premature relaxation of cervical cancer control measures already in place will bring a resurgence of the disease to the unacceptable levels of the not too distant past."[250] In other words, the need for cervical cancer screening will continue for the foreseeable future. However, for cervical cancer prevention to continue to be cost-effective, there will likely need to be changes in when to begin screening and the length of screening intervals if results are normal.

To understand when and how to effect a change to screening in the era of vaccination, internationally standardized monitoring and evaluation of prophylactic HPV vaccination programs and outcomes will be essential.[252] Integrating vaccination and screening efforts will be a critical and evolving challenge over the next decade; this will require understanding not only the impact of vaccination on reducing cervical cancer precursors but also the influence of vaccination on screening test performance.[253] Increased vaccine uptake will steadily decrease the rate of abnormal cytology reports for abnormalities associated with HPV 16 and 18, the two vaccine HPV types most commonly found in CIN 2+.[253] The number of colposcopies and cervical treatments will decline coincident with the proportion of the population vaccinated. This will decrease the number of high-grade lesions that a colposcopist may see, increasing the challenge of training and maintaining expertise in identifying and managing these lesions.[4] As high-grade cytologic abnormalities decrease, maintaining expertise in cytologic interpretation, and even in maintaining attention to detail, may become more difficult.[4,250] Organized vaccination and screening programs with good record keeping will be necessary to determine the best options for integrating the benefits of HPV vaccination with highly reduced risk of cervical cancer.[254]

18.5 ADDITIONAL OBSERVATIONS ON CERVICAL CANCER SCREENING

It is important to note that not all cervical cancer is preventable. Regardless of what test is used, screening is not likely to achieve 100% protection. Cervical cytology testing more frequent than every 12 months should be reserved for women being followed for abnormal cervical cytology results or in posttreatment follow-up.[16,219] Because most US women receive opportunistic cervical cancer screening, and frequently inaccurately recall the timing and results of prior screening, it is important for the clinician to assess, as well as possible, a new patient's screening history.[96,255] This includes, if possible, the date of her most recent cervical cytology test and the frequency and results of her prior tests, including management if abnormal.

Women treated in the past for CIN 2, CIN 3, or cancer remain at risk for persistent or recurrent disease for at least 20 years after treatment, and after initial posttreatment surveillance.[256] These women should continue to have routine screening for at least 20 years.[16,97,219,256–258] Women HIV infected or otherwise immunocompromised should be followed at intervals recommended by the CDC; that is, a Pap test should be obtained twice in the first year after diagnosis of HIV or other reason for immune suppression, and then annual screening can follow for women with normal reports on both initial screens.[259] Therefore, the routine recommendations apply only to women with normal immunity, women not previously treated for CIN 2,3 or cancer, and women not exposed to DES in utero.[97–99] Increased screening intervals are only recommended for women having normal screening results, in whom the risk of high-grade precursor disease is shown to be low prior to the next recommended screening test. Risk factors not considered important in determining screening intervals include recent acquisition of a new partner(s), the number of sexual partners, early age of first sexual intercourse, or smoking.[236]

18.5.1 Considerations and Precautions Regarding HPV Testing

Clinicians using HPV testing as a mode of primary cervical cancer screening and in abnormal cytology management must thoroughly understand the natural history of HPV and its association with cervical cancer in order to be in a position to recommend appropriate screening intervals, proper management of HPV+ test results, and deliver reassuring patient counseling messages.[260] It is imperative that cotesting be repeated only at the recommended 5-year interval for women testing

negative on both tests, as safety for at least 6 years has been demonstrated.[87,160,261] Testing more often in women with virtually no risk of having precancer adds substantial cost without comparative benefit.[262] Excessive screening all too often identifies transient HPV infections and minor cytologic abnormalities that resolve spontaneously if screening intervals are wider, adding unnecessary evaluations and procedures likely to cause patient harm.[97]

There is little reason to HPV test a woman without a cervix. No statistically significant difference has been found in the prevalence of HPV positivity between women with an intact cervix and women having had a hysterectomy (16% vs. 13.9%, respectively) or for carcinogenic HPV (6.5% vs. 4.5%, respectively).[263] Castle et al. concluded that although women with, and without, a cervix have a similar prevalence of carcinogenic HPV infection, women without a cervix have minimal risk of HPV-induced cancer and are unlikely to benefit from HPV testing or cytologic screening. Therefore, women posthysterectomy for benign disease, with no evidence of CIN 2+ or cervical cancer at the time of the hysterectomy, do not need screening per the ACS/ASCCP/ASCP and ACOG guidelines and therefore are not candidates for cotesting.[97,99] Even though the NPV of a negative HPV test in HIV+ women is very high,[264] the prevalence of HPV in immunosuppressed women is too high (up to 67% in some studies) to utilize combined HPV testing and cytology in the screening of women with HIV or other immunosuppression.[265–267] Also, higher persistence of HPV infection and progression of squamous intraepithelial lesions are well documented.[266] Extended screening intervals based upon estimates derived from women with normal immunity may be unsafe and are not recommended.[96,97] There are other situations in which HPV testing should not be utilized, and these are listed in Table 18.13.

While negative cotest results give great reassurance that a 5-year screening interval is safe,[97–99] a positive test provides much more complex information. Clinicians must understand that 5% to 15% of women ages 30 to 70 years will test positive for hrHPV, but only 0.5% to 1.0% in an already well-screened population would immediately be found to have CIN 2,3 or an extremely rare cancer at the time of the initial positive HPV test.[160] Therefore, it is imperative that clinicians not respond aggressively to a single positive HPV test in the absence of abnormal cytology reports. Because most HPV is transient, even in women over the age of 30, and only persistent hrHPV is a risk for developing CIN 2+ and cancer, testing cytology–/HPV+ women for persistence of HPV in 12 months, or immediately genotyping for HPV 16/18, and only referring women to colposcopy who retest HPV+ or abnormal cytology, or positive HPV 16/18, will minimize overevaluation and overtreatment.[13,16] This will allow time for spontaneous resolution of HPV infections and reduce colposcopic referrals to a more appropriate and manageable level.[97–99] Management options are discussed in Chapter 19.

Clinicians must understand that treating a woman with a positive HPV test in the absence of documented disease is not acceptable.[13,16,267,268] Recent evidence of an increased risk in premature rupture of the membranes, premature delivery, and low birth weight infants among women treated by cervical excisional procedures further emphasizes the importance of only treating high-grade CIN.[215–217]

18.5.2 Psychological Effects of Testing Positive for HPV and Counseling Messages

Most HPV infections, including most CIN 1 and many CIN 2 lesions, resolve spontaneously, but their detection most often causes anxiety, and may cause stigmatization from the

TABLE 18.13	WHEN AND WHERE HPV TESTING SHOULD *NOT BE* DONE

General considerations:

Testing for low-risk HPV types that do not cause cervical cancer has no clinical benefit and therefore cannot be justified or condoned.

HPV testing should never be used as a screening test for STDs, because HPV is so common and, unlike most STDs, has no treatment that would follow detection.

HPV testing should not be done as a screen prior to administering the HPV vaccine.

There is no commercially available serologic test that would identify past exposure to these 4 HPV types. The cost of prevaccination screening of all sexually active women would escalate the cost of vaccine administration.

HPV testing should never be done more often than every 12 mo.

In primary cervical screening:

Cotesting should not be done in women under the age of 30.

Cotesting should not be done more frequently than every 5 y if both tests are negative.

In management of abnormal cervical cytology (see Chapter 19):

HPV testing should be avoided as a reflex test to any abnormal Pap test other than for women >24 y with ASC-US except in postmenopausal women with LSIL.

HPV testing should not be done in the initial management of women with atypical glandular cells (AGC).

HPV testing should not be used in the initial management of LSIL, except in postmenopausal women nor in the initial management of women with ASC-H or HSIL cytology.

From Massad LS, Einstein MH, Huh WK, et al. 2012 updated consensus guidelines for the management of abnormal cervical cancer screening tests and cancer precursors. *Obstet Gynecol* 2013;121:829–846. (Also published in *J Low Genit Tract Dis* 2013;17(5 suppl 1):S1–S27.); Cox JT, Moriarty AT, Castle PE. Commentary on statement on human papillomavirus test utilization. *Arch Pathol Lab Med* 2009;133(8):1192–4.

diagnosis of a sexually transmitted disease (STD), discomfort from diagnostic procedures and treatment, and concern that procedures may eventually result in pregnancy complications.[97,215–217,222] These potential harms must be balanced against the benefit of detecting and treating true cancer precursors to prevent progression to cervical cancer. Psychological effects are a prominent group of harms to be considered. Evaluations of the psychological impact on women of having to wait up to a year for a repeat HPV test to further clarify risk have found that while women often experience considerable negative emotion when they first learn they are HPV positive, this did not generally last during the year between tests, once questions about HPV had been resolved.[269] Women appeared to be more distressed by a second HPV-positive result than a single one, and expressed a clear preference for immediate colposcopy following detection of persistent HPV. Psychological responses often noted with testing positive for HPV include negative reactions to abnormal results (which includes abnormal Pap results as well), empowerment through knowledge of results, and self-confidence to prevent future disease.[270] Most women are concerned about possible adverse social and psychological consequences, relating primarily to the sexually transmitted nature of the virus and its link to cervical cancer. Women have described feeling stigmatized, anxious, and stressed, concerned about their sexual relationships, and worried about disclosing their result to others.[271]

To destigmatize the issue of testing positive for HPV and ensure that any adverse impact of the infection on women's well-being is minimized, it is critical that HPV testing be accompanied by extensive health education about HPV, what cervical cytology and HPV are testing for, how ubiquitous HPV is, and the usually transitory nature of this viral infection.[271] Educating women about all aspects of being HPV positive, including what is known about the risk of HPV transmission to a new partner, risk of developing a treatable cervical lesion, and the source of infection, is imperative to allay as much anxiety as possible about testing positive for "high-risk" HPV (Table 18.14).[271,272] Discuss the reason that "high-risk" HPV is given this name—that, despite the association of certain HPV types with cervical precancer and cancer, the risk of developing either of these lesions is relatively low and that only persistent HPV infections or testing positive for

TABLE 18.14	KEY COUNSELING MESSAGES FOR WOMEN TESTING POSITIVE ON AN HPV TEST

- Genital HPV infections are almost always acquired through sexual contact.
- Consistent use of condoms reduces the risk of acquiring HPV by about 70%.
- Long-term persistent infection with certain types of HPV, called "high-risk" HPV, is necessary for cervical cancer to occur.
- HPV infections are so common that almost all sexually active people become infected at some point in their lifetime.
- Most HPV-positive women become HPV negative within 1–2 y due to their immune response.
- HPV-positive tests are much less common in women over the age of 30 than in younger women.
- Approximately 6%–10% of women 30 y and older will be positive for "high-risk" types of HPV, and 4%–7% will be positive for HPV but will have a normal Pap.
- Most HPV-positive women do not have CIN 2,3 or cancer, and most will not develop cervical disease.
- Women who are persistently infected with "high-risk" HPV types are at greater risk for having cervical disease, most of which is readily treatable.
- Women positive for HPV 16 or HPV 18 are at much higher risk for CIN 2,3 or cancer than women positive for other hrHPV types and should be evaluated but still are most likely to either be normal or only have readily treatable cell changes that are not yet cancer.

HPV 16 or 18 warrant further investigation. Counseling and educating patients are made even more difficult by an incomplete understanding of viral latency and whether most HPV is eventually cleared completely or just suppressed by immunity to levels below the threshold for detection by very sensitive HPV tests. Emphasize that it is usually not possible to know when a person was first exposed to HPV, nor from whom the infection was passed.[273] HPV may be detected right away, or not for many years, or even decades. Reassure that even if it is not possible to know whether HPV is completely cleared or just suppressed, once the HPV test becomes negative, the individual is not likely to continue to be infective to a new partner.

It is also imperative to reassure the patient that detectable HPV probably indicates that she shares this virus with her partner and that successful clearance or suppression of HPV by either partner is only dependent upon one's own immunity and is not affected by possible reexposure to the same HPV type through continued sexual activity with one's partner. These messages are complex and take time to discuss, but the importance of providing such education cannot be overstated. If clinicians do not feel equipped to provide this education, or do not feel that they have the time, then the anxiety generated in women testing positive will far outweigh any benefit derived by cotesting.

Anhang et al.[274] evaluated women's desired information about HPV testing. Women indicated that they wanted information about transmission, prevention, treatment, and cervical carcinoma risk and explanations of different types of tests and their results; that messages should be tailored to describe HPV susceptibility according to age and risk profile; and that clarification is needed regarding HPV types and their consequences. Additionally, it is imperative to have an accurate discussion of cancer risk, balanced by reassurance that following recommended screening practices will reduce risk to negligible levels.[274] Understanding these issues will ensure that primary screening that includes HPV testing is a success.

18.6 PROSPECTS FOR THE FUTURE OF CERVICAL CANCER PREVENTION

The escalating cost of health care in our country is moving the public and the politicians to demand that the cost of doing something is justified by the gain, a model that in one way or another much of the developed world has long embraced. As successive cohorts of young vaccinated women reach screening age, screening as we have known it will have to change to be both effective and cost-effective. Although screening will likely continue for many decades, decreasing numbers of high-grade lesions will result in increasing the screening cost to detect each precancer. Annual Pap testing, although providing significant protection for most women from getting cervical cancer, is not cost-effective, and the level of protection provided decreases for women irregularly screened. Moving to less frequent screening is the only option for improving the cost-effectiveness of cervical cancer prevention, for less frequent screening reduces not only the number of tests but also the detection of transient HPV infections that are not destined to progress. The improved test characteristics and long-term predictive value of HPV testing ensure that moving to longer intervals is not likely to put women at more risk even if the next screen exceeds 3 to 5 years.

In 2003, Crum et al. predicted that within the next 20 years, cervical cancer screening will have evolved through four phases.[11,275] The first phase, traditional screening with the Pap test, although attributed to reducing cervical cancer incidence and death by at least two-thirds, is about to end. The second phase utilizes hrHPV testing for managing cytologic abnormalities and for primary screening. We are now entering the third phase, in which HPV 16/18 detection or host or viral biomarkers (or combinations thereof) are beginning to be used to assess cancer risk and concentrate available resources on a subset of women most at risk.[275-278] The fourth and, likely, final phase will be the adjustment of screening in the era of HPV vaccines, wherein the pool of at-risk individuals and the prevalence of HPV types of greatest risk will gradually shrink.[250-254,279] This will result in further fostering the need for utilizing newer screening strategies that focus on detection of HPV alone, or of other markers for risk as they become available. Undoubtedly, improved molecular options for screening will make detection of women at risk more targeted, accurate, and cost-effective.[11] Combined with primary prevention by widespread HPV vaccination, there is at least the theoretical opportunity to make cervical cancer the first human cancer to exist only in history. What a remarkable achievement that would be.

References

1. Watson M, Saraiya M, Benard V, et al. Burden of cervical cancer in the United States, 1998–2003. *Cancer* 2008;113(10 suppl):2855–64.
2. American Cancer Society, Cancer Facts & Figures 2013. Atlanta: American Cancer Society. 2013. Available at: http://www.cancer.org/Research/CancerFactsFigures/CancerFactsFigures/cancer-facts-and-figures-2013
3. Cox JT. Management of cervical intraepithelial neoplasia. *Lancet* 1999;353:857–9.
4. Kitchener HC, Castle PE, Cox JT. Chapter 7: Achievements and limitations of cervical cytology screening. *Vaccine* 2006;24(suppl 3):S63–70.
5. Simard EP, Naishadham D, Saslow D, Jemal A. Age-specific trends in black-white disparities in cervical cancer incidence in the United States: 1975–2009. *Gynecol Oncol* 2012;127(3):611–5.
6. Dürst M, Gissmann L, Ikenberg H, zur Hausen H. A papillomavirus DNA from a cervical carcinoma and its prevalence in cancer biopsy samples from different geographic regions. *Proc Natl Acad Sci USA* 1983;80(12):3812–5.
7. Boshart M, Gissmann L, Ikenberg H, Kleinheinz A, Scheurlen W, zur Hausen H. A new type of papillomavirus DNA, its presence in genital cancer biopsies and in cell lines derived from cervical cancer. *EMBO J* 1984;3(5):1151–7.
8. Meijer CJ, van den Brule AJ, Snijders PJ, Helmerhorst T, Kenemans P, Walboomers JM. Detection of human papillomavirus in cervical scrapes by the polymerase chain reaction in relation to cytology: possible implications for cervical cancer screening. *IARC Sci Publ* 1992;(119):271–81.
9. Walboomers JM, Jacobs MV, Manos MM, et al. Human papillomavirus is a necessary cause of invasive cervical cancer worldwide. *J Pathol* 1999;189(1):12–9.
10. Zhou J, Sun XY, Davies H, Crawford L, Park D, Frazer IH. Definition of linear antigenic regions of the HPV16 L1 capsid protein using synthetic virion-like particles. *Virology* 1992;189(2):592–9.
11. Cox JT. History of the use of HPV testing in cervical screening and in the management of abnormal cervical screening results. *J Clin Virol* 2009;45(suppl 1):S3–12.
12. Wright TC Jr, Cox JT, Massad LS, Carlson J, Twiggs LB, Wilkinson EJ; American Society for Colposcopy and Cervical Pathology. 2001 consensus guidelines for the management of women with cervical intraepithelial neoplasia. *Am J Obstet Gynecol* 2003;189:295–304.
13. Wright TC Jr, Massad LS, Dunton CJ, Spitzer M, Wilkinson EJ, Solomon D; 2006 ASCCP-Sponsored Consensus Conference. 2006 consensus guidelines for the management of women with abnormal cervical screening tests. *J Low Genit Tract Dis* 2007;11(4):201–22.
14. American College of Obstetricians and Gynecologists. ACOG Practice Bulletin, Number 66. Management of abnormal cervical cytology and histology. Clinical management guidelines for the Obstetrician and Gynecologist. September, 2005.
15. American College of Obstetricians and Gynecologists. Management of abnormal cervical cancer screening test results and cervical cancer precursors. Practice Bulletin No. 140. *Obstet Gynecol* 2013;122:1338–67.
16. Massad LS, Einstein MH, Huh WK, et al. 2012 updated consensus guidelines for the management of abnormal cervical cancer screening tests and cancer precursors. *Obstet Gynecol*. 2013;121:829–846. (Also published in *J Low Genit Tract Dis* 2013;17(5 suppl 1):S1–27.)
17. Winer RL, Lee SK, Hughes JP, Adam DE, Kiviat NB, Koutsky LA. Genital human papillomavirus infection: incidence and risk factors in a cohort of female university students. *Am J Epidemiol* 2003;157:218–26.
18. Frazer IH, Cox JT, Mayeaux EJ Jr, et al. Advances in prevention of cervical cancer and other human papillomavirus-related diseases. *Pediatr Infect Dis J* 2006;25(2 suppl):S65–81.
19. Ley C, Bauer HM, Reingold A, et al. Determinants of genital human papillomavirus infection in young women. *J Natl Cancer Inst* 1991;83:997–1003.

20. Winer RL, Hughes JP, Feng Q, et al. Detection of genital HPV types in fingertip samples from newly sexually active female university students. *Cancer Epidemiol Biomarkers Prev* 2010;19(7):1682–5.

21. Cooper D, Hoffman M, Carrara H, et al. Determinants of sexual activity and its relation to cervical cancer risk among South African women. *BMC Public Health* 2007;7:341.

22. Winer RL, Hughes JP, Feng Q, et al. Condom use and the risk of genital human papillomavirus infection in young women. *N Engl J Med* 2006;354(25):2645–54.

23. Manhart LE, Koutsky LA. Do condoms prevent genital HPV infection, external genital warts, or cervical neoplasia? A meta-analysis. *Sex Transm Dis* 2002;29:725–35.

24. Kjaer SK, Svare EI, Worm AM, Walboomers JM, Meijer CJ, van den Brule AJ. Human papillomavirus infection in Danish female sex workers: decreasing prevalence with age despite continuously high sexual activity. *Sex Transm Dis* 2000;27:438–45.

25. Crochard A, Luyts D, di Nicola S, Gonçalves MA. Self-reported sexual debut and behavior in young adults aged 18–24 years in seven European countries: implications for HPV vaccination programs. *Gynecol Oncol* 2009;115(3 suppl):S7–14.

26. Zhou J, Sun XY, Stenzel DJ, Frazer IH. Expression of vaccinia recombinant HPV 16 L1 and L2 ORF proteins in epithelial cells is sufficient for assembly of HPV virion-like particles. *Virology* 1991;185:251–7.

27. Muñoz N, Castellsagué X, de González AB, Gissmann L. Chapter 1: HPV in the etiology of human cancer. *Vaccine* 2006;24(suppl 3):S3/1–10.

28. Fife KH, Wheeler CM, Koutsky LA, et al. Dose-ranging studies of the safety and immunogenicity of human papillomavirus type 11 and type 16 virus-like particle candidate vaccines in young healthy women. *Vaccine* 2004;22:2943–52.

29. Koutsky LA, Ault KA, Wheeler CM, et al. A controlled trial of a human papillomavirus type 16 vaccine. *N Engl J Med* 2002;347:1645–51.

30. Rowhani-Rahbar A, Mao C, Hughes JP, et al. Longer term efficacy of a prophylactic monovalent human papillomavirus type 16 vaccine. *Vaccine* 2009;27:5612–9.

31. Advisory Committee on Immunization Practices. Recommended adult immunization schedule: United States, 2010. *Ann Intern Med* 2010;152(1):36–9.

32. Einstein MH, Baron M, Levin MJ, et al.; HPV-010 Study Group. Comparison of the immunogenicity and safety of Cervarix and Gardasil human papillomavirus (HPV) cervical cancer vaccines in healthy women aged 18–45 years. *Hum Vaccin* 2009;5(10):705–19.

33. Garland SM, Hernandez-Avila M, Wheeler CM, et al. Quadrivalent vaccine against human papillomavirus to prevent anogenital diseases. *N Engl J Med* 2007;356:1928.

34. The FUTURE II Study Group. Quadrivalent vaccine against human papillomavirus to prevent high-grade cervical lesions. *N Engl J Med* 2007;356:1915.

35. Joura EA, Kjaer SK, Wheeler CM, et al. HPV antibody levels and clinical efficacy following administration of a prophylactic quadrivalent HPV vaccine. *Vaccine* 2008;26(52):6844–51.

36. Paavonen J, Naud P, Salmeron J, et al. Efficacy of human papillomavirus (HPV)-16/18 AS04-adjuvanted vaccine against cervical infection and precancer caused by oncogenic HPV types (PATRICIA): final analysis of a double-blind, randomized study in young women. *Lancet* 2009;374:301–14.

37. Herrero R, Hildesheim A, Rodriguez AC, et al. Rationale and design of a community-based double-blind randomized clinical trial of an HPV 16 and 18 vaccine in Guanacaste, Costa Rica. *Vaccine* 2008;26:4795.

38. Brown DR, Kjaer SK, Sigurdsson K, et al. The impact of quadrivalent human papillomavirus (HPV; types 6, 11, 16, and 18) L1 virus-like particle vaccine on infection and disease due to oncogenic nonvaccine HPV types in generally HPV-naive women aged 16–26 years. *J Infect Dis* 2009;199:926.

39. Wheeler CM, Kjaer SK, Sigurdsson K, et al. The impact of quadrivalent human papillomavirus (HPV; types 6, 11, 16, and 18) L1 virus-like particle vaccine on infection and disease due to oncogenic nonvaccine HPV types in sexually active women aged 16–26 years. *J Infect Dis* 2009;199:936.

40. Slade BA, Leidel L, Vellozzi C, et al. Postlicensure safety surveillance for quadrivalent human papillomavirus recombinant vaccine. *JAMA* 2009;302:750.

41. Gee J, Naleway A, Shui I, et al. Monitoring the safety of quadrivalent human papillomavirus vaccine: findings from the Vaccine Safety Datalink. *Vaccine* 2011;29:8279.

42. Markowitz LE, Dunne EF, Saraiya M, et al. Quadrivalent human papillomavirus vaccine: recommendations of the Advisory Committee on Immunization Practices (ACIP). *MMWR Recomm Rep* 2007;56:1–24.

43. Centers for Disease Control and Prevention (CDC). FDA licensure of bivalent human papillomavirus vaccine (HPV2, Cervarix) for use in females and updated HPV vaccination recommendations from the Advisory Committee on Immunization Practices (ACIP). *MMWR Morb Mortal Wkly Rep* 2010;59:626–9.

44. Committee opinion no. 467: Human papillomavirus vaccination. *Obstet Gynecol* 2010;116(3):800–3.

45. Saslow D, Castle PE, Cox JT, et al. American Cancer Society Guideline for human papillomavirus (HPV) vaccine use to prevent cervical cancer and its precursors. *CA Cancer J Clin* 2007;57:7.

46. The World Health Organization. Human papillomavirus and HPV vaccines: Technical information for policy-makers and health professionals.

47. http://www.who.int/vaccines-documents/DocsPDF07/866.pdf. Accessed September 10, 2011.

47. Leval A, Herweijer E, Ploner A, et al. Quadrivalent human papillomavirus vaccine effectiveness: a Swedish national cohort study. *J Natl Cancer Inst* 2013;105(7):469–74.

48. Markowitz LE, Hariri S, Lin C, et al. Reduction in human papillomavirus (HPV) prevalence among young women following HPV vaccine introduction in the United States, National Health and Nutrition Examination Surveys, 2003–2010. *J Infect Dis* 2013;208(3):385–93.

49. Advisory Committee on Immunization Practices. Recommended adult immunization schedule: United States, 2009*. *Ann Intern Med* 2009;150:40.

50. Wilkin T, Lee JY, Lensing SY, et al. Safety and immunogenicity of the quadrivalent human papillomavirus vaccine in HIV-1-infected men. *J Infect Dis* 2010;202:1246–53.

51. Levin MJ, Moscicki AB, Song LY, et al. Safety and immunogenicity of a quadrivalent human papillomavirus (types 6, 11, 16, and 18) vaccine in HIV-infected children 7 to 12 years old. *J Acquir Immune Defic Syndr* 2010;55:197.

52. Petäjä T, Keränen H, Karppa T, et al. Immunogenicity and safety of human papillomavirus (HPV)-16/18 AS04-adjuvanted vaccine in healthy boys aged 10–18 years. *J Adolesc Health* 2009;44:33–40.

53. Reisinger KS, Block SL, Lazcano-Ponce E, et al. Safety and persistent immunogenicity of a quadrivalent human papillomavirus types 6, 11, 16, 18 L1 virus-like particle vaccine in preadolescents and adolescents: a randomized controlled trial. *Pediatr Infect Dis J* 2007;26:201–9.

54. Hillman RJ, Giuliano AR, Palefsky JM, et al. Immunogenicity of the quadrivalent human papillomavirus (type 6/11/16/18) vaccine in males 16 to 26 years old. *Clin Vaccine Immunol* 2012;19(2):261–7.

55. Giuliano AR, Palefsky JM, Goldstone S, et al. The efficacy of quadrivalent HPV vaccine in preventing HPV 6/11/16/18-related external genital disease and anogenital infection in young men. *N Engl J Med* 2011;364(5):393–5.

56. U.S. Food and Drug Administration. Male indication for Gardasil. 2009. www.fda.gov/downloads/AdvisoryCommittees/CommitteesMeeting Materials/BloodVaccinesandOtherBiologics/VaccinesandRelatedBiologicalProductsAdvisoryCommittee/UCM181361.pdf. Accessed November 30, 2009.

57. Centers for Disease Control and Prevention (CDC). FDA licensure of quadrivalent human papillomavirus vaccine (HPV4, Gardasil) for use in males and guidance from the Advisory Committee on Immunization Practices (ACIP). *MMWR Morb Mortal Wkly Rep* 2010;59:630–2.

58. Dunne EF, Markowitz LE, Chesson H, et al. Centers for Disease Control and Prevention (CDC). Recommendations on the use of quadrivalent human papillomavirus vaccine in males—Advisory Committee on Immunization Practices (ACIP), 2011. *MMWR Morb Mortal Wkly Rep* 2011;60:1705.

59. Korostil IA, Ali H, Guy RJ, Donovan B, Law MG, Regan DG. Near elimination of genital warts in Australia predicted with extension of human papillomavirus vaccination to males. *Sex Transm Dis* 2013;40(11):833–5.

60. Palefsky J. Can HPV vaccination help to prevent anal cancer? *Lancet Infect Dis* 2010;10(12):815–6.

61. Gillison ML, Broutian T, Pickard RK, et al. Prevalence of oral HPV infection in the United States, 2009–2010. *JAMA* 2012;307:693.

62. Sanders GD, Taira AV. Cost-effectiveness of a potential vaccine for human papillomavirus. *Emerg Infect Dis* 2003;9:37.

63. Goldie SJ, Kohli M, Grima D, et al. Projected clinical benefits and cost-effectiveness of a human papillomavirus 16/18 vaccine. *J Natl Cancer Inst* 2004;96:604–15.

64. Kulasingam SL, Myers ER. Potential health and economic impact of adding a human papillomavirus vaccine to screening programs. *JAMA* 2003;290:781–9.

65. Kim JJ, Goldie SJ. Health and economic implications of HPV vaccination in the United States. *N Engl J Med* 2008;359:821–32.

66. Chesson HW, Ekwueme DU, Saraiya M, et al. The cost-effectiveness of male HPV vaccination in the United States. *Vaccine* 2011;29:8443.

67. Stanley M. Immunobiology of HPV and HPV vaccines. *Gynecol Oncol* 2008;109:S15–21.

68. Newall AT, Beutels P, Wood JG, et al. Cost-effectiveness analyses of human papillomavirus vaccination. *Lancet Infect Dis* 2007;7:289–96.

69. de Kok IM, Habbema JD, van Rosmalen J, van Ballegooijen M. Would the effect of HPV vaccination on non-cervical HPV-positive cancers make the difference for its cost-effectiveness? *Eur J Cancer* 2011;47(3):428–35.

70. Ali H, Donovan B, Wand H, et al. Genital warts in young Australians five years into national human papillomavirus vaccination programme: national surveillance data. *BMJ* 2013;346:f2032.

71. http://www.cdc.gov/media/releases/2013/p0619-hpv-vaccinations.html. Accessed January 12, 2013.

72. International Agency for Research on Cancer (IARC). Cancer incidence in five continents. Volume VII. *IARC Sci Publ* 1997;143:i–xxxiv, 1–1240.

73. Bray F, Loos AH, McCarron P, et al. Trends in cervical squamous cell carcinoma incidence in 13 European countries: changing risk and the effects of screening. *Cancer Epidemiol Biomarkers Prev* 2005;14:677–86.

74. Barnholtz-Sloan J, Patel N, Rollison D, Kortepeter K, MacKinnon J, Giuliano A. Incidence trends of invasive cervical cancer in the United States by combined race and ethnicity. *Cancer Causes Control* 2009;20(7):1129–38.

75. Sawaya GF, Brown AD, Washington AE, Garber AM. Clinical practice. Current approaches to cervical-cancer screening. *N Engl J Med* 2001;344(21):1603–7.

76. National Institutes of Health Consensus Development Conference Statement: cervical cancer, April 1–3, 1996. National Institutes of Health Consensus Development Panel. *J Natl Cancer Inst Monogr* 1996;21:vii–xix.

77. Sherman ME, Wang SS, Carreon J, Devesa SS. Mortality trends for cervical squamous and adenocarcinoma in the United States: relation to incidence and survival. *Cancer* 2005;103:1258–64.

78. Smith HO, Tiffany MF, Qualls CR, Key CF. The rising incidence of adenocarcinoma relative to squamous cell carcinoma of the uterine cervix in the United States: a 24-year population-based study. *Gynecol Oncol* 2000;78:97–105.

79. Kinney W, Sawaya GF, Sung HY, et al. Stage at diagnosis and mortality in patients with adenocarcinoma and adenosquamous carcinoma of the uterine cervix diagnosed as a consequence of cytologic screening. *Acta Cytol* 2003;47:167–71.

80. Henley SJ, King JB, German RR, Richardson LC, Plescia M; Centers for Disease Control and Prevention (CDC). Surveillance of screening-detected cancers (colon and rectum, breast, and cervix)—United States, 2004–2006. *MMWR Surveill Summ* 2010;59(9):1–25.

81. Kinney W, Sung HY, Kearney KA, Miller M, Sawaya G, Hiatt RA. Missed opportunities for cervical cancer screening of HMO members developing invasive cervical cancer (ICC). *Gynecol Oncol* 1998;71:428–30.

82. Feldman S. How often should we screen for cervical cancer? *N Engl J Med* 2003;349(16):1495–6.

83. U.S. Preventative Services Task Force. *Guide to Clinical Preventative Services*. Washington, DC: US Department of Health and Human Services, 2003.

84. Kulasingam SL, Myers ER, Lawson HW, et al. Cost-effectiveness of extending cervical cancer screening intervals among women with prior normal Pap tests. *Obstet Gynecol* 2006;107(2, pt 1):321–8.

85. Solomon D, Breen N, McNeel T. Cervical cancer screening rates in the United States and the potential impact of implementation of screening guidelines. *CA Cancer J Clin* 2007;57(2):105–11.

86. Mayrand MH, Duarte-Franco E, Rodrigues I, et al. Human papillomavirus DNA versus Papanicolaou screening tests for cervical cancer. *N Engl J Med* 2007;357:1579–88.

87. Dillner J, Rebolj M, Birembaut P, et al.; Joint European Cohort Study. Long term predictive values of cytology and human papillomavirus testing in cervical cancer screening: joint European cohort study. *BMJ* 2008;337: a1754.

88. Cuzick J, Szarewski A, Mesher D, et al. Long-term follow-up of cervical abnormalities among women screened by HPV testing and cytology—results from the Hammersmith study. *Int J Cancer* 2008;122:2294–300.

89. Castle PE, Fetterman B, Poitras N, et al. Five-year experience of human papillomavirus DNA and Papanicolaou test cotesting. *Obstet Gynecol* 2009;113:595–600.

90. Mayrand MH, Duarte-Franco E, Coutlée F, et al.; CCCaST Study Group. Randomized controlled trial of human papillomavirus testing versus Pap cytology in the primary screening for cervical cancer precursors: design, methods and preliminary accrual results of the Canadian cervical cancer screening trial (CCCaST). *Int J Cancer* 2006;119(3):615–23.

91. Mesher D, Szarewski A, Cadman L, et al. Long-term follow-up of cervical disease in women screened by cytology and HPV testing: results from the HART study. *Br J Cancer* 2010;102(9):1405–10.

92. Dahlström M, Ylitalo N, Sundström K, et al. Prospective study of human papillomavirus and risk of cervical adenocarcinoma. *Int J Cancer* 2010;127(8):1923–30.

93. Ronco G, Giorgi-Rossi P, Carozzi F, et al.; New Technologies for Cervical Cancer screening (NTCC) Working Group. Efficacy of human papillomavirus testing for the detection of invasive cervical cancers and cervical intraepithelial neoplasia: a randomised controlled trial. *Lancet Oncol* 2010;11(3):249–57.

94. Saslow D, Runowicz CD, Solomon D, et al.; American Cancer Society. American Cancer Society guideline for the early detection of cervical neoplasia and cancer. *CA Cancer J Clin* 2002;52:342–62.

95. ACOG Practice Bulletin. *Cervical Cytology Screening*. Washington, DC: American College of Obstetricians and Gynecologists, 2003.

96. ACOG Committee on Practice Bulletins—Gynecology. ACOG Practice Bulletin no. 109: Cervical cytology screening. *Obstet Gynecol* 2009;114(6):1409–20.

97. Saslow D, Solomon D, Lawson HW, et al. for the American Cancer Society; American Society for Colposcopy and Cervical Pathology; American Society for Clinical Pathology. American Cancer Society, American Society for Colposcopy and Cervical Pathology, and American Society for Clinical Pathology screening guidelines for the prevention and early detection of cervical cancer. *Am J Clin Pathol* 2012;137(4):516–42.

98. Moyer VA for the U.S. Preventive Services Task Force. Screening for cervical cancer. U.S. Preventive Services Task Force recommendation statement. *Ann Intern Med* 2012;156(12):880–91.

99. American College of Obstetricians and Gynecologists (ACOG). Practice Bulletin No. 131. Screening for cervical cancer. Washington, DC: November 2012.

100. Papanicolaou GN, Traut HF. *Diagnosis of uterine cancer by the vaginal smear*. New York: Commonwealth Fund, 1943.

101. Breen N, Wagener DK, Brown ML, Davis WW, Ballard-Barbash R. Progress in cancer screening over a decade: results of cancer screening from the 1987, 1992, and 1998 National Health Interview Surveys. *J Natl Cancer Inst* 2001;93:1704–13.

102. Watson M, Saraiya M, Wu X. Update of HPV-associated female genital cancers in the United States, 1999–2004. *J Womens Health (Larchmt)* 2009;18(11):1731–8.

103. Clinical laboratory Improvement Amendments of 1988, 42 C.F.R. Part 405. 1992;57:7169.

104. National Cancer Institute Workshop. The 1988 Bethesda System for reporting cervical/vaginal cytologic diagnosis. *JAMA* 1989;262:931–4.

105. Henson RM, Wyatt SW, Lee NC. The National Breast and Cervical Cancer Early Detection Program: a comprehensive public health response to two major health issues for women. *J Public Health Manag Pract* 1996;2(2):36–47.

106. Bogdanich W. Lax laboratories—the Pap test misses much cervical cancer through labs' errors. *Wall Street Journal* 1987 Nov 2; Sect A1.

107. Koss LG. The Papanicolaou test for cervical cancer detection: a triumph and a tragedy. *JAMA* 1989;261:737–43.

108. Braly P, Kinney W, Sheets E, Walton L, Farber F, Cox JT. Reporting the potential benefits of new technologies for cervical cancer screening. *J Low Genit Tract Dis* 2000;5:73–81.

109. McCrory DC, Matchar DB, Bastian L, et al. Evaluation of cervical cytology. *Evid Rep Technol Assess (Summ)* 1999;5:1–6.

110. NIH Consensus Statement Online 1996 April 1–3, cited 1999;43:1–38.

111. Fahey MT, Irwig L, Macaskill P. Meta-analysis of Pap test accuracy. *Am J Epidemiol* 1995;141:680–89.

112. Nanda K, McCrory DC, Myers ER, et al. Accuracy of the Papanicolaou test in screening for and follow-up of cervical cytologic abnormalities: a systematic review. *Ann Intern Med* 2000;132:810–9.

113. Baseman JG, Koutsky LA. The epidemiology of human papillomavirus infections. *J Clin Virol* 2005;32s:s16–24.

114. Schiffman M, Castle PE. The promise of global cervical-cancer prevention. *N Engl J Med* 2005;353(20):2101–4.

115. Stoler MH. Advances in cervical screening technology. *Mod Pathol* 2000;13:275–84.

116. Diaz-Rosario LA, Kabawat SE. Performance of a fluid-based, thin-layer Papanicolaou smear method in the clinical setting of an independent laboratory and an outpatient screening population in New England. *Arch Pathol Lab Med* 1999;123:817–21.

117. Hutchinson ML, Zahniser DJ, Sherman ME, et al. Utility of liquid-based cytology for cervical carcinoma screening: results of a population-based study conducted in a region of Costa Rica with a high incidence of cervical carcinoma. *Cancer* 1999;87:48–55.

118. Ashfaq R, Gibbons D, Vela C, Saboorian MH, Iliya F. ThinPrep Pap Test. Accuracy for glandular disease. *Acta Cytol* 1999;43:81–5.

119. Sulik SM, Kroeger K, Schultz JK, Brown JL, Becker LA, Grant WD. Are fluid-based cytologies superior to the conventional Papanicolaou test? A systematic review. *J Fam Pract* 2001;50:1040–46.

120. Chernesky M, Jang D, Smieja M, et al. Validation of the APTIMA Combo 2 assay for the detection of *Chlamydia trachomatis* and *Neisseria gonorrhoeae* in SurePath liquid-based Pap test samples taken with different collection devices. *Sex Transm Dis* 2009;36(9):581–3.

121. Cox JT. Liquid-based cytology: evaluation of effectiveness, cost-effectiveness, and application to present practice. *J Natl Compr Canc Netw* 2004;2(6):597–611.

122. Arbyn M, Bergeron C, Klinkhamer P, Martin-Hirsch P, Siebers AG, Bulten J. Liquid compared with conventional cervical cytology: a systematic review and meta-analysis. *Obstet Gynecol* 2008;111(1):167–77.

123. Davey E, Barratt A, Irwig L, et al. Effect of study design and quality on unsatisfactory rates, cytology classifications, and accuracy in liquid based versus conventional cervical cytology: a systematic review. *Lancet* 2006;367:122–32.

124. Siebers AG, Klinkhamer PJ, Grefte JM, et al. Comparison of liquid-based cytology with conventional cytology for detection of cervical cancer precursors: a randomized controlled trial. *JAMA* 2009;302(16):1757–64.

125. Siebers AG, Klinkhamer PJ, Arbyn M, et al. Cytologic detection of cervical abnormalities using liquid-based compared with conventional cytology: a randomized controlled trial. *Obstet Gynecol* 2008;112(6):1327–34.

126. Marino JF, Fremont-Smith M. Direct-to-vial experience with AutoCyte PREP in a small New England regional cytology practice. *J Reprod Med* 2001;46:353–8.

127. Lee KR, Ashfaq R, Birdsong GG, et al. Comparison of conventional Papanicolaou smears and a fluid-based thin-layer system for cervical cancer screening. *Obstet Gynecol* 1997;90:278–84.

128. Obwegeser JH, Brack S. Does liquid-based technology really improve detection of cervical neoplasia? A prospective randomized trial comparing the ThinPrep Pap Test with the conventional Pap Test including follow-up of HSIL cases. *Acta Cytol* 2001;45:709–14.

129. Bai H, Sung CJ, Steinhoff MM. ThinPrep Pap Test promotes detection of glandular lesions of the endocervix. *Diagn Cytopathol* 2000;23:19–22.

130. Hecht JL, Sheets EE, Lee KR. Atypical glandular cells of undetermined significance in conventional cervical/vaginal smears and thin-layer preparations. *Cancer* 2002;96:1–4.

131. Lee CY, Ng WK. Follow-up study of atypical glandular cells in gynecologic cytology using conventional Pap smears and liquid-based preparations: impact of the Bethesda System 2001. *Acta Cytol* 2008;52(2):159–68.

132. Cheung AN, Szeto EF, Leung BS, Khoo US, Ng AW. Liquid-based cytology and conventional cervical smears: a comparison study in an Asian screening population. *Cancer* 2003;99(6):331–5.

133. Moriarty AT, Clayton AC, Zaleski S, et al. Unsatisfactory reporting rates: 2006 practices of participants in the College of American Pathologists

133. interlaboratory comparison program in gynecologic cytology. *Arch Pathol Lab Med* 2009;133(12):1912–6.

134. Wright PK, Marshall J, Desai M. Comparison of SurePath® and ThinPrep® liquid-based cervical cytology using positive predictive value, atypical predictive value and total predictive value as performance indicators. *Cytopathology* 2010;21(6):374–8.

135. Kenyon S, Sweeney BJ, Happel J, Marchilli GE, Weinstein B, Schneider D. Comparison of BD Surepath and ThinPrep Pap systems in the processing of mucus-rich specimens. *Cancer Cytopathol* 2010;118(5):244–9.

136. Rosenthal DL. Automation and the endangered future of the Pap test. *J Natl Cancer Inst* 1998;90:738–49.

137. Wilbur DC, Parker EM, Foti JA. Location-guided screening of liquid based cervical cytology specimens: a potential improvement in accuracy and productivity is demonstrated in a preclinical feasibility trial. *Am J Clin Pathol* 2002;118:399–407.

138. Sherman ME. Chapter 11: Future directions in cervical pathology. *J Natl Cancer Inst Monogr* 2003;31:72–9.

139. Wilbur DC, Black-Schaffer WS, Luff RD, et al. The Becton Dickinson Focal Point GS Imaging System: clinical trials demonstrate significantly improved sensitivity for the detection of important cervical lesions. *Am J Clin Pathol* 2009;132(5):767–75.

140. Stoler MH, Castle PE, Solomon D, Schiffman M; American Society for Colposcopy and Cervical Pathology. The expanded use of HPV testing in gynecologic practice per ASCCP-guided management requires the use of well-validated assays. *Am J Clin Pathol* 2007;127:335–7.

141. Meijer CJ, Berkhof J, Castle PE, et al. Guidelines for human papillomavirus DNA test requirements for primary cervical cancer screening in women 30 years and older. *Int J Cancer* 2009;124:516–20.

142. Iftner T, Villa LL. Chapter 12: Human papillomavirus technologies. *J Natl Cancer Inst Monogr* 2003;(31):80–8.

143. Selvaggi SM. ASC-US and high-risk HPV testing: performance in daily clinical practice. *Diagn Cytopathol* 2006;34(11):731–3.

144. Peyton CL, Gravitt PE, Hunt WC, et al. Determinants of genital human papillomavirus detection in a US population. *J Infect Dis* 2001;183(11):1554–64.

145. Kornegay JR, Shepard AP, Hankins C, et al.; Canadian Women's HIV Study Group. Non-isotopic detection of human papillomavirus DNA in clinical specimens using a consensus PCR and a generic probe mix in an enzyme-linked immunosorbent assay format. *J Clin Microbiol* 2001;39(10):3530–6.

146. Bauer HM, Ting Y, Greer CE, et al. Genital human papillomavirus infection in female university students as determined by a PCR-based method. *JAMA* 1991;265(4):472–7.

147. Gravitt PE, Peyton CL, Apple RJ, Wheeler CM. Genotyping of 27 human papillomavirus types by using L1 consensus PCR products by a single-hybridization, reverse line blot detection method. *J Clin Microbiol* 1998;36(10):3020–7.

148. Jacobs MV, de Roda Husman AM, van den Brule AJ, Snijders PJ, Meijer CJ, Walboomers JM. Group-specific differentiation between high- and low-risk human papillomavirus genotypes by general primer mediated PCR and two cocktails of oligonucleotide probes. *J Clin Microbiol* 1995;33(4):901–5.

149. Kleter B, van Doorn LJ, Schrauwen L, et al. Development and clinical evaluation of a highly sensitive PCR-reverse hybridization line probe assay for detection and identification of anogenital human papillomavirus. *J Clin Microbiol* 1999;37(8):2508–17.

150. Einstein MH, Martens MG, Garcia F, et al. Clinical validation of the Cervista® HPV HR and 16/18 genotyping tests for use in women with ASC-US cytology. *Gynecol Oncol* 2010;118:116–22.

151. Cervista™ HPV 16/18—P080015. Brief overview of FDA-approval. http://www.fda.gov/MedicalDevices/ProductsandMedicalProcedures/DeviceApprovalsandClearances/Recently-ApprovedDevices/ucm134061.htm.

152. Castle PE, Sadorra M, Lau T, Aldrich C, Garcia FA, Kornegay J. Evaluation of a prototype real-time PCR assay for carcinogenic human papillomavirus (HPV) detection and simultaneous HPV genotype 16 (HPV16) and HPV18 genotyping. *J Clin Microbiol* 2009;47:3344–7.

153. Stoler MH, Wright TC Jr, Sharma A, Apple R, Gutekunst K, Wright TL; the ATHENA (Addressing THE Need for Advanced HPV Diagnostics) HPV Study Group. High-risk human papillomavirus testing in women with ASC-US Cytology: results from the ATHENA HPV study. *Am J Clin Pathol* 2011;135:468–75.

154. http://www.fda.gov/MedicalDevices/ProductsandMedicalProcedures/DeviceApprovalsandClearances/Recently-ApprovedDevices/ucm2545. Accessed June 12, 2014.

155. http://www.fda.gov/MedicalDevices/ProductsandMedicalProcedures/DeviceApprovalsandClearances/Recently-ApprovedDevices/ucm325771.htm. Accessed December 28, 2012.

156. Ho CM, Lee BH, Chang SF, et al. Type-specific human papillomavirus oncogene messenger RNA levels correlate with the severity of cervical neoplasia. *Int J Cancer* 2010;127(3):622–32.

157. Arbyn M, Roelens J, Cuschieri K, et al. The APTIMA HPV assay versus the Hybrid Capture 2 test in triage of women with ASC-US or LSIL cervical cytology: a meta-analysis of the diagnostic accuracy. *Int J Cancer* 2013;132:101–8.

158. Stoler MH, Wright TC, Cuzick J et al. APTIMA HPV assay performance in women with atypical squamous cells of undetermined significance cytology results. *Am J Obstet Gynecol* 2013;208(2):144.e1–8.

159. Khan MJ, Castle PE, Lorincz AT, et al. The elevated 10-year risk of cervical precancer and cancer in women with human papillomavirus (HPV) type

160. 16 or 18 and the possible utility of type-specific HPV testing in clinical practice. *J Natl Cancer Inst* 2005;97:1072–9.

160. Sherman ME, Lorincz AT, Scott DR, et al. Baseline cytology, human papillomavirus testing, and risk for cervical neoplasia: a ten year cohort analysis. *J Natl Cancer Inst* 2003;95:46–52.

161. Castle PE, Wacholder S, Lorincz AT, et al. A prospective study of high grade cervical neoplasia risk among human papillomavirus-infected women. *J Natl Cancer Inst* 2002;94:1406–14.

162. Cuzick J, Beverley E, Ho L, et al. HPV testing in primary screening of older women. *Br J Cancer* 1999;81:554–8.

163. Cuzick J, Szarewski A, Cubie H, et al. Management of women who test positive for high-risk types of human papillomavirus: the HART study. *Lancet* 2003;362:1871–6.

164. Franco EL, Ferenczy A. Assessing gains in diagnostic utility when human papillomavirus testing is used as an adjunct to Papanicolaou smear in the triage of women with cervical cytologic abnormalities. *Am J Obstet Gynecol* 1999;181:382–6.

165. Kuhn L, Denny L, Pollack A, Lorincz A, Richart RM, Wright TC. Human papillomavirus DNA testing for cervical cancer screening in low-resource settings. *J Natl Cancer Inst* 2000;92:818–25.

166. Kulasingam SL, Hughes JP, Kiviat NB, et al. Evaluation of human papillomavirus testing in primary screening for cervical abnormalities: comparison of sensitivity, specificity, and frequency of referral. *JAMA* 2002;288:1749–57.

167. Schiffman M, Herrero R, Hildesheim A, et al. HPV DNA testing in cervical cancer screening: results from women in a high-risk province of Costa Rica. *JAMA* 2000;283:87–93.

168. Cuzick J, Szarewski A, Mesher D, et al. Long-term follow-up of cervical abnormalities among women screened by HPV testing and cytology—results from the Hammersmith study. *Int J Cancer* 2008;122(10):2294–300.

169. Cuzick J, Arbyn M, Sankaranarayanan R, et al. Overview of human papillomavirus-based and other novel options for cervical cancer screening in developed and developing countries. *Vaccine* 2008;26(suppl 10):K29–41.

170. Naucler P, Ryd W, Törnberg S, et al. Efficacy of HPV DNA testing with cytology triage and/or repeat HPV DNA testing in primary cervical cancer screening. *J Natl Cancer Inst* 2009;101(2):88–99.

171. Anttila A, Kotaniemi-Talonen L, Leinonen M, et al. Rate of cervical cancer, severe intraepithelial neoplasia, and adenocarcinoma in situ in primary HPV DNA screening with cytology triage: randomized study within organized screening programme. *BMJ* 2010;340:c1804.

172. Sankaranarayanan R, Nene BM, Shastri SS, et al. HPV screening for cervical cancer in rural India. *N Engl J Med* 2009;360:1385–94.

173. Castle PE, Fetterman B, Poitras N, et al. Variable risk of cervical precancer and cancer after a human papillomavirus-positive test. *Obstet Gynecol* 2011;117(3):650–6.

174. Cuzick J, Mayrand MH, Ronco G, Snijders P, Wardle J. Chapter 10: New dimensions in cervical cancer screening. *Vaccine* 2006;S3:S90–7.

175. Castle PE, Wheeler CM, Solomon D, Schiffman M, Peyton CL; ALTS Group. Interlaboratory reliability of Hybrid Capture 2. *Am J Clin Pathol* 2004;122:238–45.

176. Ward J. Population-based mammographic screening: does 'informed choice' require any less than full disclosure to individuals of benefits, harms, limitations, and consequences? *Aust N Z J Public Health* 1999;23:301–4.

177. Marteau TM, Senior V, Sasieni P. Women's understanding of a "normal smear test result": experimental questionnaire based study. *Br Med J* 2001;322:526–8.

178. Belinson J, Qiao YL, Pretorius R, et al. Shanxi Province Cervical Cancer Screening Study: a cross-sectional comparative trial of multiple techniques to detect cervical neoplasia. *Gynecol Oncol* 2001;83:439–44.

179. Sawaya GF, Washington AE. Cervical cancer screening. Which techniques should be used, and why? *Clin Obstet Gynecol* 1999;42:922–38.

180. Sawaya GF, Brown AD, Washington AE, Garber AM. Clinical practice. Current approaches to cervical-cancer screening. *N Engl J Med* 2001;344:1603–7.

181. Brown AD, Garber AM. Cost-effectiveness of 3 methods to enhance the sensitivity of Papanicolaou testing. *JAMA* 1999;281:347–53.

182. Schiffman M, Wentzensen N, Wacholder S, Kinney W, Gage JC, Castle PE. Human papillomavirus testing in the prevention of cervical cancer. *J Natl Cancer Inst* 2011;103(5):368–83.

183. Luque JS, Tyson DM, Markossian T, et al. Increasing cervical cancer screening in a Hispanic migrant farmworker community through faith based clinical outreach. *J Low Genit Tract Dis* 2011;15(3):200–4.

184. Katz SJ, Hofer TP. Socioeconomic disparities in preventive care persist despite universal coverage. Breast and cervical cancer screening in Ontario and the United States. *JAMA* 1994;272:530–4.

185. Erwin DO, Treviño M, Saad-Harfouche FG, Rodriguez EM, Gage E, Jandorf L. Contextualizing diversity and culture within cancer control interventions for Latinas: changing interventions, not cultures. *Soc Sci Med* 2010;71(4):693–701.

186. Sambamoorthi U, McAlpine DD. Racial, ethnic, socioeconomic, and access disparities in the use of preventive services among women. *Prev Med* 2003;37:475–84.

187. Yu MY, Seetoo AD, Hong OS, Song L, Raizade R, Weller AL. Cancer screening promotion among medically underserved Asian American women: integration of research and practice. *Res Theory Nurs Pract* 2002;16:237–48.

188. Drew JA, Short SE. Disability and Pap smear receipt among U.S. Women, 2000 and 2005. *Perspect Sex Reprod Health* 2010;42(4):258–66.

189. Hawkins NA, Cooper CP, Saraiya M, Gelb CA, Polonec L. Why the Pap test? Awareness and use of the Pap test among women in the United States. *J Womens Health (Larchmt)* 2011;20(4):511–5.

190. Khan K, Curtis CR, Ekwueme DU, et al. Preventing cervical cancer: overviews of the National Breast and Cervical Cancer Early Detection Program and 2 US immunization programs. *Cancer* 2008;113(10 suppl): 3004–12.

191. United States Preventative Services Task Force. Screening for cervical cancer: Recommendations and rational. 2003. http://www.uspreventiveservicestaskforce.org/3rduspstf/cervcan/cervcanrr2.htm.

192. Cooper CP, Saraiya M, McLean TA, et al. Report from the CDC. Pap test intervals used by physicians serving low-income women through the National Breast and Cervical Cancer Early Detection Program. *Womens Health (Larchmt)* 2005;14(8):670–8.

193. Kaplan JE, Benson C, Holmes KH, Brooks JT, Pau A, Masur H; Centers for Disease Control and Prevention (CDC); National Institutes of Health; HIV Medicine Association of the Infectious Diseases Society of America. Guidelines for prevention and treatment of opportunistic infections in HIV-infected adults and adolescents: recommendations from CDC, the National Institutes of Health, and the HIV Medicine Association of the Infectious Diseases Society of America. *MMWR Recomm Rep* 2009;58(RR-4):1–207.

194. Fink DJ. Change in American Cancer Society Checkup Guidelines for detection of cervical cancer. *CA Cancer J Clin* 1988;38:127–8.

195. Sasieni P, Castanon A, Cuzick J. Effectiveness of cervical screening with age: population based case-control study of prospectively recorded data. *BMJ* 2009;339:b2968.

196. Chan PG, Sung HY, Sawaya GF. Changes in cervical cancer incidence after three decades of screening US women less than 30 years old. *Obstet Gynecol* 2003;102(4):765–73.

197. Sroczynski G, Schnell-Inderst P, Mühlberger N, et al. Decision-analytic modeling to evaluate the long-term effectiveness and cost-effectiveness of HPV-DNA testing in primary cervical cancer screening in Germany. *GMS Health Technol Assess* 2010;6:Doc05.

198. Moscicki AB, Cox JT. Practice improvement in cervical screening and management (PICSM): symposium on management of cervical abnormalities in adolescents and young women. *J Low Genit Tract Dis* 2010;14(1):73–80.

199. Gustafsson L, Ponten J, Zack M, Adami HO. International incidence rates of invasive cervical cancer after introduction of cytological screening. *Cancer Causes Control* 1997;8:755–63.

200. Sasieni P, Castanon A, Cuzick J. Screening and adenocarcinoma of the cervix. *Int J Cancer* 2009;125(3):525–9.

201. Sasieni P, Castanon A, Parkin M. How many cervical cancers are prevented by treatment of screen-detected disease in young women? *Int J Cancer* 2009;124:461–4.

202. Moscicki AB, Hills N, Shiboski S, et al. Risks for incident human papillomavirus infection and low-grade squamous intraepithelial lesion development in young females. *JAMA* 2001;285(23):2995–3002.

203. Winer RL, Feng Q, Hughes JP, et al. Risk of female human papillomavirus acquisition associated with first male sex partner. *J Infect Dis* 2008;197(2):279–82.

204. Burchell AN, Winer RL, de Sanjose S, Franco EL. Chapter 6: Epidemiology and transmission dynamics of genital HPV infection. *Vaccine* 2006;24(suppl 3):S3/52–61.

205. Munoz N, Mendez F, Posso H, et al. Incidence, duration, and determinants of cervical human papillomavirus infection in a cohort of Colombian women with normal cytological results. *J Infect Dis* 2004;190(12):2077–87.

206. Ho GY, Bierman R, Beardsley L, Chang CJ, Burk RD. Natural history of cervicovaginal papillomavirus infection in young women. *N Engl J Med* 1998;338(7):423–8.

207. Moscicki AB, Shiboski S, Hills NK, et al. Regression of low-grade squamous intra-epithelial lesions in young women. *Lancet* 2004;364(9446):1678–83.

208. Moscicki AB, Ma Y, Jonte J, et al. The role of sexual behavior and human papillomavirus persistence in predicting repeated infections with new human papillomavirus types. *Cancer Epidemiol Biomarkers Prev* 2010;19(8):2055–65.

209. Boardman LA, Stanko C, Weitzen S, Sung CJ. Atypical squamous cells of undetermined significance: human papillomavirus testing in adolescents. *Obstet Gynecol* 2005;105(4):741–6.

210. Moore K, Cofer A, Elliot L, et al. Adolescent cervical dysplasia: histologic evaluation, treatment, and outcomes. *Am J Obstet Gynecol* 2007;197(2):141,e1–6.

211. Moscicki AB, Ma Y, Wibbelsman C, et al. Rate of and risks for regression of cervical intraepithelial neoplasia 2 in adolescents and young women. *Obstet Gynecol* 2010;116(6):1373–80.

212. Forss A, Tishelman C, Widmark C, Sachs L. Women's experiences of cervical cellular changes: an unintentional transition from health to liminality? *Sociol Health Illn* 2004;26:306–25.

213. Kola S, Walsh JC. Patients' psychological reactions to colposcopy and LLETZ treatment for cervical intraepithelial neoplasia. *Eur J Obstet Gynecol Reprod Biol* 2009;146:96–9.

214. Lerman C, Miller SM, Scarborough R, Hanjani P, Nolte S, Smith D. Adverse psychologic consequences of positive cytologic cervical screening. *Am J Obstet Gynecol* 1991;165:658–62.

215. Sadler L, Saftlas A, Wang W, et al. Treatment for cervical intraepithelial neoplasia and risk of preterm delivery. *JAMA* 2004;291:2100–6.

216. Kyrgiou M, Koliopoulos G, Martin-Hirsch P, et al. Obstetric outcomes after conservative treatment for intraepithelial or early invasive cervical lesions: systematic review and meta-analysis. *Lancet* 2006;367(9509):489–98.

217. Albrechtsen S, Rasmussen S, Thoresen S, Irgens LM, Iversen OE. Pregnancy outcome in women before and after cervical conisation: population based cohort study. *BMJ* 2008;337:a1343.

218. Norman J. Cervical function and prematurity. *Best Prac Res Clin Obstet Gynaecol* 2007;21:791–806.

219. Wright TC Jr, Massad LS, Dunton CJ, et al. 2006 consensus guidelines for the management of women with cervical intraepithelial neoplasia or adenocarcinoma in situ. *Am J Obstet Gynecol* 2007;197(4):340–5.

220. U.S. Census Bureau. U.S. Interim Projections by Age, Sex, Race, and Hispanic Origin: 2000–2050. Washington, DC: USCB, 2004. Available at: http://www.census.gov/population/www/projections/usinterimproj. Accessed September 10, 2011.

221. Sawaya GF, Sung HY, Kearney KA, et al. Advancing age and cervical cancer screening and prognosis. *J Am Geriatr Soc* 2001;49:1499–504.

222. Castle PE, Schiffman M, Wheeler CM, Solomon D. Evidence for frequent regression of cervical intraepithelial neoplasia-grade 2. *Obstet Gynecol* 2009;113:18–25.

223. Stokes-Lampard H, Wilson S, Waddell C, Ryan A, Holder R, Kehoe S. Vaginal vault smears after hysterectomy for reasons other than malignancy: a systematic review of the literature. *BJOG* 2006;113:1354–65.

224. Kalogirou D, Antoniou G, Karakitsos P, Botsis D, Papadimitriou A, Giannikos L. Vaginal intraepithelial neoplasia (VaIN) following hysterectomy in patients treated for carcinoma in situ of the cervix. *Eur J Gynaecol Oncol* 1997;18:188–91.

225. Sillman FH, Fruchter RG, Chen YS, Camilien L, Sedlis A, McTigue E. Vaginal intraepithelial neoplasia: risk factors for persistence, recurrence, and invasion and its management. *Am J Obstet Gynecol* 1997;176:93–9.

226. Verloop J, van Leeuwen FE, Helmerhorst TJ, van Boven HH, Rookus MA. Cancer risk in DES daughters. *Cancer Causes Control* 2010;21:999–1007.

227. Kulasingam S, Havrilesky L, Ghebre R, Myers E. Screening for Cervical Cancer: A Decision Analysis for the US Preventive Services Task Force. AHRQ Pub. No. 11- 05157-EF-1. Rockville, MD: Agency for Healthcare Research and Quality, 2011.

228. Goldie SJ, Kim JJ, Wright TC. Cost-effectiveness of human papillomavirus DNA testing for cervical cancer screening in women aged 30 years or more. *Obstet Gynecol* 2004;103:619–31.

229. Koliopoulos G, Arbyn M, Martin-Hirsch P, Kyrgiou M, Prendiville W, Paraskevaidis E. Diagnostic accuracy of human papillomavirus testing in primary cervical screening: a systematic review and meta-analysis of nonrandomized studies. *Gynecol Oncol* 2007;104:232–46.

230. Vijayaraghavan A, Efrusy MB, Mayrand MH, Santas CC, Goggin P. Cost-effectiveness of high-risk human papillomavirus testing for cervical cancer screening in Quebec, Canada. *Can J Public Health* 2010;101:220–5.

231. International Agency for Research on Cancer Working Group on Evaluation of Cervical Cancer Screening Programmes. Screening for squamous cervical cancer: duration of low risk after negative results of cervical cytology and its implication for screening policies. *Br Med J* 1996;293:659–64.

232. Viikki M, Pukkala E, Hakama M. Risk of cervical cancer after a negative Pap smear. *J Med Screen* 1999;6:103–7.

233. Sasieni PD, Cuzick J, Lynch-Farmery E. Estimating the efficacy of screening by auditing smear histories of women with and without cervical cancer. The National Coordinating Network for Cervical Screening Working Group. *Br J Cancer* 1996;73:1001–5.

234. Miller MG, Sung HY, Sawaya GF, Kearney KA, Kinney W, Hiatt RA. Screening interval and risk of invasive squamous cell cervical cancer. *Obstet Gynecol* 2003;101:29–37.

235. ICESCC International Collaboration of Epidemiological Studies of Cervical Cancer. Comparison of risk factors for invasive squamous cell carcinoma and adenocarcinoma of the cervix: collaborative reanalysis of individual data on 8,097 women with squamous cell carcinoma and 1,374 women with adenocarcinoma from 12 epidemiological studies. *Int J Cancer* 2007;120:885–91.

236. Frame PS, Frame JS. Determinants of cancer frequency: the example of screening for cervical cancer. *J Am Board Fam Pract* 1998;11:87–95.

237. Wright TC Jr, Stoler MH, Sharma A, Zhang G, Behrens C, Wright TL; ATHENA (Addressing THE Need for Advanced HPV Diagnostics) Study Group. Evaluation of HPV-16 and HPV-18 genotyping for the triage of women with high-risk HPVþ cytology- negative results. *Am J Clin Pathol* 2011;136:578–86.

238. Bulkmans NW, Berkhof J, Rozendaal L, et al. Human papillomavirus DNA testing for the detection of cervical intraepithelial neoplasia grade 3 and cancer: 5-year follow-up of a randomized controlled implementation trial. *Lancet* 2007;370:1764–72.

239. Davies P, Arbyn M, Dillner J, et al. A report on the current status of European research on the use of human papillomavirus testing for primary cervical cancer screening. *Int J Cancer* 2006;118:791–6.

240. Petry KU, Menton S, Menton M, et al. Inclusion of HPV testing in routine cervical cancer screening for women above 29 years of age in Germany: results for 8466 patients. *Br J Cancer* 2003;88:1570–7.

241. Cuzick J, Clavel C, Petry KU, et al. Overview of the European and North American studies on HPV testing in primary cervical cancer screening. *Int J Cancer* 2006;119:1095–101.

242. Katki HA, Kinney WK, Fetterman B, et al. Cervical cancer risk for women undergoing concurrent testing for human papillomavirus and cervical

cytology: a population based study in routine clinical practice. *Lancet Oncol* 2011;12:663–72.

243. Australian Institute of Health and Welfare. Cervical Screening in Australia 2008–2009. Canberra, Australian Capital Territory, Australia: Australian Institute of Health and Welfare, 2011.

244. Bray F, Carstensen B, Moller H, et al. Incidence trends of adenocarcinoma of the cervix in 13 European countries. *Cancer Epidemiol Biomarkers Prev* 2005;14:2191–9.

245. Wang SS, Sherman ME, Hildesheim A, Lacey JV Jr, Devesa S. Cervical adenocarcinoma and squamous cell carcinoma incidence trends among white women and black women in the United States for 1976–2000. *Cancer* 2004;100:1035–44.

246. http://www.fda.gov/medicaldevices/productsandmedicalprocedures/deviceapprovalsandclearances/recently-approveddevices/ucm395694.htm. Accessed May 13, 2014.

247. Cox JT, Castle PE, Behrens CM, Sharma A, Wright TC Jr, Cuzick J; Athena HPV Study Group Comparison of cervical cancer screening strategies incorporating different combinations of cytology, HPV testing, and genotyping for HPV 16/18: results from the ATHENA HPV study. *Am J Obstet Gynecol* 2013;208(3):184.e1–11.

248. Vesco K, Whitlock E, Eder M, et al. Screening for Cervical Cancer: A Systematic Evidence Review for the US Preventive Services Task Force. Evidence Synthesis No. 86. AHRQ Pub. No. 11-05156-EF-1. Rockville, MD: Agency for Healthcare Research and Quality, 2011.

249. Centers for Disease Control and Prevention (CDC). National and state vaccination coverage among adolescents aged 13 through 17 years—United States, 2010. *MMWR Morb Mortal Wkly Rep* 2011;60:1117–23.

250. Franco EL, Harper DM. Vaccination against human papillomavirus infection: a new paradigm in cervical cancer control. *Vaccine* 2005;23:2388–94.

251. Arbyn M, Dillner J. Review of current knowledge on HPV vaccination: an appendix to the European guidelines for quality assurance in cervical cancer screening. *J Clin Virol* 2007;38(1):189–97.

252. Dillner J, Arbyn M, Unger E, Dillner L. Monitoring of human papillomavirus vaccination. *Clin Exp Immunol* 2011;163(1):17–25.

253. Castle PE, Solomon D, Saslow D, Schiffman M. Predicting the effect of successful human papillomavirus vaccination on existing cervical cancer prevention programs in the United States. *Cancer* 2008;113(10 suppl):3031–5.

254. Lynge E, Antilla A, Arbyn M, Segnan N, Ronco G. What's next? Perspectives and future needs of cervical screening in Europe in the era of molecular testing and vaccination. *Eur J Cancer* 2009;45(15):2714–21.

255. Mamoon H, Taylor R, Morrell S, Wain G, Moore H. Cervical screening: population-based comparisons between self-reported survey and registry derived Pap test rates. *Aust N Z J Public Health* 2001;25:505–10.

256. Soutter WP, Sasieni P, Panoskaltsis T. Long-term risk of invasive cervical cancer after treatment of squamous cervical intraepithelial neoplasia. *Int J Cancer* 2006;118:2048–55.

257. Flannelly G, Langhan H, Jandial L, Mana E, Campbell M, Kitchener H. A study of treatment failures following large loop excision of the transformation zone for the treatment of cervical intraepithelial neoplasia. *Br J Obstet Gynecol* 1997;104:718–22.

258. Pettersson F, Malker B. Invasive carcinoma of the uterine cervix following diagnosis and treatment of in situ carcinoma. Record linkage study within a National Cancer Registry. *Radiother Oncol* 1989;16:115–20.

259. Kaplan JE, Benson C, Holmes KH, Brooks JT, Pau A, Masur H; Centers for Disease Control and Prevention (CDC); National Institutes of Health; HIV Medicine Association of the Infectious Diseases Society of America. Guidelines for prevention and treatment of opportunistic infections in HIV-infected adults and adolescents: recommendations from CDC, the National Institutes of Health, and the HIV Medicine Association of the Infectious Diseases Society of America. *MMWR Recomm Rep* 2009;58(RR-4):1–207.

260. Berkowitz Z, Saraiya M, Benard V, Yabroff KR. Common abnormal results of Pap and human papillomavirus cotesting: what physicians are recommending for management. *Obstet Gynecol* 2010;116(6):1332–40.

261. Saraiya M, Berkowitz Z, Yabroff KR, Wideroff L, Kobrin S, Benard V. Cervical cancer screening with both human papillomavirus and Papanicolaou testing vs Papanicolaou testing alone: what screening intervals are physicians recommending? *Arch Intern Med* 2010;170(11):977–85.

262. Cox JT, Moriarty AT, Castle PE. Commentary on statement on human papillomavirus test utilization. *Arch Pathol Lab Med* 2009;133(8):1192–4.

263. Castle PE, Schiffman M, Glass AG, et al. Human papillomavirus prevalence in women who have and have not undergone a hysterectomy. *J Infect Dis* 2006;194:1702–5.

264. Keller MJ, Burk RD, Xie X, et al. Risk of cervical precancer and cancer among HIV-infected women with normal cervical cytology and no evidence of oncogenic HPV infection. *JAMA* 2012;308(4):362–9.

265. Dames DN, Ragin C, Griffith-Bowe A, Gomez P, Butler R. The prevalence of cervical cytology abnormalities and human papillomavirus in women infected with the human immunodeficiency virus. *Infect Agent Cancer* 2009;4(suppl 1):S8.

266. De Vuyst H, Lillo F, Broutet N, Smith JS. HIV, human papillomavirus, and cervical neoplasia and cancer in the era of highly active antiretroviral therapy. *Eur J Cancer Prev* 2008;17(6):545–54.

267. Wright TC Jr, Schiffman M, Solomon D, et al. Interim guidance for the use of human papillomavirus DNA testing as an adjunct to cervical cytology for screening. *Obstet Gynecol* 2004;103:304–9.

268. Wright TC, Schiffman M. Adding a test for human papillomavirus DNA to cervical-cancer screening. *N Eng J Med* 2003;348:489–90.

269. Waller J, McCaffery K, Kitchener H, Nazroo J, Wardle J. Women's experiences of repeated HPV testing in the context of cervical cancer screening: a qualitative study. *Psychooncology* 2007;16(3):196–204.

270. Kahn JA, Slap GB, Bernstein DI, et al. Psychological, behavioral, and interpersonal impact of human papillomavirus and Pap test results. *J Womens Health (Larchmt)* 2005;14(7):650–9.

271. McCaffery K, Waller J, Nazroo J, Wardle J. Social and psychological impact of HPV testing in cervical screening: a qualitative study. *Sex Transm Infect* 2006;169–74.

272. Waller J, McCaffery K, Kitchener H, Nazroo J, Wardle J. Women's experiences of repeated HPV testing in the context of cervical cancer screening: a qualitative study. *Psychooncology* 2007;16(3):196–204.

273. Thinking About Testing for HPV? Learn About Cancer. American Cancer Society. http://www.cancer.org/Cancer/CancerCauses/OtherCarcinogens/Infectious Agents/HPV/thinking-about-testing-for-hpv. Accessed April 17, 2011.

274. Anhang R, Wright TC Jr, Smock L, Goldie SJ. Women's desired information about human papillomavirus. *Cancer* 2004;100:315–20.

275. Crum CP, Abbott DW, Quade BJ. Cervical cancer screening: from the Papanicolaou smear to the vaccine era. *J Clin Oncol* 2003;21:224s–30s.

276. Schledermann D, Andersen BT, Bisgaard K, et al. Are adjunctive markers useful in routine cervical cancer screening? Application of p16(INK4a) and HPV-PCR on ThinPrep samples with histological follow-up. *Diagn Cytopathol* 2008;36(7):453–9.

277. Hesselink B, Heideman DA, Steenbergen RD, et al. Combined promoter methylation analysis of CADM1 and MAL: an objective triage tool for high-risk human papillomavirus DNA positive women. *Clin Cancer Res* 2011;17(8):2459–65.

278. Ho CM, Lee BH, Chang SF, et al. Type-specific human papillomavirus oncogene messenger RNA levels correlate with the severity of cervical neoplasia. *Int J Cancer* 2010;127(3):622–32.

279. Porras C, Rodríguez AC, Hildesheim A, et al. Human papillomavirus types by age in cervical cancer precursors: predominance of human papillomavirus 16 in young women. *Cancer Epidemiol Biomarkers Prev* 2009;18(3):863–5.

CHAPTER 7

Management of Abnormal Cervical Cancer Screening Results

19.1 INTRODUCTION
19.2 GUIDELINES FOR SPECIMEN ADEQUACY
    19.2.1 Management of Women with an Unsatisfactory Cytology Test
    19.2.2 Management of Women with Cytology Reported as Negative But with Absent or Insufficient Endocervical/Transformation Zone Component
19.3 GUIDELINES FOR THE MANAGEMENT OF WOMEN WITH ABNORMAL CERVICAL SCREENING TESTS

19.3.1 Management of Women ≥30 with Negative Cytology (NILM) and a Positive HPV Test
19.3.2 Management of ASC-US
19.3.3 Management of Women with ASC-H
19.3.4 Management of Women with LSIL
19.3.5 Management of AGC and Cytologic AIS
19.3.6 Management of HSIL
19.4 PROSPECTS FOR MANAGEMENT OF ABNORMAL CERVICAL SCREENING RESULTS IN THE FUTURE

19.1 INTRODUCTION

Prior to the 1990s, no formal guidelines for management of abnormal cervical cytology existed. In 1994, a group of experts in cervical cancer screening and abnormal cervical cytology management published "interim guidance" on the management of abnormal cervical cytology based primarily on a review of the literature and expert opinion.[1] From 1997 to 2000, a number of committee opinions on management of specimen adequacy issues and abnormal Pap test results were published by the American Society for Colposcopy and Cervical Pathology (ASCCP).[2–5] It was not until the 2001 ASCCP Consensus Guidelines Conference for the Management of Abnormal Cervical Cytology and Cervical Neoplasia that formal, evidence-based guidelines were developed and ratified by experts from the majority of organizations with interest in protecting women from cervical cancer.[6] ASCCP Consensus Conferences in 2006 and 2012 updated the 2001 guidelines based on new data published between the conferences.[7,8] In 2005, the American College of Obstetricians and Gynecologists (ACOG) published guidelines[9] almost identical to the ASCCP's 2001 guidelines and followed with a 2008 update that mirrored the ASCCP 2006 guidelines.[10] Revised ACOG guidelines consistent with the 2012 ASCCP guidelines were released in 2013.[11] Separate guidelines were developed for specimen adequacy.[12,13] These guidelines were revised and incorporated into the ASCCP recommendations at the 2012 ASCCP consensus conference.

Management of abnormal cervical cancer screening tests includes the use of human papillomavirus (HPV) testing. The 2006 ASCCP guidelines first addressed the issue that clinicians cannot assume that management decisions based on results using HPV tests not adequately validated will result in the outcomes intended by the guidelines. In fact, doing so could increase the potential for harm.[7] HPV tests used for screening or management must be analytically and clinically validated with proven acceptable reproducibility, clinical sensitivity, specificity, and positive and negative predictive values for cervical cancer and verified precancer (CIN 2,3) as documented by Food and Drug Administration (FDA) licensing and approval or publication in peer-reviewed scientific literature (Table 19.1).[7,8]

Testing should be restricted to high-risk (oncogenic) HPV types (mainly 16, 18, 31, 33, 35, 39, 45, 51, 52, 56, 58, and 59). In these guidelines and in this chapter, "HPV testing" refers only to testing for high-risk (oncogenic) HPV types. Testing for low-risk (nononcogenic) HPV types has no role in the evaluation of women with abnormal cervical cytology results as these types do not cause cervical cancer. In these guidelines, HPV testing refers only to oncogenic types.[8] Further discussion of the characteristics of each of the FDA-approved HPV tests is in Chapter 18.

This chapter discusses and outlines the most recent ASCCP recommendations for management of abnormal cervical cytology.[8] The Bethesda 2001 Workshop[14] terminology and descriptors for reporting of normal and abnormal cervical cytology used in the management guidelines are discussed in detail in Chapter 3. The ASCCP guidelines for the management of histologically confirmed cervical neoplasia can be found in Chapter 20.

19.2 GUIDELINES FOR SPECIMEN ADEQUACY

Following the National Cancer Institute (NCI) Bethesda 2001 Workshop, which updated terminology and reporting of cervical cytology,[14] an ASCCP task force published guidelines related to cytology specimen adequacy and patient management.[12] The 2002 ASCCP specimen adequacy guidelines included recommendations on the follow-up of women with either an unsatisfactory cytology test or a cytology test with quality indicators, including lack of an endocervical/transformation zone (EC/TZ) component and partially obscuring factors.[12] The adequacy guidelines were first revised in 2008[13] to accommodate liquid-based cytology (LBC) preparations and use of HPV testing as a "cotest" with cervical cytology in primary screening for women aged 30 years and older. These guidelines

TABLE 19.1	GUIDELINES FOR THE USE OF HPV TESTING IN MANAGEMENT

- Use only an HPV test that has been analytically and clinically validated with proven acceptable reproducibility and test characteristic values for cervical cancer and verified precancer (CIN 2,3), as documented by FDA approval or publication in peer-reviewed scientific literature.
- HPV testing should be restricted to high-risk (oncogenic) HPV types because low-risk HPV types are not a cause of CIN 3 or cancer. There is no clinical utility in testing for other (nononcogenic) types (AI).
- Testing for other (nononcogenic) HPV types when screening for cervical neoplasia, or during the management and follow-up of women with abnormal cervical cytology or cervical neoplasia, is unacceptable (EI).

Adapted from Massad LS, Einstein MH, Huh WK, et al. 2012 Updated consensus guidelines for the management of abnormal cervical cancer screening tests and cancer precursors. *J Low Genit Tract Dis* 2013;17:S1–27, with permission; Management of abnormal cervical cancer screening test results and cervical cancer precursors. Practice Bulletin No. 140. American College of Obstetricians and Gynecologists. *Obstet Gynecol* 2013;122:1338–67.

did not go through a national consensus conference process. The 2012 consensus conference reviewed the adequacy guidelines, adopted most, and added in new information related to adequacy when HPV test results are available. It modified the guidelines accordingly for cytology reported as negative but with an absent or insufficient EC or TZ component.[8] Presence of any detected abnormality should be fully evaluated regardless of other concerns about specimen adequacy.

19.2.1 Management of Women with an Unsatisfactory Cytology Test

Cervical cytology is reported as "unsatisfactory" when (1) specimens are rejected by the laboratory due to labeling problems, specimen vial leakage, or slide breakage or (2) specimens are completely processed but found to have insufficient squamous cells or obscuring (>75%) blood, inflammation, or other processes.[15] Bethesda 2001 provided guidance criteria on the threshold for squamous cellularity required for most patient populations and laboratory settings to designate the Pap test as "satisfactory for evaluation."[14,15] The criteria vary depending on whether the cytology test is a conventional or liquid-based specimen. For cytology obtained from liquid-based media, "insufficient squamous cells" is the most common reason for an "unsatisfactory" report. Estimating adequate cellularity of specimens with cell clusters, cytolysis, or atrophy is difficult when using representative field counts, so laboratories are advised to exercise judgment in reporting such specimens.[15] Unsatisfactory cytology tests may also be due to obscuring (>75%) blood or inflammation, although this has become less of a problem as liquid based has virtually replaced conventional cytology testing.[15]

Clinical parameters associated with unsatisfactory cytology tests include a history of pelvic malignancy, pelvic irradiation, conization, hysterectomy, pregnancy, being within 3 months postpartum, vaginal bleeding, abnormal vaginal discharge, intrauterine device, and cervical polyps.[16,17] Low cellularity and inadequate specimens are frequently found in women treated with radiation or chemotherapy for gynecologic malignancies, complicating the management of these women.[17] The authors of one study suggest that the minimum numeric threshold for cellularity can safely be reduced in women following radiotherapy without increasing the risk of missed disease.[17]

An unsatisfactory cytology test is unreliable for detecting epithelial abnormalities, as several studies reported that women with unsatisfactory results may have significant risk for disease.[18,19] Unsatisfactory Pap tests, particularly when the specimen is conventional cytology, are common in women with invasive cervical cancer. False-negative HPV tests are possible in the setting of unsatisfactory specimens, and therefore negative HPV tests should not be relied upon. Positive HPV tests should be managed as true positives.[8] Clinical correlation at the time of the initial specimen may suggest the need for additional evaluation such as colposcopy or other histologic studies. For several decades, it was believed that repeating the Pap test within a short time frame (<3 months) would decrease the adequacy and sensitivity of the Pap test. However, evaluation of Pap tests obtained in the ASCUS/LSIL Triage Study (ALTS) repeated over intervals that ranged from 15 to 120 days did not demonstrate that a short repeat interval had any adverse effect on either the quality of liquid-based repeat cytology or the HPV viral load tested from a residual liquid-based specimen.[20]

Women with an unsatisfactory cytology should have repeat cytology within 2 to 4 months.[8] (Table 19.2; Figure 19.1). Colposcopy is recommended for women with two consecutive unsatisfactory cytology tests. For women cotested who have positive HPV tests and unsatisfactory cytology, either repeat cytology or immediate colposcopy is acceptable. If HPV testing was not obtained as part of screening, it should not be done as a "reflex" to an unsatisfactory Pap test. Treatment of atrophy and specific infections prior to repeat is acceptable.

TABLE 19.2	MANAGEMENT OF WOMEN WITH UNSATISFACTORY CYTOLOGY*

- For women with an unsatisfactory cytology result and no, unknown, or a negative HPV test result, repeat cytology in 2–4 mo is recommended.
- Triage using reflex HPV testing is not recommended.
- Treatment to resolve atrophy or obscuring inflammation when a specific infection is present is acceptable.
- For women aged 30 y and older who are cotested and have unsatisfactory cytology and a positive HPV test, repeat cytology in 2–4 mo or colposcopy is acceptable.
- Colposcopy is recommended for women with two consecutive unsatisfactory cytology tests.

*Algorithm in Figure 19.1.
Adapted from Massad LS, Einstein MH, Huh WK, et al. 2012 Updated consensus guidelines for the management of abnormal cervical cancer screening tests and cancer precursors. *J Low Genit Tract Dis* 2013;17:S1–27, with permission.

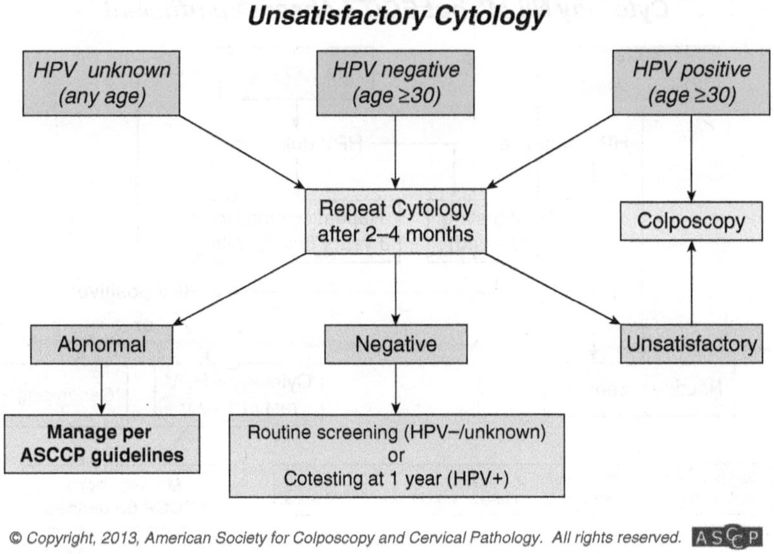

Unsatisfactory Cytology

FIGURE 19.1.   ASCCP algorithm for the management of unsatisfactory cervical cytology. (From Massad LS, Einstein MH, Huh WK, et al. 2012 Updated consensus guidelines for the management of abnormal cervical cancer screening tests and cancer precursors. *J Low Genit Tract Dis* 2013;17:S1–27, with permission.)

19.2.2 Management of Women with Cytology Reported as Negative But with Absent or Insufficient Endocervical/Transformation Zone Component

19.2.2.1 When Cytology Is the Only Screening Test

The concern regarding inadequate EC/TZ cells on the cytology specimen is the possibility that the TZ may not have been adequately sampled, thereby increasing the risk of missing cervical intraepithelial neoplasia (CIN) or adenocarcinoma in situ (AIS), typically located at the squamocolumnar junction (SCJ) in the TZ. Improved sampling technique and the use of better sampling devices have tended to increase the collection of EC/TZ cells,[3,21,22] but it is not always possible to obtain these cells. There is less frequent identification of EC/TZ cells in women on oral contraceptives and in women who are pregnant or postmenopausal.[3,23] It is more difficult to sample these cells in these groups despite good clinician technique and the use of appropriate EC sampling devices.[24] This finding is not unusual, with recent studies suggesting that it occurs in 5%[25] to nearly 20%[26] of cytology specimens.

Prior guidelines recommended early repeat cytology in patients with absent or insufficient EC/TZ component.[13] This recommendation was based on the finding in a number of studies of increased detection of cytologic abnormalities in specimens with EC cells present and a few studies that showed

false-negative cytology in women without an EC component prior to diagnosis of cancer.[27] Conversely, a number of studies comparing cytology and histology showed less frequent discordance among women with absent EC component compared to women with adequate EC component.[27] Most important, women lacking an EC/TZ component do not have an increased detection of CIN in follow-up, which would be expected if abnormalities were missed.[25,28–31] While a number of these trials were retrospective, two were prospective. Georgi Rossi showed a decreased risk over 4.5 years of follow-up when the EC component was absent on initial cytology.[25] Mitchell showed no increased risk of CIN on follow-up even when subjects had EC cells present on their follow-up cytology.[28] Women with Pap tests lacking an EC/TZ component may represent a lower-risk group as a whole because this group is skewed toward older ages.[13,21,32] This may explain the apparent inconsistency between longitudinal studies, which suggest no increase in risk, and cross-sectional studies, which report more abnormalities in samples that contain an EC/TZ component.[13] Another hypothesis is that EC cells are more accessible in patients with cervical abnormalities.[27] This lack of increased risk appears also to be present in women with no EC component on cytology performed after treatment for CIN 2,3.[13,33]

For women aged 21 to 29 years with negative cytology and absent or insufficient EC/TZ component, the updated ASCCP management guidelines recommend routine screening (Table 19.3; Figure 19.2).[8] This is an important change from prior guidelines that recommended early repeat screening.

| TABLE 19.3 | MANAGEMENT OF WOMEN WITH CYTOLOGY REPORTED AS NEGATIVE BUT WITH ABSENT OR INSUFFICIENT EC/TZ COMPONENT* |

- For women aged 21–29 y with negative cytology and absent or insufficient EC/TZ component, routine screening is recommended.
  - HPV testing is unacceptable.
- For women aged 30 y and older with cytology reported as negative and with absent or insufficient EC/TZ component and no or unknown HPV test result, HPV testing is preferred.
  - If the HPV test is done and is negative, return to routine screening is recommended.
  - If the HPV test is positive, repeating both tests (cytology and HPV) in 1 y is acceptable.
  - Genotyping is also acceptable:
    - If HPV type 16 or type 18 is present, colposcopy is recommended.
    - If HPV type 16 and type 18 are absent, repeat cotesting in 12 mo is recommended.

*Algorithm in Figure 19.2.
Adapted from Massad LS, Einstein MH, Huh WK, et al. 2012 Updated consensus guidelines for the management of abnormal cervical cancer screening tests and cancer precursors. *J Low Genit Tract Dis* 2013;17:S1–27, with permission.

FIGURE 19.2. ASCCP algorithm for the management of negative cytology and absent or insufficient EC/TZ component. (From Massad LS, Einstein MH, Huh WK, et al. 2012 Updated consensus guidelines for the management of abnormal cervical cancer screening tests and cancer precursors. *J Low Genit Tract Dis* 2013;17: S1–27, with permission.)

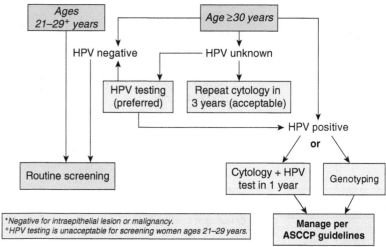

For women aged 30 years and older and with no or unknown HPV test result, HPV testing is preferred for management (see section 19.2.2.2). Repeat cytology is acceptable in 3 years if HPV testing is not performed.[8]

19.2.2.2 When Screening with a Cotest (Pap and HPV Test Combined)

Current recommendations[34–36] are that women ≥30 years of age can be screened with the combination of an HPV test and cervical cytology, called "cotesting." Evaluation of over 140,000 Pap tests demonstrated that adjunctive HPV testing is effective in stratifying risk for the presence of CIN in women with and without an EC/TZ and that HPV-positive test rates are independent of the presence or absence of an EC/TZ, confirming that HPV testing can provide an objective stratification of disease risk in women with negative Pap tests and no EC/TZ.[26] In women 30 and older having cotesting, the HPV results often guide further management. If both cytology and HPV testing are negative, the patient can continue routine screening at longer intervals than after negative cytology alone. If HPV testing is positive, immediate genotyping for HPV 16/18 or repeating cytology and HPV testing in 1 year is acceptable. If HPV 16/18 positive, colposcopy is recommended; if not, cotesting should be repeated in 12 months.

19.3 GUIDELINES FOR THE MANAGEMENT OF WOMEN WITH ABNORMAL CERVICAL SCREENING TESTS

The updated ASCCP guidelines for the management of women with abnormal cervical screening results were created by the 2012 ASCCP consensus conference[8] to update their 2006 consensus guidelines.[7] This consensus conference reviewed prior recommendations on management of abnormal cervical cancer screening tests, inadequate and limited specimens, and abnormal histologic findings and pooled all three previous separate recommendation documents into a single document. Revisions were motivated by a number of considerations. Prior recommendations were based primarily on the ALTS trial, which focused on the management of ASC-US and LSIL cytology.[38] Recommendations for other abnormalities were based on extrapolation of the data from the ALTS trial and on literature

review. Since that time, a large cervical cancer screening database from Kaiser Permanente of Northern California (KPNC) has become available with data regarding risk across all cytology results from 1.4 million women over 8 years.[39–47] The size of this KPNC database also allowed age-based stratification of data for some types of abnormalities.[8] The American Cancer Society, along with ASCCP and ASCP, revised their screening guidelines in 2012, as did the American College of OB/GYN (ACOG), considerably lengthening screening intervals with a preference for cotesting for primary screening in women 30 to 65 years of age.[34,35] Adolescents (women and girls <21) are no longer screened under current guidelines, and since it has been recognized that women aged 21 to 24 years are also at lower risk than older women, previous recommendations for managing adolescents with abnormal cervical cytology were extended to the 21- to 24-year-old age group after validation using KPNC data.[43] HPV testing has become much more widely used since the prior guidelines. Each of these issues required consideration and, ultimately, revision to previous recommendations. The consensus conference applied a principle of "similar management strategies for similar levels of risk."[8] They accepted that not all cancers were preventable, and that optimal strategies should be chosen that maximize the chance of preventing cancer while minimizing harms from overtreatment. Table 19.4 summarizes the changes from the prior guidelines related to management of screening tests. As noted at the time of the recommendation release, all of these changes entailed a great degree of complexity.[48] Computerized decision support offers great potential for following complicated algorithms. To assist providers in implementing the guidelines, "apps" have been developed for common handheld devices and are available through the ASCCP Web site (**www.ASCCP.org**). Currently the apps are available for most Apple and Android devices.

19.3.1 Management of Women ≥30 with Negative Cytology (NILM) and a Positive HPV Test

19.3.1.1 Initial Management

The revised screening guidelines from the ACS/ASCCP/ASCP[35] and ACOG,[34] though not the USPSTF,[36] specifically recommend cotesting as the *preferred* primary screening option in

TABLE 19.4	SUMMARY OF THE *PRIMARY CHANGES* FROM THE 2012 ASCCP CONSENSUS CONFERENCE FOR THE MANAGEMENT OF ABNORMAL CERVICAL CANCER SCREENING TESTS AND CANCER PRECURSORS*

- Cytology reported as negative but lacking endocervical cells can be managed without early repeat.
- Cytology reported as unsatisfactory:
  - If HPV negative, still requires repeat.
  - If HPV positive, either referral to colposcopy or repeat cytology is acceptable.
- Genotyping triages HPV-positive women with HPV type 16 or type 18 to earlier colposcopy only after negative cytology; colposcopy is indicated for all women with ASC-US/HPV-positive results, regardless of genotyping result.
- Only two options for the management of ASC-US:
  - Immediate colposcopy is no longer an option.
  - The serial cytology option for ASC-US no longer has a 6-month repeat. Instead, repeat cytology for ASC-US should be at 12 mo and then if negative, cytology every 3 y.
  - Reflex HPV testing for ASC-US should only be done on women ≥25:
    - ASC-US/HPV negative should be followed with cotesting at 3 y.
    - ASC-US/HPV negative is insufficient to allow exit from screening at age 65 y.
- More strategies incorporate cotesting for women ≥30 to reduce follow-up visits.
- Cytology as the only screening strategy is limited to women <30 y of age:
  - Cotesting can be used in women <30 y in some circumstances (i.e., where recommended in follow-up).
- Women aged 21–24 y are managed conservatively.

*Prior management guidelines were from the "2006 Consensus Guidelines for the Management of Women with Abnormal Cervical Screening Tests" (7). Prior guidelines not changed were retained.
CIN, cervical intraepithelial neoplasia; ECC, endocervical curettage; HPV, human papillomavirus; ASC-US, atypical squamous cells of undetermined significance.
Adapted from Massad LS, Einstein MH, Huh WK, et al. 2012 Updated consensus guidelines for the management of abnormal cervical cancer screening tests and cancer precursors. *J Low Genit Tract Dis* 2013;17:S1–27, with permission.

women aged 30 to 65. It is not indicated in younger women. This recommendation was primarily made on the basis of the very high sensitivity of the two tests together for CIN 2+; a woman with negative cytology and a negative HPV test has an extremely small risk of CIN 3, AIS, or cancer (CIN 3+) developing over the following 5 years (see Chapter 18). Risk of CIN 3+ is higher in women cytology negative/HPV positive than in those who are cytology negative/HPV negative. Cytology-negative/HPV-positive results occurred in 3.6% of women ages 30 to 64 in the KPNC cohort, but this rate varied significantly by age, with women aged 30 to 40 having the highest rate within this ≥30-year-old age group (Figure 19.3).[40,41] It was the most frequent positive screening result, representing a significant sized group of women requiring management. The consensus recommendations reflect the frequency of this cotest result and the relatively low risk for CIN 2+, but also reflect the continued risk of precancer and cancer in this group. In the KPNC cohort, 34% of the CIN 3+, 44% of the AIS, 29% of the total cervical cancers, and 63% of the adenocarcinomas were detected in follow-up to this cotest result.[39,41]

The ACS/ASCCP/ASCP screening guidelines document reviewed 11 studies with up to 16 years of follow-up and reported 12-month risk of CIN 3+ for cytology negative/HPV positive varying from 0.8% to 4.1%.[35] In the KPNC cohort, the 5-year risk of CIN 3+ was 4.5%, only slightly less than the 5.2% noted with LSIL, which was the threshold for colposcopy.[41] Five-year cancer risk was 0.34%, and half of the cases were adenocarcinomas.[41] Referring all women with this result for colposcopy would have required many procedures and falls below the 10% level of risk for CIN 3+ recommended for colposcopy referral.[49,50] Therefore, a strategy of early repeat testing was adopted as one option for managing this result, similar to previous guidelines.[7,51] Alternatively, genotype information may be used to immediately triage higher-risk women with cytology-negative, HPV 16/18–positive results to colposcopy, but those positive for the panel of other hrHPV types (but not 16 and/or 18) to 12-month follow-up.[8]

The rationale for early repeat testing is twofold. First, most positive HPV tests represent transient infection without risk of progression to cancer. Clearance rates of HPV in women with NILM cytology vary from 60% at 6 months in a study in France[52] to 67% by 1 year in the Guanacaste cohort.[53] In the KPNC cohort, 44% cleared at 1 year.[41] Not surprisingly,

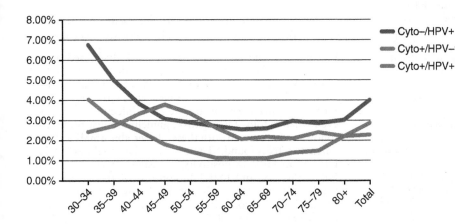

FIGURE 19.3. Rates for various combinations of HPV and Pap cotesting results per 5-year age groups in over 812,000 women in the Kaiser Permanente Northern California HMO between 2003 and 2008. The highest rate of HPV detection, that is, for women in their 30s, corresponds to the decade during which the most high-grade precancer CIN 2,3 is found in women in the Kaiser health system. (Adapted from Castle PE, Fetterman B, Poitras N, Lorey T, Shaber R, Kinney W. Five-year experience of human papillomavirus DNA and Papanicolaou test cotesting. *Obstet Gynecol* 2009;113:595–600, with permission.)

among those who did not clear, the risk of CIN 2+ increases. Of the subjects in the Guanacaste cohort who were cytology negative/HPV positive at baseline and again at 1 year, 17% developed CIN 2+ by the end of 3 years of follow-up. This compared to 1.2% in women of women HPV positive at baseline but HPV negative at 1 year.[53] CIN 2+ developed in 21% of the women remaining HPV positive throughout the 3-year follow-up. A strategy of repeat cotesting in 1 year allows many HPV infections to resolve, avoiding colposcopy in 44% to 67% of the women initially cytology negative/HPV positive, thereby reserving colposcopy for the much smaller group with persistent infection or abnormal cytology, who are at much higher risk.

Based on these considerations, colposcopy is recommended for any cytologic abnormality (≥ASC-US or HPV positive regardless of the cytology result) at the 1-year repeat. Although the risk for HPV-negative ASC-US is very small, the consensus conference delegates decided to include any abnormal cytology on repeat in the referral to colposcopy to minimize complexity. The potential for missing a cancer within the 1-year interval is very small with this strategy. In the KPNC cohort, the 1-year risk of cancer following the first cytology-negative/HPV-positive result was 0.11% compared to a 0.93% risk of CIN 3+.[41] The risk of CIN 3+ was much higher if the follow-up test (either cytology or HPV) was positive at the 12-month follow-up. For example, the 5-year risk of CIN 3+ with a repeat cytology-negative/HPV-positive result at the 12-month follow-up was 7.4% versus 4.2% at baseline.[41] Additionally, at the return visit after a baseline cytology-negative/HPV-positive result, almost every repeat cotest result predicted greater subsequent 5-year CIN 3+ risk than the same cotest result had at baseline, and these risks guided the follow-up recommendations.[41] For example, the 5-year CIN 3+ risk after cytology-negative/HPV-negative result at the return test was 0.93%. This is close to the risk after a baseline cytology-negative (alone) result (0.26%) for which a 3-year repeat cotest is recommended.[41] Therefore, a 3-year repeat cotest was chosen for management in this situation.[8] As with other algorithms, women aged 30 and over with a previous screening abnormality are recommended to continue follow-up with cotesting rather than cytology alone.[8]

Using the KNPC data, the updated ASCCP management guidelines modified the prior algorithm for managing cytology-negative/HPV-positive cotest results (Table 19.5; Figure 19.4).[8] Conceptually, it is largely unchanged from the 2006

ASCCP guidelines that proposed the option of genotyping triage to 1-year follow-up.[7] For cytology-negative/HPV-positive women managed by repeat cotesting in 12 months, colposcopy is recommended for any abnormality on repeat (≥ASC-US cytology or HPV positive). Women with cytology-negative/HPV-negative results at the 1-year follow-up should have a repeat cotest in 3 years. As discussed above, this interval is shorter than the 5-year interval recommended for women initially cytology negative/HPV negative since these women continue to have a slightly elevated CIN 3+ risk at 5 years, comparable to the CIN 3+ risk at 3 years for ASC-US/HPV negative or for a NILM report when cytology is the only screen.[8] While the risk of cancer is small with 12-month repeat cotesting, this strategy does have several drawbacks. First, it is potentially anxiety provoking for the woman to wait a year for any further analysis of risk. Second, it relies on patient adherence to return for cotesting. In a clinic-based trial of HPV testing in England, the loss to follow-up at the 1-year interval was so great that it negated the benefits of cotesting.[54,55] These limitations motivated alternative strategies.

The genotyping triage strategy is designed to identify the cytology-negative/HPV-positive women at greatest risk for CIN 3+ for referral to immediate colposcopy, thereby decreasing the risk of delayed diagnosis of CIN 3+, anxiety secondary to delayed evaluation, and loss to follow-up. Three of the FDA-approved HPV tests for cotesting include either HPV 16/18 genotyping in the initial test (Cobas) or as a reflex that can be ordered to a positive HPV test (Cervista), or as an HPV 16 and 18/45 reflex test (Aptima). They may be used to determine if a woman with a cytology-negative/HPV-positive cotest result has any of these two or three types most common in cervical cancer and is at highest risk for the development of CIN 3+ in the future.[56-58]

The 10-year cumulative incidence rates of CIN 3+ for women ages 30 and older in the long-term NCI Portland Kaiser natural history study were 20.7% among women HPV 16 positive at baseline and 17.7% among those positive for HPV 18 (Figure 19.5).[56] In contrast, only 1.5% of women positive for HPV but negative for HPV 16/18 and only 0.5% of women initially negative for HPV were found to have CIN 3+ over the same period of time. In the ATHENA trial, 11.4% of women with NILM cytology who were HPV 16 or 18 positive had CIN 2+, high enough to justify immediate colposcopy.[59]

The updated ASCCP management guidelines offer genotyping for HPV 16 and HPV 18 as an alternative to repeat cotesting for management of women who are cytology negative/HPV positive.[8] If the patient tests positive for HPV 16 or 18, she should undergo immediate colposcopy (Table 19.5; Figure 19.4). Use of HPV 16/18 testing here is in some ways analogous to reflex HPV testing for the management of ASC-US cytology.

TABLE 19.5	MANAGEMENT OF WOMEN TESTING HPV POSITIVE BUT CYTOLOGY NEGATIVE*

- For women ≥30 y of age and cytology negative/HPV positive, repeat cotesting at 1 y is acceptable.
  - At the 1-year repeat cotest, if ≥ASC-US or HPV positive, colposcopy is recommended.
  - If the 1-year repeat cotest is cytology negative/HPV negative, repeat cotesting in 3 y is recommended.
- HPV genotyping is also acceptable.
  - If HPV 16 or HPV 18 are positive, colposcopy is recommended.
  - If HPV 16 and HPV 18 tests are negative, repeat cotesting in 1 y is recommended.

*Algorithm in Figure 19.4.
Adapted from Massad LS, Einstein MH, Huh WK, et al. 2012 Updated consensus guidelines for the management of abnormal cervical cancer screening tests and cancer precursors. *J Low Genit Tract Dis* 2013;17:S1–27, with permission.

19.3.1.2 Postcolposcopy Management of Women with Cytology-Negative/HPV-Positive Results

Patients with no lesion or only CIN 1 diagnosed at colposcopy should receive follow-up according to the ASCCP postcolposcopy guidelines for the referral abnormality. Since CIN 3+ risk is elevated for women with either HPV 16 or HPV 18 or persistent oncogenic HPV infection of any type even when cytology is negative, guidelines must provide for follow-up for women with these "lesser abnormalities" even when no CIN is found.[8] These "lesser abnormalities" include HPV 16 or HPV 18 positivity, persistent untyped oncogenic HPV, ASC-US, and LSIL.[8] In contrast, if the repeat cotest cytology result was AGC or HSIL, further management should follow recommendations for the finding of ≤CIN 1 for these cytology results.

Management of Women ≥ Age 30, Who Are Cytology Negative, but HPV Positive

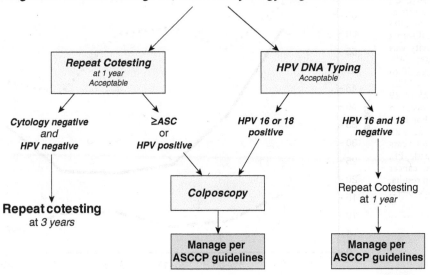

FIGURE 19.4. ASCCP algorithm for the management of women greater than or equal to age 30 who are cytology negative but HPV positive. (From Massad LS, Einstein MH, Huh WK, et al. 2012 Updated consensus guidelines for the management of abnormal cervical cancer screening tests and cancer precursors. *J Low Genit Tract Dis* 2013;17:S1–27, with permission.)

19.3.2 Management of ASC-US

19.3.2.1 General Issues with ASC-US

Atypical cells are often generated in response to events occurring in the cervicovaginal environment that have nothing to do with HPV or with neoplasia. Most of these cellular changes are difficult to differentiate from reactive and reparative changes secondary to trauma from tampon use, intercourse, bacterial and yeast infections, and other normal "life" events. The epithelial effects of aging and declining estrogen also result in cytologic changes whose meaning may be unclear. The other most frequent cause of equivocal cellular change is HPV.

ASC-US is the most common abnormal cytologic report, yet carries the lowest risk of CIN 3+.[38,42,60] The original guidelines for ASC-US triage were based on the ALTS trial that showed that immediate colposcopy, triage with HPV testing, and repeat cytology performed similarly. The ALTS trial was conducted prior to the 2001 Bethesda Workshop, which subdivided

the atypical squamous cell (ASC) category into ASC-US and "atypical squamous cells cannot exclude high-grade squamous intraepithelial lesion"(ASC-H).[14] The median rate of ASC-US most recently reported in US laboratories was 4.3%, whereas the median for ASC-H was 0.2%.[61] The recent report by Katki et al. examined the 5-year risk of CIN 3+ after an ASC-US result from the KPNC database.[42] Not surprisingly, the highest rates of HPV were found in younger women with ASC-US, with a prevalence of 54% to 56% among those under 35 years of age and 25% to 30% among those 45 years and older (Figure 19.6). Among women with HPV-positive ASC-US, the baseline risk of CIN 3+ was 3.2% and the 5-year cumulative risk was 6.8% with the highest risks among women aged 25 to 49 years.[42] Women under 25 years of age were not included because HPV testing was not considered indicated. The baseline risk of CIN 3+ among women with ASC-US, regardless of HPV status, was only 1.3%, and 5-year risk was 2.6%. Among those HPV negative, the 5-year cumulative risk was only 0.43%, which was only marginally higher

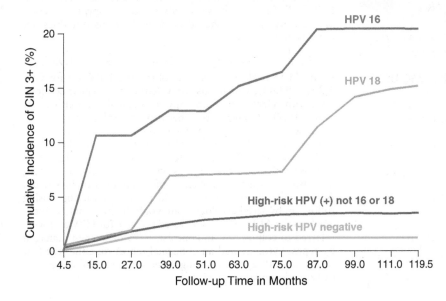

FIGURE 19.5. Cumulative incidence of CIN grade 3 and cancer (≥CIN 3) over a 10-year period in 13,229 women ≥30 years, according to oncogenic HPV status at enrollment. *Red line* for HPV 16, *orange* for HPV 18, *blue* for the panel of oncogenic (hr) HPV other than HPV 16/18, and *green* for women HPV negative for hrHPV. (Modified from Khan MJ, Castle PE, Lorincz AT, et al. The elevated 10-year risk of cervical precancer and cancer in women with human papillomavirus (HPV) type 16 or 18 and the possible utility of type-specific HPV testing in clinical practice. *J Natl Cancer Inst* 2005;97:1072–9, with permission.)

FIGURE 19.6. Positivity for HPV by age group among women with negative (dashed line), ASC-US (solid line) and LSIL (dotted line) cytology results at baseline in over 1.1 million women screened from 2003 to 2010 in the Kaiser Permanente Northern California clinics. For women with ASC-US, HPV positivity was similar for those aged 25 to 29 and 30 to 34 years (54% vs. 56%) and then declined sharply through ages 50 to 54 years (56% vs. 24%). Among women with LSIL, HPV positivity was similar for women aged 25 to 29 and 30 to 34 years (85% vs. 88%) and then declined through ages 55 to 59 years (88% vs. 69%). For Pap-negative women, HPV positivity declined over ages 25 to 29 (10%), to 30 to 34 (6.1%), to 60 to 64 years (2.1%). (From Katki HA, Schiffman M, Castle PE, et al. Five-year risks of CIN 3+ and cervical cancer among women with HPV testing of ASC-US Pap results. *J Low Genit Tract Dis* 2013;17(5 Suppl 1):S36–42, with permission.)

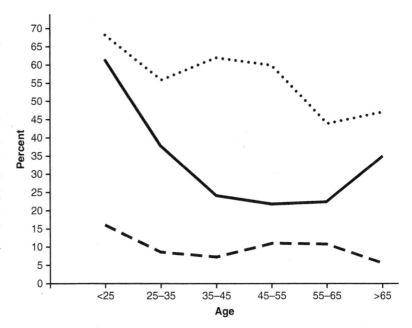

than the risk for women Pap negative but HPV unknown (0.26%). The risk of CIN 3+ for ASC-US/HPV positive was similar to that described for LSIL, which had a 5-year risk of 5.2%. These rates of HPV prevalence and CIN 3+ at baseline were similar to many other published studies suggesting that these data can be generalized.[62] The risk for CIN 3+ detection for ASC-H is substantially higher than for ASC-US; hence, these two subcategories are managed differently and will be discussed separately.

19.3.2.2 Guidelines for Initial Management of Women with ASC-US

19.3.2.2.1 WOMEN ≥25 YEARS OF AGE

Because the risk of CIN 3+ is much higher among women who are ASC-US/HPV positive than among women who are ASC-US/HPV negative or ASC-US with unknown HPV status, these women are managed differently.[39,42] The prior guidelines identified all three options (i.e., immediate colposcopy, repeat cytology, and HPV testing) for the management of women with ASC-US as safe and effective, and therefore all

TABLE 19.6	INITIAL MANAGEMENT OF WOMEN ≥25 YEARS WITH ASC-US*

- Reflex HPV testing for the initial management of ASC-US:
  - ASC-US/HPV negative, repeat cotesting at 3 y is recommended.
  - ASC-US/HPV positive (cotesting or reflex for ASC-US), colposcopy is recommended.
- Repeat cytology at 1 y is acceptable.
  - If repeat cytology is ≥ASC-US, colposcopy is recommended
  - If repeat cytology is negative, return to routine screening in 3 y.
- If colposcopy is done, an ECC is recommended if no lesion is identified.
- Immediate colposcopy is no longer recommended.

*Algorithm in Figure 19.7.
Adapted from Massad LS, Einstein MH, Huh WK, et al. 2012 Updated consensus guidelines for the management of abnormal cervical cancer screening tests and cancer precursors. *J Low Genit Tract Dis* 2013;17:S1–27, with permission.

were considered acceptable follow-up options.[6,7] If the Pap test was obtained using a liquid-based sample or the HPV test was separately obtained, HPV testing was preferred.

However, the updated ASCCP management guidelines *prefer* reflex HPV testing for the initial management of ASC-US, although repeat cytology at 1 year is acceptable. Immediate colposcopy is no longer recommended as a management option (Table 19.6; Figure 19.7).[8]

19.3.2.2.1.1 Management of ASC-US with HPV Testing
If the woman is ASC-US/HPV negative, repeat cotesting at 3 years is recommended. This is different than the 5-year recommendation made by the ACS/ASCCP/ASCP primary screening guidelines because the new data from KPNC demonstrated that although the absolute risk of CIN 3+ is low after an ASC-US/HPV-negative report, it is similar to the risk observed among women with negative cytology alone.[42] The risk for each of these is higher than for a cotest with cytology-negative/HPV-negative results. Consequently, some minimal risk for missed CIN 2,3 still exists for women with ASC-US/HPV-negative results.[38,42,60,63] If the HPV test is positive (cotesting or reflex for ASC-US), colposcopy is recommended. The rationale here is that those women with ASC-US/HPV-positive results have a risk of CIN 3+ similar to the risk in women with LSIL.[7,8] To increase the sensitivity of colposcopy, it is recommended that an ECC should be done if colposcopy does not identify any lesions.

19.3.2.2.1.2 Management of ASC-US with Repeat Cytology
In the ALTS trial, the sensitivity of the hc2 HPV test for CIN 2,3 was 92.4%, which was equivalent to two repeat cytology tests with referral to colposcopy for ≥ASC-US on either test (Table 19.7).[38,60] Therefore, when repeat cytology was used to triage women with ASC-US, the recommendation was to refer women to colposcopy at the ≥ASC-US threshold.[7] Ninety-five percent of CIN 2,3 was detected at this threshold. This level of reassurance was the same as an initial negative HPV test, but instead required an average of 12 months of follow-up. Additionally, more women would require colposcopy using follow-up by serial cytology than would be by initial HPV triage.[60] In the ALTS trial, 53% tested positive for HPV and were referred to colposcopy. In contrast, 67% of women managed by repeat cytology had an abnormal report on either the first or the second repeat requiring colposcopy in addition to one or two additional office visits.[60]

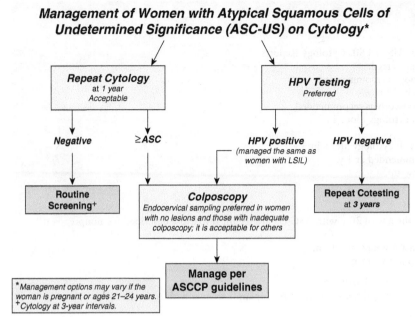

Management of Women with Atypical Squamous Cells of Undetermined Significance (ASC-US) on Cytology*

FIGURE 19.7. ASCCP algorithm for the management of women with atypical squamous cells of undetermined significance (ASC-US) on cytology. (From: Massad LS, Einstein MH, Huh WK, et al. 2012 Updated consensus guidelines for the management of abnormal cervical cancer screening tests and cancer precursors. *J Low Genit Tract Dis* 2013;17:S1–27, with permission.)

Previous guidelines recommended repeat cytology within 6 months for women with ASC-US, when no HPV testing is performed. The KPNC database analysis found that the risk for CIN 3+ within 6 months was low enough to justify annual

TABLE 19.7	ESTIMATED TRIAGE TEST PERFORMANCE IN THE ALTS TRIAL FOR THE DETECTION OF CUMULATIVE CIN 3 FROM ENROLLMENT THROUGH 2 YEARS OF FOLLOW-UP

	% SENSITIVITY FOR CIN 3	% REFERRAL
Enrollment HPV DNA test	92.4%	53.2%
HSIL cytology threshold		
One	35.5%	7.1%
Two	48.3%	10.2%
Three	60.2%	11.7%
LSIL cytology threshold		
One	59.3%	25.1%
Two	74.1%	31.7%
Three	82.0%	37.2%
ASCUS cytology threshold		
One	83.4%	58.1%
Two	95.4%	67.1%
Three	97.2%	72.7%

Estimated triage test performance in the ALTS trial for the detection of cumulative CIN 3 over the 2 y of the trial. CIN 3 diagnosis is that given by the ALTS Pathology Quality Control Group. Sensitivity for CIN 3 and percent referral to colposcopy are given for the Hybrid Capture 2 HPV test and for repeat Pap at one of three potential thresholds for referral to colposcopy: Paps interpreted as HSIL only, LSIL and above, or ASCUS and above. One, two, and three represent Paps repeated at prior ASCCP guideline recommendations of every 4–6 mo. Hence "One" is the first Pap usually repeated at 4–6 mo; "Two" is the second Pap repeated at 4–12 mo; and "Three" would be the third Pap, if three Paps were to be done, repeated at 12–18 mo. From: ASCUS-LSIL Triage Study (ALTS) Group. Results of a randomized trial on the management of cytology interpretations of atypical squamous cells of undetermined significance. *Am J Obstet Gynecol* 2003;188:1383–92, with permission.

follow-up instead of semiannual.[42] Therefore, for women with no HPV test result, the guidelines recommend that repeat cytology at 1 year is acceptable.[8] If the result is ASC-US or worse, colposcopy is recommended. If the repeat cytology is normal, it is recommended that the patient return for her next screen in 3 years, which is the current recommendation for screening with cytology alone.[34,35]

19.3.2.2.2 ASC-US in Special Populations
19.3.2.2.2.1 *Women Aged 21 to 24 Years*

Because of the low rate of cervical cancer in women <21 years of age and the significant harms that can result from screening women with a high prevalence of HPV infection, US guidelines do not recommend screening women under this age. US data demonstrate that cervical cancer risk in the 21- to 24-year-old age group is also quite low, with an estimated risk of 1.4 per 100,000 women of this age. However, this level of risk is 10-fold higher than in adolescents, and therefore screening starting at 21 years is justified.[35] Katki et al. estimated the 5-year risk of CIN 3+ among 133,947 women aged 21 to 24 years of age and compared this with 135,382 women aged 25 to 29 years and 965,360 women aged 30 to 64 years.[43] Among the 21- to 24-year-old women, the 5-year cumulative risk of CIN 3+ after HSIL was similar to the other age groups, whereas among women with LSIL and ASC-US/HPV positive, the 5-year risk of CIN 3+ was lower among the 21- to 24-year-olds than the other two age groups (3% to 4.4% vs. 5% to 7% vs. 5.2% to 6.8%, respectively). No difference was seen by age groups among the women with ASC-US/HPV-negative results. During the 5 years, only three cancers were detected in the 21- to 24-year-old women.[43]

These low CIN 3+ rates in conjunction with the low cancer rates and real potential for harm from overscreening in this group led to a consensus recommendation that the previous management guidelines for adolescents (women under 21 years of age) be applied to women aged 21 to 24 years.[8] Therefore, for women aged 21 to 24 years with ASC-US, repeat cytology alone at 12-month intervals is preferred, but reflex HPV testing is acceptable (Table 19.8; Figure 19.8).[8]

If reflex HPV testing is performed and is negative, the woman should return to routine screening with cytology alone in 3 years. If the reflex HPV test is positive, repeat

TABLE 19.8   INITIAL MANAGEMENT OF WOMEN WITH ASC-US IN SPECIAL CIRCUMSTANCES*

Management of women age 21–24 with either ASC-US or LSIL Cytology Reports
- Repeat cytology alone at 12-month intervals is preferred.
  - If ASC-H, AGC, or HSIL, referral to colposcopy is recommended.
  - If negative, ASC-US, or LSIL, repeat cytology in 12 mo:
    - If the 24-month follow-up is ≥ASC-US, colposcopy is recommended.
    - If negative, return to routine screening with cytology alone in 3 y.
- Reflex HPV testing is acceptable.
  - If HPV negative, return to routine screening with cytology alone in 3 y.
  - If HPV positive, repeat cytology alone is recommended at 1 y.
    - HPV testing should not be repeated in follow-up.
- Immediate colposcopy is not recommended.

Management of ASC-US in pregnancy
- Management options for pregnant women over the age of 20 y with ASC-US are identical to those described for nonpregnant women with the exception that
  - It is acceptable to defer colposcopy until at least 6 wk postpartum.
  - Endocervical curettage is unacceptable in pregnant women.

Management of ASC-US in women with evidence of vaginal atrophy
- Postmenopausal women with ASC-US should be managed the same as premenopausal women with ASC-US.

Management of ASC-US in the immunosuppressed**
- Either refer immediately to colposcopy
- Or repeat cytology in 6–12 mo
  - If repeat cytology is ≥ASC-US, refer to colposcopy.
- HPV testing is not recommended for triage or follow-up postcolposcopy.

*Algorithm for women <25 in Figure 19.8.
From Massad LS, Einstein MH, Huh WK, et al. 2012 Updated consensus guidelines for the management of abnormal cervical cancer screening tests and cancer precursors. *J Low Genit Tract Dis* 2013;17:S1–27, with permission.
**From The 2013 Guidelines for the Prevention and Management of Opportunistic Infections in HIV infected adolescents and adults. http://aidsinfo.nih.gov/guidelines

cytology alone is recommended at 1 year because HPV is extremely common and mostly transient at this age.[64,65] Immediate colposcopy or repeat HPV testing is not recommended. Regardless of whether an initial HPV test was performed, if repeat cytology at 12 months is ASC-H, AGC, or HSIL, referral to colposcopy is recommended. If the repeat cytology is negative, ASC-US, or LSIL, repeat cytology is recommended at 12 months. If the 24-month follow-up is ASC-US or worse, colposcopy is recommended. If negative, the woman should return to routine screening with cytology alone in 3 years.

19.3.2.2.2.2 Management of Pregnant Women with ASC-US

Performing colposcopy on women with ASC-US during pregnancy has not been shown to be helpful, and rates of cancer are relatively low.[7,66] It is reasonable to defer colposcopy in pregnant women at low risk for having cancer, as the only indication for therapy of cervical neoplasia in a pregnant woman is invasive cancer.[7] Therefore, the management options for pregnant women over the age of 20 years with ASC-US are identical to those described for nonpregnant women, with the exception that it is acceptable to defer colposcopy until at least 6 weeks postpartum.[8] Additionally, EC curettage is unacceptable in pregnant women (Table 19.8). If colposcopy is performed during pregnancy for ASC-US, women with no histologic or colposcopically suspected CIN 2+ at the initial colposcopy should have follow-up postpartum.

19.3.2.2.2.3 Management of Women ASC-US and Evidence of Vaginal Atrophy

HPV detection in postmenopausal women with ASC-US is far less than in younger women. This is partly secondary to non–HPV-related minor cellular changes being more common

in the perimenopause and postmenopause. Fortunately, ASC-US is less common in postmenopausal than in premenopausal women, and the risk of serious pathology in postmenopausal women with a history of negative cervical cancer screening is relatively low.[7,67–70] Because of the low rate of HPV positivity in this age group, HPV testing is more efficient in risk-stratifying postmenopausal women with ASC-US than in younger women, as fewer positive HPV results refers fewer to colposcopy.[71,72] In the ALTS trial, HPV was detected in only 20% of women aged ≥40 years with ASCUS.[71]

In the 2001 guidelines, the management of postmenopausal women with ASC-US differed somewhat from the general ASC-US recommendations.[6] Although all three management options, immediate colposcopy, repeat Pap, or HPV testing, were considered acceptable for the management of postmenopausal women with ASC-US, a fourth option of first treating with vaginal estrogen cream followed by repeat cytology obtained approximately 1 week after completing the regimen was provided when there was clinical or cytologic evidence of atrophy.[6] However, this recommendation was not included in the 2006 ASCCP guidelines, as there were no data supporting this approach.[7] Therefore, postmenopausal women with ASC-US should be managed in the same manner as premenopausal women with ASC-US (Table 19.8). Treatment of vaginal atrophy is reasonable if the clinician suspects that cellular changes due to atrophy are causing repeated ASC-US reports. While the literature on this subject is thin, expert opinion generally supports this approach. The usual recommendation for managing vaginal atrophy before obtaining a Pap is having the patient apply half applicator of estrogen cream in the vagina nightly for 3 weeks, ceasing the application about a week before repeating the Pap. There is currently no experience with the use of ospemifene, a newly approved selective estrogen receptor modulator (SERM) for management of atrophy symptoms for this purpose.

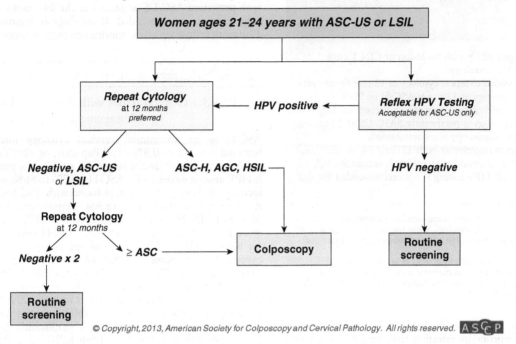

Management of Women Ages 21–24 Years with Either Atypical Squamous Cells of Undetermined Significance (ASC-US) or Low-Grade Squamous Intraepithelial Lesion (LSIL)

FIGURE 19.8.   ASCCP algorithm for the management of women ages 21 to 24 years with either atypical squamous cells of undetermined significance (ASC-US) or low-grade squamous intraepithelial lesion (LSIL). (From Massad LS, Einstein MH, Huh WK, et al. 2012 Updated consensus guidelines for the management of abnormal cervical cancer screening tests and cancer precursors. *J Low Genit Tract Dis* 2013;17:S1–27, with permission.)

19.3.2.2.2.4 *Management of Immunosuppressed Women with ASC-US*

Immunosuppressed women are known to have higher rates of HPV and HPV-associated disease, including CIN 3+ and invasive cancer.[73–76] Studies of HIV-infected women with ASC-US have shown higher rates of progression to SIL (CIN) than women not HIV infected.[77] Duerr et al.[77] found that 60% of HIV-infected women with ASC-US cytology developed SIL compared to 25% in HIV-uninfected women. Another study found no difference for CIN 2/3 in women with ASC-US by HIV status, although CIN 2/3 was correlated with low CD4 counts.[78] Because of the high rates of HPV, it has been surmised that HPV triage of ASC-US in this population would be of little benefit. Massad et al.[79] reported that in HIV-infected women with ASC-US, HPV triage had a low positive predictive value (6%). The 2013 guidelines for the Prevention and Management of Opportunistic Infections in HIV-infected adolescents and adults state that HIV-infected women with ASC-US, regardless of age, can be immediately referred either to colposcopy or to repeat cytology in 6 to 12 months (Table 19.8).[80] HPV testing is not recommended for triage or follow-up after colposcopy. If the repeat cytology is ≥ASC-US, referral to colposcopy is recommended.

19.3.2.3 Guidelines for Postcolposcopy Management of Women with ASC-US

Colposcopy did not initially detect 25% to 33% of the cumulative CIN 2,3 lesions detected over a 2-year follow-up in the ALTS trial.[60] In the KPNC database, the 5-year cumulative risk of CIN 3+ among ASC-US/HPV-positive women was 3.6% and among all women with ASC-US was 2.6%.[41] Similar risks for CIN 3+ were observed for women with LSIL or with CIN 1.[43,45] This likely reflects both newly incident CIN 2,3 occurring during follow-up and missed prevalent CIN 2,3 at the initial colposcopy.[81–83] Taking more biopsies at the initial referral colposcopy,

and doing an ECC when indicated, should decrease the number of high-grade lesions detected only at the follow-up visit.[81,83,84] Most CIN 1 also appear to regress, especially in younger women.[45] Based on this cumulative risk of CIN 3+, close monitoring is recommended for women referred to colposcopy because of either repeat ASC-US or a positive HPV test when CIN 2+ is not found at colposcopy. It is recommended that these women return in 1 year for cotesting (Table 19.9; Figure 20.5B in Chapter 20, *Management of Women with No Lesion or Biopsy-confirmed Cervical Intraepithelial Neoplasia—Grade 1 [CIN 1] Preceded by "Lesser Abnormalities"*). If ≥ASC-US cytology or a positive HPV is present, referral for repeat colposcopy is recommended.[8] If the cotest performed after colposcopy is HPV negative and

TABLE 19.9	POSTCOLPOSCOPY MANAGEMENT OF WOMEN ≥25 YEARS OF AGE WITH ASC-US CYTOLOGY NOT FOUND TO HAVE CIN 2,3

- It is recommended that these women return in 1 y for cotesting.
  - If ≥ASC-US or HPV positive, referral for repeat colposcopy is recommended.
  - If cytology negative/HPV negative, a return in 3 y for age-appropriate retesting (cotesting ≥30 y and cytology only <30 y) is recommended.
  - If the retest(s) (whether cytology with or without HPV testing) is/are negative, the woman can return to routine screening.

From Massad LS, Einstein MH, Huh WK, et al. 2012 Updated consensus guidelines for the management of abnormal cervical cancer screening tests and cancer precursors. *J Low Genit Tract Dis* 2013;17:S1–27, with permission.

TABLE 19.10	POSTCOLPOSCOPY MANAGEMENT OF WOMEN AGES 21–24 WITH ASC-US OR LSIL CYTOLOGY NOT FOUND TO HAVE CIN 2,3*

- For women aged <25 y with no lesion or CIN 1 after ASC-US (or LSIL) cytology:
  - It is recommended to repeat cytology at 12-month intervals.
    - If repeat cytology at 12 mo is ASC-H or HSIL (or AGC), referral to colposcopy is recommended.
    - If repeat cytology is persistently ≥ASC-US at 24-month follow-up, colposcopy is recommended.
    - If cytology is negative at both 12- and 24-month follow-up visits, routine screening is recommended.
  - Follow-up with HPV testing is not recommended for this age group.

---

*Although the guidelines do not recommend colposcopy for women <25 with ASC-US or LSIL cytology, some women of this age will likely get colposcopy despite the recommendation and require post-colposcopy follow-up.
From Massad LS, Einstein MH, Huh WK, et al. 2012 Updated consensus guidelines for the management of abnormal cervical cancer screening tests and cancer precursors. *J Low Genit Tract Dis* 2013;17:S1–27, with permission.

cytology negative, it is recommended that the patient return in 3 years for age-appropriate retesting (cotesting ≥30 years and cytology only if <30 years), as the risk of CIN 3+, while low, remains higher than that of women who were originally cotest negative. If the age-appropriate 3-year follow-up test is negative, then the woman can return to routine screening.

Management after colposcopy is slightly different for those 21 to 24 years of age because of the low risk for cancer, the high probability that low-grade lesions will regress without treatment, and the potential harms of overdiagnosis (Table 19.10). For women aged 21 to 24 years with no lesion or CIN 1 after ASC-US (or LSIL) cytology, it is recommended to repeat cytology at 12-month intervals.[8] Follow-up with HPV testing is not recommended in this age group. If repeat cytology at 12 months is ASC-H or HSIL, referral to colposcopy is

recommended.[8] Although not mentioned in the guidelines, this should also apply to women with AGC cytology. For women with persistent ASC-US or greater at the 24-month follow-up, colposcopy is recommended. If cytology is negative at both 12-month follow-up visits, routine screening is recommended.[8]

19.3.3 Management of Women with ASC-H

19.3.3.1 General Issues with ASC-H and Initial Management

ASC-H is an uncommon cervical cytology interpretation reported in 0.3% to 0.6% of all Pap tests, or <10% of all ASC cytology reports.[85,86] In the largest US studies, the prevalence of hrHPV among women with ASC-H is 67% to 86%, an absolute increase of about 30% over that found with ASC-US.[87–89] In the ALTS trial, 84% of women with ASC-H tested positive for HPV, 50% had CIN 2+, and 30% had CIN 3+.[88] HPV detection was more common in women <35 with ASC-H (over 85%) than for women >35 (40%), but in all age groups finding ASC-H conferred a substantially higher risk of CIN 2+ than ASC-US. Even a negative HPV result in the context of ASC-H cytology obtained on cotesting is not completely reassuring, as 20% with these results in one study were found to have CIN 2+.[90] In the largest studies, the prevalence of CIN 2,3 among women with ASC-H ranges from 26% to 68%, significantly higher than in women with ASC-US. Data from KPNC also showed that ASC-H confers a higher risk for CIN 2+ over time than do ASC-US or LSIL.[46] This was also shown to be true for women aged 21 to 24 years, although the risk for CIN 3+ in this age group is still lower than among older women.[43] The high rate of HPV detection in women with ASC-H makes reflex HPV testing unsuitable because most women will test positive and still need colposcopy, increasing cost without changing management.[8] In addition, the 5-year cancer risk among women with ASC-H/HPV-negative results is 2%, still too high to justify observation.[8,46]

Women with ASC-H are clearly at significant risk for CIN 2,3+ and should be managed by immediate colposcopy, regardless of age and HPV result obtained on cotesting (Table 19.11; Figure 19.9). In addition, the 5-year cancer risk among women

TABLE 19.11	MANAGEMENT OF WOMEN WITH ASC-H*

Initial management
- Women with ASC-H cytology should be managed by immediate colposcopy, regardless of age and HPV testing result (if cotested).
- Reflex HPV testing is not recommended.
- Further management depends on whether CIN 2,3 is detected and on age [see Table 19.21 and Figure 19.15, Management of Women <25 with ASC-H or HSIL Cytology].
- Immediate LEEP is unacceptable.

Postcolposcopy management of women ≥25 not found to have CIN 2,3
- If no CIN 2+ is found in a woman ≥25 years of age with ASC-H cytology, the guidelines recommend
  - Follow-up with cotesting in 12 and 24 months
  - A diagnostic excisional procedure
  - Observation with cotesting should only be elected if the colposcopy examination is adequate and the ECC is negative.
    - In this case, the cytology and histology should be reviewed and, if revised, management should be per the revised diagnosis.
    - If no revision, observation with cotesting is acceptable.
      - If both cotests at 12 and 24 mo are negative/negative, the woman can return in 3 y for age-specific retesting.
      - If either cotest includes a positive result, repeat colposcopy should be performed, unless cytology shows HSIL—in which case, a diagnostic excisional procedure is recommended.

Postcolposcopy management of women ages 21–24 y not found to have CIN 2,3
- Postcolposcopy management for women aged 21–24 y with ASC-H follows the same guidelines as for HSIL in this age group (Figure 19.15).
- A diagnostic excisional procedure is not recommended for this age group.

---

*Algorithm in Figure 19.9.
From Massad LS, Einstein MH, Huh WK, et al. 2012 Updated consensus guidelines for the management of abnormal cervical cancer screening tests and cancer precursors. *J Low Genit Tract Dis* 2013;17:S1–27, with permission.

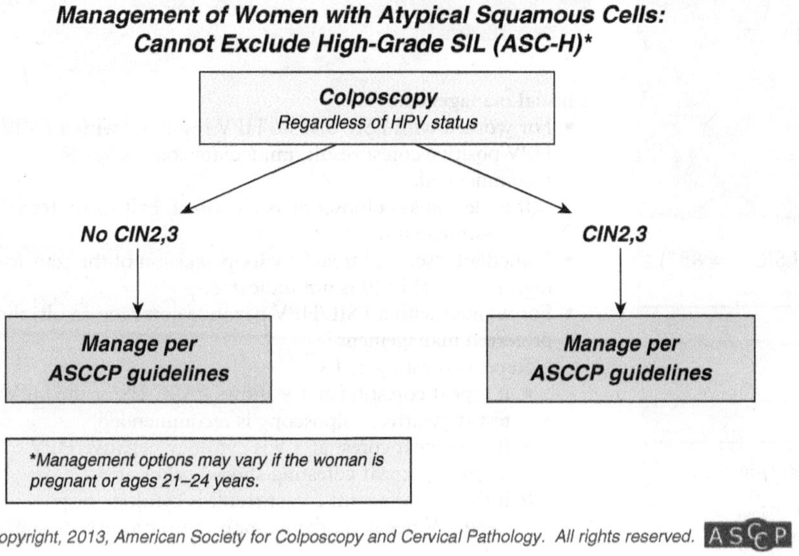

**Management of Women with Atypical Squamous Cells:
Cannot Exclude High-Grade SIL (ASC-H)***

FIGURE 19.9. ASCCP algorithm for the management of women with atypical squamous cells: cannot exclude high-grade SIL (ASC-H). (From Massad LS, Einstein MH, Huh WK, et al. 2012 Updated consensus guidelines for the management of abnormal cervical cancer screening tests and cancer precursors. *J Low Genit Tract Dis* 2013;17:S1–27, with permission.)

Colposcopy
Regardless of HPV status

No CIN2,3   *CIN2,3*

**Manage per
ASCCP guidelines**   **Manage per
ASCCP guidelines**

**Management options may vary if the woman is
pregnant or ages 21–24 years.*

with HPV-negative ASC-H is 2%, which is too high to justify observation with serial cytology.[8,46] Reflex HPV testing is not recommended. Further management depends on whether CIN 2,3 is detected and on age (Figure 19.15; Table 19.21). Immediate loop electrosurgical excision procedure (LEEP) is unacceptable.[8]

19.3.3.2 Management of Women with ASC-H after Colposcopy

If no CIN 2+ is found in a woman aged 25 or over with ASC-H, the guidelines for management of women with no lesion or biopsy-confirmed CIN 1 preceded by ASC-H or HSIL cytology should be followed. These guidelines recommend follow-up with cotesting in 12 and 24 months, a diagnostic excisional procedure, or a review of cytologic, histologic, and colposcopic findings.[8] Observation with cotesting should only be elected if the colposcopy examination is adequate and the ECC is negative. If the colposcopic, cytologic, and histologic findings are reviewed, management should be per the revised diagnosis. If no revision, observation with cotesting is acceptable. If both cotests at 12 and 24 months are negative, the woman can return in 3 years for age-specific retesting. If either cotest is abnormal (cytology ≥ ASC-US or HPV positive), repeat colposcopy should be performed unless cytology shows HSIL, in which case a diagnostic procedure is recommended. A summary of the management recommendations for ASC-H is given in Table 19.11. Management after colposcopy for women aged 21 to 24 years with ASC-H is different than that described for older women and follows the same guidelines as for HSIL in this age group. An early diagnostic excision procedure is not recommended for this age group.[8] (See Figure 20.5C *Management of Women with No Lesion or Biopsy-confirmed Cervical Intraepithelial Neoplasia—Grade 1 [CIN 1] Preceded by ASC-H or HSIL Cytology*).

19.3.4 Management of Women with LSIL

19.3.4.1 General Issues with LSIL and Initial Management

The 2001 Bethesda System classification defines LSIL as cytologic changes associated with cytopathic effects of HPV known as koilocytotic atypia and mild dysplasia/CIN 1.[14] LSIL is less common than ASC-US, and in most labs, the ASCUS:LSIL

ratio will be in the range of 2:1.[14] The College of American Pathologists (CAP) Interlaboratory Comparison Program in Cervicovaginal Cytology (PAP) collects information from participating labs on median cytology report rates. The median rate for LSIL in 1997 was 1.6%, but some laboratories serving young populations reported rates as high as 7.7%.[91] By 2003, CAP reported that the LSIL rate had increased to 2.1%, but that the rate of other cytologic abnormalities had not increased.[92] Because the median percentile reporting rate of LSIL in US laboratories in 2003 was 2.4% for LBC, but only 1.4% for conventional cytology, this increase in the LSIL rate appears to be secondary to widespread adoption of LBC during the last 12 years.[7]

The natural history of LSIL parallels that of ASC-US/HPV positive, suggesting that LSIL- and HPV-positive ASC-US should be managed similarly.[93] The majority of women with LSIL test positive for HPV, but the rate of HPV detection declines with increasing age.[93–96] A 2006 meta-analysis evaluating LSIL cytology in women of all ages reported HPV presence in 76.6%.[96] Nevertheless, the prevalence of CIN 2,3 or cancer among women with LSIL varies considerably between different series. In the ALTS trial, CIN 2+ was identified after 2 years of follow-up in 27.6% of women with LSIL, nearly identical to the 26.7% identified in women with ASC-US/HPV-positive results (Table 19.12).[93] In other studies, CIN 2,3 has been identified after a single colposcopic examination in as few as 12% of women referred with LSIL.[97]

Proponents of managing LSIL by repeating the Pap test stress that low-grade lesions most frequently regress and that repeating cytology provides time for this to occur.[98] Also, the risk that a woman with an LSIL cytology report has an existing invasive cervical cancer is very low. However, reduction in cost as a benefit of allowing lesions to regress prior to referral to colposcopy was not demonstrated in the ALTS. There, the only threshold considered safe for referral to colposcopy was ≥ASC-US.[99] At this threshold, 80.8% of women followed for LSIL cytology had a first repeat abnormal cytology necessitating colposcopy, a rate not dissimilar to that of HPV testing (Table 19.13). Other studies have reported that 53% to 76% of women with LSIL managed by repeat cytology were referred to colposcopy based on a single repeat cytology report.[100] Analysis of KPNC data showed that in women with LSIL, the prevalence of CIN 3+ was 2.5% and the cumulative 5-year risk of CIN 3+ was 5.2%.[44] The KPNC database examined LSIL/HPV-negative cotested women and showed that the risk of CIN 3+ in these women was quite low, similar to that

TABLE 19.12	CUMULATIVE DIAGNOSIS* OF TWO DISEASE END POINTS (CIN 2,3 BY CLINICAL CENTER PATHOLOGY DIAGNOSIS AND CIN 3 BY PATH QC CONSENSUS DIAGNOSIS) BY REFERRAL PAP INTERPRETATIONS, ASC HPV (+), AND LSIL	
	■ HPV + ASCUS (n = 1193)	■ LSIL (n = 897)
Clinical Center CIN 2 or 3	26.7%	27.6%
Pathology QC Group CIN 3	14.5%	15.9%

*(%) of women diagnosed with the disease end points at any time during ALTS enrollment, 2-year follow-up, or exit.
From Cox JT, Schiffman M, Solomon D; ASCUS-LSIL Triage Study (ALTS) Group. Prospective follow-up suggests similar risk of subsequent cervical intraepithelial neoplasia grade 2 or 3 among women with cervical intraepithelial neoplasia grade 1 or negative colposcopy and directed biopsy. *Am J Obstet Gynecol* 2003;188:1406–12, with permission.

observed for ASC-US.[44] Consequently, the new guidelines provide the option to repeat cotesting in 12 months in women found on cotesting to be LSIL/HPV negative.

For women with LSIL and either no HPV result or an HPV-positive result on cotesting, immediate colposcopy is

TABLE 19.13	ESTIMATED* TRIAGE TEST PERFORMANCE FOR DETECTION OF CUMULATIVE HISTOLOGIC DIAGNOSIS OF CIN 3[†] BY PATHOLOGY QUALITY CONTROL GROUP. INITIAL REFERRAL PAP LSIL	
	■ % SENSITIVITY FOR CIN 3+	■ % REFERRAL
Enrollment HPV DNA Test	95.2%	84.2%
HSIL Cytology Threshold[‡]		
One	36.0%	12.6%
Two	55.1%	16.8%
Three	65.1%	19.5%
LSIL Cytology Threshold[‡]		
One	72.8%	57.4%
Two	86.0%	64.9%
Three	93.0%	68.6%
ASCUS Cytology Threshold[‡]		
One	90.8%	80.8%
Two	98.9%	87.4%
Three	100.0%	88.9%

*For these estimates, missing test results, missed visits, and the timing of visits were ignored, in order to focus on the performance of the tests according to how many were completed.
[†]CIN 3 includes five cases of invasive cancer and one case of AIS.
[‡]Each cytology threshold reflects the finding of a cytologic abnormality greater than or equal to the cut point when cytology is performed one, two, or three times at ~6-month intervals. From ASCUS-LSIL Triage Study (ALTS) Group. A randomized trial on the management of low-grade squamous intraepithelial lesion cytology interpretations. *Am J Obstet Gynecol* 2003;188:1393–400, with permission.

TABLE 19.14	MANAGEMENT OF WOMEN ≥25 WITH LSIL CYTOLOGY*

Initial management
- For women with LSIL and no HPV result, or with a LSIL/HPV-positive cotest result, immediate colposcopy is recommended.
  - If no lesion at colposcopy is identified, ECC is preferred unless pregnant.
- Immediate "see and treat" by loop excision of the transformation zone (LEEP) is not indicated.
- For women with a LSIL/HPV negative cotesting result, the preferred management is
  - Repeat cotesting at 1 y.
    - If repeat cotesting at 1 y shows ≥ASC-US or the HPV test is positive, colposcopy is recommended.
    - If the repeat cotest at 1 y is cytology negative/HPV negative, repeat cotesting should occur at 3 y.
    - If the 3-year repeat cotest result is cytology negative/HPV negative, the woman can return to routine screening.
  - It is also acceptable to refer to colposcopy.

Postcolposcopy management
- For management of LSIL when no CIN 2,3 is diagnosed at colposcopy, management is identical to that for postcolposcopy management of ASC-US/HPV-positive results.

*Algorithm in Figure 19.10.
From Massad LS, Einstein MH, Huh WK, et al. 2012 Updated consensus guidelines for the management of abnormal cervical cancer screening tests and cancer precursors. *J Low Genit Tract Dis* 2013;17:S1–27, with permission.

recommended (Table 19.14; Figure 19.10).[8] The primary advantage of immediate colposcopy is the timely detection of CIN 2,3 or the rare cancer and reduction in the potential for loss to follow-up. Additionally, this approach reassures women without colposcopic abnormality and permits the appropriate management of women with CIN.[100,101] If cotesting is LSIL/HPV negative, the preferred management is repeat cotesting at 1 year. It is also acceptable to refer to colposcopy. If repeat cotesting at 1 year shows ≥ASC-US or the HPV test is positive, then colposcopy is recommended.[8] If the 1-year cytology and HPV test are both negative, then repeat cotesting should occur at 3 years. If all tests are negative at that time, the woman can return to routine screening. If no lesion is identified at colposcopy, ECC is preferred unless pregnant.[8]

Immediate "see and treat" by loop excision of the transformation zone (LEEP) of women with an initial LSIL cytology in the absence of biopsy-confirmed CIN 2,3 is not indicated as the yield of CIN 3+ is relatively low and the potential for harm substantial.[8,102,103]

19.3.4.2 Management of Women with LSIL after Colposcopy

Both the KPNC data and ALTS showed that the risks of CIN 2,3 were similar in women with LSIL and ASC-US/HPV positive and therefore should be managed similarly (Table 19.14).[44,93,104] For management after colposcopy, see Postcolposcopy management ASC-US/HPV positive (Table 19.9; Figure 19.7).

19.3.4.3 LSIL in Special Circumstances

For women aged 21 to 24 years and postmenopausal and pregnant women with LSIL, the ASCCP recommendations vary from those just discussed (Table 19.15).[8]

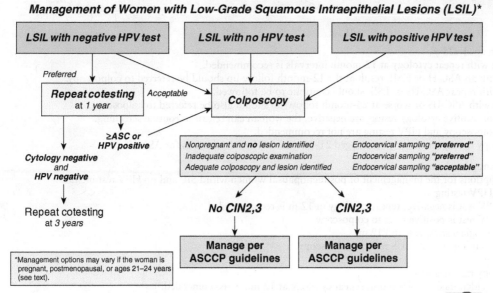

Management of Women with Low-Grade Squamous Intraepithelial Lesions (LSIL)*

FIGURE 19.10. ASCCP algorithm for the management of women with low-grade squamous intraepithelial lesion (LSIL). (From Massad LS, Einstein MH, Huh WK, et al. 2012 Updated consensus guidelines for the management of abnormal cervical cancer screening tests and cancer precursors. *J Low Genit Tract Dis* 2013;17:S1–27, with permission.)

19.3.4.3.1 LSIL IN WOMEN AGED 21 TO 24 YEARS

LSIL regresses at higher rates in women aged 21 to 24 years than older women and progression to CIN 3+ is rare.[65,105-107] Analysis of KPNC data confirmed that women with LSIL at ages 21 to 24 years have a lower prevalent and cumulative risk of CIN 3+ than older women.[43,44] The 5-year cumulative risk for CIN 3+ in this age group was 3%, a rate similar to that for ASC-US observed in women ages 30 years and older. Because of this low risk and that "reflex" HPV testing is not recommended for this age group, the guidelines recommend that women ages 21 to 24 with LSIL be observed with repeat cytology at 12-month intervals (Table 19.15).[8] Colposcopy and HPV testing are not recommended. Women with an ASC-H or HSIL result at the 12-month follow-up should be referred to colposcopy, but women with repeat ASC-US or LSIL should continue to be followed with annual cytology. After 24 months of follow-up, women with ASC-US or worse should be referred to colposcopy. If two consecutive annual cytology results are negative, the woman can return to routine screening. Management after colposcopy for women ages 21 to 24 with LSIL is the same as for women of this age group with ASC-US (Table 19.10; Figure 19.8).

19.3.4.3.2 LSIL IN POSTMENOPAUSAL WOMEN

Acceptable options for managing postmenopausal women with LSIL and no HPV test include HPV triage, repeat cytology at 6 and 12 months, or colposcopy.[8] If the HPV test is negative, repeat cytology in 12 months is recommended. If either the HPV test is positive or repeat cytology is elected and is ≥ASC-US, referral to colposcopy is recommended. If no CIN is identified at colposcopy, repeat cytology at 12 months is recommended.

The rationale for providing both repeat cytology and "reflex" HPV testing as options in addition to immediate colposcopy for management of postmenopausal women with LSIL is that progressively fewer LSIL results test HPV positive as women age; only 30% to 50% of women with LSIL age ≥40 test positive for HPV.[71,108] Because well-screened women over 40 years referred to colposcopy for LSIL are also less likely to have CIN 2,3, it is likely that misclassification of LSIL occurs with increasing frequency as women age.[109] That misclassified LSIL, rather than true HPV-related LSIL, is increasingly likely in perimenopausal and postmenopausal women is demonstrated by the declining rate of HPV positivity for LSIL in this age group. These findings support the option of "reflex" HPV testing of LSIL in postmenopausal women to determine the need for colposcopy, as well as the option of repeat cytology and immediate colposcopy (Table 19.15).[7,8]

19.3.4.3.3 LSIL IN PREGNANT WOMEN

Colposcopy is preferred for pregnant women with LSIL cytology.[8] EC curettage is unacceptable in pregnant women. Management in pregnant women aged 21 to 24 years should be the same as for management of LSIL in nonpregnant women in this age group. Deferring the initial colposcopy until at least 6 weeks postpartum is also acceptable for women of any age with LSIL. In pregnant women without cytologic, histologic, or colposcopically suspected CIN 2,3 or cancer at the initial colposcopy, postpartum follow-up is recommended. Additional colposcopic and cytologic examinations during pregnancy are unacceptable for these women (Table 19.15; Figure 19.11).

19.3.5 Management of AGC and Cytologic AIS

19.3.5.1 General Issues with AGC, Cytologic AIS, and Initial Management

The 2001 Bethesda Workshop dropped the term "of undetermined significance" because of clinical confusion generated by the similarity in the terminology of "ASCUS" and "AGUS," thereby changing AGUS to AGC.[14] The cytologic criteria for interpretation of cells as consistent with AIS were considered specific enough to list this as a separate entity.[14] All other glandular cell changes were classified into two groups.

TABLE 19.15   MANAGEMENT OF WOMEN WITH LSIL IN SPECIAL CIRCUMSTANCES*

LSIL in women aged <25 y
- Observation with repeat cytology at 12-month intervals is recommended.
  - Women with an ASC-H or HSIL result at the 12-month follow-up should be referred to colposcopy.
  - Women with repeat ASC-US or LSIL should continue to be followed.
    - Women with ASC-US or worse at 24-month follow-up should also be referred to colposcopy.
    - If two consecutive cytology results are negative, the woman can return to routine screening.
- Immediate colposcopy and HPV testing are not recommended.
- Postcolposcopy management for women aged 21–24 with LSIL is the same as for ASC-US.

LSIL in postmenopausal women
- Acceptable options for the management of postmenopausal women with LSIL and no HPV test include
  - Triage by HPV testing
    - If the HPV test is negative, repeat cytology in 12 m is recommended.
    - If the HPV test is positive refer to colposcopy
  - Repeat cytologic testing at 6 and 12 m
    - If either cytology is ≥ASC-US refer to colposcopy.
  - Colposcopy
- Postcolposcopy management:
  - If no CIN is identified at colposcopy, repeat cytology at 12 mo is recommended.

LSIL in pregnant women
- Colposcopy is preferred for pregnant women ≥25 with LSIL cytology.
  - Endocervical curettage is unacceptable in pregnant women.
  - Postpartum follow-up is recommended when no cytologic, histologic, or colposcopically suspected CIN 2,3 or cancer is found at the initial colposcopy.
    - Additional colposcopic and cytologic examinations during pregnancy are unacceptable for these women.
- Management in pregnant women aged 21–24 y should be the same as for management of nonpregnant women with LSIL in this age group.
  - Deferring the initial colposcopy until at least 6 wk postpartum is acceptable.
  - Colposcopic and cytologic examinations during pregnancy are unacceptable for these women.

---

*Algorithm in Figure 19.8 for ASC-US and LSIL in Women <25 and in Figure 19.11 for Pregnant Women with LSIL.
From Massad LS, Einstein MH, Huh WK, et al. 2012 Updated consensus guidelines for the management of abnormal cervical cancer screening tests and cancer precursors. *J Low Genit Tract Dis* 2013;17:S1–27, with permission.

The most common subclassification is AGC, which can be further designated as EC or endometrial if the cellular characteristics are well defined, or as "glandular cells, not otherwise specified (AGC-NOS)" if not. Far less common are atypical glandular cells (either endocervical or glandular cells), favor neoplasia, but this result carries a higher risk for CIN 2,3, AIS, and cancer. Grading of atypical endometrial cells has not

been successful, so no "favor neoplasia" subcategory exists for this interpretation.[14] The interpretation of AGC varies widely among cytopathologists, but interobserver agreement has been demonstrated to be better for LBC than for the corresponding conventional cytology.[110]

AGC is not a common cytologic interpretation. The median US rate reported in 2003 was 0.4%.[92] In contrast to the more

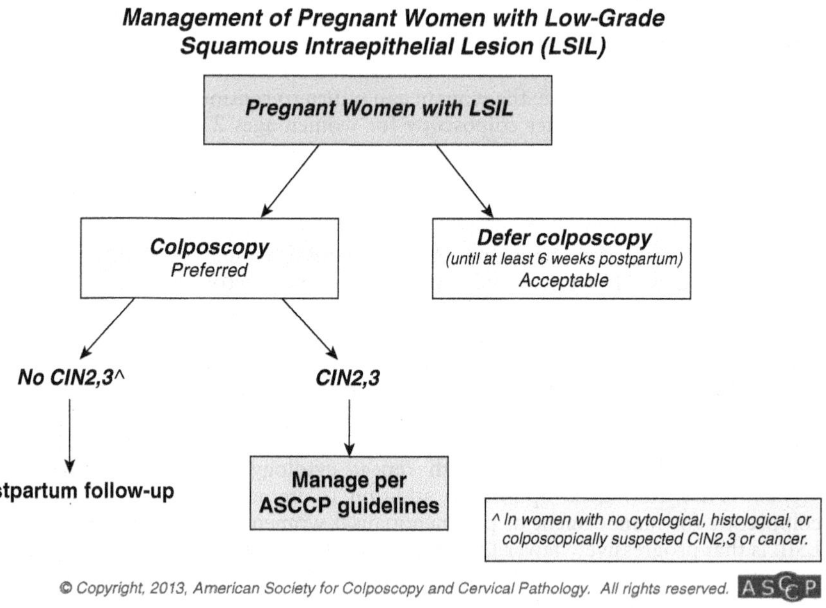

FIGURE 19.11. ASCCP algorithm for the management of pregnant women with low-grade squamous intraepithelial lesion (LSIL) on cytology. (From Massad LS, Einstein MH, Huh WK, et al. 2012 Updated consensus guidelines for the management of abnormal cervical cancer screening tests and cancer precursors. *J Low Genit Tract Dis* 2013;17:S1–27, with permission.)

Management of Pregnant Women with Low-Grade Squamous Intraepithelial Lesion (LSIL)

Pregnant Women with LSIL → Colposcopy Preferred / Defer colposcopy (until at least 6 weeks postpartum) Acceptable

Colposcopy → No CIN2,3^ → Postpartum follow-up

Colposcopy → CIN2,3 → Manage per ASCCP guidelines

^ In women with no cytological, histological, or colposcopically suspected CIN2,3 or cancer.

common findings of ASC, LSIL, and HSIL, which occur more frequently in younger women, AGC is more common in women 40 years of age and older.[105] AGC cytology, although uncommon, is important because it has more CIN 2,3 detected in follow-up than any other result except HSIL. Between 9% and 68% of women with AGC have significant neoplasia (CIN 2,3, AIS, or cancer) and from 3% to 17% have invasive cancer.[111-115] Squamous lesions are found more often than glandular lesions in the follow-up of AGC cytology. Squamous lesions are more common in younger women, glandular lesions in older women.[8,11,115] While cancer risk is lower in women with AGC who are <35 years of age, CIN 2+ risk is higher.[116] In one study, 13% of women <35 with AGC had CIN 2,3 and none had a malignancy.[111] In contrast, only 2% of women aged ≥35 years had CIN 2,3 and 3% had invasive cancer. In the KPNC cohort, 9% of women aged 30 years and older with AGC had CIN 3+ and 3% had cancer.[45] AGC is more likely than other cytologic reports to be associated with difficult-to-detect glandular lesions, including AIS and adenocarcinomas of the cervix, endometrium, ovary, and fallopian tube.[111,116] Glandular and squamous lesions are often found together, with CIN found in approximately half of women with AIS or adenocarcinoma.[111,117] However, the majority of women with AGC do not have serious lesions. It is this dichotomy that makes atypical glandular cells a cytology interpretation with so much risk for missing important disease.

CIN risk varies with cytologic interpretation. The Bethesda 2001 Workshop designated the subcategories of AGC as "not otherwise specified" (NOS) and "favor neoplasia" based on demonstration that women with ACG-NOS are at a considerably lower risk of CIN 2,3 and AIS than women with AGC "favor neoplasia."[14] CIN 2,3 has been detected in 9% to 41% of women with AGC-NOS compared to 27% to 96% of women with AGC "favor neoplasia."[95,118-121] A cytology report of AIS has the highest risk, with 48% to 69% having histologic AIS and 38% invasive cervical adenocarcinoma.[121,122] Pregnancy does not appear to change the underlying associations between AGC and gynecologic neoplasia.[7,10]

Management decisions have been made difficult by uncertainties about the natural history of glandular atypia and the sensitivity of cytology and colposcopy for detecting glandular precancer lesions. The sensitivity of cytology is diminished by the difficulty of differentiating glandular neoplasia resembling endometrial cells from the lower uterine segment, EC cells with tubal metaplasia, or reactive EC cells.[123,124] Many women with AGC cytology are found to have no abnormality on evaluation because of the difficulty differentiating these benign changes from AIS, squamous intraepithelial lesions, and carcinoma. This difficulty also explains the poor reproducibility of the AGC interpretation between observers.[110] The interpretation is further complicated because atypical glandular cells may also come from tubal, ovarian, and metastatic neoplasms in the upper genital tract or peritoneal fluid that drains into the cervicovaginal sample.

The most common benign changes found in women with AGC are cellular changes secondary to chronic endocervicitis, to ciliated cell metaplasia of the endocervix, usually seen in women who have IUDs, or to hormonal conditions such as microglandular hyperplasia.[124] More efficient capture of EC cells with the endocervical brush has resulted in cytology specimens with more endocervical cells for evaluation, which may have contributed to finding more atypical benign glandular cell changes and more squamous and endocervical neoplastic lesions.[125] Use of the endocervical brush has also been found to increase cell distortion and clumping as well as to induce "toothpick" or "brush" artifact, which may falsely inflate the category of AGC.[126]

Approximately 50% of AIS is detected at the edge of CIN, invasive squamous cell carcinoma, or adenocarcinoma.[127,128]

While most AIS is situated next to the SCJ, or to CIN, some multifocal AIS can be separate.[129,130] Consequently, the finding of AIS on histology may be unexpected because adjacent CIN 2,3 diverts attention from the colposcopically less impressive AIS lesions. Often AIS looks colposcopically similar to a normal ectopy (see Chapter 11) with only slightly accentuated acetowhitening of the columnar villi, similar to that seen among some women on hormonal contraception or during pregnancy.[131] The small size of focal AIS, its frequent location in the cervical canal, and the occasional multifocal nature of lesions can complicate detection and correct interpretation of colposcopic findings.[127]

Data suggest that the traditional management options for the follow-up of abnormal cervical cytology are all less effective in identifying AIS and small invasive cervical adenocarcinomas than similar squamous lesions.[7] However, screening with cervical cytology does detect invasive adenocarcinomas and adenosquamous carcinomas of the cervix at an earlier stage with resulting lower disease-specific mortality than glandular cancers detected among unscreened women, who usually present after they develop symptoms.[122,132] The sensitivity of the Pap test for detecting glandular lesions is low (50% to 72%), as are the reported sensitivities for identifying glandular neoplasia with both colposcopy and endocervical sampling.[114,119,123] HPV testing is highly sensitive for identifying women with CIN 2,3 and AIS, and AGC/HPV-negative women not having disease found at the initial evaluation are much less likely to have an occult CIN 2,3 or AIS lesion.[7,10,114] In one very large study, none of the AGC/HPV-negative women without disease at the initial evaluation had CIN 2,3 or AIS over 12 months of follow-up.[133] In the KPNC cohort, the CIN 3+ risk in AGC/HPV-positive women was 33.0% but when AGC/HPV negative was 0.9%.[45] The risk of cancer in the HPV-positive group was 9% compared to 0.4% in the HPV-negative group. However, non–HPV-associated neoplasia arising from the endometrium or fallopian tube would be missed by initial triage of AGC by HPV testing.[7,10,133,134] Furthermore, the risk of cancer in the AGC/HPV-negative women in the KPNC cohort was very similar to the risk of cancer among ASC-US/HPV-positive women or women with LSIL.[45] Therefore, neither repeat cytology nor HPV testing is appropriate for the initial management of women with AGC cytology, but knowledge of HPV-negative status can help identify women who may be at greater risk of endometrial than cervical disease.[117]

The broad spectrum of important findings that can be identified in women with AGC requires that the initial evaluation includes colposcopy, endocervical sampling, and endometrial evaluation when indicated (Table 19.16; Figure 19.12).[8] Endometrial evaluation is defined as endometrial biopsy, or for postmenopausal women, ultrasound assessment of endometrial thickness, with biopsy or D and C if endometrial thickness measurement >4 to 5 mm. Need for endometrial evaluation is determined by clinical risk factors such as age ≥35 or younger women with irregular bleeding or other risk factors for chronic anovulation. In instances where atypical endometrial cells are found, initial evaluation can be limited to endometrial and endocervical sampling, with colposcopy done later if no lesion is found on initial evaluation.[8]

19.3.5.1.2 BENIGN- AND ATYPICAL-APPEARING ENDOMETRIAL CELLS

While endocervical adenocarcinoma is of increasing concern in young women, endometrial cancers predominate as women age beyond 35.[134,135] Benign-appearing endometrial cells on cervical cytology are rarely of importance in asymptomatic premenopausal women.[8] Approximately 0.5% to 1.8% of cervical cytology specimens from women ≥40 years of age will contain endometrial cells, and in postmenopausal women, they may be associated with significant pathology.[136,137] Other causes for normal-appearing endometrial cells in a postmenopausal

TABLE 19.16	MANAGEMENT OF WOMEN WITH AGC OR CYTOLOGIC AIS: INITIAL WORKUP*

- For women with all subcategories of AGC and AIS except atypical endometrial cells, colposcopy with endocervical sampling is recommended regardless of HPV result.
  - Triage by reflex HPV testing is *not* recommended.
  - Triage using repeat cervical cytology is unacceptable.
- Endometrial sampling is recommended in conjunction with colposcopy and endocervical sampling:
  - In women ≥35 y of age with all subcategories of AGC and AIS.
  - In women <35 years of age with clinical indications suggesting risk for endometrial neoplasia. Risks include unexplained vaginal bleeding or conditions suggesting chronic anovulation.
- For women with atypical endometrial cells, initial evaluation limited to endometrial and endocervical sampling is preferred, with colposcopy either acceptable at the initial evaluation or deferred until the results of endometrial and endocervical sampling are known.
  - If colposcopy is deferred and no endometrial pathology is identified, colposcopy is then recommended.

*Algorithm in Figure 19.12.
From Massad LS, Einstein MH, Huh WK, et al. 2012 Updated consensus guidelines for the management of abnormal cervical cancer screening tests and cancer precursors. *J Low Genit Tract Dis* 2013;17:S1–27, with permission.

TABLE 19.17	MANAGEMENT OF BENIGN GLANDULAR CHANGES ON CYTOLOGY

- For asymptomatic premenopausal women with benign endometrial cells, endometrial stromal cells, or histiocytes, no further evaluation is recommended.
- For postmenopausal women with benign endometrial cells, endometrial assessment is recommended.
- For posthysterectomy patients with a cytologic report of benign glandular cells, no further evaluation is recommended.

Adapted from Massad LS, Einstein MH, Huh WK, et al. 2012 Updated consensus guidelines for the management of abnormal cervical cancer screening tests and cancer precursors. *J Low Genit Tract Dis* 2013;17:S1–27, with permission.

cytology specimen include endometrial polyps, endometrial hyperplasia, or endometrial carcinoma.[137] Ten (7.7%) of 130 postmenopausal women with benign-appearing endometrial cells on routine cervical cytology undergoing endometrial sampling were found to have significant pathology, including six endometrial adenocarcinomas.[137] Hence, the presence of normal endometrial cells in a postmenopausal cytology sample requires endometrial sampling even when the woman is on hormone therapy, as the prevalence of significant pathology does not appear to be reduced in this setting (Table 19.17).[8,136,137] In contrast, benign-appearing endometrial cells or endometrial stromal cells/histiocytes in normal menstruating women throughout the menstrual cycle are rarely associated with important pathology and typically do not require evaluation.[8]

The primary cellular determinant for the definition of "atypical endometrial cells" is increased nuclear size. Up to one-third of endometrial cancers are detected following an AGC cytology,[138] and cellular changes more definitive for malignancy precede detection of endometrial cancer in another 13% to 47%.[139–142] Overall, abnormal cytology correctly identifies the endometrium as the primary site in only half of cases.[138] Although cervical cytology is not intended to be a screen for endometrial neoplasia and most women with endometrial hyperplasia or cancer have irregular bleeding, any cytologic glandular abnormality in women of this age increases concern for endometrial neoplasia. Endometrial hyperplasia and endometrial cancer have been detected in the follow-up of an AGC Pap test in only 3% of women under 49 years of age but in 19% of women above that age.[138] Therefore, the ASCCP guidelines recommend endometrial sampling for all women 35 years and older with AGC or AIS cytology.[8] As noted in Section 19.3.5.1 above, endometrial sampling is recommended in women younger than 35 years with clinical indications suggesting a risk of endometrial hyperplasia or cancer (e.g., unexplained vaginal bleeding, chronic anovulation, or atypical endometrial cells).[8] When the referral was made on the basis of atypical endometrial cells, colposcopy can be deferred until the results of the initial biopsies are known, or can be done at the same time.

19.3.5.2 Subsequent Management of Women with AGC

Prior recommendations for management after initial colposcopy depended on the results of HPV testing.[7,10] These recommendations included three different pathways depending on

FIGURE 19.12. ASCCP algorithm for the initial workup of women with atypical glandular cells (AGC). (From Massad LS, Einstein MH, Huh WK, et al. 2012 Updated consensus guidelines for the management of abnormal cervical cancer screening tests and cancer precursors. *J Low Genit Tract Dis* 2013;17:S1–27, with permission.)

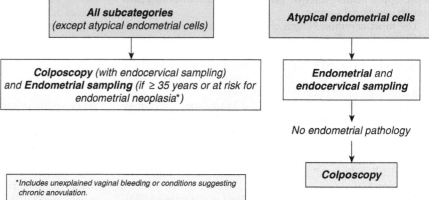

Initial Workup of Women with Atypical Glandular Cells (AGC)

All subcategories (except atypical endometrial cells) → **Colposcopy** (with endocervical sampling) and **Endometrial sampling** (if ≥ 35 years or at risk for endometrial neoplasia*)

Atypical endometrial cells → **Endometrial** and **endocervical sampling** → No endometrial pathology → **Colposcopy**

*Includes unexplained vaginal bleeding or conditions suggesting chronic anovulation.

whether the HPV test was positive, negative, or unknown, and all involved some combination of cytology with or without HPV testing at 6- or 12-month intervals. In the recently updated ASCCP management guidelines, women with no lesion found on initial evaluation are followed with cotesting at 12 and 24 months.[8] This management reflects the need for close follow-up even if HPV negative, balanced against the strong negative predictive value of a negative cotest for CIN 2+ and AIS. If any test is abnormal (defined as ≥ASC-US cytology or a positive HPV test), colposcopy should be repeated (Table 19.18; Figure 19.13). Because the data are sparse, these recommendations as in prior guidelines are based on expert opinion. Women with CIN 2+ and no glandular abnormality should be managed per the guidelines for the abnormality found (Chapter 20). The guidelines do not specify management for CIN 1 and no glandular abnormality, but these patients may be at higher risk of high-grade disease than patients with CIN 1 diagnosed after other abnormalities and should be followed closely.

The guidelines also do not address whether any additional response to repeat cytology reported as AGC or HSIL with continued negative colposcopy would be required. However, women with repeat AGC appear to be at high risk for high-grade neoplasia, including endometrial carcinoma, and HSIL cytology is always worrisome, particularly following unconfirmed AGC cytology.[120] Therefore, a diagnostic excisional procedure should be considered for women with repeat AGC or HSIL cytology reports and continued absence of detectable lesion on colposcopy, including negative vaginal colposcopy.

The significant risk for women with negative colposcopy, endocervical sampling, and endometrial sampling (when applicable) referred for a cytologic result of AGC "favor neoplasia" or AIS also warrants a cervical excisional procedure when no invasive disease is found on initial evaluation. It is recommended that the type of diagnostic excisional procedure used in this setting provides an intact specimen with interpretable

margins. When using LEEP in this setting, a large loop excising all the area at risk rather than serial passes (top-hat excision) is required to minimize the risk of thermal artifact. Concomitant endocervical sampling is preferred to assess for occult disease above the limits of excision.[8]

19.3.6 Management of HSIL

19.3.6.1 General Issues with HSIL and Initial Management

HSIL is not a common cytology interpretation. The mean HSIL reported in US laboratories is 0.7%.[92] The rate of HSIL varies with age. For example, the NCI/Kaiser Permanente Pacific Northwest study reported a rate of HSIL of 0.6% in women 20 to 29 years of age, 0.2% in women 40 to 49 years, and 0.1% in women 50 to 59 years.[105] CIN 2,3 or cervical cancer is found at colposcopy in approximately 53% to 66% of women with HSIL cytology and in 84% to 97% of women following LEEP.[143-145] Approximately 2% of women with HSIL have invasive cervical cancer. Among women 30 years and older, the 5-year risk for cancer is 8%.[45] The KPNC database demonstrated that HPV test results modify the CIN 3+ risk associated with an HSIL Pap test. HSIL/HPV-negative cotest results carried a 5-year CIN 3+ risk of 29% with 7% cervical cancer risk. In comparison, HSIL/HPV-positive results had a 5-year CIN 3+ risk of 50% and cervical cancer of 7%.[45] Both of these high risks are too high to justify reflex HPV triage in HSIL.[8] However, the slightly lower risk of HSIL/HPV-negative results may assist women in deciding whether or not to have immediate diagnostic excision or continued observation. Therefore, the initial management of most patients with HSIL regardless of HPV result is colposcopy, appropriately directed cervical biopsies and endocervical sampling or an immediate excisional procedure (Table 19.19; Figure 19.14).[8] Strategies to treat HSIL have been successful in reducing cervical cancer rates in developed countries despite limits to the sensitivity of colposcopy, biopsy, and endocervical sampling for high-grade precancer and cancer.[81,146,147]

Because colposcopy can miss CIN 2,3 lesions, failure to detect CIN 2,3 at colposcopy in a woman with HSIL cytology does not necessarily mean a CIN 2,3 lesion is not present.[146,147] As a result, most women with HSIL eventually undergo a diagnostic excisional procedure, either as treatment for proven CIN 2,3 or for colposcopic findings short of a high-grade lesion. Therefore, performing a LEEP as the initial management approach to an HSIL Pap report without prior colposcopy and biopsy confirmation of a high-grade lesion ("see-and-treat") has been advocated and is an initial management option in the guidelines.[8,148,149] This strategy has been shown to be feasible and cost-effective, as colposcopic assessment is not required prior to immediate LEEP. Nevertheless, performing LEEP under colposcopic guidance is helpful to tailor the excision to the size of the lesion and the limits of the transformation zone. However, the guidelines also take into consideration that some CIN 2,3 lesions, especially in young adults, spontaneously regress[64,150-153] and adverse pregnancy outcomes may be increased after cervical excision procedures.[154,155] Hence, the recommendation is that LEEP as an initial response to an HSIL cytology report is unacceptable in young women aged 21 to 24 years.[8]

The general recommendations of both the ASCCP and ACOG for the initial management of women ≥25 years with HSIL cytology are as follows: an immediate LEEP and colposcopy with endocervical assessment are both acceptable methods for managing women except in special populations (age 21 to 24 and in pregnancy).[8] Triage using repeat cytology alone or reflex HPV testing is unacceptable.[8,11] If

---

TABLE 19.18 MANAGEMENT OF WOMEN WITH AGC OR CYTOLOGIC AIS: POSTCOLPOSCOPY MANAGEMENT*

- For women with AGC "not otherwise specified" in whom CIN 2+ is not identified at colposcopy and biopsy, cotesting at 12 mo and 24 m is recommended.
  - If both cotests are negative/negative, return for repeat cotesting in 3 y is recommended.
  - If any cotest is abnormal, colposcopy is recommended.
- If CIN 2+ but no glandular neoplasia is identified histologically during the initial workup of a woman with atypical endocervical, endometrial, or glandular cells not otherwise specified, management should be according to the updated consensus management guidelines for the lesion diagnosed.
- For women with AGC "favor neoplasia" or endocervical AIS cytology, if invasive disease is not identified during the initial colposcopic workup, a diagnostic excisional procedure is recommended.
  - It is recommended that the type of diagnostic excisional procedure used in this setting provides an intact specimen with interpretable margins. Endocervical sampling after excision is preferred.

*Algorithm in Figure 19.13.
Adapted from Massad LS, Einstein MH, Huh WK, et al. 2012 Updated consensus guidelines for the management of abnormal cervical cancer screening tests and cancer precursors. *J Lower Gen Tract Dis* 2013;17:S1–27, with permission.

FIGURE 19.13. ASCCP algorithm for the subsequent management of women with atypical glandular cells (AGC). (From Massad LS, Einstein MH, Huh WK, et al. 2012 Updated consensus guidelines for the management of abnormal cervical cancer screening tests and cancer precursors. *J Low Genit Tract Dis* 2013;17:S1–27, with permission.)

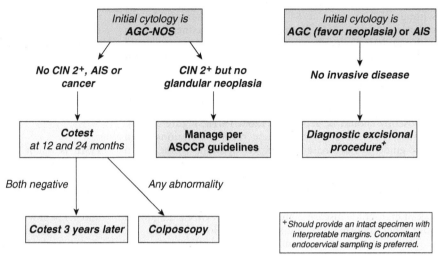

Subsequent Management of Women with Atypical Glandular Cells (AGC)

not managed by immediate excision, the woman should be referred to colposcopy regardless of the cotest HPV result. Except during pregnancy, if the colposcopic examination is inadequate, a diagnostic excisional procedure is recommended.[8] Ablation is unacceptable when colposcopy has not been performed, when CIN 2,3 is not identified histologically, and when the endocervical assessment shows CIN 2+ or ungraded CIN.

19.3.6.2 Management of Women ≥25 with HSIL after Colposcopy

There are a number of reasons why HSIL cytology may not be confirmed colposcopically. These include a lesion in the canal (endocervix) or vagina not seen by the colposcopist, poor biopsy placement, misinterpretation of cytologic or colposcopic findings, and a lesion too small to see even under

TABLE 19.19	MANAGEMENT OF WOMEN ≥25 WITH HSIL CYTOLOGY*

- The two options for the initial management of HSIL cytology in nonpregnant women ≥25 are
  - Immediate "see and treat" LEEP
  - Colposcopy with endocervical assessment
    - If the colposcopic examination is inadequate, except during pregnancy, a diagnostic excisional procedure is recommended.
- Triage using repeat cytology alone or reflex HPV testing is unacceptable.
- If not managed by immediate excisional procedure, women with HSIL cytology should be referred to colposcopy regardless of the HPV result if cotested.
- An ablation procedure is unacceptable when
  - Colposcopy has not been performed
  - When CIN 2,3 is not identified histologically
  - When the endocervical assessment shows CIN 2+ or ungraded CIN

*Algorithm in Figure 19.14.
From Massad LS, Einstein MH, Huh WK, et al. 2012 Updated consensus guidelines for the management of abnormal cervical cancer screening tests and cancer precursors. *J Low Genit Tract Dis* 2013;17:S1–27, with permission.

colposcopic magnification.[109] It is now clear that the sensitivity of colposcopy for detecting CIN 2,3 is less than previously appreciated, particularly for the small high-grade lesions often missed following ASC-US or LSIL referral.[146,147,156,157] HSIL cytology is more likely to represent larger CIN 2,3 lesions less likely to be missed at colposcopy, but misses do occur although occult carcinoma is unlikely. Atrophic change due to estrogen deficiency and small CIN 2,3 lesions within a large low-grade lesion or area of complex immature metaplasia may all make identification of the most abnormal area for biopsy difficult. Even when the biopsy specimen correctly contains an area of CIN 2,3, the lesion may not be detected in the lab due to inadequate sectioning of the tissue specimen or misclassification of the histology.

An important consideration before an excisional procedure is done for a noncorrelating HSIL Pap report is whether the high-grade cytology result is due to a vaginal lesion that could be detected by careful examination of the vagina using both 3% to 5% acetic acid and Lugol solution. When no lesion is found in the vagina and colposcopic biopsy of the cervix does not elicit the source of the HSIL Pap report in a nonpregnant woman, the choice of follow-up versus excision will depend on a number of factors: the age of the patient, likelihood of adherence with follow-up instructions, past history of screening and abnormalities, desire for future fertility, and review of cytology, colposcopy, and histology findings.[8] For many of these women, a cervical excisional procedure may be warranted.

Even with HSIL interpretations, cytology is subjective, and women with HSIL on their Pap report may not have CIN 2,3 or AIS. In a study of the reproducibility of cervical cytology, 27% of women with HSIL cytology were reclassified as LSIL on review, 23% as ASC-US, and 3% as negative.[158] Therefore, before proceeding to a cervical excision procedure, a review of the Pap report may be appropriate (Table 19.20; Figure 20.5C, *Management of Women with No Lesion or Biopsy-confirmed Cervical Intraepithelial Neoplasia—Grade 1 [CIN1] Preceded by ASC-H or HSIL Cytology* in Chapter 20). If such review leads to a revised cytologic interpretation, then management should be according to the new interpretation. However, if the Pap interpretation remains HSIL and no CIN 2,3 or cancer is found, two options are available: either a diagnostic excisional procedure or observation with cotesting at 12 and 24 months is acceptable, provided in the latter case that the colposcopy

Management of Women with High-Grade Squamous Intraepithelial Lesions (HSIL)*

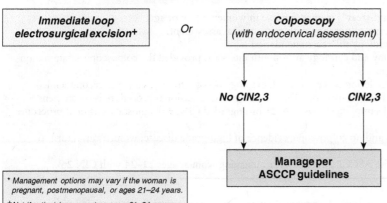

FIGURE 19.14. ASCCP algorithm for the management of women with high-grade squamous intraepithelial lesions (HSIL). (From Massad LS, Einstein MH, Huh WK, et al. 2012 Updated consensus guidelines for the management of abnormal cervical cancer screening tests and cancer precursors. *J Low Genit Tract Dis* 2013;17:S1–27, with permission.)

examination is adequate and endocervical sampling is negative.[8] Excision is required if the ECC is CIN 2+ or ungraded or if the colposcopy is inadequate. If cotesting at 12 and 24 months is elected and both tests are cytology negative/HPV negative, the woman should return for age-specific testing in 3 years. If any test is abnormal with a threshold of ≥ASC-US for cytology or positive for HPV, then repeat colposcopy is recommended. If HSIL cytology is found at either the 12- or 24-month visit, a diagnostic excision procedure is recommended.[8] A diagnostic excisional procedure is more appropriate in women not concerned about future fertility. For those desiring to avoid a procedure with any possibility of compromising pregnancy outcome,[154,155] and because some may not have CIN 2,3 or have CIN 2,3 that may spontaneously regress, the option of watchful waiting for women with adequate colposcopy and negative endocervical sampling was added in the 2006 consensus guidelines and continues with the current updated ASCCP management guidelines.[8,159]

19.3.6.3 Management of Special Populations with HSIL Cytology

19.3.6.3.1 MANAGEMENT OF WOMEN AGED 21 TO 24 YEARS WITH HSIL CYTOLOGY

Although the risks of CIN 3+ and cervical cancer are relatively low in young women, they are not negligible. In the KPNC cohort, 3 cancers occurred during follow-up of 133,947 women aged 21 to 24 years screened.[43] The 5-year cumulative CIN 3+ risk following an HSIL cytology in this age group was 28%, which was similar to the risk observed for women aged 25 to 29 years. In comparison, in women >30 years of age, the risk was 47%. Consequently, women aged 21 to 24 years with HSIL cytology should have colposcopy (Table 19.21, Figure 19.15). Immediate loop electrosurgical excision (i.e., "see-and-treat") is unacceptable in women aged 21 to 24 years of age.[8] All women of this age with HSIL cytology should have colposcopy with endocervical assessment. Post-colposcopy management is also different for these women

---

TABLE 19.20   POSTCOLPOSCOPY MANAGEMENT OF WOMEN ≥25 WITH HSIL CYTOLOGY AND NO CIN 2,3 IDENTIFIED ON COLPOSCOPY

- If CIN 2,3 or AIS is not found at colposcopy, the following are recommended:
  - Careful examination of the vagina using both 3% to 5% acetic acid and Lugol iodine solution should be done to rule out a missed high-grade vaginal lesion.
  - A review of the cytology report may be appropriate.
    - If such review leads to a revised cytologic interpretation, management should be according to the new interpretation.
    - If the cytology interpretation remains HSIL and no CIN 2,3 or cancer is found, two options are available:
      □ A diagnostic excisional procedure
      □ Observation with cotesting at 12 and 24 mo provided that the colposcopy examination is adequate and endocervical sampling is negative.
        – If cotests at both 12 and 24 mo are cytology negative/HPV negative, the woman should return for age-specific testing in 3 y.
        – If any cytology report is ≥ASC-US or any HPV test is positive, repeat colposcopy is recommended.
        – If HSIL cytology is reported at either the 12- or 24-month visit, a diagnostic excisional procedure is recommended.
      □ The choice of follow-up versus excision will depend on a number of factors:
        – The age of the patient
        – Likelihood of adherence with follow-up instructions
        – Past history of screening and abnormalities
        – Desire for future fertility
        – Review of cytology, colposcopy, and histology findings

Adapted from Massad LS, Einstein MH, Huh WK, et al. 2012 Updated consensus guidelines for the management of abnormal cervical cancer screening tests and cancer precursors. *J Low Genit Tract Dis* 2013;17:S1–27, with permission.

TABLE 19.21　MANAGEMENT OF WOMEN <25 WITH ASC-H OR HSIL CYTOLOGY*

- Immediate loop electrosurgical excision (i.e., "see-and-treat") is unacceptable in women <25 y of age.
- All women ages <25 y with HSIL cytology should have colposcopy with endocervical assessment.
- If CIN 2,3 is not diagnosed after ASC-H or HSIL cytology the recommendation is
  - Observation for up to 24 mo using both colposcopy and cytology at 6-month intervals, provided the colposcopic examination is adequate and endocervical assessment is negative.
    - If during the follow-up, a high-grade colposcopic lesion is seen or HSIL cytology persists for 1 y, biopsy is recommended.
    - If the HSIL cytology persists at 24 mo without identification of CIN 2+, a diagnostic excisional procedure is recommended.
    - When colposcopy is inadequate or endocervical sampling shows CIN 2+ or ungraded CIN, a diagnostic excisional procedure is also recommended.
    - After two consecutive negative cytology results and no colposcopic evidence of high-grade disease, women can return to routine screening.
    - If CIN 2,3 is diagnosed, manage according to the ASCCP guidelines for managing women ages 21–24 with CIN 2,3.

*Algorithm in Figure 19.15.
Adapted from Massad LS, Einstein MH, Huh WK, et al. 2012 Updated consensus guidelines for the management of abnormal cervical cancer screening tests and cancer precursors. *J Low Genit Tract Dis* 2013;17:S1–27, with permission.

when CIN 2,3 is not identified histologically after ASC-H or HSIL cytology. For these women, observation for up to 24 months using both colposcopy and cytology at 6-month intervals is recommended, provided the colposcopic examination is adequate and endocervical assessment is negative. If during the follow-up, a high-grade colposcopic lesion is seen or HSIL cytology persists for 1 year, biopsy is recommended. If the HSIL cytology persists at 24 months without identification of CIN 2+, a diagnostic excisional procedure is recommended.[8]

When colposcopy is inadequate or endocervical sampling shows CIN 2+ or ungraded CIN, a diagnostic excisional procedure is also recommended. After two consecutive negative cytology results and no colposcopic evidence of high-grade disease, women can return to routine screening.[8] If CIN 2,3 is diagnosed, manage according to the ASCCP guidelines for the management of women aged 21 to 24 years with CIN 2,3 (see Chapter 20; Figure 20.5F, Management of young women age 21–24 with CIN 2,3).

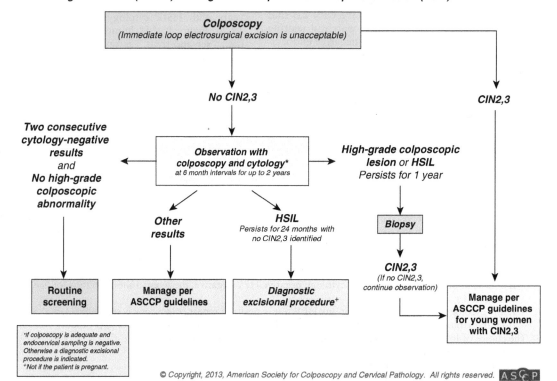

Management of Women Ages 21–24 Years with Atypical Squamous Cells, Cannot Rule Out High-Grade SIL (ASC-H) and High-Grade Squamous Intraepithelial Lesion (HSIL)

FIGURE 19.15.　ASCCP algorithm for the management of women aged 21 to 24 years with atypical squamous cells, cannot rule out high-grade SIL (ASC-H) and high-grade squamous intraepithelial lesion (HSIL) on cytology. (From Massad LS, Einstein MH, Huh WK, et al. 2012 Updated consensus guidelines for the management of abnormal cervical cancer screening tests and cancer precursors. *J Low Genit Tract Dis* 2013;17:S1–27, with permission.)

19.3.6.3.2 Management of HSIL in Pregnancy

All pregnant women with HSIL cytology should have colposcopy. The primary goal is excluding invasive cervical cancer, as this is the only diagnosis that may alter management during pregnancy.[8] Endocervical curettage is contraindicated during pregnancy because this procedure may lacerate the soft cervix with consequent hemorrhage and may also rupture the amniotic sac. Colposcopy and management of women with HSIL cytology in pregnancy are more challenging than for non-pregnant women with HSIL and ideally should be performed by a clinician experienced in seeing the colposcopic changes typical in pregnancy.[11] These include cervical hyperemia, the development of prominent normal epithelial changes that colposcopically mimic preinvasive disease, obscuring mucus, contact bleeding, prolapsing vaginal walls, and bleeding after biopsy (see Chapter 12). Biopsy is important if the colposcopic impression is high-grade disease, especially in older pregnant women at higher risk of invasive cancer. Once cancer has been excluded, management can be deferred until postpartum. CIN may regress during the interval between antenatal cytology and the postpartum examination, and progression to invasion during pregnancy is unlikely. Additionally, colposcopy becomes increasingly difficult as pregnancy proceeds. Therefore, once invasion has been ruled out, repeat colposcopy is not usually helpful until postpartum.[160,161] However, repeat colposcopy may be useful when colposcopy is inadequate or a large lesion is present that cannot be sampled thoroughly. Reassessment with cytology and colposcopy no sooner than 6 weeks after delivery are important in tailoring therapy (Table 19.22).[8]

19.4 PROSPECTS FOR MANAGEMENT OF ABNORMAL CERVICAL SCREENING RESULTS IN THE FUTURE

Management guidelines for abnormal cervical cytology have been available for only the last two decades and have evolved considerably over this short time period. Colposcopy is still the standard first-line approach for evaluating women with abnormal cytology, with reflex HPV testing of ASC-US, the standard approach for determining which women ≥25 with ASC-US cytology require immediate colposcopy. Despite the gains in efficiency with cotesting, particularly secondary to increased intervals, screening still sends many more normal women to colposcopy than is ideal. In addition, evidence-based literature that could more expertly inform postcolposcopy management scenarios is sparse. The effect of HPV vaccinations also may eventually decrease the risk associated with abnormal cytology and so alter screening and management protocols. Hence, moving to a system of screening and management that more accurately predicts the risk of CIN 3 and cancer is clearly needed. In addition, accurate tests are needed to identify the few women with CIN 1 or 2 destined to develop CIN 3 or invasive cancer.[49,50] For these reasons, the need for biomarkers that more accurately separate women at risk for disease progression from those with benign self-limited HPV infections has never been greater. Investigators are pursuing several promising avenues of research that regrettably remain investigational at present.

Certainly, type-specific HPV persistence is the key to cervical cancer development. With the availability of HPV 16/18 testing, persistence of either of these two types reflects increased risk for CIN 3+ and invasive cancer.[57] HPV 16/18 triage is already incorporated into several of the guidelines.[8] New guidelines may be revised based on long-term data from trials of assays for these types.

Higher viral load of newly detected infections and changes in viral load have been shown to predict persistence and progression of HPV infections.[162,163] However, use of viral load for risk assessment is not possible at present as quantitative assays are often not reproducible.[162,163]

Individual differences in immunologic responses to HPV play a critical role in determining infection outcomes, but markers identifying individuals most at risk due to a permissive immune response are not yet available. Certain inherited genetic polymorphisms within immune response genes (human leukocyte antigen [HLA]) associated with higher risk for CIN 3 and cervical cancer have been identified and may be useful in the future.[164] However, HLA typing for polymorphisms and testing for other genetic variants that may play a role in persistence of an HPV infection and progression of a lesion are not ready for clinical use.[165]

Variants of high-risk HPV types are another potential marker. Infections with non-European variants of HPV 16 and 18 are associated with a higher risk of persistence and development of CIN AQA3+ than infection with the European variant of HPV 16 and 18 (see Chapter 5).[166,167] HPV 35 and HPV 51 variant lineages also predict a higher risk of CIN 3+. It is known that non-European variants of HPV 16 have genomic heterogeneity in areas most responsible for up-regulation of the virus and for cellular transformation. This could help explain the dichotomy between HPV 16 being the most common hrHPV type in women found to be normal as well as in women with cervical cancer. A clinical test that could identify women with both genetic susceptibility markers and HPV 16 variants might be quite helpful in distinguishing those with increased risk from those with lesser risk.[168] Eventually, identification of markers of the immune response, of protein markers elaborated in up-regulation of the virus or in cellular dysregulation, of alterations in cellular tumor suppresser genes, or of variations in hrHPV types may be valuable markers for risk of progression.

Several protein markers elaborated in up-regulation of the virus or in cellular dysregulation have shown potential, and one (Aptima AHPV E6,E7 mRNA test, Hologic, San Diego, CA) has received FDA approval for ASC-US triage and in primary cervical screening with cytology as a cotest for women ≥30.[169] Others include testing for p16 INK4a/Ki-67 dual immunostaining and for cellular and viral methylation patterns. The AHPV tests for elaboration of messenger

---

TABLE 19.22	MANAGEMENT OF HSIL IN PREGNANCY

- All pregnant women with HSIL cytology should have colposcopy, with the primary goal of excluding the presence of invasive cervical cancer.
  - Colposcopy ideally should be performed by a clinician experienced in seeing the colposcopic changes typical in pregnancy.
  - Biopsy is important if the colposcopic impression is high-grade disease.
  - Once cancer has been excluded, cervical therapy can be deferred until postpartum.
  - Once invasion has been ruled out, repeat colposcopy is not usually helpful until postpartum.
  - Reassessment with cytology and colposcopy no sooner than 6 wk after delivery is important in tailoring therapy.
- Endocervical curettage is contraindicated during pregnancy.

Adapted from Massad LS, Einstein MH, Huh WK, et al. 2012 Updated consensus guidelines for the management of abnormal cervical cancer screening tests and cancer precursors. *J Low Genit Tract Dis* 2013;17:S1–27, with permission.

RNA from the two genetic loci (E6 and E7) most responsible for progression to CIN 3 and cervical cancer.[170,171] Sensitivity has been shown to be similar to Hybrid Capture 2, but specificity is higher. At this time, p16 is close to clinical use in screening than methylation markers.[172,173] p16 INK staining is commonly used now for histologic diagnosis of CIN 2. p16 is overexpressed with increasing up-regulation of the HPV E7 oncoprotein, making it a good biomarker for risk.[174] The combination of p16 (INK4a) and Ki-67 has been more promising in primary screening than p16 alone.

Another biomarker with potential combines two molecular markers associated with abnormal cell cycle regulation, mini-chromosome maintenance protein 2, and topoisomerase II (ProEx C, TriPath, Burlington, NC). ProEx C has been shown to be highly sensitive and specific for identification of CIN 2+ in ASC-US triage[175] and highly sensitive and specific for HPV-induced neoplastic lesions identified on evaluation of AGC cytology, while not positive for metastatic glandular lesions that were not HPV associated.[176]

The finding in cervical and other HPV-induced cancers that HPV 16 and 18 genomes are often heavily methylated, most conspicuously in the L1 gene, has heightened interest in looking at DNA methylation as a possible biomarker of risk for progression.[177] Methylation of human DNA, particularly

the cell adhesion molecule 1 (CADM1) gene and the T-lymphocyte maturation associated protein (MAL) gene, has also shown promise.[178,179]

The rate of change in cervical cancer screening and management protocols has considerably accelerated in the 21st century. The biggest change is in the introduction of HPV testing in both primary cervical cancer screening and management of equivocal and some abnormal cervical cytology results. Management and counseling of cytology-negative/HPV-positive women will continue to be a concern for some time but should be amenable to education of both the public and providers. Advances in screening and management have made it increasingly possible to prevent cervical cancer but have also made clinical decisions more complicated, with the potential for increasing costs and harms as well as benefit.[48–50] Use of decision support aids, including software integrated into electronic medical records and applications for smartphones, promises to minimize this risk. Introduction of risk modeling for cervical cancer prevention, based on appropriate clinical actions corresponding to level of risk (Figure 19.16), has played a pivotal role in the updated ASCCP management guidelines and should help better allocate resources, while at the same time protecting safety for women at greatest risk, and well-being for women at all levels of risk.[8,49,50]

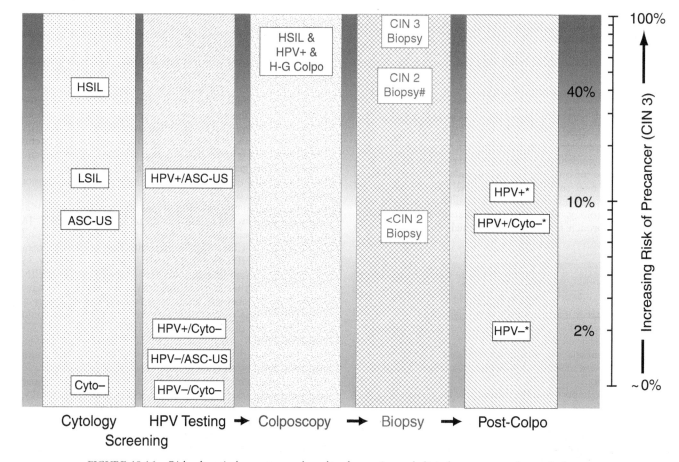

FIGURE 19.16.   Risk of cervical precancer and results of screening and clinical management for cervical cancer prevention. A graphical representation of the risk of cervical precancer at different stages and results of screening and clinical management for cervical cancer prevention. The risks for each stage and result are approximate risks for CIN 3 within the screening interval. Each stage of screening and clinical management is represented by a different pattern, with the arrows at the bottom indicating the sequence of the stages. Number sign indicates that less than half of the cases of CIN 2 on biopsy are subsequently diagnosed as CIN 3 on excisional tissue. Dagger indicates time within a screening interval. Asterisk indicates test results at the next follow-up visit (6 months or longer). (From Castle PE, Sideri M, Jeronimo J, Solomon D, Schiffman M. Risk assessment to guide the prevention of cervical cancer. *J Low Genit Tract Dis* 2008;12(1):1–7. Reprinted with permission.)

References

1. Kurman RJ, Henson DE, Herbst AL, Noller KL, Schiffman MH. Interim guidelines for management of abnormal cervical cytology. The 1992 National Cancer Institute Workshop. *JAMA* 1994;271(23):1866–9.

2. Cox JT (lead author). ASCCP practice guideline: management of glandular abnormalities in the cervical smear. *J Lower Gen Tract Dis* 1997;1:41–5.

3. Cox JT (lead author). ASCCP practice guideline: management issues related to quality of the smear. *J Lower Gen Tract Dis* 1997;2:100–106.

4. Cox JT, Wilkinson E, Lonky N, Waxman A, Tosh R, Tedeschi C. ASCCP practice guideline: management guidelines for follow-up of atypical squamous cells of undetermined significance (ASCUS). *J Lower Gen Tract Dis* 2000;4:99–113.

5. Cox JT, Massad LS, Lonky N, Tosh R, Waxman A, Wilkinson E. ASCCP practice guideline: management guidelines for follow-up of low grade squamous intraepithelial lesion (LSIL). *J Low Gen Tract Dis* 2000;4:83–92.

6. Wright TC Jr, Cox JT, Massad LS, Twiggs LB, Wilkinson EJ; ASCCP-Sponsored Consensus Conference. 2001 consensus guidelines for the management of women with cervical cytological abnormalities. *JAMA* 2002;287(16):2120–9.

7. Wright TC Jr, Massad LS, Dunton CJ, Spitzer M, Wilkinson EJ, Solomon D; 2006 ASCCP-Sponsored Consensus Conference. 2006 consensus guidelines for the management of women with abnormal cervical screening tests. *J Low Gen Tract Dis* 2007;11(4):201–22.

8. Massad LS, Einstein MH, Huh WK, et al. 2012 updated consensus guidelines for the management of abnormal cervical cancer screening tests and cancer precursors. *J Low Genit Tract Dis* 2013;17(5 Suppl 1): S1–27. Jointly published without algorithm figures as Massad LS, Einstein MH, Huh WK, et al.; 2012 ASCCP Consensus Guidelines Conference. 2012 updated consensus guidelines for the management of abnormal cervical cancer screening tests and cancer precursors. *Obstet Gynecol* 2013;121(4):829–46.

9. American College of Obstetricians and Gynecologists. ACOG Practice Bulletin number 66. Management of abnormal cervical cytology and histology. *Obstet Gynecol* 2005;106(3):645–64.

10. ACOG Practice Bulletin No. 99. Management of abnormal cervical cytology and histology. *Obstet Gynecol* 2008;112:1419–44.

11. Management of abnormal cervical cancer screening test results and cervical cancer precursors. Practice Bulletin No. 140. American College of Obstetricians and Gynecologists. *Obstet Gynecol* 2013;122:1338–67.

12. Davey DD, Austin RM, Birdsong G, et al.; American Society for Colposcopy and Cervical Pathology. ASCCP patient management guidelines: Pap test specimen adequacy and quality indicators. *Am J Clin Pathol* 2002;118:714–8.

13. Davey D, Cox JT, Austin M, et al. Cervical cytology specimen adequacy: patient management guidelines and optimizing specimen collection. *J Low Genit Tract Dis* 2008;12(2):71–81.

14. Solomon D, Davey D, Kurman R, et al.; The Forum Group Members; The Bethesda 2001 Workshop. The 2001 Bethesda System: terminology for reporting results of cervical cytology. *JAMA* 2002;287:2114–19.

15. Birdsong GG, Davey DD, Darragh TM, Elgert PA, Henry M. Specimen adequacy. In: Solomon D, Nayar R, eds. *The Bethesda System for Reporting Cervical Cytology*. New York, NY: Springer-Verlag, 2004:1–20.

16. Lu CH, Chang CC, Chang MC, et al. Clinical parameters associated with unsatisfactory specimens of conventional cervical smears. *Diagn Cytopathol* 2011;39(2):87–91.

17. Lu CH, Chang CC, Ho ES, et al. Should adequacy criteria in cervicovaginal cytology be modified after radiotherapy, chemotherapy, or hysterectomy? *Cancer Cytopathol* 2010;118(6):474–81.

18. Hock YL, Ramaiah S, Wall ES, et al. Outcome of women with inadequate cervical smears followed up for five years. *J Clin Pathol* 2003;56:592–5.

19. Ransdell JS, Davey DD, Zaleski S. Clinicopathologic correlation of the unsatisfactory Papanicolaou smear. *Cancer Cytopathol* 1997;81:139–43.

20. Jeronimo J, Khan MJ, Schiffman M, Solomon D; ALTS Group. Does the interval between Papanicolaou tests influence the quality of cytology? *Cancer* 2005;105:133–8.

21. Martin-Hirsch P, Lilford R, Jarvis G, Kitchener H. Efficacy of cervical-smear collection devices: a systematic review and meta-analysis. *Lancet* 1999;354:1763–70.

22. Curtis P, Mintzer M, Morrell D, Resnick JC, Hendrix S, Qaqish BF. Characteristics and quality of Papanicolaou smears obtained by primary care clinicians using a single commercial laboratory. *Arch Fam Med* 1999;8:407–13.

23. Hamblin JE, Brock CD, Litchfield L, Dias J. Papanicolaou smear adequacy: effect of different techniques in specific fertility states. *J Fam Pract* 1985;20:257–60.

24. Kost ER, Snyder RR, Schwartz LE, Hankins GD. The "less than optimal" cytology: importance in obstetric patients and in a routine gynecologic population. *Obstet Gynecol* 1993;81:127–30.

25. Giorgi Rossi P, Baiocchi D, Ciatto S. Risk of CIN 2 in women with a pap test without endocervical cells vs. those with a negative pap test with endocervical cells: a cohort study with 4.5 years of follow-up. *Acta Cytol* 2010;54(3):265–71.

26. Zhao C, Austin RM. Adjunctive high-risk human papillomavirus DNA testing is a useful option for disease risk assessment in patients with negative Papanicolaou tests without an endocervical/transformation zone sample. *Cancer Cytopathol* 2008;114:242–8.

27. Elumir-Tanner L, Doraty M. Management of Papanicolaou test results that lack endocervical cells. *CMAJ* 2011;183(5):563–8.

28. Mitchell HS. Longitudinal analysis of histologic high-grade disease after negative cervical cytology according to endocervical status. *Cancer (Cancer Cytopathol)* 2001;93:237–40.

29. Bos AB, van Bellegooijen M, ven den Akker-van Marle ME, et al. Endocervical status is not predictive of the incidence of cervical cancer in the years after negative smears. *Am J Clin Pathol* 2001;115:851–5.

30. Mitchell H, Medley G. Differences between Papanicolaou smears with correct and incorrect diagnoses. *Cytopathology* 1995;6:368–75.

31. O'Sullivan JP, A'Hern RP, Chapman PA, et al. A case–control study of true-positive versus false-negative cervical smears in women with cervical intraepithelial neoplasia (CIN) III. *Cytopathology* 1998;9:155–61.

32. Baer A, Kiviat NB, Kulasingam S, Mao C, Kuypers J, Koutsky LA. Liquid-based Papanicolaou smears without a transformation zone component: should clinicians worry? *Obstet Gynecol* 2002;99:1053–9.

33. Huang A, Quinn M, Tan J. Outcome in women with no endocervical component on cervical cytology after treatment for high-grade cervical dysplasia. *Aust N Z J Obstet Gynaecol* 2009;49:426–8.

34. American College of Obstetricians and Gynecologists. Practice Bulletin No. 131. Screening for cervical cancer. *Obstet Gynecol* 2012;120:1222–38.

35. Saslow D, Solomon D, Lawson HW, et al. American Cancer Society, American Society for Colposcopy and Cervical Pathology, and American Society for Clinical Pathology screening guidelines for the prevention and early detection of cervical cancer. *Am J Clin Pathol* 2012;137(4):516–42.

36. Moyer VA; for the U.S. Preventive Services Task Force. Screening for cervical cancer. U.S. Preventive Services Task Force recommendation statement. *Ann Intern Med.* 2012;156(12):880–91.

37. Zhao C, Austin RM. Human papillomavirus DNA detection in ThinPrep Pap test vials is independent of cytologic sampling of the transformation zone. *Gynecol Oncol* 2007;107:231–5.

38. Solomon D, Schiffman M, Tarone R; ALTS Study group. Comparison of three management strategies for patients with atypical squamous cells of undetermined significance: baseline results from a randomized trial. *J Natl Cancer Inst* 2001;93(4):293–9.

39. Katki HA, Kinney WK, Fetterman B, et al. Cervical cancer risk for women undergoing concurrent testing for human papillomavirus and cervical cytology: a population-based study in routine clinical practice. *Lancet Oncol* 2011;12(7): 663–72.

40. Katki HA, Schiffman M, Castle PE, et al. Benchmarking CIN 3+ risk as the basis for incorporating HPV and Pap cotesting into cervical screening and management guidelines. *J Low Genit Tract Dis* 2013;17(5 Suppl 1):S28–35.

41. Katki HA, Schiffman M, Castle PE, et al. Five-year risks of CIN 3+ and cervical cancer among women who test Pap-negative but are HPV-positive. *J Low Genit Tract Dis* 2013;17(5 Suppl 1):S56–63.

42. Katki HA, Schiffman M, Castle PE, et al. Five-year risks of CIN 3+ and cervical cancer among women with HPV testing of ASC-US Pap results. *J Low Genit Tract Dis* 2013;17(5 Suppl 1):S36–42.

43. Katki HA, Schiffman M, Castle PE, et al. Five-year risk of CIN 3+ to guide the management of women aged 21 to 24 years. *J Low Genit Tract Dis* 2013;17(5 Suppl 1):S64–8.

44. Katki HA, Schiffman M, Castle PE, et al. Five-year risks of CIN 2+ and CIN 3+ among women with HPV-positive and HPV-negative LSIL Pap results. *J Low Genit Tract Dis* 2013;17(5 Suppl 1):S43–9.

45. Katki HA, Schiffman M, Castle PE, et al. Five-year risks of CIN 3+ and cervical cancer among women with HPV-positive and HPV-negative high-grade Pap results. *J Low Genit Tract Dis* 2013;17(5 Suppl 1):S50–5.

46. Katki HA, Gage JC, Schiffman M, et al. Follow-up testing after colposcopy: five-year risk of CIN 2+ after a colposcopic diagnosis of CIN 1 or less. *J Low Genit Tract Dis* 2013;17(5 Suppl 1): S69–77.

47. Katki HA, Schiffman M, Castle PE, et al. Five-year risk of recurrence after treatment of CIN 2, CIN 3, or AIS: performance of HPV and Pap cotesting in posttreatment management. *J Low Genit Tract Dis* 2013;17(5 Suppl 1):S78–84.

48. Sawaya GF. New guidelines: it's complicated. *Obstet Gynecol* 2013;121(4): 703–4.

49. Castle PE, Sideri M, Jeronimo J, Solomon D, Schiffman M. Risk assessment to guide the prevention of cervical cancer. *J Low Genit Tract Dis* 2008; 12(1):1–7.

50. Katki HA, Wacholder S, Solomon D, Castle PE, Schiffman M. Risk estimation for the next generation of prevention programmes for cervical cancer. *Lancet Oncol* 2009;10(11):1022–3.

51. Wright TC Jr, Schiffman M, Solomon D, et al. Interim guidance for the use of human papillomavirus DNA testing as an adjunct to cervical cytology for screening. *Obstet Gynecol* 2004;103:304–9.

52. Clavel C, Masure M, Bory JP, et al. Human papillomavirus testing in primary screening for the detection of high-grade cervical lesions: a study of 7932 women. *Br J Cancer* 2001;84:1616–23.

53. Rodríguez AC, Schiffman M, Herrero R, et al.; Proyecto Epidemiológico Guanacaste Group. Rapid clearance of human papillomavirus and implications for clinical focus on persistent infections. *J Natl Cancer Inst* 2008; 100(7):513–7.

54. Kitchener HC, Almonte M, Thomson C, et al. HPV testing in combination with liquid-based cytology in primary cervical screening (ARTISTIC): a randomized controlled trial. *Lancet Oncol* 2009;10:672–82.

55. Sasieni P, Castle PE, Cuzick J. Further analysis of the ARTISTIC trial. *Lancet Oncol* 2009;10:841–2.

56. Khan MJ, Castle PE, Lorincz AT, et al. The elevated 10-year risk of cervical precancer and cancer in women with human papillomavirus (HPV) type 16 or 18 and the possible utility of type-specific HPV testing in clinical practice. *J Natl Cancer Inst* 2005;97:1072–9.

57. Kjaer SK, Frederiksen K, Munk C, Iftner T. Long-term absolute risk of cervical intraepithelial neoplasia grade 3 or worse following human papillomavirus infection: role of persistence. *J Natl Cancer Inst* 2010; 102(19):1478–88.

58. de Sanjose S, Quint WG, Alemany L, et al. Human papillomavirus genotype attribution in invasive cervical cancer: a retrospective cross-sectional worldwide study. *Lancet Oncol* 2010;11:1048–56.

59. Wright TC Jr, Stoler MH, Sharma A, Zhang G, Behrens C, Wright TL. Evaluation of HPV-16 and HPV-18 genotyping for the triage of women with high-risk HPV+ cytology-negative results. *Am J Clin Pathol* 2011; 136(4): 578–86.

60. ASCUS-LSIL Triage Study (ALTS) Group. Results of a randomized trial on the management of cytology interpretations of atypical squamous cells of undetermined significance. *Am J Obstet Gynecol* 2003;188:1383–92.

61. Eversole GM, Moriarty AT, Schwartz MR, et al. Practices of participants in the College of American Pathologists interlaboratory comparison program in cervicovaginal cytology, 2006. *Arch Pathol Lab Med* 2010;134(3):331–5.

62. Arbyn M, Sasieni P, Meijer CJ, Clavel C, Koliopoulos G, Dillner J. Chapter 9: clinical applications of HPV testing: a summary of meta-analyses. *Vaccine* 2006;24(Suppl 3):S3/78–89.

63. Castle PE, Rodriguez AC, Burk RD, et al. Short term persistence of human papillomavirus and risk of cervical precancer and cancer: population based cohort study. *BMJ* 2009;339:b2569.

64. Moscicki AB, Cox JT. Practice improvement in cervical screening and management (PICSM): symposium on management of cervical abnormalities in adolescents and young women. *J Low Gen Tract Dis* 2010;14(1):73–80.

65. Moscicki AB, Hills N, Shiboski S, et al. Risks for incident human papillomavirus infection and low-grade squamous intraepithelial lesion development in young females. *JAMA* 2001;285:2995–3002.

66. Dunn TS, Bajaj JE, Stamm CA, Beaty B. Management of the minimally abnormal Papanicolaou smear in pregnancy. *J Low Genit Tract Dis* 2001;5(3):133–7.

67. Eltoum IA, Chhieng DC, Crowe DR, Roberson J, Jin G, Broker TR. Significance and possible causes of false-negative results of reflex human papillomavirus testing. *Cancer (Cancer Cytopathol)* 2007;111:154–9.

68. Eltoum IA, Chhieng DC, Roberson J, McMillon D, Partridge EE. Reflex human papilloma virus infection testing detects the same proportion of cervical intraepithelial neoplasia grade 2–3 in young versus elderly women. *Cancer* 2005;105(4):194–8.

69. Sawaya GF, Kerlikowske K, Lee NC, Gildengorin G, Washington AE. Frequency of cervical smear abnormalities within 3 years of normal cytology. *Obstet Gynecol* 2000;96:219–23.

70. Sawaya GF, Grady D, Kerlikowske K, et al. The positive predictive value of cervical smears in previously screened postmenopausal women: the Heart and Estrogen/Progestin Replacement Study (HERS). *Ann Intern Med* 2000; 133:942–50.

71. Sherman ME, Schiffman M, Cox JT; Atypical Squamous Cells of Undetermined Significance/Low-Grade Squamous Intraepithelial Lesion Triage Study Group. Effects of age and human papilloma viral load on colposcopy triage: data from Squamous Intraepithelial Lesion Triage Study (ALTS). *J Natl Cancer Inst* 2002;94:102–7.

72. Bruner KS, Davey DD. ASC-US and HPV testing in women aged 40 years and over. *Diagn Cytopathol* 2004;31:358–61.

73. Ellerbrock TV, Chiasson MA, Bush TJ, et al. Incidence of cervical squamous intraepithelial lesions in HIV-infected women. *JAMA* 2000;283:1031–7.

74. Abraham AG, Strickler HD, Jing Y, et al. Invasive cervical cancer risk among HIV-infected women: a North American multi-cohort collaboration prospective study. *J Acquir Immune Defic Syndr* 2013;62:405–13.

75. Blitz S, Baxter J, Raboud J, et al. Evaluation of HIV and highly active antiretroviral therapy on the natural history of human papillomavirus infection and cervical cytopathologic findings in HIV-positive and high-risk HIV-negative women. *J Infect Dis* 2013;208(3):454–62.

76. Kreitchmann R, Bajotto H, Silva DA, Fuchs SC. Squamous intraepithelial lesions in HIV-infected women: prevalence, incidence, progression and regression. *Arch Gynecol Obstet* 2013;288:1107–13.

77. Duerr A, Paramsothy P, Jamieson DJ, et al. Effect of HIV infection on atypical squamous cells of undetermined significance. *Clin Infect Dis* 2006;42:855–61.

78. Boardman LA, Cotter K, Raker C, Cu-Uvin S. Cervical intraepithelial neoplasia grade 2 or worse in human immunodeficiency virus-infected women with mildly abnormal cervical cytology. *Obstet Gynecol* 2008;112(2, pt 1):238–43.

79. Massad LS, Schneider MF, Watts DH, et al. HPV testing for triage of HIV-infected women with Papanicolaou smears read as atypical squamous cells of uncertain significance. *J Women's Health (Larchmt)* 2004;13:147–53.

80. Panel on Opportunistic Infections in HIV-Infected Adults and Adolescents. Guidelines for the prevention and treatment of opportunistic infections in HIV-infected adults and adolescents: recommendations from the Centers for Disease Control and Prevention, the National Institutes of Health, and the HIV Medicine Association of the Infectious Diseases Society of America. Available at http://aidsinfo.nih.gov/contentfiles/lvguidelines/adult_oi.pdf. Accessed 9/5/2013.

81. Pretorius RG, Zhang WH, Belinson JL, et al. Colposcopically directed biopsy, random cervical biopsy, and endocervical curettage in the diagnosis of cervical intraepithelial neoplasia II or worse. *Am J Obstet Gynecol* 2004; 191(2):430–4.

82. Guido RS, Jeronimo J, Schiffman M, Solomon D; ALTS Group. The distribution of neoplasia arising on the cervix: results from the ALTS trial. *Am J Obstet Gynecol* 2005;193(4):1331–7.

83. Gage JC, Hanson VW, Abbey K, et al. Number of cervical biopsies and sensitivity of colposcopy. *Obstet Gynecol* 2006;108(2):264–72.

84. Solomon D, Stoler M, Jeronimo J, Khan M, Castle P, Schiffman M. Diagnostic utility of endocervical curettage in women undergoing colposcopy for equivocal or low-grade cytologic abnormalities. *Obstet Gynecol* 2007;110 (2, pt 1):288–95.

85. Selvaggi SM. Reporting of atypical squamous cells, cannot exclude a high-grade squamous intraepithelial lesion (ASC-H) on cervical samples: is it significant? *Diagn Cytopathol* 2003;29:38–41.

86. Alli PM, Ali SZ. Atypical squamous cells of undetermined significance—rule out high-grade squamous intraepithelial lesion: cyto-pathologic characteristics and clinical correlates. *Diagn Cytopathol* 2003;28:308–12.

87. Liman AK, Giampoli EJ, Bonfiglio TA. Should women with atypical squamous cells, cannot exclude high-grade squamous intraepithelial lesion, receive reflex human papillomavirus-DNA testing? *Cancer* 2005;105:457–60.

88. Sherman ME, Castle PE, Solomon D. Cervical cytology of atypical squamous cells-cannot exclude high-grade squamous intraepithelial lesion (ASC-H): characteristics and histologic outcomes. *Cancer* 2006;108:298–305.

89. Srodon M, Parry Dilworth H, Ronnett BM. Atypical squamous cells, cannot exclude high-grade squamous intraepithelial lesion: diagnostic performance, human papillomavirus testing, and follow-up results. *Cancer* 2006;108:32–8.

90. Galliano GE, Moatamed NA, Lee S, Salami N, Apple SK. Reflex high risk HPV testing in atypical squamous cells, cannot exclude high grade intraepithelial lesion: a large institution's experience with the significance of this often ordered test. *Acta Cytol* 2011;55(2):167–72.

91. Jones BA, Davey DD. Quality management in gynecologic cytology using interlaboratory comparison. *Arch Pathol Lab Med* 2000;124:672–81.

92. Davey DD, Neal MH, Wilbur DC, Colgan TJ, Styer PE, Mody DR. Bethesda 2001 implementation and reporting rates: 2003 practices of participants in the College of American Pathologists Interlaboratory Comparison Program in Cervicovaginal Cytology. *Arch Pathol Lab Med* 2004;128:1224–9.

93. Cox JT, Schiffman M, Solomon D; ASCUS-LSIL Triage Study (ALTS) Group. Prospective follow-up suggests similar risk of subsequent cervical intraepithelial neoplasia grade 2 or 3 among women with cervical intraepithelial neoplasia grade 1 or negative colposcopy and directed biopsy. *Am J Obstet Gynecol* 2003;188(6):1406–12.

94. Schiffman M, Solomon D. Findings to date from the ASCUS-LSIL Triage Study (ALTS). *Arch Pathol Lab Med* 2003;127:946–9.

95. Cox JT. The clinician's view: role of human papillomavirus testing in the American Society for Colposcopy and Cervical Pathology Guidelines for the management of abnormal cervical cytology and cervical cancer precursors. *Arch Pathol Lab Med* 2003;127:950–8.

96. Arbyn M, Sasieni P, Meijer CJ, Clavel C, Koliopoulos G, Dillner J. Chapter 9: clinical applications of HPV testing: a summary of metaanalyses. *Vaccine* 2006;24(suppl 3):S78–89.

97. Jones BA, Novis DA. Follow-up of abnormal gynecologic cytology: a College of American Pathologists Q-probes study of 16132 cases from 306 laboratories. *Arch Pathol Lab Med* 2000;124:665–71.

98. Cuzick J. Cervical screening. *Br J Hosp Med* 1988;39:265.

99. ASCUS-LSIL Triage Study (ALTS) Group. A randomized trial on the management of low-grade squamous intraepithelial lesion cytology interpretations. *Am J Obstet Gynecol* 2003;188:1393–400.

100. Mayeaux EJ, Harper MB, Abreo F, et al. A comparison of the reliability of repeat cervical smears and colposcopy in patients with abnormal cervical cytology. *J Fam Pract* 1995;40:57–62.

101. Ferris DG, Wright TC, Litaker MS, et al. Triage of women with ASCUS and LSIL Pap smear reports: management by repeat Pap smear, HPV DNA testing or colposcopy? *J Fam Pract* 1998;46:125–34.

102. Denny LA, Soeters R, Dehaeck K, Bloch B. Does colposcopically directed punch biopsy reduce the incidence of negative LLETZ? *Br J Obstet Gynaecol* 1995;102:545–8.

103. Howells RE, O'Mahony F, Tucker H, Millinship J, Jones PW, Redman CW. How can the incidence of negative specimens resulting from large loop excision of the cervical transformation zone (LLETZ) be reduced? An analysis of negative LLETZ specimens and development of a predictive model. *Br J Obstet Gynaecol* 2000;107:1075–82.

104. Guido R, Schiffman M, Solomon D, Burke L; ASCUS LSIL Triage Study (ALTS) Group. Postcolposcopy management strategies for women referred with low-grade squamous intraepithelial lesions or human papillomavirus DNA-positive atypical squamous cells of undetermined significance: a two-year prospective study. *Am J Obstet Gynecol* 2003;188:1401–5.

105. Insinga RP, Glass AG, Rush BB. Diagnoses and outcomes in cervical cancer screening: a population-based study. *Am J Obstet Gynecol* 2004; 191:105–13.

106. Castle PE, Solomon D, Schiffman M, Wheeler CM; for the ALTS Group. Human papillomavirus type 16 infections and 2 year absolute risk of cervical precancer in women with equivocal or mild cytologic abnormalities. *J Natl Cancer Inst* 2005;97:1066–71.

107. Sasieni P, Castanon A, Parkin M. How many cervical cancers are prevented by treatment of screen-detected disease in young women? *Int J Cancer* 2009;124:461–4.

108. Evans MF, Adamson CS, Papillo JL, St John TL, Leiman G, Cooper K. Distribution of human papillomavirus types in ThinPrep Papanicolaou tests classified according to the Bethesda 2001 terminology and correlations with patient age and biopsy outcomes. *Cancer* 2006;106:1054–64.

109. Cox JT. Evaluation of abnormal cervical cytology. In: Carr J, ed. *Clin Lab Med* 2000;20:303–43.

110. Lee KR, Darragh TM, Joste NE, et al. Atypical glandular cells of undetermined significance (AGUS): interobserver reproducibility in cervical smears and corresponding thin-layer preparations. *Am J Clin Pathol* 2002; 117(1):96–102.

111. Sharpless KE, Schnatz PF, Mandavilli S, Greene JF, Sorosky JI. Dysplasia associated with atypical glandular cells on cervical cytology. *Obstet Gynecol* 2005;105:494–500.

112. DeSimone CP, Day ME, Tovar MM, Dietrich CS III, Eastham ML, Modesitt SC. Rate of pathology from atypical glandular cell Pap tests classified by the Bethesda 2001 nomenclature. *Obstet Gynecol* 2006;107:1285–91.

113. Tam KF, Cheung AN, Liu KL, et al. A retrospective review on atypical glandular cells of undetermined significance (AGUS) using the Bethesda 2001 classification. *Gynecol Oncol* 2003;91:603–7.

114. Derchain SF, Rabelo-Santos SH, Sarian LO, et al. Human papillomavirus DNA detection and histological findings in women referred for atypical glandular cells or adenocarcinoma in situ in their Pap smears. *Gynecol Oncol* 2004;95:618–23.

115. Diaz-Montes TP, Farinola MA, Zahurak ML, Bristow RE, Rosenthal DL. Clinical utility of atypical glandular cells (AGC) classification: cyto- histologic comparison and relationship to HPV results. *Gynecol Oncol* 2007; 104(2):366–71.

116. Zhao C, Florea A, Onisko A, Austin RM. Histologic follow-up results in 662 patients with Pap test findings of atypical glandular cells: results from a large academic womens hospital laboratory employing sensitive screening methods. *Gynecol Oncol* 2009;114(3):383–9.

117. Castle PE, Fetterman M, Poitras N, Lorey T, Shaber R, Kinney W. Relationship of atypical glandular cell cytology, age and human papillomavirus detection to cervical and endometrial cancer risks. *Obstet Gynecol* 2010;115:243–8.

118. Ronnett BM, Manos MM, Ransley JE, et al. Atypical glandular cells of undetermined significance (AGUS): cytopathologic features, histopathologic results, and human papillomavirus DNA detection. *Hum Pathol* 1999;30:816–25.

119. Valdini A, Vaccaro C, Pechinsky G, Abernathy V. Incidence and evaluation of an AGUS Papanicolaou smear in primary care. *J Am Board Fam Pract* 2001; 14:172–7.

120. Chhieng DC, Elgert P, Cohen JM, Cangiarella JF. Clinical significance of atypical glandular cells of undetermined significance in postmenopausal women. *Cancer* 2001;93:1–7.

121. Veljovich DS, Stoler MH, Andersen WA, Covell JL, Rice LW. Atypical glandular cells of undetermined significance: a five-year retrospective histopathologic study. *Am J Obstet Gynecol* 1998;179:382–90.

122. Lee KR, Manna EA, St John T. Atypical endocervical glandular cells: accuracy of cytologic diagnosis. *Diagn Cytopathol* 1995;13:202–8.

123. Krane JF, Granter SR, Trask CE, Hogan CL, Lee KR. Papanicolaou smear sensitivity for the detection of adenocarcinoma of the cervix: a study of 49 cases. *Cancer* 2001;93:8–15.

124. Bose S, Kannan V, Kline TS. Abnormal endocervical cells: really abnormal? Really endocervical? *Am J Clin Pathol* 1994;101:708–13.

125. Koike N. Efficacy of the cytobrush method in aged patients. *Diagn Cytopathol* 1994;38:310.

126. Chakrabarti S. Brush versus spatula for cervical smears. *ACTA Cytol* 1994;38:315.

127. Anderson MC. Glandular lesions of the cervix. In: Jones HW, ed. *Cervical Intraepithelial Neoplasia: Baillieres Clinical Obstetrics and Gynecology*, Vol. 9. London, UK: Baillière Tindall, 1995:105–19.

128. Ostör AG, Duncan A, Quinn M, Rome R. Adenocarcinoma in situ of the uterine cervix: an experience with 100 cases. *Gynecol Oncol* 2000; 79(2):207–10.

129. Coppleson M, Atkinson KH, Dalrymple JC. Cervical squamous and glandular neoplasia: clinical features and review of management. In: Coppleson M, ed. *Gynecologic Oncology*. Edinburgh, UK: Churchill Livingston, 1992:571–607.

130. Taylor RR, Guerrieri JP, Nash JD, Henry MR, O'Connor DM. Atypical cervical cytology. Colposcopic follow-up using the Bethesda System. *J Reprod Med* 1993;38:443–7.

131. Soofer SB, Sidawy MK. Atypical glandular cells of undetermined significance: clinically significant lesions and means of patient follow-up. *Cancer* 2000;90:207–14.

132. Kinney W, Sawaya GF, Sung HY, Kearney KA, Miller M, Hiatt RA. Stage at diagnosis and mortality in patients with adenocarcinoma and adenosquamous carcinoma of the uterine cervix diagnosed as a consequence of cytologic screening. *Acta Cytol* 2003;47:167–71.

133. Fetterman B, Shaber R, Pawlick G, Kinney W. Human papillomavirus DNA testing in routine clinical practice for prediction of underlying cervical intraepithelial neoplasia 2,3 at initial evaluation and in follow-up of women with atypical glandular cell Papanicolaou tests. *J Low Genit Tract Dis* 2006;3:179.

134. Krane JF, Lee KR, Sun D, Yuan L, Crum CP. Atypical glandular cells of undetermined significance. Outcome predictions based on human papillomavirus testing. *Am J Clin Pathol* 2004;121:87–92.

135. Obenson K, Abreo F, Grafton WD. Cytohistologic correlation between AGUS and biopsy-detected lesions in postmenopausal women. *Acta Cytol* 2000;44:41–5.

136. Greenspan DL, Cardillo M, Davey DD, Heller DS, Moriarty AT. Endometrial cells in cervical cytology: review of cytological features and clinical assessment. *J Low Genit Tract Dis* 2006;10:111–22.

137. Simsir A, Carter W, Elgert P, Cangiarella J. Reporting endometrial cells in women 40 years and older: assessing the clinical usefulness of Bethesda 2001. *Am J Clin Pathol* 2005;123:571–5.

138. Eddy GL, Wojtowycz MA, Piraino PS, Mazur MT. Papanicolaou smears by the Bethesda system in endometrial malignancy: utility and prognostic importance. *Obstet Gynecol* 1997;90:999–1003.

139. Cheng RF, Hernandez E, Anderson LL, Heller PB, Shank R. Clinical significance of a cytologic diagnosis of atypical glandular cells of undetermined significance. *J Reprod Med* 1999;44:922–8.

140. Larson DM, Johnson KK, Reyes CN, Broste SK. Prognostic significance of malignant cervical cytology in patients with endometrial cancer. *Obstet Gynecol* 1994;84:399–403.

141. Demirkiran F, Arvas M, Erkun E, et al. The prognostic significance of cervicovaginal cytology in endometrial cancer. *Eur J Gynecol Oncol* 1995;16:404–9.

142. Eddy GL, Strumpf KB, Wojtowycz MA, et al. Biopsy findings in 531 patients with atypical glandular cells of undetermined significance (AGCUS) as defined by the Bethesda System (TBS). *Am J Obstet Gynecol* 1997;177:1188–95.

143. Massad LS, Collins YC, Meyer PM. Biopsy correlates of abnormal cervical cytology classified using the Bethesda system. *Gynecol Oncol* 2001; 82:516–22.

144. Dunn TS, Burke M, Shwayder J. A "see and treat" management for high-grade squamous intraepithelial lesion Pap smears. *J Low Genit Tract Dis* 2003;7:104–6.

145. Alvarez RD, Wright TC. Effective cervical neoplasia detection with a novel optical detection system: a randomized trial. *Gynecol Oncol* 2007; 104:281–9.

146. Massad LS, Jeronimo J, Schiffman M; National Institutes of Health/American Society for Colposcopy and Cervical Pathology (NIH/ASCCP) Research Group. Interobserver agreement in the assessment of components of colposcopic grading. *Obstet Gynecol* 2008;111(6):1279–84.

147. Stoler MH, Vichnin MD, Ferenczy A, et al; the FUTURE I, II and III Investigators. The accuracy of colposcopic biopsy: analyses from the placebo arm of the Gardasil clinical trials. *Int J Cancer* 2011;128(6):1354–62.

148. Holschneider CH, Ghosh K, Montz FJ. See-and-treat in the management of high-grade squamous intraepithelial lesions of the cervix: a resource utilization analysis. *Obstet Gynecol* 1999;94:377–85.

149. Numnum TM, Kirby TO, Leath CA III, HuhWK, Alvarez RD, Straughn JM Jr. A prospective evaluation of" see and treat" in women with HSIL Pap smear results: is this an appropriate strategy? *J Low Genit Tract Dis* 2005;9:2–6.

150. Peto J, Gilham C, Deacon J, et al. Cervical HPV infection and neoplasia in a large population-based prospective study: the Manchester cohort. *Br J Cancer* 2004;91:942–53.

151. Trimble CL, Piantadosi S, Gravitt P, et al. Spontaneous regression of high-grade cervical dysplasia: effects of human papillomavirus type and HLA phenotype. *Clin Cancer Res* 2005;11:4717–23.

152. Moscicki AB, Ma Y, Wibbelsman C, et al. Rate of and risks for regression of cervical intraepithelial neoplasia 2 in adolescents and young women. *Obstet Gynecol* 2010;116(6):1373–80.

153. Moscicki AB, Schiffman M, Kjaer S, Villa LL. Chapter 5: updating the natural history of HPV and anogenital cancer. *Vaccine* 2006;24(suppl 3):S42–51.

154. Jakobsson M, Gissler M, Paavonen J, Tapper AM. Loop electrosurgical excision procedure and the risk for preterm birth. *Obstet Gynecol* 2009;114(3):504–10.

155. Meirovitz M, Zlotnik A, Levy A. Obstetric outcome following cervical conization. *Arch Gynecol Obstet* 2011;283(4):765–9.

156. Zuna RE, Wang SS, Rosenthal DL, Jeronimo J, Schiffman M, Solomon D; ALTS Group. Determinants of human papillomavirus-negative, low-grade squamous intraepithelial lesions in the atypical squamous cells of undetermined significance/low-grade squamous intraepithelial lesions triage study (ALTS). *Cancer* 2005;105(5):253–62.

157. Cox JT. More questions about the accuracy of colposcopy: what does this mean for cervical cancer prevention? *Obstet Gynecol* 2008;111(6): 1266–7.

158. Sherman ME, Schiffman MH, Lorincz AT, et al. Toward objective quality assurance in cervical cytopathology. Correlation of cytopathologic diagnoses with detection of high-risk human papillomavirus types. *Am J Clin Pathol* 1994;102(2):182–7.

159. Moscicki AB, Schiffman M, Burchell A, et al. Updating the natural history of human papillomavirus and anogenital cancers. *Vaccine* 2012;30(Suppl 5): F24–33.

160. Roberts CH, Dinh TV, Hannigan EV, Yandell RB, Schnadig VJ. Management of cervical intraepithelial neoplasia during pregnancy: a simplified and cost-effective approach. *J Low Genit Tract Dis* 1998;2:67–70.

161. Boardman LA, Goldman DL, Cooper AS, Heber WW, Weitzen S. CIN in pregnancy: antepartum and postpartum cytology and histology. *J Reprod Med* 2005;50:13–8.

162. Jarboe EA, Venkat P, Hirsch MS, Cibas ES, Crum CP, Garner EI. A weakly positive human papillomavirus Hybrid Capture II result correlates with a significantly lower risk of cervical intraepithelial neoplasia 2,3 after atypical squamous cells of undetermined significance cytology. *J Low Genit Tract Dis* 2010;14(3):174–8.

163. Xi LF, Hughes JP, Castle PE, et al. Viral load in the natural history of human papillomavirus type 16 infection: a nested case–control study. *J Infect Dis* 2011;203(10):1425–33.

164. Martin MP, Borecki IB, Zhang Z, et al. HLA-Cw group 1 ligands for KIR increase susceptibility to invasive cervical cancer. *Immunogenetics* 2010;62(11–12):761–5.

165. Wang SS, Gonzalez P, Yu K, et al. Common genetic variants and risk for HPV persistence and progression to cervical cancer. *PLoS One* 2010; 5(1):e8667.

166. Sichero L, Ferreira S, Trottier H, et al. High grade cervical lesions are caused preferentially by non-European variants of HPVs 16 and 18. *Int J Cancer* 2007;120(8):1763–8.

167. Schiffman M, Rodriguez AC, Chen Z, et al. A population-based prospective study of carcinogenic human papillomavirus variant lineages, viral persistence, and cervical neoplasia. *Cancer Res* 2010;70(8):3159–69.

168. de Araujo Souza PS, Sichero L, Maciag PC. HPV variants and HLA polymorphisms: the role of variability on the risk of cervical cancer. *Future Oncol* 2009;5(3):359–70.

169. Stoler MH, Wright TC Jr, Cuzick J, et al. APTIMA HPV assay performance in women with atypical squamous cells of undetermined significance cytology results. *Am J Obstet Gynecol* 2013;208(2):144.e1–8.

170. Ho CM, Lee BH, Chang SF, et al. Type-specific human papillomavirus oncogene messenger RNA levels correlate with the severity of cervical neoplasia. *Int J Cancer* 2010;127(3):622–32.

171. Dockter J, Schroder A, Hill C, Guzenski L, Monsonego J, Giachetti C. Clinical performance of the APTIMA HPV assay for the dection of high-risk HPV and high-grade cervical lesions. *J Clin virol* 2009;45(Suppl 1):S55–61.

172. Patel DA, Rozek LS, Colacino JA, et al. Patterns of cellular and HPV 16 methylation as biomarkers for cervical neoplasia. *J Virol Methods* 2012;184(1–2):84–92.

173. Carozzi F, Gillio-Tos A, Confortini M, et al.; NTCC Working Group. Risk of high-grade cervical intraepithelial neoplasia during follow-up in HPV-positive women according to baseline p16-INK4A results: a prospective analysis of a nested substudy of the NTCC randomized controlled trial. *Lancet Oncol* 2013;14(2):168–76.

174. Schledermann D, Andersen BT, Bisgaard K, et al. Are adjunctive markers useful in routine cervical cancer screening? Application of p16(INK4a) and HPV-PCR on ThinPrep samples with histological follow-up. *Diagn Cytopathol* 2008;36(7):453–9.

175. Siddiqui MT, Hornaman K, Cohen C, Nassar A. ProEx C immunocytochemistry and high-risk human papillomavirus DNA testing in Papanicolaou tests with atypical squamous cell (ASC-US) cytology: correlation study with histologic biopsy. *Arch Pathol Lab Med* 2008; 132(10):1648–52.

176. Fletcher AH, Barklow TA, Murphy NJ, Culbertson LH, Davis AV, Hunter L. ProExC triage of atypical glandular cells on liquid-based cervical cytology specimens. *J Low Genit Tract Dis* 2011;15(1):6–10.

177. Wentzensen N, Sun C, Ghosh A, et al. Methylation of HPV18, HPV31, and HPV45 genomes and cervical intraepithelial neoplasia grade 3. *J Natl Cancer Inst* 2012;104(22):1738–49.

178. Kalantari M, Chase DM, Tewari KS, Bernard HU. Recombination of human papillomavirus-16 and host DNA in exfoliated cervical cells: a pilot study of L1 gene methylation and chromosomal integration as biomarkers of carcinogenic progression. *J Med Virol* 2010;82(2): 311–20.

179. Hesselink B, Heideman DA, Steenbergen RD, et al. Combined promoter methylation analysis of CADM1 and MAL: an objective triage tool for high-risk human papillomavirus DNA positive women. *Clin Cancer Res* 2011;17(8):2459–65.

J. THOMAS COX, FRANCISCO GARCIA,
DAVID P. CHELMOW, DARON G. FERRIS,
V. CECIL WRIGHT, EDWARD J. MAYEAUX, JR.,
RICHARD GUIDO, AND MIRIAM CREMER

Management of Lower Genital Tract Neoplasia

20.1 INTRODUCTION
20.2 MANAGEMENT OF CERVICAL INTRAEPITHELIAL
    NEOPLASIA
    20.2.1 The Role of Immunity in Successful Treatment of CIN
    20.2.2 General Principles for Managing Women with CIN
    20.2.3 Management Guidelines for Women with CIN
20.3 MANAGEMENT OF ADENOCARCINOMA *IN SITU*
    20.3.1 Management of AIS in Women Who Do Not Desire
        Fertility
    20.3.2 Management of AIS in Women Who Desire Future
        Fertility
20.4 PROCEDURES FOR TREATING CERVICAL NEOPLASIA
    20.4.1 Cryotherapy of the Cervix

20.4.2 Cold Coagulation of the Cervix
20.4.3 Carbon Dioxide Laser Surgery for the Cervix
20.4.4 Electrosurgical Procedures
20.4.5 Cold-Knife Conization of the Cervix
20.4.6 Hysterectomy for Cervical Intraepithelial Neoplasia
20.4.7 Approaches in Low-Resource Settings
20.5 TREATMENT OF EXTERNAL GENITAL WARTS
    20.5.1 Introduction
    20.5.2 Treatment Purpose and Objectives
    20.5.3 Prerequisites to Treatment of EGWs
    20.5.4 Patient-Applied Therapies
    20.5.5 Provider-Administered Therapy
    20.5.6 Other Therapies

20.1 INTRODUCTION

The modern era of outpatient diagnosis and treatment of precursor lesions of the cervix began with the popularization of colposcopy and the introduction of cryotherapy in the 1960s. This was followed in the 1970s by carbon dioxide (CO_2) laser therapy and in the early 1990s by loop electrosurgical excision procedure (LEEP). Until the mid-1990s, cervical intraepithelial neoplasia (CIN) 1, CIN 2, and CIN 3 were considered progressive lesions; therefore, all were managed by either ablative or excisional procedures. However, recognition that only most CIN 3 and some CIN 2 are true precancer lesions has fostered expectant management of women with CIN 1 and many women with CIN 2. This approach was formalized in the Consensus Guidelines Conferences for the Management of Abnormal Cervical Cytology and Cervical Cancer Precursors, sponsored by the American Society for Colposcopy and Cervical Pathology (ASCCP) in 2001,[1,2] 2006,[3] and 2012.[4] The guidelines developed from these conferences were derived through a structured consensus process utilizing an evidence-based review. They serve as a basis for discussion in this chapter of the management of women with CIN and adenocarcinoma in situ (AIS). First, it is important to understand the role that the immune response to human papillomavirus (HPV) plays in the success of any treatment approach.

20.2 MANAGEMENT OF CERVICAL INTRAEPITHELIAL NEOPLASIA

20.2.1 The Role of Immunity in Successful Treatment of CIN

Successful treatment of CIN ultimately depends upon the ability of the host immune response to prevent recurrence. Women with compromised immunity fail to respond adequately to HPV and therefore have a higher rate of recurrence following any treatment modality.[5,6] Although humoral immunity is likely to be important in the initial prevention of HPV infection, the primary immune response to tumors and viruses is cellular. The relationship between humoral and cellular immunity is exemplified by the lymphocytic population in the cervix noted in health and in disease. In the normal cervix, the primary function of the lymphocyte population is to serve as a barrier to infection by mounting a B-lymphocyte humoral immune response as the first line of defense against initial infection (Figure 20.1).[5,7] In the normal cervix, B lymphocytes predominate. By contrast, in the presence of CIN 3, B lymphocytes are a minor part of the population of immune-responsive cells, as they are replaced by natural killer cells and cytotoxic T lymphocytes, the dominant responders of local cellular immunity. In most viral infections, the foreign antigen is recognized quite rapidly, resulting in the activation of antigen-presenting cells and the release of local cytokines within only a day or two. Recognition of HPV presence is much slower and extremely variable in timing, resulting in a relative delay in HPV immune response when compared to the immune response to most other viral infections.[5]

Detection of HPV is delayed primarily because the entire HPV life cycle occurs without the virus ever crossing the epithelial basement membrane or being released outside of the protection of the infected host cell. HPV initially infects the basal epithelium.[5,8] It does not replicate until release from a variable period of viral latency results in accelerated HPV DNA production in differentiating keratinocytes above the basal layer (Figure 20.2).[9] These differentiating squamous epithelial cells are inefficient at presenting viral antigens on their surface even when the cells contain dozens of HPV genomes.[9] The protein capsule surrounding the HPV genome in infective koilocytes is reassembled in the upper layers of the epithelium as the keratinocytes mature. It is the shedding of these dead or dying cells from the surface epithelium that results in release of the infective unit.[10] Because HPV does not lyse the infected epithelial cells and these cells are not efficient at

FIGURE 20.1. The lymphocytic population of the cervix changes dramatically in the presence of CIN. B cells predominate in the normal cervix, whereas women with CIN 3 have predominantly T cells and NKCs. (Modified with permission from Cox JT. In: Lonky N, ed. Management of precursor lesions of cervical carcinoma: history, host defense, and a survey of modalities. *Obstet Gynecol Clin North Am* 2002;29:751–85.)

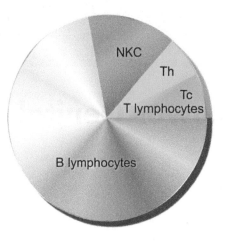

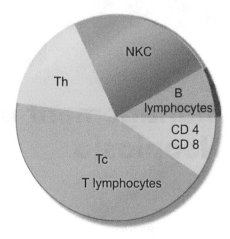

Normal Cervix

Cervical Intraepithelial Neoplasia 3

antigen presentation, the virus remains hidden during the viral productive part of its life cycle, providing the immune system little opportunity to identify its presence.

Several other mechanisms add to the efficiency of HPV in evading immune recognition. Inflammation does not occur in the absence of immune recognition, because inflammatory cytokines, such as interleukins and interferon, are not released. Additionally, HPV genes are expressed at very low levels,[11] and some gene loci have been identified that have the capability to block immune recognition.[12] For example, the HPV genomes E6 and E7 interfere with major histocompatibility complex class I presentation of antigens, and E7 can suppress both the interferon signal and the retinoblastoma gene (pRb) tumor suppression.[13,14] HPV E6 also produces a protein that suppresses the other main antioncogenic pathway (p53) that is critical in preventing accumulation of mutations that may lead to cancer.[15] Finally, antigen-detecting Langerhans cells are sparsely distributed within the epithelium.

Dead epithelial cells loaded with infective HPV DNA are shed from the surface as koilocytes

Protein capsid reassembled around HPV DNA

Accelerated production of HPV genomes in replicating cells

The virus enters the cell via an endocytic pathway and uncoats in the endosome

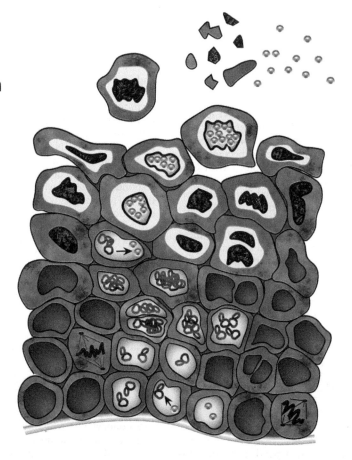

HPV Particle (Capsid Protein + DNA)

HPV Episomal DNA (Plasmid)

FIGURE 20.2. The life cycle of a HPV infection. During this entire process, HPV remains hidden within the epithelial cells. (With permission from ASCCP.)

An understanding of the HPV's capability to evade host immunity is a critical component of optimal management of HPV-associated lesions. Any treatment that results in lysis of HPV-infected cells increases the opportunity for recognizing HPV presence that will initiate a local cellular immune response comprised of HPV-specific CD4+ and CD8+ cells (Figure 20.3). Although ablative methods might seem to leave more killed HPV-infected cells exposed to immune recognition initiation by macrophages and mononuclear cells than excisional methods, clearance rates for both virus and lesions are similar, indicating that this difference is not clinically important.[16,17] Perhaps any modality for treating CIN leaves behind adequate HPV protein and DNA to initiate immune recognition (Figure 20.4). When such recognition does not occur following treatment, recurrence of HPV-induced disease is more likely.

Cervical cancer does not generally occur in the absence of long-term HPV persistence.[18,19] However, 10% to 20% of patients treated for CIN will have either persistent or recurrent disease, indicating an inability to suppress remaining HPV. The persistence of HPV is primarily secondary to inadequate destructive treatment and partially a function of the host immune response and HPV type. There are 13 to 15 known high-risk HPV types associated with cervical cancer.[18] The risk of developing CIN 3 is not the same within the high-risk types. Long-term natural history studies clearly demonstrate the importance of HPV type on the rate of persistence and the development of CIN 3. Women harboring HPV16 and 18 had a 17.2% and a 13.6% risk, respectively, of developing CIN 3 or greater over a 10-year follow-up period compared to a 0.8% risk for HPV-negative women.[20]

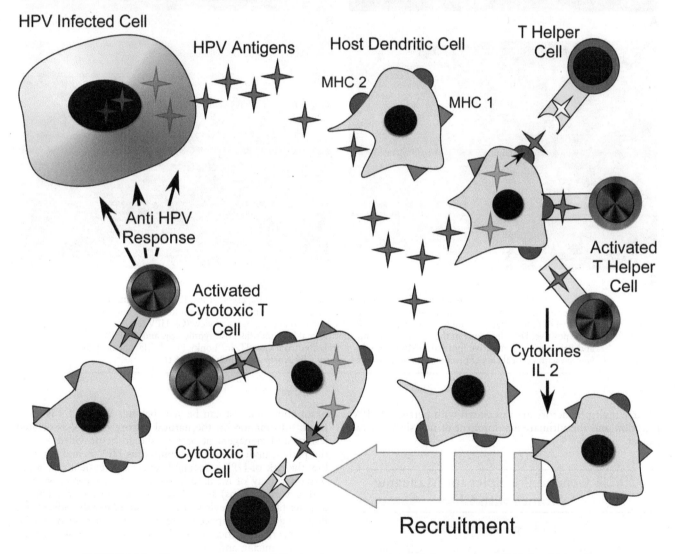

FIGURE 20.3. The sequence of events following immune recognition of the presence of HPV: Dendritic cells engulf HPV antigens and process them into bits of information that can be utilized in initiating an immune response. Dendritic cells may present both MHC Class I and MHC Class II processed antigens on their surface. The major histocompatibility complex, or MHC, is a region of the human chromosome 6 that is responsible for producing glycoproteins that are expressed on the surfaces of most cells. MHC class I processed antigens are presented in the regional lymph nodes to resting cytotoxic T cells, which become activated CD8+ cells. MHC class II processed antigens are presented to resting helper T cells, which become activated CD4+ cells. Activated CD4+ cells produce cytokines such as IL-2, interferon, and tumor necrosis factor that further promote recognition of HPV antigens and recruitment of macrophages, monocytes, and dendritic cells at the site of infection. Activated CD8+ cells also migrate back to the site of the infection to mount an anti-HPV, antitumor response. (Modified with permission from Cox JT. In: Lonky N, ed. Management of precursor lesions of cervical carcinoma: history, host defense, and a survey of modalities. *Obstet Gynecol Clin North Am* 2002;29:751–85.)

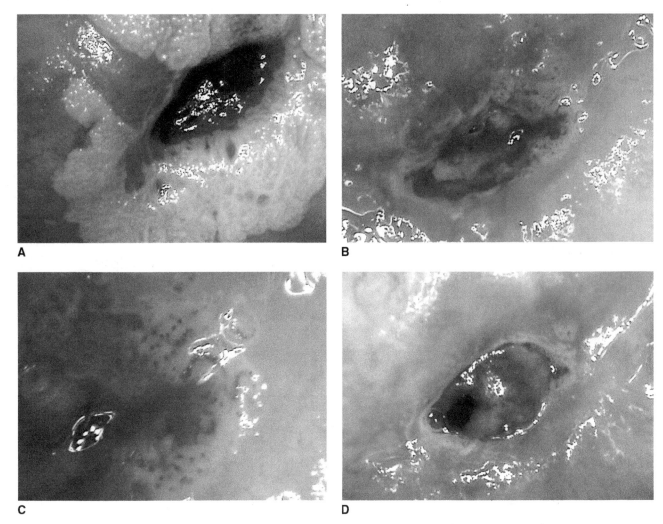

FIGURE 20.4.   A: Extensive recurrent CIN 1 can be seen 4 months following cryotherapy. Expectant management was elected in the expectation that a significant immune response could still occur. **B:** Four months later, only a very tiny area of mild acetowhite and linear punctation remains, best seen in the magnified view (**C**). HPV test continued to be positive. **D:** Colposcopy of the cervix was completely normal by 9 months postcryotherapy, and the HPV test and Pap were both negative (normal). (Modified with permission from Cox JT. In: Lonky N, ed. Management of women with cervical cancer precursor lesions. *Obstet Gynecol Clin North Am* 2002;29:787–816.)

Clearly multiple factors are associated with persistent HPV infection and the ultimate development of invasive cervical cancer.

20.2.2 General Principles for Managing Women with CIN

20.2.2.1 Preparing the Patient

The primary objective in treating women with CIN is to prevent cervical cancer, while maximizing the return of normal morphology and function to the cervix. However, in doing so, it is critical to address all her needs and concerns so as not to lose sight of her overall well-being and quality of life. Anxiety, depression, and other psychological stresses often follow an abnormal cytology test result and subsequent management. Prevention or resolution of these problems is part of any comprehensive cervical cancer prevention program. Because patient education is consistently identified as key to reducing stress related to managing women with abnormal screening results,[21,22] providing information about the nature and cause

of an abnormal test can be very helpful. When CIN is identified, information on the natural history of HPV-associated lesions and management options should be provided to help the patient understand how ubiquitous HPV is and yet how low the risk of HPV-associated cancer is.[23] Patient education using a variety of media and modalities (electronic, written, and/or verbal forms) should be provided so that the patient and her family can review at their leisure after the office visit. Providing time and space for responding to patient questions and concerns is critical in establishing a relationship of trust between clinician and patient.

20.2.2.2 Encouraging Healthful Habits

Smoking depresses the normal immune response. Women who smoke have a 60% greater risk (relative risk [RR] of 1.60) of developing cervical cancer than women who never use tobacco. In most studies, the association of smoking with increased risk of cervical cancer, and with failure to respond to CIN treatment, is fairly definitive.[24,25] Smoking's mechanism of action for this disease is likely a combination of the direct carcinogenic effects of cotinine, nicotine, and nitrosamines and local immunosuppression manifest by decreasing density and function of Langerhans (dendritic) cells.[26–28] The main function of dendritic cells is to process antigen material and present it on the surface to other cells of the immune system; that is, they function as antigen-presenting cells. Failure to clear CIN after treatment is significantly more common among smokers than nonsmokers, and heavy smokers face an increased risk of persistent HPV infection.[25] Because of the association of smoking with diminished immune function and cessation of smoking with an increase in cervical Langerhans cells,[28] it is particularly important to educate women with CIN who smoke on personalized smoking cessation strategies.

Epidemiologic data indicate that there may be an increased risk of cervical cancer in populations with inadequate dietary intake of folic acid, B_6 and B_{12}, beta-carotene, and indole-3-carbinols.[29–32] Although there are no compelling data that diets rich in these substances promote increased regression of CIN,[33–35] recommending a balanced diet is part of good general medical advice and may be beneficial.[36] A review of the literature assessing the epidemiologic role of diet and nutrition on the risk of HPV persistence and CIN has shown a possible protective effect of a diet rich in fruits, vegetables, vitamins C and E, beta- and alpha-carotene, lycopene, lutein/zeaxanthin, and cryptoxanthin.[36]

Other healthy habits that may have a positive impact on general health and prevent relative immune compromise may include avoiding excessive alcohol, drug use, and inadequate sleep. However, the most important result of providing commonsense health recommendations is the feeling of empowerment that some women will have when given an active role in controlling their disease process.[5] The as-yet-unproven health benefits of many of these measures are likely to be far less important than the psychological advantage they foster.[36]

20.2.2.3 Deciding on Active versus Expectant Management

Many women with high-grade squamous or glandular lesions will be managed actively by either an ablative or an excisional procedure since regression of CIN 2, and particularly CIN 3, is less common than with CIN 1 and the risk of progression is considerably higher. There are exceptions to this rule: Pregnant women with documented high-grade lesions are followed expectantly, and a similar option is given to young women from populations with high rates of compliance with follow-up recommendations who have CIN 2 and some with CIN 2,3.[3,4,37] Young women have high regression rates for cervical disease and low cancer risk.[38–41] The term "young women" indicates those who after counseling by their clinicians consider risk to future pregnancies from treating cervical abnormalities to outweigh risk for cancer during observation of those abnormalities.[4] No specific age threshold is intended. The management recommendations for women ≥21 with CIN 1–3 and AIS made in the ASCCP 2012 Updated Consensus Guidelines for the Management of Abnormal Cervical Cancer Screening Tests and Cancer Precursors are discussed in depth in this chapter.[4] Management of these lesions in adolescents, some of whom will get cervical screening despite recommendations that screening should not begin until age 21,[42–45] is discussed in Chapter 16.

These options were created because the risks of treatment in these circumstances outweigh the potential benefits. Treating the cervix of a pregnant woman may complicate the pregnancy, and once cancer has been ruled out, the risk of cancer developing during the short duration of a pregnancy is small.[3,4,37] Longitudinal studies of CIN 2 in adolescents and young women have demonstrated a high rate of resolution. A well-done study of 95 adolescents and young women with a mean age of 20.4 demonstrated resolution of biopsy-proven

CIN 2 in 63% of the population within 1 year and 68% by 2 years.[38] CIN 1 is managed expectantly without initial treatment, as are a majority of CIN 2 cases in these young women. This is primarily due to the extremely high rate of spontaneous resolution of CIN 1, and moderately high rate of regression of CIN 2.[39] In the ALTS trial, the majority of CIN 1 regressed spontaneously with only 10% of patients progressing to CIN 2,3 over a 2-year period.[46] The rate of resolution of CIN 1 in young women is very high, with 91% of cases resolving within 36 months.[40] Because the treatment of CIN is associated with financial cost, discomfort, and potential harm to subsequent pregnancies, treatment of CIN 1 is not recommended.[3,4,37]

A meta-analysis of 27 studies on obstetrical outcomes after conservative treatment for CIN concluded that excisional procedures (cold-knife conization [CKC], LEEP, and laser cone) are associated with preterm delivery, low birth weight, and cesarean section.[47] The results of this analysis demonstrate that CKC is associated with an increase in the RR of preterm labor (2.59 [CI: 1.80 to 3.72]) and low birth weight delivery (2.53 [CI: 1.19 to 5.36]) as defined by a weight <2500 g compared to women not treated. LEEP is also associated with an increased RR of preterm labor (1.71 [CI: 1.24 to 2.35]) and low birth weight infants (1.82 [CI: 1.09 to 3.06]) as compared to women not receiving treatment. Increased risk of preterm labor and low birth weight was also demonstrated for laser conization and laser ablation; however, the RRs did not reach statistical significance.[47] Information on the obstetrical outcomes of patients undergoing cryotherapy is lacking. While the majority of evidence demonstrates the negative impact of treatment on pregnancy, one large retrospective study of the impact of LEEP on pregnancy did not agree with this conclusion.[48] Until definitive research proves otherwise, ASCCP and American College of Obstetrics and Gynecology (ACOG) favor management algorithms that minimize the use of any ablative or excisional therapies.

The choice of observation is one that requires educating the patient, including a full explanation of the importance of close follow-up. Some women will feel treatment brings quicker closure, therefore producing less anxiety than observation does. Women who have completed childbearing or come from populations with poor rates of adherence to follow-up may be best served by treatment. This is especially true for previously unscreened women, who are at higher risk for cervical cancer and may continue to have problems accessing health care, including appropriate follow-up. The risk of nonadherence to follow-up recommendations must always be considered when expectant management is elected. In these situations, patients must assume personal responsibility for continuing to access appropriate follow-up care as recommended.

20.2.2.4 Choosing the Procedure for Women Requiring Treatment

When treatment is elected, the procedure chosen should be one that offers the best cure rate, considering the lesion characteristics and the clinician's expertise. When several options may be equally effective, operator skills, cost, availability of technology, and patient preference should also be considered. At the present time, treatment options are either ablative or excisional procedures. In the future, treatments may be available that more specifically enhance the immune response to HPV or disable regions in the HPV genome that promote viral transcription and transformation. Until then, the available options are cryotherapy, diathermy, laser ablation or excision, LEEP, and CKC. There are numerous comparative advantages and disadvantages for each procedure.[16,49] Cryotherapy requires minimal skill, is easy to use, has few complications, is reliable, and is very cost-effective. However, the effectiveness of cryotherapy is limited by certain lesion characteristics, including size and extension more than 4 to 5 mm into the cervical canal. The procedure is associated with a heavy, often odorous, watery discharge that may last several weeks. Laser vaporization is more easily tailored to lesion location and size than is either cryotherapy or LEEP but requires greater clinical expertise because of the potential for more serious injuries and is far more costly in initial outlay and ongoing maintenance. These issues have considerably reduced the availability of this modality. Lesional clearance rates following cryotherapy or laser have not been shown to be statistically different when comparing these two modalities in either nonrandomized or randomized trials (Table 20.1).[16,49–54] Marked variability in recurrence rates or CIN persistence do exist from study to study. For instance, a failure rate of 30% was reported by Kwikkel et al.[55] for laser compared to 14% for cryotherapy, whereas Wright and Davies[53] reported that 3% treated by laser failed, but 14% of women treated by cryotherapy failed. Loop excision and laser ablation have also been shown to have similar failure rates in both randomized and nonrandomized trials.[56,57] More importantly, the risk of persistent or recurrent disease in these studies was associated with three prognostic variables: endocervical gland involvement, lesion size, and lesion grade. The largest randomized trial to date for managing CIN assessed the effectiveness of all three commonly used treatment modalities (cryotherapy, laser, and LEEP) and stratified the patients by prognostic variables that may have accounted for the marked variability in clearance rates noted in previous studies.[16] Cryotherapy had a slightly higher rate of persistent or recurrent disease (24%) when compared with laser (17%) and LEEP (16%), but the difference was not statistically significant. Evaluation of the effect of lesion size, grade, location, endocervical gland involvement, HPV status, age, and smoking history determined that only the size of the lesion was statistically associated with increased failure rates, regardless of the treatment modality chosen. Lesions involving more than two-thirds of the cervical portio epithelium were 19 times more likely than were smaller lesions to persist following treatment.[16]

Other parameters that may reflect the status of host immunity, or of the infecting virus, appeared to be important in determining the patient's risk of recurrent disease following a negative posttreatment visit. For example, women older than 30 years of age, or positive for HPV 16 or 18, or with a history of prior CIN 3 treatment were more than twice as likely as others to have recurrent disease.[16] These parameters are consistent with the premise that HPV 16 and 18 have higher oncogenic risk than do other high-risk HPV types and that older women with HPV, or those having failed prior therapy, may have some decreased ability to clear HPV.[36]

Surgical complications are also reasonably comparable, occurring in only 2% post cryotherapy, 4% post laser treatment, and 8% post LEEP.[16] The difference in these complication rates was almost entirely due to the rate of postoperative bleeding—cryotherapy 0%, laser 2.3%, and LEEP 4.6% (Table 20.2). There were no significant difference in rates of infection or cervical stenosis (<1% and 1.5%, respectively, in all groups). These figures provide reassurance that the efficacy and risks of these methods are comparable and are further supported by similar findings in a meta-analysis of a much larger number of randomized and quasi-randomized trials evaluating CIN treatment modalities.[58]

Colposcopically directed biopsy does not always detect the most abnormal area.[59] In one study, 47% of women with discordant results had a more severe lesion in the excisional specimen than in the previous punch biopsy; this included one microinvasive carcinoma and three cases of AIS.[59] McIndoe found that 2 of 196 patients with CIN determined to fit the criteria for ablative treatment were subsequently found on laser conization to have microinvasive carcinoma and a third had AIS.[60] A review of 15 studies comparing the accuracy of colposcopic biopsy with later excisional treatment found that 1% to 10% of the women had lesions more severe in the excisional specimen than in the colposcopic biopsy.[61] This included 16 invasive cervical cancers missed by the pretreatment colposcopically directed biopsy of 1975 patients. Gage et al.[62] clearly demonstrated the importance of multiple biopsies for increasing the sensitivity of detecting CIN 2,3 at the time of colposcopy. Data from the ALTS trial demonstrated that the sensitivity of one cervical biopsy to detect CIN 2,3 at the time of initial colposcopy or during 2-year follow-up was 68.3%. The sensitivity improved to 81.8% when two biopsies were taken, with only marginal improvement by adding a third biopsy.[62] Additionally, biopsy of any acetowhite area has been shown to improve colposcopic accuracy to 93%.[63]

TABLE 20.1	COMPARISON OF FAILURE RATES FOR CRYOTHERAPY, LASER, AND LEEP					
STUDY	YEAR	TOTAL PATIENTS	FAILURE RATE (%)*		
			CRYO	LASER	LEEP
Nonrandomized					
Wright	1981	334	14%	3%	NA
Townsend	1983	200	7%	11%	NA
Ferenczy	1985	294	9%	4%	NA
Gunasekera	1990	199	NA	8%	5%
Randomized					
Kirwan	1985	98	17%	11%	NA
Kwikkel	1985	101	14%	30%	NA
Berget	1987	204	9%	10%	NA
Berget	1991	187	4%	8%	NA
Alvarez	1994	375	NA	4%	7%
Mitchell	1998	390	24%	17%	16%

*Persistence and recurrence combined.
From Cox JT. Management of cervical intraepithelial neoplasia. *Lancet* 1999;353:857–9, with permission.

TABLE 20.2	COMPLICATION RATES IN THE TREATMENT OF CIN BY CRYOTHERAPY, LASER, OR LEEP		
	▪ CRYO	▪ LASER	▪ LEEP
Bleeding	0%	2.3%	4.6%
Infection		All <1.0%	
Cervical stenosis		All <1.0%	

Data from Mitchell MF, Tortolero-Luna G, Cook E, Whittaker L, Rhodes-Morris H, Silva E. A randomized clinical trial of cryotherapy, loop electrosurgical excision for treatment of squamous intraepithelial lesions of the cervix. *Obstet Gynecol* 1998;92:737–44.

Hence, it is prudent to consider taking up to four biopsies and include acetowhite areas to reduce the risk of missing the most severe area of abnormality. Reports showing occult AIS or microinvasive carcinoma in 2% to 3% of biopsy documented high-grade specimens excised by LEEP have convinced many clinicians to not use ablative methods to treat any CIN 2,3.[64] However, historical experience suggests that ablation may possibly effectively address microinvasive cancers missed at colposcopy since cancer following cryotherapy is uncommon. Ablative techniques for the treatment of CIN continue to be popular and effective if used in strict observance of treatment guidelines that reduce the risk of missed occult disease.

20.2.3 Management Guidelines for Women with CIN

Evidence-based guidelines on the management of women with CIN were developed at the 2001, 2006, and 2012 ASCCP consensus workshops and are available at www.asccp.org.[2–4] These provide the basis for the following discussion of both observational and active treatment management options for CIN. The guidelines were developed using a formal structured multistep process that employed working groups that defined the important questions and conducted an initial literature review. The initial reviews were made available online for comment. The consensus process included clarification of the important clinical questions that were subsequently discussed and voted on by those attending the consensus meeting. Representatives from a large number of professional organizations were present at the meeting. A two-part rating system is used for the various recommendations.

In 2012, the Lower Anogenital Squamous Terminology Project created new terminology for HPV-related lesions of the lower genital tract that incorporates ancillary tests and other criteria to distinguish indeterminate lesions as high grade or low grade.[65] In this system, the three-tiered CIN classification is condensed into a two-tiered LSIL and HSIL classification. However, delegates to the 2012 ASCCP consensus conference determined that this classification does not yet have a sufficiently robust outcomes evidence base to allow elucidation of risk-based management guidelines. Therefore, until a comprehensive evidence review and consensus guidelines development process on the use of a two-tier terminology can be conducted, histopathology results reported as low-grade squamous intraepithelial lesions (LSIL) should be managed as cervical intraepithelial neoplasia (CIN) 1 and those reported as high-grade squamous intraepithelial lesions (HSIL) should be managed as CIN 2,3.

20.2.3.1 Management of Women with CIN 1

20.2.3.1.1 MANAGEMENT OF WOMEN WITH CIN 1 OR NO CIN FOUND AT COLPOSCOPY AFTER ABNORMAL CYTOLOGY

During recent decades, expectant management of CIN 1 without treatment has become the preferred option. Prior to the mid-1990s, the prevalent theory was that the various grades of CIN represented a progressive disease continuum and that treatment of all grades was necessary to disrupt progression.[66] However, it is now established that CIN 1 represents a histologic manifestation of HPV infection, with a natural history that is similar to LSIL or HPV-positive atypical squamous cells of undetermined significance (ASC-US). It has also become increasingly clear that high-grade lesions represent monoclonal cellular dysfunction independent of CIN 1 and that immunity will usually suppress HPV-induced low-grade lesions.[38,40,67–69] Additionally, the accuracy of a histopathologic diagnosis of CIN 1 can be challenging. In ALTS, expert review by a pathology quality control panel agreed with only 43% of the original clinical center CIN 1 histologic interpretations.[70] The majority of these discrepancies were downgraded to normal. This has led to a shift to expectant management that continues to be limited by the present inability to predict the biologic potential of a CIN 1 lesion. The risk of detecting CIN 2 and 3 during 2-year follow-up of untreated CIN 1 has been shown to be 13%.[46,71] In the past, women referred for LSIL or HPV-positive ASC-US cytology and found to have documented CIN 1 on colposcopic examination were assumed to have a higher risk for subsequent detection of CIN 2 and 3 than women with no CIN detected; however, 2-year follow-up has shown the risk to be similar (10%).[46] This similarity in risk promotes similar management depending on the degree of abnormality of the referral cytology.[2,46,71–73] The majority of CIN 1 is associated with HPV infection, and CIN 1 is most prevalent in the younger population of women. It is these women who bear the most risk of harms to future reproductive outcomes from cervical treatments.

In the ALTS trial, repeat Pap tests at 6 and 12 months cumulatively detected 85% of the CIN 3 that occurred in women with ≤CIN 1 followed over a 2-year period.[72] A single HPV test at 12 months identified 95% of the CIN 3 detected over the same time period, with slightly less referral back to colposcopy because of a positive result (55% vs. 60%, respectively). The 2006 ASCCP Guidelines incorporated these data along with evidence that only persistent HPV progresses to CIN 3[3,18] in recommending a single repeat HPV test at 12 months as a safe alternative to two repeat Pap tests (at 6 and 12 months) in the expectant management of women evaluated for HPV-positive ASC-US or LSIL and found to have CIN 1. The only cytology management strategy with acceptable sensitivity was referral to colposcopy at the threshold of ≥ASC-US, with return to routine screening for women with two consecutive negative cytology results. The alternative strategy of 12-month HPV testing provided similar reassurance, with referral back to colposcopy if HPV positive and to routine screening if negative.[3,37]

Data from Kaiser Permanente of Northern California (KPNC) demonstrated that the risk of occult CIN 3+ among women with no CIN or only CIN 1 (≤CIN 1) identified at colposcopic biopsy is linked to the risk conveyed by prior cytology.[4,73] The 5-year risk of CIN 3+ when CIN 1 or no lesion was diagnosed after ASC-US or LSIL was substantially lower than after HSIL, ASC-H, and atypical glandular cells (AGC). For example, women with CIN 1 after LSIL or HPV-positive ASC-US had a 5-year risk of CIN 3+ of 3.8%, while those with CIN 1 after HSIL had a 5-year risk of CIN 3+ of 15%.[73] Since CIN 3+ risk is elevated for women with either HPV 16 or HPV 18, or persistent oncogenic HPV infection of any type even when cytology is negative, the guidelines for follow-up of women with ≤CIN 1 referred to colposcopy for any of these "lesser abnormalities" stress the need to have continued follow-up.[4] The "lesser abnormalities" include normal cytology with a positive HPV 16 or HPV 18 genotyping test, normal cytology with persistent untyped oncogenic HPV, and ASC-US and LSIL cytology.

Recommendations in the 2012 ASCCP guidelines for the follow-up of ≤CIN 1 found on referral to colposcopy of HSIL, ASC-H, or AGC are different than those in the follow-up of "lesser abnormalities" because of the increased risk of subsequently finding a CIN 3+.[4,73] Because the natural history of HSIL cytology managed without treatment is less understood due to limited studies, management following these more major cytologic abnormalities relies primarily on expert opinion.[4] Women with HSIL cytology who do not have immediate diagnostic excision require close follow-up as discussed below.

Prior to 2001, a cervical excision procedure was the typical response to the finding of CIN 1 on endocervical sampling. Once the high spontaneous regression rate of CIN 1 was understood, and the theory of progression of CIN 1 to CIN 2,3 was discounted, guidelines began in 2001 to recommend follow-up rather than excision in this circumstance.[2-4] Additionally, endocervical samples are often contaminated by ectocervical lesions.[4] In the KPNC follow-up of women with CIN 1 on endocervical sampling, the risk of detection of CIN 2+ over the next 21 months was quite low (10.3% CIN 2 and 1.5% CIN 3).[74,75] Current guidelines on the management of CIN 1 on endocervical sampling do not apply when CIN 2, CIN 3, or CIN 2,3 is found on cervical biopsy or when the lesion seen cannot be graded, as an associated invasive cancer cannot be excluded without a diagnostic excision procedure.[4]

20.2.3.1.1.1 Management of Women With CIN 1 or No CIN Found at Colposcopy Following "Lesser Abnormalities"

Under the current 2012 ASCCP guidelines, follow-up without treatment is anticipated for the management of CIN 1 or no lesion found on colposcopy done for HPV-positive ASC-US or LSIL cytology (Table 20.3 and Figure 20.5B: Management of Women with No Lesion or Biopsy-confirmed Cervical Intraepithelial Neoplasia Grade 1 (CIN 1) Preceded by "Lesser Abnormalities").[4] The 5-year follow-up data from KPNC for women with antecedent HPV-positive/ASCUS or LSIL and ≤CIN 1 found at colposcopy demonstrated that a single negative cotest in follow-up reduced their risk to a level consistent with a 3-year return.[73] Therefore, cotesting at 1 year is the

recommended follow-up for women ≥25 years of age. If cotest results are negative/negative, repeat age-appropriate screening would occur in 3 years (cytology among women <30 and cotesting among women ≥30). If these results are negative, return to the routine age-appropriate screening is recommended.[4]

Persistence of CIN 1 beyond 2 years may be associated with a decreased likelihood of regression and viral clearance. In these instances, either continued follow-up or treatment is acceptable and will ultimately depend on patient preference and the expertise of the clinician.[4] An excisional procedure is recommended if the patient has been previously treated or if her colposcopy is inadequate and/or the endocervical sampling shows CIN 2, CIN 3, or ungraded CIN.

When CIN 1 is detected on endocervical sampling after "lesser" abnormalities but no CIN 2+ is detected in colposcopic biopsies, management should follow ASCCP management guidelines for CIN 1, with the addition of repeat endocervical sampling in 12 months (Table 20.4).[4]

Hysterectomy as the primary treatment for histologically confirmed CIN 1 is unacceptable.[4]

20.2.3.1.2 MANAGEMENT OF WOMEN WITH CIN 1 PRECEDED BY ASC-H OR HSIL CYTOLOGY

The increased risk of subsequent CIN 2,3 detection in women evaluated for HSIL or ASC-H cytology and initially found to have CIN 1 warrants a different management strategy than for CIN 1 diagnosed following ASC-US or LSIL.[3,4,37] CIN 2,3 is identified in 84% to 97% of women with HSIL cytology evaluated by a LEEP procedure.[76-78] The risk for subsequent detection of CIN 2+ in the same circumstance following an ASC-H cytology result is midway between the risk following "lesser abnormalities" and the risk following HSIL. Moreover, women with ≤CIN 1 referred for the evaluation of ASC-US/ HPV positive or LSIL had only a 0.17% 5-year cancer risk, considerably lower than the cancer risk for women referred for AGC (0.77%), ASC-H (1.6%), and HSIL+ (2.1%).[73]

In the 2001 and 2006 Guidelines, the management of women referred for AGC and only found to have ≤CIN 1 was similar to that for HSIL referral, and the management of women following ASC-H was grouped with that for women with ASC-US/ HPV positive or LSIL.[2,3] The KPNC data provided the opportunity to reexamine these earlier risk groupings, so that ASC-H and HSIL are now grouped for similar postcolposcopy management, and the management of women following AGC is in its

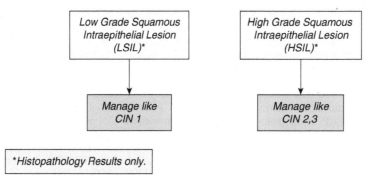

Interim Guidance for Managing Reports using the Lower Anogenital Squamous Terminology (LAST) Histopathology Diagnoses

FIGURE 20.5 A.   Interim Guidance for Managing Reports using the Lower Anogenital Squamous Terminology (LAST) Histopathology Diagnoses. (From Massad LS, Einstein MH, Huh WK, et al. 2012 Updated consensus guidelines for the management of abnormal cervical cancer screening tests and cancer precursors. *J Low Genit Tract Dis* 2013;17:S1–27, with permission.)

TABLE 20.3 MANAGEMENT OF WOMEN WITH NO LESION OR BIOPSY-CONFIRMED CERVICAL INTRAEPITHELIAL NEOPLASIA GRADE 1 (CIN 1) PRECEDED BY "LESSER ABNORMALITIES"*

- Cotesting at 1 y is recommended (BII).
  ○ Refer back to colposcopy if the 12-mo cotest is ≥ASC-US or HPV positive
  ○ If both the HPV test and cytology are negative, then age-appropriate retesting 3 y later is recommended (cytology if age is younger than 30 y, cotesting if 30 y of age or older).
    ■ If all tests are negative, then return to routine screening is recommended (BII). If any test is abnormal, then colposcopy is recommended (CIII).
- If CIN 1 persists for at least 2 y, either continued follow-up or treatment is acceptable (CII).
  ○ If treatment is selected, the ECC is negative and the colposcopic examination is adequate, either excision or ablation is acceptable (AI).
- A diagnostic excisional procedure is recommended if the colposcopic examination is inadequate; the endocervical sampling contains CIN 2, CIN 3, CIN 2,3, or ungraded CIN; or the patient has been previously treated (AIII).
  ○ Treatment modality should be determined by the judgment of the clinician and should be guided by experience, resources, and clinical value for the specific patient (A1II).
  ○ In patients with CIN 1 and an inadequate colposcopic examination, ablative procedures are unacceptable (EI).
- Podophyllin or podophyllin-related products are unacceptable for use in the vagina or on the cervix (EII).
- Hysterectomy as the primary and principal treatment for histologically diagnosed CIN 1 is unacceptable (EII).

*Algorithm in Figure 20.5B.
From Massad LS, Einstein MH, Huh WK, et al. 2012 Updated consensus guidelines for the management of abnormal cervical cancer screening tests and cancer precursors. *J Low Genit Tract Dis* 2013;17:S1–27, with permission.

own category.[4,73] Given a history of ASC-H or HSIL and CIN 2+ not identified at colposcopy, either a (1) diagnostic excisional procedure or (2) observation with cotesting at 12 and 24 months is recommended (Table 20.5 and Figure 20.5C: Management of Women with No Lesion or Biopsy-confirmed Cervical Intraepithelial Neoplasia Grade 1 (CIN 1) Preceded by ASC-H or HSIL Cytology). Alternatively, (3) review the

cytologic, histologic, and colposcopic findings and revision of the management plan based on the new interpretation. The observation option only applies if colposcopic examination is adequate and endocervical sampling is negative.[4]

The 5-year follow-up data from KPNC for women with antecedent ASC-H or HSIL cytology and ≤CIN 1 found at colposcopy demonstrated that no single negative test result

Management of Women with No Lesion or Biopsy-confirmed Cervical Intraepithelial Neoplasia - Grade 1 (CIN1) Preceded by "Lesser Abnormalities"*∞

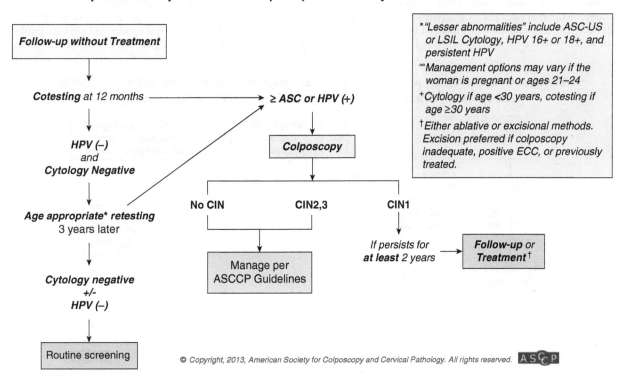

FIGURE 20.5B. Management of Women with No Lesion or Biopsy-confirmed Cervical Intraepithelial Neoplasia—Grade 1 (CIN 1) Preceded by "Lesser Abnormalities." (From Massad LS, Einstein MH, Huh WK, et al. 2012 Updated consensus guidelines for the management of abnormal cervical cancer screening tests and cancer precursors. *J Low Genit Tract Dis* 2013;17:S1–27, with permission.)

TABLE 20.4   MANAGEMENT OF WOMEN WITH CIN 1 ON ENDOCERVICAL SAMPLING

- When CIN 1 is detected on endocervical sampling after lesser abnormalities but no CIN 2+ is detected in colposcopic biopsies:
  - Management should follow ASCCP management guidelines for CIN 1, with the addition of repeat endocervical sampling in 12 mo (BII).
- For women with CIN 1 on endocervical sampling and cytology reported as ASC-H, HSIL, or AGC or with a colposcopic biopsy reported as CIN 2+, management according to the ASCCP management guidelines for the specific abnormality is recommended (BII).
  - For women not treated, repeat endocervical sampling at the time of evaluation for the other abnormality is recommended (BII).

From Massad LS, Einstein MH, Huh WK, et al. 2012 Updated consensus guidelines for the management of abnormal cervical cancer screening tests and cancer precursors. *J Low Genit Tract Dis* 2013;17:S1–27, with permission.

sufficed to reduce their risk to a level consistent with a 3-year return.[73] Therefore, if observation with cotesting is selected as the follow-up strategy, both cotests must be negative before a return to age-appropriate retesting at 3 years can be recommended.[4] Colposcopy is the recommended follow-up to any abnormal result on either cotest, except that an excisional procedure is indicated for an HSIL cytologic result during either the 12- or 24-month follow-up.[4]

If CIN 1 is detected on endocervical sampling in the setting of an ASC-H or HSIL cytology and normal or CIN 1 colposcopy, management according to the ASCCP management guidelines for the specific abnormality is recommended (Table 20.4). For example, a woman with HSIL cytology, an adequate colposcopic examination, CIN 1 on cervical biopsy, and CIN 1 on endocervical curettage may be managed by diagnostic excision or serial observation with cotesting at 12 and 24 months,

with the choice based on her balancing of risk of cancer with risk to future term delivery. If observation is elected, then endocervical sampling should be added at the 12-month visit.[4]

20.2.3.1.3 CIN 1 IN SPECIAL CIRCUMSTANCES: YOUNG WOMEN AND IN PREGNANCY

20.2.3.1.3.1 In Adolescents and in Women Aged 21 to 24 Years

Adolescents, defined as girls and women 20 years of age and younger, represent a special population. Although the latest screening guidelines recommend that women <21 years of age not receive cervical cancer screening, some women in this age group will continue to be screened and found to have CIN.[45] Adolescents with CIN have a high rate of spontaneous resolution and a very low incidence of cervical cancer.[40,79] Therefore, management of CIN 1 in adolescents is by observation and should follow the guidelines for young women aged 21–24 years.

For those women aged 21–24 years with CIN 1 after ASC-US or LSIL cytology, repeat cytology at 12-month intervals without initial colposcopy is recommended (Table 20.6 and Figure 20.5D: Management of Women Aged 21 to 24 years with No Lesion or Biopsy-confirmed Cervical Intraepithelial Neoplasia Grade 1).[4] For women in this age group, colposcopy is recommended only if at the 12-month follow-up there is an ASC-H or HSIL cytology or for any cytologic abnormality at the 24-month follow-up. By contrast, among women in this age group with CIN 1 after an ASC-H or HSIL cytology, observation for up to 24 months with colposcopy and cytology (at 6-month intervals) is recommended, provided the examination is adequate, and endocervical assessment is negative.[4] HPV testing is not recommended in this age group and if obtained inadvertently should not alter management. Also not recommended is routine treatment of CIN 1 regardless of antecedent cytology.

20.2.3.1.3.2 In Pregnant Women

Pregnant women with a histologic diagnosis of CIN 1 are at very low risk of having cervical cancer and are very unlikely to have their CIN advance to high grade during the short duration

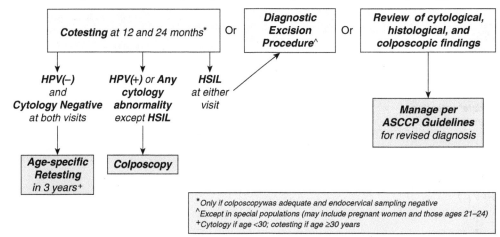

Management of Women with No Lesion or Biopsy-confirmed Cervical Intraepithelial Neoplasia - Grade 1 (CIN1) Preceded by ASC-H or HSIL Cytology

*Only if colposcopy was adequate and endocervical sampling negative
^Except in special populations (may include pregnant women and those ages 21–24)
+Cytology if age <30; cotesting if age ≥30 years

FIGURE 20.5C.   The Three Options for the Management of Women with No Lesion or Biopsy-confirmed Cervical Intraepithelial Neoplasia—Grade 1 (CIN 1) Preceded by ASC-H or HSIL Cytology. (From Massad LS, Einstein MH, Huh WK, et al. 2012 Updated consensus guidelines for the management of abnormal cervical cancer screening tests and cancer precursors. *J Low Genit Tract Dis* 2013;17:S1–27, with permission.)

TABLE 20.5   MANAGEMENT OF WOMEN WITH CIN 1 OR NO LESION PRECEDED BY ASC-H OR HSIL*

- When CIN 2+ is not identified histologically and the referral cytology was ASC-H or HSIL, the two management options recommended are
  - ○ Either a diagnostic excisional procedure
  - ○ or observation with cotesting at 12 mo and 24 mo is recommended
    - ■ Provided in the latter case that the colposcopic examination is adequate and the endocervical sampling is negative (BIII).
    - ■ In this circumstance, it is acceptable to review the cytologic, histologic, and colposcopic findings; if the review yields a revised interpretation, management should follow guidelines for the revised interpretation (BII).
    - ■ If observation with cotesting is elected and both cotests are negative, return for retesting in 3 y is recommended.
  - ○ If any test is abnormal, repeat colposcopy is recommended.
  - ○ A diagnostic excisional procedure is recommended for women with repeat HSIL cytologic results at either the 1-y or 2-y visit (CIII).

*Algorithm in Figure 20.5C.
From Massad LS, Einstein MH, Huh WK, et al. 2012 Updated consensus guidelines for the management of abnormal cervical cancer screening tests and cancer precursors. *J Low Genit Tract Dis* 2013;17:S1–S27, with permission.

of pregnancy. Therefore, follow-up without treatment is recommended in this group (BII), and repeat evaluation should occur no sooner than 6 weeks postpartum.[3,4,37] Treatment of women with CIN 1 is unacceptable during pregnancy.[4]

20.2.3.2 Management of Women with CIN 2, CIN 3, and CIN 2,3

20.2.3.2.1 MANAGEMENT OF WOMEN ≥25 WITH CIN 2, CIN 3, AND CIN 2,3

In the United States, CIN 2 and 3 have been managed similarly in adult women primarily because the reliability of histologic differentiation is only moderate,[80] and the potential for progression of CIN 2, although higher than that of CIN 1, is less than that of CIN 3 (Table 20.7 and Figure 20.5D: Management of Women with Biopsy-confirmed CIN Grade 2 and 3).[38,40,81] Numerous studies fail to demonstrate a significant difference in clearance rates for CIN 2 or 3 treated by either ablative or excisional methods.[16,49–54,57] Therefore, women with CIN 2 or 3 and an adequate colposcopic examination can receive similar successful outcomes by either ablative or excisional methods, but the risk of missed occult cancer increases with increasing lesion grade and size.[4,63,81–83] By contrast, excisional procedures are recommended for women with CIN 2 and/or CIN 3 who have an inadequate colposcopic examination, those with recurrent disease, and those for whom endocervical sampling demonstrates clinically significant disease (CIN 2, CIN 3, CIN 2,3, or CIN not graded).[3,4,37] All options (CKC, laser cone, and LEEP) have comparable success rates, but CKC more frequently results in cervical distortion and an incompetent cervix.[84,85] Because CIN 3 is a cancer precursor, concern over the increased risk of missed occult invasive disease has prompted some clinicians to use excisional procedures for large (>2 quadrant) high-grade lesions. Regardless of treatment method selected, the entire transformation zone must be included within the treatment area.[84] For most women, observation of CIN 2 or CIN 2,3 is unacceptable (except among pregnant and young women).[4] Observation of CIN 3 is always unacceptable regardless of age or concern about future fertility.[4]

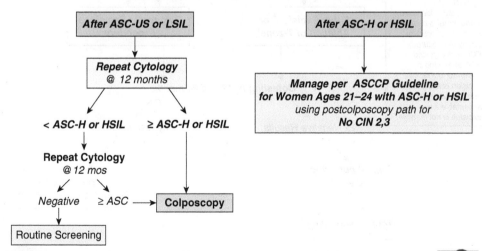

Management of Women Ages 21–24 with No Lesion or Biopsy-confirmed Cervical Intraepithelial Neoplasia - Grade 1 (CIN1)

FIGURE 20.5D.   Management of Women Aged 21–24 with No Lesion or Biopsy-Confirmed Cervical Intraepithelial Neoplasia Grade 1 (CIN 1). (From Massad LS, Einstein MH, Huh WK, et al. 2012 Updated consensus guidelines for the management of abnormal cervical cancer screening tests and cancer precursors. *J Low Genit Tract Dis* 2013;17:S1–27, with permission.)

TABLE 20.6 MANAGEMENT OF WOMEN AGED 21–24 YEARS WITH NO LESION OR BIOPSY-CONFIRMED CERVICAL INTRAEPITHELIAL NEOPLASIA—GRADE 1 (CIN 1)*

After ASC-US or LSIL cytology
- Repeat cytology at 12-mo intervals is recommended. Follow-up with HPV testing is unacceptable (EII).
  - For women with ASC-H or HSIL+ at the 12-mo follow-up, colposcopy is recommended.
  - For women with ASCUS or worse at the 24-mo follow-up, colposcopy is recommended.
  - After two consecutive negative tests, routine screening is recommended (BII).

After ASC-H or HSIL cytology
- For women aged 21–24 y with CIN 1 (or no lesion) after ASC-H or HSIL cytology, observation for up to 24 mo using both colposcopy and cytology at 6-mo intervals is recommended, provided the colposcopic examination is adequate and endocervical assessment is negative (BIII).
  - If CIN 2, CIN 3, or CIN 2,3 is identified histologically during follow-up, management should follow the guideline for the management of young women with CIN 2, CIN 3, or CIN 2,3 (BIII), see "Management of Women With CIN 2, CIN 3, and CIN 2,3."
  - If during follow-up a high-grade colposcopic lesion is identified or HSIL cytology persists for 1 y, biopsy is recommended (BIII).
  - If HSIL persists for 24 mo without identification of CIN 2+, a diagnostic excisional procedure is recommended (BIII).
  - When colposcopy is inadequate or CIN 2, CIN 3, CIN 2,3 or ungraded CIN is identified on endocervical sampling, a diagnostic excision procedure is recommended (BII).
- Regardless of antecedent cytology, treatment of CIN 1 in women aged 21–24 y is not recommended (BII).

*Algorithm in Figure 20.5D.
From Massad LS, Einstein MH, Huh WK, et al. 2012 Updated consensus guidelines for the management of abnormal cervical cancer screening tests and cancer precursors. *J Low Genit Tract Dis* 2013;17:S1–27, with permission.

Posttreatment follow-up is critical to ensure that persistence of CIN 2+ is detected. The KPNC data provide the most comprehensive 5-year evaluation of recurrence risks posttreatment for CIN 2+ and on the tests used for posttreatment evaluation.[86] Hence, the posttreatment guidelines discussed in Section 20.2.3.3 are now clearly more evidence based than previously possible.

Several retrospective studies have now demonstrated that excisional procedures by either laser or LEEP are associated with an increased risk of premature rupture of membranes,

preterm labor, particularly before 34 weeks, and low birth weight infants.[87–93] Because increasing cone depth is associated with a significant increase in the risk of preterm delivery,[92] as a general rule, the clinician should aim to remove as much tissue as needed to provide at least a 2-mm margin while preserving as much cervix as possible to reduce the risk of adverse pregnancy outcomes. However, closer margins do not require reexcision.

Hysterectomy is an unacceptable procedure for CIN 2 and 3 unless there are other indications for this procedure (i.e., symptomatic fibroid uterus, genital prolapse, etc.).[3,4,37] When

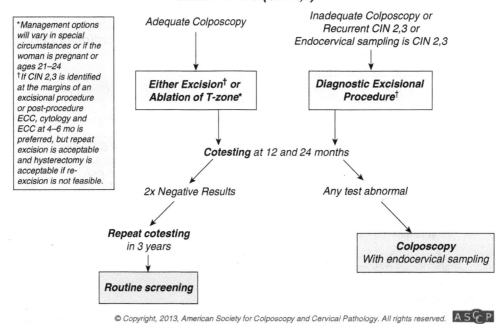

Management of Women with Biopsy-confirmed Cervical Intraepithelial Neoplasia - Grade 2 and 3 (CIN 2,3) *

*Management options will vary in special circumstances or if the woman is pregnant or ages 21–24
†If CIN 2,3 is identified at the margins of an excisional procedure or post-procedure ECC, cytology and ECC at 4–6 mo is preferred, but repeat excision is acceptable and hysterectomy is acceptable if re-excision is not feasible.

Adequate Colposcopy → Either Excision† or Ablation of T-zone*

Inadequate Colposcopy or Recurrent CIN 2,3 or Endocervical sampling is CIN 2,3 → Diagnostic Excisional Procedure†

Cotesting at 12 and 24 months

2x Negative Results → Repeat cotesting in 3 years → Routine screening

Any test abnormal → Colposcopy With endocervical sampling

FIGURE 20.5E. Management of Women with Biopsy-Confirmed Cervical Intraepithelial Neoplasia Grade 2 and 3 (CIN 2,3). (From Massad LS, Einstein MH, Huh WK, et al. 2012 Updated consensus guidelines for the management of abnormal cervical cancer screening tests and cancer precursors. *J Low Genit Tract Dis* 2013;17:S1–27, with permission.)

TABLE 20.7 MANAGEMENT OF WOMEN WITH CIN 2, CIN 3, AND CIN 2,3*

Initial Management
- For women with a histologic diagnosis of CIN 2, CIN 3, or CIN 2,3 and adequate colposcopy, both excision and ablation are acceptable treatment modalities, except in pregnant women and young women (AI).
- A diagnostic excisional procedure is recommended for women with recurrent CIN 2, CIN 3, or CIN 2,3 (AII).
- Ablation is unacceptable and a diagnostic excisional procedure is recommended for women with a histologic diagnosis of CIN 2, CIN 3, or CIN 2,3 and inadequate colposcopy or endocervical sampling showing CIN 2, CIN 3, CIN 2,3, or CIN not graded (AII).
- Observation of CIN 2, CIN 3, or CIN 2,3 with sequential cytology and colposcopy is unacceptable, except in pregnant women and young women (EII).
- Hysterectomy is unacceptable as primary therapy for CIN 2, CIN 3, or CIN 2,3 (EII).

Follow-Up After Treatment
- For women treated for CIN 2, CIN 3, or CIN 2,3, cotesting at 12 mo and 24 mo is recommended (BII).
  - If both cotests are negative, retesting in 3 y is recommended (BII).
    - If all tests are negative, routine screening is recommended for at least 20 y, even if this extends screening beyond 65 y of age (CIII).
  - If any test is abnormal, colposcopy with endocervical sampling is recommended (BII).
  - Repeat treatment or hysterectomy based only on a positive HPV test is unacceptable (EII).
- If CIN 2, CIN 3, or CIN 2,3 is identified at the margins of a diagnostic excisional procedure or in an endocervical sample obtained immediately after the procedure, reassessment using cytology with endocervical sampling at 4 to 6 mo after treatment is preferred (BII).
  - Performing a repeat diagnostic excisional procedure is acceptable (CIII).
  - Hysterectomy is acceptable if a repeat diagnostic procedure is not feasible (CIII).
- A repeat diagnostic excisional procedure or hysterectomy is acceptable for women with a histologic diagnosis of recurrent or persistent CIN 2, CIN 3, or CIN 2,3 (BII).

*Algorithm in Figure 20.5E.
From Massad LS, Einstein MH, Huh WK, et al. 2012 Updated consensus guidelines for the management of abnormal cervical cancer screening tests and cancer precursors. *J Low Genit Tract Dis* 2013;17:S1–27, with permission.

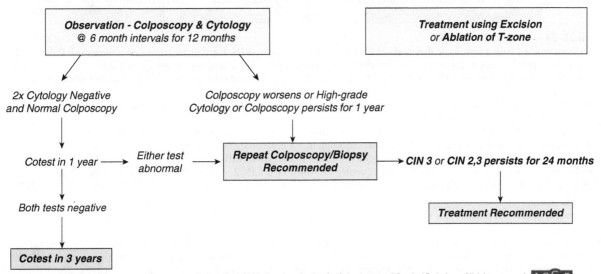

FIGURE 20.5F. Management of Young Women with Biopsy-confirmed Cervical Intraepithelial Neoplasia Grade 2,3 (CIN 2,3) in Special Circumstances. (From Massad LS, Einstein MH, Huh WK, et al. 2012 Updated consensus guidelines for the management of abnormal cervical cancer screening tests and cancer precursors. *J Low Genit Tract Dis* 2013;17:S1–27, with permission.)

hysterectomy is indicated for reasons other than CIN 2 or 3, or is indicated in a woman who has completed childbearing and has residual high-grade disease in a cervix too small to allow safe repeat conization without risk of bladder and vaginal injury, an excisional procedure should be performed to rule out invasive cancer, when possible, prior to the hysterectomy.[37,93]

20.2.3.2.2 MANAGEMENT OF YOUNG WOMEN (21 TO 24 YEARS OF AGE) WITH BIOPSY-CONFIRMED CIN 2, CIN 3, OR CIN 2,3

The ASCCP guidelines specifically separate the management of CIN 2 and CIN 2,3 (histologic HSIL) in young women from that of older women due to the more frequent resolution of CIN 2, the low risk of cancer in this population (0.000023 in the KPNC study),[41] and the greater likelihood that childbearing has not been completed.[3,4,37,41,79,94] In contrast, the management of CIN 3 is the same for young as for "older" women. Natural history studies have demonstrated spontaneous resolution of CIN 2 in 68% of adolescents and young women (mean age 20) by 12 months of follow-up.[38] It is important to note that while the age of an adolescent is clearly defined as a female 20 years of age or younger, the updated guidelines specifically pertain to women 21 to 24 years of age and assume that women <21 are not screened.[4] However, if they are and if found to have CIN 2; CIN 2,3; or CIN 3, they should be managed in the same manner as for women aged 21 to 24 years. The management algorithm is provided in Figure 20.5F (Management of Women Aged 21 to 24 years with Biopsy-confirmed Cervical Intraepithelial Neoplasia Grade 2,3).[4] For women in this age group with a histologic diagnosis of CIN 2,3 not otherwise specified, and with an adequate colposcopic examination, either treatment or observation for up to 12 months using both colposcopy and cytology (every 6 months) is acceptable (Table 20.8).[4] However, if CIN 2 is specified, observation is preferred.[3,4] When observation without treatment is elected for either CIN 2 or CIN 2,3, repeat biopsy is recommended if the appearance of the lesion worsens, or if HSIL cytology and/or a high-grade colposcopic lesion persists for 1 year. Treatment would be recommended if CIN 3 is diagnosed, or if CIN 2 or CIN 2,3 persists for

24 months.[4] Alternatively, after two negative cytology results during follow-up, cotesting is recommended at 1 year, and if negative, subsequently in 3 years.[4]

20.2.3.2.3 MANAGEMENT OF CIN 2,3 IN PREGNANCY

Treatment of CIN during pregnancy carries unacceptable risks, including excessive bleeding, premature delivery, and fetal loss.[37,95,96] Therefore, high-grade disease occurring in pregnancy is generally followed until the postpartum period because of the low risk of progression to invasion and the potential for regression as high as 69% following delivery.[3,4,95–98] Pregnant women with CIN 2 have a negligible risk, and those with CIN 3 a <10% risk of microinvasive cancer being detected at the postpartum visit.[37,99,100]

In the absence of invasive disease or advanced pregnancy, additional colposcopic and cytologic examinations are acceptable in pregnant women with a histologic diagnosis of CIN 2, CIN 3, or CIN 2,3 at intervals no more frequent than every 12 weeks.[3,4,37] Biopsy is recommended only if the lesion appears to progress or repeat cytology suggests invasion.[4] Deferring the reevaluation with cytology and colposcopy is recommended no sooner than 6 weeks postpartum.[4] A diagnostic excisional procedure should only be used if invasion is suspected.[4] Even if invasive cervical cancer is detected, treatment depends on cancer stage and the point in pregnancy when the cancer is detected.[4,101–104] The care of a woman with invasive cervical cancer during pregnancy requires consultation with a gynecologic oncologist who has the expertise to manage this very difficult situation. The stage of the cancer, the gestational age, and the health and well-being of both the mother and the fetus must be considered (see Chapter 12).

20.2.3.2.4 MANAGEMENT OF CIN 2,3 IN THE IMMUNOSUPPRESSED

Management of CIN 2,3 in immunocompromised women is challenging because of high recurrence rates posttreatment, higher prevalence of HPV, more rapid progression to CIN 2 and 3, and increased incidence of both CIN and cervical cancer.[6,105–112] Clearance rates posttreatment are less than half those seen among immunocompetent women receiving similar

---

TABLE 20.8	MANAGEMENT OF YOUNG WOMEN WITH BIOPSY-CONFIRMED CERVICAL INTRAEPITHELIAL NEOPLASIA—GRADE 2,3 (CIN 2,3) IN SPECIAL CIRCUMSTANCES*

Women 21–24
- For young women with a histologic diagnosis of CIN 2,3 not otherwise specified, either treatment or observation for up to 12 mo using both colposcopy and cytology at 6-mo intervals is acceptable, provided colposcopy is adequate (BIII).
- When a histologic diagnosis of CIN 2 is specified for a young woman, observation is preferred but treatment is acceptable.
  - If observation is elected:
    - If the colposcopic appearance of the lesion worsens or if HSIL cytology or a high-grade colposcopic lesion persists for 1 y, repeat biopsy is recommended (BIII).
    - After two consecutive negative cytology results, an additional cotest 1 y later is recommended (BIII).
    - If the additional cotest is negative, then repeat cotesting in 3 y is recommended (BIII).
    - Colposcopy is recommended if either the 2-y or 5-y cotest is abnormal (BIII).
    - Treatment is recommended if CIN 3 is subsequently identified or if CIN 2, or CIN 2,3 persists for 24 mo (BII).
- Treatment is recommended if colposcopy is inadequate, if CIN 3 is specified, or if CIN 2 or CIN 2,3 persists for 24 mo (BII).

Pregnant Women
- A diagnostic excisional procedure is recommended only if invasion is suspected (BII). Unless invasive cancer is identified, treatment is unacceptable (EII).
- In the absence of invasive disease or advanced pregnancy, additional colposcopic and cytologic examinations are acceptable in pregnant women with a histologic diagnosis of CIN 2, CIN 3, or CIN 2,3 at intervals no more frequent than every 12 wk (BII).
  - Repeat biopsy is recommended only if the appearance of the lesion worsens or if cytology suggests invasive cancer (BII).
  - Deferring reevaluation until at least 6 wk postpartum is acceptable (BII).
  - Reevaluation with cytology and colposcopy is recommended no sooner than 6 wk postpartum (CIII).

---

*Algorithm in Figure 20.5F.
From Massad LS, Einstein MH, Huh WK, et al. 2012 Updated consensus guidelines for the management of abnormal cervical cancer screening tests and cancer precursors. *J Low Genit Tract Dis* 2013;17:S1–27, with permission.

treatment, with no difference in rates for HIV-positive women treated with either cryotherapy or LEEP. Additionally, treatment of low-grade lesions does not appear to reduce the risk of progression. Hence, most immunosuppressed women with CIN 1 are followed rather than treated. However, treatment of CIN 2,3 can effectively interrupt progression to invasive cancer.[37,108,111,112] The advent of highly active antiretroviral therapy (HAART) has markedly improved the survival of women infected with HIV, but the role of HAART in the management of women with cervical precancerous lesions remains unclear.[37] Therefore, CIN 2 and 3 should be treated similarly in HIV-positive women regardless of their use of antiretroviral therapy.[37] The success rate of treating immunocompromised women with CIN 2 or 3 varies depending on the CD4 cell count and margin status.[109,113] Half of the women with a negative margin will have recurrence of their CIN, but negative margins are less common in immunocompromised women treated for CIN 2,3.[113] In some studies, recurrence after cold-knife cone is as high as 90%, and up to 100% have recurred following either LEEP or cryotherapy.[109]

No new recommendations were made in the 2012 ASCCP guidelines regarding the management of immunocompromised women. The 2006 ASCCP guidelines recommend that the management of CIN 2,3 in immunosuppressed women be the same as in the general population.[3] ACOG also states that immunocompromised women with CIN 2,3 can be treated by either standard ablative or excisional methods regardless of HIV viral load, with the selection of procedure based on the same parameters as for non–HIV-infected women.[37]

20.2.3.3 Posttreatment Follow-Up of Women Treated for CIN

Although treatment of CIN is highly successful, the long-term risk for cervical cancer remains higher than for women never having CIN. The risk appears to increase with age.[114-125] A systematic review of the literature shows that the incidence of invasive cervical cancer is 56/100,000 for at least 20 years after treatment.[123] This rate is almost 10-fold greater than in the general population. In contrast to invasive disease, the rate of posttreatment CIN falls throughout the first 10 years after treatment to a rate of about 280 per 100,000 women in the 8th year and to about 190 per 100,000 women in the 10th year.[123] Women treated for CIN 2,3 require surveillance for an extended period of time.[3,4,37,126,127]

The rate of recurrence or persistence of CIN varies from 1% to 21% regardless of the procedure used.[16,114,121,122] Large lesions have the highest treatment failure rate.[16,116,128] Positive cone margins are also indicative of a higher risk of persistent or recurrent disease.[127,129-135] In a comprehensive meta-analysis of posttreatment follow-up studies published between 1960 and 2007, the RR of posttreatment recurrence of any CIN after incomplete excision was 5.47 and for recurrent CIN 2 or 3 was 6.09 when compared to women with clear margins.[135] Margins of LEEP specimens may be difficult to interpret,[132,134] and even when margins are clearly involved, the majority will remain disease free during follow-up. Therefore, expectant management is reasonable for patients with CIN 3 and positive margins, provided these women have very careful follow-up.[3,4,37,115,132,133] Repeat conizaton is acceptable but is often not necessary.[3,4,37] Risk factors for recurrence or persistence of CIN include older age, larger lesions, and higher-grade disease, with risks as high as 50% for older women with large CIN 3 lesions.[37]

A number of follow-up approaches have been described for women treated for CIN, incorporating cytology, HPV testing, and colposcopy alone or in combination at intervals from 3 months to annually.[4] HPV testing is a very sensitive measure for posttreatment detection of CIN and may result in earlier diagnosis of persistent or recurrent disease but is less specific than is cytology.[3,4,37,136-145] The majority of women cleared of CIN posttreatment have undetectable levels of the HPV type responsible for the treated lesion within 6 months posttreatment. In contrast, women with persistent CIN continue to have detectable HPV. In one study, 94% of patients successfully treated and positive for HPV pretreatment no longer had detectable high-risk HPV DNA at the 12-month posttreatment visit.[142] Other evaluations have documented 100% negative predictive value of a posttreatment negative HPV test for recurrent or persistent CIN 2,3.[140,145] Persistently detected same-type HPV 16 or 18 six months posttreatment was demonstrated to have an increased unadjusted odds ratio of 8.0 for recurrent disease detected during 5-year follow-up.[146]

The KPNC data provide the most comprehensive 5-year evaluation of recurrence risks posttreatment for CIN 2+.[86] Risk varied both by antecedent screening test result and the histology of the treated lesion. The risk of recurrence ranged from 5% for CIN 2 preceded by ASC-US/HPV positive or LSIL to 16% for CIN 3/AIS preceded by AGC, ASC-H, or HSIL. Posttreatment negative cotests were reassuring, as this risk differential was lowered and similar regardless of antecedent screening test and histology of treated disease. The 5-year recurrent CIN 2+ risk after a single negative posttreatment cotest (2.4%) was lower than that following a single negative HPV test (3.7%) or a negative Pap result (4.2%). Two negative posttreatment tests of each kind conferred slightly lower 5-year CIN 2+ risk than one.[86] The 5-year CIN 2+ risk after two negative cotests of 1.5% was still over twice the 0.68% risk after a negative Pap test during routine screening. The authors concluded that, on the basis of the principle of "equal management of equal risks," after two negative cotest results posttreatment, the risk was still greater than for women in routine screening with a single negative cotest. Negative cotests after treatment did provide more reassurance against recurrent CIN 2+ than did either negative Pap tests or HPV tests alone.[86] The 2012 Consensus Conference recommended return to 5-year cotesting for women with negative cotests at 1, 2, and 5 years after treatment.[86] This was based on consensus opinion, not on evidence.

The ASCCP guidelines for follow-up of women posttreatment for CIN 2 or 3 are listed in Table 20.9 and in Figure 20.5E (*Management of Women with Biopsy-confirmed Cervical Intraepithelial Neoplasia Grade 2 and 3*).[4] In general, follow-up posttreatment should be with cotesting performed at 12 and 24 months. If both are negative, an additional cotest should be performed 3 years later. If the latter is also negative, the patient can return to routine age-appropriate screening for at least 20 years. Alternatively, if any of the cotests during the first three follow-ups are positive, the patient should be evaluated with colposcopy and endocervical sampling.[4]

20.3 MANAGEMENT OF ADENOCARCINOMA *IN SITU*

AIS is a relatively uncommon histologic diagnosis (<1.25 cases per 100,000 women per year). However, the incidence of AIS increased sixfold from 1970 to 1990, and incidence and mortality from adenocarcinoma increased proportionately.[126,147] AIS represents a challenge to the health care provider due to the infrequency of the diagnosis and the difficulty in detecting these lesions by both cytology and colposcopy. AIS is often almost indistinguishable from the colposcopic findings of a normal ectopy, is often hidden within the endocervical canal, is frequently next to more dramatic colposcopic changes in adjacent CIN that draw away attention from the more subtle detail of AIS, and may occasionally be buried under a squamous abnormality.[148-151] The lesions often are multifocal, that is, "skip" lesions (see Chapter 11), and therefore, negative

TABLE 20.9	MANAGEMENT OF WOMEN POSTTREATMENT CIN 2, CIN 3, AND CIN 2,3

- For women treated for CIN 2, CIN 3, or CIN 2,3, cotesting at 12 mo and 24 mo is recommended (BII).
  - If both cotests are negative, retesting in 3 y is recommended (BII). If any test is abnormal, colposcopy with endocervical sampling is recommended (BII).
  - If all tests are negative, routine screening is recommended for at least 20 y, even if this extends screening beyond 65 y of age (CIII).
  - Repeat treatment or hysterectomy based only on a positive HPV test is unacceptable (EII).
- If CIN 2, CIN 3, or CIN 2,3 is identified at the margins of a diagnostic excisional procedure or in an endocervical sample obtained immediately after the procedure, reassessment using cytology with endocervical sampling at 4–6 mo after treatment is preferred (BII).
  - Performing a repeat diagnostic excisional procedure is acceptable (CIII).
  - Hysterectomy is acceptable if a repeat diagnostic procedure is not feasible (CIII).
  - A repeat diagnostic excisional procedure or hysterectomy is acceptable for women with a histologic diagnosis of recurrent or persistent CIN 2, CIN 3, or CIN 2,3 (BII).

From Massad LS, Einstein MH, Huh WK, et al. 2012 Updated consensus guidelines for the management of abnormal cervical cancer screening tests and cancer precursors. *J Low Genit Tract Dis* 2013;17:S1–27, with permission.

margins on the cone specimen do not guarantee complete removal of the lesion.[151] A comprehensive review of the literature of 296 women with AIS treated with an excisional cone documented recurrence in 8%.[152] Despite the multifocal nature of about 6.5% to 15% of AIS,[150,151] the risk of recurrence is most strongly predicted by margin status. Women with a positive margin are found to have recurrent disease at the time of a subsequent cone biopsy or hysterectomy in 55% to 70% of cases.[153,154] In contrast, women with negative margins have residual disease in 0% to 13%. Margin status is affected by the size of the cone specimen. Therefore, there is credence in performing a cold knife cone (CKC) in women with an AIS diagnosis on cervical biopsy to provide a large specimen with margins not altered by thermal effect.[2,3,37] In 2001, knife conization was favored over loop excision because margin status and the interpretability of margins are critical to future treatment planning.[2] In 2006, wording was changed to allow diagnostic excision using any modality,[3] but care must be taken to keep the specimen intact and margins interpretable, avoiding fragmentation of the specimen, including "top-hat" serial endocervical excisions.[4] This may require use of larger loops than those employed to excise visible squamous lesions.[4] Like margin status, endocervical sampling at the time of an excisional procedure also predicts residual disease.[4,155] Also, a negative high-risk HPV test posttreatment identifies women at the lowest risk for recurrence.[4,86]

20.3.1 Management of AIS in Women Who Do Not Desire Fertility

Hysterectomy is preferred for women who have completed childbearing and have a histologic diagnosis of AIS on an excisional procedure (Table 20.10).[4] If AIS is identified on a cervical biopsy, the patient should first undergo a cone biopsy of the cervix to rule out invasive disease prior to proceeding with a hysterectomy. The ASCCP management recommendation for women with AIS who do not desire to maintain their fertility is depicted in Figure 20.5G (Management of Women Diagnosed with Adenocarcinoma in-situ during a Excisional Procedure).

Management of Women Diagnosed with Adenocarcinoma in-situ (AIS) during a Diagnostic Excisional Procedure

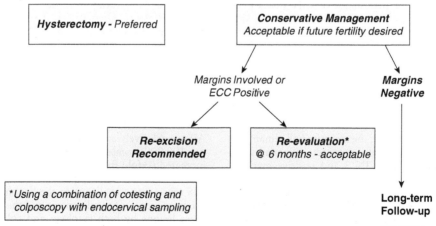

FIGURE 20.5G. Management of Women Diagnosed with Adenocarcinoma in-situ (AIS) during a Diagnostic Excisional Procedure. (From Massad LS, Einstein MH, Huh WK, et al. 2012 Updated consensus guidelines for the management of abnormal cervical cancer screening tests and cancer precursors. *J Low Genit Tract Dis* 2013;17:S1–27, with permission.)

TABLE 20.10	MANAGEMENT OF WOMEN DIAGNOSED WITH AIS DURING A DIAGNOSTIC EXCISIONAL PROCEDURE*

- Hysterectomy is preferred for women who have completed childbearing and have a histologic diagnosis of AIS on a specimen from a diagnostic excisional procedure (BIII).
- Conservative management is acceptable if future fertility is desired (AII).
  - If conservative management is planned and the margins of the specimen are involved or endocervical sampling obtained at the time of excision contains CIN or AIS, reexcision to increase the likelihood of complete excision is preferred.
    - As an alternative reevaluation at 6 mo using a combination of cotesting and colposcopy with endocervical sampling is acceptable in this circumstance.
- Long-term follow-up is recommended for women who do not undergo hysterectomy (CIII).

*Algorithm in Figure 20.5G.
From Massad LS, Einstein MH, Huh WK, et al. 2012 Updated consensus guidelines for the management of abnormal cervical cancer screening tests and cancer precursors. *J Low Genit Tract Dis* 2013;17:S1–27, with permission.

20.3.2 Management of AIS in Women Who Desire Future Fertility

Nonpregnant women identified to have AIS on a cervical biopsy require a surgical excision procedure to remove the lesion and to rule out invasive disease. Because of the difficulty in recognizing AIS cytologically and colposcopically, hysterectomy continues to be the treatment of choice for AIS when invasion is ruled out.[3,4,37] However, AIS often occurs in women who have not completed childbearing. For women who wish to maintain fertility, observation is an option, although it carries a <10% risk of persistent AIS and a small risk of cancer even when excision margins are negative.[4,156] If the margins are clear and the woman desires to maintain future fertility, and with informed consent after discussing the balance between risk and benefits for each individual patient, conservative management with cone biopsy followed by long-term follow-up with colposcopy, cytology, and HPV testing is acceptable (Table 20.10 and Figure 20.5G: Management of Women Diagnosed with Adenocarcinoma in-situ during a Diagnostic Excisional Procedure).[4] The preferred management of a patient who has positive margins for AIS on conization, or a positive endocervical sampling at the time of the cone, is a reexcision to attempt to clear the deep margin of disease.[3,4,37] An acceptable alternative in this circumstance is reevaluation at 6 months using a combination of cervical cytology, HPV testing, and colposcopy with endocervical sampling.[4] Long-term follow-up is recommended for women who do not undergo hysterectomy, but the parameters of "long-term follow-up" are not well defined.[3,4,157–159] Certainly, the more negative tests obtained, the more reassuring conservative follow-up should be.

20.4 PROCEDURES FOR TREATING CERVICAL NEOPLASIA

20.4.1 Cryotherapy of the Cervix

Cryotherapy gained popularity in the 1970s as an alternative to excisional surgery by either CKC or hysterectomy, providing the first outpatient treatment option for CIN.

A profound reduction of surgical complications was noted following the implementation of cryotherapy to treat premalignant cervical disease.[49] Furthermore, treatment failures were no more commonly encountered with cryotherapy than when compared with older excisional approaches.[58] Thus, cryotherapy earned a reputation as a safe, similarly efficacious, relatively inexpensive, easy, non–fertility-impairing procedure for treating women with lower genital tract premalignant disease. Since the 1990s, cryotherapy has been less commonly used than LEEP for treatment of intraepithelial neoplasia. However, in recent years, LEEP has been shown to have increased risk of pregnancy complications, and thus cryotherapy has been regaining popularity as an alternative treatment.

20.4.1.1 Cervical Cryotherapy Overview

Cryotherapy destroys pathologic tissues of the cervix by cryonecrosis and is used to ablate lesions and the cervical transformation zone by freezing the tissue (Figure 20.6A,B). Cryosurgical units consist of a gas cylinder usually containing either CO_2 or N_2O gas, a regulator, pressure gauge, cryogun and cryoprobe tips (Figure 20.7).[160] Failure to destroy the entire transformation zone to adequate depth is a common cause of cryotherapy failure. Theoretically, residual or recurrent neoplasia occurring in deep gland clefts not frozen to an adequate depth might be at risk for eventually progressing to invasive cancer. Hence, treatment to an adequate depth is essential. Satisfactory treatment will restore a new, normal transformation zone for the cervix. As with all other cervical therapy, destruction of the entire transformation zone, including "at-risk" epithelium in the distal part of the endocervical canal adjacent to the external os, is necessary. As with other ablative treatments for CIN, other than the initial cervical biopsies taken at colposcopy, no tissues are available to submit for histologic analysis.

20.4.1.2 Cervical Cryotherapy Objectives

The objectives of cryotherapy of the cervix are to (1) prevent the progression of CIN to cervical cancer; (2) expose all CIN to tissue lethal temperatures; (3) destroy the entire transformation zone; (4) protect surrounding normal lower genital tract tissue from thermal injury; and (5) minimize treatment side effects of patient discomfort and complications.

20.4.1.3 Prerequisites, Indications, and Contraindications

Prior to cryotherapy, the colposcopic triage guidelines for selecting candidates for ablative treatment of the cervical transformation zone must be satisfied (Table 20.11). These are as follows: (1) The complete (360 degrees) squamocolumnar junction (SCJ) must be identified. (2) The entire lesion, including both the proximal and distal margins must be seen. (3) The cytologic and colposcopic findings must be consistent. (4) The endocervical canal must be free of neoplasia as documented by a negative ECC, a negative cytobrush endocervical sample, or a normal, satisfactory endocervical colposcopy examination. (5) The presence of cancer must be excluded carefully by means of prior cytologic, colposcopic, and histologic assessment.[161,162] Before treatment, a visual triage must be performed that excludes women from cryotherapy who have suspicion for invasive cancer, a lesion larger than 75% of the cervix, or a lesion extending into the endocervical canal more than 3 to 4 mm.[161]

Invasive cervical cancer may present years following a cervical cryosurgical procedure. Cancer after cryotherapy has been found after treatment without a prior careful colposcopic examination (invasive cancer was not excluded).[162] When using a cytology or HPV test screening, colposcopy must always be performed before proceeding to cryotherapy. If women are to

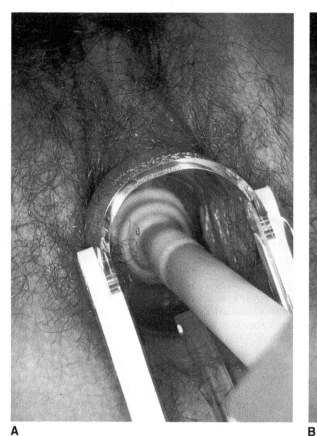
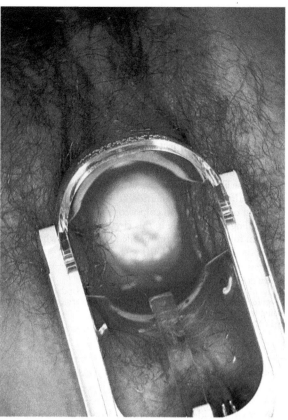

A   **B**

FIGURE 20.6. Cryotherapy of the cervix. **A:** The cryoprobe is placed on the cervix and freeze initiated. **B:** The cervix after the freeze. Most of the frozen area will undergo cryonecrosis.

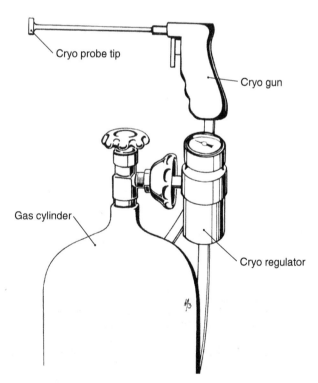

FIGURE 20.7. The cryosurgical unit, consisting of a gas cylinder, pressure gauge, cryogun, and cryoprobe tip.

Labels on figure 20.7: Cryo probe tip; Cryo gun; Gas cylinder; Cryo regulator

receive cryotherapy for reasons other than CIN, that is, for leucorrhea caused by "chronic non-STD cervicitis," cytologic and colposcopic assessment is essential prior to the procedure to exclude significant neoplasia. A normal Papanicolaou (Pap) test without colposcopic evaluation is not sufficiently sensitive to guarantee normality. No cytologic abnormality can be treated by an ablative procedure without prior colposcopic evaluation.[11,42]

The indication for cervical cryotherapy is a biopsy-confirmed CIN 2,3 or persistent CIN 1. Most women with CIN 1 should be observed as discussed previously in Section 20.2.3.1. Otherwise, women who have a CIN 1 lesion that is persistent for 2 years, or desire treatment rather than follow-up, may receive cryotherapy. Many women with small (≤2 quadrants) CIN 2 to 3 lesions also are suitable candidates for cryotherapy. Although available data do not show differences in outcomes, most women with histology read as purely CIN 3 (rather than CIN 2,3) are now treated using an excisional method.

Contraindications to cryotherapy (Table 20.12) include (1) invasive cervical cancer; (2) pregnancy; (3) *in utero* diethylstilbestrol (DES) exposure because of increased risk for cervical stenosis[163]; (4) acute cervicitis (may potentially precipitate acute salpingitis; rule out chlamydia and gonorrhea pretreatment); (5) cryoglobulinemia; (6) positive ECC; or (7) unsatisfactory colposcopic examination. Other contraindications to cervical cryotherapy include the presence of (1) lesions larger than 75% of the cervix; (2) lesions that extend more than 5 mm into the endocervical canal; and (3) exophytic, nodular, or papillary lesions or obstetrical scars that hinder proper application of the cryoprobe tip to the cervical transformation zone.

TABLE 20.11	CERVICAL ABLATION TRIAGE GUIDELINES

- Adequate colposcopic examination
- Pathologic/colposcopic diagnosis agreement
- Absence of endocervical canal neoplasia
- Cervical cancer presence excluded

Adapted from Wright TC, Cox JT, Massad LS, Carlson J, Wilkinson EJ; for the 2001 ASCCP-sponsored Consensus Workshop. 2001 Consensus Guidelines for the management of women with cervical cytological abnormalities and cervical cancer precursors—part II: histological abnormalities. *Am J Obstet Gynecol* 2003;189(1):295–304.

20.4.1.4 Patient Preparation

Women can be offered cryotherapy in an outpatient setting such as a colposcopy clinic when biopsy-confirmed lesions are present. The essence of the biopsy report, reasonable concurrence of cytology and colposcopic impression, and the potential risk for progression should be reviewed with the patient. Cryotherapy may be one of several options for treatment. Other types of management should be discussed, as appropriate. This may include careful observation, electrosurgical loop excision (LEEP), laser (excision or ablation), conization, or perhaps hysterectomy if other indications are present. Written cryotherapy patient education materials given to the patient prior to the procedure may be of benefit. Although cryotherapy is well tolerated by most women, some may wish to have a support person accompany them to the procedure. A pregnancy test should be ordered prior to cryotherapy if there is any uncertainty regarding the patient's pregnancy status. Several studies, however, have shown that cryotherapy during pregnancy does not affect pregnancy outcome.[164-166]

Explain to the patient that cryotherapy causes a "cold" burn to the skin of the cervix. A large blister develops quickly, the abnormal cells die, and a scab (eschar) appears that eventually sloughs away, typically within 1 to 3 weeks. New healthy skin will grow back to cover the treated area. She may notice mild to moderate menstrual-like cramping pain during the two-step procedure, and immediately after the cervix thaws. Use of nonsteroidal anti-inflammatory drugs prior to the procedure may help minimize discomfort. Although not commonly used, a paracervical or intracervical block just prior to the freeze blocks cramping and usually eliminates the postcryotherapy transient facial flushing and headache that some have as the cervix thaws.[167] Following treatment, a very watery, occasionally blood-tinged, malodorous vaginal discharge will be noted. Consequently, the patient will need to use

TABLE 20.12	CERVICAL CRYOTHERAPY CONTRAINDICATIONS

- Cervical cancer
- Prior in-utero DES exposure
- Pregnancy
- Acute cervicitis
- Menstruation
- Cryoglobulinemia
- Positive endocervical curettage
- Inadequate colposcopic examination
- Large cervical lesion
- Lesions extending into endocervical canal
- Lesions with irregular surface contour

sanitary napkins typically for 2 to 4 weeks.[168] Posttreatment examination compliance must be stressed, as follow-up by cytology, with or without colposcopy, at 6 and 12 months or hrHPV testing at 6 to 12 months is necessary to determine if residual disease lingers or recurrent neoplasia returns.

20.4.1.5 Equipment and Supplies

Cryotherapy equipment consists of a compressed gas cylinder that varies in size from small mobile units or large stationary tanks that can be placed on wheeled carts to increase mobility. A cryogun with a handle grip is attached via a line to the gas tank. There is a color-coded pressure gauge on the regulator of most devices to inform the operator if the pressure of the gas is too low (yellow), too high (red) or correct (green). There is a freeze button or trigger on the handle of all cryoguns and most also have a defrost button. The cryoprobe tips vary in size and shape. The operator can chose the size and contour of the tip based on the lesion and the shape of the cervix, then attach the appropriate tip to the end of the cryoprobe.

Several different cryogens (refrigerants or "freezing gases") may be used for cervical cryotherapy. The most common are nitrous oxide (N_2O) and carbon dioxide (CO_2). Liquid nitrogen (LN_2)-containing units are also available but are not widely used for treatment of the cervix. The majority of ambulatory-based cryosurgical units are designed for nitrous oxide. To date, no randomized trials have evaluated the efficacy of specific refrigerants.

Gas cylinders store the refrigerant gas used for cryotherapy. A 20-lb nonsyphon gas cylinder is preferred over a smaller, narrow "E" cylinder, because the 20-lb cylinder provides a greater volume of available gas (Figure 20.8). The larger gas reservoir provides a less rapid reduction of gas pressure and depletion of available gas; consequently, more freezes can be carried out in succession without losing pressure and less frequent cylinder refilling is required. Smaller cryosurgical cylinders carry the distinct disadvantage of only having sufficient gas for two to three patients. The efficacy of cryotherapy is directly dependent on maintaining adequate gas pressure

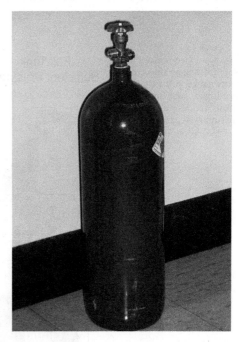

FIGURE 20.8.   A 20-lb cylinder used to store nitrous oxide is the most practical for office procedures.

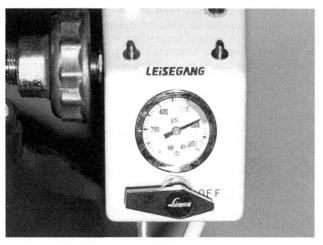

FIGURE 20.9.   A pressure gauge indicates the amount of available nitrous oxide gas for cryotherapy. On this gauge, the arrow within the "blue" zone means cryotherapy can be effectively initiated. Other gauges may indicate the "safe and effective" zone with a green area, with a "red" zone to indicate too high of a pressure, and a "yellow" zone to indicate one that is too low.

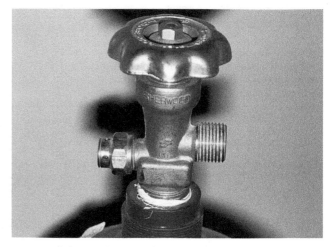

FIGURE 20.10.   The "pop off" valve on the left is designed to release before the gas pressure within the cylinder reaches a dangerously high level.

within the gas cylinder. The cylinder contains liquid refrigerant gas that subsequently produces refrigerant gas from the liquid phase. This gas is depleted from the top of the cylinder and transferred through a pressure gauge and tubing to the cryogun and cryoprobe tip during cryotherapy.

The pressure gauge monitors the pressure of refrigerant gas within the cylinder and is measured as kg per cm^2 or lbs per in^2 (Figure 20.9). There are three demarcated pressure ranges of concern: high, normal, and low pressure. When the pressure is too high, a potential disaster may be imminent. Rapidly discharging gas venting through the top of the cylinder could render the cylinder a potentially damaging missile. A "pop-off" safety valve on the cylinder yoke is designed to prevent this hazardous event from occurring (Figure 20.10). If high pressure is indicated by the needle in the red zone on the gauge, the

"closed" cylinder should be taken to an outdoor location and the pressure gauge removed from the cylinder. Cautiously opening the cylinder valve allows excess gas pressure to vent to the atmosphere. Another way to deplete slightly increased pressure is to activate the cryogun, which vents refrigerant. Otherwise, assistance can be obtained from the cylinder supplier. Gas cylinders should be stored at room temperature, ideally between 20°C to 30°C (68°F to 86°F), and should be kept away from direct sunlight, as heat increases the pressure of the gas in the cylinder. Excess pressure can damage the cryotherapy unit or break the rupture disk in the safety valve on the regulator.[169]

Cryotherapy may be safely performed when the pressure gauge indicates a normal range (Figure 20.9). However, if the pressure gauge indicates a subnormal or low range, cryotherapy should *never* be performed, as an inadequately shallow area of cryonecrosis may result even though a small amount of tissue is visibly frozen. There are two possible explanations for the low pressure indication (Figure 20.11). The first is that the essential gas phase in the top of the cylinder has been

FIGURE 20.11.   Two reasons for a low pressure reading on the cryosurgical pressure gauge: sufficient liquid but depleted gas, and insufficient liquid nitrous oxide and, thus, an inadequate supply of gas.

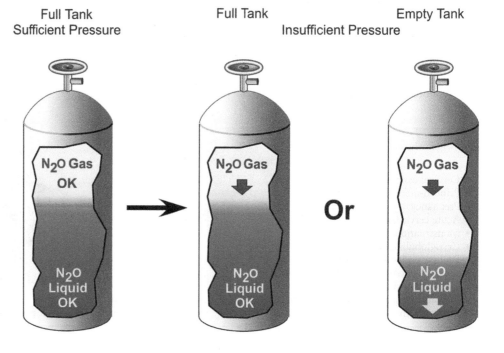

depleted to an insufficient pressure level, even though there is still sufficient liquid refrigerant gas remaining in the bottom of the cylinder. This problem can be avoided by scheduling patients requiring cryotherapy sufficiently far apart to allow ample time for regeneration of gas from the liquid phase to the upper gas phase. This will raise the gas pressure back to the normal range. The time required for gas regeneration may be reduced by placing the cylinder in a warmer environment, either directly in sunlight or near a warm radiator/vent. Careful monitoring of the pressure is essential, however, because rapid warming can generate dangerously high gas pressures. A low-level pressure can also occur when there is an inadequate amount of liquid refrigerant in the gas cylinder to generate sufficient gas. In this case, the cylinder should be refilled with nitrous oxide. It may be difficult to estimate how much usable gas remains in the cylinder, particularly when the pressure gauge indicates normal pressure prior to freezing. If sufficient pressure cannot be adequately maintained throughout a typical cryotherapy procedure, as indicated by the needle on the gauge dropping from the green to the yellow area, the cylinder should be refilled.

The cryogun, a handheld device resembling a gun with a trigger and barrel, is used to control and direct the procedure (Figure 20.12). Cryoprobe tips attach to the end of the barrel and are the part that contacts the mucosal or skin surface. The cryogun is activated by depressing a button, or trigger, or by extending a trigger forward in a locked position (depending on the design of cryotherapy equipment). Defrost is activated by releasing the trigger or, on one type of cryosurgical unit, by depressing a second button. Some units have an independent on/off switch located on the gunstock or pressure gauge housing.

Cryoprobe tips are hollow and made of a metal that conducts heat well. They come in different sizes and shapes for cervical cryotherapy (Figure 20.13). The 25- and 19-mm diameter probe tips are the most commonly used sizes for treatment of CIN. The most commonly used probe tips are flat, or are cones with, or without, a nipple-shaped tip. When a nipple shaped tip is used, the tip projection should not be more than 5 mm. Nipple-shaped probe tips with a central projection longer than 5 mm should never be used on the cervix, as this increases the risk of cervical stenosis and moves the SCJ too far up the canal for future colposcopic evaluation. Nipple-shaped probe tips do not produce better treatment outcomes. If any cervical lesion is not completely encompassed within the cryo ice ball (frozen tissue) following

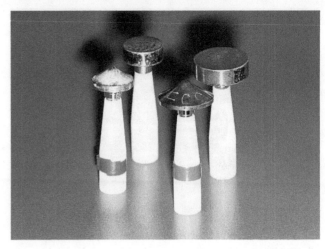

FIGURE 20.13.   19-mm and 25-mm diameter flat- and cone-shaped cryoprobe tips used for treating the cervix.

the first freeze, overlap treatment using a flat probe tip applied to lesional tissue outside the initial ice ball is required. Otherwise, the entire cervical lesion should be encompassed within the initial ice ball.

When attaching probe tips to the cryogun barrel, the tip should be fastened snugly. Some models have rubber O-rings that prevent leakage of gas between the probe and barrel joint (Figure 20.14). An extra supply of O-rings should always be available, since they occasionally dry, crack and/or rupture during use, or fall off and are lost during changing of the tip. When an O-ring is missing or damaged, a spray of gas at the joint may obscure the probe tip placement, and the freezing temperature of the spray can be painful. The long, thin, narrow tube that delivers gas through the barrel, shown in Figure 20.15 as projecting up to 2 inches beyond the end of the barrel, and located inside of the cryoprobe tip, should always be protected when not in use with a secured probe tip to prevent the fragile tube from accidental bending and breaking. Such damage would require purchase of a new cryogun and tubing. Ideally, scavenger tubing should be attached to the cryosurgical unit exhaust port (usually found on the pressure gauge) to vent the gas safely to an external location, particularly if the refrigerant is nitrous oxide.[170] This is because nitrous oxide has been

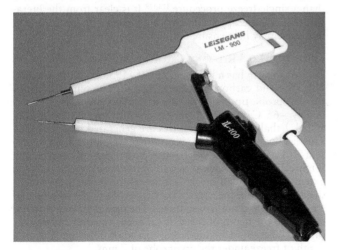

FIGURE 20.12.   Two types of cryoguns used for cryosurgery. The top unit has a single trigger, and the bottom one has two buttons—one to initiate the freeze and one to defrost.

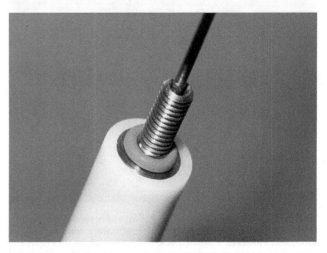

FIGURE 20.14.   Rubber "O rings" prevent leakage of gas between the barrel and cryoprobe tip joint.

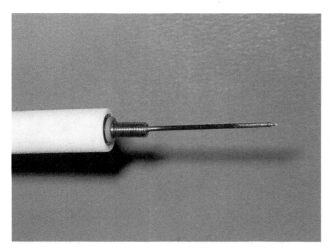

FIGURE 20.15.   The fragile narrow tube delivers gas to the cryoprobe tip. It is susceptible to damage if not properly protected.

shown to increase the risk of genetic defects in offspring of men exposed to this gas, and the risk of spontaneous abortion in females.

Supplies necessary for cryotherapy include a small amount of water-soluble gel, gloves, a vaginal speculum, vaginal side-wall retractor (when necessary), and large cotton swabs. A thin coating of water-soluble gel is applied to the cryoprobe tip prior to cryotherapy. The gel assists transfer of heat and also permits easy release of the probe tips from the frozen tissue following cryotherapy. A vaginal sidewall retractor, tongue blade, condom, or glove finger tube placed over the vaginal speculum may partially rectify obscuring vaginal sidewall prolapse, when present, and help protect the vaginal wall from inadvertent adherence to the freezing probe tip. Because the depth of the freeze can be estimated from the number of millimeters of ice ball extension around the cryoprobe tip, a measuring device such as the "freeze ball scale" depicted in Figure 20.16 is a more objective measure for determining ice ball extension.[171] However, with experience the extension of the ice ball in millimeters can usually be estimated with reasonable accuracy.

Following use, probe tips need to be disinfected, using a compatible product as recommended by the unit manufacturer.

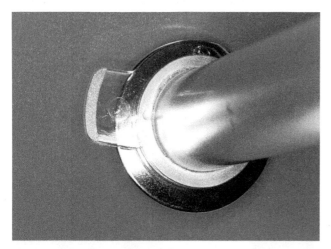

FIGURE 20.16.   A 7-mm lateral ice ball spread beyond the cryoprobe edge assures adequate depth of lethal temperature zone and can be estimated. However, a plastic freeze-ball scale, such as seen here, can be used to more accurately measure the lateral spread of freeze and determine adequate treatment termination.

When disinfecting with liquid agents, such as glutaraldehyde, keep the inside of the probe tip dry. Use of a screw-type plug in the probe tip during cleaning should prevent problems.

20.4.1.6 Principles of Cryotherapy

20.4.1.6.1 HEAT TRANSFER

An important principle of physics is that heat is transferred between entities, as opposed to cold being added to an entity. As an example, your home refrigerator's condenser removes heat from the refrigerator to lower the temperature inside and transfers the heat to the environment. During cryotherapy of the cervix, heat is removed from the cervix to the cryoprobe tip at a rate faster than heat can be delivered to the cervix through blood flow from the cervical branches of uterine arteries.

During cryotherapy, gas exits the cylinder and travels through the pressure gauge, down the tubing to the cryogun. Gas then travels through the barrel of the gun and exits through a very narrow tube positioned within the hollow cryoprobe tip (Figure 20.15) where it expands in the tip. Gas expands rapidly from the narrow tube into the hollow probe tip, causing a drop in temperature via the Joule-Thomson effect (adiabatic principle of gas expansion).[172]

20.4.1.6.2 CELLULAR INJURY AND CELL DEATH

The final temperature produced and the duration of freeze determines tissue injury. Temperatures of less than –20°C are required for tissue necrosis.[173] Tissue frozen transiently at 0°C to –20°C remains viable. The exact reason for cellular injury secondary to thermal damage from cryotherapy is not known specifically. However, it is postulated that intracellular and intercellular ice crystals form, producing dehydration in adjoining cells. The cellular membranes are pierced by the ice crystals that form, releasing the intracellular contents and causing vascular thrombosis and microcirculatory failure, anoxia, and ischemia.[174–176]

A rapid freeze with a slow defrost is the most effective means of inducing tissue damage. A slow freeze and rapid defrost technique is less effective. Modern cryosurgical equipment provides for a quick freeze as long as the pressure in the tank is adequate. The World Health Organization's recommendation for cryotherapy technique is 3 minutes freeze followed by 5 minutes of thaw followed by another 3 minutes of freeze.[177] An alternative approach to monitoring the process of cryotherapy is to continue until a 7-mm lateral spread of ice ball freeze from the margin of the cryoprobe tip is accomplished (Figure 20.16).[161] A freeze-thaw-freeze (double-freeze) treatment is more effective than a single-freeze procedure.[178,179] It is clear from the literature that cryotherapy is effective, but greater standardization in technique may help ensure optimal outcomes.

20.4.1.6.3 RELEVANT CRYOTHERAPY TEMPERATURES

Liquid nitrogen has a boiling point of –195.8°C, nitrous oxide –89.5°C, and carbon dioxide –78.5° C. The temperature of the cryoprobe tip, using a nitrous oxide system, is approximately –65°C to –75°C during cryotherapy. As previously stated, lethal tissue temperatures are generated below –20°C. The leading edge of the expanding ice ball, which represents 0°C, is the clinical reference parameter for cryotherapy (Figure 20.17). The lateral spread of freeze as measured by the extent of the ice ball on the surface of the tissue is defined as the distance from the edge of the cryoprobe to the interface of frozen tissue and nonfrozen tissue. The lateral spread of freeze equates to the depth of freeze in an approximately one-to-one ratio.[180] Thereby, a 7-mm lateral spread of freeze equates to a depth of freeze under the cryoprobe of 7 mm.

During cryotherapy, two clinically relevant temperature zones are produced within the ice ball (Figure 20.17). The lethal zone is the frozen area located between the cryoprobe

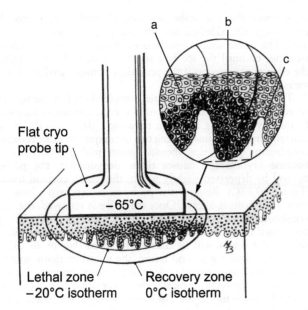

Flat cryo probe tip

−65°C

Lethal zone
−20°C isotherm

Recovery zone
0°C isotherm

FIGURE 20.17.   A cryo ice ball on squamous epithelium with CIN 2, demonstrating the visible ice-tissue interface or 0°C isotherm, the −20°C isotherm, and the temperature at the cryoprobe tip (−65°C). The lethal zone (**insert a**) represents the ice ball volume between the cryoprobe tip and the −20°C isotherm. The recovery zone (**insert b**) represents the ice ball area between the −20°C isotherm and the 0°C isotherm. Cells located in the lethal zone (**insert a**) will not remain viable, but cells located in the recovery zone (**insert b**) will be temporarily frozen but viable. Cells lateral to the 0°C isotherm (**insert c**) are not frozen and, thus, not altered by the procedure.

tip and −20°C isotherm. Tissue in this area will not survive the freeze. However, a more peripherally located recovery zone is represented by frozen tissue with temperatures between −20°C and 0°C. Tissue in the recovery zone is temporarily frozen during the procedure but will remain viable after defrosting. The recovery zone equates to frostbite. The recovery zone generated by most cryosurgical units represents the most peripheral 2-mm rim of frozen tissue adjoining the leading margin of the ice ball.[160,180]

20.4.1.6.4 CRYONECROSIS STAGES

Cervical tissue responds to the thermal insult in a characteristic fashion after cryotherapy. Erythema and hyperemia are noted immediately following cryotherapy at, and surrounding, the treatment site. Within the next 24 to 48 hours, bullae or local edema associated with vesicular formation develops. Thereafter, an eschar covers the treated site, followed by a reepithelialization and neovascularization. During the healing stages, epithelial tissue, stroma and blood vessels grow horizontally from the periphery and crater base of the wound to fill the tissue void. Loop capillaries extend vertically from the horizontal vessels to the epithelium. When viewed colposcopically from above, a fine linear or radial punctation pattern of neovascularization, extending from the periphery toward the os (much like spokes of a bicycle wheel) may be noted. This is a normal finding and can be confirmed by the lack of associated acetowhite epithelium or other colposcopic signs of neoplasia (excluding leukoplakia). Reepithelialization is complete for nearly 50% of patients at 6 weeks posttreatment. Reparative and inflammatory cytologic changes may be observed for 3 to 4 months after therapy.

20.4.1.6.5 IMMUNOLOGIC RESPONSE

The direct thermal effects of cryotherapy determine eventual treatment success. Neoplasia within the lethal zone is readily destroyed by cryonecrosis. However, adjoining tissue temporarily frozen in the recovery zone and more peripherally positioned nonfrozen residual minor neoplasia may regress following cryotherapy through the actions of the immune system. After cryotherapy debulks a large, central viral (HPV) load, the immune system may be better able to eradicate surrounding low-grade residual disease. This assumption is based on anecdotal evidence noted by many clinicians. The specifics of the immune response in relation to cryotherapy, however, are poorly understood. One recent finding in a large randomized trial in South Africa that treated all women by cryotherapy in the treatment arm of the trial who were HPV positive or had an acetowhite cervical finding on visual inspection was long-term postcryo reduction in incident (new) CIN when compared to controls not receiving cryotherapy.[181] This suggests that cryo either boosted the immune response to HPV or that maturation of the cervical transformation zone postcryo, or both, reduce the risk of new HPV exposure causing CIN.

The potential adjunctive effect of the immune system on cryotherapy outcomes is further supported by evidence that patients who are immunosuppressed (i.e., AIDS) have very poor outcomes when treated by cryotherapy, in contrast to better cure rates experienced by immunocompetent patients. Studies have found failure rates among HIV-infected women treated with cryotherapy to be as high as 40.5% at 12-month follow-up, compared to noninfected women who exhibited a 15.8% failure rate.[182] Other studies have shown similar rates of failure at 36 months after treatment with cryotherapy. As with non–HIV-infected women, complications of cryotherapy are mostly minor and do not differ in frequency between HIV-positive and HIV-negative women.[183] Moreover, immunosuppressed women treated by excisional methods, such as electrosurgical loop excision, have better cure rates than do women treated by cryotherapy.

20.4.1.7 Cryotherapy Procedure

Prior to initiating cryotherapy, one must review and satisfy the treatment triage guidelines for ablative therapy. Informed consent may be obtained once the colposcopist has fully informed the patient of the procedural details, risks, and potential complications. Prophylactic treatment with short-acting nonsteroidal anti-inflammatory drugs approximately 60 minutes prior to treatment may help block prostaglandin-mediated tissue effects and, hence, reduce cramping associated with treatment. Randomized trials have demonstrated a reduction in pain associated with the procedure with the use of an intracervical or paracervical block with local anesthesia.[167,184] Cryotherapy is best scheduled immediately following the patient's normal menstrual period to ensure the patient is not pregnant and to allow time for the majority of the eschar to slough before the next menses, thereby reducing the potential for increased cramping secondary to reduced menstrual outflow through the cervix. In general, women who are pregnant or suspected to be pregnant should have cryotherapy deferred. A precryotherapy pregnancy test may be reasonable when the patient is not on reliable birth control. Some clinicians also routinely screen for *Chlamydia trachomatis* and *Neisseria gonorrhoeae* prior to initiating treatment, as occult cervicitis due to either of these sexually transmitted diseases (STDs) can develop into pelvic inflammatory disease (PID) postcryotherapy.

Before initiating cryotherapy, sufficient gas pressure must be available within the nitrous oxide cylinder, as indicated by the pressure gauge. Following the application of acetic acid to the cervix, the cervical lesion should be visualized with the colposcope to determine size and disease distribution. Cryotherapy is best performed when the cervical mucosa is moist. Next, an appropriate, room-temperature cervix-conforming cryoprobe tip should be selected to cover the lesion and transformation zone. Lesions that are laterally positioned, or located more than 3 to 5 mm within the endocervical canal, will not be ablated by cryotherapy.[185] Once the size and distribution of the lesion has been colposcopically delineated, its use during the procedure is not necessary. In fact, attempting to visualize cryotherapy through the use of a colposcope tends to cause overestimation of the lateral spread of freeze distance and, thus, premature treatment termination.[171]

Once the cryoprobe is carefully visualized to be clear of the vaginal walls, activating a trigger or switch on the cryogun will initiate the freeze. Placement of the end of the cone or nipple projection, if present, into the cervical os will help prevent probe tip displacement during the activation of the freeze (Figure 20.18A,B). The cryoprobe position should be steadily maintained on the cervix. Once the freeze is activated, the cryoprobe tip will adhere to the cervix. When necessary, gentle retraction or forward pressure on the cervix may straighten prolapsing vaginal sidewalls to improve visualization. If the vaginal walls come in contact with the probe, gently rotate or twist the cryogun, or gently try to coax the adhering vaginal wall off the edge of the cryoprobe tip with a cotton-tipped swab or spatula. However, if it is clear that a significant area of the probe tip is adhered to the vaginal wall, or if these steps are unsuccessful, the probe should be allowed to thaw enough to dislodge the sidewall and the freeze subsequently reinitiated. The freeze should continue for 3 minutes if using timed freezing, or until the ice ball reaches at least 7 mm beyond the edge of the cryotip if the procedure is monitored by direct measurement.[161]

The probe should be defrosted completely before the tip can be removed freely from the frozen cervix. Defrost is initiated by quickly squeezing and then releasing ("flashing") the cryogun trigger several times. Using this technique, all nitrous oxide cryotherapy probe tips should defrost within 6 seconds.[160] Because cryotherapy causes tissue dehydration, the probe tip will be depressed slightly within the frozen cervical tissue (Figure 20.18C). Remove the probe from the frozen base as soon as defrosting allows. Once the probe is removed, the cervix should then be reinspected to ensure that the cryo ice ball is positioned in the intended area of treatment. A frozen depression of the cervix will be transiently noted (Figure 20.18D). Prior to initiating a second freeze, the icy-white tissue should have returned to a normal pink color and the temporary depression also be resolving. Typically, the cervix will defrost naturally over a 5-minute time span. The cryoprobe also may be activated in a defrost mode to help speed up the thawing process.

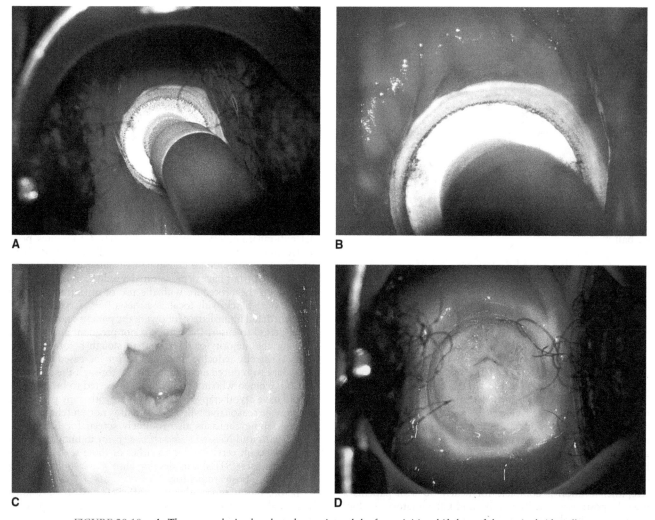

A

B

C

D

FIGURE 20.18. **A:** The cryoprobe is placed on the cervix and the freeze initiated if clear of the vaginal sidewalls. **B:** A 1–2 mm ice ball is seen shortly after beginning the freeze. **C:** The cervix immediately following cryotherapy (notice a frozen depressed area caused by the dehydration of cryotherapy). **D:** A wide 5- to 7-mm ice ball extends peripheral to the central depressed area formerly occupied by the cryoprobe tip (with partial thawing, the cervix begins to resemble its baseline appearance).

Cryotherapy should then be repeated a second time as necessary to completely cover lesions and ablate the entire transformation zone. A freeze-thaw-freeze, or double-freeze technique, is recommended for cervical cryotherapy. Researchers have demonstrated a reduced failure rate (19% from 49%) when a double-freeze method is utilized, when compared with a single freeze.[161,178,179] Because the cervical epithelium and stroma are still very cold (but not frozen), the second freeze should occur much more quickly. With large lesions or large transformation zones, multiple overlapping freeze applications may be required to ensure complete coverage (Figure 20.19A–C).

Some women will experience a transient vasomotor (vagal) symptomatology with flushing, lightheadedness, headache, bradycardia and, occasionally, tonic–clonic activity due to the transient hypoxemia. It may be prudent to have women remain in a lying position for a brief period of time following cryotherapy to prevent syncope. A simple assessment of pulse rate immediately postcryo may help to predict this occurrence. As mentioned previously, one advantage of a precryo intracervical or paracervical block is that this common postprocedure vasovagal symptomatology is usually prevented.

Debridement of the eschar 1 or 2 days postcryo was previously considered to be helpful in reducing the volume and malodor of the discharge, but subsequently has not been demonstrated to be clinically useful or cost-effective.[168]

20.4.1.8 Patient Education

Patients should be instructed that a very watery, malodorous, slightly blood-tinged vaginal discharge will be noted for the subsequent 3 to 4 weeks.[168] Patients should be instructed to wear pads, rather than tampons, to absorb this discharge, and pelvic rest should be encouraged during this healing phase. Nonsteroidal anti-inflammatory drugs may minimize immediate postoperative discomfort. If present, uterine cramping usually resolves within 24 to 48 hours. Adequate fluid intake should be advised to replace fluid lost in the excessive hydrorrhea that often follows the cervical freeze. The patient should be instructed to call or be seen if fever, unusual bleeding, or severe pelvic pain develops. Finally, the patient should clearly understand that 5% to 15% of women treated by cryotherapy will have residual disease. Therefore, follow-up visits as outlined in the ASCCP and ACOG guidelines are mandatory to determine therapeutic cure.[11,42]

20.4.1.9 Follow-Up

Unless the patient experiences one of the complications previously discussed, she does not need follow-up until that recommended posttreatment for any of the surgical procedures for CIN 2,3 (see Section 20.2.3.3 and Figure 20.5E: *Management of Women with Biopsy-confirmed Cervical Intraepithelial Neoplasia Grade 2 and 3*) (Figure 20.20A–D).

20.4.1.10 Side Effects and Complications

All women undergoing cryotherapy of the cervix experience some side effects, including a profuse, malodorous, blood-tinged hydrorrhea (watery vaginal discharge) lasting 3 to 4 weeks.[168] The volume of hydrorrhea can exceed more than 100 mL per day for some women. Most women notice

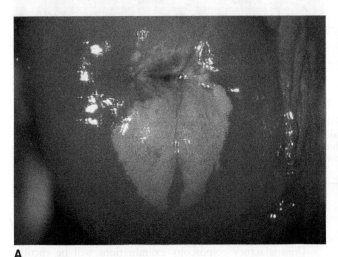

A

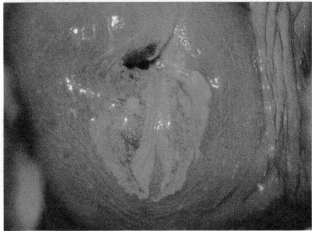

B

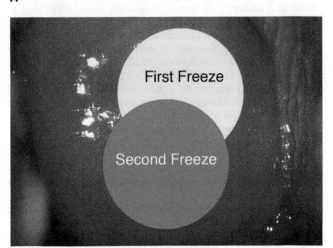

C

FIGURE 20.19. **A,B:** Cervix with large neoplasia extending to the distal ectocervix. **C:** Schematic of overlapping freezes (1 and 2) to treat the entire transformation zone and lesion.

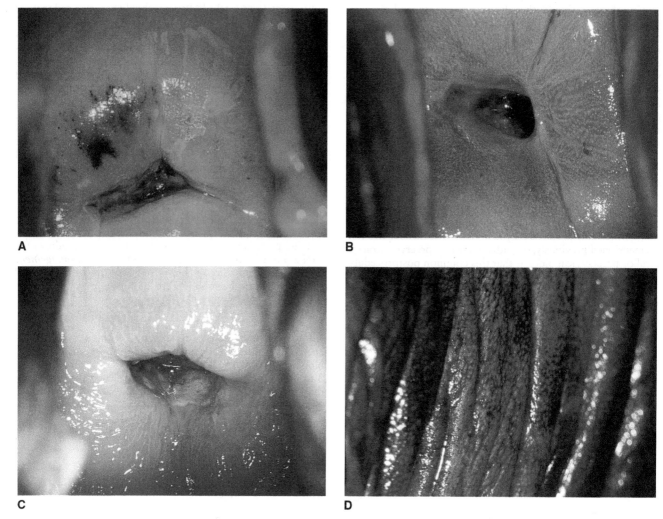

FIGURE 20.20. **A–C:** Recurrent and residual disease of the cervix is seen following cryotherapy; acetowhite areas of CIN 1 can be seen on the cervix after treatment. **D:** VaIN may be the source for an abnormal Pap smear following cryotherapy when the cervix is entirely normal. A diffusely iodine-negative area of the vagina can be seen in this woman following cryotherapy. Her biopsy diagnosis of low-grade HPV changes correlates with her LSIL Pap smear and normal cervical colposcopic findings.

menstrual-like, crampy uterine pain during cryotherapy, but if it occurs following the procedure it usually resolves within 24 to 48 hours.

Severe complications secondary to cryotherapy are quite unusual. The main complication is inadvertent injury or freezing of the adjacent vagina, which can be avoided by careful visualization, selection of a smaller (19 mm) cryoprobe tip, placement of a vaginal sidewall retraction device or condom, steady positioning, and discontinuation of cryotherapy if adhering vaginal sidewalls cannot be freed from the cryoprobe tip. Heavy bleeding is a very unusual postoperative complication, but mild bleeding/spotting may be noted approximately 7 to 10 days following treatment as the eschar sloughs from the cervix.

Although postcryotherapy PID is far less common than in the era prior to routine screening for chlamydia and gonorrhea, it may occasionally be precipitated by the procedure, particularly when asymptomatic infection with either of these organisms has not been previously identified.[161] In order to prevent salpingitis, women who are found to have acute cervicitis, or are positive on testing for either chlamydia or gonorrhea, should be first treated with an appropriate antibiotic prior to initiating cryotherapy.[186] Symptoms in the <1% who

develop postcryo PID will usually develop within 1 week of cryotherapy.

Unsatisfactory colposcopy examinations will be encountered in a minority of women following cryotherapy due to migration of the SCJ into the endocervical canal.[187] Moderate or clinically significant cervical stenosis is rare but may occur in approximately 2% or less of women (Figure 20.21).[3] Most of the literature that discusses cervical stenosis does not clearly define the term. One study did define "cervical stenosis" as a cervix requiring dilation by a provider. In this study, 1.4% of women required dilation.[3] Women exposed to DES *in utero* are especially at an increased risk for cervical stenosis.[163,188]

Cervical incompetence would be an extremely rare complication of cryotherapy. Although limited data are available, there is no evidence to support impaired fertility or other negative obstetric outcomes such as preterm labor, increased cesarean section rates, or higher spontaneous abortion rates following cryotherapy.[189]

Postoperative Pap smears and colposcopic examinations may detect parakeratosis (Figure 20.22A,B). Typically, postcryo parakeratosis is in a linear pattern with radial extension outward from the cervical os. A more diffuse fine granular texture to the area treated may also be seen.

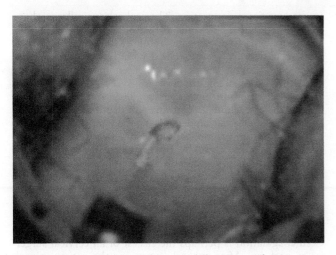

FIGURE 20.21.   Mild cervical stenosis following cryotherapy.

20.4.1.11 Outcomes

Just as with any other form of therapy, treatment failures occur with cryotherapy. Based on a meta-analysis of seven randomized controlled trials, cure rates in relation to severity of cervical dysplasia have been reported to range between 90% and 100% for CIN 1, 75% and 96% for CIN 2 and 71% and 92% for CIN 3/CIS.[161] Immunodeficient women suffer from very poor cryotherapy cure rates. Satisfactory cryotherapy outcomes correlate better with lesion size and not necessarily severity of disease, although these two parameters are proportionally related.[3,190] High-grade cervical lesions tend to be morphometrically larger in size and extend more deeply into gland clefts.[180] Therefore, larger high-grade lesions may be more effectively treated by an excisional method to ensure adequate therapeutic depth as well as to rule out occult invasion.

Treatment failure tends to arise in patients presenting with scarred, misshaped cervices from previous pregnancies, exophytic or nodular cervical lesions (poor probe/tissue adherence), or more commonly, lesions extending within the endocervical canal. Cryonecrosis is limited to no more than the distal 5 mm of the endocervical canal, although this may be variable depending on how narrow or how patulous is the os. Greater treatment failure rates have been noted for cervical lesions located at the 3 o'clock and 9 o'clock positions where the cervical branches of the uterine artery are located.[191] These areas of the cervix are relatively warmer and more resistant to cryotherapy effects than are lesions in the cooler 12 o'clock and 6 o'clock positions. Although a long-term analysis of 2839 patients treated by cryotherapy demonstrated a negligible risk for residual disease,[192] cervical cancer has been reported in women following cryotherapy of CIN.[162,193] Moderately abnormal cytologic findings after cryotherapy are worrisome, particularly when the endocervix is constricted and the SCJ is inaccessible. When recurrent or residual CIN is identified following any ablative procedure, an excisional approach to retreatment is recommended in both the ASCCP and ACOG guidelines.[11,42] Of course, this should follow proper preliminary colposcopic examination with histologic sampling.

20.4.1.12 Documentation and Coding

The specifics of the cryotherapy procedure should be fully documented. A standardized paper form or computer-based format may be helpful, so that necessary notations can be comprehensively recorded. The procedural report should include pertinent history, cytologic, colposcopic, and histologic findings; whether a single or multiple freeze were used and the duration of the freeze; dimension of ice ball(s) or more importantly, an estimation of the measurement of the lateral spread of the freeze; complications, and follow-up plans. A patient management tracking log should be maintained to ensure appropriate posttreatment follow-up. Correct documentation of cryotherapy is essential for financial purposes as well. Use proper CPT codes to minimize audit difficulties.

It is advisable to obtain informed consent prior to performing cryotherapy. As with all informed consent, the nature of the disease, the procedure to be performed, reasonable risks and complications involved, the prognosis with and without treatment, possible alternative procedures, and the opportunity to ask questions must be acknowledged in writing by the patient following explanation by the clinician. A witness should also sign and date the informed consent. A relatively small investment in time to ensure appropriate notification of potential adverse but accidental outcomes should be considered a wise and necessary obligation.

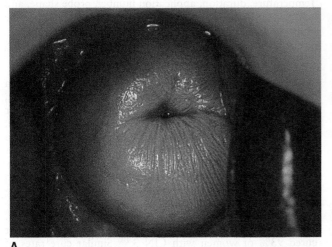

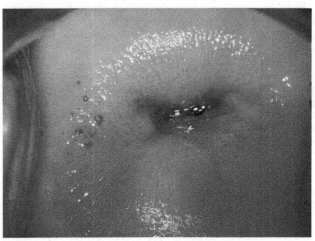

A   **B**

FIGURE 20.22.   **A,B:** Parakeratosis seen following cryotherapy of the cervix is a normal finding and may also be observed in an accompanying Pap smear. The surface appears granular and not smooth.

20.4.2 Cold Coagulation of the Cervix

20.4.2.1 Introduction

Cryotherapy and laser vaporization are the two most common cervical ablation therapies used in the United States for the treatment of CIN. Cold coagulation is another ablative procedure for the treatment of CIN, more commonly used in Europe and Australia.[194–203] As with other ablative procedures, since no tissue is available for histologic evaluation, pretreatment colposcopy and biopsy are required. Proper treatment should eradicate disease and allow the regeneration of normal healthy epithelium. Although not widely utilized in North America, this relatively simple approach expands the therapeutic options available to women. As with other ablative procedures, the objectives of cold coagulation are to (1) expose all CIN to lethal tissue temperatures; (2) eradicate the complete transformation zone; (3) minimize injury to normal tissue and posttreatment complications; and, most importantly, (4) prevent cervical cancer.

20.4.2.2 Prerequisites, Indications, and Contraindications

Because cold coagulation is an ablative therapy, specific pretreatment conditions must be met prior to initiating the procedure. These include visualizing the entire SCJ and full extent of any cervical lesion; documenting cytologic, colposcopic, and histologic concordance; ensuring an endocervical canal free of neoplasia; and excluding the presence of cervical cancer by prior clinical examination and laboratory tests. Patients who do not satisfy these triage principles are better managed by a diagnostic excision procedure.

The primary indication for cold coagulation is the presence of CIN, even though some benign conditions may be treated in the same manner. Cold coagulation is contraindicated in women with an unsatisfactory colposcopic examination, evidence of glandular neoplasia or cervical cancer, or discordant colposcopic and laboratory diagnoses.

20.4.2.3 Patient Preparation

Prior to undergoing cold coagulation, women should be informed of their condition, treatment options, pretreatment preparation, expected reaction during therapy, and posttreatment care. Patient education pamphlets are generally well accepted and serve as a printed source of information that may be reviewed at a later date. Premenopausal women are best scheduled immediately following menstruation. A urine pregnancy test may be necessary should any uncertainties arise concerning their current risk for pregnancy. An informed consent document pertaining to cold coagulation should be read and signed by the patient before surgery is initiated. Women may benefit by taking a nonsteroidal anti-inflammatory drug several hours prior to cold coagulation to minimize potential procedure-induced uterine cramping. As with other outpatient treatment procedures, pretreatment intracervical or paracervical block with local anesthetic should significantly decrease or eliminate discomfort.

20.4.2.4 Equipment and Supplies

A Semm coagulator is a medical device able to generate temperatures of 100°C in order to effectively destroy tissue.[195] "Cold coagulation" is a misnomer, as this device should not be confused with a cryosurgical unit that destroys tissue with freezing temperatures. The "cold" term implies coagulation by relatively cooler temperatures than those generated by electrocoagulation/electrocautery. The electrical device heats thermosounds (probes) to the selected temperature that is sufficient to produce tissue desiccation. The probes are similar in shape to cryotherapy probes; some are flat and others are rounded at the tip so as to achieve maximum tissue/probe adherence. These reusable probes are coated with Teflon to make posttreatment cleaning easier. No other equipment is required other than optional anesthetics.[194]

Cold coagulation causes tissue desiccation sufficient to destroy the epithelium and stroma to a depth of 3 to 4 mm.[194] The extent of desiccation depends on the temperature selected and the duration of application. In practical terms, the cold coagulator cooks tissue by invoking a rapid dehydration. Because of the high temperatures, relatively brief application times are required. Excessively prolonged application causes increased scar formation and delayed healing.

20.4.2.5 Cold Coagulation Procedure

Cold coagulation is perhaps the easiest of all cervical surgeries to perform. After properly preparing the patient, visualizing the cervical transformation zone and making sure that the vaginal walls are not in contact with the area to be treated, the coagulator is activated. Once the probe reaches 100°C, the rounded tip is placed into the vagina and onto the ectocervix, centrally positioned at the external os for approximately 20 seconds. Care must be taken to not inadvertently touch the vulva or vagina while introducing the hot probe. Therefore, lateral sidewall retractors may be necessary to protect women with prolapsing vaginal walls. Once the probe is placed on the cervix, the clinician may hear soft crackling or snapping noises as the tissue is treated. Next, a flat probe is used to treat each quadrant of the ectocervix for 20 seconds. Since the probe usually covers only 1 quadrant of the cervix at a time, four overlapping treatments are usually required to ablate the entire transformation zone.[194] However, a small cervical transformation zone may need only two or three treatments. Therefore, total treatment time should not exceed 2 minutes. Local anesthesia or paracervical blocks are not always necessary; however, it is probably safer to administer anesthetic, particularly for women with very large transformation zones.

Patients may take nonsteroidal anti-inflammatory medication for any postoperative uterine cramping or pelvic pain. Women are free to resume sexual intercourse immediately. Because postoperative vaginal discharge or bleeding is minimal, tampon use is not essential. A follow-up appointment should be scheduled before the patient is discharged from the treatment visit, or she can be placed in a follow-up notification system. The surgical procedure should be fully documented. Temperature, duration, application number, probe shape, and complications, if applicable, can be noted in the operative note. Appropriate follow-up should be discussed.

20.4.2.6 Side Effects, Complications, and Outcomes

Few side effects and complications are experienced with cold coagulation. Women may notice mild uterine cramping, although a significant number experience no side effects either during or following the treatment.[198] Mild vaginal discharge, spotting, and pelvic pain may be noted for a brief duration after the procedure.[199] Since endocervical canal lesions are not treated by cold coagulation, cervical stenosis is a rare postoperative complication. Cold coagulation appears to have no adverse effect on future fertility, although most studies are limited by inclusion of small numbers of women.

Excellent cure rates can be expected with cold coagulation. In one study based on cytologic follow-up, a single treatment cured 93% of women with CIN 3.[200] Similar cure rates of 90% to 97% for treatment of CIN 2 and 3 have been reported by other investigators.[198,201–203] These cure rates compare favorably with those experienced after loop excision, laser, and cryotherapy. An excisional technique is recommended for any primary treatment failures because of a relatively unacceptable cure rate (19%) following a repeat cold coagulation.[200]

Initial studies have examined combining loop electrosurgical excision (LLE) with cold coagulation (CC) as a treatment for CIN to increase favorable outcomes. This two-pronged approach, termed LLECC, has been shown to reduce the proportion of abnormal results at follow-up. A retrospective case-record review of over 650 women treated with LLECC found that of the 576 women initially presenting with high-grade CIN, only 4.2% had abnormal cytologic results 6 months after treatment, decreasing to 0.6% at 12 months.[203] Of the 90 women initially presenting with low-grade CIN, 3.8% had abnormal cytologic results 6 months after treatment and none (0%) at 12 months. Randomized clinical trials are required to confirm these results and to determine whether LLECC is more effective than large loop excision alone.

20.4.3 Carbon Dioxide Laser Surgery for the Cervix

20.4.3.1 Introduction

Carbon dioxide laser surgery permits precise and complete tissue eradication. However, the success of laser surgery depends upon removing all obviously diseased and potentially involved tissue. Laser surgery was widely adopted by many gynecologists in the 1970s and 1980s but began to fall out of favor following the widespread adoption of LEEP beginning in the early 1990s due to the reduced cost, upkeep, and skills required for the latter procedure. Laser, however, continues to be used by some gynecologists in routine practice in offices and, more commonly, in operating rooms. CO_2 laser surgery is a very good procedure in skilled hands.

Various substances in different physical states have been used to produce laser action. Lasers produce nonionizing electromagnetic radiation in the optical and infrared portions of the spectrum. Laser radiation is coherent (all waves are in phase in both space and time), collimated (all rays are virtually parallel), and essentially monochromatic (all waves have the same wavelength, frequency, and color). These characteristics account for the unique directionality of laser light, the predictable and uniform effect the light will have on a particular target, and the enormous intensity of the light, which is achieved by focusing the beam and, thus, concentrating the energy in a small area.

The wavelength, or its reverse, the frequency determines the effect a laser beam will have on biologic tissue. CO_2 laser energy, which is absorbed on the surfaces of tissues with high water content, vaporizes the tissue, producing steam and scattered carbonized particles. Tissue necrosis, caused by thermal denaturing of proteins, occurs within 50 to 100 μm of the crater with limited exposure time (Figure 20.23).

The development of high energy per pulse lasers permits a high maximum power output for very short periods of time. Since thermal damage is time related, even less thermal damage is seen since the high energy per pulse noted with such lasers reduces the opportunity for heat conduction. The inherent hemostatic effect is the result of heat sealing smaller blood vessels in the zone of thermal necrosis. A wider zone of injury, caused by elevated temperature, surrounds the zone of necrosis, but the tissue will recover.

20.4.3.2 Lasers in Cervical Surgery

The laser most commonly used for treating diseases of the lower female genital tract is the CO_2 laser. In order for physicians to best control laser energy, the laser is often used in

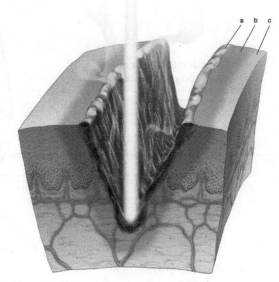

FIGURE 20.23.   The three zones of laser thermal injury. Zone 1 (*a*)—zone of vaporization. Zone 2 (*b*)—tissue necrosis usually <100 μm. Zone 3 (*c*)—further tissue necrosis, which can delay healing.

conjunction with a colposcope or an operating microscope (Figure 20.24) rather than to a pen-like handpiece. The laser beam is delivered to the microscope in one of two ways: either the laser head is attached to the scope directly or an articulated arm containing mirrors connects the laser head to the microscope (colposcope). The scope and laser lenses are parfocal and coaxial, so that the surgical beam is in focus when the microscope is in focus with a matched lens system. The beam is controlled by the surgeon using a gimbaled mirror attached by a joystick (Figure 20.24). The surgical field is unobstructed, and surgery can be performed without touching the target.[204–206]

20.4.3.3 Rationale for Employing the Carbon Dioxide Laser

When properly performed, the advantages of laser surgery over other modalities include the following: (1) microsurgical precision allowing for complete removal of diseased tissue to any depth or breadth required; (2) no-touch surgery with an unobstructed operating field; (3) minimal effect on adjacent normal tissue and rapid healing to normal or near-normal volume with a new SCJ located most often at the level of the external os; (4) quick, virtually painless treatment, which can be performed in an office or clinic in the vast majority of cases; (5) minimal side effects, causes little discharge and minimal complications; (6) in most cases, concomitant hemostasis; (7) a high success rate after first treatment; (8) early identification of persistent disease; and (9) easy retreatment, usually in the office or clinic.[204,207,208]

20.4.3.4 Disease Distribution

Laser cervical surgical procedures are based on the following disease parameters.

20.4.3.4.1 AREA OF SUSCEPTIBILITY

Tissue susceptible to developing squamous cell intraepithelial neoplasia lies between the original SCJ and the histologic os. The transformation zone (the area between the original and new SCJ) is usually transformed into normal squamous epithelium during the phase of reparative metaplasia. Once normal

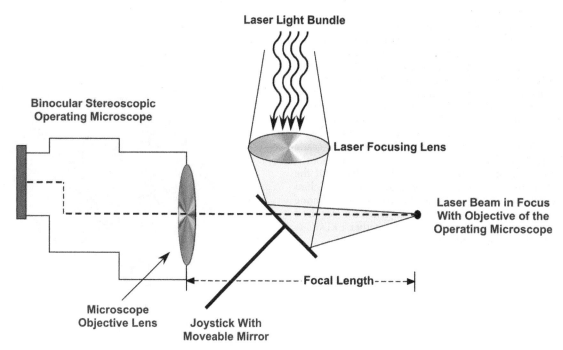

FIGURE 20.24.   Basic instrumentation for the laser for microsurgery. The laser is coupled with the optical system of the colposcope or operating microscope. (Adapted from Wright VC. Laser surgery for cervical intraepithelial neoplasia. In: Wright VC, Lickrish GM, Shier RM, eds. *Basic and Advanced Colposcopy: A Practical Handbook for Treatment* (2nd ed.). Houston, TX: Biomedical Communications, 1995:21–1.)

squamous tissue is formed, it appears to be resistant to the development of CIN and, ultimately, carcinoma. The area of susceptibility diminishes as columnar epithelium is replaced by normal squamous epithelium and as the new SCJ moves toward and, eventually, into the cervical canal. During the dynamic phases of metaplasia, however, atypical metaplastic squamous epithelium can develop in the transformation zone, creating a field of neoplastic potential. Squamous lesions begin at the caudal part of the remaining area of susceptibility and then extend cephalad, becoming histologically more severe in the process.

20.4.3.4.2 Cervical Intraepithelial Lesions Involving Cervical Crypts

CIN can extend into the underlying cervical crypts. Higher-grade lesions (severe dysplasia and CIS) extend into cervical crypts up to 5.2 mm, but in most cases, crypt depth varies between 1.24 and 1.6 mm.[209–211] In CIN 3 lesions (severe dysplasia/CIS), 85% to 95% will have some crypt extension.[204] However, 96% of these cases have depth of disease extension of <2.9 mm. It has been hypothesized that destruction of lesions to a depth of 3.8 mm will eradicate all involved crypts in 99.7% of patients.[210]

20.4.3.4.3 Radial Linear Length

The radial linear length of CIN can vary between 2 and 22 mm, but the usual linear length varies between 6 and 10 mm.[209,211–214] CIN lesions do not extend more than 22 mm up the endocervical canal when measured from the lowermost border of the lesions.[213] Therefore, when planning tissue destruction or removal for a particular patient, the surgeon must consider that the more exposed the columnar epithelium appears, the less likely it is that disease is located high within the endocervical canal. The more endocervical the columnar epithelium, the more likely there is involvement high in the canal. This is very important and helps to determine the correct procedure to remove the CIN.

20.4.3.4.4 Disease Location

The transformation zone recedes into and up the endocervical canal with age.[215,216] In women of reproductive age, CIN lesions do not extend above the level of the internal os.

20.4.3.4.5 Location of Cancer

Invasive squamous cell cancer appears on the canal side of the transformation zone. That is, the worst disease is located centrally,[217] indicating that for ectocervical CIN, sampling the innermost margin provides the most severe histologic information. To exclude invasive cancer for lesions in the canal, the upper margin must be carefully assessed regardless of the histology of the more caudal component.

20.4.3.4.6 The Geometry of CIN as a Guide to its Removal

Accepting the known dimensions of CIN, one can conceptualize the three-dimensional geometry of disease-bearing tissue in a given patient and apply appropriate operative techniques to remove or destroy it.[204,208,209,218] It is obvious that a defect resembling a cylinder best represents the solid geometry of disease regardless of its location.[207,208,212,218,219] Figure 20.25 compares volume of tissue removed with the cylindrical approach and with the cone-shaped method when all potentially involved tissue is incorporated in the specimen and when cure, not just diagnosis, is anticipated.[218] Figure 20.25A depicts ectocervical CIN. The vertical "5-mm" arrows indicate the maximum potential depth of involvement in crypts, and the heavier horizontal "1.9-cm" arrow indicates diameter of the lesion. To surround the arrows, a cone-shaped specimen would be deeper and wider and would include much more normal tissue, but a domed cylinder would match the diseased tissue and incorporate a smaller volume.

When an excision is required, the specimen must also be cylindrical in shape to incorporate lateral crypt involvement (horizontal 5-mm arrows) and the lesion along the surface of the endocervical canal (vertical 1.6-cm arrow). Figure 20.25B illustrates that a cylindrical approach removes half the volume

The Geometry of CIN

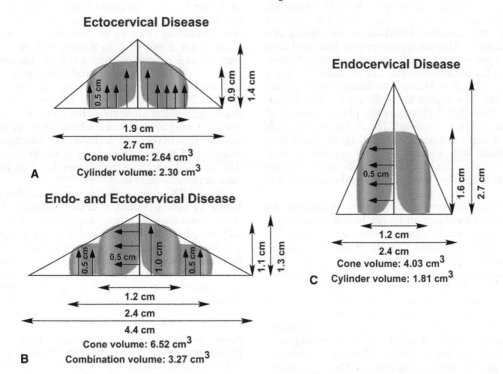

FIGURE 20.25. **A–C:** The measurements of crypt involvement and linear length provide therapeutic guidelines for eradication of CIN. Successful eradication of disease is based upon a cylindrical defect, whether vaporized or excised. The destroyed or removal volume of tissue is less than that with the conical approach. (Adapted from Wright VC. The geometry of cervical intraepithelial neoplasia: an applied guide to its removal. In: Wright VC, Lickrish GM, Shier RM, eds. *Basic and Advanced Colposcopy: A Practical Handbook for Treatment* (2nd ed.). Houston, TX: Biomedical Communications, 1995:19-1–19-7.)

of tissue required by a cone-shaped specimen when diagnosis as well as cure is intended.

Approximately 18% of CIN cases have lesions with a long length, occupying the ectocervix and extending into the endocervical canal. The principles of colposcopy dictate that the disease in the canal must be excised to rule out invasive cancer, since the worst histologic evidence is located centrally. Figure 20.25C illustrates a logical approach to these lesions, that is, a central cylinder excision plus peripheral vaporization that removes disease, establishes a diagnosis, and requires half the volume of tissue excised by a cone-shaped specimen.[207,208,218]

From these concepts, three surgical procedures account for the distribution of CIN.[207,208,218] These procedures include a shallow, dome-shaped cylinder for ectocervical CIN, a tall cylinder for canal disease, and a moderately tall central cylinder surrounded by a donut or "inner tube" configuration (similar in shape to a cowboy hat) for disease occupying the endocervical canal and extending beyond a radius of 8 mm onto the cervix.

20.4.3.5 The Laser Vaporization Procedure for Ectocervical CIN

The following criteria must be fulfilled for laser ablation: (1) cytologic, colposcopic, and histologic information must be correlated to establish an accurate cervical tissue diagnosis; (2) the entire transformation zone must be colposcopically defined; (3) the colposcopist must be certain from the qualitative assessment of the transformation zone that no cancer or AIS is present; and (4) the CIN must occupy the ectocervix at or below the level of the external os with no extension into the endocervical canal (Figure 20.26).

20.4.3.5.1 BASIC SETUP AND INSTRUMENTATION

The patient is comfortably placed in stirrups, and the cervix is exposed by using a bivalve speculum. The cervix is anesthetized with local anesthetic (intracervical block), or a paracervical block can be used. Local infiltration of 1% lidocaine (Xylocaine) with 1:100,000 dilution of epinephrine (pH 4.05) produces a stinging sensation most likely related to its

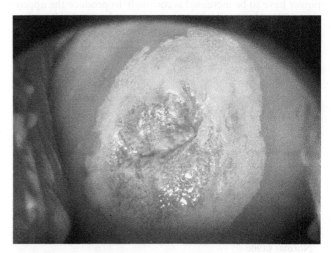

FIGURE 20.26. A colpophotograph of ectocervical CIN 2 that meets the criteria for laser ablation. (Figure reprinted with permission from Wright VC. *Color Atlas of Colposcopy—Cervix, Vagina and Vulva.* Houston, TX: Biomedical Communications, 2003.)

acid pH. The pain can be decreased by adding sodium bicarbonate (1 mEq per mL) at a dilution of 10:1. For example, 5 mL of 1% lidocaine with epinephrine is mixed in the same syringe with 0.5 mL of sodium bicarbonate. This results in a pH of 7.37 (alkaline). Alternately, vasopressin (the total dose not exceeding 1 pressor unit) can be mixed with the 1% lidocaine (pH 6.49) for local anesthesia. The purpose of using a vasoconstricting agent is to decrease the diameter of the blood vessels so that the laser beam's heat will seal them and minimize bleeding. Table 20.13 illustrates the pH of commercial local anesthetics and those modified. The author recommends local infiltration into the posterior cervical lip first, and then lateral infiltration, with injection of the anterior lip last, because the anterior cervical lip appears to be more sensitive than the posterior lip. Slow injections generally produce less discomfort.

A smoke evacuation system is necessary to remove the vapor plume. A handheld suction tip can be positioned in the vagina by an assistant, or the suction device can be attached to the upper blade of the speculum. Custom specula with suction device attachments are commercially available. A trap placed between the speculum and the filter to permit suction of both plume and blood can be helpful should bleeding occur.

The CO_2 laser is attached to a colposcope or operating microscope employing a magnification of 2.5× to 3.5×. This gives an adequate diameter of view of 57 to 80 mm. Although higher magnification offers the advantage of permitting more colposcopic detail, low magnifications allow an operator to see the entire operative field during surgery. The working distance should be 300 mm, which reflects the focal length of the microscope's main objective lens. A matched 300-mm focal lens system is used in the laser system. Thus, when the microscope is in focus, the laser beam will be in focus at the focal plane (in this case, the cervix). The main objective lens of the microscope should be at the same level as the target (cervix). A small beam diameter (0.5 mm) is effective for cutting but will produce potholes and furrowing if used for vaporization. The recommended effective laser beam diameter for laser vaporization is a minimum of 2 to 2.5 mm; this is obtained with the variable-spot-size mechanism. The laser power setting is between 25 and 40 W. A 2-mm effective laser beam diameter and 25 W results in a power density (PD) of 625 W per cm² (PD = 100 × W divided by d^2 where d is the effective laser beam diameter and W is the watts of power chosen by the surgeon). Larger beam diameters can be used, but the watts of power have to be increased accordingly to produce the appropriate PD. Alternately, high energy per pulse (200 mJ) and an average power between 25 and 40 W can be used.

The lesion on the cervix is redefined by colposcopy. The entire transformation zone including the CIN lesion is outlined with a 2-mm laser beam. This marking must be 2 to 3 mm beyond the lesion border. Most cases of CIN do not have a linear length >8 mm. The entire transformation zone, including the area of pathology, is then vaporized to a minimum depth of 6 to 8 mm, with the surgeon beginning at the 6 o'clock position and never leaving an area until proper depth is achieved. Centrally, further vaporization of 4 to 8 mm is recommended, creating the dome-shaped defect (Figures 20.25A and 20.27). The latter step takes into account the topographical anatomy of the cervix and removes part of the remaining area of susceptibility in order to prevent new disease from developing in the future. This procedure usually takes 1 to 5 minutes to perform in an office or clinic setting. The detailed operative techniques for this procedure have been previously published.[204,207,208,219]

When CIN occupies the ectocervix and has a radial linear length exceeding 8 mm, a central cylindrical dome-shaped defect measuring 10 mm centrally at the dome is vaporized. CIN peripheral to the 8-mm radial length is then vaporized to a depth of 4 to 6 mm. This results in a cowboy-hat type of configuration. These ablative methods help to preserve the cervix. Should disease extend onto the vagina, laser vaporization can be extended to encompass the disease, but vaporization depth should not exceed 1.5 mm on vaginal mucosa.

20.4.3.5.2 PITFALLS IN VAPORIZATION MANAGEMENT IN CIN

Persistent disease occurs as a result of any of three vaporization procedure errors: the initial outline of the intended defect did not include a 2- to 3-mm normal tissue border, a minimum vaporization depth of at least 6 mm was not uniformly achieved along the cervical surface, or activation of latent virus (not a procedure error) occurred. Proper depth is relatively easy to obtain at the defect's margin but harder to achieve at the external os where there is no tissue by which to judge depth. It is essential for the defect to be dome-shaped and to match the anatomical topography of the cervix and assure adequate depth at the external os (Figure 20.27).

Vaporization of larger CIN lesions (those longer than 8 mm) creating the standard dome-shaped defect can result in central or complete loss of the cervix and can produce a large central ectopy of columnar epithelium when healed. Both situations are undesirable, the first for obvious reasons and the second because metaplasia secondary to increased exposure of the columnar epithelium to the vaginal environment is newly vulnerable to oncogenic HPV. To remedy these problems, the standard procedure should be modified as described.

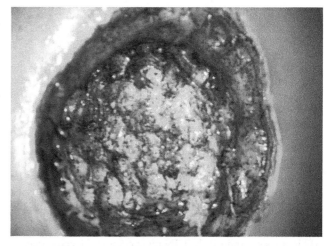

FIGURE 20.27. A colpophotograph of the laser ablation procedure using the continuous mode of the laser.

TABLE 20.13	pH OF 1% LIDOCAINE + EPINEPHRINE AND SODIUM BICARBONATE	
■ SOLUTION	■ pH
Lidocaine + commercial epinephrine	4.05
Lidocaine	6.49
Lidocaine + added epinephrine	6.39
Normal saline	6.85
Lidocaine + epinephrine + sodium bicarbonate	7.37
Lidocaine + sodium bicarbonate	7.38

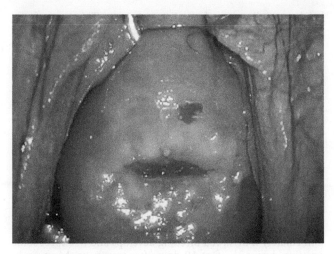

FIGURE 20.28. CIN 3 around the external os and extending into the endocervical canal. A candidate for laser cylindrical excision. (Figure reprinted with permission from Wright VC. *Color Atlas of Colposcopy—Cervix, Vagina and Vulva.* Houston, TX: Biomedical Communications, 2003.)

20.4.3.6 Cylindrical Laser Excision for Endocervical Lesions

This procedure is indicated when discrepancies exist between cytology, colposcopy, and histology; when lesions and the transformation zone are located in the endocervical canal and require tissue for histologic evaluation (Figure 20.28); when either cytologic or colposcopic results suggest possible invasive carcinoma that is not clinically visible and has not been proven by colposcopically directed biopsy; when there is a positive ECC; or when AIS is found on colpobiopsy.

Figure 20.25C illustrates the geometry of endocervical disease. In this case, the disease extends to a maximum depth of 5 mm into the underlying cervical crypts and involves the endocervical canal to a height of 1.6 cm. By removing a cylinder rather than a cone, the surgeon excises half as much tissue. This procedure is performed under anesthesia as day surgery in a hospital or surgery center. The operating requirements include a CO_2 laser attached to an operating microscope, an effective laser beam diameter of 0.5 mm, a working distance of 300 mm, and a PD >1500 W per cm^2 (usually between 1500 and 1800 W

per cm^2). To ensure a virtually bloodless operating field, hemostatic sutures are placed at the 3 o'clock and 9 o'clock positions, and then a vasopressin solution (total dose not exceeding one pressor unit) mixed in normal saline is injected into the cervical stroma. A cylindrical rather than a cone-shaped specimen is removed for histologic interpretation (Figures 20.25C and 20.29A,B). The specimen height varies from 1.5 to 1.8 cm in a reproductive woman. To proceed, the upper pole is cut with a scalpel or a tonsil snare, followed by flashing (quickly moving the beam over the apex with a 2-mm diameter laser beam to seal the blood vessels). The only thermal damaged tissue is located at the outer margin (<100 μm). The step-by-step details of this procedure have been published elsewhere.[208,219]

20.4.3.6.1 PITFALLS IN MANAGEMENT OF ENDOCERVICAL CIN

Persistent disease occurs for several reasons: (1) initial marking of the defect's periphery by the laser beam did not incorporate at least 6 mm of lateral radius; (2) adequate depth was not achieved, leaving disease in the canal; (3) the shape of the defect resembled a cone, with sloping sides cutting across crypts and leaving disease in place; or (4) latent HPV has become activated, producing condyloma or low-grade CIN during the healing process.

20.4.3.6.2 REASONS FOR AN INADEQUATE SPECIMEN

Specimens are inadequate for many reasons. Mostly they are the following: (1) inadequate PD (power density) prolonged the procedure; (2) the specimen was excised by repeated encircling of the cervix with the beam, causing excessive thermal damage; (3) it is better to achieve the desired height in one location before moving on; (4) the apex of the specimen was "coned in" and severed by the laser beam, producing a thermal effect at the upper margin and making histologic interpretation difficult (vaporization of a cone-shaped defect to correct the final defect's shape and create a cylindrical defect may destroy evidence of invasion).

20.4.3.6.3 REASON FOR POOR HEALING

The reason for poor healing is that the specimen's radius was excessive and a large central core was removed that was not restored during healing. This can result in a large central ectopy with the new SCJ located widely on the ectocervix. This is an undesirable situation because a new area of dynamic metaplasia created by exposure of the columnar epithelium of the ectopy to vaginal acidity is vulnerable to carcinogenic HPV and is therefore capable of promoting new disease. The typical

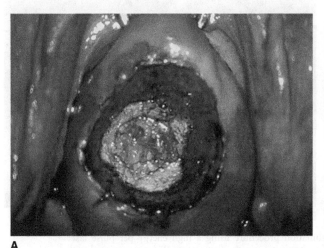 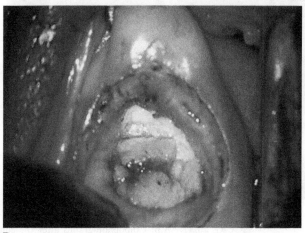

FIGURE 20.29. **A,B:** Colposcopic photographs of a cervix after the cylindrical excisional procedure; (**A**) using the laser in continuous mode and (**B**) using the laser in high energy per pulse mode.

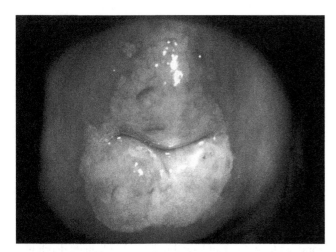

FIGURE 20.30. Ectocervical and endocervical disease. A typical candidate for the combination procedure (central excision and peripheral ablation). (Figure reprinted with permission from Wright VC. *Color Atlas of Colposcopy—Cervix, Vagina and Vulva.* Houston, TX: Biomedical Communications, 2003.)

cervix after a properly performed procedure reveals the new SCJ to be located at the level of the external os, or slightly within the endocervical canal.

20.4.3.7 Laser Excision and Vaporization (Combination Procedure)

In approximately 18% of cases, extensive disease occupies the transformation zone on the ectocervix but extends beyond colposcopic view into the endocervical canal (Figures 20.25B and 20.30). Although cytologic and colposcopic examinations indicate CIN disease, histologic examination of the endocervical tissue is necessary to completely evaluate this area. A suitable defect incorporating the ectocervix and lower endocervical canal can effectively eliminate the distribution of this disease. The combination procedure is used when the ectocervical component has a radius >8 mm.

With the patient under anesthesia, the central cylinder is removed first for histologic evaluation, as above. Specimen

heights usually range from 1.0 to 1.5 cm. This part of surgery is similar to the laser cylindrical excision. Then, using a 2-mm CO_2 laser beam, the remaining outer disease and transformation zone are vaporized to a depth of 6 mm. This results in a cowboy-hat configuration (Figure 20.31A,B). By removing a central cylinder combined with peripheral vaporization, the surgeon removes half as much tissue than if the entire disease had been included within a cone-shaped specimen (Figure 20.25B). The step-by-step operative details of this procedure have been published elsewhere.[219]

20.4.3.8 Discharge Instructions, Postoperative Complications, Healing, and Follow-Up

Patients are advised to refrain from douching, having intercourse, or using tampons for 3 weeks following laser surgery. They should be instructed to notify the physician's office immediately if brisk red bleeding develops and to expect some spotting during the first 10 days after treatment. Most problems can be managed in the office or clinic setting more easily than if the patient comes into the hospital emergency room.

Follow-up is the same as recommended following other procedures for treating CIN. Patients should be advised to return to the clinic or office for their first complete follow-up examination at 6 and 12 months following surgery if follow-up by cytology with/or without colposcopy is elected, or 6 to 12 months postsurgery if by HPV testing.[11,42] By 6 months, metaplastic cellular changes are few, and a satisfactory Pap smear can be obtained.

20.4.3.8.1 DELAYED BLEEDING

Troublesome bleeding requiring medical intervention is rarely a problem following laser ablation. It is slightly more common following laser excision (about 5% to 10% of cases). Surgical intervention is also not commonly required to control postoperative bleeding. Examination of the cervix with the colposcope will usually identify a small area of ooze or heavier bleeding. These conditions can be controlled by one, or a combination, of the following measures: application of Monsel's paste; placing a pack against the cervix and removing it 24 hours later; focal electrosurgical coagulation (very effective); laser coagulation (defocused laser beam while sucking the blood out of the operative site); suturing; arterial embolization; or if all fails, hysterectomy.

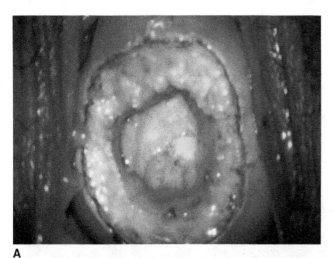

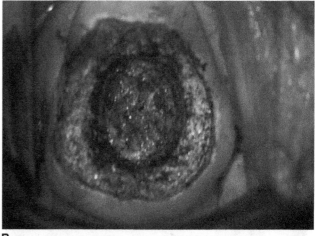

A   B

FIGURE 20.31. A,B: Colpophotographs after the combination procedure using a high energy per pulse laser (A) and using continuous mode (B). Note the absence of carbonization in the first image. (Figures reprinted with permission from Wright VC. *Color Atlas of Colposcopy—Cervix, Vagina and Vulva.* Houston, TX: Biomedical Communications, 2003.)

The last two would be very unusual methods necessary to stop the bleeding. Further, it is important not to soak a pack in Monsel's paste and leave it in the cervix for any period of time, since considerable sloughing of cervical tissue could result. If an inflammatory process is present, appropriate cultures should be taken and appropriate antibiotics prescribed. The maximum probability of encountering bleeding, hence the greatest chance of difficulty, occurs between the 6th and 10th postoperative day.

20.4.3.8.2 INFECTION

Infection is virtually nonexistent, probably because of the sterilized wound, the absence of necrotic debris, and the sealing of lymphatics and blood vessels. Antibiotics, therefore, are unnecessary except as prophylaxis, for example in patients with a history of previous PID.

20.4.3.8.3 HEALING

Healing patterns are well documented. Some sloughing of necrotic tissue and carbon residue occurs during the first 2 days with extensive acute inflammatory cells in the exudate. By day 3, squamous epithelium begins to proliferate in the defect, and specks of carbonized debris on the crater surface can be seen through the colposcope and within the new epithelium as it begins to fill the cavity. Soon the inflammatory reaction subsides. When the cervical procedure is appropriately planned, cervical tissue loss is minimized, and normal topography is usually restored by day 21. Mature epithelium with normal tensile strength has been documented cytologically, histologically, and by scanning electron microscopy.[220,221]

20.4.3.8.4 STENOSIS

Cervical stenosis after excisional procedures on the cervix is not common. While some narrowing of the cervix after these procedures is frequently seen, symptomatic cervical stenosis only occasionally presents as a problem in management. When stenosis occurs, it usually involves only the cervical os and does not exceed 2 mm. In most cases, a small membrane of tissue covers the external os. Regardless, prevention is better than cure. Cervical stenosis can occur in the following circumstances: women of reproductive age group with oligomenorrhea or amenorrhea, women on low-dose birth control pills who have oligomenorrhea or amenorrhea, women who are postpartum and lactating, postmenopausal women who are not on hormone replacement therapy, women who are on estrogen and progesterone therapy with amenorrhea and women using progestin-only contraception.

In any of these circumstances reflecting a hypoestrogen state, cyclic systemic estrogen and progesterone at doses that cause menstruation will likely prevent stenosis. This should occur before, during, and after the excisional procedure and can be achieved by prescribing conjugated estrogen and progestin for three or four cycles. In lactating women, topical vaginal estrogen can be prescribed for use before and after the procedure. Alternately, the procedure may be postponed, provided there is no concern about cancer, until breast-feeding is discontinued and menstrual periods resume. For medroxyprogesterone patients, the procedure can be delayed until the medication has cleared and cycles have resumed. However, this could delay treatment for an indefinite period of time and increase the risk of intercurrent pregnancy. Alternatively, vaginal estrogen cream can be prescribed to be applied twice daily for 14 days before the procedure and posttreatment until healing is achieved. Patients at high risk for stenosis should be examined every 2 weeks for at least 6 to 8 weeks following excision, and their endocervical canal probed to maintain patency. Stenosis cannot be completely prevented, but the incidence can be reduced.[222]

20.4.3.9 Results of Laser Surgery

In one series, a single operator treated 2327 patients with CIN by the CO_2 laser (1454 by laser vaporization and 873 by cylindrical excision or the combination procedure).[204] Vaporization produced cure rates of 94.8% and the excisional and/or the combination procedure 95.1% after one surgery. Pregnancy outcome in 195 patients within the whole group (142 laser vaporizations and 53 laser excisions) indicated no increase in the premature delivery rate or cesarean rate.[204,223,224] Similar cure rates have been published elsewhere.[225-230] The first follow-up examination performed at the recommended interval, including colposcopic and cytologic evaluation, was very accurate in predicting persistent disease. That is, 90% of all patients who were shown to have persistent disease were identified at the first follow-up visit, with the remaining noted at the second visit, except for one case, whose persistence was not identified until the third visit (9 months postprocedure). After laser surgery, the new SCJ formed at the external os in 90% of cases, and in all cases, the cervix appeared to regenerate to its original or near-original mass.[204]

20.4.4 Electrosurgical Procedures

20.4.4.1 Introduction

Electrosurgery was first introduced in the late 1920s by William Bovie and Harvey Cushing. They invented the first electrosurgical generator (ESG) that produced high-frequency energy for surgical cutting and coagulation of biologic tissue. Since that time, safer and more flexible equipment has been developed, and electrosurgery has become popular in a variety of disciplines.[231-238] Electrosurgery can be defined as the use of radio frequency current to cut tissue or achieve hemostasis. The primary rules of electricity pertain to the following: (1) electricity flows to ground; (2) electricity follows the path of least resistance; (3) impedance to electric current produces heat.

Human tissue resists the flow of electrical current. This impedance creates the heat required for tissue cutting or coagulation. Modern electrosurgical units (ESUs) apply an alternating current to the tissue at frequencies much higher than the 60 Hz of an alternating current used in household electronics. Electrosurgery requires high voltage, high frequency, and low current density, as opposed to the standard 110 V, low frequency, and high current density provided by standard power sources used in household electricity. ESUs increase the typical 60-Hz household current to between 500 kHz and 4 million Hz. These frequencies employed in electrosurgery are within the frequencies of AM radio. Hence, electrosurgery is at times referred to as radiofrequency surgery. Frequencies below 100 kHz can stimulate muscles and nerves (faradic effect). Should this occur, surgery must be discontinued and the cause of the low frequency investigated. However, modern ESUs have safeguards that should prevent this.

20.4.4.2 Stages of Thermal Destruction

The utilization of thermal energy permits the physician to perform electrosurgical cutting (flash boiling or vaporization) and electrosurgical dehydration of tissue (coagulation, desiccation, and fulguration). Table 20.14 illustrates the stages of thermal destruction in tissue.

20.4.4.3 Waveforms Produced by Electrosurgical Generators

The basic waveforms employed in electrosurgery are pure sine waves (Figure 20.32), damped sine waves (Figure 20.33), and modulated sine waves (Figure 20.34). In each figure, the horizontal axis represents time.

TABLE 20.14	STAGES OF THERMAL DESTRUCTION*
■ TEMPERATURE	■ EFFECT
Up to ~40°C	No significant effect
Above ~40°C	Reversible cell damage depending upon duration of exposure
Above 40°C	Irreversible cell damage (denaturing of protein occurs)
Above ~70°C	Coagulation. Collagen is converted to glucose
At 100°C	Flash boiling, vaporization
Above 100°C	Desiccation occurs
Above ~200°C	Carbonization occurs

*The most severe thermal effects in electrosurgery pertain to coagulation. Electrosurgical cutting produces the least thermal effect.

20.4.4.3.1 THE PURE SINE WAVE

If the voltage output of an ESG is plotted over time, a pure cut waveform is representative of a continuous sine wave alternating from positive to negative at the frequency of the generator (Figure 20.32). The amplitude of the waveform is the voltage (Figure 20.32). The peak voltage is the highest voltage when measured from zero, and the peak-to-peak voltage represents the voltage to the highest positive voltage, the RMS (root mean square) being the mathematical average of the waveform (Figure 20.32). The ratio of peak voltage to RMS voltage (average voltage) of a periodic waveform is termed the *Crest Factor*.

Clinically, the Crest Factor is a method of indicating the potential degree of thermal effect (providing hemostasis) in an electrosurgical waveform. The lower the Crest Factor, the less is the thermal effect. Hence, pure sine waves have the lowest Crest Factor (1.4). Crest factors for the individual settings (like cut, blend 1, Coag) are different from one generator to the other.

20.4.4.3.2 THE BLENDED CUT

Blend is cutting waveform with more hemostatic effect than a pure sine wave (has a higher Crest Factor than a pure sine wave). Basically, this is achieved by employing a damped (Figure 20.33) or a modulated waveform (Figure 20.34). The latter consists of on and off periods producing a duty cycle (e.g., 80% on and 20% off). The duty cycle is the ratio of the duration of output bursts to the time between the initiation of the bursts. For example, a pure sine wave has a duty cycle of 100%. A modulated waveform is <100%.

20.4.4.3.3 INCREASING VOLTAGE WHILE MAINTAINING A PURE SINE WAVE

Some ESGs are designed to maintain a pure sine wave in the face of increasing voltage (Constant Voltage™, ERBE). In this setting, a pure sine wave is employed (Crest Factor 1.4) for all tissue mode settings (Figure 20.32). The voltage can be selected between 200 and 500 peak volts and is kept relatively constant during the cutting process regardless of the variations in tissue impedance. Increasing the voltage while maintaining a pure sine wave will uniformly increase the thermal effect. The sparking to tissue increases in direct proportion to the voltage. This is the principle of constant voltage technology (Figure 20.35).[239]

20.4.4.4 INSTANT RESPONSE™ ELECTROSURGICAL GENERATORS

Tissue impedance is not uniform. In the Instant Response System™ (Valleylab), a computer-controlled feedback system is incorporated so that the unit can respond to changing tissue impedances while maintaining a constant power and controlling the current density. The current density around the tissue electrode varies by the formula $j = I/\text{Area}$, where j = current density and I = current. In electrosurgery, tissue electrodes are used to deliver current to the body. Tissue electrodes vary in length and diameter: they are usually in the configuration of a wire loop, a needle or spatula, and ball electrode. Since current density varies directly with the amount of current and inversely with the cross-sectional area, or in the case of the ball electrode, the surface area, it follows that PD varies with the configuration of the tissue electrode. Watts being constant, thin wires have more PD than do thick ones and, therefore, produce less thermal damage. Long wires have less PD than shorter ones, and big balls less than smaller ones.

20.4.4.5 Monopolar Electrosurgical Cutting

Unless the voltage is kept constant, the alternating current flows from the ESG under a variable voltage to the active tissue electrode and through the patient to a return electrode, termed the *dispersive plate or electrode*. The dispersive plate provides an electrical contact over a very large area on the patient. The current density at the dispersive plate is small in comparison to the current density at the active tissue electrode. In modern ESGs, an isolation transformer inside the unit isolates the therapeutic current from ground (isolated ESG, which protects against current division); hence, the generator, not the ground, completes

FIGURE 20.32. A pure sine wave. (Image provided courtesy of Dr. Wright VC. *Understanding Electrosurgery*. Houston, TX: Biomedical Communications, 1995.)

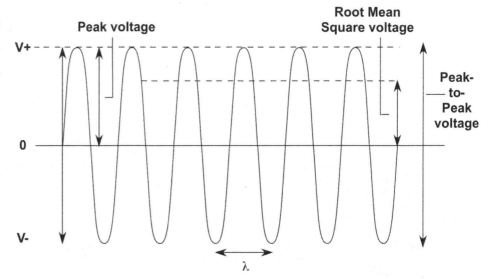

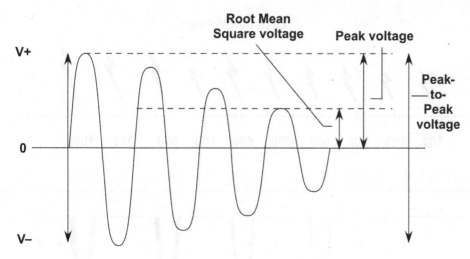

FIGURE 20.33. A damped sine wave. (Image provided courtesy of Dr. Wright VC. *Understanding Electrosurgery*. Houston, TX: Biomedical Communications, 1995.)

the circuit (Figure 20.36A). In the isolated system used in all modern ESUs, there is no alternative pathway through which the electricity can flow. Hence, modern ESUs eliminate the risk of burns through other pathways. Return electrode monitoring (REM) systems also help reduce, or eliminate, the risk of burns at the site of the dispersive plate (Figure 20.36B) by disabling the system if the dispersive pad is partially detached.

The following parameters appear to be of surgical importance: a voltage >200 peak volts is required to produce the electric spark between a metal tissue electrode and biologic tissue; with a voltage >200 peak volts, electric sparks increase in length and strength in proportion to the voltage; the radial extent of coagulation along the cut increases with voltage and with the length and intensity of the electric spark; at more than 500 peak volts, carbonization occurs; control of thermal damage and carbonization is maximized when the voltage in the active tissue electrode is between 200 and 500 peak volts, irrespective of tissue impedance while employing a pure sine wave (Figure 20.32). Many commercial ESGs used for general surgery greatly exceed 1000 peak volts in the cut mode, but these units are rarely used now for LEEP procedures as they are less than ideal.

20.4.4.5.1 CORE CONCEPTS FOR MONOPOLAR ELECTROSURGICAL CUTTING

1. The active tissue electrode must be in contact with the tissue.
2. The tissue is cut by moving the electrode through tissue.

3. Low-amplitude continuous sinusoidal waveforms produce the least thermal effect (lowest Crest Factor).
4. To provide better hemostasis and minimal thermal effect to the tissue, a blend (mixed mode), damped, or modulated waveform is used. This is accomplished by adjusting the amplitude and degree of modulation of the high-frequency voltage. The degree of this alteration is reflected in the Crest Factor.
5. The higher the Crest Factor, the greater the tissue coagulation.
6. The Crest Factor is not equal for the same setting on different generators, so modern ESUs come with instructions on the power setting for that generator ideal for the size loop or ball, and for cutting, blend, and coag modes.
7. A duty cycle is expressed as a ratio of the burst duration of the sine wave to the time between the initiation of the bursts.

20.4.4.6 Monopolar Electrosurgical Coagulation

A coagulation (Coag) waveform consists of short bursts (microseconds) of radiofrequency sine waves (Figures 20.33 and 20.34). The Coag waveform has a considerably greater peak-to-peak voltage (higher Crest Factor) than the cut waveform. The energy (heat per second) is less because the

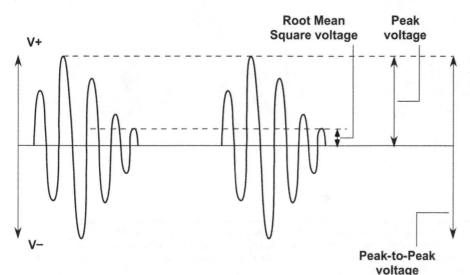

FIGURE 20.34. A modulated sine wave (RMS, root mean square). (Image provided courtesy of Dr. Wright VC. *Understanding Electrosurgery*. Houston, TX: Biomedical Communications, 1995.)

FIGURE 20.35. In constant voltage technology, the increased thermal effect (K) occurs due to increasing the peak voltage (Vp). (Image provided courtesy of Dr. Wright VC *Understanding Electrosurgery*. Houston, TX: Biomedical Communications, 1995.)

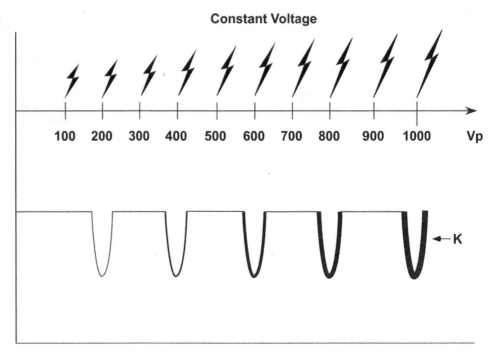

Constant Voltage

Coag is turned off most of the time. Figures 20.37 and 20.38 indicate that Coag waveforms vary in frequency and duration between different ESGs. Therefore, the tissue effect per unit of time will not be the same for similar power settings. The three methods used surgically to produce coagulation are desiccation, fulguration, and puncture coagulation.

20.4.4.6.1 Monopolar Electrosurgical Desiccation

Desiccation occurs with the active tissue electrode (ball electrode) in contact with the tissue. Heat is generated in the tissue as a result of current moving against tissue impedance. Steam forms as the energized tissue evaporates, resulting in dehydration and increased tissue impedance to current flow. If the voltage is sufficient (>200 peak volts), electric sparking will occur to the nearest moist tissue. Desiccation can be accomplished in any waveform. The amount of sparking lateral to the site of desiccation that occurs depends on the peak voltage of the waveform.

Soft coagulation (no spark coagulation) is the term applied when no sparking is produced between the coagulating electrode and tissue during the coagulation process. This is achieved by employing a pure sine wave; however, the voltage must be <200 peak volts. Forced coagulation occurs when the spark is intentionally generated between the coagulation electrode and the tissue. Intense sparking is produced when the peak voltage is the highest (Coag waveform, highest Crest Factor).

20.4.4.6.1.1 Core Concepts of Monopolar Desiccation

For desiccation to occur, the tissue electrode is held in contact with the tissue.

1. Tissue desiccation can occur in any waveform.
2. Dehydration of tissue occurs, followed by sparking to the nearest moist tissue, if the voltage is >200 peak volts. The sparks are finer than those produced by fulguration (noncontact coagulation).

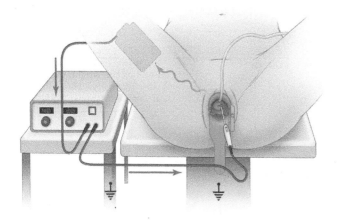

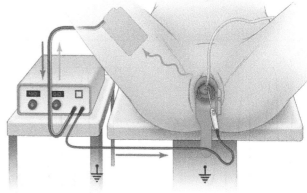

A

B

FIGURE 20.36. **A:** The flow of alternating current in an isolated ESU. Such a unit prevents current division and alternate site burns (except at the potential site of the dispersive plate if improperly attached). **B:** The REM system. The REM circuitry recognizes the quality of the return electrode's pats; that is, any reduction of surface area contact between patient and dispersive plate (increased current concentration) or lack of conductivity between patient's skin and the dispersive plate surface deactivates the generator.

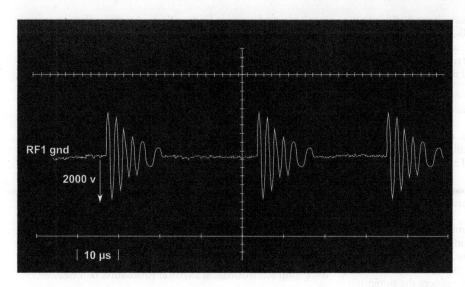

FIGURE 20.37. An oscilloscope tracing of a Coag waveform of a conventional ESG. (Image provided courtesy of Dr. Wright VC. *Understanding Electrosurgery.* Houston, TX: Biomedical Communications, 1995.)

3. The intensity of the sparking to the adjacent moist tissue increases proportionally with increase in voltage; thus, the greatest sparking is observed when desiccating in the Coag waveform.
4. The PD varies inversely with the contact surface area of the coagulating electrode, that is, PD = watts (volts × amps)/contact surface area.
5. The larger the electrode contact area, the more current is required to produce the same effective current density.
6. The higher the power setting (watts), the greater the amount of current delivered and the quicker the desiccation.

20.4.4.6.2 MONOPOLAR ELECTROSURGICAL FULGURATION (SPRAYING)

Fulguration is produced with nontissue contact by the tissue electrode. High voltage is required (Coag waveform). If the peak voltage is insufficient, the operator will touch the tissue electrode to the tissue, causing desiccation, not fulguration. The sparks produced cause superficial tissue necrosis. Excessive fulguration can char tissue and cause excessive damage once the tissue has become dehydrated. The sparks produced by each cycle of voltage have a high current density. The greater the frequency of the ESG, the more frequent is the sparking to tissue.

20.4.4.6.2.1 Core Concepts of Monopolar Fulguration

1. In fulguration, the tissue electrode is not in contact with the tissue.
2. There is long sparking to tissue across the electrode-tissue gap.
3. Fulguration occurs with relatively high voltage and low amperage current.
4. Superficial dehydration of tissue results.
5. With fulguration, in contrast to desiccation, only one-fifth of the amount of current enters the tissue.
6. High voltage (Coag waveform) with sparking to tissue raises the possibility of neuromuscular stimulation resulting from production of low-frequency waveforms.

20.4.4.7 Bipolar Electrosurgery

Bipolar electrosurgery can be used for tissue cutting and desiccation. Both require two similar active tissue electrodes. This bipolar (two-pole) tissue electrode provides one tip as the active electrode and the other as the return electrode; therefore, no separate dispersive plate is required. The current flows from the bipolar connection port to one of the tips of the bipolar forceps, through the grasped tissue between the forceps tips and returns to the ESG via the other tip. A high-frequency, low-voltage unmodulated waveform (sine wave) is employed

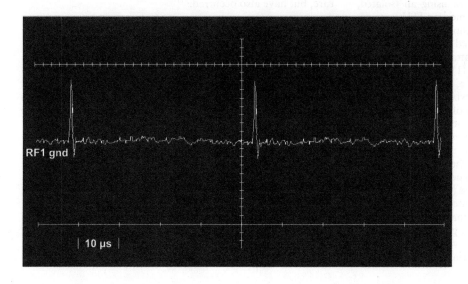

FIGURE 20.38. An oscilloscope tracing of a Coag waveform from a constant voltage generator. This varies considerably from the one shown in Figure 20.37. (Image provided courtesy of Dr. Wright VC. *Understanding Electrosurgery.* Houston, TX: Biomedical Communications, 1995.)

(Figure 20.32). The high frequency flows through the tissue (between electrode tips) within a well-defined area; lateral spread of tissue coagulation does not occur. The amount of tissue desiccation depends on the volume of tissue grasped. Bipolar units are not commonly used for cervical excision procedures.

20.4.4.7.1 CORE CONCEPTS OF BIPOLAR ELECTROSURGERY

1. Bipolar electrodes are combined with a bipolar instrument.
2. The high-frequency, low-voltage current (sine waveform) flows through the tissue within a well-defined area between two similar electrodes. Thus, lateral spread of thermal damage does not occur.
3. Because of low voltage, there is less risk of interference with the electronic circuits simultaneously connected to the patient.
4. Bipolar desiccation potentially eliminates sparking, lowering the risk of inadvertent burning to adjacent tissue.
5. Because there is no dispersive plate, alternate site burns, as seen in monopolar electrosurgery, do not occur.
6. The reduction of generator power reduces the potential of nerve and muscle stimulation.
7. Bipolar instruments can be used in a normal saline bathing solution (a urologic advantage).

20.4.4.8 Electrosurgery versus Electrocautery

The term *electrocautery* is often confused with the term *electrosurgery*. In electrocautery, no current is passed to the patient because the tissue effects are caused by heat transference. The electrocautery tip is a resistance wire similar to that used in an electric stove or toaster. It is important not to confuse the methods or the terms.

20.4.4.9 Electrosurgical Systems

There are three basic components to all electrosurgical systems: the ESG, the patient return electrode (dispersive plate), and the active tissue electrode. As previously discussed, the isolated ESG (Figure 20.36A) has replaced the grounded unit (Bovie ESG). The addition of REM circuitry has helped eliminate burns at the site of the dispersive plate. This mechanism monitors the quality of the electrical contact between the return electrode (dispersive plate) and the patient during electrosurgery. Specifically, it measures the electro-patient impedance. Any imbalance or poor dispersive plate contact signals an alarm system and shuts down the generator (Figure 20.36B).

20.4.4.10 Electrosurgical Safety

Most electrosurgical injuries relate to not using an isolated, REM system or accidental burns. With modern ESU systems, accidental burns should not occur from improper use of the dispersive plate, since the REM system should shut off the generator if the dispersive plate is not properly attached to the patient. However, injuries could still occur with (1) unintentional activation of the ESU when the loop, needle, or ball electrode is touching any body part other than the cervix; (2) unsuitable and or defective accessories; and (3) ignition of flammable liquids, gases, and/or vapors. Modern ESUs come with a "standby" switch. In order to prevent accidental burns it is very important to keep the unit switched to standby until the operator is ready to proceed with the procedure. Other safety issues may develop from stimulation of muscles and nerves (faradic effect) and interference with electrical equipment (e.g., pacemakers).

Policies and procedures for the maintenance and safe use of the ESG should be written by the biomedical engineering department staff or safety committee. In general, the instructions that come with modern ESUs can serve as the technologic basis for the use of the unit. The material should be readily available and reviewed annually within the office or institution. Factors to be considered include verifying that clinicians using the equipment have received training in the procedure, and testing new equipment before employing it surgically, frequently testing equipment, and accurately recording mishaps, equipment maintenance, and repairs.

20.4.4.11 Electrosurgical Approaches to Treatment of CIN

Electrosurgical excision is the most common modality being used to treat CIN. With electrosurgery, a straight-needle electrode or a curved- or square-loop electrode is used to excise the abnormal transformation zone, followed by a ball electrode (3 or 5 mm in diameter) to coagulate vessels.[231,240–250] Loop excision is sometimes referred to as large loop excision of the transformation zone (LLETZ), a term coined in England by investigators who first studied the techniques.[231,242] In North America, the use of smaller electrodes led to naming the procedure loop electrosurgical excision procedure, or LEEP.[240,243,246]

20.4.4.11.1 RATIONALE FOR EXCISION OF CIN

Electrosurgical techniques produce one or more specimens of cervical tissue for histologic interpretation. These procedures reduce the chance of potential diagnostic errors by minimizing the possibility of missing an invasive squamous cell cancer, AIS or an adenocarcinoma. They are used to confirm the complete removal of diseased tissue. Ideally, these electrosurgical procedures could replace other excisional methods, such as scalpel, CO_2 laser conization, and many ablative procedures.

Each specimen is examined in the same manner as a traditional cone specimen. Reported studies demonstrate that loop specimens are adequate for thorough evaluation of cervical dysplasia in most specimens.[244–246] In evaluating and reporting on these specimens, the pathologist needs to report both margin status and severity of disease. However, in reality, specimens are often far from ideal. In some cases, the pathologic interpretation is insufficient for adequately grading the lesion, excluding malignancy, or predicting persistent disease because of excessive thermal effects or having to report on multiple bits of excised tissue.[135,247–251] In reviewing LLETZ specimens, Ioffe et al.[247] found that the presence of tissue artifacts interfering with interpretation was only rarely mentioned within the original pathology report. Furthermore, the status of margins was a better predictor of abnormal follow-up in CKC than in the LLETZ specimens. The worst thermal effect occurs at the upper margin (base of specimen or apex of defect), where the worst disease potentially exists. Significant injuries to adjacent normal anatomical structures such as bladder and bowel are rare, but have also occurred.[250]

20.4.4.11.2 EVALUATING THE PATIENT PRIOR TO ELECTROSURGERY

Even in "see and treat," colposcopic evaluation of the cervix and vagina is necessary before any excisional procedure. This evaluation, in part, determines the location and size of the lesion and its potential grade. It further helps the practitioner decide which electrode should be chosen and what electrosurgical technique should be used to encompass the lesion.[252] Two options exist for management of women with lesions: immediate "see and treat" or colposcopy, biopsy, and triage to treatment.

20.4.4.11.3 ONE- OR TWO-VISIT APPOINTMENT TO REMOVE LESIONS

The electrosurgical method has been used for both diagnosis and treatment at the same visit. This one-visit approach is termed *see and treat LEEP*. In this approach, the colposcopic examination is performed based on a HSIL cytologic result, a colposcopic identification of an ectocervical lesion, and informed consent that the patient would prefer to proceed directly with treatment.[11,42] Because the loop procedure supplies a specimen for pathologic interpretation, no preliminary biopsies or ECC is necessary. This quick approach is only considered appropriate when the patient has been referred for evaluation of a HSIL Pap result and a colposcopic lesion is identified. "See and treat" is not appropriate for LSIL, ASC-US, ASC-H or AGC, nor is "see and treat" LEEP to be used for HSIL in adolescents and young women.[11,42] It is inappropriate in these other circumstances because the risk of CIN 2,3 is not high enough to justify the risk of the procedure without prior histologic confirmation. "See and treat" is a particularly appropriate choice for patients with a significant lesion who are not expected to be compliant.[240]

The two-step approach is the more traditional approach, consisting of standard colposcopic examination, directed biopsies, and ECC (when appropriate). This approach relies on subsequent correlation of the three diagnoses—cytologic, colposcopic, and histologic—followed by treatment at the next patient visit or further investigation, if warranted. Thus, the strategy of patient management is influenced by the grade of the cytologic specimen, the reliability and age of the patient, the location of the lesion, the colposcopic impression, and the confidence of the colposcopist.

20.4.4.11.4 Contraindications for LEEP

Regardless of the number of visits, there are contraindications for the loop procedure, including the presence of a cervical inflammatory process, bleeding disorders, an obvious cancer, the need to differentiate between microinvasive cancer on biopsy and advanced disease, disease within the endocervical canal that could not be encompassed by a single pass or LEEP conization, pregnancy, and DES abnormality. When glandular disease (i.e., AIS) has been documented on biopsy, CKC is favored as the excisional procedure of choice because a long endocervical canal excision without a central burn margin can be obtained with CKC, but not with a "top hat" LEEP. However, the ASCCP guidelines now simply state that, irrespective of conization method, clinicians should remember that margin status and interpretability of the margins are important for future treatment planning and management.[11] Caution should be used when treating women who are in a state of amenorrhea (e.g., patients in the postpartum period or menopause, and patients who are breast-feeding or using medroxyprogesterone). In the amenorrhea group, hypoestrogenic atrophy can lead to posttreatment cervical stenosis unless remedied.

20.4.4.11.5 The LEEP Procedure

20.4.4.11.5.1 Preparing the Room and the Patient for LEEP

As with any other operative procedure, it is imperative to fully discuss with the patient before the procedure the pros and cons of the treatment chosen, alternative options for treating the disease, possible complications, and a description of what to expect during, and following, the procedure. An informed consent should be read and signed by the patient and witnessed.

All materials necessary for the procedure should ideally be set up before the patient enters the procedure room. The ESU should have been recently checked as described previously, and the smoke evacuator should have been checked to make sure that it is appropriately suctioning air. A tray should be prepared with anesthetic, a fine long needle that can attach to a dental syringe (a Potocky needle is ideal because it combines a strong shaft with a 27-gauge needle on the end), local anesthetic combined with vasopressin (in the ratio of 10 units of vasopressin per 30 mL of 1% lidocaine), Monsel's paste or gel, acetic acid, half-strength Lugol's solution, large cotton swabs, and specimen bottles with 10% neutral buffered formulin. Appropriate-sized loop and ball electrodes should

be available, as well as an insulated electrode handle, smoke evacuator tubing, and smoke evacuator filter. Also available should be appropriate-sized insulated specula and an insulated vaginal wall retractor. These can be made out of either nonconductive material or metal coated with a nonconductive material. Although rarely needed, it is also prudent to have a 12-inch needle holder with 2-0 absorbable suture available.

Once the room supplies, ESU, and smoke evacuator have all been checked and affirmed to be ready, the ESU connected to an appropriate dispersive grounding pad and the smoke evacuator tubing connected to the smoke evacuator, the patient can assume the dorsal lithotomy position. The dispersive pad should then be placed on the patient's thigh as close as possible to the surgical site. If the speculum has a smoke evacuator port, the end of the suction tube can be placed in this port before inserting the speculum.

The cervix is exposed with the insulated bivalve speculum with appropriate smoke evacuator suction apparatus. It is important to have the cervix in the midposition and as perpendicular to the operator as possible. This may require the placement of a large swab or dental cylindrical cottonoid (a long string attached for removal and reminder purposes) in order to relocate its position. If the vaginal walls are lax and at risk for thermal injury, a condom cut at the end can be put over the speculum prior to insertion, or an insulated vaginal retractor can be inserted through the speculum. The cervix should be inspected through the colposcope both before and after the application of acetic acid. The location and size of the lesion and extent of endocervical involvement should again be checked and the prerequisites for LEEP again verified. Half-strength Lugol's solution can then be applied to further verify the extent of the cervix requiring excision. The local anesthetic (usually from 1.8 to 3.6 mL, or one to two dental syringe vials of 1% to 2% lidocaine and 1:100,000 epinephrine) should then be injected with a fine needle of 27 gauge or less, inserted just under (~2 mm) the mucosal surface. Inject at 3 o'clock, 6 o'clock, 9 o'clock, and 12 o'clock until blanching is seen. This intracervical block is generally more effective in preventing pain during the procedure than a paracervical block and less painful to administer. Occasionally, a large cervix may require additional injections placed between the four described above.

The loop size should be chosen on the basis of the size of the lesion and the extent of endocervical involvement, if any. An appropriate-sized 3- or 5-mm ball electrode should also be available for fulguration. The manufacturer usually suggests power settings appropriate to their specific conventional ESU and the size of the electrode, so the ESU should be set to the recommended power setting for the size of the loop electrode and the type of current being selected. For the excisional part of the procedure, some clinicians prefer to use the pure cutting mode, which employs a pure sine wave (Figure 20.32). Others prefer the blend mode, which employs a modulated sine wave (Figures 20.33). In general, the loop is less likely to stall in the cutting mode and less likely to produce significant "burn artifact" than the blend mode. However, the blend mode is better at coagulating vessels as it cuts, and therefore less likely to be accompanied by significant bleeding. During the procedure (see below) it may be necessary to change the size of the loop, requiring readjusting the ESU power setting. Readjusting the power setting is also necessary when switching from the excisional part of the procedure to the coagulation mode (Coag waveform) needed for coagulation of any bleeding sites. (Figures 20.33, 20.37, and 20.38) Fulguration is preferred over desiccation to any remaining bleeding points because fulguration reduces current delivered to the tissue and produces only superficial thermal injury.

From this point on, the procedure will be dictated by the size and location of the cervical neoplasia. Various surgical approaches have been previously described in detail.[63,231,252,253] The approach chosen is that required to best eradicate the disease with the smallest volume of tissue removed. There are four primary procedure types, each determined by these parameters. These are (1) removal of ectocervical tissue with a single pass; (2) removal of ectocervical tissue with a multiple passes (required for large ectocervical lesions); (3) excision of primarily endocervical CIN; and (4) excision when there is both extensive ectocervical and endocervical disease.

20.4.4.11.5.2 Selecting the Surgical Approach

The operator chooses the desired loop or needle electrode with intention to remove all lesional tissue, while at the same time sparing as much normal tissue as possible. In doing so, the linear length of disease, the location of disease, and the potential for crypt involvement must be considered. When the canal is involved, the specimen removed must be cylindrical rather than conical in configuration. The resulting defect must spare as much peripheral cervical stroma as possible to minimize cervical volume loss during the healing and regenerative process.

20.4.4.11.5.2.1 Removal of Ectocervical Tissue with a Single Pass
A single-pass LEEP is ideal in excising an ectocervical lesion not encroaching the endocervical canal.[252] The operator selects an appropriate loop electrode, ideally one that can remove the lesion and the transformation zone in a single pass to a depth of about 8 mm. Some operators prefer to monitor the surgical procedure while looking through the colposcope. Others find this awkward and use the colposcope as a light source. A good compromise is to mark the start and stop location of the LEEP using the wire loop under direct colposcopic guidance. The colposcope can then be moved out of the way, and the procedure can be done under direct vision. The handpiece to be employed can be activated by switches on the handpiece ("cut" or "coag") or by a footswitch. Some generators come with both activation sources, others with only a footswitch.

The operator positions the upper arc of the semicircular loop just outside the active transformation zone or the outer boundary of the lesion, whichever is most distal from the os. The current is applied just before tissue contact. The probe is directed straight ahead into the cervical stroma up to the crossbar or to a depth of 7 to 10 mm. After reaching the desired depth in the stroma and using the same smooth, continuous motion, the operator moves the handpiece to the opposite transformation zone or lesion border, keeping the same depth throughout the cut by touching or almost touching the surface of the cervix with the crossbar as it moves over the lesion. A backstop (a large swab or wooden tongue blade) can be placed to protect the exit side in the vagina for extra protection should the upper electrode's wire arc come in contact with the vaginal wall during removal of the loop from the cervical tissue. This is helpful because resistance against motion at that point drops dramatically. When the crossbar is at the exit point, the operator pulls the handpiece straight out, continuing in the same smooth motion, and when the upper arc cuts through the tissue surface, the current is shut off by releasing the switch on the handpiece or releasing the footswitch.

Most operators have the entrance point at 3 o'clock and the exit point at 9 o'clock or the reverse. Others find a beginning point of 6 o'clock and exiting point at 12 o'clock to be effective. However, when beginning at the 12 o'clock position and approaching the 6 o'clock exit point, the partially excised specimen may fall forward as the cutting process continues, obscuring the procedure before the exit point is achieved. This may require stopping the procedure until the situation is remedied. Frequently the specimen remains in place and needs to be removed with forceps and placed in fixative.

Any bleeding sites are fulgurated using a ball electrode in the Coag waveform. Unfortunately, it is impossible to fulgurate through blood, particularly the blood pool that accumulates in the cavity of the posterior cervix. In order to avoid desiccation, which destroys too much tissue, the ball electrode should not be pushed into the blood mass. Removal of blood from the operative site permits fulguration. This can be accomplished by having a smoke evacuation system that includes a blood trap, or by using a plastic suction device that handles both smoke and blood simultaneously. A plastic suction device can also serve as an insulated retractor. Alternatively, large cotton swabs can be used to blot blood from the excised cavity and to apply pressure to blood vessels until fulgurated. Monsel's paste is applied to the crater bed to complete the procedure.

Figures 20.39A–G illustrate the removal of tissue with one pass of the tissue electrode. Problems encountered during any of the three basic LEEP procedures are discussed in Section 20.4.4.11.6.

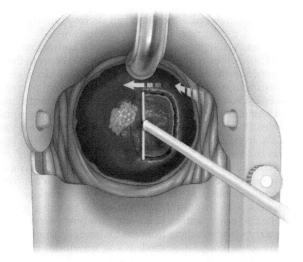

A

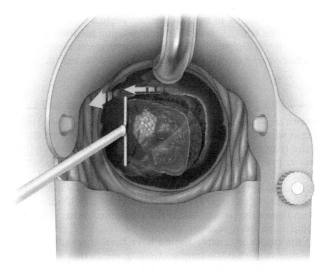

B

FIGURE 20.39.   Tissue removal with one pass of the tissue electrode. **A:** For a one-pass loop excision, the activated loop tissue electrode is pushed into the cervical stroma at the 3 o'clock position up to the level of its crossbar. **B:** With current continuing to flow through it, the loop electrode is slowly and deliberately moved laterally, keeping the crossbar at or just slightly above the surface as it moves towards the 9 o'clock exit position. There it is pulled straight out, and afterwards the cylindrical severed specimen is removed with forceps.

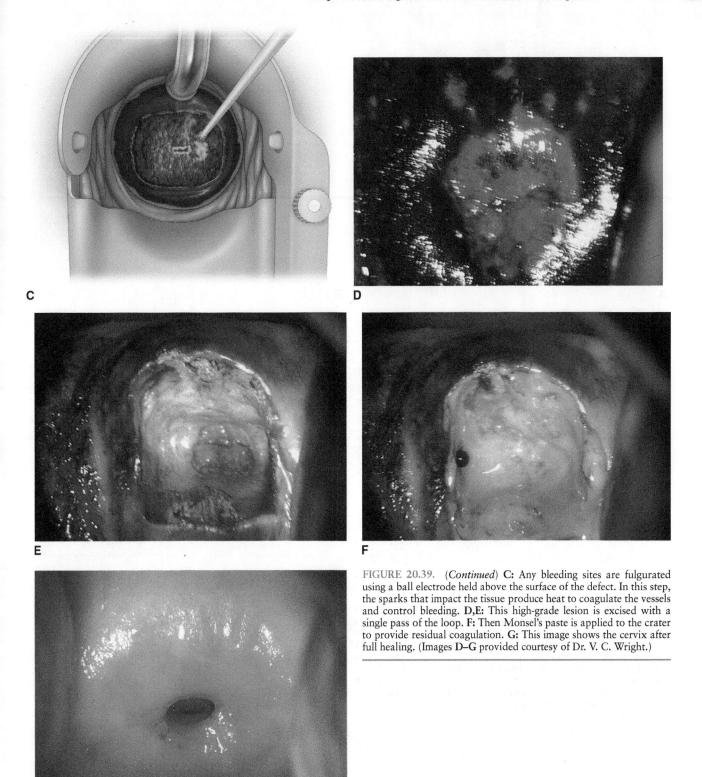

FIGURE 20.39. (*Continued*) **C:** Any bleeding sites are fulgurated using a ball electrode held above the surface of the defect. In this step, the sparks that impact the tissue produce heat to coagulate the vessels and control bleeding. **D,E:** This high-grade lesion is excised with a single pass of the loop. **F:** Then Monsel's paste is applied to the crater to provide residual coagulation. **G:** This image shows the cervix after full healing. (Images **D–G** provided courtesy of Dr. V. C. Wright.)

20.4.4.11.5.2.2 Removal of Ectocervical CIN with Multiple Passes   Approximately 10% of cases will require more than one pass of the loop electrode because of the extent of disease. Multiple passes using one or two different loops can excise the diseased tissue. This approach produces two or more specimens, each of which must be pathologically evaluated. The central portion of the lesion, which potentially has the worst disease, is usually removed first. Further passes are

made to remove the remaining disease (Figure 20.40A–E). This method of excision is similar to that for the single-pass approach already described. After each pass, the specimen is picked up with forceps, and placed in containers with fixative for pathologic interpretation.

20.4.4.11.5.2.3 Excision of Endocervical CIN   Disease confined to the endocervical canal can potentially extend as far

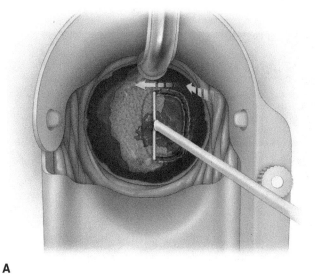

A

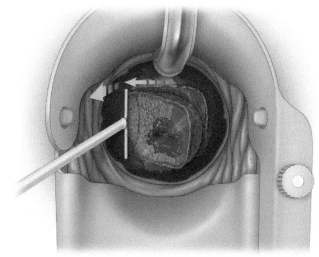

B

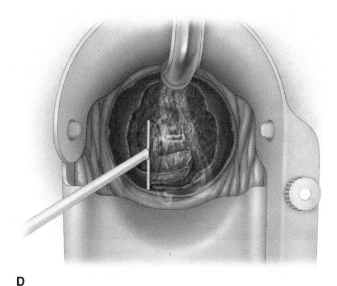

C

D

FIGURE 20.40. Excision of disease requiring more than one pass of the tissue electrode. **A:** When more than one pass is required to remove ectocervical disease, the central portion is first removed by beginning at the 3 o'clock position. **B:** The loop exists at the 9 o'clock position; after the central disease is removed, residual disease can be seen peripheral to the excision defect. **C:** The anterior residual disease is removed. **D:** The posterior disease is removed. Each specimen is placed in fixative in different marked containers. **E:** The procedure is completed by fulguration to any bleeding areas.

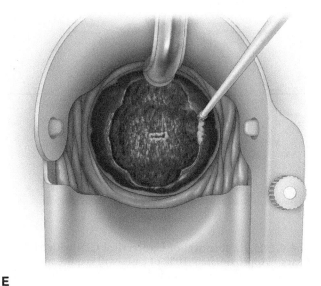

E

as 22 mm from its lowermost border, but 86% of CIN 3 lesions have a length of 10 mm or less. Because of this, most endocervical lesions can be entirely removed with one pass of the loop electrode using the same technique as described for ectocervical disease. Longer lesions or those that extend

beyond the limits of view require more than one pass, or a cylindrical excision using the needle electrode. Older patients and those with a large CIN 3 lesion are more likely to require this procedure. If two specimens are taken from the canal, it is important for pathologic identification that the upper margin of the second specimen be marked (e.g., using India ink or suture) to define final margin status. The two procedures for excising endocervical disease extending >10 mm in the canal are needle excision of endocervical CIN and the "top hat" LEEP procedure.

20.4.4.11.5.2.3.1 Needle Excision of Endocervical CIN Needle excision can be performed on an outpatient basis by working through a bivalve speculum, although it is probably better performed under local or general anesthesia in an operating room (Figure 20.41A–G).[241,253] In the operating room,

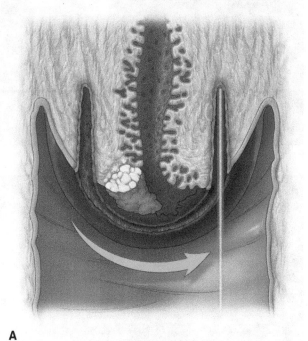

A

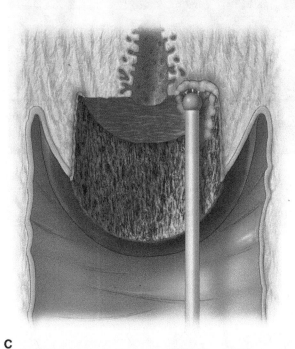

C

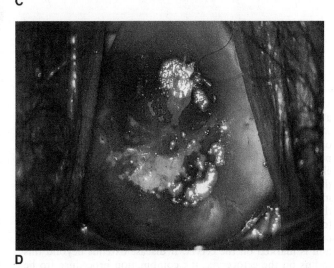

D

FIGURE 20.41.   Operative schematics for endocervical disease. **A:** When disease is confined to the endocervical canal, needle electrode excision is performed similar to the laser cylindrical excision procedure. The circular incision is developed around the os using forceps for traction as the line of incision is developed parallel to the canal. **B:** After sufficient depth is achieved, the specimen is severed at the apex with a scalpel or tonsil snare, producing a cylinder of tissue that is removed by forceps and fixed. **C:** The base of the defect is fulgurated using a ball electrode for hemostasis. **D:** A CIN lesion before needle electrode excision.

B

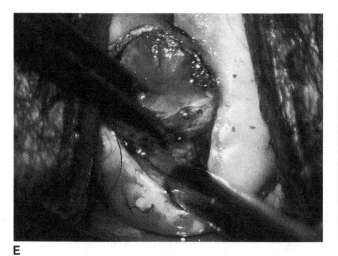

E

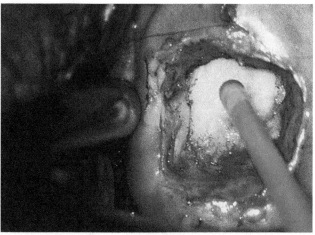

F

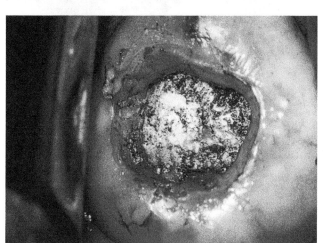

G

FIGURE 20.41. (*Continued*) **E:** A tonsil snare is used to cut the apex of the specimen. **F,G:** Fulguration of the base of the excision. (Images **D–G** provided courtesy of Dr. V. C. Wright.)

a weighted speculum is placed along the posterior vaginal wall, and an insulated tenaculum grasps the anterior cervix outside the tissue to be excised. The tenaculum can be used to position the cervix so that the canal is parallel to the needle electrode angle. A vasoconstrictive solution is infiltrated into the cervix to decrease blood flow to the surgical site. Viewing directly or through the colposcope, the operator positions the long needle electrode and activates it in the blend mode (conventional ESG) just before the needle tip comes into contact with the tissue. A circle with a radius not exceeding 8 mm is marked on the cervix. If disease extends beyond this radius on the ectocervix, the combination procedure (to be described next) is recommended, which would remove any remaining transformation zone and disease. Insulated forceps are positioned within the developing specimen, pulling inward from the incision being developed by the needle tip. The incision will be made to a height (depth) of approximately 15 mm, or deeper if necessary. When the circular incision is completed to the anticipated height, the cylindrical specimen is severed transversely at the apex using a scalpel or a tonsil snare. This provides a specimen with an upper nonthermal edge for accurate histologic reporting of diseased margins. Following the excision, acetic acid can be applied to the canal and the canal can be colposcopically inspected with an endocervical speculum in place to identify disease beyond the excision, if any, as acetowhite rather than pink epithelium. If desired, more tissue can be removed and identified for pathologic examination accordingly. Alternatively, an ECC can be done beyond the canal excision. Following this,

the defect's base is fulgurated with the ball electrode in the Coag mode.

20.4.4.11.5.2.3.2 The "top hat" LEEP for Endocervical CIN The "top hat" procedure can be used instead of needle excision for extensive endocervical preinvasive neoplasia. It is also a good option when there is both extensive canal and portio involvement. In each circumstance, the procedure is the same except that the loop chosen for the exocervical excision portion of the "top hat" procedure for women with only endocervical involvement will typically be smaller (12 to 15 mm wide) than that chosen when the lesion extends significantly onto the portio. Since the procedure is otherwise the same, they will both be discussed in the following section.

20.4.4.11.5.2.4 Excision of Combined Ectocervical and Endocervical CIN with a "top hat LEEP" Approximately 18% of CIN lesions have both endocervical canal extension and wide involvement of the ectocervix. The ectocervical portion usually can be excised by one pass of a large loop (Figure 20.42A–C). The remaining disease in the canal is excised with a smaller loop (Figure 20.42D) or using the technique of long needle excision as previously described (Figure 20.41A–G). The base is then fulgurated as needed (Figure 20.42E). It is important to mark the upper margin of the second specimen for pathologic orientation. Figures 20.42E and 20.43 demonstrate the cervical defect following the combination procedure and Figure 20.44 the healed cervix with good restoration of cervical tissue margin.

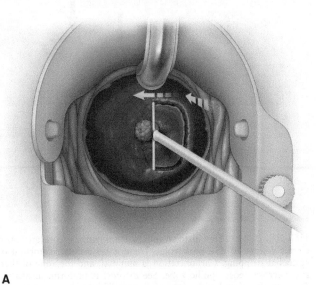

A

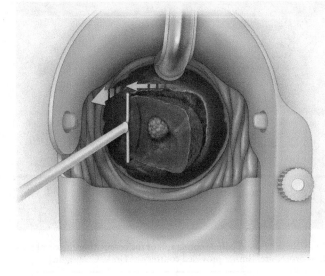

B

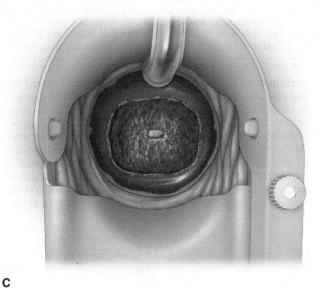

C

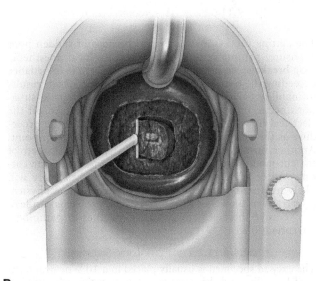

D

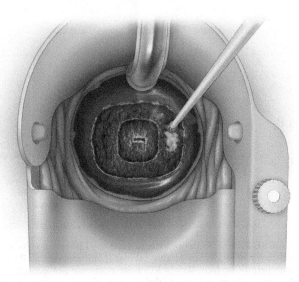

E

FIGURE 20.42.   The combination procedure for extensive ectocervical disease involvement with canal extension. **A:** When a combination procedure is required to deal with ectocervical disease as well as endocervical disease, the ectocervical disease is first removed using the same approach as for the simple ectocervical disease starting at 3 o'clock. **B:** The loop electrode exits the ectocervical tissue at the 9 o'clock. **C:** The defect in the cervix appears after the specimen is removed with forceps. **D:** Using a smaller loop, the endocervical canal component is removed. **E:** The final two-tiered defect appears after the smaller specimen is removed. Any bleeding or ooze is controlled by fulguration with the ball electrode followed by the application of Monsel's paste.

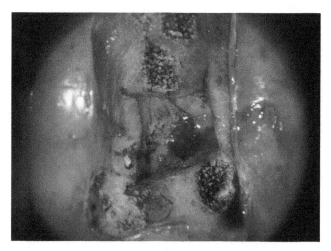

FIGURE 20.43.   A colpophotograph of the cervix after the combination procedure. (Image provided courtesy of Dr. V. C. Wright.)

20.4.4.11.6 PROBLEMS ENCOUNTERED DURING THE LEEP PROCEDURE

The cutting process may be halted because of sudden poor exposure, painful stimuli requiring more local anesthetic, loop breakage, equipment malfunction, or tissue impedance exceeding the output power of the generator, which results in inability to advance the loop. When any of these situations occur, immediately release the switch to turn off the electrical flow, remedy the situation, and restart the procedure at the exit point and end at the initial cut stop point. Another mistake is activating the Coag mode instead of the cut mode when cutting. If this happens, very little cutting will occur, the wire loop will drag, and the wire will likely fracture because of the high voltage and the physical properties of the Coag waveform. These problems can lead to excessive thermal damage and difficulties in pathologic interpretation.

20.4.4.11.7 THE PATHOLOGIC SPECIMEN

The excised specimen is usually placed in a 10% neutral buffered formalin, and the usual radial sections are processed at the laboratory for conventional microscopy. The pathologist should study three zones: the attachment of squamous

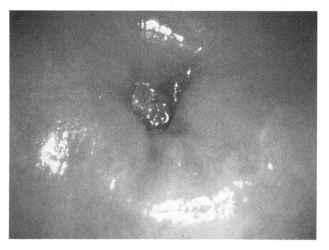

FIGURE 20.44.   The cervix as shown in Figure 20.43 nicely healed with good restoration of volume and an appropriately located SCJ. (Image provided courtesy of Dr. V. C. Wright.)

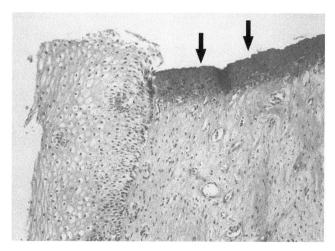

FIGURE 20.45.   The histopathology employing a constant open circuit voltage of 250 peak volts. There is no cellular distortion or epithelial stripping. Carbonization is minimal, and the zone of thermal necrosis (eosinophilic zone, See *arrows*) is uniform, measuring 200 μm. (Reprinted with permission from Wright VC. Loop electrosurgical procedures for treatment of cervical intraepithelial neoplasia: Principles and results. In: Wright VC, Lickrish GM, Shier RM, eds. *Basic and Advanced Colposcopy: A Practical Handbook for Treatment* (2nd ed.). Houston, TX: Biomedical Communications, 1995.)

epithelium to the underlying stroma, the lateral (deep) thermal cut, and the base of the excised specimen. The degree of thermal artifact is studied further according to the (1) degree of detachment of the epithelium or denudation and stripping of the squamous epithelium; (2) degree of cellular distortion; (3) degree of charring; and (4) amount of coagulation necrosis (eosinophilia of the connective tissue stroma). Figure 20.45 demonstrates an ideal LEEP specimen without histologic artifact, whereas Figures 20.46 to 20.48 illustrate some classical undesirable features of loop histology secondary to thermal damage.

20.4.4.11.8 POSTOPERATIVE INSTRUCTIONS

Patient management after LEEP is similar to that after laser surgery. The methods for management of complications

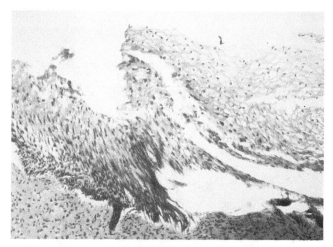

FIGURE 20.46.   With open circuit voltage >1200 peak volts, epithelial stripping and considerable cellular distortion occur. (Reprinted with permission from Wright VC. Loop electrosurgical procedures for treatment of cervical intraepithelial neoplasia: Principles and results. In: Wright VC, Lickrish GM, Shier RM, eds. *Basic and Advanced Colposcopy: A Practical Handbook for Treatment* (2nd ed.). Houston, TX: Biomedical Communications, 1995.)

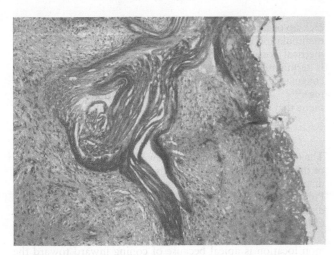

FIGURE 20.47. Electric current has completely destroyed the cellular structure of an endocervical gland. (Image provided courtesy of Dr. V. C. Wright.)

following any excisional procedure are identical, including those for bleeding management discussed previously in the section on laser surgery. Patients are evaluated by cytology, with or without colposcopy, at 6 and 12 months or with HPV DNA testing at least 6 months after treatment.[11,42] Persistent disease is usually discovered at one of these intervals (usually the first). After two normal and satisfactory examinations, or a single negative HPV test, the patient can have routine cytologic surveillance for at least 20 years.[11,42]

20.4.4.11.9 THERAPEUTIC EFFECTIVENESS

In general, loop specimens using the one-pass technique are smaller than the traditional CKC specimens. Some authors state that both procedures are equally effective. The main difference is the nonthermal effect and the better histologic interpretation in the cold-knife group.[108,123,252,254,255] Studies indicate that the overall disease eradication rate after a

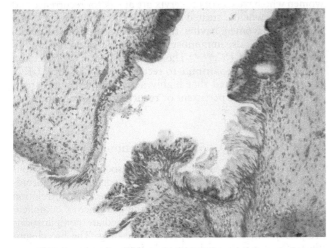

FIGURE 20.48. AIS involves the upper part of the cervical crypt. The epithelium below the disease shows distortion and pseudostratification making pathological assessment difficult. (Reprinted with permission from Wright VC. Loop electrosurgical procedures for treatment of cervical intraepithelial neoplasia: Principles and results. In: Wright VC, Lickrish GM, Shier RM, eds. *Basic and Advanced Colposcopy: A Practical Handbook for Treatment* (2nd ed.). Houston, TX: Biomedical Communications, 1995.)

single treatment ranges from 63% to 95%. The most common complication is bleeding (perioperative and postoperative) in 4% to 6% of patients. Most patients with bleeding are managed on an outpatient basis with 2% requiring hospitalization.[63,108,231,241,242,256]

Women with HIV often experience lower cure rates with LEEP treatment of CIN than do noninfected women treated similarly. Retrospective cohort studies of women with HIV treated by LEEP have shown that treatment failure at initial follow-up was common, occurring in 51% of women with a diagnosis of CIN 1 and 55% in women with CIN 2 or greater.[257] Most lesions detected posttreatment were high grade, regardless of the classification of the initial lesion. Among these women, LEEP is a significant risk factor compared to CKC (RR 1.76, CI: 1.15 to 2.64), as was a low CD4 count.[257] Another significant risk factor for recurrence was positive margins (hazard ratio 6.12, CI: 1.90 to 20.73). Because of high risk of recurrence, frequent follow-up for women with HIV treated for CIN was recommended.[257] Future studies should work to identify the relationship between HAART and CIN as well as the impact of the HPV vaccine among HIV-infected women.

20.4.4.11.10 LONG-TERM CONSEQUENCES OF LEEP

LEEP has become the most widely used method in the United States for treatment of CIN 2,3. As LEEP has become more popular, there have been concerns about increased risk from the procedure of low birth weight infants, PROM, preterm labor, shortened cervical length, and cervical stenosis. A review of the literature by Crane et al. in 2003 evaluated pregnancy outcomes in five cohort studies of women who had received LEEP versus those who had not undergone the procedure.[258] Women having LEEP were more likely to have preterm birth (<37 weeks) as well as birth weight <2500 g, with one extra case of preterm birth demonstrated for every 18 LEEPs. Another meta-analysis of 27 studies by Kyrgiou et al. in 2006 reached a similar conclusion.[47] The OR for preterm birth (<34 weeks) for women having LEEP versus those who did not was 1.70 (1.24 to 2.35), for lower birth weight 1.82 (1.09 to 3.06) and for risk of preterm PROM was 2.69 (1.69 to 4.46). With few exceptions, the majority of other recent studies on the effect of excisional procedures on pregnancy outcome have reported similar results, with the greatest risk being for preterm birth before 34 weeks.[85–91]

20.4.4.11.11 POSTTREATMENT FOLLOW-UP

Posttreatment follow-up is the same as for any other procedure for treatment of cervical precancer and is discussed in this chapter in Sections 20.2.3.3 and 20.3.

20.4.5 Cold-Knife Conization of the Cervix

20.4.5.1 Introduction

Traditionally, CKC was used for investigation of abnormal cytology and for the definitive treatment of CIS, once it was determined in the 1970s that hysterectomy was not necessary as the primary treatment for this precancer.[5,256,259–261] The CKC procedure was usually performed as an inpatient procedure (average 3 to 6 days of hospital stay) rather than as day surgery. With the proliferation of LEEP, there has been a marked decrease in the need for CKC, so much so that training in the procedure is often now lacking. CKCs are almost exclusively performed in an operating room setting because of the potential of bleeding and the need for adequate exposure that is not tolerated well by patients without anesthesia. Patients can be discharged the same day.

20.4.5.2 Changing the Trend

Early publications correlating cytopathology, colposcopy, and histopathology as well as the development and widespread use of outpatient treatment by cryotherapy, and later by laser and LEEP, brought to a close, in most cases, the era of mandatory conization for significantly abnormal cervical cytology.[53,262–265] However, there are still valid indications for the CKC. The operative technique is described in any modern operative gynecologic textbook.

20.4.5.3 Current Indications for Conization

With the 2006 ASCCP and 2008 ACOG guidelines, many of the treatment pathways that were listed as conization became "diagnostic excision procedure" since there was little evidence to recommend one procedure over another.[11,42] However, CKC is the prototypical excisional procedure and at the provider's discretion may be used for this purpose. The following are indications for conization: (1) lack of correlation between cytology (typically HSIL, AGC "favor neoplasia," AIS or cancer), colposcopy, and histology; (2) a positive endocervical sampling; (3) when any portion of a high-grade lesion is located within the endocervical canal requiring tissue to be submitted for histologic evaluation; (4) when cytologic or colposcopic findings suggest invasive carcinoma that has not been proven by colposcopically directed biopsy; (5) when colposcopic biopsy or cytologic findings indicate AIS, since colposcopic and cytologic examinations cannot differentiate between AIS and adenocarcinoma; (6) when colposcopic biopsy indicates microinvasive squamous cell carcinoma; and (7) when colposcopy is unsatisfactory, particularly in the presence of high-grade cytologic findings.

A cold-knife cone can be used for any of the indications listed above for conization; however, with the advent of the LEEP conization procedure, CKC is more commonly used in situations where there is a significant concern for malignancy, when AIS is found on colpobiopsy, or when the patient is not a good candidate for outpatient electrosurgery. The CKC can provide an excellent specimen for pathologic evaluation without thermal artifact on the margins. This is especially important with glandular lesions and situations where cancer must be ruled out.

20.4.5.4 Basic Operative Technique

Regional or general anesthesia can be used for the procedure. The cervix and the vagina should be prepped after a careful colposcopic examination is conducted to plan the outline of the cone. A vasoconstricting agent should be injected into the cervical stroma. Some surgeons recommend the use of sutures placed at the lateral aspect of the cervix at the vaginal fornix. This technique is helpful for traction on the cervix and may reduce blood loss at the time of the CKC. The margins of the excision are planned according to lesion topography. The depth of the CKC should be determined by the endocervical involvement of the disease. The average length of most CKCs is approximately 2 cm; however, the cone length (height) can be customized based on the depth of the disease. The procedure should remove the lesion "completely," but cone dimensions vary considerably. A shallow cone is done for ectocervical disease (wide base, short height), but an increase in excisional length (height) with a corresponding decrease in base is used for more centrally located lesions that extend into the cervical canal.

A number 11 scalpel is typically used, as it provides the most precise incision and easily cuts through the cervical tissue. The incision is begun by cutting into the cervix to a depth of 5 to 8 mm. Following the completion of the initial incision, the scalpel is used to continue the depth of the cone by putting traction on the surgical specimen and angling the incision toward the cervical canal. Traction on the specimen is required. Either a

pick up or lateral stay sutures can be used for the all-important manipulation of the cervix that is required to produce a symmetrical cone specimen. Once the canal is reached the cone is terminated. Bleeding can be controlled by electrosurgical coagulation, sutures, (including Sturmdorf type, and/or packing).[266,267] There are a variety of surgical variations to this technique that can be best obtained from a gynecologic surgery text.

20.4.5.5 Results of Cold-Knife Conization

The older literature must be reviewed to appreciate the results of this procedure, since it was historically performed for both diagnostic and therapeutic purposes, mostly for CIS lesions. Publications between 1956 and 1995 reported that residual disease was found at subsequent hysterectomy or repeat CKC in 12% to 47% (average 23.8%) of women undergoing CKC.[214,256,267–277] When margins are positive, the most common location is apical because of coning inward toward the internal os; hence, the high persistent disease rate. Performing colposcopy before the procedure decreased the persistent disease rate somewhat.[260,278] Relatively more recent studies indicate that 2.8% to 7.7% of CIN 3 cases have squamous cell carcinoma, half of which will be microinvasive.[274,279–281] Therefore, CIN 3 patients with postcone-positive apical margins are at risk of harboring more advanced disease.

It is difficult to predict residual disease after CKC, as there are no consistent predictive factors.[130,274,282,283] Some studies indicate margin status failed to predict residual neoplasia in the excised cervix.[130,274,282,283] One study demonstrated similar residual disease (32%) whether the margins were negative or positive.[282] However, the cancers were found in the women with CIN 3 and positive margins, not in the women with negative margins. Some authors indicate that the only predictors of residual dysplasia are increased age and severity of disease in the cone specimen.[282] Other investigators disagree.[130]

Despite the conservative approach of CKC, invasive squamous cell cancer develops in the cervix in 0.9% and recurrent CIS in 2.3% of patients,[261] while after hysterectomy 1.2% of women develop CIS and 2.1% invasive cancer in the vaginal vault. Although these statistics may at least partially reflect the role that extent of disease played in determining whether conization or hysterectomy was chosen, there is little doubt that women who have CIS of the cervix are at risk for recurrence and malignancy whether treated conservatively or more radically.[261]

As with women having treatment for cervical neoplasia by other methods, immunosuppression increases the risk of recurrence post-CKC.[284,285] The degree of immunosuppression and the viral load contribute to recurrence of CIN after CKC. It has been suggested that highly active antiretroviral treatment may decrease persistent or recurrent squamous intraepithelial lesion (SIL).[285]

20.4.5.6 Complications

CKC is a major operative procedure associated with complications that are significant in both incidence and morbidity.[270] There does not appear to be any appreciable correlation between the technique of CKC and the incidence of complications.[276,284,286] The most major and immediate complications are perioperative and postoperative bleeding. The blood supply to the cervix is predominantly from the uterine artery (a branch of the internal iliac artery). The overall blood supply to the cervix involves anastomotic pelvic and extrapelvic sources (Figure 20.49). Hemorrhage, defined as blood loss >100 mL or heavy bleeding requiring suturing, packing, or other procedures, varies between 9.3% and 15% of all CKCs.[256,267,271,272,276,287]

The hospital readmission rate for supervision and bleeding control is 2.2%.[269,270] The transfusion rate in those who bled varied between 10.0% and 78.5%.[256,267,269,270,276] In older

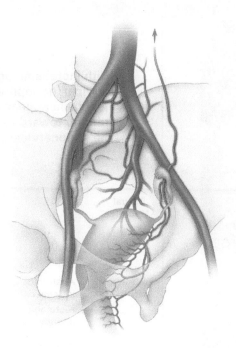

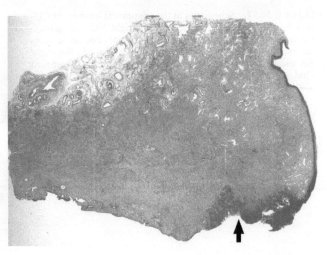

FIGURE 20.50.   Cervical histology specimen demonstrating CIN 3 lesion peripherally and invasive cancer centrally (see *arrow*) in the endocervical canal. (Reprinted with permission from Wright VC. *Color Atlas of Colposcopy: Cervix, Vagina, Vulva, and Adjacent Sites* (2nd ed.). Houston, TX: Biomedical Communications, 2010.)

FIGURE 20.49.   The pelvic superfluous blood supply to the cervix.

studies, when transfusion was necessary, so was hysterectomy as a life-saving procedure in 14.3% to 18.3% of these cases.[270,276]

Symptomatic cervical stenosis occurs in 1.0% to 3.2% of CKC cases[267,271] and uterine perforation in 0.4% to 1.9%.[267,269,271,277] Measurement of the cone dimensions showed that the factor most responsible for these complications was the length of the cone biopsy (specimen height > 25 mm) rather than the overall volume of tissue removed.[256,260,268,276]

Adverse pregnancy outcomes have also been associated with CKC. Meta-analyses have shown that CKC is associated with a significantly higher risk of severe preterm delivery (RR 2.78, CI: 1.72 to 4.51) and extreme preterm delivery (RR 5.33, CI: 1.63 to 17.40), as well as a significantly increased risk of perinatal mortality (RR 2.87, 95% CI: 1.42 to 5.81), and low birth weight (defined as weighing <2000 g) (RR 2.86, CI: 1.37 to 5.97).[165] It is quite clear that adverse pregnancy outcomes are associated with treatment of CIN with CKC. The actual cause of adverse pregnancy outcomes appears to be related to the amount of cervix that is removed by any surgical treatment, although one study questioned whether having CIN itself, without cervical treatment, increased risk for preterm labor.[288]

20.4.5.7 Modifying the Procedure to Account for Disease Distribution

The main advantage that CKC has over LEEP is that there are no thermal effects. This can be critical in managing patients with one of three indications for excision: (1) differentiating microinvasive squamous carcinoma from more advanced disease; (2) differentiating AIS from adenocarcinoma; and (3) sorting out the abnormal glandular Pap test. In these three situations, a cylindrical specimen without burn margins as described accounts best for the distribution of disease. In addition, a small AIS or microinvasive carcinoma could be missed if it fell within the area at the base of the first pass of the loop electrode in a top hat LEEP. In squamous disease, any peripheral CIN can be managed by loop excision or laser ablation. If the excised specimen (which includes the entire transformation zone) demonstrates cancer, the patient is staged and treated accordingly. If the histology of the central disease is CIN, the patient is routinely followed as with any patient treated for CIN.

Because glandular disease (AIS) can exist as skip lesions and can significantly extend up the canal, an excision for glandular disease should ideally be cylindrical and remove the majority of the canal in a single piece. Its dimensions vary according to the distribution of disease similar to squamous. The loop procedure is less ideal in these situations because the high probability of thermal injury to the specimen may result in the pathologist being unable to grade the lesion and exclude malignancy.[247] As with squamous, the worst disease potentially lies centrally (apically, Figure 20.50). Figure 20.51 illustrates the anatomical location of CIN as a function of age. Figure 20.52 illustrates that a single cylinder or a combination of cylinders compared with a conical defect removes far less tissue but still encompasses the distribution of disease.[208,218] The processing of a cone specimen is illustrated in Figure 20.53.

20.4.6 Hysterectomy for Cervical Intraepithelial Neoplasia

20.4.6.1 Introduction

Before 1970, hysterectomy was the definitive method for the management of cervical CIS.[5] Since then, the more conservative, mostly outpatient treatment modalities have supplanted hysterectomy as the main treatments for cervical dysplasia, including CIN 3/CIS.

20.4.6.2 Indications for Hysterectomy

Hysterectomy is employed only in special circumstances, including the following[11,42,229,260,261,270,273,276,289]:

1. Persistent or recurrent high-grade CIN lesion for which conization has failed and reexcision is either not deemed possible or the patient prefers to proceed to hysterectomy.
2. Extensive high-grade disease occupying the cervix with vaginal extension for which conservative management may be difficult. Vaginal extension occurs in 4% of CIS cases.[261] In this situation, the involved vagina is removed as a cuff attached to the hysterectomy specimen. Alternately, laser ablation of the vaginal involvement plus hysterectomy may be appropriate.

FIGURE 20.51.   Schematics of the anatomical location of CIN as a function of age. (Adapted from Wright VC. The geometry of cervical intraepithelial neoplasia: An applied guide to its removal. In: Wright VC, Lickrish GM, Shier RM, eds. *Basic and Advanced Colposcopy: A Practical Handbook for Treatment* (2nd ed.). Houston, TX: Biomedical Communications, 1995.)

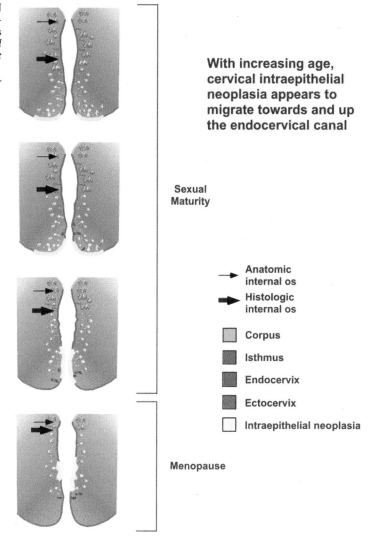

With increasing age, cervical intraepithelial neoplasia appears to migrate towards and up the endocervical canal

Sexual Maturity

→ Anatomic internal os

➡ Histologic internal os

☐ Corpus

☐ Isthmus

☐ Endocervix

☐ Ectocervix

☐ Intraepithelial neoplasia

Menopause

3. The presence of coexisting gynecologic conditions necessitating hysterectomy, such as large symptomatic fibroids, uterine prolapse, endometriosis, or intractable menorrhagia. Because of advances in endoscopic surgery, some of these cases can now be managed by hysteroscopic and laparoscopic methods. Each case must be considered on an individual basis.

4. Technical difficulties (exposure problems) for conservative management. An example of this circumstance is a nulliparous, postmenopausal, nonestrogenized woman. It may be easier to remove the cervix and its lesion (usually in the canal) by hysterectomy rather than risking major complications, such as uncontrolled hemorrhage and/or injury to adjacent organs.

5. Unresolved stenosis after conservative treatment, particularly when a positive upper margin exists. This circumstance inhibits long-term posttreatment assessment and detection of postmenopausal bleeding, induced by either malignancy or hormones.

6. Definitive management for AIS when fertility is no longer an issue.[11,42]

7. To control intractable hemorrhage postconization.[11,42]

The ASCCP and ACOG guidelines both definitively state that hysterectomy is unacceptable as primary therapy for CIN.[11,42]

20.4.6.3 Operative Methods

A Class I hysterectomy (extrafacial) is advised to ensure removal of all cervical tissue.[290] Reflection and retraction of the ureters laterally without actual dissection from the ureteral bed allows clamping of the adjacent paracervical tissue without cutting the side of the cervical tissue. This procedure is recommended primarily for CIS, true microinvasive carcinoma, and AIS.

The various options for operative approach are vaginal hysterectomy, laparoscopically assisted vaginal hysterectomy, total abdominal hysterectomy with or without salpingo-oophorectomy, and total abdominal hysterectomy plus vaginal cuff if there is vaginal extension. A more modified radical hysterectomy will be required for extensive vaginal involvement since the ureters must be isolated to ensure safe excision of the upper third of the vagina (Class II hysterectomy without pelvic lymphadenectomy).[290] The approach must be chosen on an individual case basis, taking into consideration other associated disease states and medical conditions.

20.4.6.4 Posthysterectomy Assessments

Hysterectomy offers no assurance that the patient will be free from disease. Vaginal intraepithelial neoplasia (VaIN) seen at the vaginal vault immediately posthysterectomy indicates that there was unrecognized disease at the time of the hysterectomy. Prior to a hysterectomy, vaginal colposcopy should always be carried out using iodine staining in the estrogenized patient. Post-hysterectomy, disease noted at the vaginal vault suture line may reflect buried disease (hidden disease), which requires a more complicated plan of management.

VaIN that develops many years after hysterectomy likely represents disease missed by screening, inadequate screening,

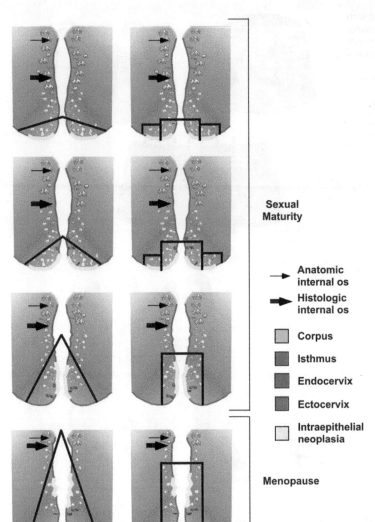

FIGURE 20.52. Schematics of a cone-shaped specimen versus a cylindrical configuration. The cylindrical excisional method removes less tissue when accounting for the distribution of disease (linear length and crypt involvement). (Adapted from Wright VC. The geometry of cervical intraepithelial neoplasia: An applied guide to its removal. In: Wright VC, Lickrish GM, Shier RM, eds. *Basic and Advanced Colposcopy: A Practical Handbook for Treatment* (2nd ed.). Houston, TX: Biomedical Communications, 1995.)

Sexual Maturity

→ Anatomic internal os

➤ Histologic internal os

▢ Corpus

▣ Isthmus

▣ Endocervix

▣ Ectocervix

▢ Intraepithelial neoplasia

Menopause

or new disease (Figures 20.54 and 20.55). Kolstad and Valborg[261] found CIS of the vaginal vault developing after conization for CIS in 1.2% and invasive carcinoma in 2.1%. Creasman and Parker[291] reported recurrent CIS in 1.5% and invasive disease in 0.5%, and Boyes et al.[292] noted recurrent CIS in 0.7% and cancer in 0.1%. Because of these findings, all women undergoing hysterectomy for CIN require initial surveillance with Pap tests from the vaginal vault and upper third of the vagina since these are the frequent sites of recurrence/persistence (Figures 20.54 and 20.55). Granulation tissue can develop at the site of the excision line at the vaginal vault in hysterectomy cases (Figure 20.56A,B). Although it has colposcopic visual characteristics, biopsy may be required to differentiate it from malignancy.

The American Cancer Society recommends that women treated for CIN 2,3 by hysterectomy have follow-up cytology every 4 to 6 months.[293] Cytology screening can be discontinued following three documented, consecutive, technically satisfactory normal/negative vaginal cytology tests and no abnormal/positive cytology tests achieved within an 18- to 24-month period following hysterectomy. These recommendations suggest that lesions found years later are related to initial inadequate screening posthysterectomy.

Occasionally, the pathologist will report invasive cancer in the extirpated specimen. If it is microinvasive by standard definition and all margins are clear, surgery is sufficient. If advanced disease is reported, a referral to an appropriate cancer specialist is necessary.

20.4.7 Approaches in Low-Resource Settings

Heretofore, Chapter 20 has discussed treatment of CIN and AIS in high-resource settings. While serial cytology screening has significantly reduced cervical cancer incidence and mortality in the developed world, cervical cancer remains one of the leading causes of cancer mortality among women in low- and middle-income countries, with more than 80% of the estimated 500,000 new cases and 275,000 deaths each year occurring in the developing world.[294] Many developing countries lack the required infrastructure to develop successful cytology programs, which require multiple visits before treatment is administered, as well as trained providers, high-quality laboratories, reliable transportation of specimens, and quality control metrics.[295,296] Given these requirements, there are few examples of successful cytology-based programs in low- and middle-income countries. An implementation of screening programs could identify and treat precancerous lesions before they progress to cervical cancer, thereby saving the lives of millions of vulnerable women. Cryotherapy is the main treatment option for use in resource-poor areas. Cryotherapy does not need electricity or running water and has been shown to be effective for treating CIN with good cure rates.

A long-term randomized "screen and treat" trial in South Africa demonstrated that screening previously unscreened

FIGURE 20.53. The cylindrical specimen is opened and pinned with the stromal side down. The larger tissue pieces are cut into smaller serial cross sections—termed bread loafing. Single 5-micron sections from each slice are placed on a glass slide for histologic diagnosis and to establish whether or not the margins are free of disease.

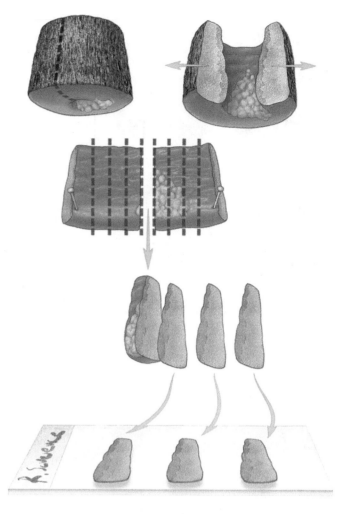

women with a HPV test, followed by treatment of all HPV-positive women by cryotherapy, significantly decreased subsequent detection of CIN 2+ when compared to women receiving no initial screening or treatment.[181] Only 1.5% of women receiving cryotherapy were found to have CIN 2+

over a period of 36+ months of follow-up versus 5.6% of controls. Prior to cryotherapy, the risk of freezing a cervical cancer was reduced by visual inspection after application of acetic acid. This is the most conclusive evidence that in certain low-resource settings where screening is limited,

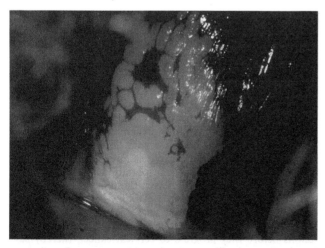

FIGURE 20.54. VaIN 3 of the vaginal vault after Lugol's staining of the estrogenized epithelium. The lesion is multifocal, and the diseased areas fail to retain the iodine solution because of a lack of glucose in the intraepithelial lesion. A previous hysterectomy for CIN 3 was done 5 years earlier. (Reprinted with permission from Wright VC. *Color Atlas of Colposcopy: Cervix, Vagina and Vulva.* Houston, TX: Biomedical Communications, 2003.)

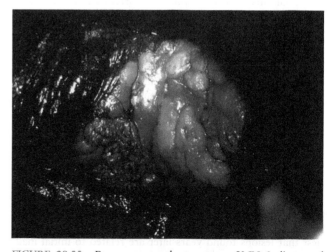

FIGURE 20.55. Four years posthysterectomy, VaIN 3 disease of the left upper third of the lateral vaginal wall is identified by a positive Lugol's iodine test. (Reprinted with permission from Wright VC. *Color Atlas of Colposcopy: Cervix, Vagina and Vulva.* Houston, TX: Biomedical Communications, 2003.)

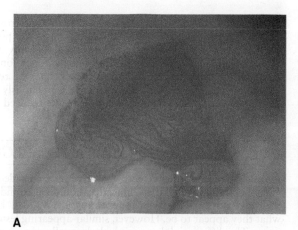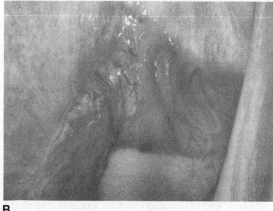

FIGURE 20.56.   A,B: Two presentations of posthysterectomy granulation tissue of the vaginal vault. The angioarchitecture is classic. Biopsy is acceptable to exclude malignancy if there is a concern. (Reproduced with permission from Wright VC. *Comprehensive Colposcopy Review: Cervix, Vagina, Vulva and Adjacent Sites CD-ROM.* Houston, TX: Biomedical Communications, 2008.)

treatment without biopsy by a simple low-cost method such as cryotherapy of women between the ages of 35 to 65 positive for hrHPV should reduce the risk of cervical cancer.

In world areas with low-resource settings, industrial-grade CO_2 from a beverage bottling facility may be the only refrigerant available or the most inexpensive. In countries with low resources, it may not be necessary to perform a pregnancy test prior to treatment with cryotherapy, and where the patient is at high risk for loss to follow-up it may be reasonable to perform cryotherapy on patients <20 weeks.[297]

20.5 TREATMENT OF EXTERNAL GENITAL WARTS

20.5.1 Introduction

External genital warts (EGWs), caused by various types of HPV, are seen primarily in young, sexually active people, although they can be seen at any age. They affect approximately 1% of the population at any time, and the lifetime risk of getting identifiable genital warts (GWs) is about 10%.[298] In many cases, these warts are quite small and, because of their anatomical location, remain unnoticed. In immunocompetent patients, these lesions frequently regress without therapeutic intervention. However, in some cases, GWs multiply in number, expand in size, and do not resolve spontaneously. Rarely, they produce symptoms of itching, irritation, bleeding, or a mass effect that can interfere with hygiene, function, and sexual activity (Figure 20.57). Psychologic sequelae often arise from typical concerns about sexually transmitted infection, including embarrassment, worry about infecting the partner, where it came from and when, and whether the warts will ever go away.[299] Evaluation and therapy are usually sought once individuals notice the lesions or otherwise become symptomatic.

Diagnosis of EGWs is usually clinical, made by gross visual inspection. GWs can be confirmed by biopsy, which might be indicated if (1) the diagnosis is uncertain; (2) the lesions do not respond to standard therapy; (3) the disease worsens during therapy; (4) the lesion is atypical appearing; (5) the patient is immunocompromised and the lesions are not classic condyloma; or (6) the warts are pigmented, indurated, fixed, bleeding, or ulcerated.[300] EGWs are usually asymptomatic, but depending on the size and anatomic location, they might be painful or pruritic. The use of HPV DNA testing for GW diagnosis is not recommended since test results would not alter management.[300] The application of 3% to 5% acetic acid is not recommended for screening to detect mucosal changes attributed to HPV infection because acetowhitening on external genitalia is not specific for HPV-induced changes.[301]

The advent of prophylactic HPV vaccines in 2006 was a major breakthrough for the prevention of not only cervical cancer but also EGWs. At present, only the quadrivalent HPV vaccine (Gardasil) contains virus-like particles that are designed to prevent the accusation of HPV type 6 and 11, which are responsible for 90% of GWs.[302,303] Women and girls receiving all three doses of the quadrivalent HPV vaccine and naïve to HPV 6 and 11 when given the vaccine have up to a 99% reduction in EGWs caused by these two types.[302] The quadrivalent HPV vaccine was also 90.4% effective in decreasing the incidence of vaccine-related EGWs in the HPV 6– and 11–naïve population of males aged 16 to 26 years.[304] Despite this important development in the prevention of HPV, by the end of 2010 <40% of the eligible population of women and girls age 9 to 26 in the United States had been vaccinated.[305] Therefore, clinicians will need a variety of treatment options for GWs for the foreseeable future.

Clinicians have a wide variety of treatment options available that allow therapy to be tailored for each patient. A rational

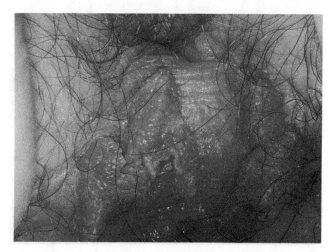

FIGURE 20.57.   This perineal condyloma caused itching followed by a self-inspection that detected a growth.

and selective treatment plan will maximize optimal outcomes and may minimize side effects even though cure rates are quite similar for the different approaches. This section describes the various methods for treating GWs. The treatment options are divided into patient-applied and provider therapies to reflect the various delivery methods for EGW therapy. Specifically, the composition and mechanism of action, indications and contraindications, application or delivery techniques, advantages and disadvantages, and effectiveness of each option will be discussed.

20.5.2 Treatment Purpose and Objectives

Patients want GWs treated for many reasons. Because EGWs pose few serious risks, treatment should be considered elective in most cases, and observation may be a reasonable alternative, although patients rarely choose this option. The main purpose for treating EGWs is to eliminate the lesion(s) and allow the restoration of healthy epithelium. Current understanding of "successful treatment" is that active expression of HPV is eliminated, but that latent (unexpressed) HPV may indefinitely persist in infected epithelium. Consequently, all forms of treatment are associated with a certain risk for recurrent disease that, however, diminishes as time goes by. It is clear that some individuals remain at risk for recurrence long-term, as the rate of expression of GWs after severe immune suppression, such as posttransplantation surgery, is very high.[5]

The objectives of GW management are to (1) destroy clinically evident GWs, when desired, (2) minimize the possibility of disease recurrence, (3) address psychologically related concerns, and (4) provide appropriate patient education.[301] By reducing the viral load an additional benefit may be reduced likelihood of transmission of the virus to a previously unexposed partner, but the definitive timing of this reduced risk is not possible to predict or document.

20.5.3 Prerequisites to Treatment of EGWs

Prior to treating patients with GWs, certain considerations must be entertained. First, clinicians should be confident of their diagnosis. Most typical-appearing EGWs will be just what they appear to be. However, similar-appearing lesions do occur. The differential diagnosis includes molluscum contagiosum, nevi, seborrheic keratosis, and other papular or plaque-like benign dermatologic conditions, and very rarely, verrucous carcinoma (Buschke-Löwenstein tumor) and condyloma lata (syphilis). Normal anatomic findings may also mimic EGWs; micropapillomatosis labialis in women (see Chapter 15) and pearly penile papules in men (see Chapter 17). EGWs that do not respond as expected to conventional therapy, present in the elderly, or are pigmented, hard, or ulcerated should be biopsied to confirm the diagnosis.

The distribution and site of disease must be considered (Figure 20.58A–D). Diffuse anogenital warts may present

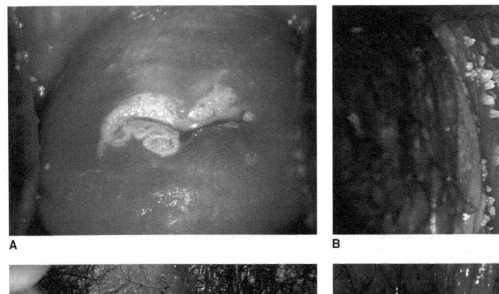

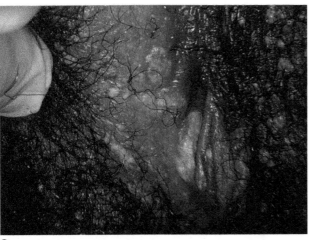

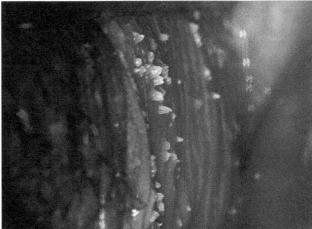

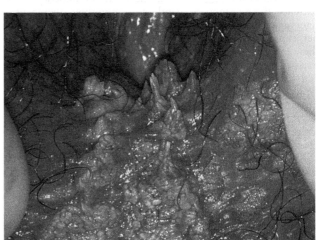

FIGURE 20.58.   A–D: This young woman has cervical, vaginal, vulvar, and perirectal condylomas that require different therapies.

TABLE 20.15	THE CENTERS FOR DISEASE CONTROL AND PREVENTION TREATMENT OPTIONS FOR GENITAL WARTS

Patient-Applied
Podofilox 0.5% solution or gel
Imiquimod 5% cream
Sinecatechins 15% ointment

Provider-Administered
Cryotherapy with liquid nitrogen or cryoprobe
Podophyllin resin 10%–25% in a compound tincture of
  benzoin
Trichloroacetic acid (TCA) or bichloroacetic acid (BCA)
  80%–90%
Surgical removal: scissor excision, shave excision, curettage,
  electrosurgery, or laser ablation.

Modified from Workowski KA, Berman S; Centers for Disease Control and Prevention (CDC). Sexually transmitted diseases treatment guidelines, 2010. *MMWR Recomm Rep* 2010;59(RR-12):1–110.

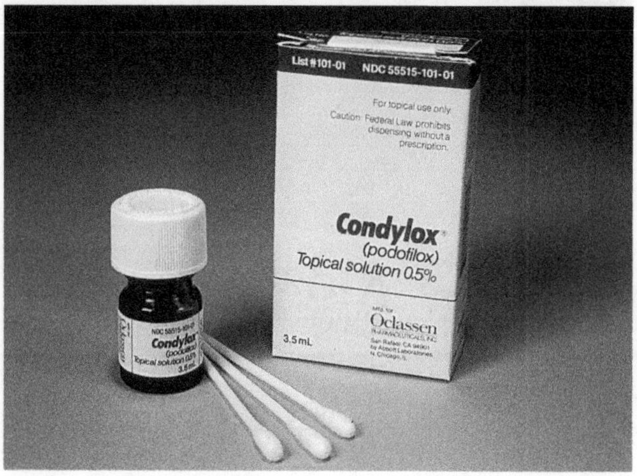

FIGURE 20.59. Commercially available podofilox used to treat external genital condyloma.

different implications for therapy when compared with unifocal disease. Likewise, choice of treatment may be influenced by whether disease is located on mucosal or keratinized epithelium. External genital lesions may extend internally within the vagina, urethra, minor vestibular glands, or rectum, necessitating two or more different treatment approaches. GWs involving "sensitive" areas, such as the clitoris or glans penis, require tissue-sparing therapy that avoids excessive treatment of normal epithelium and reduces the risk of postoperative discomfort. Cervical condylomas and CIN 1 are not routinely treated unless they persist for 2 or more years.[11,42] Management is also influenced by the number, size, and shape of the EGWs. For instance, simple excision may be preferred for treating large, solitary, pedunculated warts, while topical application or vaporization may be more appropriate for multiple small sessile or papular warts.

Clinicians must also consider the patient's age, immune status including reduced immune response due to use of tobacco, other associated medical conditions, history of response to past therapy, history of getting rid of warts in general, drug allergies, and pregnancy status. Because each type of treatment is associated with potentially bothersome side effects, full patient disclosure of the anticipated cure rate, average length of treatment, potential adverse reactions and cost is necessary prior to initiating therapy. Patients who use tobacco should be encouraged to discontinue its use because cotinine, nicotine, and nitrosamine by products of tobacco use are thought to suppress the immune response to HPV.[5]

The Centers for Disease Control and Prevention (CDC) treatment options for EGWs can be divided into patient-applied modalities and provider-administered therapies. The 2010 CDC recommendations for the treatment are listed in Table 20.15.[301]

20.5.4 Patient-Applied Therapies

20.5.4.1 Podofilox 0.5% Solution or Gel

Podofilox 0.5% is a purified form of podophyllin (Figure 20.59) Podofilox works by arresting cellular division in mitosis. Both solution and gel forms of the drug are commercially available. Podofilox is indicated for use on small EGWs that cover a limited area and reside primarily on keratinized epithelium. Podophyllotoxin is absorbed quite readily through mucosal epithelium. Therefore, care should be exercised to prevent

potential drug-induced toxicity by limiting the extent of GW treatment involving this tissue and not applying internally or on occluded epithelium. The safety of podofilox has not been established in pregnant women (Pregnancy class C). Its parent drug, podophyllin resin, is pregnancy class X.

Podofilox is a patient-applied product. Patients apply podofilox to warts twice a day for 3 successive days followed by a rest period of 4 days. This sequence is repeated on a weekly basis for as long as 4 weeks or until wart resolution occurs. The total wart area treated should not exceed 10 cm², and the total volume of podofilox should be limited to 0.5 mL per day.[298]

Podofilox has two main advantages when compared with podophyllin resin. It is a purified form of podophyllin that is prepared at a standardized concentration. This allows it to be a patient-applied form of treatment, providing easy home application in a confidential setting. Mild to moderate pain or local irritation might develop after treatment, but it is generally well tolerated. Since podofilox is self-applied, improper application risks treatment failure, so the provider should apply the initial treatment to demonstrate the proper application technique and identify which warts should be treated.[301] Epidermal erythema, ulceration, irritation, and pain may accompany its use.[300]

The cure rate expected with podofilox varies between 45% and 80%.[306–308] Recurrence has been reported in 0% to 90% of the patients. Depending upon the spectrum of disease, a 4-week course of treatment may be necessary to completely eradicate the lesions treated.

20.5.4.2 Imiquimod

Imiquimod is an immune response modifying agent with properties that induce alpha-interferon, tumor necrosis factor, IL-6, and other cytokines. The exact mechanism of action on warts is not yet completely understood, but it does clearly result in an immune response that has been shown to decrease the amount of HPV DNA in affected tissues. It is commercially formulated as a 5% cream (Figure 20.60).

Patients with diffusely located EGWs are ideal candidates. This scenario is very conducive to a regional cream application, instead of a precise site-specific application. However, patients with focal or a solitary GW can also be treated with imiquimod. The safety of imiquimod has not been established in pregnant women (Pregnancy class C). Even though off-label use of this drug occurs, imiquimod is not FDA approved to treat condylomas of the cervix, vagina, urethra, or rectum,

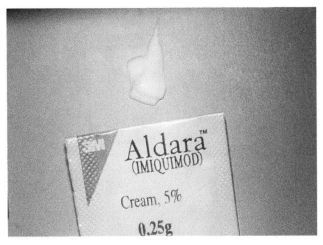

FIGURE 20.60. Commercially available imiquimod cream used to treat external genital condylomas. Imiquimod is an immune-response modifying agent.

primarily because of lack of adequate studies. Imiquimod cream is applied to GWs three times a week (i.e., Monday, Wednesday, Friday). The cream is washed off after each application 8 hours later.[301] Although complete resolution of warts may be achieved in a much shorter interval, application for up to 16 weeks may be necessary to clear some EGWs.

There are several therapeutic advantages observed with imiquimod. Imiquimod works by boosting the local immune system.[5] Therefore, some regional antiviral effect may be noted. As a consequence, warts distant from the area(s) of application, such as in the vagina or anus, have at times been noted to spontaneously resolve coincident with resolution of the treated EGWs, and areas not adjacent to treated warts will occasionally erode, suggesting an immune response to HPV-induced subclinical disease. Like other self-applied products, imiquimod is applied by the patient in the privacy of their own home. This is particularly appealing to embarrassed individuals or those otherwise inconvenienced by multiple health care appointments. Imiquimod use may precipitate erythema, ulceration, and discomfort at the treatment site.

Between 40% to 80% of patients treated with imiquimod are cured following treatment (Figure 20.61A,B).[309–314] GWs in women may respond more favorably than those in men,[310] although cure rates in men may actually be equivalent.[311] Because of its mechanism of action, imiquimod is not as effective in treating immunosuppressed individuals, as demonstrated by a 1999 study in which imiquimod was no more effective than placebo when treating HIV-infected patients.[308] However, more recent studies in the era of HAART have demonstrated imiquimod to be useful as an adjunct to other treatments for genital-induced HPV lesions.[313,314] In the general population, recurrence rates are low and vary between 10% to 20%. The low recurrence rates may be explained by the regional effect on the immune system.

20.5.4.3 Sinecatechins 15% Ointment

Sinecatechins are a standardized extract of green tea leaves from Camellia sinensis that contains mainly tea polyphenols, particularly catechins (more than 85%).[300] The green tea catechins have multiple biologic activities including a potent antiviral effect and antioxidant activity. Catechins bind to a variety of proteins, including enzymes involved in the generation of inflammatory mediators, proteases promoting tumor invasion, and kinases needed in tumor signaling, cell cycle modification, and induction of apoptosis, thereby contributing to the therapeutic effect of the extract.[315–320]

Excellent results have been demonstrated in randomized placebo-controlled trials when sinecatechin 15% ointment has been applied to EGWs by the patient three times daily for up to 16 weeks.[319] As compared to the control, 15% ointment produced complete clearance of baseline and newly obtained warts in 57.2% as compared to 33.7% for the control group in a study population of both men and women. The clearance of the warts was found to be significant at the 4-week follow-up time period. Women had a higher rate of complete clearance (64.6% compared to 45.8% for the control group).[319,321] The treatment was well tolerated with local skin reaction being the most common side effect. The majority of skin reactions occurred within the first 4 weeks of treatment and generally decreased thereafter during continued use. Some local skin reaction was experienced by 87% compared to 72% in the control group, with most being mild to moderate. Reported local skin reactions are erythema, pruritus/burning, pain, ulceration, edema, induration, and vesicular rash.[301,319,321]

Sinecatechin 15% should be applied three times daily (0.5 cm strand of ointment to each wart) using a finger to ensure coverage with a thin layer of ointment until complete clearance of warts, but no longer than 16 weeks.[301] The medication should not be washed off after use. Sexual (i.e., genital,

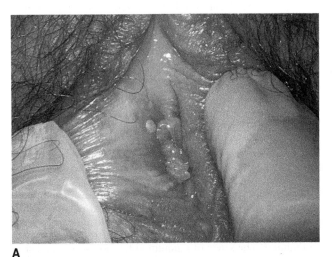

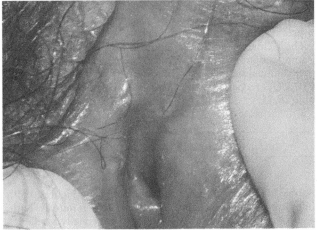

A **B**

FIGURE 20.61. **A:** A small vulvar condyloma (**B**) cleared following several applications of topical imiquimod.

anal, or oral) contact should be avoided while the ointment is on the skin. The medication may weaken condoms and diaphragms. The medication is not recommended for HIV-infected persons, immunocompromised persons, or persons with clinical genital herpes because the safety and efficacy of therapy in these settings has not been established.[301] The safety of sinecatechins during pregnancy also is unknown.

20.5.5 Provider-Administered Therapy

20.5.5.1 Podophyllin Resin 10% to 25%

Podophyllin resin is derived from the root of the "may apple plant," *Podophyllum peltatum*. The solution is commonly formulated as a 25% concentration in tincture of benzoin, although the actual concentration may vary considerably. Podophyllin arrests cellular replication of warts by inhibiting mitosis. This effect is noted particularly in rapidly growing tissue.

Podophyllin resin is used infrequently because newer, safer, and perhaps more effective forms of treatment are now available. However, podophyllin resin 10% to 25% can be used on small EGWs that cover a limited area and reside primarily on keratinized epithelium. Podophyllin is absorbed quite readily through mucosal epithelium. Systemic reactions, neurotoxicity, and death are documented in the literature with extensive application, application to mucous membranes, or if left on the skin for long periods of time. Reactions include nausea, vomiting, fever, confusion, coma, renal failure, ileus, and leukopenia.[300] Because podophyllin is a teratogen, its use is contraindicated in pregnant women (Figure 20.62).[301]

The solution containing podophyllin resin 10% to 25% should be applied directly to GWs using a cotton-tip applicator or the wooden end of an applicator stick and allowed to dry before coming into contact with cloths (Figure 20.63). Approximately 1 to 4 hours following application, patients should wash the treated area with soap and water even though the tincture of benzoin is water insoluble. Although latent HPV can be found in the normal-appearing epithelium surrounding warts, care should be exercised to treat only the warts and not the normal adjoining tissues. Therefore, some advocate covering the adjoining normal epithelium with a protective barrier of petrolatum before applying podophyllin to the wart, but this is not widely practiced. Podophyllin can be reapplied weekly for 4 to 6 weeks or until wart resolution.

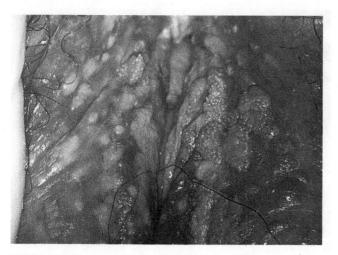

FIGURE 20.62. Several vulvar condyloma were noted on this pregnant woman. Podophyllin, podofilox, 15% sinecatechin ointment, 5-FU, and imiquimod would be contraindicated for use.

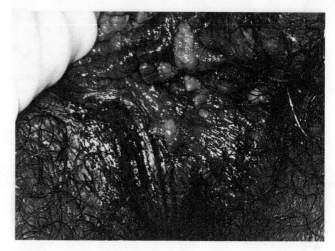

FIGURE 20.63. Podophyllin applied to external genital condyloma.

If warts do not respond within this interval, biopsy confirmation of the original diagnosis and/or treatment with another modality is advised.

To avoid the possibility of complications associated with systemic absorption and toxicity, two guidelines should be followed: (1) application should be limited to <0.5 mL of podophyllin or an area of <10 cm² of warts per session and (2) the area to which treatment is administered should not contain any open lesions or wounds.[301]

Because podophyllin is fairly inexpensive, it has historically been an attractive therapeutic option. Furthermore, some patients prefer its painless application. However, podophyllin acts relatively slowly, and many patients require multiple clinician-applied treatments. Consequently, it may not be the best treatment for impatient or noncompliant patients. If a GW must be biopsied following recent unsuccessful podophyllin use, clinicians should inform the pathologist. By promoting mitotic cells, podophyllin may produce histopathologic changes that mimic epithelial atypia.[300] Podophyllin should not be used to treat warts located within the urethra, vagina, or rectum. Podophyllin can precipitate skin erythema, ulceration, and pain.

Wart cure rates reported for podophyllin vary between 20% and 80%, depending on the clinical trial.[306,322,323] Because some study endpoints for cure were defined at six treatments, greater cure rates may be expected with longer treatment. Unfortunately, 25% to 70% of patients have a recurrence of condylomas following use of podophyllin.

20.5.5.2 Trichloroacetic Acid or Bichloroacetic Acid

Bichloroacetic acid (BCA) and trichloroacetic acid (TCA) 70% to 90% are potent caustic solutions commonly used to treat EGWs. These acids can also be applied to GWs within the vagina or anus or those on the ectocervix if located outside the transformation zone. However, care must be taken when using these products to treat internal GWs because depth of tissue destruction may be more difficult to control. Patients who have a limited number of GWs are ideal candidates for BCA/TCA. Multiple, diffusely distributed lesions may be better treated using other agents. BCA and TCA can be used safely to treat EGWs in pregnant women.

When treating small solitary GWs, BCA and TCA are best applied using a small-caliber wood stick or the end of a wooden-shaft cotton-tip applicator (Figure 20.64A,B). Larger lesions may be treated using a cotton-tip applicator soaked in TCA. The surface of the GW will assume a white color

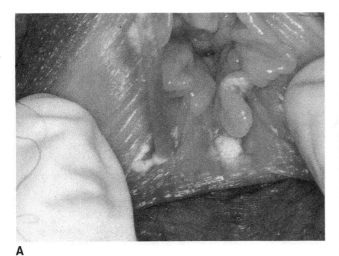 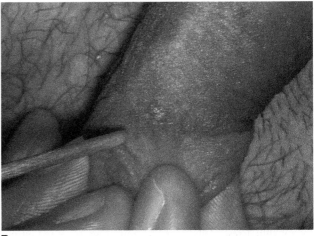

A   B

FIGURE 20.64.   Use of a wood stick to apply BCA/TCA to external genital condyloma on the vulva (A) and penis (B).

following proper application (Figure 20.65A,B). Patients do not need to rinse the treated areas following treatment. Several days later, the affected desiccated tissues will slough, sometimes leaving a slight erosion. Care must be exercised to keep the wooden application device perpendicular to the surface of the epithelium so as to treat only the warts. Wooden-shaft applicators have inherent capillary action that tends to draw solutions up the shaft from the immersed tip. If the wet applicator is held parallel and touches the surface of the skin, some linear trauma to normal adjoining tissue is possible. Some advocate applying petrolatum to the normal epithelium surrounding warts prior to using BCA/TCA, but this additional effort is not usually necessary if the BCA/TCA is applied cautiously only to the wart. Because of its low viscosity, large drops of BCA/TCA tend to flow easily off warts and onto surrounding tissue. Therefore, before removing the wooden shaft applicator from the vial of BCA/TCA, tap the drop that usually adheres at the end of the stick against the container to dislodge it prior to wart application. This simple "flick" prevents acid runoff (Figure 20.66). Alternatively, if the TCA/BCA in the bottle is kept at a level of only about ½ inch in depth, the amount that could run off the stick is kept to a manageable amount. TCA/BCA is considered a clinician-applied form of treatment for GWs. Potentially extensive and deep burns may occur if the product is applied improperly. Sodium bicarbonate can be used to neutralize TCA/BCA, if necessary.

BCA/TCA works quite effectively for most patients. It is comparatively inexpensive, and reasonable outcomes can be expected. The solutions may cause immediate mild-to-moderate burning, which can be more severe if normal epithelium is treated accidentally. Usually this discomfort resolves within 5 to 10 minutes or less. When present, posttreatment erosion may also cause some pain for several days (Figure 20.67). Deeper ulcerations can occur following aggressive treatment. In this case, healed tissue may be depigmented if the melanocytes are permanently damaged. Small warts often resolve following a single application. Particularly large or heavily keratinized GWs may be reduced in size or in some cases completely eradicated following a single application. Multiple applications may be necessary (Figure 20.68). Patients are often treated on a bimonthly basis to allow interval healing, but can be repeated weekly, if necessary.[301] Therapeutic response depends on the host immune status, size of the lesions, viral load, type of epithelium, and spectrum of HPV disease. Cure rates of between 50% and

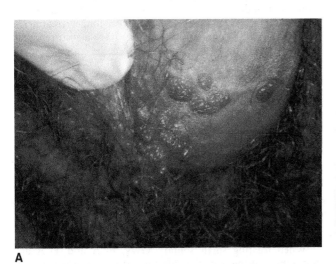 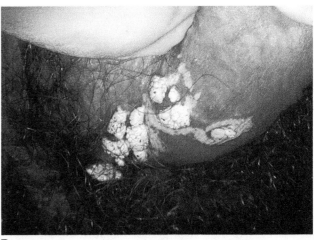

A   B

FIGURE 20.65.   Penile condyloma before (A) and after (B) application of TCA. Note the immediate white discoloration of treated epithelium.

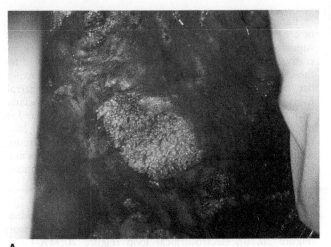
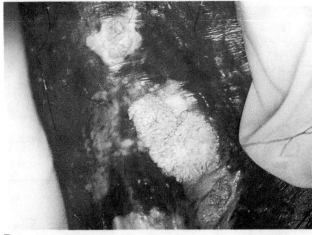

A   **B**

FIGURE 20.66.   Vulvar condyloma before (**A**) and following treatment (**B**). Notice some runoff of the TCA onto normal surrounding epithelium.

100% may be expected with the use of BCA/TCA.[306,324] GW recurrence rates vary between 5% and 50% (Figure 20.69).

20.5.5.3 Cryotherapy

Nitrous oxide, liquid nitrogen, and carbon dioxide cryogens can be used to treat GWs. Each cryogen generates tissue temperatures below –20°C that are sufficient to cause cell death. Initially, cryotherapy produces an intracellular dehydration. Thereafter, ice crystals pierce the cell membranes, releasing vasoactive substances that cause small vessel thrombosis, leading to anoxia and ischemia.

Cryotherapy is an ablative method used to treat GWs. Each cryogen may be better suited to treat certain warts based on their size and shape, and cryogen delivery method (i.e., spray, probe, etc.). Liquid nitrogen is the most common refrigerant used to treat all types of warts. There are four ways that liquid nitrogen may be used to treat EGWs. The cryogen may be applied directly to the wart using large or small cotton-tip applicators that have been dipped in liquid nitrogen. Liquid nitrogen may also be applied by a device that directs a focal spray onto the wart. Cryo-tweezers that are placed in liquid nitrogen may be used to grasp and freeze isolated warts. Finally, a metal probe that contains liquid nitrogen can be placed against the warts to complete a freeze.

Nitrous oxide systems should have available several different probe tips of different sizes and shapes in order to better conform to the size and shape of the wart. Cryoprobe tips used for cervical cryotherapy are typically too large to be used on most GWs. Because of the difficulty controlling depth of freeze, vaginal GWs are not usually treated by cryotherapy using cryoprobes, although the use of liquid nitrogen is acceptable.[301] When used to treat EGWs, a thin film of water-soluble lubricant gel is first applied to the nitrous oxide probe tip, and then the tip is applied to the GW. Freezing is initiated by depressing a trigger located on a cryogun. Once the GW is completely frozen, including a surrounding 1- to 2-mm rim of normal tissue, the freeze may be discontinued for any cryotherapy method. When using a nitrous oxide cryoprobe to freeze EGWs, care should be taken to not freeze neurovascular tissue that may lie directly beneath GW. To prevent this from occurring, once the cryoprobe tip adheres to the wart, the wart should be gently retracted away from deeper

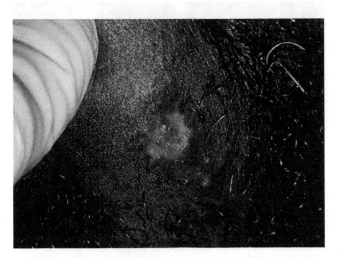

FIGURE 20.67.   Healing ulceration on base of penis 2 weeks after treating a condyloma with TCA.

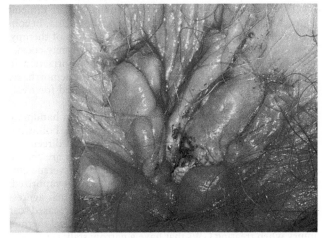

FIGURE 20.68.   Residual perianal warts after a prolonged course of treatment. Notice the smooth contour of these incompletely eradicated warts.

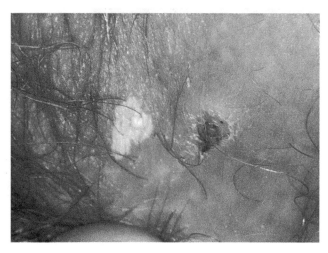

FIGURE 20.69.   Healing penile site after condyloma treatment with TCA. Notice a new condyloma (after application of TCA) has become apparent since the past treatment.

structures. A double-freeze (freeze, thaw, repeat freeze) technique may improve cryotherapy efficacy.

Cryotherapy is a clinician-directed treatment that causes minimal to moderate operative discomfort. Patients with solitary or a limited number of GWs are perhaps the best candidates. Aggressive treatment may cause postoperative ulceration, pain, and depigmentation. Many patients respond to a single treatment provided are of a smaller size and adequately frozen. Cryotherapy successfully treats EGWs in 60% to nearly 100% of cases.[302] Treatment technique greatly determines outcome. Many clinicians have a tendency to undertreat using an abbreviated approach. Recurrence rates vary between 20% and 80%. Treatment should be repeated every 1 to 2 weeks until clear. Cryotherapy is contraindicated in patients with cryoglobulinemia. Pregnant women with EGWs may be treated using cryotherapy.

20.5.5.4 Laser Vaporization

Carbon dioxide (CO_2) laser is another way to ablate GWs. The depth and extent of vaporization is determined by the power of the laser, diameter of the beam, duration of laser activation, and skill of the surgeon. Laser vaporization is best indicated for widely distributed, recalcitrant, or heavily keratinized GWs. Laser vaporization is also a very effective form of treatment for GWs found in anatomical locations that are difficult to reach. These sites include the rectum and the vagina. In contrast with some of the previously mentioned types of therapy, laser effectively treats noninvasive neoplasia that may coexist with GWs. It is contraindicated to use laser vaporization in patients who are fully anticoagulated or have a hemorrhagic diathesis. Laser vaporization is not contraindicated for treating EGWs in pregnant women.

The surgeon guides the laser beam with either a handpiece instrument or a joystick mounted on a colposcope. Following either local or general anesthesia, the laser beam is directed at the GW. A laser beam spot size and watts of power are chosen that meet the criteria for effective laser ablation versus cutting. The treatment continues until the entire GW is vaporized. Caution must be taken to not treat too deeply. Such aggressive treatment may cause prolonged healing and increased scar formation. A useful technique that may reduce lateral thermal injury when treating GWs that have a narrow stalk is to grasp the wart at is base with a laser-safe straight clamp. The laser can then be directed at the wart until ablation occurs to the level of the clamp. The clamp acts as a backstop to reduce thermal spread and seals the vessel leading up to the GW.

Patients with GWs that are numerous and spread diffusely, or are recalcitrant to prior therapy, are best managed by laser vaporization. Because of the high cost and moderate postoperative morbidity, laser vaporization is generally reserved for these select cases. Furthermore, laser requires surgical expertise and, for many clinicians, this means patient referral. Even properly performed laser vaporization may be associated with significant postoperative discomfort and pain, scar formation, and postoperative bleeding. GW cure rates using laser vaporization vary between 60% and 100%.[306,325] Furthermore, recurrence rates vary between 0% and 80%. These figures may reflect the more difficult cases reserved for laser vaporization.

20.5.5.5 Excisional Procedures

Simple excision procedures easily remove raised or pedunculated GWs. Excision can be accomplished using scissors (Figure 20.70), electrosurgical loop (Figure 20.71A–C) or needle, or scalpel. There are usually few complications, limited to pain, infection, scar formation, and bleeding. Preoperative local anesthesia is usually necessary unless a pedunculated wart's stalk is quite narrow or general anesthesia is given. Surgical excision is best reserved for patients with a limited number of raised GWs. Lesions are excised to or just above the level of the papillary dermis. Surgical excision cure and recurrence rates vary between 10% and 35%.[306]

20.5.6 Other Therapies

Historically, 5-flurouracil (5-FU), a chemotherapeutic agent that inhibited DNA synthesis, and interferon alpha, beta, and gamma were used for the treatment of GWs. In the 1980s, 5-FU was used extensively to treat vaginal HPV-induced lesions, but the frequent occurrence of vaginal ulcerations, the difficulty in subsequent healing of these lesions, and the development of adenosis in previously ulcerated areas discouraged use.[326] Once rare cases of clear cell carcinoma were described that appeared to arise in areas of post–5-FU adenosis,[327] the use of 5-FU vaginally essentially ceased.

Alternative regimens include treatment options that might be associated with more side effects and/or less data on efficacy. They include intralesional interferon, photodynamic therapy, and topical cidofovir. With today's wide array of therapeutic options, these agents are infrequently used as they have moderate side effects and limited data on treatment benefit.[301]

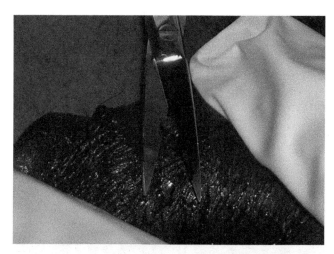

FIGURE 20.70.   Single wart removal using scissors. After the lesion is anesthetized, the scissors are advanced until they engage the lesion and then lifted slightly above the surrounding skin, and the lesion is quickly excised. (Dr. EJ Mayeaux Jr, MD, used with permission.)

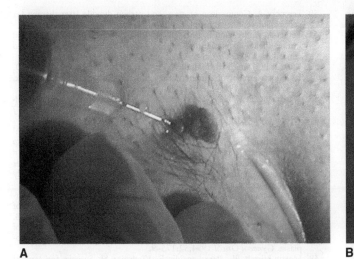

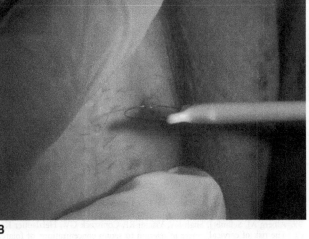

FIGURE 20.71. Single wart removal using electrosurgery. **A:** The lesion is anesthetized with lidocaine with epinephrine, **(B)** the loop is passed through the base of the lesion at the level of the papillary dermis, **(C)** the edges of the excision are smoothed or "feathered" to produce a smooth shallow crater. (Dr. EJ Mayeaux Jr, MD, used with permission.)

References

1. Wright TC, Cox JT, Massad LS, Twiggs LB, Wilkinson EJ; for the 2001 ASCCP-sponsored Consensus Workshop. 2001 Consensus Guidelines for the management of women with cervical cytological abnormalities and cervical cancer precursors—part I: cytological abnormalities. *JAMA* 2002;287:2120–9.

2. Wright TC Jr, Cox JT, Massad LS, Carlson J, Twiggs LB, Wilkinson EJ; American Society for Colposcopy and Cervical Pathology. 2001 Consensus Guidelines for the management of women with cervical intraepithelial neoplasia. *Am J Obstet Gynecol* 2003;189:295–304.

3. Wright TC, Massad LS, Dunton CJ, Spitzer M, Wilkinson EJ, Solomon D; For the American Society for Colposcopy and Cervical Pathology. 2006 Consensus Guidelines for the management of women with cervical intraepithelial neoplasia or adenocarcinoma in situ. *Am J Obstet Gynecol* 2007;197(4):340–5.

4. Massad LS, Einstein MH, Huh WK, et al.; 2012 ASCCP Consensus Guidelines Conference. 2012 updated consensus guidelines for the management of abnormal cervical cancer screening tests and cancer precursors. *Obstet Gynecol* 2013;121(4):829–46.

5. Cox JT. Management of precursor lesions of cervical carcinoma: history, host defense, and a survey of modalities. *Obstet Gynecol Clin North Am* 2002;29(4):751–85.

6. Tate DR, Anderson RJ. Recurrence of cervical dysplasia in the human immunodeficiency virus-seropositive patient. *Obstet Gynecol* 2001;97(suppl 1):S60.

7. Crowley-Nowick PA, Bell M, Edwards RP, et al. Normal uterine cervix: characterization of isolated lymphocyte phenotypes and immunoglobulin secretion. *Am J Reprod Immunol* 1995;34:241–7.

8. Schiller JT, Day PM, Kines RC. Current understanding of the mechanism of HPV infection. *Gynecol Oncol* 2010;118(1 suppl):S12–7.

9. Chow LT, Broker TR. Papillomavirus DNA replication. *Intervirology* 1994;37:150–8.

10. Cheng S, Schmidt-Grimminger D-C, Murant T, et al. Differentiation dependent up-regulation of the human papillomavirus gene reactivates cellular DNA replication in suprabasal differentiated keratinocytes. *Genes Dev* 1995;9:2335–49.

11. Dollard SC, Wilson JL, Demeter LM, et al. Production of human papillomavirus and modulation of the infectious program in epithelial raft cultures. *Genes Dev* 1992;6:1131–42.

12. Flores ER, Lambert PF. Evidence for a switch in the mode of human papillomavirus type 16 DNA replication during the viral life cycle. *J Virol* 1997;71:7167–79.

13. Jian Y, Schmidt-Grimminger D-C, Chien W-M, et al. Post-transcriptional induction of p21cip 1 protein by human papillomavirus E7 inhibits unscheduled DNA synthesis reactivated in differentiated keratinocytes. *Oncogene* 1998;17:2027–38.

14. Dyson N, Howley PM, Munger K, et al. The human papillomavirus-16 E7 oncoprotein is able to bind to the retinoblastoma gene product. *Science* 1989;243:934–6.

15. Werness BA, Levine AJ, Howley PM. Association of human papillomavirus types 16 and 18 E6 proteins with p53. *Science* 1990;248:76–9.

16. Mitchell MF, Tortolero-Luna G, Cook E, Whittaker L, Rhodes-Morris H, Silva E. A randomized clinical trial of cryotherapy, laser vaporization, and loop electrosurgical excision for treatment of squamous intraepithelial lesions of the cervix. *Obstet Gynecol* 1998;92(5):737–44.

17. Nuovo GJ, Banbury R, Calayag PT. Human papillomavirus types and recurrent cervical warts in immunocompromised women. *Mod Pathol* 1991;4:632–5.

18. Nobbenhuis M, Walboomers JM, Helmerhorst TJ, Rozendaal L. Relation of human papillomavirus status to cervical lesions and consequences for cervical-cancer screening: a prospective study. *Lancet* 1999;354:20–5.

19. Hopman EH, Rozendaal L, Voorhorst FJ, Walboomers JM, Kenemans P, Helmerhorst TJ. High risk human papillomavirus in women with normal cervical cytology prior to the development of abnormal cytology and colposcopy. *BJOG* 2000;107:600–4.

20. Khan MJ, Castle PE, Lorincz AT, et al. The elevated 10-year risk of cervical precancer and cancer in women with human papillomavirus (HPV) type 16 or 18 and the possible utility of type-specific HPV testing in clinical practice. *J Natl Cancer Inst* 2005;97(14):1072–9.

21. Bjork S, Hagstrom HG. Of what significance is abnormal result of smear test? Anxiety because of insufficient information in connection with abnormal result of cervical smear test. *Lakartidningen* 2001;98:2796–800.
22. Jones MH, Singer A, Jenkins D. The mildly abnormal cervical smear: patient anxiety and choice of management. *J R Soc Med* 1996;89:257–60.
23. Wilkinson C, Jones JM, McBridge J. Anxiety caused by abnormal result of a cervical smear test: a controlled trial. *Br Med J* 1990;300:440.
24. Moore TO, Moore AY, Carrasco D, et al. Human papillomavirus, smoking, and cancer. *J Cutan Med Surg* 2001;5:323–8.
25. Acladious NN, Sutton C, Mandal D, Hopkins R, Zaklama M, Kitchener H. Persistent human papillomavirus infection and smoking increase risk of failure of treatment of cervical intraepithelial neoplasia (CIN). *Int J Cancer* 2002;98:435–9.
26. Schiffman MH, Haley NJ, Felton JS, et al. Biochemical epidemiology of cervical neoplasia: measuring cigarette smoke constituents in the cervix. *Cancer Res* 1987;47:3886–8.
27. Hellberg D, Nilsson S, Haley NJ, Hoffman D, Wynder E. Smoking and cervical intraepithelial neoplasia: nicotine and cotinine in serum and cervical mucus in smokers and nonsmokers. *Am J Obstet Gynecol* 1988;158:910–3.
28. Szarewski A, Maddox P, Royston P, et al. The effect of stopping smoking on cervical Langerhans' cells and lymphocytes. *BJOG* 2001;10:295–303.
29. Alberg AJ, Selhub J, Shah KV, Viscidi RP, Comstock GW, Helzlsouer KJ. The risk of cervical cancer in relation to serum concentrations of folate, vitamin B_{12}, and homocysteine. *Cancer Epidemiol Biomarkers Prev* 2000;9:761–4.
30. Thomson SW, Heimburger DC, Cornwell PE, et al. Effect of total plasma homocysteine on cervical dysplasia risk. *Nutr Cancer* 2000;37:128–33.
31. Weinstein SJ, Ziegler RG, Frongillo EA Jr, et al. Low serum and red blood cell folate are moderately, but nonsignificantly associated with increased risk of invasive cervical cancer in U.S. women. *J Nutr* 2001;131:2040–8.
32. Garcia-Closas R, Castellsague X, Bosch X, Gonzalez CA. The role of diet and nutrition in cervical carcinogenesis: a review of recent evidence. *Int J Cancer* 2005;117:629–37.
33. Palan PR, Chang CJ, Mikhail MS, Ho GY, Basu J, Romney SL. Plasma concentrations of micronutrients during a nine-month clinical trial of beta-carotene in women with precursor cervical cancer lesions. *Nutr Cancer* 1998;30:46–52.
34. Bell MC, Crowley-Nowick P, Bradlow HL, et al. Placebo-controlled trial of indole-3-carbinol in the treatment of CIN. *Gynecol Oncol* 2000;78:123–9.
35. Comerci JT Jr, Runowicz CD, Fields AL, et al. Induction of transforming growth factor beta-1 in cervical intraepithelial neoplasia in vivo after treatment with beta-carotene. *Clin Cancer Res* 1997;3(2):157–60.
36. Cox JT. Management of women with cervical cancer precursor lesions. *Obstet Gynecol Clin North Am* 2002;29:787–816.
37. American College of Obstetricians and Gynecologists. ACOG Practice Bulletin number 99. Management of abnormal cervical cytology and histology. *Obstet Gynecol* 2008;112:1419–44.
38. Moscicki AB, Ma Y, Wibbelsman C, et al. Rate of and risks for regression of cervical intraepithelial neoplasia 2 in adolescents and young women. *Obstet Gynecol* 2010;116(6):1373–80.
39. Bansal N, Wright JD, Cohen CJ, Herzog TJ. Natural history of established low grade cervical intraepithelial (CIN 1) lesions. *Anticancer Res* 2008;28(3B):1763–6.
40. Moscicki AB, Shiboski S, Hills NK, et al. Regression of low-grade squamous intraepithelial neoplasia in young women. *Lancet* 2004;364:1678–83.
41. Katki HA, Schiffman M, Castle PE, et al. Five-year risk of CIN 3+ to guide the management of women aged 21 to 24 years. *J Low Genit Tract Dis* 2013;17(5 suppl 1):S64–68.
42. Moscicki AB, Cox JT. Practice improvement in cervical screening and management (PICSM): symposium on management of cervical abnormalities in adolescents and young women. *J Low Genit Tract Dis* 2010;14(1):73–80.
43. Moyer VA; for the U.S. Preventive Services Task Force. Screening for cervical cancer. U.S. Preventive Services Task Force recommendation statement. *Ann Intern Med* 2012;156(12):880–91.
44. Saslow D, Solomon D, Lawson HW, et al. American Cancer Society, American Society for Colposcopy and Cervical Pathology, and American Society for Clinical Pathology screening guidelines for the prevention and early detection of cervical cancer. *Am J Clin Pathol* 2012;137(4):516–42.
45. American College of Obstetricians and Gynecologists (ACOG). ACOG Practice Bulletin Number 131: Screening for cervical cancer. Committee on Practice Bulletins-Gynecology. *Obstet Gynecol* 2012;120(5):1222–38.
46. Cox JT, Schiffman M, Solomon D; ASCUS-LSIL Triage Study (ALTS) Group. Prospective follow-up suggests similar risk of subsequent cervical intraepithelial neoplasia grade 2 or 3 among women with cervical intraepithelial neoplasia grade 1 or negative colposcopy and directed biopsy. *Am J Obstet Gynecol* 2003;188:1406–12.
47. Kyrgiou M, Koliopoulos G, Martin-Hirsch P, Arbyn M, Prendiville W, Paraskevaidis E. Obstetrical outcomes after conservative treatment for intraepithelial or early invasive cervical lesions: systematic review and meta-analysis. *Lancet* 2006;367:489–98.
48. Werner CL, Lo JY, Heffernan T, Griffith WF, McIntire DD, Leveno KJ. Loop electrosurgical excision procedure and risk of preterm birth. *Obstet Gynecol* 2010;115(3):605–8.
49. Townsend DE, Richart RM. Cryotherapy and carbon dioxide laser management of cervical intraepithelial neoplasia: a controlled comparison. *Obstet Gynecol* 1983;61:75–8.
50. Ferenczy A. Comparison of cryo- and carbon dioxide laser therapy for cervical intraepithelial neoplasia. *Obstet Gynecol* 1985;66:793–8.
51. Berget A, Andreasson B, Bock JE, et al. Outpatient treatment of cervical intraepithelial neoplasia: the CO_2 laser versus cryosurgery, a randomized clinical trial. *Acta Obstet Gynecol Scand* 1987;66:531–6.
52. Kirwan PH, Smith IR, Naftalin NJ. A study of cryosurgery and the CO_2 laser in treatment of carcinoma in situ (CIN III) of the uterine cervix. *Gynecol Oncol* 1985;22:195–200.
53. Wright VC, Davies EM. The conservative management of cervical intraepithelial neoplasia: the use of cryosurgery and the carbon dioxide laser. *Br J Obstet Gynaecol* 1981;88:663–8.
54. Berget A, Andreasson B, Bock JE. Laser and cryosurgery for cervical intraepithelial neoplasia: a randomized trial and long-term follow-up. *Acta Obstet Gynecol Scand* 1991;70:231–5.
55. Kwikkel HJ, Helmerhorst TJM, Bezemer PD, Quaak MJ, Stolk JG. Laser or cryotherapy for cervical intraepithelial neoplasia: a randomized study to compare efficacy and side effects. *Gynecol Oncol* 1985;22:23–31.
56. Gunasekera PC, Phipps JH, Lewis BV. Large-loop excision of the transformation zone (LLETZ) compared to carbon dioxide laser in the treatment of CIN: a superior mode of treatment. *Br J Obstet Gynaecol* 1990;97:995–8.
57. Alvarez RD, Helm CW, Edwards RP, et al. Prospective randomized trial of LLETZ versus laser ablation in patients with cervical intraepithelial neoplasia. *Gynecol Oncol* 1994;52:175–9.
58. Martin-Hirsch PL, Paraskevaidis E, Kitchener H. Surgery for cervical intraepithelial neoplasia. *Cochrane Database Syst Rev* 2000;2:13–18.
59. Buxton EJ, Luesley DM, Shafi MI, Rollason M. Colposcopically directed punch biopsy; a potentially misleading investigation. *Br J Obstet Gynaecol* 1991;98:1273–6.
60. McIndoe A, Robson M, Tidy J, Mason P, Anderson M. Laser excision rather than vaporization: the treatment of choice for cervical intraepithelial neoplasia. *Obstet Gynecol* 1989;74:165–8.
61. Sze E, Rosenzweig B, Birenbaum D, et al. Excisional conization of the cervix-uteri. *J Gynecol Surg* 1989;5:325–31.
62. Gage JC, Hanson VW, Abbey K, et al.; The ASCUS LSIL Triage Study (ALTS) Group. Number of cervical biopsies and sensitivity of colposcopy. *Obstet Gynecol* 2006;108(2):264–72.
63. Massad LS, Jeronimo J, Katki HA, Schiffman M; National Institutes of Health/American Society for Colposcopy and Cervical Pathology Research Group. The accuracy of colposcopic grading for detection of high-grade cervical intraepithelial neoplasia. *J Low Genit Tract Dis* 2009;13(3):137–44.
64. Ferenczy A, Choukroun D, Arseneau J. Loop electrosurgical excision procedure for squamous intraepithelial lesions of the cervix: advantages and potential pitfalls. *Obstet Gynecol* 1996;87:332–7.
65. Darragh TM, Colgan TJ, Cox JT, et al.; Members of LAST Project Work Groups. The Lower Anogenital Squamous Terminology Standardization Project for HPV-associated lesions: background and consensus recommendations from the College of American Pathologists and the American Society for Colposcopy and Cervical Pathology. *J Low Genit Tract Dis* 2012;16:205–42.
66. Richart RM, Barron BA. A follow-up study of patients cervical dysplasia. *Am J Obstet Gynecol* 1969;105:386–92.
67. Ostor AG. Natural history of CIN: a critical review. *Int J Gynecol Pathol* 1993;12:186–92.
68. Nasiell K, Roger V, Nasiell M. Behavior of mild cervical dysplasia during long-term follow-up. *Obstet Gynecol* 1986;67:665–69.
69. Nasiell K, Nasiell M, Vaclavinkova V. Behavior of moderate cervical dysplasia during long-term follow-up. *Obstet Gynecol* 1983;61:609–14.
70. Stoler MH, Schiffman M. Interobserver reproducibility of cervical cytologic and histologic interpretations: realistic estimates from the ASCUS LSIL Triage Study. *JAMA* 2001;285:1500–5.
71. Cox JT. The clinician's view: role of human papillomavirus testing in the American Society for Colposcopy and Cervical Pathology Guidelines for the management of abnormal cervical cytology and cervical cancer precursors. *Arch Pathol Lab Med* 2003;127:950–8.
72. Guido R, Schiffman M, Solomon D, Burke L.; for The ASCUS LSIL Triage Study (ALTS) Group. Post-colposcopy management strategies for patients referred with LSIL or HPV DNA positive ASCUS: a two-year prospective study. *Am J Obstet Gynecol* 2003;188:1.
73. Katki HA, Gage JC, Schiffman M, et al. Follow-up testing after colposcopy: five-year risk of CIN 2+ after a colposcopic diagnosis of CIN 1 or less. *J Low Genit Tract Dis* 2013;17(5 suppl 1):S69–77.
74. Fukuchi E, Fetterman B, Poitras N, Kinney W, Lorey T, Littell RD. Risk of cervical precancer and cancer in women with cervical intraepithelial neoplasia grade 1 on endocervical curettage. *J Low Genit Tract Dis* 2013;17(3):255–6.
75. Gage JC, Duggan MA, Nation JG, Gao S, Castle PE. Comparative risk of high-grade histopathology diagnosis following a CIN1 finding in endocervical curettage vs. cervical biopsy. *J Low Genit Tract Dis* 2012;17:137–41.
76. Massad LS, Collins YC, Meyer PM. Biopsy correlates of abnormal cervical cytology classified using the Bethesda system. *Gynecol Oncol* 2001;82:516–22.
77. Alvarez RD, Wright TC. Effective cervical neoplasia detection with a novel optical detection system: a randomized trial. *Gynecol Oncol* 2007;104:281–9.
78. Dunn TS, Burke M, Shwayder J. A "see and treat" management for high grade squamous intraepithelial lesion pap smears. *J Low Genit Tract Dis* 2003;7104–6.

79. Ries LA, Melbert D, Krapcho M, et al., eds. *SEER Cancer Statistics Review, 1975–2006*. Bethesda, MD: National Cancer Institute, 2009. Available at: http://seer.cancer.gov/csr/1975_2006

80. Ismail SM, Colelough AB, Dinnen JS, et al. Observer variation in histopathological diagnosis and grading of cervical intraepithelial neoplasia. *BMJ* 1989;298:707–10.

81. Tidbury P, Singer A, Jenkins D. CIN 3: the role of lesion size in invasion. *Br J Obstet Gynaecol* 1992;99:583–6.

82. Andersen ES, Nielsen K, Pedersen B. The reliability of preconization diagnostic evaluation in patients with cervical intraepithelial neoplasia and microinvasive carcinoma. *Gynecol Oncol* 1995;59:143–7.

83. Burke L, Covell L, Antonioli D. Carbon dioxide laser therapy of cervical intraepithelial neoplasia: factors determining success rate. *Lasers Surg Med* 1980;1:113–22.

84. Duggan BD, Felix JC, Muderspach LI, et al. Cold-knife conization versus conization by the loop electrosurgical excision procedure: a randomized, prospective study. *Am J Obstet Gynecol* 1999;180:276–82.

85. Naumann RW, Bell MC, Alvarez RD, et al. LLETZ is an acceptable alternative to diagnostic cold-knife conization. *Gynecol Oncol* 1994;55:224–8.

86. Katki HA, Schiffman M, Castle PE, et al. Five-year risk of recurrence after treatment of CIN2, CIN3, or AIS: performance of HPV and Pap cotesting in post treatment management. *J Low Genit Tract Dis* 2013;17 (5 suppl 1):S78–84.

87. Samson SL, Bentley JR, Fahey TJ, McKay DJ, Gill GH. The effect of loop electrosurgical excision procedure on future pregnancy outcome. *Obstet Gynecol* 2005;105:325–32.

88. Sadler L, Saftlas A, Wang W, Exeter M, Whittaker J, McCowan L. Treatment for cervical intraepithelial neoplasia and risk of preterm delivery. *JAMA* 2004;291:2100–6.

89. Jakobsson M, Gissler M, Sainio S, Paavonen J, Tapper AM. Preterm delivery after surgical treatment for cervical intraepithelial neoplasia. *Obstet Gynecol* 2007;109:309–13.

90. Jakobsson M, Gissler M, Paavonen J, Tapper AM. Loop electrosurgical excision procedure and the risk for preterm birth. *Obstet Gynecol* 2009;114(3):504–10.

91. Armarnik S, Sheiner E, Piura B, Meirovitz M, Zlotnik A, Levy A. Obstetric outcome following cervical conization. *Arch Gynecol Obstet* 2011;283(4):765–9.

92. Noehr B, Jensen A, Frederiksen K, Tabor A, Kjaer SK. Depth of cervical cone removed by loop electrosurgical excision procedure and subsequent risk of spontaneous preterm delivery. *Obstet Gynecol* 2009;114(6):1232–8.

93. Bevis KS, Biggio JR. Cervical conization and the risk of preterm delivery. *Am J Obstet Gynecol* 2011;205:19–27.

94. Moscicki AB, Schiffman M, Kjaer S, Villa LL. Chapter 5: Updating the natural history of HPV and anogenital cancer. *Vaccine* 2006;24(suppl 3):S42–51.

95. Connor JP. Noninvasive cervical cancer complicating pregnancy. *Obstet Gynecol Clin North Am* 1998;25:331–42.

96. Robinson WR, Webb S, Tirpack J, Degefu S, O'Quinn AG. Management of cervical intraepithelial neoplasia during pregnancy with LOOP excision. *Gynecol Oncol* 1997;64:153–5.

97. Economos K, Perez Veridiano N, Delke I, Collado ML, Tancer ML. Abnormal cervical cytology in pregnancy: a 17-year experience. *Obstet Gynecol* 1993;81:915–8.

98. Fader AN, Alward EK, Niederhauser A, et al. Cervical dysplasia in pregnancy: a multi-institutional evaluation. *Am J Obstet Gynecol* 2010;203(2):113, e1–6.

99. Roberts CH, Dinh TV, Hannigan EV, Yandell RB, Schnadig VJ. Management of cervical intraepithelial neoplasia during pregnancy: a simplified and cost-effective approach. *J Low Genit Tract Dis* 1998;2:67–70.

100. Boardman LA, Goldman DL, Cooper AS, Heber WW, Weitzen S. CIN in pregnancy: antepartum and postpartum cytology and histology. *J Reprod Med* 2005;50:13–8.

101. Nguyen C, Montz FJ, Bristow RE. Management of stage I cervical cancer in pregnancy. *Obstet Gynecol Surv* 2000;55:633–43.

102. Norstrom A, Jansson I, Andreasson B. Carcinoma of the uterine cervix in pregnancy. A study of the incidence and treatment in the western region of Sweden 1973 to 1992. *Acta Obstet Gynecol Scand* 1997;76:5

103. Duggan B, Madersbach LL, Roman LD, Curtin JP, d'Ablaing G, Morrow CP. Cervical cancer in pregnancy: reporting on planned delay in therapy. *Obstet Gynecol* 1993;82:598–602.

104. Hunter MI, Tewari K, Monk BJ. Cervical neoplasia in pregnancy. Part 2: current treatment of invasive disease. *Am J Obstet Gynecol* 2008;199(1):10–8.

105. Wright TC, Ellerbock TV, Chiasson MA, Van De Vanter N, Sun XW. Cervical intraepithelial neoplasia in women infected with human immunodeficiency virus: prevalence, risk factors, and validity of Papanicolaou smears. New York Cervical Disease Study. *Obstet Gynecol* 1994;84:591–7.

106. Sun XW, Kuhn L, Ellerbrock TV, Chiasson MA, Bush TJ, Wright TC Jr. Human papillomavirus infection in women infected with the human immunodeficiency virus. *N Engl J Med* 1997;337:1343–9.

107. Palefsky JM, Minkoff H, Kalish LA, et al. Cervicovaginal human papillomavirus infection in human immunodeficiency virus-1 (HIV)-positive and high-risk HIV-negative women. *J Natl Cancer Inst* 1999;91:226–36.

108. Holcomb K, Matthews RP, Chapman JE, et al. The efficacy of cervical conization in the treatment of cervical intraepithelial neoplasia in HIV-positive women. *Gynecol Oncol* 1999;74:428–31.

109. Ellerbrock TV, Chiasson MA, Bush TJ, et al. Incidence of cervical squamous intraepithelial lesions in HIV-infected women. *JAMA* 2000;283:1031–7.

110. Massad LS, Ahdieh L, Benning L, et al. Evolution of cervical abnormalities among women with HIV-1: evidence from surveillance cytology in the women's interagency HIV study. *J Acquir Immune Defic Syndr* 2001;27(5):432–42.

111. Maiman M, Fruchter RG, Serur E, Levine PA, Arrastia CD, Sedlis A. Recurrent cervical intraepithelial neoplasia in human immunodeficiency virus-seropositive women. *Obstet Gynecol* 1993;82:170–4.

112. Fruchter RG, Maiman M, Sedlis A, Bartley L, Camilien L, Arrastia CD. Multiple recurrences of cervical intraepithelial neoplasia in women with the human immunodeficiency virus. *Obstet Gynecol* 1996;87:338–44.

113. Boardman LA, Peipert JF, Hogan JW, Cooper AS. Positive cone biopsy specimen margins in women infected with the human immunodeficiency virus. *Am J Obstet Gynecol* 1999;181:1395–9.

114. Reich O, Pickel H, Lahousen M, Tamussino K, Winter R. Cervical intraepithelial neoplasia III: long-term outcome after cold-knife conization with clear margins. *Obstet Gynecol* 2001;97:428–30.

115. Reich O, Lahousen M, Pickel H, Tamussino K, Winter R. Cervical intraepithelial neoplasia III: long-term follow-up after cold-knife conization with involved margins. *Obstet Gynecol* 2002;99:193–6.

116. Kolstad P, Klem V. Long-term follow-up of 1121 cases of carcinoma in situ. *Obstet Gynecol* 1976;48:125–9.

117. Anderson MC. Invasive carcinoma of the cervix following local destructive treatment for cervical intraepithelial neoplasia. *Br J Obstet Gynaecol* 1993;100:657–63.

118. Brown JV, Peters WA, Corwin DJ. Invasive carcinoma after cone biopsy for cervical intraepithelial neoplasia. *Gynecol Oncol* 1991;40:25–8.

119. Gornall RJ, Boyd IE, Manolitsas T, Herbert A. Interval cervical cancer following treatment for cervical intraepithelial neoplasia. *Int J Gynecol Cancer* 2000;10:198–202.

120. Flannelly G, Bolger B, Fawzi H, De Lopes AB, Monaghan JM. Follow up after LLETZ: could schedules be modified according to risk of recurrence? *BJOG* 2001;108:1025–30.

121. Gardeil F, Barry-Walsh C, Prendiville W, Clinch J, Turner MJ. Persistent intraepithelial neoplasia after excision for cervical intraepithelial neoplasia grade III. *Obstet Gynecol* 1997;89:419–22.

122. Giacalone PL, Laffargue F, Aligier N, Roger P, Combecal J, Daures JP. Randomized study comparing two techniques of conization: cold knife versus loop excision. *Gynecol Oncol* 1999;75:356–60.

123. Soutter WP, Sasieni P, Panoskaltsis T. Long-term risk of invasive cervical cancer after treatment of squamous cervical intraepithelial neoplasia. *Int J Cancer* 2006;118:2048–55.

124. Melnikow J, McGahan C, Sawaya GF, Ehlen T, Coldman A. Cervical intraepithelial neoplasia outcomes after treatment: long-term follow-up from the British Columbia Cohort Study. *J Natl Cancer Inst* 2009;101(10):721–8.

125. Nieminen P, Dyba T, Pukkala E, Anttila A. Cancer free survival after CIN treatment: comparisons of treatment methods and histology. *Gynecol Oncol* 2007;105(1):228–33.

126. Wang SS, Sherman ME, Hildesheim A, Lacey JV Jr, Devesa S. Cervical adenocarcinoma and squamous cell carcinoma incidence trends among white women and black women in the United States for 1976–2000. *Cancer* 2004;100:1035–44.

127. Chan KS, Yu KM, Lok YH, Sin SY, Tang LC. Conservative management of patients with histological incomplete excision of cervical intraepithelial neoplasia after large loop excision of transformation zone. *Chin Med J (Engl)* 1997;110:617–9.

128. Paraskevaidis E, Lolis ED, Koliopoulos G, Alamanos Y, Fotiou S, Kitchener HC. Cervical intraepithelial neoplasia outcomes after large loop excision with clear margins. *Obstet Gynecol* 2000;95(6 pt 1):828–31.

129. Narducci F, Occelli B, Boman F, Vinatier D, Leroy JL. Positive margins after conization and risk of persistent lesion. *Gynecol Oncol* 2000;76:311–4.

130. Felix JC, Muderspach LI, Duggan BD, Roman LD. The significance of positive margins in loop electrosurgical cone biopsies. *Obstet Gynecol* 1994;84:996–1000.

131. Zaitoun AM, McKee G, Coppen MJ, Thomas SM, Wilson PO. Completeness of excision and follow up cytology in patients treated with loop excision biopsy. *J Clin Pathol* 2000;53:191–6.

132. Murdoch JB, Morgan PR, Lopes A, Monaghan JM. Histological incomplete excision of CIN after large loop excision of the transformation zone (LLETZ) merits careful follow up, not retreatment. *Br J Obstet Gynaecol* 1992;99:990–3.

133. Lapaquette TK, Dinh TV, Hannigan EV, Doherty MG, Yandell RB, Buchanan VS. Management of patients with positive margins after cervical conization. *Obstet Gynecol* 1993;82:440–3.

134. Mathevet P, Dargent D, Roy M, Beau G. A randomized prospective study comparing three techniques of conization: cold knife, laser, and LEEP. *Gynecol Oncol* 1994;54:175–9.

135. Ghaem-Maghami S, Sagi S, Majeed G, Soutter WP. Incomplete excision of cervical intraepithelial neoplasia and risk of treatment failure: a meta-analysis. *Lancet Oncol* 2007;8(11):985–93.

136. Kocken M, Uijterwaal MH, de Vries AL, Berkhof J, Ket JC, Helmerhorst TJ, et al. High-risk human papillomavirus testing versus cytology in predicting post-treatment disease in women treated for high-grade cervical disease: a systematic review and meta-analysis. *Gynecol Oncol* 2012;125:500Y7.

137. Kreimer AR, Guido RS, Solomon D, et al. Human papillomavirus testing following loop electrosurgical excision procedure identifies women at risk for posttreatment cervical intraepithelial neoplasia grade 2 or 3 disease. *Cancer Epidemiol Biomarkers Prev* 2006;15(5):908–14.

138. Paraskevaidis E, Koliopoulos G, Alamanos Y, Malamou-Mitsi V, Lolis ED, Kitchener HC. Human papillomavirus testing and the outcome of treatment for cervical intraepithelial neoplasia. *Obstet Gynecol* 2001;98:833–6.

139. Strand A, Wilander E, Zehbe I, Rylander E. High risk HPV persists after treatment of genital papillomavirus infection but not after treatment of cervical intraepithelial neoplasia. *Acta Obstet Gynecol Scand* 1997;76:140–4.

140. Jain S, Tseng CJ, Horng SG, Soong YK, Pao CC. Negative predictive value of human papillomavirus test following conization of the cervix uteri. *Gynecol Oncol* 2001;82:177–80.

141. Lin CT, Tseng CJ, Lai CH, et al. Value of human papillomavirus deoxyribonucleic acid testing after conization in the prediction of residual disease in the subsequent hysterectomy specimen. *Am J Obstet Gynecol* 2001;184:940–5.

142. Kucera E, Sliutz G, Czerwenka K, Breitenecker G, Leodolter S, Reinthaller A. Is high-risk human papillomavirus infection associated with cervical intraepithelial neoplasia eliminated after conization by large-loop excision of the transformation zone? *Eur J Obstet Gynecol Reprod Biol* 2000;100:72–6.

143. Kjellberg L, Wadell G, Bergman F, Isaksson M, Angstrom T, Dillner J. Regular disappearance of the human papillomavirus genome after conization of cervical dysplasia by carbon dioxide laser. *Am J Obstet Gynecol* 2000;183:1238–42.

144. Arbyn M, Paraskevaidis E, Martin-Hirsch P, Prendiville W, Dillner J. Clinical utility of HPV-DNA detection: triage of minor cervical lesions, follow-up of women treated for high-grade CIN: an update of pooled evidence. *Gynecol Oncol* 2005;99(3 suppl 1):S7–11.

145. Heymans J, Benoy IH, Poppe W, Depuydt CE. Type-specific HPV genotyping improves detection of recurrent high-grade cervical neoplasia after conization. *Int J Cancer* 2011;129(4):903–9.

146. Cruikshank ME, Sharp L, Chambers G, Smart L, Murray G. Persistent infection with human papillomavirus following the successful treatment of high-grade cervical intraepithelial neoplasia. *BJOG* 2002;109:579–81.

147. Sherman ME, Wang SS, Carreon J, Devesa SS. Mortality trends for cervical squamous and adenocarcinoma in the United States: relation to incidence and survival. *Cancer* 2005;103:1258–64.

148. Lickrish GM, Colgan TJ, Wright VC. Colposcopy of adenocarcinoma in situ and invasive adenocarcinoma of the cervix. *Obstet Gynecol Clin North Am* 1993;20:111–22.

149. Wright VC. Colposcopic features of cervical adenocarcinoma *in situ* and adenocarcinoma and management of preinvasive disease. In: Apgar B, Bronztman GL, Spitzer M, eds. *Colposcopy—Principles and Practice*. Philadelphia, PA: WB Saunders, 2001:301–20.

150. Bertrand M, Lickrish GM, Colgan TJ. The anatomical distribution of cervical adenocarcinoma *in situ*. *Am J Obstet Gynecol* 1987;1:21–26.

151. Östör AG, Paganor, Davoran AM, et al. Adenocarcinoma in situ of the cervix. *Int J Obstet Gynecol Path* 1984;3:179–90.

152. Soutter WP, Haidopoulos D, Gormail RJ, et al. Is conservative treatment for adenocarcinoma in situ of the cervix safe? *BJOG* 2001;108(11):1184–9.

153. Srisomboon J, Kietpeerakool C, Suprasert P, Siriaunkgul S, Khunamornpong S, Prompittayarat W. Factors affecting residual lesion in women with cervical adenocarcinoma in situ after cone excisional biopsy. *Asian Pac J Cancer Prev* 2007;8(2):225–8.

154. Young JL, Jazaeri AA, Lachance JA, et al. Cervical adenocarcinoma in situ: the predictive value of conization margin status. *Am J Obstet Gynecol* 2007;197(2):195, e1–7.

155. Lea JS, Shin CH, Sheets EE, et al. Endocervical curettage at conization to predict residual cervical adenocarcinoma in situ. *Gynecol Oncol* 2002;87:129–32.

156. van Hanegem N, Barroilhet LM, Nucci MR, Bernstein M, Feldman S. Fertility-sparing treatment in younger women with adenocarcinoma in situ of the cervix. *Gynecol Oncol* 2012;124:72–7.

157. Hwang DM, Lickrish GM, Chapman W, Colgan TJ. Long-term surveillance is required for all women treated for cervical adenocarcinoma in situ. *J Low Genit Tract Dis* 2004;8:125–31.

158. Shin CH, Schorge JO, Lee KR, Sheets EE. Conservative management of adenocarcinoma in situ of the cervix. *Gynecol Oncol* 2000;79:6–10.

159. McHale MT, Le TD, Burger RA, Gu M, Rutgers JL, Monk BJ. Fertility sparing treatment for in situ and early invasive adenocarcinoma of the cervix. *Obstet Gynecol* 2001;98:726–31.

160. Ferris DG, Ho JJ. Cryosurgical equipment: a critical review. *J Fam Pract* 1992;35:185–93.

161. Castro W, Gage J, Gaffikin L, et al. *Effectiveness, Safety, and Acceptability of Cryotherapy: A Systematic Literature Review. Cervical Cancer Prevention Issues in Depth #1*. Seattle, WA: PATH, 2003.

162. Schmidt C, Pretorius RG, Bonin M, Hanson L, Semrad N, Watring W. Invasive cervical cancer following cryotherapy for cervical intraepithelial neoplasia or human papillomavirus infection. *Obstet Gyencol* 1992;180:797–800.

163. Kalstone C. Cervical stenosis in pregnancy: a complication of cryotherapy in diethylstilbestrol-exposed women. *Am J Obstet Gynecol* 1992;166:502–3.

164. Hemmingsson E. Outcome of third trimester pregnancies after cryotherapy of the uterine cervix. *Br J Obstet Gynaecol* 1982;89(8):675–7.

165. Arbyn M, Kyrgiou M, Simoens C, et al. Perinatal mortality and other severe adverse pregnancy outcomes associated with treatment of cervical intraepithelial neoplasia: meta-analysis. *BMJ* 2008;337:a1284.

166. Loizzi P, Carriero C, Di Gesù A, Resta L, Nappi R. Rational use of cryosurgery and cold knife conization for treatment of cervical intraepithelial neoplasia. *Eur J Gynaecol Oncol* 1992;13(6):507–13.

167. Harper DM. Paracervical block diminishes cramping associated with cryosurgery. *J Fam Pract* 1997;44(1):71–5.

168. Harper DM, Mayeaux EJ, Daaleman T, Woodward LD, Ferris DG, Johnson CA. The natural history of cervical cryosurgical healing. *J Fam Pract* 2000;49:694–700.

169. McIntosh N, Blumenthal PD, Blouse A, JHPIEGO. *Cervical Cancer Prevention Guidelines for Low-resource Settings*. Baltimore, MD: JHPIEGO, 2001.

170. http://whqlibdoc.who.int/publications/2011/9789241502856_eng.pdf. Accessed May 17, 2014.

171. Ferris DG, Crawley GR, Baxley EG, Line R, Ellis KE, Wagner P. Cryotherapy precision: clinician's estimate of cryosurgical iceball lateral spread of freeze. *Arch Fam Med* 1993;2:269–75.

172. Garamy G. Engineering aspects of cryosurgery. In: Rand RW, Rinfret AP, von Leden H, eds. *Cryosurgery*. Springfield, IL: Charles C. Thomas, 1968:92–132.

173. Gage AA. What temperature is lethal for cells? *J Dermatol Surg Oncol* 1979;5:459–64.

174. Cooper IS. Cryogenic surgery. *N Engl J Med* 1963;268:743–9.

175. Daniels F. Some of the cryobiology behind cryosurgery. *Cutis* 1975;16:421–4.

176. Rubinsky B, Lee CY, Bastacky J, Onik G. The process of freezing and the mechanism of damage during hepatic cryosurgery. *Cryobiology* 1990;27:85–97.

177. World Health Organization, Department of Reproductive Health and Research and Department of Chronic Diseases and Health Promotion. *Comprehensive Cervical Cancer Control: A Guide to Essential Practice*, 2006. Accessed September 16, 2011 http://www.who.int/reproductivehealth/publications/cancers/9241547006/en/index.html

178. Creasman WT, Weed JC Jr, Curry SL, Johnston WW, Parker RT. Efficacy of cryosurgical treatment of severe cervical intraepithelial neoplasia. *Obstet Gynecol* 1973;4:501–6.

179. Schantz A, Thormann L. Cryosurgery for dysplasia of the uterine ectocervix: a randomized study of the efficacy of the single- and double-freeze techniques. *Acta Obstet Gynecol Scand* 1984;63:417–20.

180. Torre D. Understanding the relationship between lateral spread of freeze and depth of freeze. *J Dermatol Surg Oncol* 1979;5:51–3.

181. Denny L, Kuhn L, Hu CC, Tsai WY, Wright TC Jr. Human papillomavirus based cervical cancer prevention: long-term results of a randomized screening trial. *J Natl Cancer Inst* 2010;102(20):1557–67.

182. Chirenje ZM, Rusakaniko S, Akino V, Munjoma M, Mlingo M. Effect of HIV disease in treatment outcome of cervical squamous intraepithelial lesions among Zimbabwean women. *J Low Genit Tract Dis* 2003;7(1):16–21.

183. Kuhn L, Wang C, Tsai WY, Wright TC, Denny L. Efficacy of human papillomavirus-based screen-and-treat for cervical cancer prevention among HIV-infected women. *AIDS* 2010;24(16):2553–61.

184. Sammarco MJ, Hartenbach EM, Hunter VJ. Local anesthesia for cryosurgery on the cervix. *J Reprod Med* 1993;38(3):170–2.

185. Rothenborg HW, Fraser J. "Third generation" cryotherapy. *J Dermatol Surg Oncol* 1977;3:408–13.

186. Hillard PA, Biro FM, Wildey L. Complications of cervical cryotherapy in adolescents. *J Reprod Med* 1991;36:711–6.

187. Ostergard DR, Townsend DE, Hirose FM. The long-term effects of cryosurgery of the uterine cervix. *J Cryosurg* 1969;2:17–22.

188. Weed JC, Curry SL, Duncan ID, Parker RT, Creasman WT. Fertility after cryosurgery of the cervix. *Obstet Gynecol* 1978;52:245–6.

189. Jacob M, Broekhuizen FF, Castro W, Sellors J. Experience using cryotherapy for treatment of cervical precancerous lesions in low-resource settings. *Int J Gynaecol Obstet* 2005;89(suppl 2):S13–20.

190. Townsend DE. Cryosurgery for CIN. *Obstet Gynecol Surv* 1979;34:828.

191. Boonstra H, Koudstaal J, Oosterhuis JW, Wymenga HA, Aalders JG, Janssens J. Analysis of cryolesions in the uterine cervix: application techniques, extension and failures. *Obstet Gynecol* 1990;75:232–9.

192. Richart RM, Townsend DE, Crisp W, et al. An analysis of "long-term" follow-up results in patients with cervical intraepithelial neoplasia treated by cryotherapy. *Am J Obstet Gynecol* 1980;137:823–6.

193. Sevin BU, Ford JH, Girtanner RD, et al. Invasive cancer of the cervix after cryosurgery: pitfalls of conservative management. *Obstet Gynecol* 1979;53:465–71.

194. Duncan ID. Cold coagulation. *Bailliers Clin Obstet Gynecol* 1995;9:145–55.

195. Semm K. New apparatus for the "cold coagulation" of benign cervical lesions. *Am J Obstet Gynecol* 1966;95:963–6.

196. Loobuyck HA, Duncan ID. Destruction of CIN 1 and 2 with the Semm cold coagulator: 13 years' experience with a see-and-treat policy. *Br J Obstet Gynaecol* 1993;100(5):465–8.

197. Vukosavic´-Cimic´ B, Kraljevic´ Z, Pirkic´ A, Grbavac I, Bolanca I. Cytologic follow-up in patients with CIN treated by LLETZ, cold knife conization and Semm's cold coagulation. *Coll Antropol* 2010;34(1):13–7.

198. Staland B. Treatment of premalignant lesions of uterine cervix by means of moderate heat thermosurgery using the Semm coagulator. *Ann Chir Gynaecol* 1978;67:112–6.

199. Duncan ID. The Semm cold coagulator in the management of cervical intraepithelial neoplasia. *Clin Obstet Gynecol* 1983;26:996–1006.

200. Gordon HK, Duncan ID. Effective destruction of cervical intraepithelial neoplasia (CIN) 3 at 100°C using the Semm cold coagulator: 14 years experience. *Br J Obstet Gynecol* 1991;98:14–20.

201. Smart GE, Livingstone JRB, Gordon A, et al. Randomized trial to compare laser with cold coagulation therapy in the treatment of CIN II and III. *Colp Gynecol Laser Surg* 1987;3:47.

202. Signh P, Lokr KL, Hii JHC, et al. Cold coagulation versus cryotherapy for treatment of cervical intraepithelial neoplasia: results of a prospective randomized trial. *J Gynecol Surg* 1988;4(4):211–21.

203. Allam M, Paterson A, Thomson A, Ray B, Rajagopalan C, Sarkar G. Large loop excision and cold coagulation for management of cervical intraepithelial neoplasia. *Int J Gynaecol Obstet* 2005;88(1):38–43.

204. Wright VC. Carbon dioxide laser surgery for the cervix and vagina: indications, complications, and results. *Compr Ther* 1988;14:54–64.

205. Wright VC, Riopelle MA. Laser physics for surgeons. *Acta Obstet Gynecol Scand* 1984;63(125 suppl):5–15.

206. Fisher JC. Qualitative and quantitative tissue effects of light from important surgical lasers: optimal surgical principles. In: Wright VC, Fisher JC, eds. *Laser Surgery in Gynecology*. Philadelphia, PA: WB Saunders Company, 1993;73–8.

207. Wright VC, Davies E, Riopelle MA. Laser surgery for cervical intraepithelial neoplasia: principles, and results. *Am J Obstet Gynecol* 1983;145:181–4.

208. Wright VC, Davies E, Riopelle MA. Laser cylindrical excision to replace conization. *Am J Obstet Gynecol* 1984;150:704–9.

209. Abdul-Karim FH, Fu YS, Reagan JW, Wentz WB. Morphometric study of intraepithelial neoplasia of the uterine cervix. *Obstet Gynecol* 1982;60:210–4.

210. Anderson MC, Hartley RB. Cervical crypt involvement by intraepithelial neoplasia. *Am J Obstet Gynecol* 1980;55:546–9.

211. Boonstra H, Aalders JG, Koudstaal J, et al. Minimum extension and appropriate topographic position of tissue destruction for treatment of cervical intraepithelial neoplasia. *Obstet Gynecol* 1990;75:227–31.

212. Reagan JW, Patten SF Jr. Dysplasia: a basic reaction to injury in the uterine cervix. *Ann N Y Acad Sci* 1962;97:662–7.

213. Przybora LA, Plutowa A. Histological topography of carcinoma in situ of the uterine cervix. *Cancer* 1959;12:268–73.

214. Scott RB, Reagan JW. Diagnostic cervical biopsy technique for the study of early cancer. Value of the cold-knife conization procedure. *JAMA* 1956;160:343–8.

215. Hanperl H, Kaufman C. The cervix uteri at various stages. *Obstet Gynecol* 1959;14:621–5.

216. Bertelsen B, Tande T, Sandvei R, et al. Laser conization of cervical intraepithelial neoplasia grade 3: free resection margins indicative of lesion survival. *Acta Obstet Gynecol Scand* 1999;78:54–9.

217. Holzer E. Localization of dysplastic epithelium. In: Burghardt E, Holzer E, Jordan JA, eds. *Cervical Colposcopy and Pathology*. Stuttgart, Germany: Georg Thieme Publishers, 1978.

218. Wright VC, Riopelle MA. The geometry of cervical intraepithelial neoplasia as a guide to its eradication. *Cervix* 1986;4:21–38.

219. Wright VC. CO$_2$ laser surgery for cervical intraepithelial neoplasia. In: Wright VC, Fisher JC, eds. *Laser Surgery in Gynecology: A Clinical Guide*. Philadelphia, PA: WB Saunders Company, 1993.

220. Holmquist ND, Bellina JH, Danol ML. Vaginal and cervical cytologic changes following laser treatment. *Acta Cytol* 1976;20:290–4.

221. Bellina JH, Seto YJ. Pathological and physiological investigations into CO$_2$ laser-tissue interactions with specific emphasis on cervical intraepithelial neoplasia. *Lasers Surg Med* 1980;1:47–55.

222. Lickrish GM. Colposcopy in the management of cervical intraepithelial neoplasia: problems and solutions. *J Soc Obstet Gynaecol Can* 2000;22:429–34.

223. Larsson G, Grundell H, Gullberg H, et al. Outcome of pregnancy after conization. *Surg Gynecol Obstet* 1982;54:59–61.

224. Anderson MC, Howell DH, Broby Z. Outcome of pregnancy after laser vaporization conization. *Colp Gynecol Laser Surg* 1984;1:35–9.

225. Baggish MS. High-power density carbon dioxide laser therapy for early cervical dysplasia. *Am J Obstet Gynecol* 1980;136:117–21.

226. Baggish MS. Management of cervical intraepithelial neoplasia by carbon dioxide laser. *Obstet Gynecol* 1982;60:379–83.

227. Bertelsen B, Tande T, Sandvei R, et al. Laser conization of cervical intraepithelial neoplasia grade 3: free resection margins indicative of lesional survival. *Acta Obstet Gynecol Scand* 1999;78:54–9.

228. Dorsey JH, Diggs ES. Microsurgical conization of the cervix by carbon dioxide laser. *Obstet Gynecol* 1979;54:565–70.

229. Hagen B, Skjeldestad FE, Tingulstad S, et al. CO$_2$ laser conization for cervical intraepithelial neoplasia grade II–III: complications and efficacy. *Acta Obstet Gynecol* 1998;77:558–63.

230. Fevalli G, Lomini M, Schreiber C, et al. The use of carbon-dioxide laser surgery in the treatment of intraepithelial neoplasia of the uterine cervix. *Przegl Lek* 1999;56:58–64.

231. Prendiville W, Cullimore J, Norman S. Large loop excision of the transformation zone (LLETZ): a new method of management for women with intraepithelial neoplasia. *Br J Obstet Gynecol* 1989;96:1054–60.

232. Pearce JA. *Electrosurgery*. London, UK: Chapman & Hall, 1986.

233. Soderstrom R. Principles of electrosurgery as applied to gynecology. In: Rock JA, Thompson JD, eds. *Te Linde's Operative Gynecology* (8th ed.). Philadelphia, PA: Lippincott-Raven, 1997:321–36.

234. Ferris DG, Saxena S, Hainer BL, et al. Gynecologic and dermatologic electrosurgical units. *J Fam Pract* 1994;39:160–6.

235. Ferenczy A. Management of patients with high grade squamous intraepithelial lesions. *Cancer* 1995;76:1828–33.

236. Sebben JE. Electrosurgical principles. Cutting current and cutaneous surgery—Part I. *J Dermatol Surg Oncol* 1988;14:29–35.

237. Tucker Rd, Schmitt OH, Sievert CE, et al. Demodulated low frequency currents from electrosurgical procedures. *Surg Gynecol Obstet* 1984;159:39–42.

238. Bennett RG. *Fundamentals of Cutaneous Surgery*. St. Louis, MO: C. V. Mosby Company, 1988: Chapter 16.

239. Nunns D, Yates W, Stanbridge C, Lee S. A comparison of the ERBE Erbotom ICC 200 generator and the Valleylab Force 2 electrosurgical generator in performing large loop excision of the transformation zone. *Int J Gynecol Cancer* 2000;10(2):100–4.

240. Spitzer M, Chernys AE, Seltzer VL. The use of large loop excision of the transformation zone in an inner city population. *Obstet Gynecol* 1993;82:731–5.

241. Sadek AL. Needle excision of the transformation zone: a new method for treatment of cervical intraepithelial neoplasia. *Am J Obstet Gynecol* 2000;182:866–71.

242. Murdoch JB, Grimshaw RN, Monaghan JM. Loop diathermy excision of the abnormal transformation zone. *Int J Gynecol Cancer* 1991;1:105–9.

243. Wright TC, Richart RM, Ferenczy A. *Electrosurgery for HPV Related Diseases of the Anogenital Tract*. New York: Arthur Vision, 1992.

244. Huang L-W, Huang J-L. A comparison between loop electrosurgical excision procedure and cold knife conization for the treatment of cervical dysplasia: residual disease in a subsequent hysterectomy specimen. *Gynecol Oncol* 1999;73:12–5.

245. Baggish MS, Barash F, Noel Y, et al. Comparison of thermal injury zone in loop electrical and laser excisional conization. *Am J Obstet Gynecol* 1992;166:545–8.

246. Wright TC, Richart RM, Ferenczy A, et al. Comparison of specimens removed by CO$_2$ laser conization and loop electrosurgical procedures. *Obstet Gynecol* 1991;79:147–53.

247. Ioffe OB, Brooks SE, De Rezende RB, et al. Artifact in cervical LLETZ specimens: correlation with follow-up. *Int J Gynecol Pathol* 1999;18:115–21.

248. Messing MJ, Otken L, King LA, et al. Larger loop excision of the transformation zone (LLETZ): a pathological evaluation. *Gynecol Oncol* 1994;52:207–11.

249. Montz FJ, Holschneider CH, Thompson LDR. Large-loop excision of the transformation zone: effect on the pathological interpretation of resection margins. *Obstet Gynecol* 1993;81:976–82.

250. Krebs H, Pastor L, Helmkamp BF. Loop electrosurgical procedures for dysplasia. Experience in a community hospital. *Am J Obstet Gynecol* 1993;169:289–95.

251. Thomas PA, Zaleski MS, Ohlhausen WW, et al. Cytomorphologic characteristics of thermal injury related to endocervical brushing following loop electrosurgical procedure. *Diagn Cytopathol* 1996;14:212–5.

252. Darwish A, Gadallah H. One step management of cervical lesions. *Int J Gynaecol Obstet* 1998;61:261–7.

253. Wright VC. Loop electrosurgical procedures for treatment of cervical intraepithelial neoplasia: principles and results. In: Wright VC, Lickrish GM, Shier RM, eds. *Basic and Advanced Colposcopy—Part Two: A Practical Handbook for Treatment* (2nd ed.). Houston, TX: Biomedical Communications, 1995:20/1–20/31.

254. Takac I, Gorisek B. Cold knife conization and loop excision for cervical intraepithelial neoplasia. *Tumori* 1999;85:243–6.

255. Simmons JR, Anderson L, Hernadez E, et al. Evaluating cervical neoplasia. LEEP as an alternative to cold knife conization. *J Reprod Med* 1998;43:1007–13.

256. Bjerre B, Eliasson G, Linell F. Conization as only treatment of carcinoma in situ of the uterine cervix. *Am J Obstet Gynecol* 1976;125:143–52.

257. Reimers LL, Sotardi S, Daniel D, et al. Outcomes after an excisional procedure for cervical intraepithelial neoplasia in HIV-infected women. *Gynecol Oncol* 2010;119(1):92–7.

258. Crane JM. Pregnancy outcome after loop electrosurgical excision procedure: a systematic review. *Obstet Gynecol* 2003;102(5 pt 1):1058–62.

259. Kreiger JS, McCormack LJ. The indications for conservative therapy for carcinoma in situ of the cervix. *Am J Obstet Gynecol* 1963;76:312–20.

260. Jordan JA. Symposium on cervical dysplasia I. Excisional methods. *Colp Gynecol Laser Surg* 1984;4:271–4.

261. Kolstad P, Valborg K. Long term follow-up of 1121 cases of carcinoma in situ. *Obstet Gynecol* 1976;48:125–9.

262. Thompson BH, Woodruff JD, Davis HJ, et al. Cytopathology, histopathology, and colposcopy in the management of cervical neoplasia. *Am J Obstet Gynecol* 1972;114:329–34.

263. Hovadhanakul P, Mehra U, Terragno A, et al. Comparison of colposcopy directed biopsies and cold knife conization in patients with abnormal cytology. *Surg Gynecol Obstet* 1976;142:333–6.

264. Townsend DE, Ostergard DR. Cryocauterization for preinvasive cervical dysplasia. *J Reprod Med* 1971;6:171–3.

265. Creasman WT, Weed JC Jr. Conservative management of cervical intraepithelial neoplasia. *Clin Obstet Gynecol* 1980;43:281–5.

266. Rubin S, Battistini M. Endometrial curettage at the time of cervical conization. *Obstet Gynecol* 1986;67:663–4.

267. Berkus M, Daly JW. Cone biopsy: an outpatient procedure. *Am J Obstet Gynecol* 1980;137:953–8.

268. Larsson G, Alm P, Grundell H. Laser conization verses cold knife conization. *Surg Gynecol Obstet* 1982;154:59–61.

269. McCann S, Mickal A, Crapazano JT. Sharp conization of the cervix. *Obstet Gynecol* 1969;33:470–5.

270. Van Nagell JR, Parker JC, Hicks LP, et al. Diagnostic and therapeutic efficacy of cervical conization. *Am J Obstet Gynecol* 1976;124:134–9.

271. Hester LL, Read RA. An evaluation of cervical conization. *Am J Obstet Gynecol* 1960;80:715–21.

272. Bostofte E, Berget A, Larsen JF, et al. Conization by carbon dioxide laser or cold knife in the treatment of cervical intraepithelial neoplasia. *Acta Obstet Gynecol Scand* 1986;65:199–202.

273. Burghardt E, Holzer E. Treatment of carcinoma in situ. Evaluation of 1609 cases. *Am J Obstet Gynecol* 1980;55:539–45.

274. Ostegard DR. Prediction of clearance of cervical intraepithelial neoplasia by conization. *Obstet Gynecol* 1980;56:77–80.

275. Adelman HC, Hajdee SI. Role of conization in the treatment of cervical carcinoma in situ. *Am J Obstet Gynecol* 1967;56:173–9.

276. Villasanta U, Durkan JP. Indications and complications of cold conization of the cervix. Observation on 200 consecutive cases. *Obstet Gynecol* 1965;27:717–23.

277. Davis RM, Cooke JK, Kirk RF. Cervical conization—an experience with 400 patients. *Obstet Gynecol* 1972;40:23–7.

278. Holdt DG, Jacobs AJ, Scott J, et al. Diagnostic significance and sequelae of cone biopsy. *Am J Obstet Gynecol* 1982;143:312–5.

279. Killackey MA, Jones WB, Lewis J Jr. Diagnostic conization of the cervix: review of 460 consecutive cases. *Obstet Gynecol* 1986;67:766–70.

280. Jafari K, Ravindranaths S. Role of endocervical curettage in colposcopy. *Am J Obstet Gynecol* 1978;131:83–87.

281. Benedet JL, Anderson GH, Boyes DA. Colposcopic accuracy in the diagnosis of microinvasive and occult invasive carcinoma of the cervix. *Obstet Gynecol* 1985;65:551–61.

282. Moore BC, Higgins RV, Laurent SL, et al. Predictive factors from cold knife conization for residual intraepithelial neoplasia in subsequent hysterectomy. *Am J Obstet Gynecol* 1995;173:361–8.

283. Murta EF, Resende AV, Adad SJ, et al. Importance of surgical margins in conization for cervical intraepithelial neoplasia grade III. *Arch Gynecol Obstet* 1999;263:42–4.

284. Fogle RH, Spann CO, Easley KA, Basil JB. Predictors of cervical dysplasia after the loop electrosurgical excision procedure in an inner-city population. *J Reprod Med* 2004;49(6):481–6.

285. Robinson WR, Hamilton CA, Michaels SH, Kissinger P. Effect of excisional therapy and highly active antiretroviral therapy on cervical intraepithelial neoplasia in women infected with human immunodeficiency virus. *Am J Obstet Gynecol* 2001;184(4):538–43.

286. Claman AD, Lee N. Factors that relate to complications of cone biopsy. *Am J Obstet Gynecol* 1974;120:124–8.

287. Larsen G. Conization for cervical dysplasia and carcinoma in situ: long term follow-up of 1013 women. *Ann Chir Gynaecol* 1981;70:79–85.

288. Bruinsma F, Lumley J, Tan J, Quinn M. Precancerous changes in the cervix and risk for subsequent preterm birth. *BJOG* 2007;114(1):70–80.

289. Lickrish GM. Hysterectomy for cervical intraepithelial neoplasia. In: Wright VC, Lickrish GM, Shier RM, eds. *Basic and Advanced Colposcopy—A Practical Handbook for Treatment* 2nd ed. Houston, TX: Biomedical Communications, 1995:23-1 to 23-4.

290. Piver MS, Rutledge FN, Smith PJ. Five classes of hysterectomy of extended hysterectomy of women with cervical cancer. *Obstet Gynecol* 1974;44:265–9.

291. Creasman WT, Parker RT. Management of early cervical neoplasia. *Clin Obstet Gynecol* 1975;18:233–8.

292. Boyes DA, Worth J, Fidler HK. The results of treatment of 4389 cases of pre-clinical cervical squamous carcinoma. *J Obstet Gynaecol Br Commwlth* 1979;77:769–13.

293. Saslow D, Runowicz CD, Solomon D, et al. American Cancer Society Guidelines for the early detection of cervical neoplasia and cancer. *J Lower Gen Tract Dis* 2003;7:67–79.

294. Ferlay J, Shin HR, Bray F, Forman D, Mathers C, Parkin DM. Estimates of worldwide burden of cancer in 2008: GLOBOCAN 2008. *Int J Cancer* 2010;127(12):2893–917.

295. Franceschi S, Denny L, Irwin KL, et al. Eurogin 2010 roadmap on cervical cancer prevention. *Int J Cancer* 2011;128(12):2765–74.

296. Schiffman M, Wentzensen N, Wacholder S, Kinney W, Gage JC, Castle PE. Human papillomavirus testing in the prevention of cervical cancer. *J Natl Cancer Inst* 2011;103(5):368–83.

297. Gaffikin L, Blumenthal PD, Emerson M, Limpaphayom K; Royal Thai College of Obstetricians and Gynaecologists (RTCOG)/JHPIEGO Corporation Cervical Cancer Prevention Group. Safety, acceptability, and feasibility of a single-visit approach to cervical-cancer prevention in rural Thailand: a demonstration project. *Lancet* 2003;361(9360):814–20.

298. Gunter J. Genital and perianal warts: new treatment opportunities for human papillomavirus infection. *Am J Obstet Gyencol* 2003;189(3 suppl):S3–11.

299. Woodhall S, Ramsey T, Cai C, et al. Estimation of the impact of genital warts on health-related quality of life. *Sex Transm Infect* 2008;84(3):161–6.

300. Mayeaux EJ Jr, Dunton C. Modern management of external genital warts. *J Low Genit Tract Dis* 2008;12(3):185–92.

301. Workowski KA, Berman S; Centers for Disease Control and Prevention (CDC). Sexually transmitted diseases treatment guidelines, 2010. *MMWR Recomm Rep* 2010;59(RR-12):1–110.

302. FUTURE I/II Study Group, Dillner J, Kjaer SK, et al. Four year efficacy of prophylactic human papillomavirus quadrivalent vaccine against low grade cervical, vulvar, and vaginal intraepithelial neoplasia and anogenital warts: randomised controlled trial. *BMJ* 2010;341:c3493.

303. Garland SM, Steben M, Sings HL, et al. Natural history of genital warts: analysis of the placebo arm of 2 randomized phase III trials of a quadrivalent human papillomavirus (types 6, 11, 16, and 18) vaccine. *J Infect Dis* 2009;199:805–14.

304. Garnock-Jones KP, Giuliano AR. Quadrivalent human papillomavirus (HPV) types 6, 11, 16, 18 vaccine: For the prevention of genital warts in males. *Drugs* 2011;71(5):591–602.

305. Pruitt SL, Shootman M. Geographic disparity, area poverty and human papillomavirus vaccination. *Am J Prev Med* 2010;38(5):525–33.

306. Beutner KR, Wiley DJ, Douglas JM, et al. Genital warts and their treatment. *Clin Inf Dis* 1999;28:S37–56.

307. Greenberg MD, Rutledge LH, Reid R, Berman NR, Precop SL, Elswick RK. A double-blind, randomized trial of 0.5% podofilox and placebo for the treatment of genital warts in women. *Obstet Gynecol* 1991;77:735–9.

308. Beutner KR, Friedman-Kien AE, Artman NN, et al. Patient-applied podofilox for treatment of genital warts. *Lancet* 1989;1:831–4.

309. Fife KH, Ferenczy A, Douglas JM Jr, Brown DR, Smith M, Owens ML. Treatment of external genital warts in men using 5% imiquimod cream applied three times a week, once daily, twice daily or three times a day. *Sex Transm Dis* 2001;28:226–31.

310. Edwards L, Ferenczy A, Eron L, et al. Self-administered topical 5% imiquimod cream for external genital warts. *Arch Dermatol* 1998;134:25–30.

311. Gollnick H, Barrasso R, Jappe U, et al. Safety and efficacy of imiquimod 5% cream in the treatment of penile genital warts in uncircumcised men when applied three times weekly or once per day. *Int J STD AIDS* 2001;12:22–8.

312. Gilson RJ, Shupack JL, Friedman-Kien AE, et al. A randomized, controlled, safety study using imiquimod for the topical treatment of anogenital warts in HIV-infected patients. *AIDS* 1999;13:2397–404.

313. Fox PA, Nathan M, Francis N, et al. A double-blind, randomized controlled trial of the use of imiquimod cream for the treatment of anal canal high-grade anal intraepithelial neoplasia in HIV-positive MSM on HAART, with long-term follow-up data including the use of open-label imiquimod. *AIDS* 2010;24(15):2331–5.

314. Mahto M, Nathan M, O'Mahony C. More than a decade on: review of the use of imiquimod in lower anogenital intraepithelial neoplasia. *Int J STD AIDS* 2010;21(1):8–16.

315. Khan N, Afaq F, Saleem M, Ahmad N, Mukhtar H. Targeting multiple signaling pathways by green tea polyphenol (-)-epigallocatechin-3-gallate. *Cancer Res* 2006;66:2500–5.

316. Ahmad N, Cheng P, Mukhtar H. Cell cycle dysregulation by green tea polyphenol epigallocatechin-3-gallage. *Biochem Biophys Res Commun* 2000;257:328–34.

317. Li HC, Yashiki S, Sonoda J, et al. Green tea polyphenols induce apoptosis in vitro in peripheral blood T lymphocytes of adult T-cell leukemia patients. *JPN J Cancer Res* 2000;91:34–40.

318. Yang GY, Liao J, Kim K, Yurkow EJ, Yang CS. Inhibition of growth and induction of apoptosis in human cancer cell lines by tea polyphenols. *Carcinogenesis* 1998;19:611–6.

319. Tatti S, Swinehart JM, Thielert C, Tawfik H, Mescheder A, Beutner KR. Sinecatechins, a defined green tea extract, in the treatment of external anogenital warts. *Obstet Gynecol* 2008;111:1371–9.

320. Tzellos TG, Sardeli C, Lallas A, Papazisis G, Chourdakis M, Kouvelas D. Efficacy, safety and tolerability of green tea catechins in the treatment of external anogenital warts: a systematic review and meta-analysis. *J Eur Acad Dermatol Venereol* 2011;25(3):345–53.

321. Tatti S, Stockfleth E, Beutner KR, et al. Polyphenon E®: a new treatment for external anogenital warts. *Br J Dermatol* 2010;162:176–184.

322. von Krogh G, Lacey CJN, Gross G, Barrasso R, Schneider A. European course on HPV associated pathology: guidelines for primary care physicians for the diagnosis and management of anogenital warts. *Sex Transm Inf* 2000;76:162–8.

323. Simmons PD. Podophyllin 10 percent and 25 percent in the treatment of anogenital warts: a comparative double-blind study. *Br J Vener Dis* 1981; 57:208–9.

324. Abdullah AN, Walzman M, Wade A. Treatment of external genital warts comparing cryotherapy (liquid nitrogen) and trichloroacetic acid. *Sex Transm Dis* 1993;30:544–5.

325. Baggish MS. Improved laser techniques for the elimination of genital and extragenital warts. *Am J Obstet Gynecol* 1985;153:545–50.

326. Krebs HB, Helmkamp F. Chronic ulcerations following topical therapy with 5-fluorouracil therapy for vaginal human papillomavirus associated lesions. *Obstet Gynecol* 1991;78:205–8.

327. Goodman A, Zukerberg LR, Nikrui N, Scully RE. Vaginal adenosis and clear cell carcinoma after 5-fluorouracil treatment for condylomas. *Cancer* 1991;68(7):1628–32.

Preventing Errors during Colposcopy and Management of Lower Genital Tract Neoplasia

21.1 INTRODUCTION
21.2 ERRORS PRIOR TO THE COLPOSCOPY EXAMINATION
21.3 ERRORS DURING THE COLPOSCOPY EXAMINATION
    21.3.1 Visualization Errors
    21.3.2 Assessment Errors
    21.3.3 Sampling Errors

21.4 ERRORS AFTER THE COLPOSCOPY EXAMINATION
    21.4.1 Correlation Errors
    21.4.2 Management Errors

21.1 INTRODUCTION

Performing effective colposcopy requires specialized knowledge and sophisticated skills. Because the colposcopy processes demand more complex cognitive skills than psychomotor skills, a greater risk for assessment and management errors exists. Technical and procedural complications can also occur. Structured training, ample experience, reasonable dexterity, problem-solving capabilities, and sufficient knowledge collectively determine a colposcopist's procedural proficiency.[1] Mastery of all of these areas is required to perform colposcopy effectively and determine an appropriate plan for patient care.

Colposcopic errors may result from ignorance, carelessness, misinterpretation, deviation, or omission of basic colposcopic processes. Proficiency with a series of four colposcopic steps must be achieved and maintained: visualization, assessment, sampling, and correlation (VASC). *Visualization* involves identifying normal anatomical landmarks and lower genital tract neoplasia. *Assessment* involves determining the extent of disease and selecting biopsy site(s). *Sampling* involves removing representative portions of the disease present and tissue from other areas with high potential for containing neoplasia. *Correlation* involves associating cytologic, colposcopic, and histologic findings to determine an accurate diagnosis and proper patient management. Adhering to these four colposcopic steps minimizes untoward outcomes. Errors can certainly occur from educational deficiencies, whether in initial training or in continuing education. This includes not knowing or applying the knowledge that taking more than one biopsy is at least as important for identifying neoplasia as is colposcopic assessment, even for experts.

Judgment errors occur most commonly, whether related to diagnosis or management. Neglecting the therapeutic triage guidelines increases the chance that improper care will occur. Learning from others' mistakes or recognizing possible traps may minimize problems. This chapter provides insight into potential colposcopic and management errors and suggests ways to prevent them.

21.2 ERRORS PRIOR TO THE COLPOSCOPY EXAMINATION

Many errors, primarily decisional, occur prior to the patient's colposcopic examination. In most cases, abnormal cytology, persistent HPV positivity or testing positive for HPV 16 or 18 are the reasons women are referred for colposcopy. The insensitivity and subjectivity of the Papanicolaou (Pap) test is well known.[2] Interpretive errors and lack of interobserver agreement are particularly frequent with cervical cytology, especially when equivocal or minimal abnormalities exist (e.g., atypical squamous cells of undetermined significance [ASC-US]).[3]

Cytologic results may either overrepresent or underrepresent the true state of cervical epithelial change (Figure 21.1). False-negative Pap tests are particularly troublesome when a high-grade neoplasia or cancer is missed (Figure 21.2). Simple awareness of the difficulty in reaching cytologic agreement among pathologists should prompt the colposcopist to seek further cytopathologic consultation when the preliminary cytology reports do not agree with relevant clinical findings. This may involve requesting the initial pathologist to review her or his findings or consulting with another pathologist with gynecologic pathology expertise. The advice or second opinion of pathology experts, when necessary, may provide a more complete understanding of difficult, perplexing cases.

Guidelines have been developed to help clinicians appropriately manage abnormal cervical cytology, HPV test results, and specimen adequacy issues.[4,5] The guidelines have greatly improved clinician adherence to appropriate patient management[6,7] when compared to the pre-guideline era,[8] but guidelines continue to not always be followed or easily understood by clinicians, with some failing to act effectively when confronted with an abnormal screening test result. Because most high-grade cervical neoplasia progresses slowly, cases involving missed early management opportunities are frequently discovered before serious outcomes occur, especially if the patient adheres to standard recommendations for screening and follow-up. In contrast, omitting colposcopic evaluation after a high-grade cytologic abnormality may result in considerable morbidity. As noted in the guidelines, clinicians must recognize the cytologic indications for colposcopy—ASC-US/high-risk human papillomavirus (hrHPV) DNA+ in women aged ≥25 years, atypical squamous cells rule out high grade (ASC-H), low-grade squamous intraepithelial lesion (LSIL) in women aged ≥25 years, high-grade squamous intraepithelial lesion (HSIL), and atypical glandular cells (AGC).[4] Performing colposcopy when not clearly indicated may lead to overdiagnosis of unimportant lesions and morbidity from overtreatment.

Consideration of noncytologic indications for colposcopy is an important aspect of error prevention. Women ≥30 years

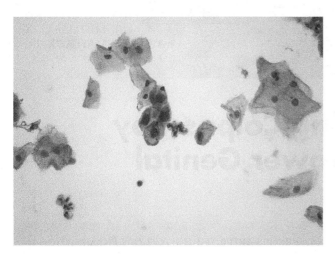

FIGURE 21.1. Cervical cytology showing ASC-US initially diagnosed as normal (Papanicolaou stain, high-power magnification).

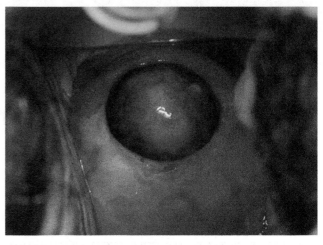

FIGURE 21.3. A cervical mass discovered by palpation and subsequently examined by colposcopy. The mass was a prolapsed uterine leiomyoma that was soon passed by the patient.

with normal cytology but testing positive for HPV 16 and/ or 18 or persistently positive for a panel of high-risk HPV at 12 month follow-up should have colposcopy. Any cervical or vaginal mass or persistent ulceration seen or palpated during a routine gynecologic examination should be evaluated by colposcopy or biopsied (Figures 21.3 and 21.4). Any patient with unexplained chronic cervical or vaginal bleeding should be referred for colposcopy to rule out the presence of a lower genital tract malignancy. Unexplained vaginal bleeding during pregnancy may also require colposcopic evaluation after more common pregnancy-associated causes like abruption and placenta previa are excluded. Women with vulvar or anal intraepithelial neoplasia are at increased risk for having a coexisting cervical or vaginal neoplasia. These women may benefit from a colposcopic examination (Figure 21.5A,B).

Even though most women exposed to diethylstilbestrol in utero have already been identified, and at a minimal age of over 40 years are likely to have fully mature transformation zones, colposcopic examination remains the foundation for assessment of these patients, along with conducting a pelvic examination and serial cervicovaginal cytology.[9] However, another option is to do Pap tests more often than recommended routinely, supplemented as appropriate by application of Lugol solution, inspection and palpation of the vaginal wall,

and colposcopic evaluation if any of these raises concerns (see Section 13.2.4 in Chapter 13). The 2008 ASCCP Guidelines for Specimen Adequacy suggested that lateral vaginal Paps are also appropriate,[5] although this was not mentioned in the most recent ASCCP guidelines update.[4]

Other sources of potential errors can occur due to lapses in patient tracking—scheduling, recall, and follow-up. If a patient does not return for indicated evaluation or treatment, she is at risk for developing more severe disease (Figure 21.6). Commercially available electronic medical record tracking systems may help minimize unintentional nonadherence.

21.3 ERRORS DURING THE COLPOSCOPY EXAMINATION

21.3.1 Visualization Errors

21.3.1.1 Causes of Poor Visualization

Obtaining good visualization of pertinent lower genital tract anatomy is the first step in performing colposcopy; the remainder of the examination depends on this. That which is not seen cannot be diagnosed. Interpretation errors can occur when blood, debris, mucus, discharge, or spermicides or other

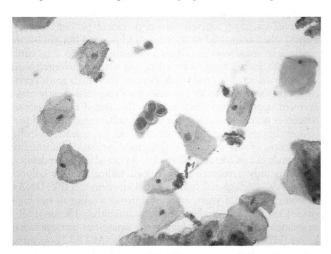

FIGURE 21.2. Cervical cytology findings originally interpreted as negative, but on review reported as HSIL (Papanicolaou stain, high-power magnification).

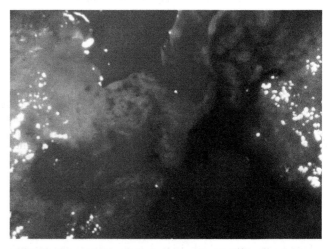

FIGURE 21.4. A cervical ulceration associated with an occult cancer.

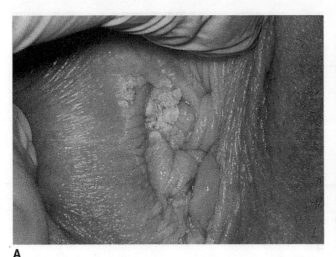

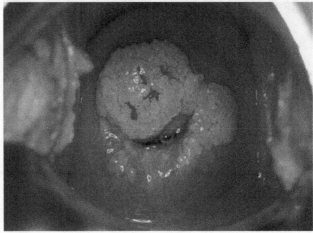

A   **B**

FIGURE 21.5.   During a routine annual examination, condylomas were noted on this young woman's vulva (**A**). Her Pap test was normal but a colposcopic examination done later because of a palpable cervical mass showed this very large cervical lesion (**B**).

chemicals obscure cervical or vaginal lesions or when other anatomic structures obstruct the colposcopist's view. If this occurs, lesions may not be identified, inspected, or biopsied.

21.3.1.1.1 BLEEDING

Traumatic bleeding points, occurring de novo or induced inadvertently by minor trauma, may be controlled by applying firm pressure with a cotton swab. Bleeding from the cervix is of concern for cancer or cervicitis. Excessive abrasive manipulation of the cervix can cause traumatic bleeding. When the source of of the bleeding is clearly traumatic, hemostasis can be obtained by application of Monsel paste or silver nitrate sticks. When the cause of the bleeding is not definitively traumatic, cultures and antibiotics for cervicitis and/or biopsies are indicated. The source of the bleeding must be pursued until either resolved or the diagnosis is established. Care must be exercised when using hemostatic agents (Monsel paste or silver nitrate sticks) that can obscure proper visualization of surrounding features. Moistening cotton swabs before using them to maneuver the cervix can prevent bleeding (Figure 21.7). Using cotton balls or large swabs to apply acetic acid to the cervix also minimizes trauma. Avoid using gauze pads, which can be abrasive. Using a scouring or

rotary motion with a dry cotton swab against columnar epithelium can cause bleeding and also should be avoided.

21.3.1.1.2 MUCUS, DEBRIS, AND DISCHARGE

Cervical mucus can be thin and watery or thick and cloudy depending on the phase of the patient's menstrual cycle. The latter type of mucus may especially hinder visualization. Thick, opaque mucus can be removed, pushed to the side, or positioned deeper within the endocervical canal using a cotton swab. Endocervical mucus can also be removed using an endocervical brush; however, this frequently causes bleeding. Debris or discharge can be gently removed with a large cotton swab.

21.3.1.1.3 PROLAPSING VAGINAL WALLS

In pregnant, elderly, or obese patients, laxity of vaginal tissue may cause the sidewalls to protrude into the vagina between the speculum blades. Prolapsing vaginal sidewalls can be retracted using a vaginal speculum covered by a condom or the finger from a latex glove (Figure 21.8A,B). A lateral sidewall retractor also works well but should be used cautiously to prevent pinching that can occur when the sidewall prolapses between the retractor and speculum blades. Small cotton swabs, tongue blades, or ring forceps also can be used to retract the vaginal walls. A tenaculum is not an instrument

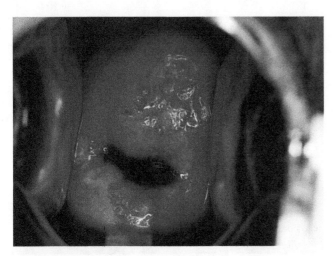

FIGURE 21.6.   This 35-year-old woman failed to return for treatment after a cervical biopsy showed CIN 3. She presented 3 years later with cervical cancer, seen here on the anterior portion of the cervix at 12–2 o'clock.

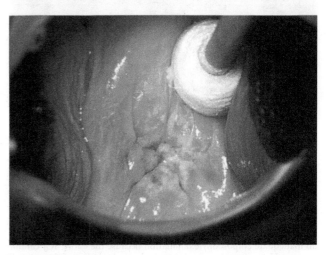

FIGURE 21.7.   Large moistened cotton swab used to atraumatically maneuver the cervix.

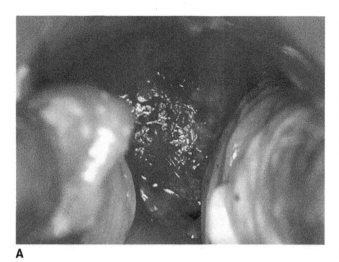 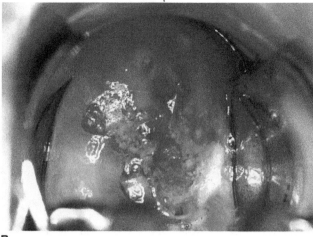

A   B

FIGURE 21.8.   **A:** Prolapsed vaginal sidewalls hinder proper colposcopic evaluation of this woman's cervix. Colposcopists should not discontinue their inspection if this occurs. **B:** Vaginal sidewall retractors help to show the source (seen at 3 o'clock) of her abnormal cytology report.

typically used during colposcopy because it may traumatize tissue and cause bleeding, obscuring inspection. Often, gentle manipulation of the vaginal speculum will enhance visualization. For instance, applying downward pressure against the anterior cervix with the anterior vaginal speculum blade can align an anteriorly oriented ectocervix so that it is perpendicular to the colposcopist's line of sight. In addition, proper illumination from the colposcope's light source is essential for identifying necessary anatomy and disease. Adjusting the light rheostat to maximum, directing the light beam down toward the central axis of the vagina, and opening the yoke of the vaginal speculum as wide as the patient can tolerate can maximize proper illumination and visibility.

Using the colposcope at a low-power magnification setting provides greater illumination, depth of field, and field of view than does using a high-power magnification setting. The external genitalia are also best examined with the colposcope at low magnification so subtle lesions are not missed. Dust and dirt on the colposcope lenses can impair visualization as well. Covering the colposcope when not in use and routinely cleaning lenses and eyepieces are of great value.

21.3.1.2 Inadequate Visualization of the Squamocolumnar Junction

A potentially serious error of colposcopy is to assume the entire squamocolumnar junction (SCJ) has been examined when only a portion is observed (Figures 21.9 and 21.10). If a woman is referred for colposcopy because of an abnormal Pap result, no colposcopic abnormality is found, and only part of the SCJ is seen, the source of neoplasia may be in the unvisualized portion of the SCJ. Every effort should be taken to view the unseen SCJ section. By opening the vaginal speculum blades in both planes as widely as the patient can tolerate, the resulting cervical eversion may allow the obscured areas of the SCJ to be inspected. If this step does not permit adequate SCJ visualization, the cervical os may be gently opened by applying pressure to the vaginal fornices or directly on the ectocervix in opposing directions using moistened cotton swabs. Alternatively, a closed endocervical speculum or ring forceps can be placed gently within the canal and carefully opened to permit viewing. These instruments should be used cautiously since the thin, fragile columnar epithelium of the endocervix can be easily sheared, resulting in

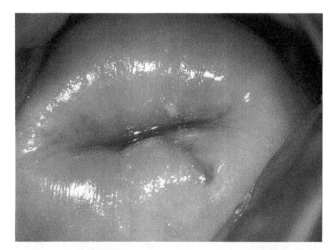 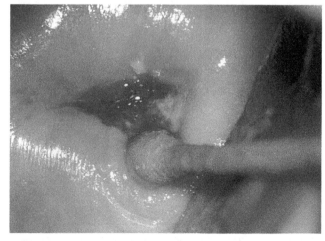

FIGURE 21.9.   Examining only the area visible here would result in an inadequate colposcopy examination because the entire SCJ cannot be seen. However, this may change with manipulation of the cervical os with a Q-tip or an endocervical speculum.

FIGURE 21.10.   The same patient as seen in Figure 21.9. Now the entire SCJ is seen along with the previously undetected high-grade neoplasia located at 3 o'clock.

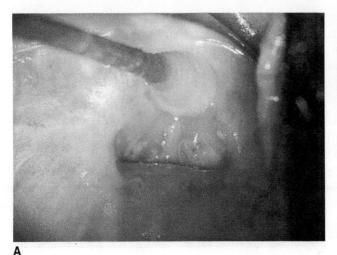 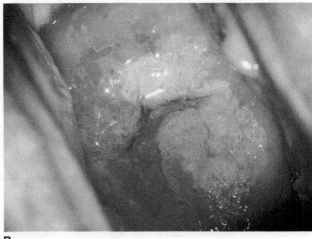

A   **B**

FIGURES 21.11.   A small CIN 1 lesion is seen on the anterior lip of the cervix (**A**). The lesion extends into the endocervical canal beyond colposcopic view. The patient may have a more severe lesion along the SCJ. In (**B**), a large two-quadrant lesion is seen. This examination would also be considered inadequate because the lesion extends into the endocervical canal beyond view.

bleeding, which will obscure visibility. Although usually well tolerated, use of an endocervical speculum can cause the patient to experience some discomfort or mild cramping. Endocervical canal bleeding considerably compromises inspection of an area that is already difficult to examine. As described in the section on bleeding, tamponade with a cotton swab moistened with a 5% acetic acid solution will sometimes help if the etiology of the bleeding is only minor trauma. When acute cervicitis or menstruation is the source of the bleeding, it is often necessary to reschedule the examination after treatment or completion of menses. Pregnant women with inadequate colposcopic examinations during the first 12 weeks of pregnancy should be reexamined after 20 weeks' gestation when cervical eversion and os dilation facilitate identification of the SCJ.

21.3.1.3 Inadequate Visualization of Lesions Extending Deep into the Cervical Canal

Colposcopists may be unable initially to identify the margin of a lesion that extends deep into the endocervical canal (Figure 21.11A,B). The same visualization maneuvers described in the previous section may be used to identify the deep margin

of an endocervical lesion. If unable to identify the margin deep in the canal, the evaluation qualifies as an inadequate colposcopic examination. If the woman is elderly and/or estrogen deficient, a 2- to 3-week course of vaginal estrogen cream may facilitate an adequate colposcopic examination about 1 month later. If the woman is well estrogenized, the colposcopy should be considered inadequate, endocervical sampling should be done, and appropriate guidelines-based follow-up should be ordered.

21.3.1.4 Special Situations in Which Comprehensive Colposcopic Visualization of the Vagina and Vulva Is Necessary

When no lesions are seen on the cervix of a woman with an abnormal Pap test, the entire vagina should be carefully inspected since an occult lesion may found in the vagina (Figure 21.12A,B). Vaginal neoplasia may also be the cause of abnormal cytology in women who have an inadequate colposcopy examination (Figure 21.13A,B). Cervical and vaginal sites should be assessed to determine the location of the disease, since the cervix, the vagina, or both sites may be involved. The cervix may be gently manipulated toward the opposite side to view

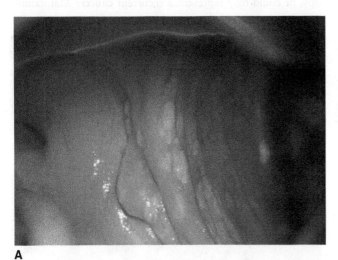 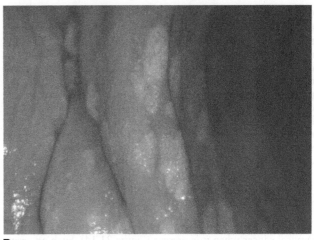

A   **B**

FIGURES 21.12.   This woman's Pap report was LSIL. Although colposcopy of her cervix was normal, acetowhite lesions were found on the left proximal vaginal wall (**A,B**). **A:** A vaginal biopsy revealed a low-grade HPV lesion.

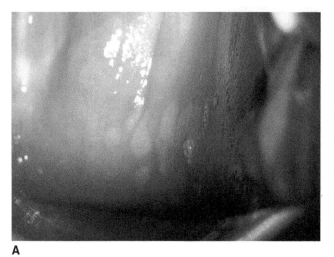

A

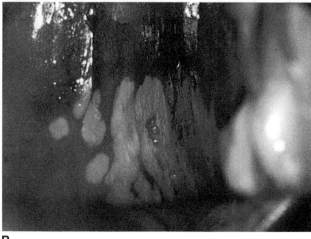

B

FIGURE 21.13.   This woman had normal colposcopy of the cervix. Acetowhite (**A**) and corresponding iodine-negative lesions (**B**) can be seen on the right vaginal wall. This biopsy was interpreted as VaIN 2.

the entire vaginal fornix. In most cases of vaginal neoplasia, disease is located in the vagina near the cervix. Use of a 3% to 5% acetic acid solution and/or dilute Lugol iodine solution is necessary for adequately identifying most vaginal neoplasia. Confluent iodine-negative yellow areas represent sites of potential vaginal neoplasia and contrast well with the surrounding mahogany brown staining normal vaginal squamous epithelium. Visualizing some vulvar lesions may be difficult because of their anatomic position. Identifying vulvar neoplasia and condylomas may be challenging when these are hidden within the urethra, beneath the clitoral hood, protruding from minor vestibular glands, or behind redundant hymeneal tissue. Applying a 5% acetic acid solution directly to these areas and using low-power colposcopic magnification or a handheld magnifying glass to inspect them may be helpful. It must be kept in mind that acetowhitening on the vulva can be a very nonspecific finding (see Chapter 15). Regular cursory examinations of the external genitalia at the conclusion of cervicovaginal colposcopy may prevent overlooking vulvar neoplasia in these areas.

21.3.2 Assessment Errors

21.3.2.1 Developing Colposcopic Assessment Skills

Once proper visualization of the lower genital tract is achieved, the colposcopist must critically assess each area. Visualization primarily involves psychomotor skills readily learned by most novice colposcopists. In contrast, colposcopic assessment demands cognitive skills learned and then continuously refined through years of experience. Skills can be improved by comparing the final colposcopic impression of a patient with the cytologic and histologic findings from biopsies taken. Only by critical feedback can these important assessment skills be maintained and improved. Routine use of a colposcopic index with standardized assessment categories may provide objective criteria for deriving a colposcopic impression.

21.3.2.2 Common Errors in Recognizing Cervical Cancer

The most detrimental assessment error is failing to recognize cervical cancer when it is present (Figure 21.14). Such an error may harm the patient if it causes a significant delay in diagnosis. In a retrospective study, Shumsky et al.[10] evaluated the outcomes of women who developed invasive cervical cancer following

treatment of cervical intraepithelial neoplasia (CIN). The mean interval between the treatment of CIN and the diagnosis of cancer was approximately 24 months. Most of the cancers were detected at an early stage. In 13% of these cases, however, Shumsky et al. concluded that the invasive disease may have been present prior to ablative therapy but was not detected.

Certainly, cancers within the endocervical canal can be overlooked by clinicians with considerable expertise. However, colposcopists should be aware of and vigilant for the warning signs of cervical cancer (see Chapters 10 and 11), even in women referred for colposcopy because of low-grade cytologic abnormalities. Colposcopists fail to diagnose microinvasive and invasive cancer at significant rates of 15.9% and 10.4%, respectively.[11]

As noted above, the site of the lesion also influences the colposcopist's success in detecting cancer. Even the most novice colposcopist is expected to recognize atypical blood vessels and to biopsy the involved tissue. However, if the atypical blood vessels are in an area of very immature squamous metaplasia or are present in a patient after radiation therapy, even an experienced colposcopist may mistakenly decide that the involved tissues are benign (Figures 21.15 and 21.16A,B). The latter case presents a difficult challenge for all colposcopists: Are the atypical vessels the result of successful radiation therapy, or could they represent a recurrent cancer? Maintaining

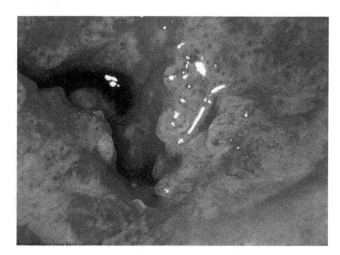

FIGURE 21.14.   An occult cervical cancer not readily detected.

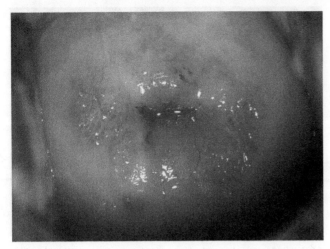

FIGURE 21.15. This atypical blood vessel in a field of normal immature metaplasia is benign but mimics atypical blood vessels of invasive cancer. Cervical biopsy is usually warranted to define the status of the epithelium.

a low threshold for biopsying any atypical vessels minimizes errors in diagnosing new or recurring cancers. Similarly, ulcerations thought to be iatrogenic, viral, or bacterial in etiology could be due to a malignancy. Large vaginal ulcerations may also be caused by a retained or overused tampons. Biopsy, especially when ulcers are of a chronic nature, and careful observation and reexamination at a later date are reasonable management options for ulcers (see Chapter 13). However, when they are accompanied by warning signs of cancer, or adjoin intact acetowhite or non–iodine-staining epithelium, immediate biopsy is indicated (Figure 21.17).

Microglandular hyperplasia, both associated with the use of progestins in oral contraceptives and in decidual tissue seen in women during pregnancy, can be mistaken for a malignancy. In both cases, the women affected are mostly young, and the risk for cancer is low. If in doubt, a biopsy should be taken to eliminate cancer as the etiology for the finding. Even experienced colposcopists can overlook small high-grade lesions or occult areas of microinvasive cancer positioned within larger low-grade lesions. Establishing a regimen of checking for internal margins within acetowhite lesions will help to reduce the probability of this error occurring. One of the most difficult lesions

to discriminate from cancer is a large, four-quadrant, exophytic cervical condyloma (Figures 21.18A,B and 21.19). Generally, condylomas will be symmetrical and papillary in contour. The presence of ulcerations, yellow necrotic epithelium, irregular surface contour, and atypical vessels would suggest cancer. Fine central capillary vessels may be observed within the papillary projections of condylomas when viewed colposcopically at high magnification. Obtaining biopsies for histologic analysis is indicated to establish the true etiology since differentiating condylomas from cancer can be very challenging, even for an expert colposcopist. Discriminating between cancer and benign mimics during colposcopy is even more difficult when the patient has a history of prior abnormal cervical cytology results.

Insufficient and infrequent application of 5% acetic acid solution to the cervix during the examination will adversely affect the colposcopist's ability to assess disease. Lesions will either not be detected or, if seen, appear to be less significant levels of neoplasia than they actually are (Figures 21.20 and 21.21). The color and opacity of the lesion(s) are important features to note when attempting to correctly identify and classify cervical neoplasia. The use of contrast agents greatly facilitates the colposcopic examination; however, they may also hinder assessment. For example, use of Lugol iodine solution may help in discriminating between neoplasia and benign tissue changes; however, if it is applied prematurely, the resulting brown and yellow staining may obscure important colposcopic features, such as atypical vessels. Applying topical benzocaine gel or a solution of 10% sodium hypochlorite to the area can reverse iodine uptake by glycogen-containing epithelium. The green filter accentuates vessel appearance and aids with vessel recognition, particularly by the novice colposcopist. However, the green filter may modify the appearance of the epithelium by darkening the field of view.

Failure to evaluate the true caliber of blood vessels prior to applying an acetic acid solution or as the acetic acid effect is diminishing also may lead to incorrect assessment. Acetic acid exerts a vasoconstrictive effect that narrows the caliber of the vessels, sometimes causing the colposcopist to underestimate the presence of disease. This error can be prevented by applying a saline solution to the cervix and evaluating colposcopically prior to applying the 5% acetic acid solution. The colposcopist should also assess the vessels as the acetic acid effect is waning.

21.3.2.3 Failing to Form a Colposcopic Impression

Finally, the primary goal of the assessment process is to formulate a colposcopic impression in order to locate the best sites to

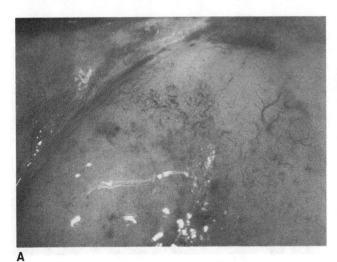

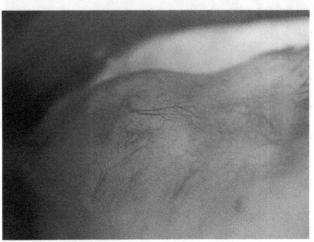

A   B

FIGURE 21.16. Atypical blood vessels noted in this elderly woman following radiation therapy for cervical cancer. These vessels are benign and induced by her therapy (A,B). However, discrimination from recurrent disease can be exceedingly difficult.

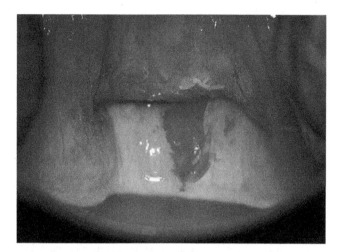

FIGURE 21.17. A large vaginal ulceration and opaque thickened acetowhite epithelium are seen, raising the suspicion of vaginal cancer. A biopsy of the area was interpreted as VaIN 3.

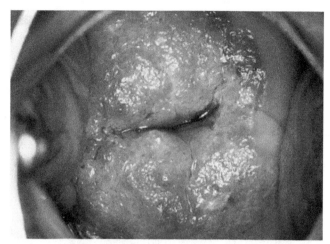

FIGURE 21.19. A cervical cancer that appears strikingly similar to the large condyloma seen in Figure 21.18. (Photo courtesy of Dr. Vesna Kesic.)

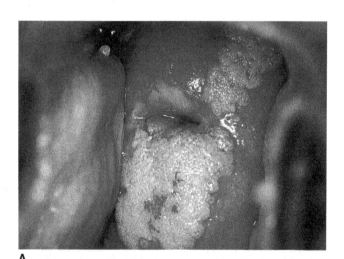

A

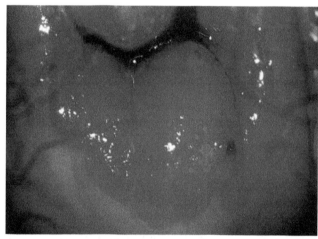

FIGURE 21.20. The cervix of a woman with a HSIL Pap report seen with insufficient 5% acetic acid application. Her lesion is not clearly seen.

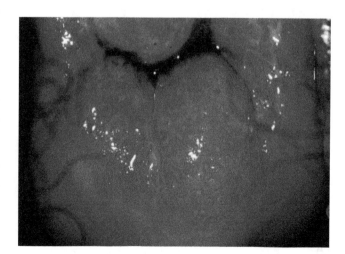

B

FIGURE 21.18. A large exophytic cervical condyloma that mimics an invasive lesion is seen (A,B). The irregular surface contour is apparent.

FIGURE 21.21. The same cervix in Figure 21.20 after sufficient acetic acid application. Now a CIN 2–3 lesion can be readily appreciated.

biopsy. An objectively derived colposcopic impression should be formulated at the completion of each colposcopic examination. Only in this way can a good colposcopist compare her or his colposcopic impressions with the cytologic and histologic reports. Furthermore, disease may not be properly managed if the colposcopist overlooks the important step of making a clinical diagnosis. Many novice colposcopists are uncomfortable initially with their ability to form a colposcopic impression.

Yet, failure to derive a clinical diagnosis prevents the colposcopist from determining whether important clinical findings and the overall colposcopic impression correlate with laboratory findings, cytology reports, and histologic diagnoses. Colposcopists should realize that pathologists commonly fail to agree among themselves about findings on cytologic tests and, more importantly, their findings on histopathologic specimens; that is, cytologic and histologic interpretations suffer from subjectivity and human error just as colposcopic interpretation does.[12,13] Nevertheless, when findings from histology and colposcopy are considered collectively, diagnostic error is minimized.

21.3.3 Sampling Errors

An obligatory component of colposcopy is retrieving representative histologic specimens from lesions following assessment of the most severe areas of change. Cognitive skills are required to select potential abnormal epithelium for histologic sampling. Identification of which areas to biopsy is one of the most difficult parts of colposcopy. Procedurally speaking, this phase also involves psychomotor skills that can be achieved with moderate practice. Biopsying inanimate materials that simulate cervical anatomy and neoplasia may allow the novice colposcopist to gain confidence and become more competent prior to performing a biopsy on a patient.[14] In addition to developing proper technique, proper sampling equipment should be selected and carefully maintained. Biopsy instruments must be kept sharp to minimize the amount of crushing artifact resulting from a biopsy and to insure retrieval of an adequate specimen. Moreover, dull biopsy instruments are probably the main cause of patient discomfort.[15]

It is difficult to collect too deep of a cervical biopsy when using commercially available instruments intended for that purpose (Figure 21.22). However, too conservative superficial sampling may result in a biopsy of inadequate depth and, because the basement membrane of the tissue was not included in the specimen, may prevent a pathologist from properly assessing whether or not an invasive process exists. Such biopsies are infrequent and usually result from inexperience. A shallow biopsy also can result when the colposcopist samples a lesion located on a flat epithelial surface such as the cervix or the vagina. A satisfactory vaginal biopsy is more easily obtained when the speculum blades are released slightly, which reduces the tautness of sidewalls and increases tissue folding, allowing the colposcopist to grasp the tissue with little resistance. Use of a dull instrument is more likely to obtain a thin, superficial specimen that may exhibit "crush" artifact. When dull, the jaws tend to slip from the surface before grasping an adequate specimen. Opening the sharp jaws of a biopsy instrument widely and pushing the cervix backward until the cardinal ligaments prevent further cephalad motion will prevent the biopsy instrument from slipping.

Occasionally, biopsy specimens will be "lost" immediately after sampling the tissue. Sometimes when the biopsy is taken, the movable upper jaw of the instrument will force the specimen through the bottom jaw and the specimen retention grid of the biopsy forceps. A search of the posterior, proximal vaginal fornix or posterior speculum blade will usually locate the missing specimen. Tissue may also fall out of the jaws when the closed jaws are accidentally opened prior to placing the tissue into formalin. Some colposcopists use biopsy forceps that

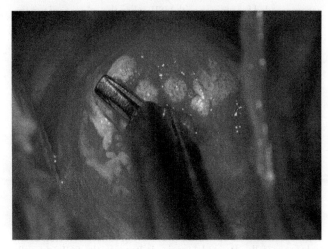

FIGURE 21.22. An adequate cervical biopsy is necessary to gain an accurate histologic diagnosis. Using modern biopsy forceps, taking too deep or too large of a cervical biopsy is unlikely. The risk is of taking too small or too shallow a sample.

have a locking device, which is easily activated by turning a thumbscrew, limiting the possibility of losing a specimen.

Retrieving an insufficient amount of tissue from the cervix following endocervical curettage (ECC) is a more common sampling problem. Using a sharp curette and applying firm pressure when scraping the tissue of the endocervical canal and assuring that all of the contents of the canal resulting from the curettage (i.e., blood, mucus, and cellular material) are evacuated are crucial for obtaining sufficient tissue. It may not be readily apparent upon clinical inspection that an ample specimen has been obtained because of the large volume of blood and mucus collected. Using an endocervical brush to evacuate the contents of the endocervical canal after metal curettage may help to increase the amount of endocervical tissue in the specimen (Figure 21.23). Even more important is recognizing when collection of an endocervical specimen is necessary to reach an accurate diagnosis.

In nonpregnant patients referred for the evaluation of ASC-US or LSIL cytology, endocervical sampling is preferred when no lesion is identified or when colposcopy is inadequate but is acceptable for women with an adequate colposcopy and a lesion identified in the transformation zone.[4] An immediate loop electrosurgical excision procedure (LEEP) and colposcopy with endocervical assessment are both acceptable options for managing women with HSIL, except in adolescents and young women, and in pregnant patients.[4] A diagnostic excisional procedure is

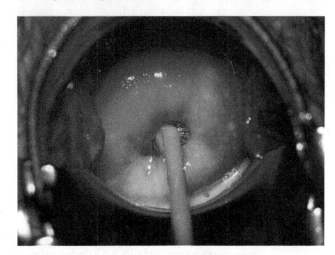

FIGURE 21.23. An endocervical brush can effectively remove cellular contents of the endocervical canal following ECC.

recommended for women with HSIL when the colposcopic examination is inadequate, except during pregnancy.[4] In nonpregnant patients with AGC, initial evaluation should include colposcopy, endocervical evaluation and sampling, and possibly endometrial evaluation. ECC is always unacceptable in pregnant women.[4] Certainly, if the patient has cytologic evidence of cervical neoplasia and an inadequate colposcopic examination, an ECC must be performed unless the patient is pregnant, even if the findings from the colposcopic examination are normal and further evaluation is imperative unless cancer is found on the endocervical sample, prompting referral to a gynecologic oncologist (Figure 21.24).

Lack of an ECC or inadequate tissue on an ECC can be reason that cervical cancer is missed on colposcopy.[16,17] Cytologic or histologic evaluation of the products of an ECC is very likely to detect cervical cancer if present in the endocervical sample. In one study in which colposcopic biopsy and ECC were performed in 2304 women, neoplastic epithelium was found in the ECC specimens of 15 women not having cancer detected in the colposcopically directed biopsies.[18] Because the SCJ generally recedes into the cervical canal as women age, as do high-grade lesions, endocervical sampling becomes increasingly important in older women as demonstrated in the ALTS study.[19]

Most studies demonstrate a 3% to 5% increase detection of CIN 2+ with ECC and improved opportunity to detect subtle adenocarcinoma in situ (AIS) or adenocarcinoma (Figure 21.25A–D).[19–21] Although skip lesions in the endocervical canal

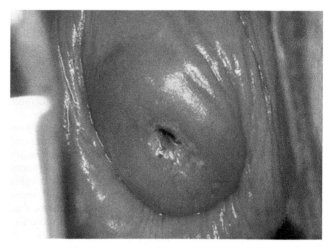

FIGURE 21.24. The colposcopic examination is inadequate in this woman with a HSIL Pap report. The SCJ is not visualized. If the vagina is free of disease, the source of the cytologic abnormality is likely hidden in the canal.

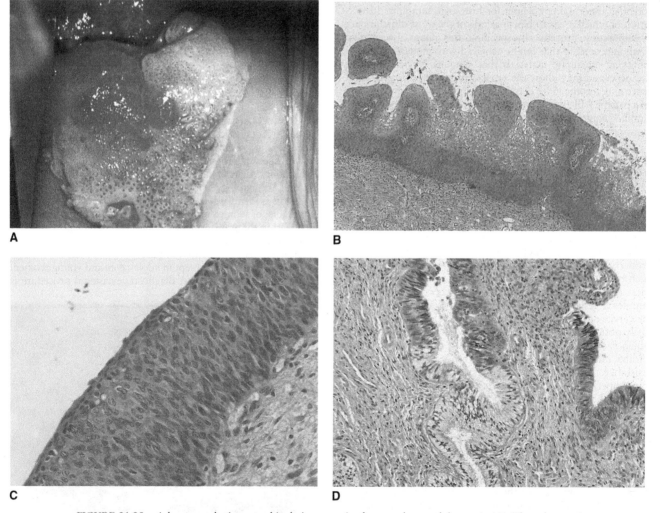

A

B

C

D

FIGURE 21.25. A large exophytic acetowhite lesion occupies four quadrants of the cervix (**A**). The colposcopic examination was inadequate. Cervical biopsies demonstrate condyloma (**B**) (hematoxylin-eosin stain; medium-power magnification) and CIN 3 (**C**) (hematoxylin-eosin stain; high-power magnification). A loop electrosurgical excision procedure (LEEP) conization also detected occult adenocarcinoma in situ in the endocervical canal (**D**) (hematoxylin-eosin stain; medium-power magnification).

are very rare and found primarily in women with a history of prior cervical procedures and in some women with AIS, when present, they are more likely to be detected by ECC. Skip lesions are usually occult endocervical lesions separated from more readily apparent ectocervical lesions by normal epithelium. The ectocervical lesion may explain the previous abnormal cytology result. However, the skip lesion may be more severe histologically. All nonpregnant women with a history of prior procedures of the cervix and abnormal cytologic results on a recent or current test should have an endocervical specimen collected. No colposcopist will ever be criticized for performing an ECC, except when contraindicated during pregnancy.

Errors made in sampling result in submitting nonrepresentative specimens for histologic evaluation. Preventing such errors depends on the cervix being properly assessed and the site of suspected most severe disease being accurately identified, particularly when a large complex lesion is present. In general, the most severe lesions are located along or near the SCJ. Recognition of this principle can help guide biopsy site selection, particularly if a large, seemingly homogeneous lesion is present. Therefore, the ideal location for obtaining biopsies is along the SCJ and usually within the center of uniformly appearing lesions. When normal immature metaplasia and cervical neoplasia coexist, frequently the larger benign tissue is mistakenly biopsied because it is more visible (Figure 21.26A–C). Failing to biopsy the most severe disease present is perhaps the most critical error that can be made during colposcopy. Collecting multiple biopsies improves detection of CIN 3 and thus should be done whenever possible.[4,21,22] Occasionally, during the biopsy, the jaws of the forceps will slip from the intended sampling site. Quickly examining the site using the colposcope immediately

following the biopsy, before bleeding obscures visualization, will allow the colposcopist to determine whether the desired specimen was obtained. If the site was missed, another biopsy should be performed to assure that the tissue desired is sampled. Mucus, debris, or blood may obscure an area of severe disease. Excessive bleeding also may be encountered when performing biopsies in pregnant women or women with acute cervicitis or cancer. A potential for hemorrhage should not preclude a biopsy when indicated since rapid application of Monsel or silver nitrate sticks will typically curtail bleeding. By anticipating possible complications and having hemostatic agents readily available to control the bleeding, excessive blood loss is unlikely; very rarely a suture will need to be placed. Limiting the number of biopsies taken because of typical tolerable patient discomfort, additional cost, or extra time required to identify the best sites to sample is not wise. Large lesions or multiple distinct lesions may require several biopsies to insure that tissue representative of the disease is obtained. Even aggressive use of biopsy forceps will never remove as much tissue as is removed during cervical conization. Obtaining deep or wedge-shaped biopsies is indicated when cancer is suspected.

Unintentional trauma inflicted while inserting or removing biopsy instruments can also jeopardize care. For example, while using the endocervical curette, an ectocervical lesion located on the external os could be "nicked" accidentally (Figure 21.27). Usually, when this occurs, a single fragment of abnormality is found in the ECC, and if the ECC is performed under direct colposcopic visualization, often the nicking of the lesion at the os can be identified at the time it is done. When a specimen obtained by ECC is found in a woman ≥25 to contain high-grade cells, a cervical excision procedure is usually done to

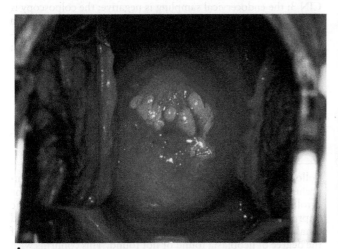

A

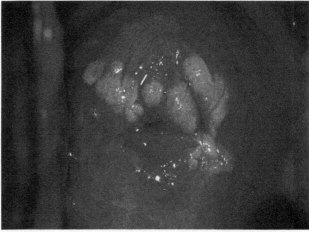

B

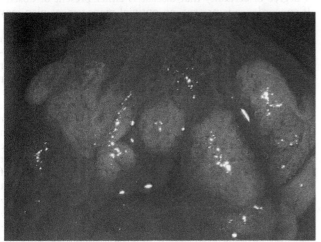

C

FIGURE 21.26. Acetowhite epithelium is noted on the anterior and posterior lips of the cervix (**A**). A cervical biopsy of the posterior lip showed benign immature metaplasia. A biopsy of the anterior lip detected CIN 3. An internal margin marking the more proximally positioned CIN 3 from the less severe, peripherally located CIN is clearly seen (**B,C**). Hence, three different acetowhite areas of different densities are observed.

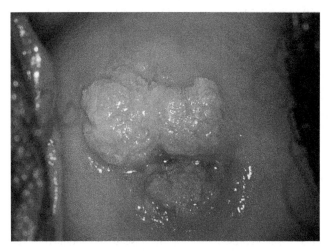

FIGURE 21.27.   A cervical neoplasia extending into the endocervical canal that could be sampled accidentally by a careless ECC.

properly diagnose (and possibly treat) endocervical neoplasia even if the colposcopist felt it likely came from "nicking" the lesion at the external os. Some colposcopists argue that if properly documented, a cervical excision procedure would be unnecessary under this "accidental" circumstance. However, such an assumption is most often difficult to substantiate. Sound colposcopy practice dictates that a positive ECC is reason for concern and dictates further histologic evaluation or reliable follow-up. In contrast the finding of CIN1 on ECC is typically followed, although the option to do a cervical excision procedure or to follow by cotesting at 12 and 24 months is provided for women ≥25 with a referral cytology of HSIL or ASC-H.

Passing the endocervical brush or curette through a protective straw or tube-like device placed in the cervical os can prevent the colposcopist from accidentally scraping the vagina or ectocervix and contaminating the instrument. Otherwise, endocervical sampling should be carefully performed under direct visualization through the colposcope, and the curette should be withdrawn with the cutting edge turned away from any observed lesions to limit the possibility of contaminating the instrument being used to acquire the sample.

Colposcopy has resulted in a reduction in the number of cervical conizations performed during the past 40 years. However, a diagnostic excisional procedure or cervical conization should

always be performed when the procedure is clearly indicated to insure a comprehensive evaluation of the lower genital tract.

Conization usually provides an adequately deep specimen for thorough pathologic analysis of the endocervical canal, including the detection of cancer (Figure 21.28). A diagnostic excisional procedure is typically indicated in nonpregnant women in the following circumstances: (1) when preliminary histology, cytology, or colposcopy results indicate the possible presence of microinvasion or invasive cancer; (2) when the biopsy result is CIN 3, AIS or microinvasion; (3) when recurrent CIN 2, CIN 3, or CIN 2,3 is identified posttreatment; (4) when an HSIL Pap is not confirmed by biopsy or ECC in a woman aged 25 years or over two options are available: A diagnostic excisional procedure or observation with cotesting at 12 and 24 mo provided that the colposcopy examination is adequate, or in a woman aged 21 years and over when colposcopy is inadequate; (5) when CIN 2, CIN 3, CIN 2,3, or ungraded CIN is identified on endocervical sampling; (6) when cancer is not found on colposcopic biopsy in the evaluation of women with cytology interpreted as AGC "favor neoplasia" or AIS; or (7) when the cervical biopsy indicates AIS.[4] Observation of CIN 3 with sequential cytology and colposcopy is unacceptable, except in pregnant women. Observation of CIN 2 and CIN2,3 with sequential cytology and colposcopy is unacceptable, except in pregnant women and young women, with the proviso that the term "young women" be applied to "those who after counseling by their clinicians consider risk to future pregnancies from treating cervical abnormalities to outweigh risk for cancer during observation of those abnormalities. No specific age threshold is intended."[4] Ablation is an acceptable alternative to excision when the histology is reported as CIN 2, CIN 2,3, or CIN 3; the endocervical sampling is negative; the colposcopy is adequate and the entire lesion can be seen; and cancer has been ruled out.[4] An immediate LEEP or colposcopy with endocervical assessment are acceptable methods for managing women with HSIL, except in adolescents and young women.

21.4 ERRORS AFTER THE COLPOSCOPY EXAMINATION

21.4.1 Correlation Errors

Following careful visualization, critical assessment, and comprehensive sampling, the colposcopist must correlate the cytology report and histologic diagnosis with the colposcopic impression. Ideally, these laboratory and clinical results should "make sense" by being concordant or very similar in terms of the degree of neoplasia found or not found. This confirms with a degree of certainty that disease is either present or absent. If concordance is present, an optimal management plan may then be pursued with reasonable confidence.

Lack of agreement within one degree of severity (i.e., between normal and CIN 1 or between CIN 2 and CIN 3) among cytologic, histologic, and colposcopic results does occur and is not necessarily a failure on the part of the colposcopist, clinician, or pathologist (Figure 21.29A–C). Lack of correlation within one degree most often does not significantly impact management. However, lack of correlation within 2 degrees is of concern, for management may be appreciably impacted. For example, when the cytology and colposcopic impression are high grade but the biopsy is normal or CIN 1, the colposcopist should attempt to determine why discrepancy exists. Imprecise selection of the biopsy site, misinterpretation of pathology results, patient identification errors, or faulty reasoning in formulating the colposcopic impression may lead to discordant results. When this occurs, having the pathologist review the cytology and histology may solve the discrepancy, but if it does not, the colposcopy may need to be repeated and additional specimens obtained.

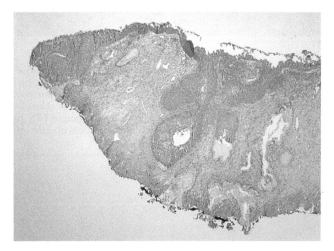

FIGURE 21.28.   A histologic section from a cervical conization demonstrating CIN 3 (hematoxylin-eosin stain; medium-power magnification). The conization was necessary because of colposcopic and cytologic discordance.

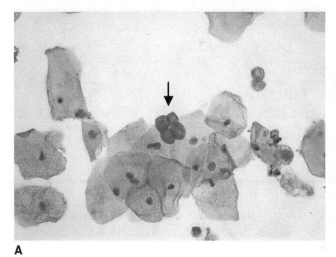

A

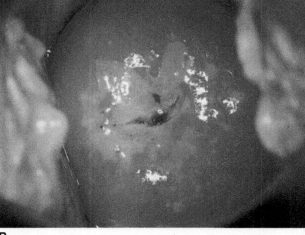

B

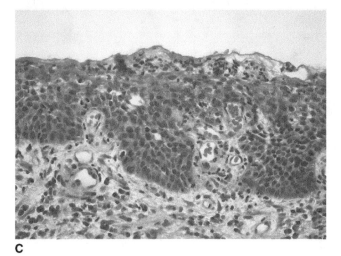

C

FIGURE 21.29. Lack of agreement of cytology, histology, and colposcopic impression. The cytology was HSIL (**A**) (Papanicolaou stain, high-power magnification), the colposcopy was normal but inadequate (**B**), and the histology report was immature metaplasia (**C**) (hematoxylin-eosin stain; medium-power magnification). Further evaluation is necessary to achieve a diagnosis and determine proper management.

If resolution of disagreement does not readily occur, clinicians may be tempted to disregard their colposcopic impression despite the severity of the discrepancy. However, the value of the colposcopic impression, especially if arrived at using appropriate colposcopic methods, should not be underestimated or quickly dismissed. Nevertheless, errors may be made in formulating a colposcopic impression. Of particular concern are cases in which the colposcopic impression is notably more severe than indicated by the laboratory findings (Figure 21.30A–C). In those cases, the colposcopist should consider reexamining the patient or referring the woman to an expert colposcopist for a second opinion. Many times, reevaluation by another colposcopist and further histologic sampling will help to resolve discordance. As a last resort, the colposcopist should consider a diagnostic excision, if indicated by the severity of the discrepancy, since laboratory findings from the greater amount of tissue obtained might provide an explanation for the diagnostic discrepancy.

Subjecting a patient to therapy prior to establishing a level of certainty about a diagnosis risks improper management and the possibility of overtreatment that may not be in the best interest of the patient. However, when at least one of several findings suggests the presence of invasive cancer, contradictory findings cannot be ignored (Figure 21.31). A pathology report that suggests even the "possibility of cancer" should always be considered seriously, and follow-up testing should be diligently pursued, regardless of what the colposcopic impression was. Women who have previously received cervical radiation treatment present the added challenge of delineating the SCJ and transformation zone. Consequently, the results of the colposcopic examination will frequently remain inadequate and

cytology and histology alone must be used to determine appropriate management. However, if ectocervical or vaginal disease is observed during colposcopy, additional histologic assessment is imperative. Invariably, women with colposcopic or histologic evidence of neoplasia located deep within the endocervical canal should undergo cervical conization. In such cases, further colposcopic evaluation or histologic testing of specimens from ECC will not likely provide a more accurate or specific diagnosis. When evidence of significant endocervical disease is present, the diagnosis ultimately resides in the hands of the pathologist. Management is then usually directed by the histologic results from the diagnostic excision. Because the area excised often includes the entire site of diseased tissue, conization is sometimes considered a therapeutic as well as a diagnostic procedure.

21.4.2 Management Errors

As stated previously, the procedure of colposcopy consists of four unique and sequential steps: visualization, assessment, sampling, and correlation (VASC). Patient management evolves from the last step of correlating the cervical cytology and histology results with the colposcopic impression. The patient's characteristics, relevant history, and personal desires also influence the decision-making process regarding therapy. These factors collectively form the basis on which a proper strategy for management of cervical neoplasia is built.

Determining a plan for optimum patient care is usually straightforward and relatively easy; however, it can be intimidating if discordant or confusing data are presented,

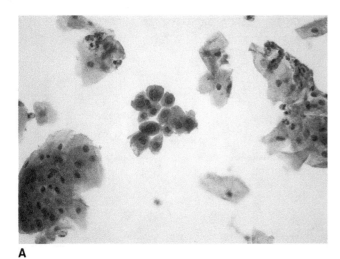

A

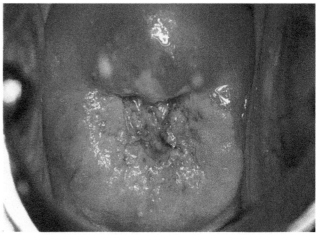

B

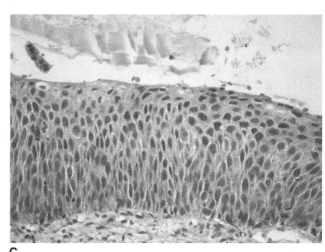

C

FIGURE 21.30.   Discordance of the Pap test (**A**) (Papanicolaou stain, high-power magnification), biopsy report, and colposcopic impression. A colposcopically visible cervical cancer appears present (**B**), but the Pap was interpreted as reactive versus ASC-US and the biopsy as CIN 2 (**C**) (hematoxylin-eosin stain; medium-power magnification). Repeat sampling (wedge biopsy or diagnostic excision) should help resolve the disagreement. (Colposcopic photograph courtesy of Dr. Vesna Kesic.)

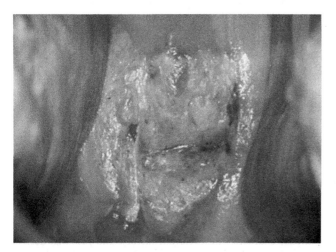

FIGURE 21.31.   Regardless of cytology or histology results, a diagnostic excision is mandatory for this woman with colposcopic suspicion of microinvasion. The cone specimen showed <4 mm of invasion. (Photo courtesy of Dr. Vesna Kesic.)

extraneous influences arise, seemingly equivalent therapeutic techniques are considered, or dilemmas concerning balance of risks and benefits emerge. Tailoring management plans to suit the patient when multiple therapeutic options are available requires an extensive understanding of the disease process and of the likely outcomes associated with each treatment

option. Furthermore, patient management is frequently a dynamic process since unexpected events may alter the original treatment plans. Consequently, the process of selecting an appropriate management plan may sometimes seem extremely complex. A structured and systematic approach that considers all relevant information optimizes the likelihood of achieving satisfactory patient outcomes.

Prior to embarking upon any cervical treatment, a comprehensive colposcopy examination should be performed. Normal, large cervical ectropions, with their beefy red color, have been confused by clinicians as representing important cervical pathology. A clinician may erroneously diagnose a copious, clear vaginal discharge as "cervicitis" or a cervical "erosion" and perform an ablative procedure without first conducting a colposcopic examination, only to later discover that the patient actually had invasive cancer.[16] Cervical friability may be a sign of acute cervicitis in most cases, but this same inflammatory, necrotic tissue could be caused by invasive cancer (Figure 21.32). A careful colposcopist will biopsy every large cervical wart and review the pathology report prior to making a definitive decision on management to eliminate the possibility that a benign-looking finding is actually malignant.

All colposcopists should be able to properly evaluate at least 90% of patients seen in normal practice. However, a greater level of colposcopic expertise may be necessary to evaluate patients with more challenging conditions. As colposcopic expertise increases, the spectrum of diseases and challenging cases that the colposcopist can effectively manage will also increase. However, during the early learning phase, questions concerning colposcopic technique or management

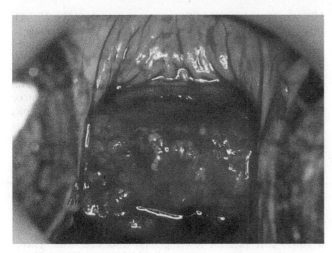

FIGURE 21.32.   Cervical friability and bleeding seen on this patient's cervix can be misdiagnosed as cervicitis. Instead, this woman was found to have invasive cervical cancer.

will arise and consultation should be obtained. Pregnant patients, particularly those in the late second and third trimesters of pregnancy, are extremely difficult to evaluate because of normal, hormonally mediated lower genital tract responses to pregnancy (Chapter 12). Many of these physiologic changes can make proper visualization of the cervix difficult. Normal cervical changes during pregnancy, such as the development of decidual tissue and dilated vessels, may have an appearance that mimics that of severe cervical neoplasia. Immunosuppressed patients also present unique challenges, particularly in regard to choosing effective treatment and managing neoplasia, which is notoriously persistent in these patients. Patients who have received prior cervical treatment may have grossly deformed cervices or cervical stenosis, which make performing an adequate evaluation almost impossible (Figure 21.33).

Postmenopausal women or women who are estrogen deficient can be challenging to evaluate because of the resulting epithelial changes and anatomical modifications. Women with cytologic evidence of glandular disease can be extremely difficult to evaluate colposcopically, particularly when the anatomical location of the neoplasia is within the endocervical canal. Furthermore, glandular neoplasia may be very subtle

and difficult to recognize because it does not have the same colposcopic signs as those seen with squamous disease (Chapter 11). Finally, women with microinvasive or invasive cancer require the care of a gynecologic oncologist.

The triage guidelines for determining ablative versus excisional therapy of the cervix also must be considered prior to embarking on definitive treatment. In review, the guidelines for ablative treatment are (1) no cytologic, colposcopic, or histologic evidence of cancer; (2) adequate findings from a thorough colposcopic examination that included full visualization of the SCJ and transformation zone, as well as evaluation of any cervical lesions (Figure 21.34); and (3) a normal or negative test result on an endocervical sample. If these guidelines are met, an ablative therapy (cryotherapy, laser ablation, etc.) may be performed for women with high-grade CIN. Ablation should never be performed for AIS. Otherwise, excisional treatment must be done. Failing to perform a diagnostic excision in patients who have a positive test result from a specimen obtained by ECC risks failing to diagnose cancer.[17,18] Ablation performed for the wrong indication risks providing only partial treatment or, in the case of cancer, improper therapy. Thus, invasive cancer must be ruled out during the preliminary colposcopic evaluation and prior to performing any definitive treatment.[4]

In an evaluation of the treatment histories of patients discovered to have cervical cancer following therapy, a frequent error identified was treating the cervix based only on the cytology result and the findings from a colposcopic examination.[16] Performing one or more cervical biopsies is essential to histologically defining the severity of disease and to rule out the presence of cancer whenever possible. As stated earlier, using ablative therapy to treat cervical disease without first obtaining biopsies and a histology report is contraindicated. However, obtaining a histologic specimen and treatment can be performed in a single visit if a high suspicion of severe preinvasive disease exists. Since most women with HSIL eventually undergo a diagnostic excisional procedure, many have advocated "see and treat" by LEEP as the initial management of women ≥25 referred for the evaluation of HSIL cytology. The ASCCP guidelines state that an immediate LEEP and colposcopy with endocervical assessment are acceptable methods for managing women referred for the evaluation of HSIL cytology.[4] However, for women aged 21 to 24 years with HSIL cytology, colposcopy is recommended and immediate

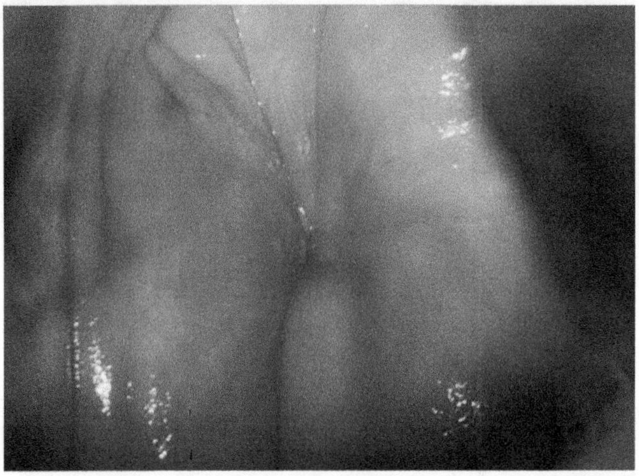

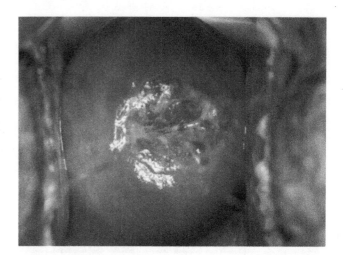

FIGURE 21.34.   The cervix of a young woman now aged 25 years who had an initial ASC-US Pap report and a 12-month follow-up Pap report of ASC-US. Adherence to the ASC-US triage threshold facilitated her clinician identifying this subtle high-grade cervical lesion. Cryotherapy was elected since her cervical findings correlated with the guidelines for ablative treatment.

FIGURE 21.33.   Complete cervical stenosis following LEEP conization in a young woman treated for CIN 3. She required a procedure to open the canal to allow menstrual flow and follow-up cytologic sampling.

treatment (i.e., see and treat) is unacceptable as it would also be for adolescents.[4] Also, for "young women" as defined previously in Section 21.3.3, "see and treat" may not be a good option.[4]

Similarly, a hysterectomy should not be performed prior to conducting a preliminary evaluation. Among 148 women who underwent a simple hysterectomy in the presence of undiagnosed invasive cervical cancer, in 21% a previously obtained abnormal Pap test or cervical biopsy result had been inadequately evaluated; in 11%, a grossly apparent cancer had been overlooked, and in 2%, a gross cervical lesion had not been biopsied.[23] Preoperative colposcopy with biopsy of gross lesions and conization consistent with the ASCCP guidelines would have prevented the majority of these errors and triaged these patients to appropriate treatment for invasive cervical cancer. Several other treatment errors are more common than most colposcopists believe. During any cervical treatment, the entire abnormal transformation zone must be treated and not just the cervical lesion(s). Then, new, healthy tissue can be expected to replace the diseased epithelium in approximately 90% of cases. Incomplete treatment of the abnormal transformation zone risks leaving residual disease that may later give rise to neoplasia. Of equal importance, the treatment should penetrate to a depth sufficient to eliminate all neoplasia that may extend to the depths of the gland clefts, whether on the portio epithelium or within the endocervical canal. Performing a narrow conization risks leaving behind a "positive" margin and residual disease (Figure 21.35).

Women with CIN 1 should not be treated unless progression to high-grade disease is documented during follow-up. The exception to this statement is that when only CIN 1 is identified histologically in follow-up to ASC-H or HSIL cytology in a woman ≥25, then either a diagnostic excisional procedure or observation with cotesting at 12 and 24 months is recommended, provided in the latter case that the colposcopic examination is adequate and the endocervical sampling is negative.[4] The other exception is when CIN 1 is the only histologic finding at colposcopy for AGC "favor neoplasia" or cytologic AIS, for these women should have an excisional procedure.[4] The recommendations for conservative management of CIN 1 reflect the high rate of spontaneous regression of CIN 1 found on evaluation of women who are cytology negative/ HPV positive, ASC-US/HPV positive, repeat ASC-US, ASC-H, or LSIL.[4] In contrast, CIN 3 has a real risk of progressing to cervical cancer and should be treated. CIN 2 may be followed or treated as discussed in Chapter 20. There is always a risk that residual disease is present following treatment of the cervix. Disease may remain in the periphery of the treated area or, more commonly, deep within gland clefts when the ablation or excision was not sufficiently deep. If cytologic, colposcopic, and histologic evidence of significant cervical neoplasia is found in a woman post- either ablative or excisional therapy, repeat treatment must be by excision to provide a histologic specimen, verify the margin status, and ensure that the areas at risk for recurrence are adequately treated (Figure 21.36). Here, the risk of occult cancer is real; therefore, margin status in the excised specimen is extremely important.

Comprehensive patient follow-up is critical. No form of cervical treatment, including hysterectomy, guarantees a 100% cure rate for lower genital tract neoplasia. Therefore, follow-up posttreatment should be cotesting at 12 mo and 24 mo, to screen for and detect residual disease, which recurs in 5% to 15% of women following treatment of CIN (Figure 21.37A,B). The rate of recurrence is even greater among women who are immunosuppressed and in women with or without normal immunity but excision margins positive for high-grade CIN.[24] Therefore, when the excisional

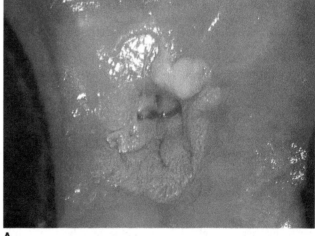

A

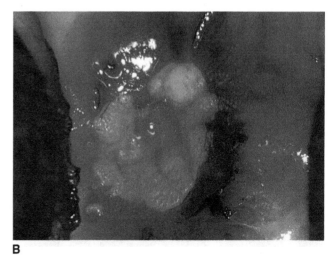

B

FIGURE 21.36. Residual CIN 2 identified 8 months following cryotherapy (**A,B**). An excisional treatment modality would be preferred for this circumstance.

FIGURE 21.35. A positive endocervical margin is noted in this conization specimen (hematoxylin-eosin stain; medium-power magnification). The patient should have serial endocervical sampling postoperatively to identify residual disease that occurs in 15% to 20% of these cases.

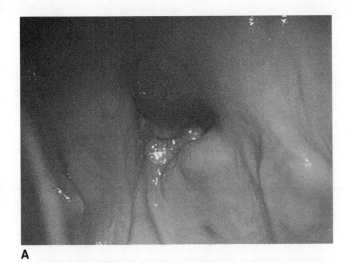

A

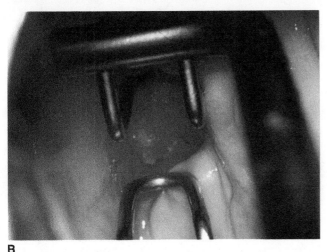

B

FIGURE 21.37. Woman lost to follow-up for 2 years following a cervical LEEP. A high-grade cervical lesion within the endocervical canal can be seen using the endocervical speculum (**A,B**).

margin or immediately post-procedure ECC is positive for CIN 2, CIN 3, or CIN 2,3 follow-up is more intense, that is, reassessment using cytology with endocervical sampling at 4–6 mo after treatment is preferred but reexcision is acceptable.[4] Clearly, postoperative follow-up is also necessary for women following treatment for invasive cervical cancer. Recurrence rates and survival will vary depending on the stage of disease at the time of detection. Patient nonadherence challenges the effectiveness of otherwise rational follow-up strategies. Therefore, the importance of careful follow-up must be effectively communicated to and accepted by women prior to discharge following therapy. Tracking systems help to monitor and limit the frequency of subsequent "no-shows." In summary, errors occur in colposcopy and the management of women with lower genital tract neoplasia. The wise clinician must be aware of these potential pitfalls in order to minimize poor outcomes.

References

1. Ferris DG, Miller NM. Colposcopic accuracy in a residency program: defining competency and proficiency. *J Fam Pract* 1993;36:515–20.
2. Koss LG. The Papanicolaou test for cervical cancer detection. *JAMA* 1989;261:737–43.
3. Sherman ME, Schiffman MH, Lorincz AT, et al. Toward objective quality assurance in cervical cytopathology: correlation of cytopathologic diagnosis with detection of high risk Human papillomavirus types. *Am J Clin Pathol* 1994;102:182–7.
4. Massad LS, Einstein MH, Huh WK, et al. 2012 updated consensus guidelines for the management of abnormal cervical cancer screening tests and cancer precursors. *J Low Genit Tract Dis* 2013;17(5 suppl 1):S1–27. Jointly published without algorithm figures as Massad LS, Einstein MH, Huh WK, et al.; 2012 ASCCP Consensus Guidelines Conference. 2012 updated consensus guidelines for the management of abnormal cervical cancer screening tests and cancer precursors. *Obstet Gynecol* 2013;121(14):829–46.
5. Davey D, Cox JT, Austin M, et al. Cervical cytology specimen adequacy: patient management guidelines and optimizing specimen collection. *J Low Genit Tract Dis* 2008;12(2):71–81.
6. Keehbauch J, Green L, Lugo N, Pepe J. The influence of ASCCP guideline changes on family medicine residency colposcopy training. *Fam Med* 2012;44(9):650–3.
7. Ancheta E, Perry J, Bernard-Pearl L, Paul S, Darragh T, Smith-McCune K. Participants at the ASCCP 2000 Biennial meeting adhere to published guidelines in their management of atypical squamous cells and atypical glandular cells on Pap test. *J Low Genit Tract Dis* 2003;7:279–84.
8. Ferris DG, Miller MD, Wagner P, Walaitis E, Lawler FH. Clinical decision making following abnormal Papanicolaou smear reports. *Fam Pract Res J.*1993;13:343–53.
9. Noller KL. Role of colposcopy in the examination of diethylstilbestrol exposed women. *Obstet Gynecol Clin North Am* 1993;20(1):165–76.
10. Shumsky AG, Stuart GCE, Nation J. Carcinoma of the cervix following conservative management of cervical intraepithelial neoplasia. *Gynecol Oncol* 1994;53:50–4.
11. Benedet JL, Anderson GH, Boyes DA. Colposcopic accuracy in the diagnosis of microinvasive and occult invasive carcinoma of the cervix. *Obstet Gynecol* 1985;65:557–62.
12. Stoler MH, Schiffman M. Interobserver reproducibility of cervical cytologic and histologic interpretations: realistic estimates from the ASCUS LSIL triage study. *JAMA* 2001;285:1500–5.
13. Ismail SM, Colclough AB, Dinnen JS, et al. Observer variation in histopathological diagnosis and grading of cervical intraepithelial neoplasia. *BMJ* 1989;298:707–10.
14. Ferris DG, Waxman AG, Miller NM. Colposcopy and cervical biopsy educational training models. *Fam Med* 1994;26:30–5.
15. Ferris DG, Harper DM, Callahan B, et al. The efficacy of topical benzocaine gel in providing anesthesia prior to cervical biopsy and endocervical curettage. *J Low Genit Tract Dis* 1997;1:221–6.
16. Townsend DE, Richart RM. Diagnostic errors in colposcopy. *Gynecol Oncol* 1981;12:S259–64.
17. Townsend DE, Richart RM, Marks E, Nielsen J. Invasive cancer following outpatient evaluation and therapy for cervical disease. *Obstet Gynecol* 1981;57:145–9.
18. Hatch KD, Shingleton HM, Orr JW, Gore H, Soong SJ. Role of endocervical curettage in colposcopy. *Obstet Gynecol* 1985;65:403–8.
19. Solomon D, Stoler M, Jeronimo J, Khan M, Castle P, Schiffman M. Diagnostic utility of endocervical curettage in women undergoing colposcopy for equivocal or low grade cytologic abnormalities. *Obstet Gynecol* 2007;110:288–95.
20. Mogensen ST, Bak M, Dueholm M, Frost L, Knolblaugh NO, Praest J, et al. Cytobrush and endocervical curettage in the diagnosis of dysplasia and malignancy of the uterine cervix. *Acta Obstet Gynecol Scand* 1997;76:69–73.
21. Pretorius RG, Zhang WH, Belinson JL, et al. Colposcopically directed biopsy, random cervical biopsy, and endocervical curettage in the diagnosis of cervical intraepithelial neoplasia II or worse. *Am J Obstet Gynecol* 2004;191(2):430–4.
22. Cox JT. More questions about the accuracy of colposcopy: what does this mean for cervical cancer prevention? *Obstet Gynecol* 2008;111(6):1266–7.
23. Roman LD, Morris M, Eifel PJ, Burke TW, Gershenson DM, Wharton JT. Reasons for inappropriate simple hysterectomy in the presence of invasive cancer of the cervix. *Obstet Gynecol* 1992;79:485–9.
24. Ghaem-Maghami S, Sagi S, Majeed G, Soutter WP. Incomplete excision of cervical intraepithelial neoplasia and risk of treatment failure: a meta-analysis. *Lancet Oncol* 2007;8(11):985–93.

Page numbers in italics indicate tables, figures, and photographs.

A

Abnormal cervical epithelium. *See* Colposcopic signs
Abnormal cervix
  acetowhite epithelium, 170–77, *171–77*
  clinical significance, 180–82, *180–81*, 224
  colposcopic appearance, 180, *180*
  leukoplakia
    clinical significance, 167–68, *169*
    colposcopic appearance, 164, 166–67, *167–69*
    etiology, 164
Abnormal Pap management guidelines, 6–8. *See* ASCCP Consensus Guidelines
  history of, 6–8
Abnormal transformation zone (ATZ), 155, 160
Abortion, cervical neoplasia and, 372–73
Acanthosis, 433
Acetic acid solution
  application of, 125, 127, *127–28*
    abnormal cervix and, 227, 231–32, *231–32*
    epithelial color and, 169–77, *171–77*
  naked-eye examination, 121
Acetowhite epithelium
  clinical significance, 176–77, *179*
  colposcopic appearance, 171, 173–76, *173–76*
  definition, 170–71, *171*
  etiology, 171, *173*
Acetowhitening, 436, *437*
Actinomyces, *42*
Active *vs.* expectant management, 603
Adenocarcinoma in situ and adenocarcinoma, 46, 47, 322–40
  atypical blood vessels, 330, *336–40*
  columnar epithelium, 322–23
    fate of, 322, 323
    neoplastic transformation of, 323, *323, 324*
  confirming the diagnosis, 331, 332, 333, 334
    management of the patient who desires fertility, 332
    significance of negative margins in the excised specimen, 333
    significance of positive margins in the excised specimen, 333, 334
  invasive, 46, *47–48*
  morphologic spectrum of glandular intraepithelial lesions, 325
  problems detecting, 325–26
    buried disease, *324*, 326
    colposcopic inexperience, 326
    cytologic screening, 325
    lesion size and location, 326
    mixed disease, 326, *326–27*
    skip (multifocal) lesions, 326
  stimulus of disease development, 324, *324*
  surface patterns
    elevated lesions, *323, 324, 327, 328, 328*
    epithelial budding, 329, *333, 334*
    lesions with a patchy (variegated) red and white surface, *328, 329, 330, 330, 334–36*
    lesions with large crypt openings, *328, 329, 330*
    papillary lesions, *323, 324, 326, 327, 329, 329, 331–33*
  three colposcopic presentations, 327, *327–29*
  vaginal, *425*
  vulvar, *467*
Adenosis, vaginal, 411
Adolescents
  ASC-US, *579*
  HPV infections
    cervical cancer screening, 479
    cervical squamous neoplasia, 472–73
    CIN 1, 480

    CIN 2, 3, 481
    colposcopic findings, 479, *480, 481*
    histology, 480–81
    management, 480, 481
    risks, 473–78, *474–78*
    squamous intraepithelial lesion, 478–79
  HSIL, 473
  LSIL, *586*
Advisory Committee on Immunization Practice (ACIP), 535, 536
AGC. *See* Atypical glandular cells
American Cancer Society (ACS)
  cervical screening recommendations, *559*
  HPV test with the Pap in primary screening, *563*
  screening after hysterectomy, 558, *559*
  screening intervals, *560*
American College of Obstetricians and Gynecologists (ACOG)
  cervical screening recommendations, *559*
  HPV test with the Pap in primary screening, *563*
  screening after hysterectomy, *559*
  screening intervals, *560*
American Society for Colposcopy and Cervical Pathology (ASCCP), 571, *599*
  ASCCP Consensus Conference, 575, *575*
  ASCCP Consensus Guidelines
    guidelines for biopsy confirmed CIN 2, 3, follow-up treatment, *614*
    guidelines for CIN 2, 3, *611*
    guidelines for management of AGC, 585–87, *588*
    guidelines for management of ASC, *581, 581–82*
    guidelines for management of ASC-H, *582*
    guidelines for management of HSIL, *589–593*
    guidelines for management of LSIL, *584*
    recommendations for biopsy-confirmed CIN 1, *607*
    recommendations for CIN 2,3-special circumstances, *612*
    specimen adequacy guidelines, 571–72, *572*
Anal canal and perianus
  anatomy, *495, 495*
  anorectal region, examining, 143–44, *144*
  evaluation
    abnormal anal transformation zone, 503–4, *503–16, 511–12*
    anal cytology collection, 496, 497, *497*
    assessment of new patients, 492, *493–94, 495*
    biopsies, 500
    digital anorectal examination, 497
    examination, *495, 495–96, 497*
    high-resolution anoscopy, 497–99, *497–99*
    HRA *vs.* cervical colposcopy, 499–500
    normal anal transformation zone, 503
  management and treatment
    anal neoplasia, 522
    cancer, 529–30, *530–32*
    HGAIN and condyloma, 522, 530, 533
    office-based treatment of AIN, 522–29, *523–29*
    UCSF experience, 529
  pathology
    anal cytology, 488–90, *490, 491, 496, 497, 497*
    histopathology, 490, *491, 491–92, 492*
  squamous epithelium, *491, 491*
Anal cancer
  age-adjusted incidence rate, 485
  epidemiology, *486, 486–87*
  screening, 488, *489*
  staging and management, 533–34, *534*

Anal cytology
  benign findings and specimen adequacy, 489–90, *490*
  Candida, 489, *490*
  collection, 496, 497, *497*
  HSIL, 490, *491*
  LSIL, 490, *490*
  sensitivity and specificity, 488, 489
  squamous cell abnormalities, 490, *490, 491*
Anal intraepithelial neoplasia (AIN)
  epidemiology, 487–88
  office-based treatment
    patient-applied topical treatments, 523, *524–25*
    provider-applied therapy, 522–23, *523–24*
    surgical excision and ablative techniques, 525, *525–29, 526–29*
Anal squamous epithelium, 498, *498*
Anal squamous metaplasia, 498, *498*
Anal transformation zone (AnTZ)
  abnormal
    high-resolution anoscopy
      high-grade anal intraepithelial neoplasia, 504, *508–12*
      invasive squamous cell carcinoma, 504, 511, *512–16*
      low-grade anal intraepithelial neoplasia, 503, 504, *505–8*
  normal, 503
Anesthetics, *116*, 116–17
Antepartum management. *See* Pregnancy
Anti bacterial solutions for instrument care, 117
ASCUS-LSIL Triage Study (ALTS), 236, *236*
Assessment. *See* Colposcopic examination
Assessment errors
  common mistakes in failing to recognize cervical cancer, 672–73, *673, 674*
  failing to form colposcopic impression, *673, 675*
  see also Errors
Atypical blood vessels, 201, 202–11, *202–11*
  clinical significance, 208, *209–11*
  colposcopic appearance, 204–5, 207–8, *207–8*
  definition, 201, *205–6*
  etiology, 201, 204
  see also Colposcopic signs; Vessels
Atypical glandular cells (AGC), 46
  initial management, 585–87, *588*
    atypical endometrial cells, 587, *588*
    benign-appearing endometrial cells, 587, *588, 588*
    postcolposcopy management, 588, *589, 589*
Atypical glandular cells/adenocarcinoma in situ, 46, *47*
Atypical squamous cells, 44, *44*
Atypical squamous cells cannot rule out high grade (ASC-H), *592*
Atypical squamous cells of undetermined significance (ASC-US), 44
  adolescents, *579, 580, 581*
  age trend, *578*
  ALTS trial data, 577
  management of women, 578, *579*
    and evidence of vaginal atrophy, 580, *580*
    HPV testing, 578
    immediate colposcopy, *578, 578, 579*
    immunosuppression, *580*, 581
    pregnant women, 580
    repeat cytology, 578–79
  postcolposcopy management, 581–82, *581–82*
  risk, *578, 578–79*
Atypical transformation zone, 2
Automated screening, 549–50

B

Bacterial desquamative disorders, 406–7
Bacterial vaginosis, 41, *41*
Bartholin's glands and ducts, 432
Bethesda system, 6–8
  cervicovaginal abnormalities
    atypical squamous cells, 44, *44*
    high-grade squamous intraepithelial lesions,
      45, *45*
    invasive adenocarcinoma, 46, *47–48*
    invasive squamous cell carcinoma, 45–46,
      46
    low-grade squamous intraepithelial lesions,
      44–45, *45*
    organisms, 39, 41, *41*
    reactive/reparative changes, 41–43, *42*
    specimen quality, 39
    squamous intraepithelial lesions/malignancy,
      39
    typical glandular cells/adenocarcinoma *in
      situ*, 46, *47*
    vaginal glandular/or normal endometrial
      cells, 43, *43*
Biologic markers, human papillomavirus (HPV),
  95, 97
Biopsies
  anal and perianal, 500
  cervical, 138–40, *139*
  specimen collection, processing, and interpreta-
    tion, 30–34, *30–34*
  vaginal, 403, *403*
  vulvar, 434–36, *435*
Biopsy forceps, 111–13, *112–13*
Blood vessels
  atypical blood vessels, 201, 202–11, *202–11*
  mosaic, 193, 194, 198–201, *198–204*
  punctation, 186, 188–93, *189–97*
British Columbia cytology-colposcopy program,
  234, *235*
Buried disease, *324*, 326
Burke grading system, 242, *242*

C

Cancer
  cervical cancer. *See* Cervical cancer
  glandular cancer, 467, 587
  invasive adenocarcinoma, 46, *47–48*
  invasive anal cancer, 533, *534*
  invasive carcinoma, 52–53, *53–54*
  invasive cervical cancer, worldwide incidence, 61
  invasive squamous cell carcinoma, 45–46, *46*,
    316, 318–20, *318–20*
  squamous cell carcinoma, 79, *79*, 306–20
    circumstances that warrant concern
      atypical vessels, 314, *315–17*
      color, *313*, 313, 314
      cytology, 311
      high-grade lesions with complete or
        partial canal involvement, *312*,
        312–13, *313*
      linear length, surface area of lesions, and
        cervical diameter, 311–12, *312*
      patient age, *311*, 311
      persistence or recurrence of high-grade
        lesions after treatment, 314, 317, 318
      surface contour, *313*, 313
    colposcopic mimics, 316, *318–20*
    correlation process, 309
    differentiating normal from abnormal, 307,
      308–10
    disparities, 306–7
    effect of screening, 307
    etiology, 306
    excision, 310–11
    incidence and mortality, 306
    adequate vs. inadequate colposcopic
      examination, 307, 309
    superficially invasive squamous cell carcinomas
      of the anus, 534
    when excision is required because of suspected
      cancer, 310–11
    why cancer is missed, 311
Candida, 490
  maintenance regimens, 447, *449*
  recurrent vulvovaginal candidiasis, 447

  treatments, 446–47, *448*
  vulvovaginal candidiasis, 446, *446*
Carbon dioxide laser ablation, *427–26*, 427–28
  see also Cervical intraepithelial neoplasia (CIN)
    treatment
Carbon dioxide laser surgery. *See* Cervical intraep-
    ithelial neoplasia (CIN) treatment
Carcinomas, invasive, 52–53, *53–54*
Cervex-brush®, 34–35
Cervical ablation triage guidelines, *617*
Cervical anomalies, *392, 393*
Cervical biopsy, 30, *33*, 111, 113, 138–40, *139*
  benign immature metaplasia, *677*
  CIN 1, 253
  CIN 3, 283, 294
  condyloma, *676*
  forceps, 112
  postprocedure instructions, 146–48, *147–48*
  squamous metaplasia, 50, *50*
Cervical cancer
  cofactors to HPV-induced oncogenesis
    cigarette smoking, 71
    genetic factors, 70–71
    high parity, 69–70
    immunosuppression and HIV, 70
    oral contraceptive pills, 70
    by race, 66, *66*
    STD, 69
  colposcopy
    accuracy, 10–11
    birth of, 1–3
    21st century, role of, 11
    growth and acceptance, 5–6
    integration, 6–9
    practice, 9
  common mistakes in failing to recognize,
    672–73, *673, 674*
  epidemiologic evidence, 71
  factors affecting geographic variations, 65–67,
    66
  pregnancy and. *See* Pregnancy
  prevalence of invasive cervical cancer
    worldwide, 61, *62*
  risk factors
    human papillomavirus, 67–69, *68*
    sexual behavior, 65
  screening, 3–5
  time trends and impact of screening, 61–65,
    63–66
Cervical cancer screening
  adolescents, 479
  ASC-H
    initial management, 582–83, *582–83*
    postcolposcopy management, 582–83, *582–83*
  ASC-US
    adolescents, 579, 580, *581*
    age trend, 578
    ALTS trial data, 577
    management of women, *578, 579*
      and evidence of vaginal atrophy, 580, *580*
      HPV testing, 578
      immediate colposcopy, 578, *578, 579*
      immunosuppression, *580*, 581
      pregnant women, 580
      repeat cytology, 578–79
    postcolposcopy management, 581–82,
      581–82
    risk, 578, *578–79*
  atypical glandular cells
    initial management, 585–87, *588*
      atypical endometrial cells, 587, *588*
      benign-appearing endometrial cells, 587,
        588, 588
    postcolposcopy management, 588, *589, 589*
  automated, 549–50
  conventional cervical cytology, 547, 548, *549*
  developing methods, 3–5
  future prospects, 565, 593–94, *594*
  high-grade squamous intraepithelial lesion
    adolescents, 591, *592, 592*
    initial management, 589, *590, 591*
    postcolposcopy management, 590, *591, 591*
    pregnancy, *593, 593*
  HPV vaccination, 562–63
  human papillomavirus (HPV) testing, 575–76,
    575, 577

  impediments to, 553
  liquid-based cytology, 548, 549
  low-grade squamous intraepithelial lesion
    adolescents, 585, *586*
    initial management, 583–84, *584, 585*
    postcolposcopy management, 584, *584*
    postmenopausal women, 585, *586*
    pregnant women, 585, *586*
  molecular-based technologies, 550–53
  with a Pap lacking an endocervical/
    transformation zone component,
    572, *573*, 573–74
  with a Pap that has partially obscuring blood,
    inflammation, other limiting quality
    indicators, 572
  primary guidelines
    after hysterectomy, 558, *559*
    screening interval
      cotesting overview and guideline
        recommendations, 560–62
      HPV positive results and counseling
        messages, 563, *564*, 564–65
      with HPV testing, 562
      not using HPV test, 564
    screening interval (ACS, USPSTE, ACOG),
      559–62
    when to begin (ACS, USPSTE, ACOG),
      554–58, *555–57*
    when to discontinue (ACS, USPSTE,
      ACOG), 558, *559*
  primary prevention
    abstinence, 539–40
    condoms, 540
    HPV vaccination, 540–47
  secondary prevention, 547–53
  specimen adequacy guidelines, 571–74
  unsatisfactory cytology test, 572, *572, 573*
Cervical duplication, 391–92, *392*
Cervical intraepithelial neoplasia (CIN), 2
  CIN 1, 51–52, *52*
  CIN 2, 52, *52*
  CIN 3, 52, *53*
  colposcopic accuracy
    age, 236, *237*
    biopsies, 237, 238, *238*
    epithelial thickness, 236, 237, *237*
    HPV type, 236, *237*
    lesion size, 236, *237*
    sensitivity and specificity, 235–36
    variability, 239
Cervical intraepithelial neoplasia (CIN) treatment,
  480, 481, 559–61
  active *vs.* expectant management, 603
  adenocarcinoma *in situ* (AIS) management
    who desire fertility, 615
    who do not desire fertility, 614, *615*
  carbon dioxide laser surgery, 627–33
    combining excision and vaporization, 632,
      632
    cylindrical excision for endocervical, *631*,
      631–32
    delayed bleeding, 632–33
    discharge instructions, post-operative com-
      plications, healing and follow-up,
      632–33
    disease distribution, 627–29
    excision, *631*, 631–32
    geometry of CIN as a guide for its removal,
      628–29, *629*
    healing, 633
    infection, 633
    laser energy, 627, *628*
    rationale for using, 627
    results of, 633
    stenosis, 633
    vaporization, 629–30, *629–30*
  choosing the procedure, 603–05, *604–05*
  CIN 2 and 3 management, 609–13, *609–12*
    in adolescents, 609–12, *609, 611*
    in the immunosuppressed, 612, *613*
    in pregnancy, 612
  CIN 1 colposcopy, 259–72
    color, 260, 264, *264, 265, 265*
    contour, 259, 260, 261–62
    iodine staining of, 265, *268–70*
    location, 259, *259–61*

margins, 260, *263*
size and distribution, 265, *270–73, 272*
vessels, 265, *266–68*
CIN 2 colposcopy, 272–77
  color, 275, *277*
  contour, 273, *275, 276*
  iodine staining of, 275, *279–80*
  location, 272, *274–75*
  margins, 273, *275, 276, 277*
  size and distribution of, 275, *277, 280, 281*
  vessels, 275, *278, 279*
CIN 3 colposcopy, 277, 278, 281–3
  color, 287, *291–92*
  contour, 278, *285–87*
  iodine staining of, 297, *299–301*
  location, 278, *282–84*
  margins, 281, *283, 287, 287–91*
  size and distribution of, 297, *302–3, 303*
  vessels, 288, *292–99*
CIN 1 management by, 605–9
  adolescents and pregnancy, 608, *609*
  HPV-positive ASC-US and LSIL, 605–6,
    606
  HSIL or ASC-H cytology, 606–8, *608–9*
cold coagulation, 626–27
  documentation, 625
  equipment and supplies, 626
  objectives, 626
  outcomes, 626–27
  patient preparation, 626
  prerequisities, indications and
    contraindications, 626
  procedure, 626
  side-effects and complications, 626–27
cold-knife conization, 613, 651–53
  complications, 648–49, *649*
  indications for, 648
  modifying the procedure to account for
    disease distribution, 649, *649*
  operative technique, 648
  results, 648
  trend, changing the, 648
colposcopic grading
  Burke system, 242, *242*
  Coppleson system, 241, *241*
  Hinselmann system, 241
  importance of, 240
  impression, 240–41, *241*
  rationale, 240
  Reid colposcopic index, 242
    color, 244, *248, 249*
    correlation, 253, *254, 255*
    design, 242, *243*
    iodine, 249, *250, 253–55*
    margin, 242, *244–48*
    reproducibility of, 258
    scores, 242, *243, 250, 252*
    special considerations concerning, *253,
      254, 254, 255, 256–57, 258*
    vessels, 244, *246, 249, 250–52*
  Stafl system, 241, *242*
comparison of failure rates for, *604*
complication rates, *605*
cryotherapy, 603, 615–25
  cellular injury and death, 620, *620*
  cryonecrosis stages, 621
  cryoprobe tips, 615, *616*
  determining freeze termination, 620, *620*
  documentation, 625
  equipment and supplies, 617–20, *617–20*
  follow-up, 623
  heat transfer, 620, *620*
  immunologic response, 621
  induction and defrost, 620
  Joule-Thomson effect, 620, *620*
  outcomes, 625
  patient education, 623
  patient preparation, 623
  prerequisites, indications and contraindica-
    tions, 615–16, *617*
  procedural and diagnostic codes, 625
  procedure, 621–23, *622, 623*
  side effects and complications, 623–24, *625*
  temperatures, 620–21, *621*
hysterectomy, 610, 649–51
  indications, 649–50

operative methods, *650*
post-hysterectomy assessments, 650–51, *652*
immunity role in, 559–62, 600–2
loop electrosurgical excision procedure (LEEP),
  633–47
  bipolar electrosurgery, *635, 637–38*
  complications, 646
  contraindications for, 639
  electrosurgery *vs.* electrocautery, 638
  electrosurgical safety, 638
  electrosurgical systems, 638
  instant response, 634
  long-term consequences of, 647
  monopolar electrosurgical coagulation, *635,
    635–37*
  monopolar electrosurgical cutting, *634,
    634–35, 636*
  one-or-two visit approach, 638–39
  pathological specimen, 646, *646, 647*
  patient prior evaluation, 638
  post-treatment follow-up, 647
  postoperative management, 646, *647*
  procedure, *628*, 635–36, *637*, 639–44,
    640–46
  rationale for using, 638
  stages of thermal destruction, 633, *634*
  surgical approaches, 638
  therapeutic effectiveness, 647
  waveforms, 633, *634–35*
low-resource settings, approaches in, 651–53
post-treatment follow-up, 613, *614*
pregnancy and. *See* Pregnancy
trichloroacetic acid, 657–59, *658–59*
Cervical lesions, determining size, shape, contour,
  location and extent of, *133–34,
  135, 135–36*
Cervical neoplasia, 678
Cervical polyps, 385–87, *385–87*
Cervical squamous neoplasia, 472–73
Cervical stenosis, 390, *390*, 633
Cervicography, 8
Cervicovaginal abnormalities
  Bethesda system
    atypical squamous cells, 44, *44*
    cytologic evidence of vaginal glandular cells
      or endometrial cells, 43, *43*
    high-grade squamous intraepithelial lesions,
      45, *45*
    invasive adenocarcinoma, 46, *47–48*
    invasive squamous cell carcinoma, 45–46, *46*
    low-grade squamous intraepithelial lesions,
      44–45, *45*
    negative for squamous intraepithelial lesions
      or malignancy, 39
    organisms, 39, 41, *41*
    quality of specimen, 39
    reactive/reparative changes, 41–43, *42*
    specimen quality, 39
    squamous intraepithelial lesions/malignancy,
      39
    typical glandular cells/adenocarcinoma *In
      Situ,* 46, *47*
    vaginal glandular/or normal endometrial
      cells, 43, *43*
  glandular abnormalities
    biomarkers, cervical squamous and glandu-
      lar neoplasias, 55–56
    intraepithelial lesions, 54, *55*
    invasive adenocarcinoma, 54–55, *55*
    reactive changes, 54, *54*
  intraepithelial lesions
    grade 1 cervical/vaginal intraepithelial neo-
      plasia, 51–52, *52*
    grade 2 cervical/vaginal intraepithelial neo-
      plasia, 52, *52*
    grade 3 cervical/vaginal intraepithelial neo-
      plasia, 52, *53*
  new technologies
    computer analysis, 49–50, *50*
    digital imaging systems, 49, *49*
    processing systems, 47–49
    reporting systems, 49–50, *50*
  reactive and reparative change, 51
  squamous abnormalities
    intraepithelial lesions, 51–52, *51–52*
    invasive carcinoma, 52–54, *53–54*

Cervicovaginal abnormalities
  squamous intraepithelial lesions, 56–59
    lower anogenital tract, 56, *57*
    LSIL, 56, *58*
    SISCCA, 57, *58–59*
Cervix
  anatomy, 14–15
  cytology, 22–23
  embryology, 14
  histology
    columnar epithelium, *18*, 18–19
    squamous epithelium, 15, *17*, 17–18
  transformation zone
    formation of squamous metaplasia, 19–20, *20*
    histology of squamous metaplasia, 20–22,
      20–22
Chancroid, 444, *445, 445*
Chemical agents
  acetic acid solution, 114, *115*
  bactericidal solutions for instrument care, 117
  disposable supplies, 117
  Lugol's solution, 115, *116*
  Monsel's solution, 115–16, *116*
  saline, 114, *115*
  silver nitrate sticks, 116, *116*
  topical and local anesthetics, *116*, 116–17
Chlamydia, *445*, 445–46, *446*
Chlamydia trachomatis, 21, 69
Chronic follicular cervicitis, 21
Cigarette smoking, 70
CIN. *See* Cervical intraepithelial neoplasia (CIN)
Cold coagulation of the cervix. *See* Cervical
  intraepithelial neoplasia (CIN)
  treatment
Cold knife conization. *See* Cervical intraepithelial
  neoplasia (CIN) treatment
Color
  of CIN 1, 260, *264, 264, 265, 265*
  of CIN 2, 275, *277*
  of CIN 3, 287, *291–92*
  squamous cell carcinoma, 313, *314*
Colpophotography, *117*, 117–18
Colposcopes
  birth of, 1–3
  care of, 108
  colpophotography, 117–18
  cost of, 107–8
  examination table and instrument stand, 110
  focus controls, 107, *110*
  glandular neoplasia, 9–10
  growth and acceptance, 5–6
  illumination and filters, 103–4, *104*
  instruments
    biopsy forceps, 111–13, *112–13*
    endocervical curette, 113, *114–15*
    endocervical specula, 111, *111*
    lateral sidewall retractors, 111, *111*
    long scissors, needle driver, and pickups,
      113–14, *115*
    vaginal specula, 110–11
  magnification, 104–5, *106*
  mounting, 106–7, *108–9*
  objective lenses and focal length, 103, *104*
  oculars, video, and monocular observation
    tubes, 106–7, *106–7*
  practice expansion, broader clinical base, 9
  role of, 11
  video, 108–10, *109–10*
  video systems, 117, *117*
Colposcopic accuracy
  age, 236, *237*
  biopsies, 237, *238, 238*
  epithelial thickness, 236, 237, *237*
  HPV type, 236, *237*
  lesion size, 236, *237*
  sensitivity and specificity, 235–36
  variability, 239
Colposcopic examination
  anorectal region examination, 143–44, *144*
  application of acetic acid, 125–27, *128–29*
  application of diluted Lugol's iodine solution,
    127–31, *130–32*
  application of normal saline, 125, *126–27*
  assessment
    concept of the "adequate" colposcopic
      examination, 131–32

Colposcopic examination (*Continued*)
  epithelial abnormalities identification, 133–35
  size, shape, contour, location, and extent of
      cervical lesions, 135, *135–36*
  transformation zone identification, 132–33,
      132–34
  complications during, 140
  documentation
    colposcopic findings, 145–46
    correlation of cytology, histology, and col-
        poscopy findings, 146, *146, 147*
  focusing the colposcope, 123–25, *124*
  objectives, 120, *121*
  Papanicolaou and microbiologic test
      collection, 125
  patient preparation, 121–22, *122*
  postprocedure instructions, 146–48, *147–48*
  purpose, 120
  removing obscuring blood and mucus, 125
  sampling
    cervical biopsy, 138–40, *139*
    endocervical sampling, 136–38, *136–38*
    vaginal examination, 140–41, *140–41*
    visualizing the cervix, 122–23
    vulvar, perineal, perianal, and bimanual
        examinations, 141–43, *141–43*
Colposcopic findings, 479, *480*
Colposcopic mimics, 316, *318–20*
Colposcopic signs
  abnormal transformation zone, 155, 160
  after application of acetic acid, 169–77, *171–77*
  after application of Lugol's iodine solution
    abnormal cervix, 180–82, *180–81*
    background, 177
    normal cervix, 177, 179, *179*
  critical considerations, 160–61
  epithelial color
    before application of acetic acid and Lugol's
        iodine solution
      leukoplakia, 163–68, *163–68*
      neoplasia, 168–69
  identification, 161
  margin characteristics of abnormal cervical
      epithelium
    after application of acetic acid and Lugol's
        iodine solution, 227–32, *231–32*
    before application of acetic acid and Lugol's
        iodine solution, 227
  normal transformation zone, 150–56
    neoplastic alteration, 156
  surface topography
    epithelial elevations, 215–27
    ulceration/erosion, 209–15, *212–13*
  vasculature
    atypical blood vessels, 201, 202–11,
        202–11
    mosaic, 193, 194, 198–201, *198–204*
    normal cervix, 183–86, *183–88*
    punctation, 186, 188–93, *189–97*
Colposcopists, job and skill requirements, 667
Colposcopy during pregnancy. *See* Pregnancy
Colposcopy of vagina. *See* Vagina
Columnar epithelium, *18,* 18–19
  histology, 18–19, *18–19*
  neoplastic transformation of, 323, *323, 324*
Complications, during colposcopy, 140
Computer analysis and reporting systems,
    49–50, *50*
Condoms, 540
Condylomas, 440, 441–42, *441–43,* 522,
    530, 533
  Condylomas treatment. *See* Genital wart
      treatment
Condylomata acuminata, 417–19, *418, 419*
Congenital transformation zone (CTZ), 409, 410,
    410, 411
Conization, 6
  see also Cervical intraepithelial neoplasia (CIN)
      treatment
Conization-related complications, cervical neopla-
    sia and pregnancy, 373
Contour
  CIN 1, 259, 260, *261–62*
  CIN 2, 273, *275, 276*
  CIN 3, 278, *285–87*

squamous cell carcinoma, 313, *313*
Conventional cervical cytology (CC), 547,
    548, *549*
Coppleson grading system, 241, *241*
Corneum epidermidis, 432
Corps ronds, 433, *434*
Correlation errors, 678–79, *679, 680*
Correlation process, 309
Crest factor, 634
Cryosurgery. *See* Cervical intraepithelial neoplasia
    (CIN) treatment
Cryotherapy, 522, *523*
  freeze-ball scale, 620, *620*
  see also Cervical intraepithelial neoplasia (CIN)
      treatment
CTZ. *See* Congenital transformation zone
Curettage, endocervical, 32, 136–38, 675
Cusco speculum, 110
Cytobrush®, 34
Cytologic atypias, 41–42
Cytology
  adenocarcinoma in situ and adenocarcinoma,
      325
  cervicovaginal abnormalities
    Bethesda system, 37, 39–47
    new technologies, 47–50
  cervix, 22–23
  specimen collection, processing, and interpreta-
      tion, 34, *34–36, 35*

D
Data management, *118,* 118–19
Desquamative disorders
  bacterial, 406–7
  non bacterial, 407–9, *407–9*
Developing countries, cervical cancer, 65
Developmental malformations
  cervical anomalies, 392, *393*
  transverse vaginal septum, 391, *391*
  vaginal and cervical duplication, 391–92, *392*
Di-or tri-chloroacetic acid, 657–59, *657–60*
Diaphragms, 412
Digital anorectal examination (DARE),
    488, 497
Digital imaging systems, 49, *49*
Disposable supplies, 117
Documentation, colposcopic findings, 145–46
Dysesthetic vulvodynia, 449
Dyskeratosis, 433, *434*

E
ECC. *See* Endocervical curettage
Electrodiathermy, 7
Electrosurgical procedures. *See* Cervical
    intraepithelial neoplasia (CIN)
    treatment
Elevated lesions, 328, *328–29*
Emphysematous vaginitis, 412
Endocervical cells, *23*
Endocervical curettage (ECC), 32, 136–38, 675
Endocervical curette, 113, *114–15*
Endocervical specula, 111, *111*
Endometrial cells, 43, *43*
Endometriosis, vaginal, 413
Eosinophilic molluscum, *440*
Epidemiology
  cervical cancer. *See* Cervical cancer
  cervical intraepithelial neoplasia (CIN),
      347, *347*
  human papillomavirus, 343–44, *344*
Epithelial abnormalities, identification of,
    133–35
Epithelial budding, 329, *333–34*
Epithelial color
  before application of acetic acid and Lugol's
      iodine solution
    abnormal cervix
      leukoplakia
        clinical significance, 167–68, *169*
        colposcopic appearance, 164, 166–67,
            167–69
        etiology, 164
      neoplasia, 168–69
      normal cervix, 162–63, *163–64*

Epithelial elevations
  clinical significance, 224, *228*
  colposcopic appearance, 220–24, *222–27*
  definition, 215, *215–20*
  etiology, 215, 220, *220–23*
Epithelial honeycombing (EH), *503, 505*
Erosion. *See* Colposcopic signs
Errors
  assessment
    common mistakes in failing to recognize
        cervical cancer, 672–73, *673, 674*
    failing to form colposcopic impression,
        673, *675*
  during the colposcopy examination
    visualization
      bleeding, 669
      inadequate of lesions extending deep into
          cervical canal, 671
      inadequate of squamocolumnar junction,
          670–71
      mucus, debris, and discharge, 669
      prolapsing vaginal walls, 669–70
      vagina and vulva, 671–72, *671–72*
  errors after the colposcopy exam
    correlation, 678–79, *679, 680*
    management, 679–83, *680–83*
  prior to the colposcopy examination, 667–68
  sampling, 675–78, *675–78*
Estrogen deficiency, 381–84, *383*
Examination tables, 110, *110*
Excision
  significance of negative margins in the speci-
      men, 333
  significance of positive margins in the specimen,
      333–34
  see also Cervical intraepithelial neoplasia (CIN)
      treatment
Extensive circumferential lesions, 530, *533*
Extragenital transmission, of human
    papillomavirus (HPV), 85

F
False negative Pap smears, 667
Follicular cervicitis, 21, *22*
Fordyce's spots, 29, 437, *438*
Fungi, 446–48, *447, 448*

G
Gartner's duct cysts, 413, *414*
Genital wart treatment
  chemical agents
    di-or tri-chloroacetic acid (DCA, TCA),
        657–59, *657–60*
    imiquimod, 655–56, *656*
    interferon, 660
    podofilox, 655, *655*
    podophyllin, 657, *657*
    podophyllotoxin, 655
    sinecatechins, 656, *657*
  diagnosis, 653
  prerequisites, 654–55, *654–55*
  purpose and objectives, 654
  surgical approaches
    cryotherapy, 659, 660
    excisional procedures, 660, *660–661*
    laser vaporization, 660
  symptoms, 653, *653*
  therapeutic vaccines, 653
Genital warts, 77, 84, *84*
  see also Genital wart treatment
Genitalia
  ambiguous, 28, *28*
  development of external genitalia, 27
Giant condyloma, 77, 466
Glandular abnormalities
  biomarkers, cervical squamous and glandular
      neoplasias, 55–56
  histology of, 54–56, *54–56*
  intraepithelial lesions, 54, *55*
  invasive adenocarcinoma, 54–55, *55*
  reactive changes, 54, *54*
Glandular lesions. *See* Adenocarcinoma in situ and
    adenocarcinoma
Glandular neoplasia, 9–10

Grading of cervical neoplasia. *See* Cervical intraepithelial neoplasia (CIN) treatment; Squamous cell carcinoma
Granular cell tumor, 462, 463, *463*
Granulation tissue, 415, 416, *416*
Granuloma inguinale, 444, *444*
Granulosum epidermidis, 432

H

Hart's line, 27, 152, 432
Hemangioma, 414, 415, *415*
Hematocolpos, *29*, 432
Hemorrhage, cervical neoplasia while pregnant, 373, *373*
Herpes simplex virus infection, 8, 69, 489, *490*
High-grade anal intraepithelial neoplasia (HGAIN)
   acetowhite coloring, *501*
   coarse punctation, *502*
   extensive circumferential lesions, 530, *533*
   flat contour, *501*
   medium and small-volume disease, *533*
   mosaic pattern, *502*
High-grade squamous intraepithelial lesion (HSIL), 45, *45*
   cervical cancer screening
      adolescents, 591, 592, *592*
      initial management, 589, 590, *590, 591*
      postcolposcopy management, 590, 591, *591*
      pregnancy, 593, *593*
      with complete or partial canal involvement, 312, 312–13, *313*
   during pregnancy. *See* Pregnancy
High-resolution anoscopy (HRA), 497–99, *497–99*
   vs. cervical colposcopy, 499–500
   color, 500, *500, 501*
   contour, 500, *501*
   high-grade anal intraepithelial neoplasia, 504, *508–12*
   invasive squamous cell carcinoma, 504, 511, *512–16*
   low-grade anal intraepithelial neoplasia, 503, 504, *505–8*
   Lugol's staining, 500, *503*
   margins, 500, *501*
   role of, 522
   vascular patterns, 500, *502*
Hinselmann colposcopic grading system, 241
Histology
   columnar epithelium, 18–19, *18–19*
   glandular abnormalities
      biomarkers, cervical squamous and glandular neoplasias, 55–56
      intraepithelial lesions, 54, *55*
      invasive adenocarcinoma, 54–55, *55*
      reactive changes, 54, *54*
   squamous abnormalities
      intraepithelial lesions, 51–52, *51–52*
      invasive carcinoma, 52–54, *53–54*
   squamous epithelium, 15, *17,* 17–18
   squamous metaplasia, 20–22, *20–22*
   vagina, 26, *26*
   vulva, 30, *32*
HIV. *See* Human immunodeficiency virus
Hormonally induced changes
   due to estrogen-progestin-releasing contraceptives, 376–77, *377*
   due to progestin-only contraceptives, 377
   estrogen deficiency, 381, 382, *383,* 383–84
   microglandular hyperplasia, 377, 378, *378*
   vaginal adenosis and *in utero* diethylstilbestrol exposure, 378–81, *379–83*
Hormone replacement therapy (HRT), 42
HPV. *See* Human papillomavirus
HSIL. *See* High-grade squamous intraepithelial lesion
Human immunodeficiency virus (HIV), 70, 485
Human leukocyte antigen (HLA), 71
Human papillomavirus (HPV), 74–97
   adenocarcinoma in situ and adenocarcinoma, 324
   adolescents
      cervical cancer screening, 479
      colposcopic findings, 479, *480, 481*

epidemiology, 472–73
   risks, 473–78, *474–78*
   squamous intraepithelial lesion, 478–79
anal canal and perianus
   abnormal anal transformation zone, 503–4, *503–16,* 511–12
   anal cytology, 488–90, *490, 491,* 496, 497, *497*
   anal neoplasia, 522
   assessment of new patients, 492, *493–94,* 495
   biopsies, 500
   digital anorectal examination, 497
   examination, *495,* 495–96, *496*
   high-resolution anoscopy, 497–99, *497–99,* 522
   histopathology, 490, *491,* 491–92, *492*
   normal anal transformation zone, 503
cervical cancer, risk factor, 67–71, *68*
cervical disease
   clinical utility, 8–9
   colposcopic triage, 9
   discovery of, 8
   vaccine impact, 10–11
epidemiology, 484–88, *486*
HPV genes, 74, 75
HPV types, 76, 77
   distribution of HPV types worldwide, 79
   functional differences between low-risk and high-risk HPV types, 81–82, *82, 83*
   high-risk viral types, 78–81, *79, 80*
   immunity and, 599–602, *600–2*
   infections with multiple HPV types, 81
   life cycle of, 599, *600*
   low-risk viral types, 78, *78*
life cycle of, 86–91
   host containment, 89, *90, 91, 91*
   productive viral infection, 88–89, *88–89*
   viral entry, 86, 86–88, *87*
major clinical association of genital tract and other mucosal HPVs, 77
natural history of cervical intraepithelial neoplasia, 91–95
   low-grade disease, 91–92, *92, 93*
   progression to high-grade CIN, 92–94, *94*
   progression to invasion, 94, *95,* 95–97
   tumor suppressor gene inactivation, 94
natural history of genital HPV infection, 82, 84–86
new biologic markers, 95, 97
transmission, 82, *84,* 84–86
   extragenital and fomite, 85
   sexual, 84, 85
   vertical, 85–86
vaccination
   cost-effectiveness, 546
   cross-protection evidence with closely related HPV types, 544
   immunosuppression, 546
   male immunization, 546
   pregnant women, 545–46
   principles, 540, 541, *541–42*
   recommendations, 545
   safety and efficacy trials, 542–45
   see also Cervical cancer screening
Hymen, 432
Hymenal perforations, 29
Hymenal ring, 29, 391, 395, *395,* 432
Hyperkeratosis, 42
Hysterectomy
   screening after, 558, *558*
   see also Cervical intraepithelial neoplasia (CIN) treatment

I

IARC. *See* International Agency for Research on Cancer
Image management systems, 119
Imiquimod, 523, *523,* 524–25, 655–56, *656, 657*
Immunity, treating CIN and, 599–602, *600–2*
Immunosuppression, 70, *580,* 581
In situ hybridization (ISH), 69, 409, 440
Inflammation
   bacteria-induced desquamative disorders, 406, 407

candida, *404,* 404–5, *405*
   trichomonas, 405, 406, *406*
Instrument stands, 110
Interferon, 442, 451
International Agency for Research on Cancer (IARC), 7, 67
International Society for the Study of Vulvovaginal Disease (ISSVD), 449
Intradermal nevus, 463
Invasive adenocarcinoma, 46, *47–48*
Invasive anal cancer, 533, *534*
Invasive carcinoma, 52–54, *53–54*
   during pregnancy. *See* pregnancy
Invasive cervical cancer, worldwide incidence, 61
Invasive squamous cell carcinoma, 45–46, *46,* 316, 318–20, *318–20*
Iodine staining
   of CIN 1, 265, 268–70
   of CIN 2, 275, 279–80
   of CIN 3, 297, 299–301

J

Junctional nevi, 463

K

Keratinization, 491
Keratinocytes, 30, 432, *435, 456, 459,* 492

L

Labia minora and majora, 28, 29
Large loop excision of transformation zone (LLETZ), 638
Laser vaporization. *See* Cervical intraepithelial neoplasia (CIN) treatment
Lateral sidewall retractors, 111, *111*
Lentigo formation, 433
Lesions
   elevated, 328, *328–29*
   with large crypt openings, 329, *330*
   papillary, *324–25,* 329, *329,* 331–32
   with a patchy (variegated) red and white surface, 328, 329–30, *330,* 334–35
   see also High-grade squamous intraepithelial lesion (HSIL); Low-grade squamous intraepithelial lesion (LSIL)
Leukoplakia, 1
   clinical significance, 167–68, *169*
   colposcopic appearance, 164, 166–67, *167–69*
   etiology, 164
Lichen planus, 407–9, *409*
Lichen sclerosus, 452–53, *453, 454*
Lichen simplex chronicus, 453, *456*
Lichenoid change, 433
Liquid-based cytology (LBC), 548, 549
Location
   of CIN 1, 259, *259–61*
   of CIN 2, 272, *274–75*
   of CIN 3, 278, *282–84*
Long-handled scissors, 113–14, *115*
Loop electrosurgical excision procedure (LEEP), 50, 310, 332, 427, *427,* 481, 599, 603, 604, 605, 613, 633–47, 676, 681
   bipolar electrosurgery, *634,* 637–38
   buttoning, 389, *390*
   complications, 644, 646, 647
   contraindications for, 639
   electrosurgery vs. electrocautery, 638
   electrosurgical safety, 638
   electrosurgical systems, 638
   instant response, 634
   long-term consequences of, 647
   monopolar electrosurgical coagulation, 635–36, *635–37*
   monopolar electrosurgical cutting, *634,* 634–35, *636*
   one-or-two visit approach, 638–39
   pathological specimen, 647
   patient prior evaluation, 638
   postoperative management, 646, 647
   post-treatment follow-up, 647
   procedure, 627, 633–34, 637, 639–44, *645, 646*
   rationale for using, 638
   sine waves, 634, *634, 635*

Loop electrosurgical excision procedure (LEEP)
(*Continued*)
   stages of thermal destruction, 633, *634*
   surgical approaches, 638
   therapeutic effectiveness, 647
   waveforms, 634
Low-grade anal intraepithelial neoplasia
     (LGAIN), 491
   Lugol's partial staining, *508*
   micropapillae, *505*
Low-grade squamous intraepithelial lesion (LSIL),
     44–45, *45*, 490, *490*
   adolescents, 591, 592, *592*
   initial management, 582–84, *584, 585*
   postcolposcopy management, 590, 591, *591*
   postmenopausal women, 585, *586*
   pregnant women, 585, *586*
Lugol's negative staining, *507, 508*
Lugol's solutions
   applications
     abnormal cervix, 163–69, *163–69,*
       180–82, *180*
     background, 177
     normal cervix, 162–63, *163–64*, 177, 179
Lugol's stain, 500, *503, 504, 504*
Lymphogranuloma venereum (LGV), *445,*
     445–46, *446*

M
Management errors, 679–83, *680–83*
Management guidelines, 605–14, *607–15*
Margins
   of CIN 1, 260, *263*
   of CIN 2, 273, 275, *276, 277*
   of CIN 3, 281, 283, 287, *287–91*
Matrix area of carcinoma, 2
Melanocytic carcinoma (melanoma), 466–67, *467*
Melanoma *in situ*, 462, *462*
Melanosis, vaginal, 413–14
Metaplastic cells, *23*
Microglandular hyperplasia, 19
Microinvasive carcinoma, during pregnancy.
     See Pregnancy
Micropapillations, 436, *436*
Mixed disease, 326, *326–27*
Molluscum contagiosum, 439–40, *440, 441*
Mons pubis, 28
Monsel's solution, 115–16, *116*
Mosaic, 193, 194, 198–201, *198–204*
   clinical significance, 200–1
   colposcopic appearance, 199–200, *202–4*
   definition, 193, 198, *198*
   etiology, 193, 194, 198, 199, *198–99*
Multiparity, 69
Myrtiform caruncles, 29

N
Naked eye examination, 1, *2*
National Cancer Institute, Surveillance
     Epidemiology and End Results
     (SEER), 554
Native or original squamocolumnar junction
     (SCJ), 14
Needle drivers, 113, *115*
Neoplasia, 168–69
Nevi, 463, *464*
Normal and abnormal cervix. *See* Colposcopic
     signs
Normal endometrial cells, 43, *43*
Normal micropapillae, 30
Normal transformation zone, 150–56
   neoplastic alteration, 156

O
Oral contraceptive pills (OCPs), 70
   changes due to, 377
Organisms, 39, 41, *41*

P
Paget's disease, *461,* 461–62
Pap tests, 489, 490
   false negative, 667

preparation, 47–49, *48*
repeating, 125
see also Abnormal Pap management; Cervical
     cancer screening
Papette®, 34–35
Papillary dermis, 30, 432
Papillary hidradenoma, 462, *462–63*
Papillary lesions, *327–29, 329, 331–32*
Papillomatosis, 433
   vaginal, 409
Parabasal cells, 22
Parakeratosis, 42, 433, *435*
Patient preparation, for colposcopy, 121–22, *122*
Patient tracking systems, 118, *118–19*
PCR. *See* Polymerase chain reaction
Pearly penile papules, 654
Penile condyloma, *658*
Penile intraepithelial neoplasia, 80
Perianal examination, 495–96, *495–96*, 512, 516,
     516–22, 521
Perianal fissures, *516*
Perianal hemorrhoid, *517*
Perianal hyperkeratosis, *517*
Perianal hyperpigmentation, *517*
Podofilox, 655, *655*
Podofilox gel, 523, *523, 655*
Podophyllin, 657, *657*
Polymerase chain reaction (PCR), 8, 67, 68,
     91, 439
Polyps, 224, 385–87
Post procedure instructions, colposcopy, 146,
     147–48
Postpartum management. *See* pregnancy
Posttreatment findings
   mimics of cervical neoplasia, 387–89, *387–89*
   other, *389–90, 389–91*
Pregnancy
   antepartum management
     ASC and LSIL Pap results, 369, *370, 371*
     ASC-H, AGC, and HSIL Pap results, 369,
       371, 372
     Pap test report, 372
   cervical cancer and
     epidemiology of, 348, 349, *349*
     natural history of, 349
     potential complications, 349–50
   cervical intraepithelial neoplasia
     complications of, 348, *348*
     epidemiology of, 347, *347*
     natural history of, 347–48, *347*
   colposcopic findings
     high-grade cervical lesions (CIN 2,3), 363,
       364, *366–67, 368*
     low-grade cervical and vaginal lesions, 363,
       364, *363–66*
   colposcopy during
     assessment, 356, *357–62, 358–61*
     correlation, 363
     indications for, 353, *354, 355*
     objectives of, 355
     sampling, 361, 362, 363, *363*
     visualization, 355–56, *355–57*
   human papillomavirus (HPV) and, 343–47
     epidemiology of, 343–44, *344*
     natural history of, 344, *345*
     potential complications from HPV
       infections, 344–47, *345–46*
   invasive carcinoma, 366, 367, *369*
   lower genital tract modifications
     cytology, 352, 353, *354*
     histology, 353, *354, 355*
     physiology, 350–52, *350–52, 353, 354*
   management
     CIN 1, 372
     CIN 2, 3, 372
     complications
       abortion, 372–73
       conization-related, 373
       hemorrhage, 373, *373*
       invasive cervical cancer, 372
     microinvasive cancer, 365, *368*
     postpartum management, 373–74
Productive viral infection (HPV), *88,* 88–89
Prolapsing vaginal walls, 669–70
Proximal margin, 135

Psoriasis, 456–57, *457–58*
Punctation, vasculature, 186, 188–93, *189–97*
   clinical significance, 193, *197*
   colposcopic appearance, 191–93, *191–96*
   definition, 186
   etiology, 186, 188–91, *188–90*

R
Radiation-induced changes, *384,* 384–85
Reactive and reparative changes, 41–42, *42*
Rectal columnar epithelium, 498, *498*
Recurrent vulvovaginal candidiasis (RVVC), 447
Reid colposcopic index (RCI), 242
   color, 244, *248, 249*
   correlation, 253, 254, *255*
   design, 242, *243*
   iodine, 249, 250, *253–55*
   margin, 242, *244–48*
   reproducibility of, 258
   scores, 242, *243,* 250, 252
   special considerations concerning, *253, 254,*
     254, 255, 256–57, 258
   vessels, 244, 246, 249, *250–52*
Reserve cells, 23
Rete pegs, 30, 432
Reticular dermis, 432
Risk factors for invasive cervical cancer
   cofactors to HPV-induced oncogenesis, 69–71
   human papillomavirus, 67–69

S
Saline, 114
   applications of, *203, 204, 289*
Sampling error, 675–78, *675–78*
Satisfactory colposcopic examination. *See* Native
     or original squamocolumnar
     junction
Schiller's test, 4–5
Sebaceous hyperplasia, 437
Sexual assault victims, 392, 393–96
   colposcopy findings in consensual intercourse
     and nonintercourse-related trauma,
     394–95, *394–95*
   colposcopy findings in sexual assault,
     396, *396*
   use of colposcopy in sexual assault examina-
     tion, 393–94, *393–94*
Sexual behaviors, invasive cervical cancer, 67
Sexual partners, 66
Sexual transmission, of human papillomavirus
     (HPV), 84–85
Silver nitrate sticks, 116, *116*
Simple atypical, 2
Sine waves, 634, *634, 635*
Sinecatechins, 525, 656, *657*
Size and distribution
   of CIN 1, 265, 270–73, *272*
   of CIN 2, 275, 277, *280, 281*
   of CIN 3, 297, *302–3, 303*
Skene's glands and ducts, 29, 30, 432
Skip (multifocal) lesions, 326
Smoking, 67, 70, 86, 324, 347, 460, *461,* 472,
     474, 485, 495, 507, 508, 560
Specimen adequacy guidelines, *572*
Spongiosis, 433
Squamocolumnar junction (SCJ), 14
   inadequate visualization, 670–71
Squamous abnormalities
   anal cytology, 490, *490,* 491
   intraepithelial lesions, 51–52, *51–52*
   invasive carcinoma, 52–54, *53–54*
   reactive and reparative change, 51
Squamous cell carcinoma, 79, *79,* 306–20
   circumstances that warrant concern
     atypical vessels, 314, *315–17*
     color, 313, *313, 314*
     cytology, 311
     high-grade lesions with complete or par-
       tial canal involvement, *312,*
       312–13, *313*
     linear length, surface area of lesions, and
       cervical diameter, 311–12, *312*
     patient age, 311, *311*

persistence or recurrence of high-grade lesions after treatment, 314, 317, 318
surface contour, 313, 313
colposcopic mimics, 316, 318–20
correlation process, 309
differentiating normal from abnormal, 307, 308–10
disparities, 306–7
effect of screening, 307
etiology, 306
excision, 310–11
incidence and mortality, 306
adequate vs. inadequate colposcopic examination, 307, 309
Squamous epithelium, 15, 16–18, 17, 17–18
histology, 15, 17, 17–18
Squamous intraepithelial lesion (SIL), 39, 478–79
Squamous metaplasia
formation of, 19–20, 20
histology of, 20–22, 20–22
Stafl grading system, 241, 242
Stratum spinosum, 432
Superficially invasive squamous cell carcinomas of the anus (SISCCA), 534
Supplies, disposable, 117
Surface contour. See Contour
Surface patterns in adenocarcinoma in situ and adenocarcinoma. See Adenocarcinoma in situ and adenocarcinoma
Surface topography
epithelial elevations, 215–27
ulceration/erosion
clinical significance, 214–15, 214
colposcopic appearance, 213–14, 212, 213
definition, 209–10, 212
etiology, 210–11, 213, 213
Syphilis, 442–44, 443–44

T

Telangiectasia, 414–15, 415
Thermal destruction, 633, 634
Tinea cruris, 447–48, 449
Tobacco, 85
Transformation zone
abnormal, 155, 160
congenital, 409–11, 410–11
endocervical/transformation zone, 572–73
formation of squamous metaplasia, 19–20, 20
identification of, 132–33, 132–34
normal, 150–56
neoplastic alteration, 156
Transverse vaginal septum, 391, 391
Traumatic vaginal lesions, 411–12, 411–12
Trichloroacetic acid (TCA), 522, 523, 523–24, 657–59, 658–59
Trichomonas, 41, 405–6, 406
Tumor suppressor gene inactivation, 94
Typical glandular cells, 46, 47

U

UCSF Anal Neoplasia Clinic New Patient Questionnaire, 493–94
Ulceration (erosion)
clinical significance, 214–15, 214
colposcopic appearance, 213–14, 212, 213
definition, 209–10, 212
etiology, 210–11, 213, 213
United States Public Services Task Force (USPSTF)
cervical screening recommendations, 559
screening after hysterectomy, 559
screening intervals, 560
Unsatisfactory colposcopy examinations, 624, 670
Urethral meatus, 28
U.S. Food and Drug Administration, 535

V

Vaccines, 653
human papillomavirus
cost-effectiveness, 546
cross-protection evidence with closely related HPV types, 544

immunosuppression, 546
male immunization, 546
pregnant women, 545–46
principles, 540, 541, 541–42
recommendations, 545
safety and efficacy trials, 542–45
Vagina, 399–428
anatomy, 24, 24–25
biopsy, 403, 403
colposcopy indications, 399–400, 400
colposcopy of benign vaginal epithelial changes, 403, 404–16
congenital transformation zone, 409, 410, 410, 411
endometriosis, 413, 414
Gartner's duct cysts, 413, 414
granulation tissue, 415, 416, 416
inflammation
bacteria-induced desquamative disorders, 406, 407
candida, 404, 404–5, 405
trichomonas, 405, 406, 406
nonbacterial desquamative disorders
desquamative inflammatory vaginitis, 407, 407, 408
lichen planus, 407, 408–9, 409
radiation changes, 416
traumatic vaginal lesions, 411–12, 412
vaginal adenosis, 411
vaginal hemangioma and telangiectasia, 414, 415, 415
vaginal melanosis, 413, 414
vaginal papillomatosis, 409, 409, 410
vaginitis emphysematosa, 412, 413, 413
colposcopy technique, 400–2, 400–3, 404
cytology, 26–27
embryology, 24, 24
examination of, 140–41, 140–41
histology, 26, 26
neoplastic disorders, 416–28
colposcopy of
vaginal cancers, 423, 424–25, 425
adenocarcinoma, 425
malignant melanoma, 425
squamous cell carcinoma, 424, 425
VAIN 2-3 high-grade intraepithelial neoplasia, 423, 423, 424
VAIN 1/low-grade HPV expression, 417–22
condylomatous vaginitis, 419, 420, 420–21, 421
flat vaginal warts/VAIN 1, 421, 422, 422
vaginal condylomata acuminata, 417–19, 418, 419
epidemiology and natural history of VAIN and vaginal cancer, 417
pathology, 417
treatment
high-grade VAIN, 426–28, 427, 428
low-grade VAIN and condyloma, 426
visualization, error, 671–72, 671–72
Vaginal adenosis, 26, 378–81, 411
Vaginal and cervical duplication, 391–92, 392
Vaginal cancer, 417, 423–25
see also Vagina
Vaginal glandular cells, 43, 43
Vaginal intraepithelial neoplasia (VAIN), 131, 650
Vaginal lesions, traumatic, 411–12, 412
Vaginal melanosis, 413–14
Vaginal papillomatosis, 409, 409–10
Vaginal specula, 110–12
Vaginismus, 449
VAIN. See Vaginal intraepithelial neoplasia
VASC. See Visualization, assessment, sampling and correlation (VASC)
Vascular ectasia, 436–37, 437–38
Vasculature
atypical blood vessels, 201, 202–11, 202–11
clinical significance, 208, 209–11
colposcopic appearance, 204–5, 207–8, 207–8
definition, 201, 205–6
etiology, 201, 204

of CIN 1, 265, 266–68
of CIN 2, 275, 278, 279
of CIN 3, 288, 292–99
mosaic, 193, 194, 198–201, 198–204
clinical significance, 200–1
colposcopic appearance, 199–200, 202–4
definition, 193, 198, 198
etiology, 193–94, 199, 198–99
normal cervix, 183–86, 183–88
punctation, 186, 188–93, 189–97
clinical significance, 193, 197
colposcopic appearance, 191–93, 191–96
definition, 186
etiology, 186, 188–91, 188–90
Verrucous carcinoma, 467
Vertical transmission, of human papillomavirus (HPV), 85–86
Vestibular papillae, 436
Vestibule, 28, 432
Video colposcope, 108–10, 110
Viral entry (HPV), 86, 86–88, 87–88
Visualization, assessment, sampling and correlation (VASC), 667, 679
see also Errors
Visualization errors
bleeding, 669
lesions extending deep into cervical canal, 671
inadequate of squamocolumnar junction, 670–71
mucus, debris, and discharge, 669
prolapsing vaginal walls, 669–70
vagina and vulva, 671–72, 671–72
Vulva
anatomy, 28, 28–30
embryology, 27–28, 28
examinations, 141–43, 141–43
histology, 30, 32
visualization, error, 671–72, 671–72
Vulvar abnormalities
anatomy and histology, 432–33, 433, 434, 435
differentiation of definite disease from normal, 436–37
acetowhitening, 436, 437
Fordyce's spots, 437, 438
micropapillations, 436, 436
vascular ectasia, 436, 437, 437, 438
examination and biopsy techniques, 434, 435, 435, 436
infections
bacterial
chancroid, 444–45, 445
granuloma inguinale, 444, 444
syphilis, 442–44, 443, 444
chlamydia, lymphogranuloma venereum (LGV), 445, 445–46, 446
fungi
candidiasis, 446, 446–47, 447, 448
tinea cruris, 447, 448, 449
viral
condyloma, 440, 441–42, 441–43
genital herpes in pregnancy, 439
herpes simplex virus, 438, 439, 439
molluscum contagiosum, 439–40, 440, 441
invasive carcinoma
adenocarcinoma, 467
melanocytic carcinoma (melanoma), 466, 467, 467, 468
squamous cell, 464–66, 464–67
noninvasive neoplastic abnormalities
other
granular cell tumor, 462, 463, 463
melanosis, 464
nevi, 463, 464
papillary hidradenoma, 462, 462, 463
vulvar intraepithelial neoplasia (VIN)
nonsquamous
melanoma in situ, 462, 462
Paget's disease, 461, 461–62
squamous
clinical appearance, 458, 458, 459
histology, 458, 459, 459, 461
treatment, 459, 460, 461

Vulvar abnormalities (*Continued*)
  nonneoplastic conditions
    ISSVD classification, 452, *453*
    lichen sclerosus, 452, 453, *455, 456*
    other
      lichen planus, 454, 455, 456, *456, 457*
      psoriasis, 456, 457, *457, 458*
    squamous cell hyperplasia, 453, *456*
  vulvodynia
    etiologic theories, 449, *451*
    historical information, 449

    localized vulvar pain, 449, 450–52, *452, 453*
    vaginismus, 449
    vestibular erythema, *451*
Vulvar intraepithelial neoplasia (VIN)
  nonsquamous
    melanoma in situ, 462, *462*
    Paget's disease, *461*, 461–62
  squamous
    clinical appearance, 458, *458, 459*
    histology, 458, 459, *459, 461*
    treatment, 459, 460, 461

Vulvar vestibulitis, 449
Vulvodynia
  etiologic theories, 449, *451*
  historical information, 449
  localized vulvar pain
    topical medications, 450
    tricyclic antidepressants, 450–52, *452, 453*
    vulvar care measures, 450
  vaginismus, 449
  vestibular erythema, *451*
Vulvovaginal candidiasis (VVC), 446, *446, 449*